Differential Diagnosis in Surgical Pathology

Differential Diagnosis in Surgical Pathology

Second Edition

Paolo Gattuso, MD
Professor of Pathology
Director of Anatomic Pathology
Rush Medical College of Rush University
Chicago, Illinois

Vijaya B. Reddy, MD
Professor and Associate Chair of Pathology
Rush Medical College of Rush University
Senior Attending
Rush University Medical Center
Chicago, Illinois

Odile David, MD
Director of Cytopathology
Department of Pathology
University of Illinois at Chicago
Chicago, Illinois

Daniel J. Spitz, MD
Chief Medical Examiner
Macomb County, Michigan
Clinical Assistant Professor of Pathology
Wayne State University School of Medicine
Detroit, Michigan

Meryl H. Haber, MD
Borland Professor and Chairman of Pathology,
    Emeritus
Rush Medical College of Rush University
Chicago, Illinois

SAUNDERS

ELSEVIER

1600 John F. Kennedy Blvd.
Ste 1800
Philadelphia, PA 19103-2899

Notices

Knowledge and best practice in this field are constantly changing. As new research and experience
broaden our understanding, changes in research methods, professional practices, or medical treatment
may become necessary.

Practitioners and researchers must always rely on their own experience and knowledge in
evaluating and using any information, methods, compounds, or experiments described herein. In
using such information or methods they should be mindful of their own safety and the safety of others,
including parties for whom they have a professional responsibility.

With respect to any drug or pharmaceutical products identified, readers are advised to check the
most current information provided (i) on procedures featured or (ii) by the manufacturer of each
product to be administered, to verify the recommended dose or formula, the method and duration of
administration, and contraindications. It is the responsibility of practitioners, relying on their own
experience and knowledge of their patients, to make diagnoses, to determine dosages and the best
treatment for each individual patient, and to take all appropriate safety precautions.

To the fullest extent of the law, neither the publisher nor the authors, contributors, or editors,
assume any liability for any injury and/or damage to persons or property as a matter of products
liability, negligence or otherwise, or from any use or operation of any methods, products, instructions,
or ideas contained in the material herein.

Library of Congress Cataloging-in-Publication Data
   Differential diagnosis in surgical pathology. — 2nd ed. / [edited by] Paolo Gattuso ... [et al.].
        p. ; cm.
   Includes bibliographical references and index.
   ISBN 978-1-4160-4580-9
   1. Pathology, Surgical.   2. Diagnosis, Differential.   I. Gattuso, Paolo.
   [DNLM: 1. Pathology, Surgical.   2. Diagnosis, Differential.   WO 142 D5695 2009]
   RD57.D535 2009
   617′.075—dc22   2008048839

Publishing Director: Linda Belfus
Acquisitions Editor: William Schmitt
Developmental Editor: Katie DeFrancesco
Publishing Services Manager: Tina Rebane
Project Manager: Amy Norwitz
Design Direction: Louis Forgione

Printed in China

Last digit is the print number: 9   8   7   6   5   4   3

To my wife Nancy and my children Vincent and Francesca.

Paolo Gattuso

To my son Vikram, for the nineteen years of life, love, and memories.

Vijaya B. Reddy

For my family, to whom I owe my appreciation of life and learning.

Odile David

To my parents for setting me on the right track, and to my wife Jodi
for her continuous support and encouragement.

Daniel J. Spitz

This book is dedicated to all of my former students, residents,
fellows, and physician associates who I have always learned more
from than I have been able to teach.

Meryl H. Haber

List of Contributors

Sylvia L. Asa, MD, PhD
Professor of Laboratory Medicine and Pathobiology
University of Toronto Faculty of Medicine
Pathologist-in-Chief
Medical Director, Laboratory Medicine Program
Senior Scientist, Ontario Cancer Institute
Toronto, Ontario
Canada
Adrenal Gland

Pincas Bitterman, MD
Professor of Pathology and Obstetrics and Gynecology
Rush Medical College of Rush University
Chicago, Illinois
Female Reproductive System

Jean E. Blair, MD
Assistant Professor of Pathology
Northeastern Ohio Universities College of Medicine
Rootstown, Ohio
Staff Pathologist
AmeriPath Youngstown
Youngstown, Ohio
Gastrointestinal System

Elizabeth J. Cochran, MD
Associate Professor of Pathology and Neurological Sciences
Rush Medical College of Rush University
Attending Physician
Rush University Medical Center
Chicago, Illinois
Central Nervous System

Kumarasen Cooper, MBChB, FRCPath, DPhil
Professor of Pathology
University of Vermont College of Medicine
Director of Anatomic Pathology and Vice-Chair of Pathology
Fletcher Allen Health Care
Burlington, Vermont
Special Diagnostic Techniques in Surgical Pathology

Byron E. Crawford, MD
Professor of Pathology
Director of Anatomic Pathology
Assistant Dean of Academic Affairs
Tulane University School of Medicine
New Orleans, Louisiana
Bones and Joints

Magdalena Czader, MD, PhD
Assistant Professor
Director, Division of Hematopathology
Director, Clinical Flow Cytometry Laboratory
Indiana University School of Medicine
Indianapolis, Indiana
Spleen

Michael J. Davis, MD
Instructor, Department of Ophthalmology
Rush Medical College of Rush University
Chicago, Illinois
Eye and Orbit

Adel K. El-Naggar, MD, PhD
Professor of Pathology and Head and Neck Surgery
Program Director, Head and Neck Pathology Fellowship
University of Texas M.D. Anderson Cancer Center
Houston, Texas
Head and Neck

Mark F. Evans, PhD
Research Assistant Professor, Department of Pathology
University of Vermont College of Medicine
Burlington, Vermont
Special Diagnostic Techniques in Surgical Pathology

Sandra E. Fischer, MD
Assistant Professor
University of Toronto Faculty of Medicine
Staff Pathologist
University Health Network
Toronto, Ontario
Canada
Adrenal Gland

Table 1-3. Filaments and Tubules

Component	Diameter	Location
Microfilaments (actin, nonmuscle myosin)	6-8 nm	Cytoskeleton of all cells
Intermediate filaments	10 nm	
Cytokeratin	>19 proteins 40-68 kd	Epithelial cells
Glial fibrillary acid protein	55 kd	Astrocytes
Neurofilament	68, 160, 200 kd	Neural tissue
Vimentin	57 kd	Mesenchymal tissues
Desmin	53 kd	Muscle
Microtubules	25 nm	Neural derivatives (e.g., neuroblastoma)

kD, kilodaltons; nm, nanometers; 50 kD = ~4 nm

Figure 1-10. Electron microscopy. Short villi lining an intracytoplasmic lumen in adenocarcinoma of the breast.

- Junctions are seen in virtually all cells except those of hematopoietic origin
- Basal lamina is seen surrounding all endodermal and ectodermal derivatives; cells with muscle differentiation also may have a basal lamina, which may be incomplete

Extracellular Matrix

- Collagen shows a regular structure
- Amyloid
  - Fibrils measuring approximately 10 nm in diameter, with an electron-lucent core
  - Fibrils are straight, nonbranching, and arranged randomly

Selected References

Ghadially FN: Diagnostic Ultrastructural Pathology, 2nd ed. Boston, Butterworth-Heinemann, 1998.

Ghadially FN: Ultrastructure of the Cell and Matrix, 4th ed. Boston, Butterworth-Heinemann, 1997.

Ghadially FN: Diagnostic Electron Microscopy of Tumors. Boston, Butterworth-Heinemann, 1986.

Immunohistochemistry

Introduction

IHC combines anatomic, immunologic, and biochemical techniques to identify specific tissue components using a specific antigen-antibody reaction labeled with a visible reporter molecule. This binding is then visualized through the use of various enzymes that are coupled to the antibodies being used. The enzyme acts on a chromogenic substrate to cause deposition of a colored material at the site of antibody-antigen bindings. Hence, IHC permits the visualization and localization of specific cellular components within a cell or tissue while importantly preserving the overall morphology and structure of the tissue section. During the past several decades, major improvements in protein conjugation, antigen preservation and antigen retrieval methods, and enhanced immunodetection systems have enshrined IHC as a major adjunctive investigative tool for both surgical and cytopathology. IHC is not only critical for the accurate diagnosis of malignancies but also plays a pivotal role in prognostic evaluation (e.g., estrogen and progesterone receptors in breast cancer) and treatments strategies (e.g., c-kit protein for gastrointestinal stromal tumors and *HER-2-neu* in certain breast cancers).

Technical Overview

- Formalin cross-links proteins in tissues; success of immunohistochemical staining depends on the availability of an antigen after fixation
  - Various techniques may unmask antigens, such as digestion by enzymes (e.g., trypsin) or antigen retrieval using heat, metallic mordants, or alkaline buffers
  - Commonly used enzymes include peroxidase, alkaline phosphatase, and glucose oxidase
  - Most commonly used chromogen substrates produce brown (DAB) or red (AEC) reaction products
- Definition of terms
  - **Polyclonal antibody:** Conventional antiserum produced by multiple plasma cells of an animal that had been injected with an antigen; a polyclonal antibody may have multiple determinants (binding sites)
  - **Monoclonal antibody:** Produced by fusion of a malignant cell with a plasma cell producing antibody to a specific epitope; antibodies may be grown in tissue culture
- Antibodies for the detection of cellular components
  - Intermediate filaments (see Table 1-3)
  - Other cellular and tissue components: (e.g., α_1-antitrypsin, myeloperoxidase, synaptophysin and chromogranin, myoglobin)
  - Leukocyte antigens and immunoglobulin components commonly used in paraffin-embedded tissues

List of Contributors

Sylvia L. Asa, MD, PhD
Professor of Laboratory Medicine and Pathobiology
University of Toronto Faculty of Medicine
Pathologist-in-Chief
Medical Director, Laboratory Medicine Program
Senior Scientist, Ontario Cancer Institute
Toronto, Ontario
Canada
Adrenal Gland

Pincas Bitterman, MD
Professor of Pathology and Obstetrics and Gynecology
Rush Medical College of Rush University
Chicago, Illinois
Female Reproductive System

Jean E. Blair, MD
Assistant Professor of Pathology
Northeastern Ohio Universities College of Medicine
Rootstown, Ohio
Staff Pathologist
AmeriPath Youngstown
Youngstown, Ohio
Gastrointestinal System

Elizabeth J. Cochran, MD
Associate Professor of Pathology and Neurological Sciences
Rush Medical College of Rush University
Attending Physician
Rush University Medical Center
Chicago, Illinois
Central Nervous System

Kumarasen Cooper, MBChB, FRCPath, DPhil
Professor of Pathology
University of Vermont College of Medicine
Director of Anatomic Pathology and Vice-Chair of Pathology
Fletcher Allen Health Care
Burlington, Vermont
Special Diagnostic Techniques in Surgical Pathology

Byron E. Crawford, MD
Professor of Pathology
Director of Anatomic Pathology
Assistant Dean of Academic Affairs
Tulane University School of Medicine
New Orleans, Louisiana
Bones and Joints

Magdalena Czader, MD, PhD
Assistant Professor
Director, Division of Hematopathology
Director, Clinical Flow Cytometry Laboratory
Indiana University School of Medicine
Indianapolis, Indiana
Spleen

Michael J. Davis, MD
Instructor, Department of Ophthalmology
Rush Medical College of Rush University
Chicago, Illinois
Eye and Orbit

Adel K. El-Naggar, MD, PhD
Professor of Pathology and Head and Neck Surgery
Program Director, Head and Neck Pathology Fellowship
University of Texas M.D. Anderson Cancer Center
Houston, Texas
Head and Neck

Mark F. Evans, PhD
Research Assistant Professor, Department of Pathology
University of Vermont College of Medicine
Burlington, Vermont
Special Diagnostic Techniques in Surgical Pathology

Sandra E. Fischer, MD
Assistant Professor
University of Toronto Faculty of Medicine
Staff Pathologist
University Health Network
Toronto, Ontario
Canada
Adrenal Gland

Richard J. Grostern, MD
Assistant Professor of Ophthalmology and Pathology
Rush Medical College of Rush University
Chicago, Illinois
Eye and Orbit

Mehmet Guler, MD, PhD
GI/Liver Fellow, Department of Pathology
Johns Hopkins Medical Institutions
Baltimore, Maryland
Pancreas

Ralph H. Hruban, MD
Professor of Pathology and Oncology
Johns Hopkins University School of Medicine
Attending Pathologist
The Johns Hopkins Hospital
Baltimore, Maryland
Pancreas

Aliya N. Husain, MD
Professor of Pathology
University of Chicago Pritzker School of Medicine
Chicago, Illinois
Lung and Pleura

Alexandra N. Kalof, MD
Assistant Professor of Pathology
University of Vermont College of Medicine
Attending Physician, Department of Pathology
Fletcher Allen Health Care
Burlington, Vermont
Special Diagnostic Techniques in Surgical Pathology

Robin D. LeGallo, MD
Assistant Professor of Pathology
University of Virginia Medical Center
Charlottesville, Virginia
Soft Tissue

Jerome M. Loew, MD
Associate Professor of Pathology
Rush Medical College of Rush University
Assistant Attending
Rush University Medical Center
Chicago, Illinois
Lymph Nodes

Alexander Craig MacKinnon, Jr., MD, PhD
Fellow, Molecular Genetic Pathology and Cardiovascular
  Pathology
University of Chicago Medical Center
Chicago, Illinois
Lung and Pleura

William R. Macon, MD
Professor of Laboratory Medicine and Pathology
Mayo College of Medicine
Consultant in Pathology, Department of Laboratory Medicine
  and Pathology
Mayo Clinic Foundation
Rochester, Minnesota
Lymph Nodes

Cristina Magi-Galluzzi, MD, PhD
Assistant Professor
Cleveland Clinic Lerner College of Medicine of Case Western
  Reserve University
Director of Genitourinary Pathology
Cleveland Clinic Foundation
Cleveland, Ohio
Ureter, Urinary Bladder, and Kidney

Maria J. Merino, MD
Chief, Translational Surgical Pathology
National Institutes of Health
National Cancer Institute
Bethesda, Maryland
Breast

Cesar A. Moran, MD
Professor of Pathology and Deputy Chairman of Anatomic
  Pathology
University of Texas M.D. Anderson Cancer Center
Houston, Texas
Thymus and Mediastinum

Attilio Orazi, MD
Professor of Pathology and Laboratory Medicine
Weill Cornell Medical College of Cornell University
Attending Pathologist
Director, Division of Hematopathology
New York-Presbyterian Hospital
New York, New York
Spleen

Robert E. Petras, MD
Associate Clinical Professor of Pathology
Northeastern Ohio Universities Colleges of Medicine
Rootstown, Ohio
AmeriPath Gastrointestinal Institute
Oakwood Village, Ohio
Gastrointestinal System

Michael R. Pins, MD
Professor of Clinical Pathology
University of Illinois at Chicago College of Medicine
Medical Director, Anatomic Pathology
Advocate Lutheran General Hospital
Park Ridge, Illinois
Male Genitourinary System

Jose A. Plaza, MD
Assistant Professor of Pathology
Medical College of Wisconsin
Milwaukee, Wisconsin
Thymus and Mediastinum

Martha M. Quezado, MD
Staff Pathologist
Laboratory of Pathology
National Cancer Institute
National Institutes of Health
Bethesda, Maryland
Breast

Vijaya B. Reddy, MD
Professor and Associate Chair of Pathology
Rush Medical College of Rush University
Senior Attending
Rush University Medical Center
Chicago, Illinois
Skin and Adnexal Structures

E Rene Rodriguez, MD
Adjunct and Professor
Johns Hopkins University School of Medicine
Baltimore, Maryland
Staff, Department of Anatomic Pathology
Cleveland Clinic Foundation
Cleveland, Ohio
Heart, Pericardium, and Blood Vessels

Saul Suster, MD
Chairman and Professor, Department of Pathology and
    Laboratory Medicine
Medical College of Wisconsin
Milwaukee, Wisconsin
Thymus and Mediastinum

Paul E. Swanson, MD
Professor of Pathology
University of Washington School of Medicine
Director of Anatomic Pathology
Director of Immunocytochemistry
University of Washington Medical Center
Seattle, Washington
Hepatobiliary System

Carmela D. Tan, MD
Staff, Section of Cardiovascular Pathology
Department of Anatomic Pathology
Cleveland Clinic Foundation
Cleveland, Ohio
Heart, Pericardium, and Blood Vessels

Mark R. Wick, MD
Professor of Pathology
University of Virginia School of Medicine
Associate Director of Virginia Health System
Charlottesville, Virginia
Soft Tissue

Michelle D. Williams, MD
Assistant Professor of Pathology
University of Texas M.D. Anderson Cancer Center
Houston, Texas
Head and Neck

Matthew M. Yeh, MD, PhD
Associate Professor of Pathology
University of Washington School of Medicine
Staff Pathologist
Gastrointestinal and Hepatic Pathology
University of Washington Medical Center
Seattle, Washington
Hepatobiliary System

Ming Zhou, MD, PhD
Assistant Professor
Cleveland Clinic Lerner College of Medicine of Case Western
    Reserve University
Staff Pathologist
Cleveland Clinic Foundation
Cleveland, Ohio
Ureter, Urinary Bladder, and Kidney

Preface

It has been nearly seven years since the publication of the first edition of this textbook. Who knew then that *Differential Diagnosis in Surgical Pathology* would become a textbook widely used by residents and fellows in pathology departments in the United States, as well as around the world, and by innumerable practicing pathologists. As a result of this widespread acceptance the authors began the process of updating and revising the text and illustrations while making certain to continue the successful features of the first edition, especially the organization by systems; the use of an outline format for text; and integration of the photomicrographic images with corresponding subject matter. This process took over three years.

Writing a new textbook is an immense undertaking; writing a second edition is, perhaps, an even greater undertaking. In this cost-containment environment an important consideration was to keep the book's price affordable for its audience, primarily by not increasing the number of pages (over 1000) while updating the content. This was achieved with cautious and careful editing. It was also of primary importance to fill obvious gaps and revise subject matter where needed with contributions from additional acknowledged expert pathologists. Another significant change from the first edition is the inclusion of almost all color images in this edition.

The editors, aware of the success of the book, became even more aware of some of its deficiencies or inadequacies. Every attempt to rectify any shortcomings has been made in this edition. The use of algorithms, a prominent feature of the first edition, has been dropped. Instead, each chapter outline follows a logical algorithmic approach to arriving at a correct diagnosis. The reason for this change relates to the uneven quality of several of the original algorithms and the fact that not all were useful in reaching an accurate diagnosis, mostly because of the complexity of the diagnostic problem.

The first edition's concept of brevity of each topic, not encyclopedic coverage, and outline text format accompanied by integrated illustrative examples of the pathology and limited references is maintained. It is hoped that this textbook will find its way into the hands of residents and practicing pathologists because of its concise format, excellent representative illustrations, and immediate usefulness.

Meryl H. Haber

Acknowledgments

The second edition of this textbook has greatly benefited from the expertise and experience of its many contributors throughout the United States of America and Canada. We thank them all wholeheartedly for placing their confidence in this book and sharing their knowledge so freely.

The editors gratefully acknowledge the work of authors who have contributed to this book in its previous edition.

We thank Irma Parker, Mira Davis, and Rachel Martin for their secretarial assistance. We are thankful to our publisher, Elsevier, and William R. Schmitt, Executive Editor, for his support and encouragement in the production of a second edition. A special thanks to Katie DeFrancesco, Development Editor at Elsevier, for her patience and competence in keeping the book on course over the last three years, and to Amy Norwitz, Senior Project Manager at Elsevier, who oversaw with great skill and tenacity the excruciating details that go into the final stages of the publication process.

Vijaya B. Reddy, MD

Contents

Alexandra N. Kalof, Mark F. Evans, and Kumarasen Cooper

Special Diagnostic Techniques in Surgical Pathology

Light Microscopy

Tissue Processing Overview

- Fixation
  - Preserves tissues in situ as close to the lifelike state as possible
  - Ideally, fixation will be carried out as soon as possible after removal of the tissues, and the fixative will kill the tissue quickly, thus preventing autolysis
- Dehydration
  - Fixed tissue is too fragile to be sectioned and must be embedded first in a nonaqueous supporting medium (e.g., paraffin)
  - The tissue must first be dehydrated through a series of ethanol solutions
- Clearing
  - Ethanol is not miscible with paraffin, so nonpolar solvents (e.g., xylene, toluene) are used as clearing agents; this also makes the tissue more translucent
- Embedding
  - Paraffin is the usual embedding medium; however, tissues are sometimes embedded in a plastic resin, allowing for thinner sections (required for electron microscopy [EM])
  - This embedding process is important because the tissues must be aligned, or oriented, properly in the block of paraffin
- Sectioning
  - Embedded in paraffin, which is similar in density to tissue, tissue can be sectioned at anywhere from 3 to 10 μm (routine sections are usually cut at 6 to 8 μm)
- Staining
  - Allows for differentiation of the nuclear and cytoplasmic components of cells as well as the intercellular structure of the tissue
- Cover-slipping
  - The stained section on the slide is covered with a thin piece of plastic or glass to protect the tissue from being scratched, to provide better optical quality for viewing under the microscope, and to preserve the tissue section for years

Fixation

- There are five major groups of fixatives, classified according to mechanism of action
  - Aldehydes
    - Formalin
      - ◇ Aqueous solution of formaldehyde gas that penetrates tissue well but relatively slowly; the standard solution is 10% neutral buffered formalin
      - ◇ A buffer prevents acidity that would promote autolysis and cause precipitation of formol-heme pigment in the tissues
      - ◇ Tissue is fixed by cross-linkages formed in the proteins, particularly between lysine residues
      - ◇ This cross-linkage *does not harm the structure of proteins greatly, preserving antigenicity,* and is therefore good for immunoperoxidase techniques
    - Glutaraldehyde
      - ◇ The standard solution is a 2% buffered glutaraldehyde and must be cold, buffered, and not more than 3 months old
      - ◇ *Fixes tissue quickly and therefore is ideal for EM*
      - ◇ Causes deformation of α-helix structure in proteins and therefore *is not good for immunoperoxidase staining*
      - ◇ Penetrates poorly but gives best overall cytoplasmic and nuclear detail
      - ◇ Tissue must be as fresh as possible and preferably sectioned within the glutaraldehyde at a thickness of no more than 1 mm to enhance fixation
  - Mercurials
    - B-5 and Zenker
      - ◇ Contain mercuric chloride and must be disposed of carefully
      - ◇ Penetrate poorly and cause tissue hardness but are fast and give excellent nuclear detail
      - ◇ Best application is for *fixation of hematopoietic and reticuloendothelial tissues*
  - Alcohols
    - Methyl alcohol (methanol) and ethyl alcohol (ethanol)
      - ◇ Protein denaturants
      - ◇ Not used routinely for tissue because they dehydrate, resulting in tissues' becoming brittle and hard
      - ◇ *Good for cytologic smears because they act quickly and give good nuclear detail*
  - Oxidizing agents
    - Permanganate fixatives (potassium permanganate), dichromate fixatives (potassium dichromate), and osmium tetroxide cross-link proteins
    - Cause extensive denaturation
    - Some of these have specialized applications but are used infrequently
  - Picrates
    - Bouin solution has an unknown mechanism of action
    - It does almost as well as mercurials with nuclear detail but does not cause as much hardness

- Picric acid is an explosion hazard in dry form
- Recommended for fixation of tissues from testis, gastrointestinal tract, and endocrine organs
- Factors affecting fixation
  - Buffering
    - Fixation is optimal at a neutral pH, in the range of 6 to 8
    - Hypoxia of tissues lowers the pH, so there must be buffering capacity in the fixative to prevent excessive acidity; acidity causes formation of formalin-heme pigment that appears as black, polarizable deposits in tissue
    - Common buffers include phosphate, bicarbonate, cacodylate, and veronal
  - Penetration
    - Fixative solutions penetrate at different rates, depending on the diffusibility of each individual fixative
    - In order of decreasing speed of penetration: formaldehyde, acetic acid, mercuric chloride, methyl alcohol osmium tetroxide, and picric acid
    - Because fixation begins at the periphery, thick sections sometimes remain unfixed in the center, compromising both histology and antigenicity of the cells (important for immunohistochemistry [IHC])
    - It is important to section the tissues thinly (2 to 3 mm)
  - Volume
    - Should be at least a 10:1 ratio of fixative to tissue
  - Temperature
    - Increasing the temperature, as with all chemical reactions, increases the speed of fixation
    - Hot formalin fixes tissues faster, and this is often the first step on an automated tissue processor
  - Concentration
    - Formalin is best at 10%; glutaraldehyde is generally made up at 0.25% to 4%
  - Time interval
    - Formalin should have 6 to 8 hours to act before the remainder of the processing is begun
- Decalcification
  - Tissue calcium deposits are extremely firm and do not section properly with paraffin embedding because of the difference in densities between calcium and paraffin
  - Strong mineral acids such as nitric and hydrochloric acids are used with dense cortical bone because they remove large quantities of calcium at a rapid rate
  - These strong acids also damage cellular morphology and thus are not recommended for delicate tissues such as bone marrow

- Organic acids such as acetic and formic acid are better suited to bone marrow because they are not as harsh; however, they act more slowly on dense cortical bone
- Formic acid in a 10% concentration is the best all-around decalcifier

Pearls

- Prolonged fixation can affect immunohistochemical results owing to alcohol precipitation of antigen at the cell surface; to optimize antigenicity of the tissue for IHC, the American Society of Clinical Oncology/College of American Pathologists (ASCO/CAP) guidelines recommend fixation of tissue destined for IHC in neutral buffered formalin for a minimum of 6 hours and a maximum of 48 hours (see Wolff et al, 2007)
- Urate crystals are water soluble and require a nonaqueous fixative such as absolute alcohol
- If tissue is needed for *immunofluorescence* (e.g., kidney or skin biopsies) or *enzyme profiles* (e.g., muscle biopsies), the specimen must be frozen without fixative; enzymes are rapidly inactivated by even brief exposure to fixation
- For rapid intraoperative analysis of tissue specimens, tissue can be frozen, and frozen sections can be cut with a special freezing microtome ("cryostat"); the pieces of tissue to be studied are snap-frozen in a cold liquid or cold environment ($-20°$ to $-70°C$); freezing makes the tissue solid enough to section with a microtome

Histologic Stains

- The staining process makes use of a variety of dyes that have been chosen for their ability to stain various cellular components of tissue
- Hematoxylin and eosin (H&E) stain
  - The most common histologic stain used for routine surgical pathology
  - Hematoxylin, because it is a basic dye, has an affinity for the nucleic acids of the cell nucleus
  - Hematoxylin does not directly stain tissues but needs a "mordant" or link to the tissues; this is provided by a metal cation such as iron, aluminum, or tungsten
  - The hematoxylin-metal complex acts as a basic dye, and any component that is stained is considered to be *basophilic* (i.e., contains the acid groups that bind the positively charged basic dye), appearing blue in tissue section
  - The variety of hematoxylin stains available for use is based partially on choice of metal ion used, which can vary the intensity or hue
  - Conversely, eosin is an acid aniline dye with an affinity for cytoplasmic components of the cell

— Eosin stains the more basic proteins within cells (cytoplasm) and in extracellular spaces (collagen) pink to red *(acidophilic)*

Connective Tissue

- Elastin stain
  — Elastin van Gieson (EVG) stain highlights elastic fibers in connective tissue
  — EVG stain is useful in demonstrating pathologic changes in elastic fibers, such as reduplication, breaks or splitting that may result from episodes of vasculitis, or connective tissue disorders such as Marfan syndrome
  — Elastic fibers are blue to black; collagen appears red; and the remaining connective tissue is yellow
- Masson trichrome stain
  — Helpful in differentiating between collagen fibers (blue staining) and smooth muscle (bright red staining)
- Reticulin stain
  — A silver impregnation technique stains reticulin fibers in tissue section black
  — Particularly helpful in assessing for alteration in the normal reticular fiber pattern, such as can be seen in some liver diseases or marrow fibrosis
- Jones silver stain
  — A silver impregnation procedure that highlights basement membrane material; used mainly in kidney biopsies

Fats and Lipids

- Oil red O stain
  — Demonstrates neutral lipids in frozen tissue

Figure 1-1. Elastin/Alcian blue stain. Aortic cystic medial degeneration in Marfan syndrome. Elastin stain highlights fragmentation of elastic fibers (*brown-black*) and pooling of mucopolysaccharides (*blue*) within the media.

Figure 1-2. Masson trichrome stain. Cirrhosis of the liver characterized by bridging fibrosis (*blue*) and regenerative nodule formation (*red*).

- Sudan black stain
  — Demonstrates neutral lipids in tissue sections
  — Mainly used in hematologic preparations such as peripheral blood or bone marrow aspirations for demonstration of primary granules of myeloid lineage

Carbohydrates and Mucoproteins

- Congo red stain
  — Amyloid is a fibrillar protein with a β-pleated sheath structure
  — Amyloid deposits in tissue exhibit a deep red or salmon color, whereas elastic tissue remains pale pink
  — When viewed under polarized light, amyloid deposits exhibit apple-green birefringence
  — The amyloid fibril–Congo red complex demonstrates green birefringence owing to the parallel alignment of dye molecules along the β-pleated sheath
  — The thickness of the section is critical (8 to 10 μm)
- Mucicarmine stain
  — Demonstrates epithelial mucin in tissue sections
  — Also highlights mucin-rich capsule of *Cryptococcus* species
- Periodic acid–Schiff (PAS) stain
  — Glycogen, neutral mucosubstances, basement membranes, and fungal walls exhibit a positive PAS (bright rose)
  — *PAS with diastase digestion*: diastase and amylase act on glycogen to depolymerize it into smaller sugar units that are then washed out of the section
  — Digestion removes glycogen but retains staining of other substances attached to sugars (i.e., mucopolysaccharides)

Figure 1-3. Membranous glomerulopathy. A, Jones silver stain highlighting basement membrane "spikes" (*arrow*) along glomerular capillary loops corresponding to basement membrane material surrounding intramembranous immune complexes. **B,** Direct immunofluorescence showing diffuse, granular staining of the glomerular capillary basement membranes with goat antihuman immunoglobulin G. This technique requires fresh-frozen tissue sections. **C,** Electron microscopy showing intramembranous electron-dense immune complexes within the glomerular capillary basement membranes. (Courtesy of Pamela Gibson, MD, University of Vermont/ Fletcher Allen Health Care, Department of Pathology, Burlington, VT.)

Figure 1-4. Alzheimer disease. A, Congo red–positive core of Alzheimer disease plaque. **B,** Apple-green birefringence of amyloid core under polarized light. **C,** Bielschowsky stain highlighting Alzheimer disease plaque (*arrow*) and neurofibrillary tangle within neuronal cell bodies (*arrowhead*).

- Alcian blue stain
  - May be used to distinguish various glandular epithelia of the gastrointestinal tract and in the diagnosis of Barrett epithelium
    - ◆ pH 1.0: acid sulfated mucin positive (colonic-like)
    - ◆ pH 2.5: acid sulfated mucin (colonic-like) and acid nonsulfated mucin (small intestinal-like) positive
    - ◆ Neutral mucins (gastric-like) negative at pH 1.0 and 2.5

Pigments and Minerals

- Ferric iron (Prussian blue), bilirubin (bile stain), calcium (von Kossa), copper (rhodanine), and melanin (Fontana-Masson) are the most common pigments and minerals demonstrated in surgical pathology specimens

Nerves and Fibers

- Bielschowsky stain
  - A silver impregnation procedure that demonstrates the presence of neurofibrillary tangles and senile plaques in Alzheimer disease
  - Axons stain black
- Luxol fast blue stain
  - Demonstrates myelin in tissue sections
  - Loss of staining indicates myelin breakdown secondary to axonal degeneration
  - Gray matter and demyelinated white matter should be almost colorless and contrast with the blue-stained myelinated white matter

Hematopoietic and Nuclear Elements

- Toluidine blue stain
  - Demonstrates mast cells in tissue

- Giemsa, Wright, and May-Grünwald stains
  - For cellular details, including hematopoietic (peripheral blood or bone marrow) and cytology preparations
- Leder stain (chloracetate esterase)
  - Identification of cytoplasmic granules of granulocytes and myeloid precursors

Microorganisms: Bacteria, Fungi, Parasites

- Brown and Brenn Gram stain
  - Demonstration of gram-negative (red) and gram-positive (blue) bacteria in tissue
- Giemsa stain
  - Demonstration of bacteria, rickettsia, and *Toxoplasma gondii* in tissue sections
- Grocott methenamine silver (GMS) stain
  - Demonstration of fungi or *Pneumocystis* organisms (fungi may also be demonstrated by PAS-amylase stain)
- Warthin-Starry and Steiner stains
  - Silver impregnation technique for spirochetes (e.g., *Borrelia burgdorferi*, *Treponema pallidum*) in tissue sections
  - *Note:* all bacteria are nonselectively blackened by silver impregnation methods such as the Warthin-Starry and Steiner stains
  - These methods are more sensitive for small gram-negative bacteria (e.g., *Legionella* species, *Helicobacter pylori*, and *Bartonella* species) than tissue Gram stain
- Ziehl-Neelsen method for acid-fast bacteria (AFB)
  - Detect the presence of acid-fast mycobacteria (bright red) in tissue sections (background light blue)
  - Fite method should be used to demonstrate *Mycobacterium leprae* or *Nocardia* species, both of which are weakly acid fast

Figure 1-5. Luxol fast blue stain. Demyelination in multiple sclerosis (*colorless regions*).

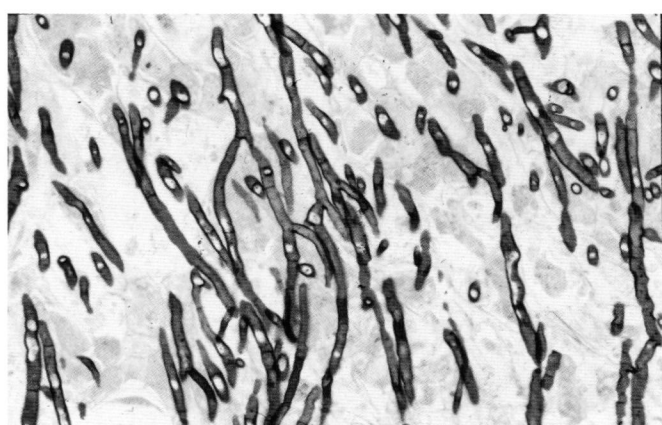

Figure 1-6. *Aspergillus* organisms in the lung stained by Grocott methenamine silver stain.

Figure 1-7. Ziehl-Neelsen stain for acid-fast bacilli. Abundant *Mycobacterium avian intracellulare* organisms (*red*) within macrophages in the lung.

Selected References

Wolff AC, Hammond ME, Schwartz JN, et al: American Society of Clinical Oncology/College of American Pathologists Guideline Recommendations for Human Epidermal Growth Factor Receptor 2 Testing in Breast Cancer. Arch Pathol Lab Med 131:18-43, 2007.

Bancroft JD, Gamble M: Theory and Practice of Histochemical Techniques, 5th ed. Philadelphia, Elsevier, 2001.

Carson FL: Histotechnology: A self-instructional text, 2nd ed. Chicago, American Society for Clinical Pathology (ASCP) Press, 1997.

Fluorescence Microscopy

- Tissue is exposed to short-wavelength ultraviolet (UV) light (2500 to 4000 angstroms) through a mercury or halogen lamp; the energy is absorbed by molecules that then release the energy as visible light (4000 to 8000 angstroms)
- In immunofluorescence techniques, antibodies are labeled with a fluorescent dye such as fluorescein isothiocyanate (FITC)
- Direct immunofluorescence
  — Fluorescein-labeled antihuman globulin primary antibodies are applied to frozen, unfixed tissue sections to locate and combine with antibodies, complement, or antigens deposited in tissue
- Indirect immunofluorescence
  — Unlabeled primary antibody is applied to the tissue section, followed by application of an FITC-labeled antibody that is directed against a portion of the unlabelled primary antibody
  — More sensitive and more expensive
  — Primary application in surgical pathology is detection of autoimmune diseases involving the skin and kidney (Table 1-1)

Table 1-1. Immunofluorescence Patterns and Disease Associations

Disease	Antibodies	Pattern	Histologic Manifestation
Skin			
Pemphigus vulgaris	Antidesmosomal	Intercellular chicken-wire IgG in epidermis	Suprabasal vesiculation
Bullous pemphigoid	Antiepithelial BM; anti-hemidesmosome [collagen XVII (BP180)]	Linear IgG along BM; in salt-split skin, reactivity along roof	Subepithelial vesiculation
Epidermolysis bullosa acquisita (EBA)	EBA Ag	Linear IgG along BM; in salt-split skin, reactivity along floor	Subepithelial vesiculation
Dermatitis herpetiformis	Anti-gluten	Granular IgA, especially in tips of dermal papillae	Subepithelial vesiculation
Kidney			
Anti–glomerular basement membrane (anti-GBM) disease	Anti-GBM COL4-A3 antigen	Linear GBM staining for IgG, corresponding granular staining for C3	Crescentic GN
Membranous glomerulopathy	Subepithelial deposits secondary to in situ immune complex formation (antigen unknown; associated with lupus nephritis, hepatitis B, penicillamine, gold, malignancy)	Diffuse, granular GBM staining for IgG and C3	Diffusely thickened glomerular capillary loops with lace-like splitting and "spikes" identified on Jones silver stain
IgA nephropathy	Deposited IgA polyclonal: possible increased production in response to exposure to environmental agents (e.g., viruses, bacteria, food proteins such as gluten)	IgA ± IgG, IgM, and C3 in mesangium	Focal proliferative GN; mesangial widening
Membranoproliferative glomerulonephritis	Type I: immune complex	Type 1: IgG + C3; C1q + C4	Mesangial proliferation; GBM thickening; splitting
	Type II: autoantibody to alternative complement pathway	Type II: C3 ± IgG; no C1q or C4	

BM, basement membrane; GBM, glomerular basement membrane; GN, glomerulonephritis; Ig, immunoglobulin.

Selected References

Kalaaji AN, Nicolas MEO: Mayo Clinic Atlas of Immunofluorescence in Dermatology: Patterns and Target Antigens. Informa Healthcare, New York, NY, 2006.

D'Agati VD, Jennette JC, Silva FG: Non-neoplastic Kidney Diseases. AFIP Atlas of Nontumor Pathology, vol 4. Washington, DC, Armed Forces Institute of Pathology, 2005.

Electron Microscopy

- The electron microscope has a magnification range of 1,000 to 500,000 diameters (×) (the upper limit of light microscopy is about 1,000 diameters), thereby allowing for analyzing the ultrastructure of a cell
- There are two types of EM:
  — Transmission EM
    ◆ Two-dimensional (2D) black-and-white image is produced
    ◆ Tissue either transmits electrons (producing "lucent" or clear areas in the image) or deflects electrons (producing electron "dense" or dark areas in the image)
    ◆ Useful in the diagnosis of non-neoplastic diseases of the kidney
  — Scanning EM
    ◆ Three-dimensional (3D) black-and-white image results as an electron beam sweeps the surface of the specimen and releases secondary electrons
    ◆ Lower resolution than transmission EM and used primarily in the research setting to study cell surface membrane changes
- Application in surgical pathology: EM is a useful diagnostic technique to supplement morphologic, immunohistochemical, cytogenetic, and molecular analysis of tissues
- Immunoperoxidase techniques have largely replaced EM for tumor diagnosis in surgical pathology
- EM is useful in
  — Renal, skin, myocardial, nerve, and muscle biopsies
  — Undifferentiated or poorly differentiated neoplasms
  — Diagnosis of lysosomal storage disorders
  — Ciliary dysmorphology
  — Visualization of infectious agents

Technical Overview

- The main fixative used for EM is glutaraldehyde, which penetrates tissues more slowly than formalin; cubes of tissue 1 mm or smaller are needed
- Processing postfixation with osmium tetroxide, which binds to lipids in membranes for better visualization; dehydration with graded alcohols; infiltration with propylene oxide and epoxy resin; embedding in epoxy resin
- 1-μm sections (semithin) are cut and stained with toluidine blue to verify that the area of interest has been selected for EM
- 100-nm sections (ultrathin) are cut and collected on copper grids
- Tissues are stained with heavy metals (uranyl acetate and lead citrate)
- *Electron dense*: darker in color as a result of heavy impregnation with heavy metal
- *Electron lucent*: lighter in color

Ultrastructure of a Cell

Nucleus

- Nuclear membrane
- Nuclear pore
- Nucleolus
  — Dense, rounded basophilic structure that consists of 80% to 90% protein
  — Produces most of the ribosomal RNA
  — Mitotically or metabolically active cells have multiple nucleoli
- Chromatin
  — Heterochromatin: stainable, condensed regions of chromosomes seen as intensely basophilic nuclear material in light microscopy
  — Euchromatin: nonstainable, extended portions of the chromosomes that consist of genetically active DNA

Cytoplasm

- Plasma membrane
  — Appears as two electron-dense (dark) layers with an intervening electron-lucent (light) layer
- Basement membrane = basal lamina (lamina densa + lamina lucida) + lamina reticularis + anchoring fibrils + microfibrils
  — Lamina densa
    ◆ Electron-dense membrane made up of type IV collagen fibers coated by a heparan sulfate proteoglycan
    ◆ About 30 to 70 nm thick with an underlying network of reticular collagen (type III) fibrils, which average 30 nm in diameter and 0.1 to 2 μm in thickness
- Mitochondria
  — The energy-producing component of the cell; these membrane-bound organelles undergo oxidative reactions to produce energy
  — Energy generation occurs on the cristae, which are composed of the inner mitochondrial membrane
  — Most cells contain shelflike mitochondrial cristae
  — Steroid-producing cells (i.e., adrenal cortex) contain tubular cristae
  — Mitochondrial crystals are always pathologic

— Hürthle cell change occurs when the cytoplasm of a cell becomes packed with mitochondria
- Ribosomes
  — Sites of protein synthesis
  — Usually responsible for the basophilic staining of the cytoplasm on H&E-stained sections
- Endoplasmic reticulum
  — Membrane-bound channels responsible for the transport and processing of secretory products of the cell
  — Granular or rough endoplasmic reticulum is abundant in cells that actively produce secretory products destined to be released to other cells (e.g., plasma cells producing immunoglobulin and pancreatic acinar cells producing digestive enzymes); the granular appearance is due to attached ribosomes
  — Smooth endoplasmic reticulum is abundant in cells that synthesize steroids (i.e., adrenal cortex, Sertoli-Leydig cells) and in tumors derived from these types of cells
- Golgi apparatus
  — Concentrates and packages proteins into secretory vesicles for transport to the cell surface
  - Prominent in cells that secrete proteins

Single Membrane–Bound Structures

- Cytoplasmic granules are classified based on size and morphology (Table 1-2)
- Lysosomes
  — Contain enzymes that assist in digesting material to be disposed of in the cell
  — Endogenous and exogenous pigments can be collected in lysosomes; can be large and filled with undigested cellular components in lysosomal storage disorders
- Dense core granules: seen in cells and tumors with neuroendocrine differentiation
- Melanosomes and premelanosomes are specific single membrane–bound structures
- Weibel-Palade bodies are specific for endothelial cells
- Birbeck granules are seen in Langerhans cell histiocytosis

Filaments and Tubules

- Filaments are classified based on size (Table 1-3)
- Microtubules are seen in association with the mitotic spindle and in cells or tumors of neural origin (e.g., neuroblastoma)

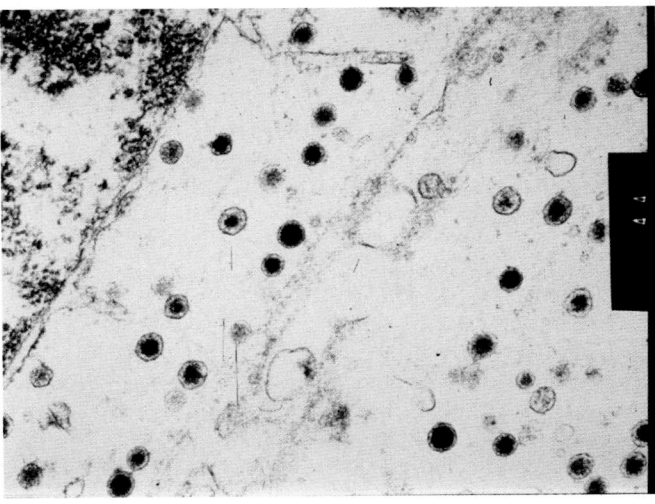

Figure 1-8. Electron microscopy. Neuroendocrine granules in small cell carcinoma of the lung.

Figure 1-9. Electron microscopy. Birbeck granules (*arrow*) in Langerhans cell histiocytosis. (Photo courtesy of Janet Schwarz, Senior Research Technician, Microscopy Imaging Center, University of Vermont, Burlington, VT.)

Cell Surface

- Cell processes are seen in cells that are capable of movement; some tumors, such as schwannomas and meningiomas, demonstrate interdigitating processes
- Villi are prominent and regular in cells or tumors of glandular origin
- Terminal web and rootlets in villi are seen in foregut derivatives (e.g., colon)

Table 1-2. Cytoplasmic Granules

Type	Size	Morphology	Product	Cell Type/Tumor
Mucigen	0.7-1.8 μm	Electron lucent	Glycoprotein	Mucin secreting
Serous, zymogen	0.5-1.5 μm	Electron dense	Proenzyme/enzyme	Example: acinar cells of pancreas
Neuroendocrine	100-300 nm	Dense core	Example: biogenic amines	Neuroendocrine cells

Table 1-3. Filaments and Tubules

Component	Diameter	Location
Microfilaments (actin, nonmuscle myosin)	6-8 nm	Cytoskeleton of all cells
Intermediate filaments	10 nm	
Cytokeratin	>19 proteins 40-68 kd	Epithelial cells
Glial fibrillary acid protein	55 kd	Astrocytes
Neurofilament	68, 160, 200 kd	Neural tissue
Vimentin	57 kd	Mesenchymal tissues
Desmin	53 kd	Muscle
Microtubules	25 nm	Neural derivatives (e.g., neuroblastoma)

kD, kilodaltons; nm, nanometers; 50 kD = ~4 nm

Figure 1-10. Electron microscopy. Short villi lining an intracytoplasmic lumen in adenocarcinoma of the breast.

- Junctions are seen in virtually all cells except those of hematopoietic origin
- Basal lamina is seen surrounding all endodermal and ectodermal derivatives; cells with muscle differentiation also may have a basal lamina, which may be incomplete

Extracellular Matrix

- Collagen shows a regular structure
- Amyloid
  - Fibrils measuring approximately 10 nm in diameter, with an electron-lucent core
  - Fibrils are straight, nonbranching, and arranged randomly

Selected References

Ghadially FN: Diagnostic Ultrastructural Pathology, 2nd ed. Boston, Butterworth-Heinemann, 1998.

Ghadially FN: Ultrastructure of the Cell and Matrix, 4th ed. Boston, Butterworth-Heinemann, 1997.

Ghadially FN: Diagnostic Electron Microscopy of Tumors. Boston, Butterworth-Heinemann, 1986.

Immunohistochemistry

Introduction

IHC combines anatomic, immunologic, and biochemical techniques to identify specific tissue components using a specific antigen-antibody reaction labeled with a visible reporter molecule. This binding is then visualized through the use of various enzymes that are coupled to the antibodies being used. The enzyme acts on a chromogenic substrate to cause deposition of a colored material at the site of antibody-antigen bindings. Hence, IHC permits the visualization and localization of specific cellular components within a cell or tissue while importantly preserving the overall morphology and structure of the tissue section. During the past several decades, major improvements in protein conjugation, antigen preservation and antigen retrieval methods, and enhanced immunodetection systems have enshrined IHC as a major adjunctive investigative tool for both surgical and cytopathology. IHC is not only critical for the accurate diagnosis of malignancies but also plays a pivotal role in prognostic evaluation (e.g., estrogen and progesterone receptors in breast cancer) and treatments strategies (e.g., c-kit protein for gastrointestinal stromal tumors and *HER-2-neu* in certain breast cancers).

Technical Overview

- Formalin cross-links proteins in tissues; success of immunohistochemical staining depends on the availability of an antigen after fixation
  - Various techniques may unmask antigens, such as digestion by enzymes (e.g., trypsin) or antigen retrieval using heat, metallic mordants, or alkaline buffers
  - Commonly used enzymes include peroxidase, alkaline phosphatase, and glucose oxidase
  - Most commonly used chromogen substrates produce brown (DAB) or red (AEC) reaction products
- Definition of terms
  - **Polyclonal antibody:** Conventional antiserum produced by multiple plasma cells of an animal that had been injected with an antigen; a polyclonal antibody may have multiple determinants (binding sites)
  - **Monoclonal antibody:** Produced by fusion of a malignant cell with a plasma cell producing antibody to a specific epitope; antibodies may be grown in tissue culture
- Antibodies for the detection of cellular components
  - Intermediate filaments (see Table 1-3)
  - Other cellular and tissue components: (e.g., α_1-antitrypsin, myeloperoxidase, synaptophysin and chromogranin, myoglobin)
  - Leukocyte antigens and immunoglobulin components commonly used in paraffin-embedded tissues

- ◆ T-cell
  - ◇ CD1a: thymocyte; also marks Langerhans cells
  - ◇ CD3: Pan–T-cell marker that shows cytoplasmic and membrane staining
  - ◇ CD5: Pan–T-cell marker also expressed by some B-cell lymphomas
  - ◇ CD43: Pan–T-cell marker also expressed by some B-cell lymphomas
  - ◇ CD45RO (UCHL-1), CD4, CD8: T-cell markers
- ◆ B-cell
  - ◇ CD20: Pan–B-cell marker
  - ◇ Immunoglobulin heavy and light chains: used for demonstration of clonality in B-cell neoplasms
- ◆ Myeloid
  - ◇ CD15 (Leu-M1): pan-myeloid antigen that also marks Reed-Sternberg cells of Hodgkin lymphoma
- ◆ Monocyte and histiocyte
  - ◇ CD163, CD68
- ◆ Natural killer cell
  - ◇ CD57 (Leu-7)
  - ◇ CD56 (neural cell adhesion molecules, NCAM, Leu-19)
- ◆ Megakaryocyte
  - ◇ CD41
  - ◇ Factor VIII–von Willebrand factor (vWF)
  - ◇ *Ulex europaeus* agglutinin-1 (UEA-1)
- • Hormones and hormone receptors
  - — Presence may have prognostic significance
  - — Estrogen and progesterone receptors in breast carcinomas
  - — Androgen receptors
- • Infectious agents
- • Oncogenes and oncogene products
  - — May correlate with prognosis
  - — *bcl-1*, *bcl-2*, *bcl-6* in lymphoid neoplasms
  - — *HER-2-neu* and *C-erbB2* in breast carcinomas
  - — *p53* tumor suppressor gene: mutations are seen in a variety of malignant tumors

Ground Rules for Quality Application of Immunohistochemistry in Surgical Pathology

- • Technique
  - — It is imperative that the pathologist work closely with the immunohistotechnologist to optimize, validate, and interpret the IHC assay for any particular antibody reagent
  - — Adequate fixation of tissue or specimen in 10% buffered formalin is essential to high-quality IHC; it is probably better to overfix (because modern antigen retrieval systems can unmask epitopes) rather than underfix (because inadvertent alcohol fixation during tissue processing precipitates and masks epitopes)
  - — It is best to use a polymer-based detection system, which has the advantage of being avidin-biotin free, thereby avoiding false immunoreactivity with endogenous biotin
  - — Appropriate antigen retrieval systems should be optimized for each antibody (noting that different antibodies require unique systems, and some require none)
- • Antibody choice
  - — A generic screening panel of antibodies should be chosen initially, followed algorithmically by a specific panel to further characterize a neoplasm
  - — Avoid using a single antibody in isolation (because this may result in a potentially erroneous diagnosis), and always use more than one antibody to target a specific antigen
  - — The choice of a panel of antibodies to target a specific antigen should always be made in the context of the morphology and clinical presentation of any neoplasm; avoid use of the "buckshot" approach in hope that an IHC assay returns a positive reaction
  - — Avoid preordering an IHC panel of antibodies before previewing the morphology; remember that IHC is an ancillary or adjunctive technique to the quality practice of surgical pathology and not vice versa
- • Interpretation
  - — Interpretation of IHC should always be made in the context of the known subcellular localization or distribution of the targeted antigen (e.g., membranous, cytoplasmic, nuclear, or perinuclear "Golgi pattern" of immunoreactivity)
- • Controls
  - — Finally, the importance of adequate incorporation of appropriate tissue and reagent (both positive

Figure 1-11. Immunohistochemistry for *HER-2-neu* in a breast adenocarcinoma showing (3+) membranous staining.

and negative) controls in every run of IHC cannot be overemphasized; this is ultimately the highest form of quality control of the IHC assay and should be reviewed daily to avoid false-positive and false-negative interpretation

Figure 1-12. **Immunohistochemistry for HepPar-1** highlighting strong cytoplasmic staining of normal hepatic parenchyma.

A Practical Tabular Approach to Using Immunohistochemistry for Common Diagnostic Problems

- Because a complete technical overview of IHC and comprehensive listing of available antibodies is beyond the scope of this chapter, our goal is to provide a practical approach to IHC application in surgical pathology; the following tables are presented as guidelines to assist with the choice of an antibody panel when confronted with certain differential diagnoses (Tables 1-4 through 1-29)

Pearls

- Tumors are not 100% specific or sensitive to a particular immunoreagent; interpretation of these tables should be used in this context to avoid diagnostic pitfalls.
- Always target the IHC panel in the context of the morphologic differential diagnosis

Figure 1-13. **Immunohistochemistry for TTF-1. A,** Nuclear immunoreactivity in normal thyroid parenchyma. **B,** Nuclear immunoreactivity in pulmonary adenocarcinoma.

Table 1-4. Immunohistochemistry Approach to Undifferentiated Tumors

	Pan-CK	**EMA**	**S-100**	**PLAP**	**LCA**	**CD138**
Carcinoma	+	+	−	−/v	−	−
Melanoma	−/v	−	+	−	−	−
Germ cell	v	−	−	+	−	−
Lymphoma	−	−	−	−	+	−
Anaplastic plasmacytoma/myeloma	−	+	−	−	−/+	+

EMA, epithelial membrane antigen; LCA, leukocyte common antigen; Pan-CK, pan-cytokeratin; PLAP, placental alkaline phosphatase; v, variable; +, positive; −, negative; −/+, rarely positive.

Table 1-5. Immunophenotypic Distribution of Cytokeratins 7 and 20

Carcinoma Type*	CK7	CK20
Colorectal and Merkel cell	−	+
Hepatocellular	−	−
Salivary gland	+	−
Lung, non–small cell carcinoma	+	−
Lung, neuroendocrine carcinoma	−	−
Breast, ductal	+	−
Ovarian, serous, and endometrioid	+	−
Endometrial and endocervical	+	−
Renal cell	−	−
Prostatic	−	−
Urothelial	+	+
Pancreas	+/−	+/−
Mesothelioma	+	−

*Only about 70% to 90% of these tumors follow the given CK7/20 immunoprofile; therefore, reliance solely on this profile to determine the primary site of carcinomas is not recommended.

CK, cytokeratin; +, positive; −, negative; +/−, variably positive.

Table 1-6. Specific Antibody Reagents to Identify Primary Site of Metastatic Carcinoma

Carcinoma Type	Antibody	Signal Localization	Other Tumors Identified
Breast	GCDFP-15	Cytoplasmic	Salivary, sweat gland
Breast	Mammoglobin	Cytoplasmic	Salivary, sweat gland
Colon	CDX2	Nuclear	Subset of pancreas, gastric
Hepatocellular	HepPar-1 Ag	Cytoplasmic	Hepatoid carcinomas of stomach, ovary
Hepatocellular	pCEA or CD10	Bile canaliculi	Hepatoid carcinomas
Hepatocellular	GPC-3	Membranous and cytoplasmic	Melanoma, a subset of chronic active hepatitis
Lung and thyroid except mucinous BAC	TTF-1	Nuclear	Neuroendocrine carcinoma extrapulmonary
Ovarian serous	WT-1, p16	Nuclear	Mesothelioma (WT-1)
Prostate	PSA, PAP	Cytoplasmic	
Squamous, urothelial, thymic	p63	Nuclear	Salivary gland, neuroendocrine, subset prostate
Thyroid	Thyroglobulin	Cytoplasmic	—
Urothelial	Uroplakin III	Membranous	—
Renal, clear	RCC	Membranous	

BAC, bronchoalveolar carcinoma; GCDFP-15, gross cystic disease fluid protein-15; GPC-3, glypican 3; PAP, prostatic acid phosphatase; pCEA, polyclonal carcinoembryonic antigen; PSA, prostate-specific antigen; RCC, renal cell carcinoma; TTF-1, thyroid transcription factor-1; WT-1, Wilms' tumor gene protein 1.

Modified from Gown et al: Arch Pathol Lab Med 2009, in press.

Table 1-7. Immunohistochemistry Panel for Interpretation of Lung Mesothelioma and Adenocarcinoma

Antibody	Epithelioid Mesothelioma (Percentage Positive)	Sarcomatoid Mesothelioma (Percentage Positive)	Adenocarcinoma (Percentage Positive)
Epithelial marker			
mCEA	3	—	81
Ber-Ep4	10	0	80
B72.3	7	0	80
CD15 (Leu-M1)	7	0	72
MOC-31	7	0	93
TTF-1	Negative	0	72 (lung)
Mesothelial marker			
Cytokeratin 5/6	83	13	15
Calretinin	82	88	15
WT-1	77	13	4
D2-40	86-100	0	36 (weak)
Mesothelin	100	0	—

mCEA, monoclonal carcinoembryonic antigen; TTF-1,thyroid transcription factor; WT-1, Wilms' tumor gene protein 1.

Modified from Marchevsky AM: Application of immunohistochemistry to the diagnosis of malignant mesothelioma. Arch Pathol Lab Med 132:397-401, 2008.

Table 1-8. Immunohistochemistry Panel for Lung Adenocarcinoma and Breast Adenocarcinoma

Immunostain	Lung Adenocarcinoma (Percentage Positive)	Breast Adenocarcinoma (Percentage Positive)
TTF-1	77	0
Mammoglobin	17	85
GCDFP-15	2	53
ER	4	72

ER, estrogen receptor; GCDFP-15, gross cystic disease fluid protein-15; TTF-1, thyroid transcription factor.

Data from Takeda Y, Tsuta K, Shibuki Y, et al: Analysis of expression patterns of breast cancer-specific markers (mammaglobin and gross cystic disease fluid protein 15) in lung and pleural tumors. Arch Pathol Lab Med 132:239, 2008; and Striebel JM, Dacic S, Yousem SA: Gross cystic disease fluid protein-(GCDFP-15): Expression in primary lung adenocarcinoma. Am J Surg Pathol 32:426, 2008.

Table 1-9. Immunohistochemistry Comparison of Spindle Cell Areas in Metaplastic Carcinoma, Phyllodes Tumor, and Fibromatosis of the Breast

	CD34	SMA	34βe12	Pan-CK	Desmin	p63
Metaplastic carcinoma	–	+/–	+/–	–/+	–/+	+
Phyllodes	+/–	+/–	–	–	–/+	–
Fibromatosis	–	+/–	–	–	–	–
Myofibroblastoma	+	+/–	–	–	+	–
Myoepithelial tumor	–	+/–	+/–	+	–/+	+/–

Pan-CK, pan-cytokeratin; SMA, smooth muscle actin; +, positive; –, negative; +/–, often positive; –/+, rarely positive.

Modified from Dunne B, Lee AH, Pinder SE, et al: An immunohistochemical study of metaplastic spindle cell carcinoma, phyllodes tumor and fibromatosis of the breast. Hum Pathol 34:1009-1015, 2003.

Table 1-10. Useful Antibody Panel to Demonstrate Myoepithelial and Basal Cells in Breast Lesions to Distinguish Benign (+) from Invasive (−) Carcinoma

	Myoepithelial/Basal Cells	Stromal Myofibroblasts
Smooth muscle heavy-chain myosin	+ (Cytoplasmic)	−/+
p63	+ (Nuclear)	−
α-SMA	+ (Cytoplasmic)	+/−
S-100	+ (Nuclear and cytoplasmic)	v
Calponin	+ (Cytoplasmic)	−/+
D2-40*	−/+	−

*D2-40 is a useful marker to highlight lymphatic endothelium in lymphovascular invasion (LVI) by carcinoma but may in addition occasionally stain myoepithelial and basal cells—hence the use of D2-40 to demonstrate that LVI should always be accompanied by p63/SMHCM immunohistochemistry.

SMA, smooth muscle actin; v, variable; +, positive; −, negative; −/+, rarely positive.

Modified from Rabban JT, Chen YY: D2-40 expression by breast myoepithelium: Potential pitfalls in distinguishing intralymphatic carcinoma from in situ carcinoma. Hum Pathol 39:175-183, 2008.

Table 1-11. Immunohistochemical Panel Approach to Differential Diagnosis of Hepatocellular Carcinoma

	HepPar-1	CK19	MOC-31	GPC-3	pCEA	CDX-2	TTF-1	RCC	Inhibin/Melan-A/D2-40
Hepatocellular carcinoma	+	−	−/+	+	+	−	−*	−	−
Cholangiocarcinoma	−	+/−	+/−	−	−		−	−	−
Metastatic adenocarcinoma									
Colon	−			−	−	+	−	−	
Thyroid, lung	−			−	−	−	+	−	−
Tumors with polygonal cells									
RCC	−		+			−	−	+	−
Adrenocortical carcinoma	−				−	−	−		+
Neuroendocrine tumors†	−		+		−		v		
Hepatoid carcinoma, e.g., gastric, ovary	+								

*Certain TTF-1 antibody reagents may highlight the cytoplasm of liver cells (only nuclear immunoreactivity should be interpreted as being of thyroid or lung origin in the correct clinical setting).

†Strong synaptophysin and chromogranin support neuroendocrine tumor; TTF-1 may notoriously highlight extrapulmonary neuroendocrine tumors.

CK, cytokeratin; p-CEA, canalicular pattern of staining; RCC, renal cell carcinoma; TTF-1, thyroid transcription factor; v, variable; +, positive; −, negative; +/−, often positive; −/+, rarely positive.

Modified from Kakar S, Gown AM, Goodman ZD, Ferrell LD: Best practices in diagnostic immunohistochemistry: Hepatocellular carcinoma versus metastatic neoplasms. Arch Pathol Lab Med 131:1648-1654, 2007.

Table 1-12. Immunohistochemistry Panel Interpretation for Gastrointestinal and Abdominal Spindle Cell Tumors

	CD117	CD34	SMA	Desmin	S-100 Protein	β-Catenin
Leiomyoma	−	−	+	+	−	
Leiomyosarcoma (LMS)*	−	−/+*	+	+	−	
Inflammatory myofibroblastic tumor	−	−	+/−	−	−	
Inflammatory fibroid polyp	−	+	+/−	−	−	
Solitary fibrous tumor	−	+	−	−	−	
Desmoid fibromatosis	−	−	+	−/+	−	+ (Nuclear)
Gastrointestinal schwannoma	−	−	−	−	+	
Metastatic melanoma	+/−	−	−	−	+	
Desmoplastic small round cell tumor	−	−	−	+	−	
GIST	+	+	+/−	−/+	−/+	

*Retroperitoneal LMS may be positive.

GIST, gastrointestinal stromal tumor; SMA, smooth muscle actin; +, positive; −, negative; +/−, often positive; −/+, rarely positive.

Modified from Miettinen M, Sobin LH, Sarlomo-Rikala M: Immunohistochemical spectrum of GISTs at different sites and their differential diagnosis with a reference to CD117 (KIT). Mod Pathol 13:1134-1142, 2000.

Table 1-13. Immunophenotype of Primary Ovarian and Metastatic Colorectal Adenocarcinoma

	Mucinous Ovarian Tumors		Endometrioid Adenocarcinoma	Metastatic Colorectal Adenocarcinoma
	Intestinal Type	Endocervical Type		
CK7	+++/+	+++	+++	−
CK20	−/+/+++	−	−	+++
mCEA	+	−	−	++
CDX2	+	−	−/+	++
ER	−	+	+	−

ER, estrogen receptor; mCEA, monoclonal carcinoembryonic antigen; +++, diffusely positive; +, focally positive; −, negative.

Modified from McCluggage WG: My approach to and thoughts on the typing of ovarian carcinomas. J Clin Pathol 61:152-163, 2008.

Table 1-14. Immunohistochemistry Panel for Primary and Metastatic Adenocarcinoma of the Ovary

	CK7	CK20	CDX2	DPC4
Primary mucinous, intestinal type	+	+	+/−	+
Primary endometrioid	+	−	−	+
Metastatic colorectal	−	+	+	+
Metastatic pancreas	+/−	+/−	−	−

CK, cytokeratin; DPC, deleted in pancreatic carcinoma; +, positive; −, negative; +/−, often positive; −/+, rarely positive.

Modified from Ji H, Isacson C, Seidman JD, et al: Cytokeratins 7 and 20, Dpc4, and MUC5AC in the distinction of metastatic mucinous carcinomas in the ovary from primary ovarian mucinous tumors: Dpc4 assists in identifying metastatic pancreatic carcinomas. Int J Gynecol Pathol 21:391-400, 2002.

Table 1-15. Immunohistochemistry: High-Grade Serous Carcinoma and Poorly Differentiated Endometrioid Adenocarcinoma of the Ovary and Endometrium

	Serous	Endometrioid
WT-1	+++	−/+
p53	+++	−/+/+++*
p16	+++	−/+
β-Catenin	membranous	membranous/nuclear

*The +++ expression corresponds to some high-grade carcinomas.

WT-1, Wilms' tumor gene protein 1; +++, diffusely positive; +, focally positive; −, negative.

Modified from McCluggage WG: My approach to and thoughts on the typing of ovarian carcinomas. J Clin Pathol 61:152-163, 2008.

Table 1-16. Immunohistochemistry Approach to Ovarian Sex Cord–Stromal Tumors and Endometrioid Adenocarcinoma

	Inhibin	Calretinin	CD99	EMA	Pan-cytokeratin
Granulosa cell tumor	+	+	+	−	−/+
Sertoli-Leydig cell tumor	+	+	+	−	+/−
Endometrioid adenocarcinoma	−	−	−	+	+

EMA, epithelial membrane antigen; +, positive; −, negative; +/−, often positive; −/+, rarely positive.

Modified from Mount SL, Cooper K: Tumours with divergent müllerian differentiation of the uterine corpus. Curr Diagn Pathol 11:349-355, 2005.

Table 1-17. Immunohistochemistry Approach to Endocervical Adenocarcinoma and Endometrioid Endometrial Adenocarcinoma

	mCEA	Vimentin	ER/PR	p16	HPV DNA
Endocervical	+	−	−	+	+
Endometrial	−	+	+	−/+	−

ER/PR, estrogen/progesterone receptor; HPV, human papillomavirus; mCEA, monoclonal carcinoembryonic antigen; +, positive; −, negative; −/+, rarely positive.

Modified from Staebler A, Sherman ME, Zaino RJ, Ronnett BM: Hormone receptor immunohistochemistry and human papillomavirus in situ hybridization are useful for distinguishing endocervical and endometrial adenocarcinomas. Am J Surg Pathol 26:998-1006, 2002.

Table 1-18. Immunohistochemistry in the Differential Diagnosis of Squamous and Glandular Lesions of the Uterine Cervix

	p16*	MIB-1 (Ki-67)
LSIL (CIN I)	+/−	Increased
HSIL (CIN II-III)	+	Increased (full thickness)
Adenocarcinoma in situ	+	+
Atypical immature metaplasia	−	−/+
Reactive squamous or glandular atypia	−	+
Tubal metaplasia	+/−	−

*Expression of p16 (nuclear and cytoplasmic) is a surrogate marker for high-risk human papillomavirus (HPV), for example, HPV-16 and HPV-18. In LSIL, the p16 expression may be confined to the lower one third or one half of the squamous epithelium or show focal immunoreactivity (the latter being a pattern of expression, albeit cytoplasmic only, that may be seen in reactive squamous epithelia). HSIL p16 immunoexpression usually involves two thirds or full thickness of the squamous epithelium.

CIN, cervical intraepithelial neoplasia; HSIL, high-grade squamous intraepithelial neoplasia; LSIL, low-grade squamous intraepithelial neoplasia; +, positive; −, negative; +/−, often positive; −/+, rarely positive.

Modified from Kalof AN, Cooper K: p16INK4a immunoexpression: Surrogate marker of high-risk HPV and high-grade cervical intraepithelial neoplasia. Adv Anat Pathol 13:190-194, 2006.

Table 1-19. p57^KIP2 Immunoreaction and *HER-2* Fluorescence In Situ Hybridization (FISH) Analysis in Molar Pregnancy

	Villous Cytotrophoblasts	Villous Stroma	Syncytiotrophoblasts	*HER-2* FISH Analysis
Complete hydatidiform molar pregnancy	−	−	+	diploid
Partial hydatidiform molar pregnancy	+	+	+	triploid
Hydropic abortion	+	+	+	diploid

Note: p57^KIP2 Is a paternally imprinted, maternally expressed gene protein. Hence, complete moles comprising only paternal genes will not express this protein.

Modified from Hoffner L, Dunn J, Esposito N, et al: p57^KIP2 Immunostaining and molecular cytogenetics: combined approach aids in diagnosis of morphologically challenging cases with molar phenotype and in detecting androgenetic cell lines in mosaic/chimeric conceptions. Hum Pathol 39:63, 2008; and LeGallo RD, Stelow EB, Ramirez NC, et al: Diagnosis of hydatidiform moles using p57 immunohistochemistry and her2 fluorescent in situ hybridization. Am J Clin Pathol 129:749, 2008.

Table 1-20. Immunohistochemical Approach for Trophoblastic Lesions

Trophoblastic Lesion	CK18	p63	hPL	MIB-1 LI (%)
Exaggerated placental site	+++	−	+++	<1
Placental site trophoblastic tumor	+++	−	+++	>1
Placental site nodule	+++	+++	−/+	<10
Epithelioid trophoblastic tumor	+++	+++	−/+	>10
Choriocarcinoma	+++	−/+	++	

Note: Expression of p63 highlights mononucleated trophoblasts corresponding to cytotrophoblasts, and human chorionic gonadotropin selectively stains syncytiotrophoblasts; this combination is indicative of choriocarcinoma.

CK, cytokeratin; hPL, human placental lactogen; LI, labeling index; MIB-1, Ki-67 proliferation marker; +++, diffusely positive; +, focally positive; − negative.

Modified from Shih IM, Kurman RJ: p63 Expression is useful in the distinction of epithelioid trophoblastic and placental site trophoblastic tumors by profiling trophoblastic subpopulations. Am J Surg Pathol 28:1177-1183, 2004.

Table 1-21. Immunohistochemistry for Selected Germ Cell Tumors

	PLAP	c-kit	OCT3/4	CD30	AFP	GPC-3	D2-40	β-hCG
Germinoma	+	+	+	−	−	−	+	−*
Embryonal carcinoma	+	−	+	+	−	−	−	v
Yolk sac tumor	+	−	−	−	v	+	−	−
Choriocarcinoma	+	−	−	−	−	−	−	+

*Except for syncytiotrophoblastic giant cells in seminoma.

AFP, α-fetoprotein; β-hCG, β−human chorionic gonadotropin; GPC-3, glypican-3; PLAP, placental alkaline phosphatase; +, positive; −, negative; v, variable.

Modified from Ulbright TM: The most common, clinically significant misdiagnoses in testicular tumor pathology, and how to avoid them. Adv Anat Pathol 15:18-27, 2008; and Young RH: Testicular tumors: Some new and a few perennial problems. Arch Pathol Lab Med 132:548-564, 2008.

Table 1-22. Immunohistochemistry Panel to Distinguish Renal Cell Neoplasms

	RCC	CD10	CK7	AMACR	CD117	PAX2
Clear cell carcinoma	+/−	+	−	−	−	+
Chromophobe carcinoma	−	−	+/−	−	+	−
Papillary carcinoma	+/−	−/+	+/−	+	−	−/+
Oncocytoma	−	−	−/+	−	+/−	−

AMACR, α-methylacyl coenzyme A racemase (P504S); CK, cytokeratin; PAX2, paired box gene-2; RCC, renal cell carcinoma; +, positive; −, negative; +/−, often positive; −/+, rarely positive.

Modified from Hammerich AH, Ayala GE, Wheeler TM: Application of immunohistochemistry to the genitourinary system (prostate, urinary bladder, testis, and kidney). Arch Pathol Lab Med 132:432-440, 2008.

Table 1-23. Immunohistochemistry Approach to Atypical Glandular Proliferative Lesion in the Prostate*

Lesion	Basal Cell Markers (HMWCK 34βE12, CK5/6, p63)	AMACR (p504S)
Atrophic glands	+	−
Post–atrophic hyperplasia	+	−
Basal cell hyperplasia	+	−
Atypical adenomatous hyperplasia (adenosis)	+/− (patchy)	−/+
Prostatic intraepithelial neoplasia	+	+
Prostate carcinoma	−†	+

*See Fig. 1-14.

†Rarely, p63 may demonstrate immunoreactivity in prostate carcinoma (see Ali TZ, Epstein JI: False positive labeling of prostate cancer with high molecular weight cytokeratin: p63 a more specific immunomarker for basal cells. Am J Surg Pathol 32:1890-1895, 2008.).

AMACR, α-methylacyl coenzyme A racemase; CK, cytokeratin; HMWCK, high-molecular-weight cytokeratin; +, positive; −, negative; +/−, often positive; −/+, rarely positive.

Modified from Paner GP, Luthringer DJ, Amin MB: Best practices in diagnostic immunohistochemistry: Prostate carcinoma and its mimics in needle core biopsies. Arch Pathol Lab Med 132:1388-1396, 2008.

Table 1-24. Immunohistochemistry Panel to Distinguish Prostate and Urothelial Carcinomas

	CK7	CK20	PSA	Uroplakin	p63
Prostate carcinoma	−/+	−/+	+	−	−/+
Urothelial carcinoma	+/−	+/−	−	+/−	+

CK, cytokeratin; PSA, prostate-specific antigen; +, positive; −, negative; +/−, often positive; −/+, rarely positive.

Notes:

- Only CK7/20 negativity (prostate carcinoma) and CK7/20 positivity (urothelial carcinoma) reliably distinguish between these two carcinomas. Any other permutation is unreliable.
- Uroplakin is highly specific for urothelial carcinoma but has a low sensitivity, being focally present in about 50% to 60% of tumors.
- Expression of p63 is used more often to highlight basal cells in benign prostate glands but may rarely be positive in the prostate carcinoma itself (see Ali TZ, Epstein JI: False positive labeling of prostate cancer with high molecular weight cytokeratin: p63 a more specific immunomarker for basal cells. Am J Surg Pathol 32:1890-1895, 2008.).

Modified from Hammerich AH, Ayala GE, Wheeler TM: Application of immunohistochemistry to the genitourinary system (prostate, urinary bladder, testis, and kidney). Arch Pathol Lab Med 132:432-440, 2008.

Figure 1-14. Immunohistochemistry in prostate adenocarcinoma. Both p63 (**A**) and 34βE12 (**B**) highlight an intact basal cell layer surrounding benign glands and loss around small acini of invasive adenocarcinoma. **C,** P504S immunohistochemistry shows strong, granular luminal staining in invasive adenocarcinoma and prostatic intraepithelial neoplasia. Normal glands are negative.

Table 1-25. Recommended Antibody Panel for Common Pleomorphic Cutaneous Spindle Cell Tumors

	Cytokeratins (Pan, HMW, CK5/6)	S-100 Protein	Melanocytic (HMB-45, Melan-A)	Smooth Muscle Actin	Desmin	Endothelial (CD31, CD34)
Sarcomatoid squamous cell carcinoma	+	−	−	−	−	−
Melanoma	−/+	+	+/−	−	−/+	−
Atypical fibroxanthoma	−	−	−	−/+	−	−
Leiomyosarcoma	−/+	−/+	−	+	+/−	−/+
Angiosarcoma	−/+	−	−	−	−	+

+, Positive; −, negative; +/−, often positive; −/+, rarely positive.

Modified from Folpe AL, Cooper K: Best practices in diagnostic immunohistochemistry: Pleomorphic cutaneous spindle cell tumors. Arch Pathol Lab Med 131:1517, 2007.

Table 1-26. Immunohistochemistry Panel for the Interpretation of Low-Grade (Small) B-Cell Lymphoma

	CD23 (%)	CD5 (%)	Cyclin D1 (%)	CD10 (%)	bcl-1 (%)
SLL/chronic lymphocytic leukemia	85	80	0	0	2
Mantle	2	80	75-100	2	85
Marginal zone	8	0	0	2	0
Lymphoplasmacytic	0-30	5	0	3	0
Follicular	0-25	0	0	85	0
Extranodal marginal	0	0	0	0	0

SLL, small lymphocytic lymphoma.

Modified from http://surgpathcriteria.stanford.edu.

Table 1-27. Antibody Panel for Differential Diagnosis of Hodgkin Lymphoma

	CD30	CD15	CD20	CD45 (LCA)	ALK
Hodgkin lymphoma	+	+	−/+	−	−
ALCL	+	−	−	−/+	+
DLBCL	−/+	−	+	+	−

ALCL, anaplastic large cell lymphoma; ALK, alkaline kinase; DLBCL, diffuse large B-cell lymphoma; EMA, epithelial membrane antigen; LCA, leukocyte common antigen; +, positive; −, negative; +/−, often positive; −/+, rarely positive.

Table 1-28. Immunoprofile of Small Round Cell Tumors

	Pan-CK	CD99	Desmin	Myogenin	WT-1	CD56
Ewing sarcoma, primitive neuroectodermal tumor	v	+	−	−	−	v
Rhabdomyosarcoma	−	v	+	+	−	+
Poorly differentiated synovial sarcoma†	+	+	−	−	−	+
Desmoplastic small round cell tumor	+	v	+	−	+	v
Neuroblastoma	−	−	−	−	−	+
Lymphoblastic lymphoma‡	−	+	−	−	−	−
Wilms' tumor	v	v	+	v*	+	+

*In rhabdomyomatous Wilms tumor.

†Epithelial membrane antigen is frequently positive.

‡Frequently leukocyte common antigen negative.

Pan-CK, pan-cytokeratin; WT-1, Wilms' tumor gene protein 1; + positive; −, negative; v, variable.

Modified from Barami A, Truong LD, Ro JY: Undifferentiated tumor: True identity by immunohistochemistry. Arch Pathol Lab Med 132:326-348, 2008.

Table 1-29. Immunohistochemistry Panel to Distinguish Follicular Variant of Papillary Thyroid Carcinoma (FCPTP) from Follicular Adenoma (FA)

	HBME1 (%)	CK19 (%)	Galectin-3 (%)
FVPTC	96	91-100	98
FA	7-11	44-68	30

Note: The combination of HBME1 and CK19 has the greatest utility in differentiating FVPTC from benign follicular lesions.

From Erickson LA, Lloyd RV: Utility of a panel of immunohistochemical markers in the diagnosis of follicular variant of papillary thyroid carcinoma. Adv Anat Pathol 15:59-60, 2008.

Selected References

Jagirder J: Immunohistochemistry: Then and now. Arch Pathol Lab Med 132:323-509, 2008.

Dabbs D: Diagnostic Immunohistochemistry, 2nd ed. Philadelphia, Churchill Livingstone, 2006.

Yaziji H, Barry T: Diagnostic immunohistochemistry: What can go wrong? Adv Anat Pathol 13:238-246, 2006.

Leong AS-Y, Leong TY-M: Newer developments in immunohistology. J Clin Pathol 59:1117-1126, 2006.

Flow Cytometry

Introduction

- Flow cytometry is widely used to immunophenotypically detect clonal hematopoietic populations (e.g., leukemia and lymphoma)
- When performed on peripheral blood, bone marrow, and lymph nodal tissue, single-cell suspensions are required

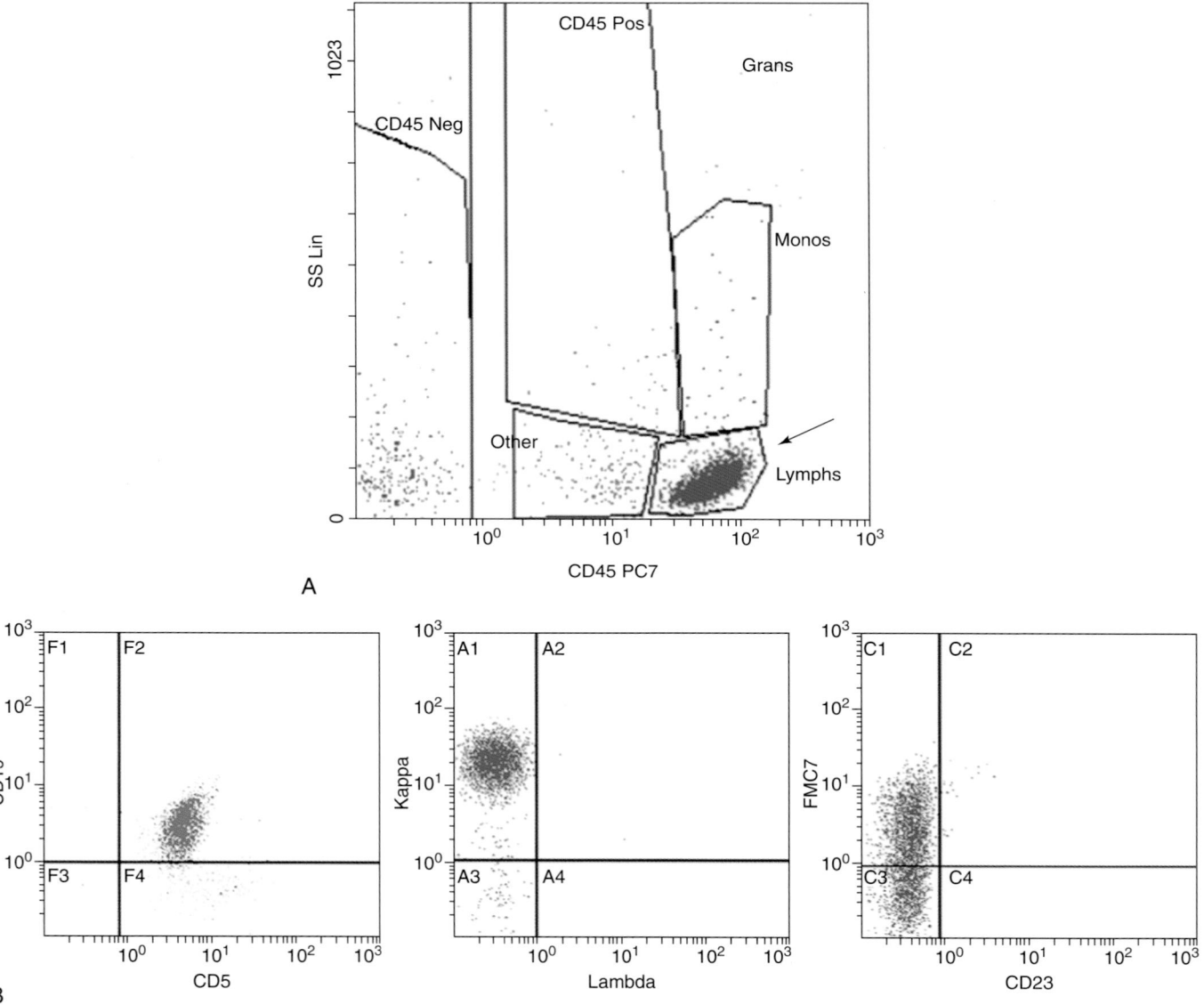

Figure 1-15. Flow cytometry. A, Gating for lymphocytes (CD45 vs. side scatter, linear scale [SS Lin]) shows the relative locations of granulocytes (Grans), monocytes (Monos), and lymphocytes (Lymphs) (*arrowhead*). **B,** Mantle cell lymphoma. Flow cytometric analysis of a lymph node specimen shows that nearly all of the lymphocytes express CD19, CD5, and kappa immunoglobulin light chains. A subset coexpresses FMC7, while the cells are negative for CD23. Expression of CD20 is not dim (data not shown). This immunophenotypic profile fits with involvement by mantle cell lymphoma. (Courtesy of Michael R. Lewis, MD, MBA, Department of Pathology, University of Vermont/Fletcher Allen Health Care, Burlington, VT.)

- Manipulation of solid tissue samples into single-cell suspensions can sometimes compromise the integrity of the cell surface

Technical Overview

- Single-cell suspension is split into multiple tubes
- Various fluorescent-labeled antibodies against different cell surface antigens (each with a different attached fluorochrome) are added to each tube
- One by one, the cells are run through the flow cytometer; as the cells pass through the counting chamber, multiple data points are collected
  — Degree of forward light scatter (FSC): indicator of cell size
  — Degree of 90-degree light scatter or side scatter (SSC): indicator of nuclear complexity and cytoplasmic granularity
  — Intensity of fluorochrome on the cell surface: detects expression of cell surface antigens (e.g., CD45, leukocyte common antigen)
- Gating: the cell of interest are digitally selected for interpretation; for example, if lymphocytes are to be examined, one would "gate" around the cells that exhibit low side scatter (little cytoplasmic granularity) and strong CD45 (leukocyte common antigen) expression

- Typical findings in mantle cell lymphoma would include a CD20-positive population (B cells) exhibiting coexpression of CD19 and CD5 (narrowing the differential to small lymphocytic lymphoma and mantle cell lymphoma), with light chain restriction supporting clonality. Lack of CD23 expression helps to exclude small lymphocytic lymphoma, which would have an immunophenotype similar to that of mantle cell lymphoma, except for CD23 expression and dimmer light chain expression. Follicular lymphoma would also consist of a population of CD20-positive B cells that express CD10 and lack CD5.

Selected Reference

Carey JL, McCoy P, Keren DF: Flow Cytometry in Clinical Diagnosis, 4th ed. Chicago, ASCP Press, 2007.

Cytogenetic Analysis

- Technical overview
  — Fresh tissue is incubated in short-term culture, and metaphase chromosomes are spread on glass slides
  — After staining of the chromosomes, specific chromosomal abnormalities can be detected

Figure 1-16. Well-differentiated liposarcoma. Karyotype analysis of a deep retroperitoneal lesion revealed a giant ring chromosome. (Courtesy of Mary Tang, MD, Cytogenetic Laboratory, University of Vermont/ Fletcher Allen Heath Care, Burlington, VT.)

- In surgical pathology practice at University of Vermont/Fletcher Allen Health Care, we routinely submit fresh tissue in Hanks solution for cytogenetics in the following cases
  - All renal tumors (except for urothelial carcinomas of the renal pelvis)
  - Any soft tissue tumor larger than 5 cm (including adipocytic neoplasms)
  - In addition, a portion of fresh tissue (1 cm^3, if available) is snap-frozen for potential molecular analyses for tumor-specific translocations or for potential treatment protocols
- Oncogenes (Table 1-30) and tumor suppressor genes (Table 1-31) of importance in surgical pathology

- Cytogenetic abnormalities of importance in surgical pathology (Table 1-32)

Selected References

Richmond JA, Tang M, Cooper K: Cytogenetic and clinicopathologic analysis of benign lipomatous tumors. Arch Pathol Lab Med 129:553, 2005.

Gersen SL, Keagle MB: The Principles of Clinical Cytogenetics, 2nd ed. Totowa, Humana Press, 2004.

Korf B: Molecular medicine: Molecular diagnosis (part I). N Engl J Med 332:1218-1220, 1995.

Korf B: Molecular medicine: Molecular diagnosis (part II). N Engl J Med 332:1499-1502, 1995.

Table 1-30. Oncogenes of Importance in Surgical Pathology

Oncogene	Location (Chromosome)	Association
Abl	9q34	Chronic myeloid leukemia translocation to 22q forming bcr-abl protein with tyrosine kinase activity
bcl-1 (PRAD-1)	11q13	Parathyroid adenomatosis; mantle zone lymphomas with translocation to 14q32
bcl-2	18q21	Block of apoptosis; translocation to 14q in follicular lymphomas
bcl-6	3q27	Diffuse large cell lymphoma
erbA	17	Erythroleukemia
erbB1	7p11-12	Squamous cell carcinoma
neu (erbB2, HER-2)	17q11-12	Breast carcinoma
fes (fps)	15q25-26	Acute promyelocytic leukemia
c-myc	8q24	Burkitt lymphoma
Ras	6q16-22	Pancreatic, lung, colonic, bladder carcinomas; neuroblastoma, leukemia
Ret	10q11.2	Medullary and papillary thyroid carcinomas
Myb	6q22-24	Colon carcinoma
L-myc	1p32	Small cell carcinoma of lung
N-myc	2p23-24	Neuroblastoma

Table 1-31. Tumor Suppressor Genes of Importance in Surgical Pathology

Gene	Location (Chromosome)	Association
RB (retinoblastoma)	13q14	Retinoblastoma, childhood osteosarcoma
p53	17p13.1	Mutations in cancers of colon, breast, lung, leukemia, sarcoma; progression to diffuse large cell lymphoma (germline mutation of p53 forms the basis for Li-Fraumeni syndrome)
WT-1	11p13	Wilms' tumor; desmoplastic small round cell tumor
EWS	22q12	Ewing/primitive neuroectodermal tumor, soft tissue clear cell sarcoma, desmoplastic small round cell tumor, myxoid liposarcoma, acute myelogenous leukemia
BRCA1	17q21	Breast carcinoma
APC	5q21	Familial adenomatous polyposis coli; carcinomas of colon, stomach, pancreas
DCC	18q21	Carcinomas of colon, stomach
NF1	17q11	Schwannomas, neurogenic sarcomas
NF2	22q12	Central schwannomas, meningiomas

Table 1-32. Cytogenetic Abnormalities of Importance in Surgical Pathology

Tumor	Chromosomal Abnormality	Fusion Transcript, Involved Genes
Hematopoietic Neoplasms		
Acute myelogenous leukemia (AML)		
AML-M1	t(9;22)	*BCR-ABL*
AML-M2	t(8;21) (favorable)	*CBFα-ETO*
AML-M3	t(15;17)	*RARα/PML*
AML-M4eo	inv(16) (favorable)	*CBFβ/MYH11*
Chronic myelogenous leukemia	t(9;22)(q34;q11)	*BCR-ABL*
B-cell acute lymphoblastic leukemia	t(12;21)	*CBFα-ETV6*
Chronic lymphocytic leukemia	Trisomy 12, deletions of 11q, 13q and 17p	
Burkitt lymphoma	t(8;14), t(8;22), t(4;8)	Involving *c-myc* and Ig loci
Follicular lymphoma	t(14;18)	*BCL2* gene
Mantle zone lymphoma	t(11;14)	*BCL1* (cyclin D1) and immunoglobulin H
Primitive Precursor Cell Neoplasms		
Ewing sarcoma/primitive neuroectodermal tumor	t(11;22)(q24;q12)	*EWS-FLI1* fusion
Medulloblastoma	del 17q	
Neuroblastoma	del 1p (poor prognosis); double minute chromosomes	*N-myc* amplification
Retinoblastoma	del 13q (band q14)	
Wilms' tumor	del 11p (band p13)	
Epithelial Neoplasms		
Colorectal carcinoma	del 17p	
Mesothelioma	del of 1p, 3p, 22p	
Renal cell carcinoma (RCC)		
Clear cell carcinoma	del 3p	
Papillary RCC	Trisomy 7 and 17	
Chromophobe RCC	Loss of chromosome 1, 2, 6, or 10	
Oncocytoma	Loss of chromosome 1; translocation involving 11q13	
Small cell carcinoma	del 3p	
Soft Tissue Neoplasms		
Alveolar soft part sarcoma	t(X;17)(p11;q25)	*TFE3-ASPL* fusion
Chondrosarcoma, extraskeletal myxoid	t(9;22)(q22;q12)	*EWS-NR4A3* fusion
Clear cell sarcoma	t(12;22)(q13;q12)	*EWSR1-ATF1* fusion
Desmoplastic small round cell tumor	t(11;22)(q24;q12)	*EWSR1-WT-1* fusion
Dermatofibrosarcoma protuberans	Ring form of chromosomes 17 and 22	*COL1A1-PDGFB* fusion
Fibrosarcoma, infantile	t(12;15)(p13;q26)	*ETV6-NTRK3* fusion
Hibernoma	Translocation at 11q13	
Inflammatory myofibroblastic tumor	t(1;2)(q22;p23)	*TPM3-ALK* fusion
Leiomyoma	t(12;14), del 7q	
Leiomyosarcoma	del 1p	
Lipoma	Rearrangement of 12q15	*HMGIC* fusion
Liposarcoma (myxoid)	t(12;16)(q13;p11)	*TLS/CHOP*
Liposarcoma (well differentiated)	Ring chromosome 12	

Table 1-32. *Continued*

Tumor	Chromosomal Abnormality	Fusion Transcript, Involved Genes
Rhabdoid tumor	Deletion of 22q	*INI1* inactivation
Rhabdomyosarcoma (alveolar)	t(2;13)(q35;q14)	*PAX3-FKHR*
Rhabdomyosarcoma (embryonal)	Trisomies 2q, 8, and 20	
Synovial sarcoma	t(X;18)(p11;q11)	*SYT-SSX1/SYT-SSX2*
Central Nervous System Neoplasms		
Atypical teratoid rhabdoid tumor	Deletion of 22q	*INI1* inactivation
Oligodendroglioma	del 1p, 19q (improved response to chemotherapy)	
Schwannoma	Deletion of 22q	*NF-2* inactivation

Molecular Pathology Methods

Introduction

Molecular-based methods are now standard aids in the diagnosis of a variety of pathologic conditions. Ongoing advances in molecular pathology, genomics, epigenomics, proteomics, and infectious diseases research, as well as technologic developments, will serve to further the battery of molecular assays available for improved disease characterization and patient care. This section reviews a wide range of molecular pathology techniques that can be adaptable for application in surgical pathology practice. The polymerase chain reaction (PCR) and in situ hybridization (ISH) have widespread clinical use.

Nucleic Acid Extraction Methods

- The extraction of nucleic acids from pathology samples involves cell lysis followed by selective DNA or RNA isolation, and a quantity and quality assessment relative to the requirements of the end-diagnostic test
- Pathology samples that can be used for molecular analysis include tissue samples (fresh or formalin-fixed, paraffin-embedded [FFPE]); bodily fluids—amniotic fluid, saliva, stools, urine, buccal and cervical scrapes; fine-needle aspirates; hair root; peripheral blood; and cell cultures
- DNA extraction methods
  - Classic methods were time-consuming (about 3 days) and required relatively large quantities of tissues (100 mg to >1 g)
  - Numerous extraction kits are now available that use glass-fiber filters that selectively bind DNA after tissue treatments with a protease and chaotropic buffers (which disrupt protein and DNA secondary structures). The glass fibers, typically loaded in mini-columns, are washed to rinse away cellular debris, extraction solution reagents, and pathology tissue processing chemicals. The DNA is then recovered from the resin or glass-fiber by low-salt buffer rinses. Pure DNA recovery from diverse pathology samples is possible within several hours by these procedures

  - Automated DNA extraction platforms are available for the processing of multiple patient samples
- RNA extraction methods
  - Classic methods required the rapid homogenization of large quantities of fresh tissues in protease and guanidinium thiocyanate solution to denature ubiquitous endogenous RNases that otherwise degrade cellular RNA
  - Current methods allow the relatively rapid (1-day) recovery of RNA, again after tissue homogenization in a chaotropic guanidinium salt solution that leaves RNA contained in an aqueous phase and protein and DNA in an organic phase. Admixture of the aqueous phase with nucleic acid–binding glass filters allows recovery of pure total RNA by elution from the glass filters with a low-salt buffer. Messenger RNA (mRNA) can be purified from total RNA by passage through oligo(dT) cellulose spin columns. Mini-columns have been developed for the extraction of RNA from all types of pathology samples
- DNA and RNA quantification, purity, and integrity assay
  - High-integrity nucleic acids are best extracted from fresh tissue specimens. Extraction from tissues preserved in liquid nitrogen is the next best option. Commercially available storage reagents (e.g., RNA*later*, Ambion, Inc., Foster City, CA) preserve tissue morphology and nucleic acid integrity
  - DNA and RNA extracts from FFPE tissues tend to be degraded. In general, the quality of nucleic acids extractable from FFPE blocks decreases with block age
  - The concentration of extracted nucleic acids is assessed spectrophotometrically. Both DNA and RNA absorb UV light, with peak absorbance at a wavelength of 260 nm; an absorbance (A_{260}) reading of 1.0 demonstrates a DNA concentration of 50 µg/mL or an RNA concentration of 40 µg/mL
  - The purity of extracted DNA or RNA is also determined spectrophotometrically. Readings taken at A_{230} and at A_{270} are indicators of contamination with organics (such as guanidinium salts) and phenol, respectively.

Contamination with proteins can be inferred from an A_{280} reading, at which peak protein absorbance occurs. Particulate matter contamination can be gauged from an A_{320} reading. Typically, an $A_{(260-320)}:A_{(280-320)}$ ratio is calculated; a value of 1.7 to 2.0 indicates pure DNA or RNA
— Nucleic acid integrity can be estimated by comparing nucleic acid fragment size against a molecular weight ladder after agarose gel electrophoresis. The presence of a smear extending to smaller fragments indicates degraded DNA. Total RNA integrity is gauged in terms of the presence of 28S (about 5 kb) and 18S (about 2 kb) ribosomal RNA (rRNA). Discrete 28S and 18S bands, with minimal smearing, indicate intact RNA species, whereas partial or absent bands and smeared rRNA indicate a degraded sample
— Instruments such as the NanoDrop spectrophotometer (Thermo Fisher Scientific, Wilmington, DE) and the Agilent 2100 Bioanalyzer (Agilent Technologies Inc., Santa Clara, CA) have facilitated rapid DNA and RNA quantitation and purity analyses, and RNA integrity assay, respectively
• Nucleic acids storage
— DNA is generally stored at 4°C for assays performed within 1 week to 1 month of extraction, and in aliquots at −20°C or −80°C for longer-term storage; repeated freeze-thawing may lead to DNA degradation
— RNA is more labile than DNA and is susceptible to degradation by RNases that are a pervasive laboratory hazard. For short-term use, RNA is stored at −20°C, and at −80°C or under liquid nitrogen for longer-term use

Tissue Microdissection Methods

• Background
— Microdissection enables the targeted collection of cells or tissues from slide-mounted cytologic specimens or frozen or FFPE tissues sections
— Sample tissues may be treated for nucleic acids or protein extraction
• Methods
— In the simplest approach, lightly stained tissues sections are viewed by dissecting microscope, and after dampening the tissues with 70% ethanol, the tissues are selectively scraped off the slides using a syringe needle. DNA is extracted from the collected tissues after digestion with proteinase K. A glass-fiber mini-column method allows further purification
— Laser capture microdissection (LCM) requires a specialized microscopy apparatus such as the ArcturusXT system (MDS Analytical Technologies, Sunnyvale, CA)

1. Place cap on tissue

2. Pulse laser at target cells

3. Remove cap with adhered target cells

4. Extract molecules from target cells

Figure 1-17. Laser capture technology. Target tissues are overlaid with a cap using microscope guidance. Cells are adhered to the thermoplastic film of the cap by laser pulsing. Lifting the cap removes the target cells for nucleic acids or protein extraction. (Courtesy of Molecular Devices, Sunnydale, CA.)

— The procedure involves overlaying the tissue of interest with a thermoplastic film contained in a cap. LCM can be applied to frozen or FFPE tissues, to blood smears, or to cytologic or cell culture samples. Tissues can be unstained or histochemically or immunohistochemically stained (chromogenic or fluorescence). A pulsed laser beam is targeted against the selected cells, which fuses them to the thermoplastic film. The cap is then removed from the tissue section surface, and nucleic acids are recoverable from the cells adhered there after cell lysis treatments applied directly to the cap film
• Applications
— Microdissection is primarily a research application but is useful in surgical pathology practice when there is a suspicion of patient sample cross-contamination. PCR-based identity testing comparing the known patient samples with the queried tissue supports verification of a patient's diagnosis

Amplification Methods

Nucleic Acids Amplification Methods
• PCR
— Background: PCR is a method for the in vitro amplification of DNA involving automated cycles of denaturation, annealing, and extension or synthesis performed in a thermocycler

Figure 1-18. Polymerase chain reaction (PCR). A PCR cycle consists of denaturation, primer annealing, and DNA synthesis or extension steps. Following the first PCR cycle, there is (theoretically) a per-cycle doubling in the number of copies of the PCR product. (Modified from Leonard DGB [ed]: Diagnostic Molecular Pathology. Philadelphia, WB Saunders, 2003.)

— Basic PCR method
  ◆ During the denaturation stage, sample specimen DNA is rendered single-stranded by heating to 94° to 98°C
  ◆ In the annealing step, oligonucleotide primers hybridize with the target sequences they have been designed to complement. The annealing temperature depends on deoxyribonucleoside triphosphate (dNTP) composition of the primers and is typically in the range of 40° to 60°C
  ◆ During the extension step (72°C), the annealed primer or target DNA seeds the ($5' \rightarrow 3'$) synthesis by thermostable DNA polymerase of a new DNA strand
  ◆ DNA amplification is accomplished by repetition of the denaturation, annealing, and extension cycle, 30 to 50 more times
  ◆ The time period for each of the denaturation, annealing, and extension steps can vary from 10 seconds to more than 1 minute and depends on reaction volume size, amplicon base composition and length, thermostable DNA polymerase activity (about 1000 bp are extended per minute), and thermal cycler hardware specifications
— The essential ingredients in a PCR include
  ◆ DNase or RNase free pure water: final PCR reaction volumes vary from 10 to 50 μL

  ◆ Buffer: pH is typically maintained using a Tris-HCl–based buffer. Other ingredients include KCl, which can aid primer template annealing; nonionic detergents; and bovine serum albumin (BSA) to aid Taq DNA polymerase enzyme stability
  ◆ Magnesium cations: Mg^{2+} is an essential ingredient and stabilizes the interaction between the oligonucleotide primer, template DNA, and Taq DNA polymerase enzyme
  ◆ dNTPs: 2′-deoxyadenosine 5′-triphosphate (dATP), 2′-deoxycytidine 5′-triphosphate (dCTP), 2′-deoxyguanosine, 5′-triphosphate (dGTP), and thymidine 5′-triphosphate (TTP, also referred to as dTTP)
  ◆ Oligonucleotide primers: 18 to 25 bases in length
  ◆ Template DNA: the amount of sample in a reaction can range from 1 ng to 1 μg, with about 100 ng representing a standard quantity for many applications
  ◆ Thermostable DNA polymerase enzymes such as Taq DNA polymerase extracted from Thermus aquaticus isolated from a hot-springs dwelling bacterium of the Deinococcus-Thermus phylum
— PCR efficiency
  ◆ Optimization experiments are required to ensure that the PCR test efficiency approaches ideal efficiency and to avoid false-negative data. Potentially, each component of the PCR setup can be manipulated for improved PCR specificity and sensitivity. A variety of reagents can be added to enhance a PCR
— PCR method variations
  ◆ The PCR technique is a highly adaptable technique enabling its applicability in a wide range of research and clinical niches
  ◆ Modifications centered on primer design and use
    ◇ Multiplex PCR supports the simultaneous detection of more than one target by use of multiple primer pair sets
    ◇ Consensus PCR can be used to amplify a single target that has variable sequences or multiple targets that have similar (common) sequences
    ◇ Degenerate PCR is also used in the amplification of a variable sequence target
    ◇ Nested PCR is a method for improved PCR sensitivity and specificity
  ◆ Reverse transcription PCR (RT-PCR)
    ◇ RT-PCR allows the investigation of RNA expression through PCR
    ◇ Thermostable DNA polymerases require DNA as a substrate; the first step in RT-PCR is thus the conversion of (DNA-free) total RNA or mRNA into single-stranded complementary DNA (cDNA)

Figure 1-19. Reverse transcription polymerase chain reaction (RT-PCR).
Complementary DNA (cDNA) is synthesized from an RNA sample by a reverse transcriptase enzyme; thereafter, the cDNA is available for PCR amplification. (Modified from Leonard DGB [ed]: Diagnostic Molecular Pathology. Philadelphia, WB Saunders, 2003.)

◇ The two most commonly used reverse transcriptase enzymes are the avian myeloblastoma virus (AMV) and Moloney murine leukemia virus (M-MuLV) reverse transcriptases

◇ In addition to the general determinants of standard PCR success, RT-PCR efficiency depends on RNA sample quality and the effectiveness of the reverse transcriptase step

◆ Real-time quantitative PCR (qPCR)

◇ In standard PCR, also referred to as end-point PCR, the final product obtained after 30 to 50 PCR cycles is the object of data interpretation. Although end-point PCR can be semiquantitative, it is essentially a qualitative assay. qPCR is used for the accurate quantification of a DNA or RNA and cDNA target in a sample

— Other PCR methods

◆ Amplification refractory mutation system (ARMS), allele-specific PCR (AS-PCR), PCR amplification of specific alleles (PASA)

◆ LA PCR: long and accurate PCR; allows the amplification of sequences 5 to >20 kb in length

— PCR contamination control

◆ The sensitivity of PCR incurs the potential defect of false-positive data owing to the amplification of cross-contaminating DNA from an exogenous source. Strict measures are required from patient sample collection through PCR assay to ensure authentic data

◆ Ideally, laboratory space should be arranged such that DNA sample extraction, PCR setup, and post-PCR manipulations all occur in physically distinct areas, and using PCR-grade reagent aliquots, dedicated equipment, and laboratory coats specific for each area. PCR products from previous rounds of PCR represent the major potential source for contamination

— PCR tests in pathology practice

◆ PCR is highly adaptable for use in a wide variety of clinical applications, including

◇ Infectious pathogens detection

◇ Genetic diseases diagnosis

◇ Hematologic diseases diagnosis, for example, chimeric RNA transcripts detection such as the *bcr-abl* translocation product characteristic of chronic myelogenous leukemia

◇ Sarcoma diagnosis by signature gene fusions detection, for example, *EWS/FLI1* in Ewing sarcoma or peripheral neuroectodermal tumor

◇ Solid tumor characterization, for example, hereditary nonpolyposis colorectal cancer (HNPCC) mutation analyses
◇ Identity testing
◇ Detection of circulating tumor or pathogen nucleic acids signatures
◆ Table 1-33 details current U.S. Food and Drug Administration (FDA)-cleared or FDA-approved PCR-based tests
◆ There are many non–FDA-approved tests in widespread clinical diagnostics use. The Mayo Medical Laboratories *MayoAccess Test Catalog* lists more than 200 PCR-based tests, including
◇ Infectious pathogen detection: adenovirus (qPCR), *Bartonella henselae*, BK virus, cytomegalovirus (CMV), enterovirus, hepatitis B virus (HBV), human herpesvirus-6, human metapneumovirus (hMPV), JC virus, *Legionella* RNA, Lyme disease, malaria, parvovirus B19, varicella-zoster virus
◇ Genetic diseases diagnosis: Bloom syndrome mutation analysis, Fabry disease known mutation, factor IX gene known mutation, familial amyloidosis DNA sequence, familial dysautonomia, fragile X syndrome, Gaucher disease mutation, Fanconi anemia mutation analysis, galactosemia gene analysis, hemochromatosis, Prader-Willi and Angelman syndromes, spinobulbar muscular atrophy, Tay-Sachs disease

Table 1-33. Food and Drug Administration–Approved* and Cleared† Molecular Diagnostic Polymerase Chain Reaction–Based Assays

Test	Method	Tissue Sample	Test Name	Supplier
Avian flu	qRT-PCR	Nasopharyngeal swab, washes	†Influenza A/H5	Centers for Disease Control and Prevention
Bacillus anthracis	qPCR	Blood	†Joint Biological Agent Identification and Diagnostic System (JBAIDS) Anthrax Detection kit	Idaho Technology, Inc., Salt Lake City, UT
Breast cancer: detection of breast cancer spread to lymph nodes	qRT-PCR	FFPE sections	*GeneSearch Breast Lymph Node (BLN) Assay (screens for mammoglobin [MG] and cytokeratin 19 [CK19] in lymph nodes)	Veridex, LLC, Warren, NJ
Chlamydia trachomatis	PCR	Swab, urine	†AMPLICOR CT/NG (test for *Chlamydia trachomatis*)	Roche Molecular Diagnostics, Pleasanton, CA
Cystic fibrosis	Multiplex PCR	Blood, amniotic fluid, chorionic villus	†Tag-It Mutation Detection Kit CFTR 40+4	Luminex Molecular Diagnostics, Toronto, Canada
			†eSensor Cystic Fibrosis Carrier Detection System	Osmetech Molecular Diagnostics, Pasadena, CA
Drug metabolizing enzymes	qPCR	Saliva	†Gentris Rapid Genotyping Assay: CYP2C9, VKORC1 warfarin sensitivity assay	ParagonDx, LLC, Morrisville, NC
Enteroviral meningitis detection	qRT-PCR	CSF	†Xpert EV	Cepheid, Sunnyvale, CA
Francisella tularensis	qPCR	Blood, bodily fluids	†Joint Biological Agent Identification and Diagnostic System (JBAIDS) Tularemia Detection kit	Idaho Technology, Inc., Salt Lake City, UT
Factor II (prothrombin)	PCR	Blood	†INFINITI System Assay for Factor II	AutoGenomics Inc., Carlsbad, CA
	qPCR	Blood	*Factor II (prothrombin) G20210A kit	Roche Diagnostics, Pleasanton, CA
Factor V Leiden	PCR	Blood	†INFINITI System Assay for Factor V	AutoGenomics Inc., Carlsbad, CA
	qPCR	Blood	*Factor V Leiden kit	Roche Diagnostics, Pleasanton, CA
Group B streptococci detection	qPCR	Vaginal, rectal swabs, LIM broth	†Smart GBS Xpert GBS	Cepheid, Sunnyvale, CA
			†IDI-Strep B Assay	Becton, Dickinson & Company, Sparks, MD

Table 1-33. *Continued*

Test	Method	Tissue Sample	Test Name	Supplier
HBV for blood donations	PCR	Blood	*COBAS AmpliScreen HBV Test	Roche Molecular Diagnostics Pleasanton, CA
HCV for blood donations	RT-PCR	Blood	*HCV RT-PCR assay	BioLife Plasma Services, L.P., Deerfield, IL
		Blood	*COBAS AmpliScreen HCV Test, v2.0	Roche Molecular Diagnostics, Pleasanton, CA
		Blood	*UltraQual HCV RT-PCR assay	National Genetics Institute, Los Angeles, CA
HCV qualitative detection	PCR	Blood	*AMPLICOR HCV Test, v2.0	Roche Molecular Diagnostics, Pleasanton, CA
HIV for blood donations	RT-PCR	Blood	*UltraQual HIV-1 RT-PCR assay	National Genetics Institute, Los Angeles, CA
			*HIV-1 RT-PCR assay	BioLife Plasma Services, L.P., Deerfield, IL
HIV quantitation	qRT-PCR	Blood	*Abbott real-time HIV-1	Abbott Molecular, Inc., Des Plaines, IL
	RT-PCR	Blood	*AMPLICOR HIV-1 MONITOR Test, v1.5	Roche Molecular Diagnostics, Pleasanton, CA
			COBAS AmpliPrep/COBAS TaqMan HIV-1 Test	
HLA typing	PCR	Blood	†Biotest HLA SSP	Biotest Diagnostics Corp., Denville, NJ
			†Dynal Reli SSO typing kits: HLA-A, HLA-B, HLA-Cw, HLA-DQB1, HLA-DRB3/4/5	Invitrogen, Carlsbad, CA
			†GTI PAT HPA-1 (P1) genotyping kit	GTI, Brookfield, WI
			†Micro SSP HLA class II DNA typing kit	One Lambda, Inc., Canoga Park, CA
MRSA for *Staphylococcus aureus*—screening assay	qPCR	Nasopharyngeal swab, washes	†IDI-MRSA assay	Becton, Dickinson & Company, Sparks, MD
	qPCR		†Xpert MRSA	Cepheid, Sunnyvale, CA
MRSA for *Staphylococcus aureus*—diagnostic assay	qPCR		†GeneOhm StaphSR	Becton, Dickinson & Company, Sparks, MD
Mycobacterium tuberculosis detection	PCR	Respiratory swabs	*AMPLICOR *Mycobacterium tuberculosis* test	Roche Molecular Diagnostics, Pleasanton, CA
Neisseria gonorrhoeae detection (single organism)	PCR	Swab, urine	†AMPLICOR CT/NG test for *Neisseria gonorrhoeae*	Roche Molecular Diagnostics, Pleasanton, CA
			†COBAS AMPLICOR CT/NG test for *Neisseria gonorrhoeae*	
Respiratory virus panel (strains of influenza A and B, and respiratory syncytial virus)	Multiplex qPCR	Respiratory swabs	†ProFlu+ assay	Prodesse, Waukesha, WI
West Nile virus for blood donations	qPCR	Blood	†Procleix WNV	Gen-Probe, Inc., San Diego, CA
	PCR		†Cobas Taq Screen WNV	Roche Molecular Diagnostics, Pleasanton, CA
Yersinia pestis	qPCR	Blood	†Joint Biological Agent Identification and Diagnostic System (JBAIDS) Plague Detection kit	Idaho Technology, Inc., Salt Lake City, UT

CSF, cerebrospinal fluid; FFPE, formalin-fixed, paraffin-embedded; HBV, hepatitis B virus; HCV, hepatitis C virus; HIV, human immunodeficiency virus; HLA, human leukocyte antigen; MRSA, methicillin-resistant *Staphylococcus aureus*; PCR, polymerase chain reaction; qPCR, quantitative PCR; qRT-PCR, quantitative RT-PCR; RT-PCR, reverse transcription PCR.

*Approved.

†Cleared.

◇ Tumor characterization and diagnosis: *BCR/ABL* (qRT-PCR), DSRCT (RT-PCR), Ewing sarcoma (RT-PCR), HNPCC, *JAK2* V617F mutation detection, microsatellite instability, *PML/RARA* (qPCR), *RET/PTC* rearrangements (RT-PCR), synovial sarcoma (RT-PCR)

- Other nucleic acids amplification methods
  — Transcription-mediated amplification (TMA)
    ◆ TMA supports the amplification of RNA targets, including species-specific rRNA sequences
    ◆ The method involves an isothermal reaction containing the following ingredients
      ◇ RNA sample
      ◇ A target-specific "forward" primer with an RNA polymerase promoter sequence at the 5′-end
      ◇ Reverse transcriptase with active RNase H activity (e.g., AMV reverse transcriptase)
      ◇ A target-specific "reverse" primer
      ◇ RNA polymerase (e.g., SP6, T3, or T7 RNA polymerase)
    ◆ Applications
      ◇ TMA is a proprietary technique of Gen-Probe Inc., San Diego, CA. FDA-cleared TMA tests are available for the detection of *Chlamydia trachomatis*, *Neisseria gonorrhoeae*, and *Mycobacterium tuberculosis* (APTIMA CT, APTIMA GC, and, AMPLIFIED *Mycobacterium tuberculosis* Direct Test [MTD] assays, respectively)
      ◇ An FDA-approved TMA qualitative assay for hepatitis C virus (HCV) is also available (VERSANT HCV RNA [distributed by Siemens Healthcare Diagnostics, Deerfield, IL])
  — Nucleic acid sequence–based amplification (NASBA)
    ◆ NASBA is an isothermal amplification technique and can be used for the amplification of a DNA or RNA target. The technique requires an initial heat denaturation step when DNA is the sample to render the target sequences single-stranded
    ◆ The technique is essentially identical to TMA but uses a separate RNase H enzyme and fluorescence resonance energy transfer (FRET)-based detection technology. NASBA amplifies its target by a factor of 109 in a 90-minute reaction at 41°C
    ◆ Applications: proprietary NASBA assays have been developed by bioMérieux, Inc. (Durham, NC) for the detection of CMV and human immunodeficiency virus (HIV) RNA (NucliSENS CMV pp67 [FDA cleared] and NucliSENS HIV-1 QT [FDA-approved], respectively)

— Strand displacement amplification (SDA)
  ◆ The SDA technique requires the use of a DNA polymerase that has "strand displacement" activity, for example, Bst DNA polymerase (derived from *Bacillus stearothermophilus*) or Phi29 DNA polymerase (derived from the *Bacillus subtilis* phage phi29 [Φ29])
  ◆ As with other DNA polymerases, these enzymes synthesize DNA in the 5′ → 3′ direction; unlike other polymerases, these enzymes, having initiated DNA polymerization from an upstream (proximal) primer binding site, displace a double-stranded DNA region resulting from synthesis initiated at a downstream (distal) region. This property supports isothermal DNA amplification because it is not necessary to (cyclically) heat-denature DNA to produce a single-stranded template
  ◆ Applications: FDA-cleared proprietary tests, based on SDA, have been developed for the detection of *Chlamydia trachomatis*, *Neisseria gonorrhoeae*, and *Legionella pneumophila* (BD ProbeTec ET systems for each microorganism [Becton, Dickinson and Company, Sparks, MD])
  ◆ The method involves generating a target-specific sequence that uses primers specific to the microorganism and also incorporates a restriction enzyme site into the polymerized product; exponential amplification of these targets then occurs
  ◆ In excess of 109 copies of the target may be produced within 15 minutes
— Ligase chain reaction (LCR)
  ◆ LCR involves cycles of DNA denaturation and annealing and uses a thermostable DNA ligase, which catalyzes nicotinamide adenine dinucleotide (NAD)-dependent ligation of adjacent 3′-hydroxylated and 5′-phosphorylated termini in duplex DNA structures
  ◆ Applications: FDA-approved proprietary LCR tests were available for the detection of *Chlamydia trachomatis* and *Neisseria gonorrhoeae* (Abbott LCx tests, Abbott Laboratories, Chicago, IL) but were withdrawn in 2003 after test standardization issues. In a manner analogous to ARMS, LCR can be used to detect mutant sequences by designing a primer to mismatch the mutant (or wild type) at an appropriate primer terminus

Signal Amplification Techniques

- The assays described previously directly amplify target nucleic acid sequences to a threshold of detection

- An alternative strategy is to employ amplification technology at the level of detection; a (nonamplified) nucleic acid is targeted using a probe, and an amplified signal is generated from the probe
- Signal amplification techniques may be less susceptible to false-positive data resulting from patient sample cross-contamination than PCR-based methods
- Branch DNA (bDNA)
  — This method involves the capture of specimen RNA or DNA in a microtiter plate well, followed by a sequential four-step detection procedure
  — bDNA technology allows highly specific and quantitative nucleic acid assays
  — Applications: FDA-approved bDNA tests are available for HCV and for HIV quantitation (VERSANT HCV RNA 3.0 assay and VERSANT HIV-1 RNA 3.0 assay, respectively [Siemens Healthcare Diagnostics, Deerfield, IL]). bDNA research applications are available from Panomics, Inc., Fremont, CA
- Invader chemistry
  — Invader chemistry is a proprietary technique developed by Hologic Inc. (Bedford, MA) for the specific and accurate detection of single-base changes, insertions, deletions, and changes in gene and chromosome number
  — The method involves two simultaneous isothermal reactions: a primary reaction detects the DNA target of interest, and a second reaction generates detectable signal
  — Invader chemistry can be adapted for combined use with PCR for even greater detection sensitivity
  — Applications
    ◆ An FDA-cleared Invader chemistry assay screens for 46 cystic fibrosis mutations (InPlex Molecular Test). An FDA-cleared assay is also available to identify patients homozygous for abnormal uridine diphosphate glucuronosyltransferase 1A1 (UGT1A1) genes (Invader UGT1A1 molecular assay). Patients with seven instead of six TA repeats in the TATA box region of the gene metabolize the chemotherapeutic agent irinotecan (CAMPTOSAR, Pfizer Corporation) poorly and require lowered dosages to avoid a toxic response
    ◆ Invader-based assays for high-risk human papillomaviruses (HPV) (Cervista HPV HR [high-risk] and Cervista HPV 16/18) are FDA approved
    ◆ Mutation and variant screening Invader tests have been developed for factor V Leiden, factor II, methylenetetrahydrofolate reductase 677 (MTHRFR 677), MTHRFR 1298, cytochrome P-450, and vitamin K genes. A kit to detect the six major hepatitis C virus genotypes is also available

- Multiple ligation-dependent probe amplification (MLPA)
  — MLPA is a proprietary technology of MRC-Holland, Amsterdam, The Netherlands
  — The technique involves the ligation of two oligonucleotides that have hybridized immediately adjacent to each other at the target of interest (i.e., similar to primer annealing in ARMS PCR or LCR). The ligation product is then amplified by PCR
  — Applications: MLPA is applicable for the detection of mutations and single nucleotide polymorphisms (SNPs), deletions, and amplifications. Nonamplification with a particular probe indicates the presence of a mutation, SNP, or deletion; excess amplification demonstrates an amplification event. MLPA tests (none is currently FDA cleared or approved) are available for the diagnosis of a large variety of pathologic conditions, including
    ◆ Familial cancers: ataxia telangiectasia, BRCA1 and BRCA2 testing, colon polyposis (APC), MLH1/MSH1/MSH2/MSH6/PMS2 testing, Li-Fraumeni syndrome, multiple endocrine neoplasia, neurofibromatosis types 1 and 2, Peutz-Jeghers syndrome, retinoblastoma, von Hippel-Lindau syndrome, Wilms tumor
    ◆ Tumor analyses: melanoma (uveal), mismatch repair genes, neuroblastoma, oligodendroma, phosphatase and tensin homologue (PTEN), rhabdoid tumors, tumor suppressor genes
    ◆ Prenatal and postnatal screening: aneuploidy (Down, Edwards, Patau syndromes), mental retardation syndromes, microdeletion syndromes (Prader-Willi and Angelman syndromes; RETT/Xq28 duplication, and others)
    ◆ Pharmacogenetics: dihydropyrimidine dehydrogenase (DPD) deficiency
    ◆ Specific syndromes: cystic fibrosis, Turner and Klinefelter syndromes, typical uremic syndrome, and Wilson disease
- Hybrid capture
  — The hybrid capture assay (QIAGEN, Germantown, MD) involves an in vitro solution hybridization of a target DNA sequence with an RNA probe, followed by a signal amplification step
  — Applications: the FDA-approved Digene HPV Test uses hybrid capture (hc2) technology. The test screens for 13 high-risk HPV genotypes (16, 18, 31, 33, 35, 39, 45, 51, 52, 56, 58, 59, and 68). The hc2 assay uses cells left over after routine cytology screening and can detect 1000 to 5000 copies of HPV DNA per test sample. FDA-cleared hybrid capture assays are also available for the detection and quantitation of CMV, Chlamydia trachomatis, and Neisseria gonorrhoeae. Assays are also available for HBV and herpes simplex virus (HSV)

Gel Electrophoresis Methods

- Background
  - Gel electrophoresis, as a method for separating, identifying, or purifying nucleic acids, was conceived in the mid-1960s by Vin Thorne (Institute of Virology, Glasgow, UK), who was interested in analyzing different forms of the polyomavirus
  - Nucleic acids are negatively charged at neutral pH owing to the phosphate in the sugar-phosphate backbone of DNA or RNA. Accordingly, in the presence of an electrical field, nucleic acids migrate from the cathode to the anode; migration through a sieving matrix (gel) depends on the size of the nucleic acid molecule, its conformation (secondary folding) and net charge (dependent on the pH of the gel buffer), and the pore size of the gel
  - Agarose gel and polyacrylamide gel are the basic forms of electrophoresis. Variations on these methods include pulsed-field gel electrophoresis (PFGE), capillary gel electrophoresis (CGE), denaturing gradient gel electrophoresis (DGGE), and temperature gradient gel electrophoresis (TGGE)
- Agarose gel electrophoresis
  - Agarose is manufactured from seaweed such as Rhodophyta. It consists of multiple linked repeat units of the disaccharide agarobiose (D-galactose and 3,6-anhydro-L-galactose)
  - Applications
    - Agarose gel electrophoresis is commonly used for the analysis of end-point PCR or RT-PCR assays in which the presence or absence of amplicons defines the interpretation of the test; for example, the detection a fusion transcript or a pathogen
    - The analysis of restriction fragment length polymorphism (RFLP) assays (discussed under "Hybridization Methods: Southern Blotting") generally requires agarose gel electrophoresis
    - The technique is used routinely in molecular biology for the analysis of recombinant DNA experiments and can be used for the purification of probes for ISH and blot hybridization by excision of DNA fragments from a gel followed by mini-column purification
- Pulsed-field gel electrophoresis (PFGE)
  - PFGE is an electrophoresis method for the improved resolution of high-molecular-weight DNA
  - The improved resolution of PFGE is accomplished by alternating the direction of the electrical field. In the simplest approach, the direction of field is constantly reversed so that the DNA spends some time moving backward. More refined techniques alternate the field so that the DNA moves through the gel in a zigzag pattern
  - Applications: PFGE can be used for the identification of microorganism strains such as *Escherichia coli* O157:H7 and *Salmonella*, *Shigella*, *Listeria*, or *Campylobacter* species. High-molecular-weight DNA extracts (from culture) are digested with a restriction enzyme (see "Southern Blotting"). The PFGE electrophoretic DNA "fingerprint" helps identify the infective strain. The Centers for Disease Control and Prevention (CDC) maintains databases of PFGE-standardized molecular subtypes for the identification of microorganisms. In combination with Southern blot analysis, PFGE can be used in the evaluation of autosomal dominant ataxia
- Polyacrylamide gel electrophoresis
  - Polyacrylamide is produced from monomers of acrylamide in a reaction initiated by free radicals generated by reduction of ammonium persulfate by TEMED (N,N,N',N'-tetramethylene diamine). These linear strands of polyacrylamide form into a gel after cross-linkage by N,N'-methylenebisacrylamide. The higher the concentration of acrylamide, the finer the resolution of DNA fragments
  - The advantage of polyacrylamide over agarose is that size differences at the base-pair level can be distinguished
  - Applications: end-point PCR fragment analysis in which fragment size differences are slight. Polyacrylamide slab gels are used for sequencing assays and for microsatellite marker–based assays using autoradiography or fluorescence-labeled fragments
- Capillary gel electrophoresis
  - Capillary gel electrophoresis supports automated DNA sequencing and fragment analyses
  - Applications: capillary gel electrophoresis is widely used for sequencing and microsatellite assay data analyses

Hybridization Methods

- Southern blotting
  - Dr. E. M. Southern developed the Southern blot technique in 1975 as a method for transferring DNA out of an agarose slab gel onto a solid support (a nitrocellulose or nylon membrane)
  - The method involves the use of restriction endonucleases to cut (restrict) genomic DNA into differently sized fragments that are size-fractionated by gel electrophoresis. After transfer, the membrane is hybridized with a labeled probe specific to the target sequence of interest
  - Can be used to detect chromosomal rearrangements, DNA amplifications, deletions,

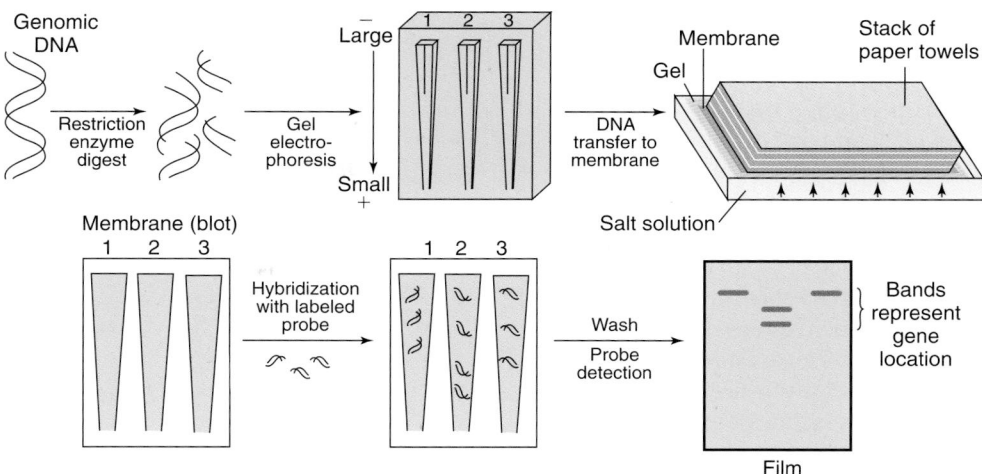

Figure 1-20. Southern blot analysis. Following agarose gel electrophoresis of restriction endonuclease-treated genomic DNA, alkali-denatured DNA is transferred onto a nylon membrane by capillary action. The recovered membrane is screened for target sequences by hybridization with a labeled probe. (Modified from Leonard DGB [ed]: Diagnostic Molecular Pathology. Philadelphia, WB Saunders, 2003.)

and loss of heterozygosity and to assess clonal status
— The technique generally requires relatively large quantities of high-molecular-weight DNA (5- to 10-µg per restriction endonuclease–treated sample)
— Applications
   ◆ The Southern blot method is widely used in RFLP analysis. The number of restriction sites for a given restriction endonuclease in the site of a gene may vary because of normal (polymorphic) variation between individuals or due to sequence mutations. These differences can result in altered restriction fragment patterns. Altered fragment sizes between individuals may also result when the restriction fragment contains variable number of tandem repeat (VNTR) sequences. VNTR regions contain microsatellite or mini-satellite repeats comprising about <6-bp or 10- to 100-bp repeat sequences, respectively. Differences in the number of these repeat units may be detectable as altered fragment sizes
   ◆ Despite the requirement for relatively large quantities of DNA and time-consuming procedures, Southern blotting may have advantages over PCR in certain applications— for example, when available sequence data are insufficient to design PCR primers specific to the site of a chromosomal rearrangement or when competition from normal cells in a sample masks the detection of an anomaly by PCR
   ◆ The detection of clonality by immunoglobulin (Ig) gene rearrangements in B-cell lymphoproliferative disorders can aid the diagnosis of minimal residual disease. PCR tests

for B-cell clonality may have a false-negative rate of up to 30%, and the gold standard test for the detection of Ig clonal rearrangements may be Southern blot analysis
   ◆ Southern blotting can also have an advantage over PCR in the detection of fragile X syndrome
   ◆ Southern blotting can be combined with PCR. Hybridization with a target-specific probe can be used to confirm that PCR amplicons represent the target and are not anomalous products resulting from incidental primer annealing events. PCR amplicon RFLP analyses may also be performed by Southern blotting
   ◆ Examples of Southern blot clinical applications include
      ◇ Autosomal dominant ataxia evaluation (in combination with PFGE)
      ◇ Beckwith-Wiedemann syndrome
      ◇ Myotonic dystrophy evaluation
      ◇ Epstein-Barr virus clonality assay
      ◇ Fragile X syndrome
      ◇ Hemophilia A analysis for inversion, deletion, and carrier
      ◇ Ig gene rearrangement
      ◇ *MLH1* deletion/duplication screen
      ◇ *MSH2* deletion/duplication screen
      ◇ *MSH6* deletion/duplication screen
      ◇ Partial Duchenne muscular dystrophy (DMD) deletion/duplication assay
      ◇ T-cell receptor gene rearrangement
● Northern blotting
   — The northern blot technique is used in the analysis of mRNA expression
   — mRNA constitutes up to 5% of the total cellular RNA. Extracted mRNA is denatured with formaldehyde or glyoxal to prevent the formation

of secondary RNA structures. Digestion of the RNA into smaller fragments is not required because native mRNA fragment sizes range from about 300 to 12,000 nucleotides; the average size is 1000 to 3000 nucleotides

— After agarose gel electrophoresis, RNA is transferred to a membrane by a capillary, vacuum, or electrotransfer process, and the membrane is hybridized with a labeled probe to the gene target

— The resulting data indicate whether a gene is overexpressed or underexpressed, or if an abnormally sized transcript is expressed

— The method requires relatively large amounts of high-integrity RNA, is time-consuming, and requires a high level of laboratory skill, all of which limit the clinical utility of northern blotting

● Dot blotting

— Dot blot hybridization involves spotting denatured DNA or RNA onto a membrane for hybridization with a labeled probe

— The method allows confirmation that a genomic DNA or RNA sample or a PCR product is positive for the probe target

— Can also be used semiquantitatively to assess or compare target sequence load within a sample

— Reverse-line dot blot hybridization: an alternative approach to the standard dot blot is to fix an array of unlabeled probes onto the membrane and hybridize this with labeled nucleic acids or PCR products

— Applications

◆ A variety of "line probe assays" (LiPA) have been developed. These include screening tests for apolipoprotein E mutations, cystic fibrosis mutations, HBV and HPV genotyping, HLA typing, and *Mycobacteria* species detection

◆ Outside the United States, Conformité Européenne (CE)-marked LiPA tests are available for PCR-based HPV clinical screening

◆ The SPF_{10}-INNO LiPA HPV genotyping test (Innogenetics, Ghent, Belgium) allows the specific genotyping of 25 different HPV types

◆ The Roche Linear Array (LA) HPV genotyping test (Roche Molecular Systems, Inc., Branchburg, NJ) detects 37 different HPV types

◆ With both systems, biotinylated PCR product is hybridized with a membrane strip affixed with a line of HPV genotype-specific probes. Detection of the PCR product label indicates the HPV genotypes for which the patient is positive

● ISH

— ISH enables the direct visualization of nucleic acid targets in relation to cytologic, histologic, or karyotypic features

— ISH was first described in 1969 using radiolabeled probes and slide autoradiography to assess hybridization data. ISH methods employing ^{3}H-, ^{125}I-, ^{32}P-, ^{33}P-, or ^{35}S-labeled probes are still used

Figure 1-21. In situ hybridization (ISH). Slide-mounted tissues are pretreated/protease digested to facilitate labeled probe access to nucleic acid targets for hybridization. Chromogenic ISH involves the detection of a hapten-labeled probe with enzyme-labeled secondary reagents and a chromogenic substrate. Fluorescence ISH involves the use of fluorophore-labeled probes or fluorescence-labeled secondary detection reagents. (Modified from Leonard DGB [ed]: Diagnostic Molecular Pathology. Philadelphia, WB Saunders, 2003.)

in a research setting but are hazardous and may require long exposures

— Chromogenic ISH (CISH) techniques were first developed during the 1980s using biotin, 2,4-dinitrophenyl (DNP), digoxigenin, or fluorescein hapten-labeled probes

— Fluorescence ISH (FISH) techniques were developed during the 1990s; labels include cyanine compounds, fluorescein isothiocyanate (FITC), rhodamine, Texas Red (sulforhodamine 101 acid chloride), and a wide range of proprietary fluorophores such as the Alexa Fluor (Invitrogen Corporation), Cy (GE Healthcare), DyLight (ThermoFisher Scientific), MFP (MoBiTech), and Spectrum (Abbott Molecular, Inc.) dye series. FISH techniques can be practiced using fluorophore-labeled nucleic acid probes or using fluorophore-labeled secondary reagents against hapten-labeled probes

— ISH is applicable to all pathology sample preparations, including cytologic samples, primary cell cultures, chromosome spreads, fine-needle aspirations, ThinPrep smears, frozen tissue sections, and FFPE specimens

— Method: the ISH method consists of pretreatments, hybridization, posthybridization washes, and probe label detection

— Applications

◆ ISH techniques are amenable to a wide range of applications, including investigation of genetic instability, gene amplification, gene expression, and chromosomal rearrangements

Figure 1-22. Chromogenic in situ hybridization (CISH). Human papillomavirus (HPV) detected by CISH in cervical tissue; low-grade lesion (**A**), high-grade lesion (**B**), and squamous cell carcinoma (**C**). "Diffuse" signals (*blue arrows*) are indicative of episomal HPV, and "punctuate" signals (*red arrows*) are indicative of HPV integrated into the cell genome.

◆ The extensive list of pathogens that can be detected by FISH includes CMV, Epstein-Barr virus (DNA or mRNA), HCV RNA, HSV, HPV, hantavirus, influenza virus, parvovirus B19, and varicella-zoster virus

◆ FISH is used in the diagnosis of diverse hematologic and sarcomatoid disorders, in the diagnosis of breast and bladder cancer, in prenatal screening, and in assessing sex-mismatched bone marrow transplantation success

◆ FDA-approved FISH tests include the UroVysion for bladder cancer and the PathVysion for HER-2 amplification in breast cancer (Abbott Molecular Inc., Des Plaines, IL). An FDA-approved CISH test for HER-2 amplification is also available, the SPOT-Light HER2 CISH kit (Invitrogen, Carlsbad, CA)

Figure 1-23. Fluorescence in situ hybridization (FISH). FISH assay (PathVysion, Abbott Molecular Inc., Des Plaines, IL) of breast carcinoma tissues for *HER-2* gene amplification. Nonamplification (**A**) is indicated by a balanced ratio of green signals (chromosome 17 centromere) (*green arrows*) to orange signals (*HER-2* locus-specific probe [17q11.2-q12] (*red arrows*)). Amplification (**B**) is indicated by a relative excess of *HER-2* signals.

◆ There are many non-FDA cited tests in widespread clinical diagnostics use; for example, the Mayo Medical Laboratories *MayoAccess Test Catalog* lists more than 40 available FISH tests, including tests for acute lymphocytic leukemia (B-cell, T-cell), acute myeloblastic leukemia, *BCR/ABL*, Ewing sarcoma, 22q12 rearrangement, biliary tract malignancy, cri-du-chat, 5p del, and N-*myc* amplification

● DNA microarray technology
— DNA microarrays comprise a solid support (a silicon chip) imprinted with sequence-specific oligonucleotide probes. Fluorescence-labeled sample DNA or cDNA is hybridized with the microarray, and the detected emissions demonstrate qualitatively or quantitatively the nucleic acid species present in the sample
— DNA microarrays can be used to examine gene expression by simultaneously hybridizing the array with cDNA from normal and diseased tissues; each cDNA preparation is labeled with a different fluorophore. Analysis of the intensities of the different labels demonstrates genes that are underexpressed, overexpressed, or unchanged in expression
— A similar assay using labeled DNAs and chromosome-specific probes can be performed to infer chromosome losses or gains. DNA microarrays can also be used to screen for SNPs

— Potentially, thousands of sequences can be screened using a single microarray. Limited target (<100) set arrays designed toward cell pathways (e.g., apoptosis, angiogenesis, cell cycle, cytokines, signal transduction) or tumor nucleic acid signatures have also been developed
— Microarray assay affordability, standardization, and clinical interpretability are issues limiting clinical array applications
— Applications: FDA-cleared microarray tests include
◆ The MammaPrint test (Agendia BV, Amsterdam, The Netherlands) screens 70 genes to assess the likelihood of recurrence in patients who have undergone breast cancer surgery. The expressed gene data indicate high or low risk for disease recurrence. The test is applicable to lymph node–negative patients younger than 61 years with stage I or II tumors 5 cm or smaller
◆ The Pathwork Tissue of Origin Test (Pathwork Diagnostics, Sunnyvale, CA) aids identification of the origin of a tumor. The test measures the expression pattern of more than 1500 genes in the "uncertain" tumor. This pattern is compared with expression patterns of a panel of 15 known tumor types, representing 60 morphologies overall. An objective, probability-based score is generated relative to each of the 15 potential tumor types supporting assignment or exclusion of the uncertain tumor to each panel type

Nucleic Acid Sequencing

- The most widely used nucleic acid sequencing technique has been the chain termination method originated by Frederic Sanger in the mid-1970s. This technique has since been adapted to include PCR technology and fluorescently labeled nucleotides leading to the development of dye terminator sequencing that allows routine automated sequence analyses
- Applications: DNA sequencing represents the gold-standard confirmation of a mutation. Clinical applications generally involve PCR amplification of a defined target region followed by sequencing; available tests include
  - Autosomal recessive polycystic kidney disease (*ARPKD*) mutation screen
  - Biotinidase deficiency (*BTD*) gene analysis
  - *CFTR* gene analysis
  - 21-Hydroxylase (*CYP21A2*) gene analysis
  - Dentatorubral-pallidoluysian atrophy (*DRPLA*) gene analysis
  - Fabry disease gene analysis
  - Galactose-1-phosphate uridyltransferase gene (*GALT*) gene analysis
  - *MLH1* HNPCC mutation screen
  - *MLH1/MSH2* mutation screen
  - *MSH2* mutation screen
  - *MSH6* mutation screen
  - Niemann-Pick type C (NPC) mutation screen
  - Progranulin (*GRN*) gene analysis
  - Von Hippel-Lindau disease (*VHL*) gene analysis
  - FDA-cleared sequencing assays are available for HIV drug resistance testing (ViroSeq HIV-1 Genotyping System, Celera Diagnostics, CA, and TruGene HIV-1 Genotyping and Open Gene DNA Sequencing System, Siemens Healthcare Diagnostics, Deerfield, IL)

Protein Analytical Methods

- Aberrant protein expression consequent to disrupted nucleic acids or infective pathogens is detectable by protein analytical techniques
- IHC (see "Immunohistochemistry") demonstrates protein expression at the morphologic level; genogenic IHC supports the detection of chimeric proteins, such as the EWS-FLI1 protein (Ewing sarcoma), which can arise after translocation events
- Western blotting consists of polyacrylamide gel electrophoresis of proteins followed by electroblotting onto a nitrocellulose membrane; the membrane is incubated with labeled antibodies directed against the protein of interest, and expression is measured by the detection of the label
- The enzyme immunoassay (EIA) technique involves the capture of a specimen antigen (or antibody) in an antibody- (or antigen-) coated microtiter plate well. Secondary enzyme-labeled (e.g., horseradish peroxidase [HRP]) antibodies are applied, and the label is detected by a colorimetric substrate reaction that can be qualitative or quantitative
- Line immunoassays (LIA, Innogenetics, Ghent, Belgium) involve incubation of patient serum or plasma with a membrane strip prefixed with a range of purified recombinant, or synthetic antigens. CE-approved INNO-LIA assays are available for the detection of HCV, HIV, human T-cell lymphotrophic virus, and syphilis
- Membrane immunochromatographic (ICT) tests for infectious agents have been developed (NOW-Technologies by Binax, Inc., Scarborough, ME). FDA-cleared tests are available for *Legionella pneumophila* serogroup 1 antigen in urine specimens, malaria (*Plasmodium falciparum* [P.f.] antigen, and the antigen common to all to pan-malarial species: *Plasmodium vivax* [P.v.], *Plasmodium ovale* [P.o.], and *Plasmodium malariae* [P.m.] in whole blood.), reparatory syncytial virus (RSV) fusion protein antigen in nasal wash and nasopharyngeal swab, *Streptococcus pyogenes* group A antigen from throat swab specimens, and *Streptococcus pneumoniae* antigen test for urine of patients with pneumonia and in the cerebral spinal fluid of patients with meningitis

Emerging Methodologies

- DNA methylation assays are likely to increase in significance as more is discovered about the importance of epigenetic factors in disease etiology. Abnormal methylation, which can result in gene silencing, is a recognized diagnostic factor for Angelman, Prader-Willi, and Beckwith-Wiedemann syndromes and is implicated as a general tumor

TCTGATCTTGGTCGCTGGATAGTCGTCTGTGTTTCTTCGGTGCCCAA

Figure 1-24. Nucleic acid sequencing data output.

characteristic. Methylation can be detected by Southern blot RFLP analysis using methylation-sensitive restriction endonucleases (as in the current assays for Beckwith-Wiedemann syndrome, etc.) or by PCR in combination with sample DNA treatment with bisulfite. Bisulfite converts dCTP residues to dUTP; during PCR, the dUTP is replaced with dTTP. Methylated cytosine is unaffected by bisulfite treatment. A comparison of bisulfite-treated and -untreated PCR amplicon sequences (by direct sequencing or restriction endonuclease analysis) reveals the methylation status of investigated sequences. The pyrosequencing technique also supports DNA methylation characterization

- MicroRNA (miRNA), short single-stranded RNA that can bind complementary mRNA preventing protein translation, is emerging as potential biomarker of pathologic conditions. Array technology may also prove useful in screening for pathology defining miRNA species expression. For example, Rosetta Genomics (Philadelphia, PA) has developed several miRNA microarray clinical assays. These include tests for the tissue-of-origin of metastatic tumors using miRNA extracted from FFPE specimens, and a blood-based miRNA diagnostic for colon cancer.

- Mass Spectrometry (MS) can distinguish proteins on the basis of the mass/charge (m/z) ratio profile of ions derived from a fragmented parent molecule. Tumors and other pathologic conditions may be identifiable by a characteristic protein signature detectable by MS. Clinical assays may emerge from ongoing developments in proteomics research

Web Resources

General Methods

An animation of LCM is accessible at: http://www.moleculardevices.com/pages/instruments/microgenomics.html

Max Animations Genetics (http://www.maxanim.com/genetics/index.htm) includes or has planned animations on DNA restriction, microarrays, PCR, RFLP, and Southern blotting

Davidson College, NC, has prepared an animation of RT-PCR, available at: http://www.bio.davidson.edu/courses/Immunology/Flash/RT_PCR.html

Animated expositions of real-time PCR techniques are available at Biocompare's website (http://www.biocompare.com/Documents/tutorialqPCR/qPCR/flash_go.html)

Proprietary Methods

An animation of the Transcription-Mediated Amplification (TMA) assay is available at: http://www.gen-probe.com/science/amplification.aspx

The Nucleic Acid Sequence-Based Amplification (NASBA) technique is shown at: http://biomerieux-usa.com/clinical/nucleicacid/nasba.htm. A PowerPoint presentation is available at: http://www.ibi.cc/nasba%20step%20by%20step.htm and http://www.ibi.cc/NASBA_automation.ppt

Details of the Strand Displacement Amplification (SDA) techniques are available at: http://www.bd.com/ds/productCenter/BdProbetecEtSystem.asp

The branch DNA (bDNA) method is illustrated at: http://www.panomics.com/downloads/QG2_Bro_RevB_121707B.pdf.

The Invader chemistry assay is illustrated at: http://www.twt.com/invader/invader.html

Details of the Multiple Ligation-dependent Probe Amplification (MLPA) assay, including a PowerPoint presentation, are available at: http://www.mrc-holland.com/pages/support_mlpa_infopag.html

Hybrid Capture technology is shown at: http://www1.qiagen.com/hpv/hc2Technology.aspx

The Pathwork Tissue of Origin Test microarray details are at: http://www.pathworkdx.com/TissueofOrigenTest/Technology

The MammaPrint Microarray is described at: http://usa.agendia.com/index.php?option=com_content&task=view&id=27&Itemid=271

Rosetta Genomics miRNA microarray clinical tests are detailed at: http://www.rosettagenomics.com/index.asp

Details of Line Probe Assay (LiPA) applications are available at: http://www.innogenetics.com/platform.html?id=2

Details of Line Immunoassays (LIA) are at: http://www.innogenetics.com/platform.html?id=3

Details of the immunochromatographic (ICT) technique are available at: http://www.binax.com/default.aspx

Association for Molecular Pathology (AMP): the AMP (http://www.amp.org/index.htm) is a not-for-profit scientific society dedicated to the advancement, practice, and science of clinical molecular laboratory medicine and translational research based on the applications of genomics and proteomics. Carol A. Holland, Ph.D., maintains an updated list of FDA-cleared/approved molecular techniques at the website.

Selected References

Cheng L, Zhang, DY (eds): Molecular Genetic Pathology. Totowa, Humana Press, 2008.

Leonard, DGB (ed): Molecular Pathology in Clinical Practice. Springer, New York, 2007.

Coleman BC, Tsongalis GJ (eds): Molecular Diagnostics for the Clinical Laboratorian, 2nd ed. Totowa, Humana Press, 2006.

McPerson M, Møller S: PCR, 2nd ed. New York, Taylor & Francis Group, 2006.

Van de Rijn J. Fletcher: Genetic of soft tissue tumors: Expression profiling studies. In Annual Review of Pathology: Mechanisms of Disease, vol 1. Palo Alto, Annual Reviews, 2006, pp 448-449.

Killeen AA: Principles of Molecular Pathology. Totowa, Humana Press, 2004.

Roulston JE, Bartlett JMS (eds): Molecular Diagnosis of Cancer: Methods and Protocols, 2nd ed. Totowa, Humana Press, 2004.

Leonard DGB (ed): Diagnostic Molecular Pathology. Philadelphia, WB Saunders, 2003.

Sambrook J, Russell DW: Molecular Cloning: A Laboratory Manual, 3rd ed. New York, Cold Spring Harbor Laboratory Press, 2001.

Acknowledgments

The authors would like to thank Lisa Kapoor for her assistance and support during the preparation of the chapter.

Vijaya B. Reddy

2 Skin and Adnexal Structures

Inflammatory Conditions

Superficial Perivascular Dermatitis

Dermatitis with Minimal Epidermal Changes

Superficial Dermatophytosis (Tinea)

Clinical Features

- Caused by three genera of imperfect fungi—*Epidermophyton*, *Trichophyton*, and *Microsporum*—that cause superficial infections involving keratinized tissues such as the cornified layer of epidermis, the hair, and the nails
- Dermatophytosis involving different anatomic sites are named with site-specific terms such as *tinea capitis* (scalp), *tinea barbae* (beard area), *tinea faciei* (face), *tinea corporis* (trunk), *tinea cruris* (intertriginous areas), *tinea pedis et manus* (feet and hands), and *tinea unguium* (nails)
- Typical lesions of superficial dermatophytosis present as sharply demarcated patches with an arcuate border
- Tinea capitis and tinea barbae present as folliculitis; tinea unguium is characterized by yellow-gray discoloration of nails

Histopathology

- Focal parakeratosis with neutrophils and mild epidermal spongiosis
- Mild, superficial perivascular lymphocytic infiltrate
- Fungi are present as filamentous hyphae, spores, or yeast forms in the cornified layer and in the hair shafts in cases of tinea capitis and tinea barbae

Special Stains and Immunohistochemistry

- Periodic acid–Schiff (PAS) reaction stains fungi deep red to pink, and Gomori methenamine silver (GMS) stains fungi black

Figure 2-1. Dermatophytosis. A, Hematoxylin and eosin–stained section shows focal parakeratosis with neutrophils and mild superficial perivascular inflammation. **B,** Periodic acid–Schiff stain shows the presence of fungal hyphae within the cornified layer.

Other Techniques for Diagnosis

- Microbiologic cultures are useful in identifying the genera and species of the fungal organisms
- In folliculitis pattern, fluorescein-labeled *Trichophyton mentagrophytes* antiserum may be helpful in demonstrating fungal infection

Differential Diagnosis

▮ Vitiligo and urticaria
- Should be considered in cases with minimal histologic changes
- Demonstration of the fungal organisms with special stains confirms the diagnosis of dermatophytosis
▮ Disseminated candidiasis
- Can be considered in patients with impaired host response, especially patients with hematologic malignancies
- Histologic sections show spongiotic or subcorneal pustules in which budding yeast forms can be demonstrated with PAS or GMS stain
▮ Pityriasis (tinea) versicolor caused by genus *Malassezia*
- Affects upper trunk with brownish discoloration that may become hypopigmented
- Histologic sections show slight hyperkeratosis, round spores, and thick, short hyphae recognizable as faintly basophilic, refractive structures in routine hematoxylin and eosin (H&E)–stained sections
- Folliculitis pattern of dermatophytosis may be similar to *Malassezia (Pityrosporum)* folliculitis

Pearls

- Identification of fungal organisms on routine H&E-stained sections may be aided by lowering the microscope condenser, which enhances the refractile nature of the fungi
- Fungi in the cornified layer are sandwiched between a lower zone of parakeratosis and an upper zone of orthokeratosis ("sandwich sign"); diagnosis can be confirmed by demonstration of fungi with special stains
- The presence of neutrophils in a slightly parakeratotic cornified layer and mild superficial perivascular dermatitis should always prompt a PAS stain in search of fungal elements

Selected References

Havlickova B, Czaika VA, Frieddrich M: Epidemiologic trends in skin mycosis worldwide. Mycoses 51(Suppl 4):2-15, 2008.

Vermout S, Tabart J, Baldo A, et al: Pathogenesis of dermatophytosis. Mycopathologia 166:267-275, 2008.

Howard RM, Frieden IJ: Dermatophyte infections in children. Adv Pediatr Infect Dis 14:73-107, 1999.

Noble SL, Forbes RC, Stamm PL: Diagnosis and management of common tinea infections. Am Fam Physician 58:163-174, 177-178, 1998.

Gottlieb GJ, Ackerman AB: The "sandwich sign" of dermatophytosis. Am J Dermatopathol 8:347, 1996.

Vitiligo

Clinical Features

- Acquired, possibly autoimmune disease with strong familial association
- Characterized by patches of pigment loss in skin
- Localized disease may show linear, segmental pattern
- Generalized vitiligo involves face, upper trunk, dorsa of hands, periorificial areas, and genitalia; scalp and eyelashes are not typically affected
- Stable patches of vitiligo are sharply demarcated and may be surrounded by a zone of hyperpigmentation; in active lesions, areas of total depigmentation may be surrounded by a zone of partial depigmentation and have a slight rim of erythema at the border

Histopathology

- Low-power examination shows mostly unremarkable skin or mild superficial perivascular inflammation with scattered melanophages
- With silver stain, total absence of melanocytes is seen in well-established lesions and in the depigmented center of expanding lesions of vitiligo

Figure 2-2. A, Vitiligo. Fontana-Masson stain shows loss of pigmentation at the basal cell layer. **B, Normal skin.** Fontana-Masson stain shows normal pigmentation at the basal cell layer.

- A few dopa-positive melanocytes may be seen in the hypopigmented areas; in the outer border of the patches, prominent melanocytes with long dendritic processes filled with melanin granules and a mild superficial perivascular inflammation are present
- Mild superficial perivascular and patchy lichenoid lymphocytic infiltrate and vacuolar alteration of the basal cell layer can be seen in normal-appearing skin adjacent to the vitiliginous patches

Special Stains and Immunohistochemistry

- Silver stains or the dopa reaction (Fontana-Masson) are used in demonstrating absence of melanocytes and melanin pigmentation
- Immunohistochemical stains for S-100 protein or pan-melanocytic marker may also be helpful in demonstrating melanocytes

Other Techniques for Diagnosis

- Noncontributory

Differential Diagnosis

- On routine H&E-stained sections, other diseases manifesting with minimal histologic alterations (apparently normal-appearing skin), such as tinea versicolor, urticaria, and macular variant of urticaria pigmentosa, should be considered

Pearls

- Studies show that autoimmune mechanisms and genetic predisposition are the most likely causative factors
- Additional evidence for autoimmune mechanism includes the coexistence of vitiligo and idiopathic uveitis and the occurrence of vitiligo in Vogt-Koyanagi-Harada syndrome

Selected References

Le Poole IC, Luiten RM: Autoimmune etiology of generalized vitiligo. Curr Dir Autoimmun 10:227-243, 2008.

Attili VR, Attili SK: Lichenoid inflammation in vitiligo: A clinical and histopathologic review of 210 cases. Int J Dermatol 47:663-669, 2008.

Halder RM, Young CM: New and emerging therapies for vitiligo. Dermatol Clin 18:79-89, ix, 2000.

Halder RM: Childhood vitiligo. Clin Dermatol 15:899-906, 1997.

Le Poole IC, Das PK: Microscopic changes in vitiligo. Clin Dermatol 15:863-873, 1997.

Urticaria

Clinical Features

- Presents with pruritic, raised, erythematous, and edematous areas known as *wheals*
- In acute urticaria, episodes last for only several hours
- In chronic urticaria, episodes last up to 24 hours or longer and recur over a period of at least 6 weeks

Figure 2-3. Urticaria. Histologic section shows mild superficial perivascular mixed inflammatory cell infiltrate and interstitial edema.

Figure 2-4. Urticaria pigmentosa, macular type. A, Hematoxylin and eosin–stained section shows dilated blood vessels in the superficial dermis surrounded by a mild perivascular infiltrate of cells. Without a high degree of suspicion and special stains, it might be difficult to notice that the cells are predominantly mast cells. **B,** Giemsa stain highlights the mast cells in the infiltrate.

- An underlying predisposing condition can be identified in up to 25% of patients; certain foods, drugs, contact allergens, and physical stimuli such as pressure, cold temperature, and occult infections may be factors

- Urticarial vasculitis is a syndrome consisting of recurrent urticaria, arthralgia, and abdominal pain; individual cutaneous lesions persist for more than 24 hours
- In angioedema, dermal edema extends into subcutaneous fat and presents with large wheals

Histopathology

- Acute urticaria is characterized by interstitial edema, dilated vessels, and a sparse perivascular inflammatory cell infiltrate
- In chronic urticaria, in addition to dermal edema, there is a perivascular and interstitial mixed inflammatory cell infiltrate composed of lymphocytes, eosinophils, and neutrophils
- Urticarial vasculitis shows an early leukocytoclastic vasculitis with a perivascular infiltrate of neutrophils, neutrophilic nuclear dust, and extravasated red blood cells; minimal or absent fibrin deposits in the vessel walls

Special Stains and Immunohistochemistry

- Noncontributory

Other Techniques for Diagnosis

- Hypocomplementemia is seen in 32% of patients with urticarial vasculitis; measurements of CH50 and C1q binding assays are helpful
- Electron microscopy: degranulation of mast cells and eosinophils may be seen in urticaria
- Patients with hereditary angioedema have a low serum level of esterase inhibitor of first component of complement
- Direct immunofluorescence: vascular deposits of immunoglobulins, complement, or fibrin are seen in one third of patients with urticarial vasculitis

Differential Diagnosis

- ▌ Macular variant of urticaria pigmentosa (telangiectasia macularis eruptiva perstans)
  - Generally occurs as an extensive eruption of brownish-red macules with only little urtication
  - Histologic sections show dilated blood vessels in the upper dermis and a mild superficial perivascular mononuclear cell infiltrate composed mostly of mast cells; eosinophils are generally absent; dermal edema is not prominent
  - Giemsa, toluidine blue, Leder, or immunohisto-chemical stain for mast cell tryptase can help demonstrate the increased number of mast cells
- ▌ Other causes of leukocytoclastic vasculitis should be considered in the differential diagnosis of urticarial vasculitis

Pearls

- In hereditary angioedema, a form of dominantly inherited angioedema, recurrent attacks of edema involve skin and oral, laryngeal, and gastrointestinal mucosa; death due to laryngeal edema can occur if not treated
- Urticarial vasculitis may be associated with infectious mononucleosis, infectious hepatitis, and autoimmune diseases such as systemic lupus erythematosus

Selected References

Cugno M, Castelli R, Cicardi M: Angioedema due to acquired C1-inhibitor deficiency: A bridging condition between autoimmunity and lymphoproliferation. Autoimmun Rev 8:156-159, 2008.

Młynek A, Maurer M, Zalewska A: Update on chronic urticaria: Focusing on mechanisms. Curr Opin Allergy Clin Immunol 8:433-437, 2008.

Greaves M: Chronic urticaria. J Allergy Clin Immunol 105:664-672, 2000.

Wisnieski JJ: Urticarial vasculitis. Curr Opin Rheumatol 12:24-31, 2000.

Gibbs NF, Friedlander SF, Harpster EF: Telangiectasia macularis eruptiva perstans. Pediatr Dermatol 17:194-197, 2000.

Black AK: Urticarial vasculitis. Clin Dermatol 17:565-569, 1999.

Beltrani VS: Urticaria and angioedema. Dermatol Clin 14:171-198, 1996.

Interface Dermatitis

Lichen Planus

Clinical Features

- Disorder of unknown etiology involving skin, mucous membranes, hair follicles, and nails
- Typically presents as pruritic, flat-topped violaceous papules with a fine scale
- Predilection for flexor surfaces of extremities, lower back, and glans penis
- Surface of lesions may show a network of white lines known as *Wickham striae*

Figure 2-5. Lichen planus. Histologic section shows hyperkeratosis, hypergranulosis, irregular epidermal hyperplasia, and a bandlike, predominantly lymphocytic infiltrate that obscures the dermoepidermal junction. Melanophages are present in the dermal infiltrate.

- Oral lesions may be seen as sole manifestation or in association with skin involvement and consist of lacy, reticular network of papules involving buccal mucosa or tongue

Histopathology

- Compact hyperkeratosis and wedge-shaped hypergranulosis that corresponds to the openings of follicles and acrosyringia
- Irregular epidermal hyperplasia with a sawtooth appearance, and a bandlike, predominantly lymphocytic infiltrate in the superficial dermis that obscures the dermoepidermal junction
- Eosinophilic colloid bodies or Civatte bodies are present at the dermoepidermal junction and usually represent damage to the basal cell layer
- Small clefts known as *Max-Joseph spaces* may be seen between the epidermis and dermis
- Chronic lesions show hyperkeratosis and papillomatous epidermal hyperplasia (hypertrophic lichen planus)
- Oral lesions show parakeratosis, less epithelial hyperplasia, and frequent ulceration
- Lichen planus of hair follicles (lichen planopilaris) shows a dense lymphocytic infiltrate surrounding the follicular epithelium; in later stages, there is perifollicular fibrosis with advanced stages resulting in scarring alopecia

Special Stains and Immunohistochemistry

- Lymphoid infiltrate is composed predominantly of T cells

Other Techniques for Diagnosis

- Noncontributory

Differential Diagnosis

▌ Lichenoid drug eruption
- Focal parakeratosis and necrotic keratinocytes particularly at and above the dermoepidermal junction
- Presence of eosinophils in the inflammatory cell infiltrate favors a diagnosis of lichenoid drug eruption

▌ Lichen planus–like keratosis (benign lichenoid keratosis)
- Solitary lesion that shows parakeratosis in addition to lichenoid pattern of inflammation
- Adjacent areas may show changes of solar lentigo

▌ Lichenoid graft-versus-host disease (GVHD)
- Generally the inflammatory cell infiltrate is sparse and more perivascular
- Foci of parakeratosis and thinning of epidermis may be present

▌ Lichen striatus
- More common in children than adults and presents as a unilateral eruption along Blaschko lines on extremities, trunk, or neck

- Histologic features may be similar to those of lichen planus
- Distinguishing features include the presence of inflammatory cell infiltrate deep in the reticular dermis around hair follicles and sweat glands
- Epidermal spongiosis and an admixture of histiocytes in the inflammatory cell infiltrate can be present

▌ Lichen nitidus
- Asymptomatic dermatosis of childhood, characterized by round, flat-topped papules that measure only a few millimeters
- Histologically, the inflammatory infiltrate is bandlike but small and discrete; infiltrate is confined to widened dermal papillae and enclosed by elongated rete, which give an appearance of a claw clutching a ball
- Presence of numerous histiocytes in the infiltrate and focal parakeratosis are helpful in differentiating lichen nitidus from lichen planus

▌ Lichen planopilaris versus alopecia areata
- The presence of lymphocytes mostly at the base of the follicular bulb rather than along the infundibulum favors alopecia areata
- Scarring is not a feature of alopecia areata

Pearls

- Parakeratosis is not a feature of cutaneous lichen planus and should prompt consideration of other causes of lichenoid inflammation
- Koebner phenomenon (formation of a linear configuration of lesion due to scratching) can be seen in lichen planus

Selected References

Johnson H, Soldano AC, Kovich O, Long W: Oral lichen planus. Dermatol Online J 14:20, 2008.

Kang H, Alzolibani AA, Otberg N, Shapiro J: Lichen planopilaris. Dermatol Ther 21:249-256, 2008.

Katta R: Lichen planus. Am Fam Physician 61:3319-3324, 3327-3328, 2000.

Shai A, Halevy S: Lichen planus and lichen planus-like eruptions: Pathogenesis and associated diseases. Int J Dermatol 31:379-384, 1992.

Boyd AS, Neldner KH: Lichen planus. J Am Acad Dermatol 25:593-619, 1991.

Shiohara T: The lichenoid tissue reaction: An immunological perspective. Am J Dermatopathol 10:252-256, 1988.

Camisa C: Lichen planus and related conditions. Adv Dermatol 2:47-70, 1987.

Erythema Multiforme

Clinical Features

- Erythema multiforme is an acute cytotoxic cell-mediated hypersensitivity reaction to infections, most

Figure 2-6. A, Erythema multiforme. Vacuolar alteration of the basal cell layer is seen, above which there are necrotic keratinocytes. **B, Toxic epidermal necrolysis.** Full-thickness epidermal necrosis with separation at the dermoepidermal junction is seen. The cornified layer is unaltered, attesting to the acute nature of the process, and there is only a minimal inflammatory cell infiltrate.

commonly herpes simplex virus infection, and drugs, in particular sulfonamides
- The eruption is multiform and consists of macules, papules, vesicles, and occasionally large flaccid bullae; often associated with fever
- Herpesvirus-associated erythema multiforme involves the extremities and presents with typical target-like lesions, whereas that associated with drugs shows truncal involvement and a purpuric type of macular eruption; mucosal involvement (Stevens-Johnson syndrome) is characteristic
- In the most severe form, toxic epidermal necrolysis, a widespread blotchy erythema, is soon followed by large flaccid bullae with detachment of epidermis; this is most often caused by drugs, including sulfonamides, β-lactam antibiotics, and nonsteroidal anti-inflammatory drugs; associated with a high mortality rate

Histopathology

- Cornified layer is unaltered, attesting to the acute nature of the disease
- Vacuolar alteration of the basal cell layer and a sparse superficial perivascular lymphocytic infiltrate may focally obscure the dermoepidermal junction
- The hallmark of erythema multiforme is the presence of necrotic keratinocytes, initially as single cells and later as small clusters; the necrosis is more widespread in drug-induced erythema multiforme; in bullous lesions and toxic epidermal necrolysis, there is full-thickness epidermal necrosis resulting in subepidermal bullae
- In late lesions, the papillary dermis may contain melanophages (a sign of damage to the basal cell layer)

Special Stains and Immunohistochemistry

- Noncontributory

Other Techniques for Diagnosis

- Immunofluorescence studies show immunoglobulin M (IgM) and C3 in the walls of superficial dermal vessels
- Herpes simplex virus DNA has been detected within lesions of erythema multiforme using polymerase chain reaction (PCR) and in situ hybridization (ISH)

Differential Diagnosis

▌ Staphylococcal scalded-skin syndrome
- Can be clinically similar to toxic epidermal necrolysis
- Microscopically, staphylococcal scalded-skin syndrome shows a split in the granular layer, whereas in toxic epidermal necrolysis, there is separation at the dermoepidermal junction, a feature most helpful in distinguishing the two entities
▌ Acute GVHD disease
- May be histologically indistinguishable from early erythema multiforme
▌ Drug eruptions, including fixed drug eruptions
- Characterized by the presence of necrotic keratinocytes
- Presence of eosinophils and deeper infiltrate in fixed drug eruption

Pearls

- Erythema multiforme, Stevens-Johnson syndrome, and toxic epidermal necrolysis are best regarded as a spectrum of the same disease process
- The presence or absence of mucosal lesions in bullous forms of erythema multiforme does not appear to correlate with severity or prognosis

Selected References

Borchers AT, Lee JL, Naguwa SM, et al: Stevens-Johnson syndrome and toxic epidermal necrolysis. Autoimmun Rev 7:598-605, 2008.

Pereira FA, Mudgil AV, Rosmarin DM: Toxic epidermal necrolysis. J Am Acad Dermatol 56:181-200, 2007.

Wolkenstein PE, Roujeau JC, Revuz J: Drug-induced toxic epidermal necrolysis. Clin Dermatol 16:399-408, 1998.

Roujeau JC: Stevens-Johnson syndrome and toxic epidermal necrolysis are severity variants of the same disease which differs from erythema multiforme. J Dermatol 24:726-729, 1997.

Duarte AM, Pruksachatkunakorn C, Schachner LA: Life-threatening dermatoses in pediatric dermatology. Adv Dermatol 10:329-370, 1995.

Brady WJ, DeBehnke D, Crosby DL: Dermatological emergencies. Am J Emerg Med 12:217-237, 1994.

Ackerman AB, Ragaz A: Erythema multiforme. Am J Dermatopathol 7:133, 1985.

Graft-versus-Host Disease

Clinical Features

- Occurs when immunodeficient patients receive immunocompetent lymphocytes through either bone marrow transplantation or blood products
- Occurs in 70% of bone marrow transplant recipients; a rare congenital form also exists
- Acute phase
  - Occurs in 75% of patients and typically presents with the triad of skin lesions, hepatic dysfunction, and diarrhea; skin eruption develops between 11 and 16 days (peak at 18 days)
  - Skin lesions are characterized by extensive erythematous macules, purpuric to violaceous papules and plaques, and in severe cases, toxic epidermal necrolysis–like eruption; oral lesions may be present
- Chronic phase
  - Occurs in 10% of patients and begins several months to a year after transplantation
  - In the early lichenoid stage, the eruption is similar to lichen planus

Figure 2-7. Acute graft-versus-host disease. Vacuolar alteration of the basal cell layer is seen with scattered necrotic keratinocytes within the epidermis. Lymphocytes are present at the basal cell layer and extending into the epidermis, where they may surround the necrotic keratinocytes (satellite necrosis).

- Late sclerotic stage is characterized by dermal sclerosis and atrophy

Histopathology

- Acute phase
  - Grade I: vacuolar alteration of the basal cell layer, which may be focal or diffuse
  - Grade II: necrotic keratinocytes occasionally surrounded by lymphocytes (satellite necrosis) are seen in the epidermis
  - Grade III: more widespread necrosis of keratinocytes with separation at the dermoepidermal junction
  - Grade IV: full-thickness necrosis and loss of epidermis
  - Sparse superficial perivascular lymphocytic infiltrate is usually present in acute GVHD
  - Occasionally follicular papules are seen clinically, and histologic changes similar to those of epidermis can be seen in the follicular epithelium
- Chronic phase
  - Early lichenoid phase shows histologic features of lichen planus; satellite necrosis may still be seen in GVHD
  - Late sclerotic phase shows changes similar to scleroderma with dermal sclerosis extending into subcutaneous fat and loss of adnexal structures; however, epidermal atrophy is present in GVHD

Special Stains and Immunohistochemistry

- Noncontributory

Other Techniques for Diagnosis

- Noncontributory

Differential Diagnosis

❚ Erythema multiforme
- Acute GVHD shows histologic changes and a spectrum of severity indistinguishable from that of erythema multiforme

❚ Lichen planus
- Lichenoid phase of GVHD may be indistinguishable from lichen planus

❚ Scleroderma
- Epidermal atrophy, if present, helps in differentiating sclerotic phase of GVHD from scleroderma

Pearls

- Acute phase of GVHD is caused by the attack of donor immunocompetent T lymphocytes against histocompatibility antigens exposed on recipient cells
- Chronic phase of GVHD is caused by immunocompetent lymphocytes that differentiate in the recipient
- Target cells in GVHD are the stem cells in the regenerating compartment, that is, the basal keratinocyte in skin and the epithelial cells at the base of the crypts in the gastrointestinal tract

Selected References

Martí N, Martin JM, Monteagudo C, et al: Follicular graft-versus-host disease: A rare manifestation of chronic cutaneous graft versus host disease. Am J Dermatopathol 30:620-621, 2008.

Häusermann P, Walter RB, Halter J, et al: Cutaneous graft-versus-host disease: A guide for the dermatologist. Dermatology 216:287-304, 2008.

Zhou Y, Barnett MJ, Rivers JK: Clinical significance of skin biopsies in the diagnosis and management of graft-vs-host disease in early post-allogeneic bone marrow transplantation. Arch Dermatol 136:717-721, 2000.

Flowers ME, Kansu E, Sullivan KM: Pathophysiology and treatment of graft-versus-host disease. Hematol Oncol Clin N Am 13:1091-1112, viii-ix, 1999.

Aractingi S, Chosidow O: Cutaneous graft-versus-host disease. Arch Dermatol 134:602-612, 1998.

Marcellus DC, Vogelsang GB: Graft-versus-host disease. Curr Opin Oncol 9:131-138, 1997.

Vogelsang GB: Graft-versus-host disease: Implications from basic immunology for prophylaxis and treatment. Cancer Treat Res 77:87-97, 1997.

Dinulos JG, Levy ML: Graft-versus-host disease in children. Semin Dermatol 14:66-69, 1995.

Chaudhuri SPR, Smoller BR: Acute cutaneous graft versus host disease: A clinicopathologic and immunophenotypic study. Int J Dermatol 31:270, 1992.

Cutaneous Lupus Erythematosus

Clinical Features

- Lupus erythematosus is a chronic multisystem autoimmune disease that affects the connective tissue and vasculature of various organs
- Cutaneous changes may be subdivided according to the clinical appearance as discoid, verrucous, tumid, or lupus panniculitis; the lesions can be acute, subacute, or chronic
- Classic discoid lesions of cutaneous lupus erythematosus appear as mildly scaling, erythematous, edematous, sharply demarcated plaques measuring up to 15 cm, involving scalp, face, upper trunk, and upper extremities; follicular plugging may be seen
- Older lesions appear atrophic with variable pigmentation
- Tumid form of lupus presents as indurated plaques and nodules without overlying erythema or atrophy
- Verrucous lesions due to epidermal proliferation are seen in 2% of patients with chronic cutaneous lupus erythematosus
- Panniculitis may be seen in some patients with chronic cutaneous or systemic forms of lupus erythematosus

Histopathology

- Histologic features of discoid lupus erythematosus are characteristic and include hyperkeratosis with follicular plugging, atrophy of epidermis, vacuolar alteration of the basal cell layer, and marked thickening of the basement membrane
- Variable amount of lymphocytic infiltrate obscures the dermoepidermal junction and surrounds the adnexal structures and dermal blood vessels
- Interstitial deposits of mucin are noted in many cases
- Epidermal hyperplasia with papillomatosis is seen in the verrucous form of lupus
- In the dermal form of lupus erythematosus known as *tumid lupus erythematosus*, there is superficial and deep perivascular and periadnexal lymphocytic infiltrate with interstitial mucin but no epidermal changes
- In lupus panniculitis, there is a lobular lymphocytic panniculitis with hyaline fat necrosis and interstitial mucin, with or without epidermal changes

Special Stains and Immunohistochemistry

- PAS stain is helpful in demonstrating the thickened basement membrane
- Colloidal iron stain can highlight interstitial mucin deposits

Other Techniques for Diagnosis

- Direct immunofluorescence shows a continuous granular deposition of IgG, IgM, and C3 in a band along the dermoepidermal junction

Differential Diagnosis

▌ Dermatomyositis
- May show histologic changes similar to those of subacute lesions of cutaneous lupus erythematosus
- Immunofluorescence studies show no deposits at the dermoepidermal junction

▌ Lichen planus
- The epidermal changes of discoid lupus erythematosus may resemble lichen planus
- Presence of hypergranulosis, irregular epidermal hyperplasia with sawtooth appearance, and absence of interstitial mucin deposits favors a diagnosis of lichen planus

▌ Polymorphous light eruption
- Superficial and deep perivascular lymphocytic infiltrates of lupus (especially tumid form) must be differentiated from polymorphous light eruption, which usually shows marked edema of papillary dermis

▌ Lymphoma
- Superficial and deep dense lymphocytic infiltrate of lupus, when seen in the absence of changes at the dermoepidermal junction (tumid form), may raise the possibility of lymphoma or leukemia; interstitial deposits of mucin are present in lupus, and the lymphoid cells are small and mature

Figure 2-8. Cutaneous lupus erythematosus. A, Hematoxylin and eosin–stained section demonstrates hyperkeratosis with follicular plugging, atrophy of the epidermis, marked vacuolar alteration of the basal cell layer, and a thickened and smudged basement membrane. Perifollicular lymphocytic infiltrate is present. **B,** Periodic acid–Schiff stain demonstrates the thickening of the basement membrane. **C,** Direct immunofluorescence studies show granular positivity along the basement membrane of the epidermis and the adnexal epithelium. Positive fluorescence may be seen with immunoglobulin G (IgG) or IgM and C3. **D,** Lupus profundus. Section shows a predominantly lobular pattern of lymphocytic panniculitis with associated hyaline fat necrosis.

- In the differential diagnosis of lupus profundus panniculitis, cytophagic panniculitis (T-cell lymphoma) may be considered; the lymphoid cells in T-cell lymphoma panniculitis are atypical, and atypical nuclei are also present within the cytoplasm of histiocytes

Pearls

- Subacute cutaneous lupus erythematosus and neonatal lupus erythematosus show prominent changes at the dermoepidermal junction but less prominent hyperkeratosis and inflammatory cell infiltrate than discoid lupus erythematosus
- Cutaneous manifestations of subacute lupus erythematosus include malar erythema, photosensitivity, and bullous lesions

- Well-defined lesions of discoid lupus erythematosus occur in 15% of patients with subacute lupus erythematosus

Selected References

Patel P, Werth V: Cutaneous lupus erythematosus: A review. Dermatol Clin 20:373-385, 2002.

Magro CM, Crowson AN, Kovatich AJ, et al: Lupus profundus, indeterminate lymphocytic lobular panniculitis and subcutaneous T-cell lymphoma: A spectrum of subcuticular T-cell lymphoid dyscrasia. J Cutan Pathol 28:235, 2001.

Callen JP: New and emerging therapies for collagen-vascular diseases. Dermatol Clin 18:139-146, 2000.

Lee LA, Weston WL: Cutaneous lupus erythematosus during the neonatal and childhood periods. Lupus 6:132-138, 1997.

Eng AM: Cutaneous expressions of antiphospholipid syndromes. Semin Thromb Hemost 20:71-78, 1994.

Hochberg MC, Petri M: Clinical features of systemic lupus erythematosus. Curr Opin Rheumatol 5:575-586, 1993.
Jerdan MS, Hood AF, Moore GW, et al: Histopathologic comparison of the subsets of lupus erythematosus. Arch Dermatol 126:52, 1990.

Dermatomyositis

Clinical Features

- Dermatomyositis is a connective tissue disease characterized by inflammatory myositis involving the proximal muscles and cutaneous lesions consisting of heliotrope rash, Gottron papules, and erythematous-edematous lesions
  — *Heliotrope rash* refers to violaceous, slightly edematous periorbital patches involving the eyelids
  — *Gottron papules* are discrete red-purple papules over bony prominences of knuckles, knees, and elbows
- The disease has two peaks—one in childhood and one between the ages of 45 and 65 years

Histopathology

- Histologic changes of the erythematous-edematous lesions of the skin may be similar to those seen in subacute lupus erythematosus and consist of epidermal atrophy, vacuolar alteration of the basal cell layer, and a sparse superficial perivascular lymphocytic infiltrate
- Interstitial mucin deposits may be present
- Subepidermal fibrin deposits can be seen
- Sections of Gottron papules show epidermal hyperplasia in addition to interface changes
- Panniculitis and calcification of the subcutaneous tissue may be seen at a later stage

Special Stains and Immunohistochemistry

- Noncontributory

Figure 2-9. Dermatomyositis. Vacuolar alteration of the basal cell layer, epidermal atrophy, and a mild perivascular inflammatory cell infiltrate are seen.

Other Techniques for Diagnosis

- Negative direct immunofluorescence studies are helpful in differentiating dermatomyositis from lupus erythematosus

Differential Diagnosis

▌ Subacute cutaneous or systemic lupus erythematosus
- Histologic changes of dermatomyositis are indistinguishable from those of lupus
- A negative lupus band test is generally helpful, especially in early stages of dermatomyositis when the muscular weakness is not apparent

Pearls

- Dermatomyositis has been shown to be associated with malignancy, particularly ovarian carcinoma; exact incidence, however, is controversial

Selected References

Hill CL, Zhang Y, Sigurgeirsson B, et al: Frequency of specific cancer types in dermatomyositis and polymyositis: A population-based study. Lancet 357:96-100, 2001.
Callen JP: Dermatomyositis. Lancet 355:53-57, 2000.
Krajnc I: Dermatomyositis: Diagnosis and evaluation of dermatomyositis, polymyositis, and inclusion-body myositis. Adv Exp Med Biol 455:181-186, 1999.
Sontheimer RD: Cutaneous features of classic dermatomyositis and amyopathic dermatomyositis. Curr Opin Rheumatol 11:475-482, 1999.
Kovacs SO, Kovacs SC: Dermatomyositis. J Am Acad Dermatol 39:899-920; quiz, 921-922, 1998.
Stonecipher MR, Callen JP, Jorizzo JL: The red face: Dermatomyositis. Clin Dermatol 11:261-273, 1993.

Epidermal Spongiosis

Spongiotic Dermatitis

Clinical Features

- *Spongiotic dermatitis* refers to a heterogeneous group of disorders, characterized histologically by the presence of intercellular edema (spongiosis) in the epidermis. In this group are included allergic contact dermatitis, photoallergic dermatitis, nummular dermatitis, atopic dermatitis, dyshidrotic dermatitis, and Id reaction
▌ Allergic contact dermatitis
- Most commonly caused by poison ivy, nickel, and rubber compounds
- Presents with pruritic, edematous, erythematous papules and occasional vesicles usually within 1 to 3 days after exposure
▌ Photoallergic dermatitis
- Due to topical application (photocontact) or ingestion of an allergen

Figure 2-10. Spongiotic dermatitis. A, Marked epidermal spongiosis with formation of spongiotic vesicles and a superficial perivascular mixed inflammatory cell infiltrate are seen. **B,** Higher-power view shows abundant eosinophils within the spongiotic vesicle, which favors a diagnosis of contact dermatitis.

- Shows pruritic and erythematous papulovesicular lesions on sun-exposed skin; usually on face, arms, and neck
- Nummular dermatitis
  - Disease of unknown etiology characterized by coin-shaped, pruritic, erythematous, scaly, crusted plaques on exterior aspects of extremities
- Atopic dermatitis
  - Inherited chronic, pruritic, scaly eruption affecting face and extensor aspects of extremities in children
- Dyshidrotic dermatitis
  - Characterized by numerous pruritic vesicles along sides of fingers and toes and palms and soles

- Autoeczematization or Id reaction
  - Refers to a sudden localized or generalized eruption of pinhead-sized vesicles developing in association with a defined local dermatitis or with infection
  - Most common cause is a remote dermatophyte infection

Histopathology
  - Spongiotic dermatitis, irrespective of the specific type, may be acute, subacute, or chronic
- Acute spongiotic dermatitis
  - Shows variable degree of epidermal spongiosis with vesiculation in extreme cases
  - Mild papillary dermal edema and a superficial perivascular lymphohistiocytic inflammation are present
  - In allergic contact dermatitis, eosinophils may be present in the dermis and spongiotic foci
- Subacute spongiotic dermatitis
  - Shows parakeratosis with plasma, mild to moderate spongiosis, epidermal hyperplasia, and superficial perivascular lymphohistiocytic infiltrate
- Chronic spongiotic dermatitis
  - Spongiosis is mild or absent, but changes of chronicity include a hyperkeratotic cornified layer, marked epidermal hyperplasia, and fibrosis of papillary dermis
  - Dermal inflammatory cell infiltrate is mild

Special Stains and Immunohistochemistry
  - PAS stain may be useful in excluding dermatophytosis with spongiosis

Other Techniques for Diagnosis
  - Noncontributory

Differential Diagnosis
- Includes many causes of dermatitis that show foci of spongiosis such as seborrheic dermatitis, pityriasis rosea, insect bite reactions, and dermatophyte infections
- Seborrheic dermatitis
  - Spongiosis is mild and associated with a parakeratotic scale at the openings of the follicular infundibula
- Pityriasis rosea
  - Spongiosis is focal and associated with mounds of parakeratosis and extravasated red cells
  - Identical changes are also seen in superficial form of erythema annulare centrifugum
- Spongiotic drug eruptions and insect bite reactions
  - Show deeper infiltrate of inflammatory cells that also include eosinophils
- Psoriasis
  - Chronic spongiotic dermatitis (lichen simplex chronicus) may resemble psoriasis but generally lacks confluent parakeratosis with neutrophils and thinning of suprapapillary plates

Pearls

- The term *eczema* is a nonspecific term used clinically to describe erythematous vesicular lesions with scaly crust that show spongiotic dermatitis on histologic examination

Selected References

Weedon D: Skin Pathology, 2nd ed. New York, Churchill Livingstone, 2002, p 112.

Ackerman AB, Chongchitnant N, Sanchez J, et al: Histologic Diagnosis of Inflammatory Skin Diseases. Baltimore, Williams & Wilkins, 1997.

Ackerman AB, Ragaz A: A plea to expunge the word "eczema" from the lexicon of dermatology and dermatopathology. Am J Dermatopathol 4:315, 1982.

Incontinentia Pigmenti

Clinical Features

- Incontinentia pigmenti is an X-linked–dominant dermatosis that affects mostly females
- Characteristic cutaneous manifestations seen at birth include crops of vesicles and bullae on extremities arranged in a linear or whorled pattern
- Lesions heal with hyperkeratosis and verrucous epidermal hyperplasia; the verrucous lesions heal with streaks and whorls of hyperpigmentation that are later replaced by faint hypochromic patches

Histopathology

- Vesicular stage is characterized by marked epidermal spongiosis with eosinophils
- Verrucous stage is characterized by hyperkeratosis and papillomatous epidermal hyperplasia
- Hyperpigmented stage is characterized by numerous melanophages in the dermis

Figure 2-11. Incontinentia pigmenti. Intraepidermal spongiosis and collections of eosinophils both within the epidermis and in the dermal inflammatory cell infiltrate are seen.

Special Stains and Immunohistochemistry

- Noncontributory

Other Techniques for Diagnosis

- Noncontributory

Differential Diagnosis

- Spongiosis with eosinophils can be seen in allergic contact dermatitis and in the early stages of pemphigus and bullous pemphigoid; clinical history is essential
- Toxic erythema of newborn
  - Eosinophils are typically abundant, but spongiosis is much less prominent

Pearls

- Eosinophilic chemotactic activity has been shown in the blister fluid of patients with incontinentia pigmenti
- In up to 80% of patients, systemic findings with involvement of the central nervous system and eye may be seen; teeth abnormalities may be present
- Extent of systemic involvement determines the clinical course

Selected References

Ackerman AB, Chongchitnant N, Sanchez J, et al: Histologic Diagnosis of Inflammatory Skin Diseases. Baltimore, Williams & Wilkins, 1997.

Ashley JR, Burgdorf WHC: Incontinentia pigmenti: Pigmentary changes independent of incontinence. J Cutan Pathol 14:263, 1987.

Sulzberger MB: Incontinentia pigmenti (Bloch-Sulzberger). Arch Dermatol Syph 38:57, 1938.

Psoriasiform Dermatitis

Psoriasis

Clinical Features

- Chronic dermatosis of unknown etiology affecting up to 2% of the population
- Males and females affected equally
- Predilection for areas with trauma, including scalp, lumbosacral skin, and extensor surfaces of elbows and knees
- Variably sized well-demarcated plaques covered by thick, silvery white scale
- Localized or generalized pustular psoriasis, eruptive or guttate psoriasis, and erythrodermic psoriasis are other manifestations of the disease
- Involvement of nails, oral mucosa, and tongue can occur

Histopathology

- Parakeratosis that is often confluent and contains neutrophilic collections (Munro microabscesses)

Figure 2-12. Psoriasis. Confluent parakeratosis with collections of neutrophils, diminished granular layer, regular (psoriasiform) epidermal hyperplasia with thinning of suprapapillary plates, dilated blood vessels in the papillary dermis, and mild superficial perivascular inflammation are seen.

- Hypogranulosis corresponding to zones of parakeratosis
- Regular epidermal hyperplasia with elongation of rete ridges and thinning of suprapapillary plates
- Dilated tortuous blood vessels in the dermal papillae
- Mild superficial perivascular lymphocytic infiltrate
- In pustular psoriasis, there are prominent spongiform pustules (pustules of Kogoj)
- In guttate psoriasis, the changes are those of early lesion of psoriasis with less pronounced epidermal hyperplasia
- In erythrodermic psoriasis, the histologic changes may be nonspecific

Special Stains and Immunohistochemistry

- PAS stain is helpful in excluding the possibility of dermatophytic infections

Other Techniques for Diagnosis

- Noncontributory

Differential Diagnosis

▌ Chronic spongiotic dermatitis such as contact or nummular dermatitis should be considered in the differential diagnosis of psoriasiform dermatitis; presence of spongiosis and eosinophils in spongiotic dermatitis may be helpful in differentiation
▌ Dermatophytes and bacterial impetigo
  - Parakeratosis with neutrophils and spongiform pustules should prompt PAS and Gram stains to rule out dermatophytes and bacterial impetigo

▌ Pityriasis rubra pilaris
  - Shows epidermal hyperplasia and parakeratosis and may resemble psoriasis
  - However, in pityriasis rubra pilaris, the suprapapillary plates are thick, the granular layer is prominent, and neutrophils are absent in the parakeratotic cornified layer

Pearls

- Removal of the scale on a psoriatic plaque results in a tiny bleeding point (Auspitz sign)
- Psoriatic arthritis characteristically involves terminal interphalangeal joints

Selected References

Nestle FO: Psoriasis. Curr Dir Autoimmun 10:65-75, 2008.

Drew GS: Psoriasis. Prim Care 27:385-406, 2000.

Barker JN: Pathogenesis of psoriasis. J Dermatol 25:778-781, 1998.

Linden KG, Weinstein GD: Psoriasis: Current perspectives with an emphasis on treatment. Am J Med 107:595-605, 1999.

Nickoloff BJ: The immunologic and genetic basis of psoriasis. Arch Dermatol 135:1104-1110, 1999.

Feldman SR, Clark AR: Psoriasis. Med Clin N Am 82:1135-1144, 1998.

Stern RS: Psoriasis. Lancet 350:349-353, 1997.

Ragaz A, Ackerman AB: Evolution, maturation, and regression of lesions of psoriasis. Am J Dermatopathol 1:199, 1979.

Pityriasis Rubra Pilaris

Clinical Features

- Pityriasis rubra pilaris is a chronic follicular-based erythematous papular eruption of unknown etiology that progresses to form orange-red scaly plaques that contain islands of normal-appearing skin
- With progression, a generalized erythroderma may occur
- Palmoplantar keratoderma and scales on face and scalp may be seen

Histopathology

- Sections of fully developed erythematous lesions show alternating orthokeratosis and parakeratosis in horizontal and vertical directions
- Epidermal hyperplasia with broad and short rete, thick suprapapillary plates
- Mild superficial perivascular lymphocytic infiltrate
- Sections of follicular papules show dilated follicular infundibula with follicular plugging

Special Stains and Immunohistochemistry

- Noncontributory

Other Techniques for Diagnosis

- Noncontributory

Figure 2-13. Pityriasis rubra pilaris. A, Alternating layers of hyperkeratosis and parakeratosis in both vertical and horizontal patterns, psoriasiform epidermal hyperplasia, and mild superficial perivascular inflammation are seen. **B,** High-power view shows alternating hyperkeratosis and parakeratosis with a normal granular layer.

Differential Diagnosis

▌ Psoriasis
  - Pityriasis rubra pilaris resembles psoriasis clinically
  - Characteristic histologic changes of psoriasis such as parakeratosis with neutrophils, hypogranulosis, regular epidermal hyperplasia, and thin suprapapillary plates are not seen in pityriasis rubra pilaris

Pearls

  - A familial form of pityriasis rubra pilaris inherited as an autosomal dominant trait is recognized

Selected References

Mobini N, Toussaint S, Kamino H: Noninfectious erythematous, papular, and squamous diseases. In Elder DE, Elenitsas R, Johnson BL Jr, et al (eds): Lever's Histopathology of Skin, 10th ed. Philadelphia, Lippincott Williams & Wilkins, 2008, p. 169.

Albert MR, Mackool BT: Pityriasis rubra pilaris. Int J Dermatol 38:1-11, 1999.

Piamphongsant T, Akaraphant R: Pityriasis rubra pilaris: A new proposed classification. Clin Exp Dermatol 19:134-138, 1994.

Barr RJ, Young EM Jr: Psoriasiform and related papulosquamous disorders. J Cutan Pathol 12:412-425, 1985.

Superficial and Deep Perivascular Dermatitis

Dermatitis with Minimal Epidermal Changes
Lymphocytes Predominant

Polymorphous Light Eruption

Clinical Features

  - Pruritic papules and plaques that occur in young women mostly during summer, induced by ultraviolet radiation (UVR)
  - Eruption starts few minutes to few hours after exposure and lasts for hours to days

Histopathology

  - Epidermis is mostly unremarkable or shows small foci of spongiosis
  - Prominent papillary dermal edema is present
  - Superficial and deep perivascular, predominantly lymphocytic infiltrate

Special Stains and Immunohistochemistry

  - Noncontributory

Other Techniques for Diagnosis

  - Noncontributory

Differential Diagnosis

▌ Cutaneous lupus erythematosus
  - Typically the subacute and tumid forms should be considered in the differential diagnosis
  - Polymorphous light eruption lacks changes at the dermoepidermal junction, has less prominent periadnexal infiltrate, and lacks interstitial mucin deposits, features typically seen in cutaneous lupus

Figure 2-14. Polymorphous light eruption. A superficial and deep perivascular lymphocytic infiltrate is associated with marked papillary dermal edema.

- Papillary dermal edema is more prominent in polymorphous light eruption than in subacute cutaneous lupus erythematosus

▌ Jessner lymphocytic infiltrate

- Shows changes similar to tumid form of lupus erythematosus and may be related

Pearls

- Treatment is mostly prophylactic
- Limitation of UVR exposure, proper clothing, and application of sunscreens during exposure are helpful

Selected References

Lipsker D, Mitschler A, Grosshans E, Cribier B: Could Jessner's lymphocytic infiltrate of the skin be a dermal variant of lupus erythematosus? An analysis of 210 cases. Dermatology 213:15-22, 2006.

Boonstra HE, van Weelden H, Toonstra J, van Vloten WA: Polymorphous light eruption: A clinical, photobiologic, and follow-up study of 110 patients. J Am Acad Dermatol 42:199-207, 2000.

Hasan T, Ranki A, Jansen CT, Karvonen J: Disease associations in polymorphous light eruption: A long-term follow-up study of 94 patients. Arch Dermatol 1998; 134(9):1081-1085.

Eosinophils Predominant

Insect Bite Reaction (Papular Urticaria)

Clinical Features

- An allergic reaction induced by bites from mosquitoes, fleas, and bedbugs
- Papules and papulovesicles that are intensely pruritic and often become excoriated

Histopathology

- Epidermis and cornified layer may show changes of excoriation
- A superficial and deep perivascular and interstitial mixed inflammatory cell infiltrate containing frequent eosinophils and arranged in a V- or wedge-shaped pattern is the characteristic finding

Special Stains and Immunohistochemistry

- Noncontributory

Other Techniques for Diagnosis

- Noncontributory

Differential Diagnosis

- The histologic changes may be similar in hypersensitivity reactions caused by some drugs and scabies

Pearls

- In the case of tick bites, parts of the tick mouth parts may be found in the dermis

Figure 2-15. Insect bite reaction. A, A superficial and deep perivascular and interstitial infiltrate is arranged in a wedge shape. **B,** High-power view shows the presence of frequent eosinophils within the infiltrate.

- A dense chronic lymphoid response (persistent arthropod bite reaction) can be seen with tick bites and stings of bees, wasps, and hornets

Selected References

Kain KC: Skin lesions in returned travelers. Med Clin N Am 83:1077-1102, 1999.

Ackerman AB, Chongchitnant N, Sanchez J, et al: Histologic Diagnosis of Inflammatory Skin Diseases: An Algorithmic Method Based on Pattern Analysis, 2nd ed. Baltimore, Williams & Wilkins, 1997, p 202.

Howard R, Frieden IJ: Papular urticaria in children. Pediatr Dermatol 13:246-249, 1996.

Interface Dermatitis

Pityriasis Lichenoides

Clinical Features

- Self-limited cutaneous eruption of unknown cause that affects young adults and children
- Two forms are recognized
  — Mucha-Habermann disease
    ◆ An acute, more severe form also known as *pityriasis lichenoides et varioliformis acuta*

Figure 2-16. Pityriasis lichenoides acuta. Parakeratosis containing collections of neutrophils, vacuolar alteration of the basal cell layer, and patchy lichenoid and perivascular lymphocytic inflammation are seen. Scattered necrotic keratinocytes and extravasated red cells are present.

— Pityriasis lichenoides chronica
  ◆ Chronic, milder form
— Occasional transitional forms with changes between the two extremes occur
- In pityriasis lichenoides et varioliformis acuta, a papular, papulonecrotic, and occasionally vesiculopustular eruption occurs on trunk and proximal extremities and usually resolves in a few weeks; crops of new lesions can continue to appear, and the disease process itself may have a chronic course
- In pityriasis lichenoides chronica, recurrent crops of reddish-brown papules with adherent scales occur on trunk and extremities and resolve in a few weeks

Histopathology

- Parakeratosis and a scale crust with neutrophils in severe cases
- Epidermal spongiosis and necrotic keratinocytes with eventual erosion and ulceration
- Vacuolar alteration of the basal cell layer
- Papillary dermal edema and extravasated red cells
- Superficial and deep perivascular, predominantly lymphocytic infiltrate
- In pityriasis lichenoides et varioliformis acuta, the infiltrate is denser and deeper than in pityriasis lichenoides chronica, and it obscures the dermoepidermal junction, where there is also marked vacuolar alteration
- In ulceronecrotic variant of pityriasis lichenoides et varioliformis acuta, there may be lymphocytic vasculitis

Special Stains and Immunohistochemistry

- Noncontributory

Other Techniques for Diagnosis

- Noncontributory

Differential Diagnosis

▮ Lymphomatoid papulosis
  - May show histologic overlap with pityriasis lichenoides
  - Presence of atypical lymphoid cells in lymphomatoid papulosis is helpful in differentiating the two conditions
▮ Vesicular insect bite reactions
  - Can be differentiated from pityriasis lichenoides et varioliformis acuta by the presence of frequent eosinophils in the inflammatory cell infiltrate
  - A spongiotic vesicle may be present at the site of the bite

Pearls

- Inflammatory cell infiltrate consists mostly of lymphocytes with a predominance of CD8-positive T-lymphoid cells

Selected References

Ersoy-Evans S, Greco MF, et al: Pityriasis lichenoides in childhood: A retrospective review of 124 patients. J Am Acad Dermatol 56:205, 2007.

Bowers S, Warshaw EM: Pityriasis lichenoides and its subtypes. J Am Acad Dermatol 55:557-572, 2006.

Magro CM, Morrison C, Kovatich A, et al: Pityriasis lichenoides is a cutaneous T-cell dyscrasia: A clinical, genotypic, and phenotypic study. Hum Pathol 33:788, 2002.

Tsuji T, Kasamatsu M, Yokota M, et al: Mucha-Habermann disease and its febrile ulceronecrotic variant. Cutis 58:123-131, 1996.

Fixed Drug Eruption

Clinical Features

- Well-defined, circumscribed patches occur at the same site in response to repeated intake of the drug
- Lesions are slightly edematous and erythematous and may develop dusky centers and become bullous
- Lesions heal with pigmentation

Histopathology

- Vacuolar alteration of the basal cell layer and scattered necrotic keratinocytes; changes identical to those in erythema multiforme
- Bullae result from full-thickness epidermal necrosis, similar to that seen in toxic epidermal necrolysis
- Superficial and deep perivascular and occasionally lichenoid inflammatory cell infiltrate with lymphocytes, neutrophils, and eosinophils
- Melanophages in upper dermis

Special Stains and Immunohistochemistry

- Noncontributory

Figure 2-17. Fixed drug eruption. Necrotic keratinocytes in the epidermis, vacuolar alteration of the basal cell layer, and patchy lichenoid inflammatory cell infiltrate that obscures the dermoepidermal junction are seen. Histologic changes are similar to those seen erythema multiforme.

Other Techniques for Diagnosis

- Noncontributory

Differential Diagnosis

▮ Erythema multiforme and toxic epidermal necrolysis
- May have histologic changes similar to those of fixed drug eruption
- Clinical information is essential
- Superficial and deep perivascular and occasionally lichenoid inflammatory cell infiltrate with lymphocytes, neutrophils, and eosinophils, when present, favor fixed drug eruption

Pearls

- Fixed drug eruptions occur most commonly with trimethoprim-sulfamethoxazole, acetylsalicylic acid, and phenolphthalein
- Increasing number of lesions can occur with each successive administration of the offending drug

Selected References

Shiohara T, Mizukawa Y: Fixed drug eruption: A disease mediated by self-inflicted responses of intraepidermal T cells. Eur J Dermatol 17:201-208, 2007.

Sehgal VN, Srivastava G: Fixed drug eruption (FDE): Changing scenario of incriminating drugs. Int J Dermatol 45:897-908, 2006.

Roujeau JC: Neutrophilic drug eruptions. Clin Dermatol 18:331-337, 2000.

Crowson AN, Magro CM: Recent advances in the pathology of cutaneous drug eruptions. Dermatol Clin 17:537-560, viii, 1999.

Wolkenstein P, Revuz J: Allergic emergencies encountered by the dermatologist: Severe cutaneous adverse drug reactions. Clin Rev Allergy Immunol 17:497-511, 1999.

Lymphomatoid Papulosis

Clinical Features

- Presents as multiple, small papules that are most often short lived but usually recurrent

Histopathology

- Sections show a superficial and deep mixed cell infiltrate that is wedge shaped and also lichenoid
- In addition to neutrophils, eosinophils, and plasma cells, significant number of atypical lymphocytes are present
- Surface ulceration may be present

Special Stains and Immunohistochemistry

- The atypical lymphocytes are positive for CD30 (Ki-1)

Other Techniques for Diagnosis

- Clonal rearrangement of T-cell receptor gene may be present

Differential Diagnosis

▮ Insect bite reaction
- Activated lymphocytes may be present
- Atypical cells of lymphomatoid papulosis are CD30 positive
▮ Pityriasis lichenoides acuta
- Histologic patterns of both conditions may be similar
- Demonstration of CD30-positive lymphoid cells in lymphomatoid papulosis is helpful in the differential diagnosis

Pearls

- Progression of lymphomatoid papulosis to large cell anaplastic lymphoma (CD30 positive) can occur, suggesting that lymphomatoid papulosis may represent the benign end in the spectrum of CD30-positive T cell lymphoproliferative disorders

Figure 2-18. Lymphomatoid papulosis. Section shows a dense perivascular and interstitial infiltrate consisting predominantly of lymphocytes. A significant number of the lymphocytes are large and contain enlarged hyperchromatic and irregular nuclei.

Selected References

Werner B, Massone C, Kerl H, Cerroni L: Large CD30-positive cells in benign, atypical lymphoid infiltrates of the skin. J Cutan Pathol 35:1100-1107, 2008.

Wang HH, Myers T, Lach LJ, et al: Increased risk of lymphoid and nonlymphoid malignancies in patients with lymphomatoid papulosis. Cancer 86:1240-1245, 1999.

Cerroni L: Lymphomatoid papulosis, pityriasis lichenoides et varioliformis acuta, and anaplastic large-cell (Ki-1+) lymphoma. J Am Acad Dermatol 37:287, 1997.

Demierre MF, Goldberg LJ, Kadin ME, Koh HK: Is it lymphoma or lymphomatoid papulosis? J Am Acad Dermatol 36:765-772, 1997.

LeBoit PE: Lymphomatoid papulosis and cutaneous CD30+ lymphoma. Am J Dermatopathol 18:221-235, 1996.

Psoriasiform Dermatitis

Secondary Syphilis

Clinical Features

- Hematogenous dissemination of causative organism, *Treponema pallidum*, results in cutaneous eruption that can be macular, papular, papulosquamous, or rarely, pustular
- Associated constitutional symptoms such as fever and lymphadenopathy may be present; other manifestations include condyloma lata, syphilis cornee, lues maligna, and alopecia

Histopathology

- Patchy or confluent parakeratosis containing neutrophils
- Regular (psoriasiform) epidermal hyperplasia with focal spongiosis
- Epidermal hyperplasia is least in macular lesions and most in condylomata lata
- Vacuolar alteration of the basal cell layer, occasional necrotic keratinocytes, and edema of papillary dermis
- Superficial and deep perivascular and periadnexal infiltrate that can also be lichenoid with obscuring of the dermoepidermal junction; plasma cells may be present around nerves
- Infiltrate can be lymphocytic, lymphoplasmacytic, or lymphohistiocytic with rare granuloma formation

Special Stains and Immunohistochemistry

- Silver stain (Warthin-Starry) may show spirochetes within the epidermis in one third of cases
- Immunohistochemistry with monoclonal antibody to *T. pallidum* is more specific

Other Techniques for Diagnosis

- Immunofluorescence shows positivity for spirochetes in some cases

Figure 2-19. Secondary syphilis. A, Histologic section shows parakeratosis with neutrophils, epidermal hyperplasia, and a dense bandlike inflammatory cell infiltrate that obscures the dermoepidermal junction. **B,** On high-power view, the infiltrate contains a large number of plasma cells.

Differential Diagnosis

- Mycosis fungoides
  - Shows psoriasiform lichenoid pattern in which atypical lymphoid cells are present within the dermal infiltrate and in the mildly spongiotic epidermis
  - Plasma cells are not frequent
- Subacute and chronic spongiotic dermatitis, including photoallergic dermatitis
  - May show some psoriasiform hyperplasia and spongiosis
  - In general, plasma cells are not prominent
- Pityriasis lichenoides
  - Can simulate secondary syphilis but shows predominantly a lymphocytic infiltrate without plasma cells
- Psoriasis and psoriasiform drug eruption
  - Inflammatory infiltrate is not deep
  - Suprapapillary plate thinning is not a feature of secondary syphilis

- Sarcoid and other conditions with a prominent granulomatous pattern
  - May appear similar to the granulomatous pattern of secondary in syphilis

Pearls

- An unusual variant of secondary syphilis is lues maligna, which is an ulcerative form characterized by thrombotic endarteritis of vessels in the deep dermis resulting in ischemic necrosis

Selected References

Hoang MP, High WA, Molberg KH: Secondary syphilis: A histologic and immunohistochemical evaluation. J Cutan Pathol 31:595-599, 2004.

Goens JL, Janniger CK, De Wolf K: Dermatologic and systemic manifestations of syphilis. Am Fam Physician 50:1013-1020, 1994.

Johnson RA, White M: Syphilis in the 1990s: Cutaneous and neurologic manifestations. Semin Neurol 12:287-298, 1992.

Hira SK, Patel JS, Bhat SG, et al: Clinical manifestations of secondary syphilis. Int J Dermatol 26:103-107, 1987.

Abell E, Marks R, Wilson Jones E: Secondary syphilis: A clinicopathological review. Br J Dermatol 93:53, 1975.

Jeerapaet P, Ackerman AS: Histologic patterns of secondary syphilis. Arch Dermatol 107:373, 1973.

Nodular and Diffuse Dermatitis

Neutrophils Predominant

Sweet Syndrome

Clinical Features

- Acute febrile neutrophilic dermatosis, or Sweet syndrome, is characterized by fever, leukocytosis, and a cutaneous eruption that consists of violaceous

Figure 2-20. Sweet syndrome. Histologic section shows a diffuse dermal infiltrate consisting predominantly of neutrophils and extravasated red blood cells. Intact blood vessels help in differentiating this from leukocytoclastic vasculitis.

plaquelike lesions involving face and extremities and, rarely, trunk
- It is chiefly a disease of middle-aged women and in some an underlying malignancy or inflammatory disease may be detected
- Sweet syndrome–like eruption is reported with many drugs

Histopathology

- Dense, diffuse, upper dermal infiltrate of predominantly neutrophils and neutrophilic nuclear dust with scattered lymphocytes, histiocytes, and eosinophils
- Edema of the papillary dermis
- Dilated blood vessels with plump endothelial lining and extravasated red blood cells

Special Stains and Immunohistochemistry

- Noncontributory

Other Techniques for Diagnosis

- Noncontributory

Differential Diagnosis

- Leukocytoclastic vasculitis
  - Vascular damage with fibrin deposition in the vessel wall is not a feature of Sweet syndrome
- Pyoderma gangrenosum
  - Inflammatory infiltrate (predominately neutrophilic) is deeper and denser than in Sweet syndrome
  - Surface ulceration and secondary vasculitis may be present

Pearls

- Sweet syndrome is believed to be a hypersensitivity reaction of unknown etiology
- Potential infectious etiology should be considered and excluded in all cases of neutrophilic dermatoses

Selected References

Buck T, González LM, Lambert WC, Schwartz RA: Sweet's syndrome with hematologic disorders: A review and reappraisal. Int J Dermatol 47:775-782, 2008.

Roujeau JC: Neutrophilic drug eruptions. Clin Dermatol 18:331-337, 2000.

Cohen PR, Kurzrock R: Sweet's syndrome: A neutrophilic dermatosis classically associated with acute onset and fever. Clin Dermatol 18:265-282, 2000.

Huang W, McNeely MC: Neutrophilic tissue reactions. Adv Dermatol 13:33-64, 1997.

Cohen PR, Kurzrock R: Sweet's syndrome and cancer. Clin Dermatol 11:149-157, 1993.

Sweet RD: Acute febrile neutrophilic dermatosis. Br J Dermatol 74:349, 1964.

Pyoderma Gangrenosum

Clinical Features

- Idiopathic ulceronecrotic skin disease that begins as follicular papules and pustules that eventually ulcerate

Figure 2-21. Pyoderma gangrenosum. Histologic section shows a dense diffuse dermal infiltrate of predominantly neutrophils. Blood vessels show plump endothelial lining. The infiltrate is generally denser than that seen in Sweet syndrome.

- Lower extremities and trunk are often involved
- Fully developed lesions show necrotic center with a raised, undermined border with a dusky-purple hue
- Pyoderma gangrenosum may be the cutaneous manifestation of underlying systemic diseases such as inflammatory bowel disease, connective tissue disease, hematopoietic malignancies, and liver diseases

Histopathology

- Features are nonspecific and vary according to the area biopsied
- The center of the lesion shows ulcer with necrosis, neutrophilic infiltrate, and occasionally secondary vasculitis
- Biopsy of the undermined border shows mixed inflammatory cell infiltrate in addition to neutrophils
- Periphery of the lesions shows primarily a lymphocytic and histiocytic reaction

Special Stains and Immunohistochemistry

- Special stains and microbiologic cultures are helpful in excluding an infectious etiology

Other Techniques for Diagnosis

- Noncontributory

Differential Diagnosis

❚ Sweet syndrome
- Less prominent neutrophilic infiltrate that is typically more superficial
❚ Bacterial cellulitis
- Should always be considered in the differential diagnosis
- Requires demonstration of bacteria by special stains or microbiologic cultures

Pearls

- Areas of granulomatous inflammation may be seen in pyoderma gangrenosum associated with Crohn disease

Selected References

Powell FC, Collins S: Pyoderma gangrenosum. Clin Dermatol 18:283-293, 2000.
Callen JP: Pyoderma gangrenosum. Lancet 351:581-585, 1998.
Takvorian T, Skarin A, Johnson R: Pyoderma gangrenosum. J Clin Oncol 15:407, 1997.
Powell FC, Su WP, Perry HO: Pyoderma gangrenosum: Classification and management. J Am Acad Dermatol 34:395-409, 1996.
Su WP, Schroeter AL, Perry HO, et al: Histopathologic and immunopathologic study of pyoderma gangrenosum. J Cutan Pathol 13:323, 1986.

Eosinophils Predominant

Eosinophilic Cellulitis

Clinical Features

- Eosinophilic cellulitis (Wells syndrome) is a rare, recurrent dermatosis of uncertain pathogenesis, characterized by sudden onset of erythematous patches that evolve into painful plaques
- May be associated with insect bites, parasitosis, infections, and drug reactions
- Usually associated with peripheral blood eosinophilia

Histopathology

- Spongiotic intraepidermal vesicles may be present
- Diffuse and dense dermal infiltrate of eosinophils occasionally extending into the subcutaneous tissue
- Eosinophil degranulation is more prominent in older lesions and may impregnate the collagen bundles (flame figures)
- Palisading histiocytes with central necrobiosis may be seen in florid lesions

Special Stains and Immunohistochemistry

- Noncontributory

Other Techniques for Diagnosis

- Noncontributory

Differential Diagnosis

- Consider other dermal hypersensitivity reactions, including reactions to insect bites, parasites, and drugs

Pearls

- Eosinophilic cellulitis most likely represents an exaggerated dermal hypersensitivity reaction rather than a specific disease, and a search for inciting stimuli is warranted

Selected References

Fujii K, Tanabe H, Kanno Y, et al: Eosinophilic cellulitis as a cutaneous manifestation of idiopathic hypereosinophilic syndrome. J Am Acad Dermatol 49:1174-1177, 2003.

Espana A, Sanz ML, Sola J, Gil P: Wells' syndrome (eosinophilic cellulitis): Correlation. J Dermatol 140:127-130, 1999.
Goh CL: Eosinophilic cellulitis (Wells' syndrome). Int J Dermatol 31:429-430, 1992.

Scabies

Clinical Features

- Scabies is a contagious, pruritic, papulovesicular and pustular eruption caused by the mite *Sarcoptes scabiei*
- The eruption is most pronounced on the abdomen, buttocks, and anterior axillary folds
- Burrows produced by the female mite typically involve the palms, web spaces between fingers, and male genitalia
- Persistent pruritic nodules or nodular scabies involving most commonly the scrotum can be seen up to several months after treatment

Histopathology

- Sections taken from the burrow show a tunnel-like space between layers of parakeratosis; the mite or its products such as eggshells and fecal deposits need to be demonstrated for a definite diagnosis
- Spongiosis and vesiculation may be present in the epidermis
- Superficial and deep dermal infiltrate containing varying numbers of eosinophils
- Persistent nodular lesions show dense, diffuse, mixed inflammatory cell infiltrate containing eosinophils, thick-walled blood vessels, and occasionally atypical mononuclear cells; pseudolymphomatous pattern may also be seen (the mite is generally absent in these lesions)

Figure 2-22. Scabies. Histologic section shows a parakeratotic burrow containing body parts of the mite of scabies. The dermal inflammatory cell infiltrate typically contains frequent eosinophils.

Special Stains and Immunohistochemistry

- Noncontributory

Other Techniques for Diagnosis

- A suspected burrow can be shaved, placed on a glass slide, and examined under oil immersion

Differential Diagnosis

- In the absence of the mite or its products in the cornified layer, the histologic changes cannot be distinguished from other hypersensitivity reactions such as those caused by arthropod bites

Pearls

- Norwegian scabies is a rare variant in which an immeasurable number of mites is present within the cornified layer; generally seen in patients with congenital or iatrogenic impairment of immune responses, the mentally deficient, and physically debilitated patients

Selected References

Brites C, Weyll M, Pedroso C, et al: Severe and Norwegian scabies are strongly associated with retroviral (HIV-1/HTLV-1) infection in Bahia, Brazil. AIDS 16:1292, 2002.
Angel TA, Nigro J, Levy ML: Infestations in the pediatric patient. Pediatr Clin N Am 47:921-935, 2000.
Chosidow O: Scabies and pediculosis. Lancet 355:819-826, 2000.
Orkin M: Scabies: What's new? Curr Prob Dermatol 22:105-111, 1995.
Fernandez N, Torres A, Ackerman AB: Pathological findings in human scabies. Arch Dermatol 113:320, 1977.

Histiocytes Predominant

Xanthogranuloma

Clinical Features

- Typically occurs during infancy (within first 6 months of life)
- About 20% are congenital
- Usually presents as single or multiple tan to pink-red nodules that almost always regresses over time to a tan macule or depression
- Occasionally found in the deep soft tissue
- Infrequent association with neurofibromatosis and urticaria pigmentosa (mastocytosis)

Histopathology

- Well-defined or focally infiltrative margins
- Characterized by uniform-appearing histiocytes with an eosinophilic, vacuolated, or xanthomatous cytoplasm
- Touton giant cells are typically seen
- Scattered acute and chronic inflammatory cells are commonly present

Figure 2-23. Xanthogranuloma. Histologic section shows dermal infiltrate of predominantly histiocytes, including multinucleated histiocytes containing foamy cytoplasm and nuclei arranged at the periphery in a wreathlike pattern (Touton giant cells). Lymphocytes are present in the background.

Special Stains and Immunohistochemistry

- Oil red O highlights intracytoplasmic neutral lipids
- CD68 positive in the histiocytes

Other Techniques for Diagnosis

- Noncontributory

Differential Diagnosis

- Langerhans cell histiocytosis (eosinophilic granuloma)
  - Characterized by the presence of histiocytes and eosinophils
  - Histiocytes positive for CD1a and S-100 protein
  - Electron microscopy demonstrates Birbeck granules
- Fibrous histiocytoma
  - Found in adults (usually third to fifth decades)
  - Composed of spindle-shaped fibroblasts and histiocytic cells arranged in a storiform pattern
  - Typically lacks Touton giant cells
- Xanthoma
  - Typically associated with hyperlipidemia
  - Characterized by the presence of sheets of histiocytes containing abundant intracytoplasmic lipid
  - Cholesterol clefts and multinucleated giant cells are typical

Pearls

- Pathogenesis remains uncertain; believed to be a reactive rather than neoplastic process
- Not associated with a lipid abnormality
- Skin lesions almost always regress with time and ultimately appear as a slight depression on the skin surface
- Overall prognosis is excellent

Selected References

Janssen D, Harms D: Juvenile xanthogranuloma in childhood and adolescence: A clinicopathologic study of 129 patients from the Kiel pediatric tumor registry. Am J Surg Pathol 29:21, 2005.

Burgdorf WH, Zelger B: JXG, NF1, and JMML: Alphabet soup or a clinical issue? Pediatr Dermatol 21:174, 2004.

Dehner LP: Juvenile xanthogranulomas in the first two decades of life: A clinicopathologic study of 174 cases with cutaneous and extracutaneous manifestations. Am J Surg Pathol 27:579, 2003.

Hernandez-Martin A, Baselga E, Drolet BA, Esterly NB: Juvenile xanthogranuloma. J Am Acad Dermatol 36:355-367; quiz, 368-369, 1997.

Freyer DR, Kennedy R, Bostrom BC, et al: Juvenile xanthogranuloma: Forms of systemic disease and their clinical implications. J Pediatr 129:227-237, 1996.

Reticulohistiocytic Granuloma

Clinical Features

- Typically occurs in adults
- Most frequently presents as red-brown cutaneous nodules
- Typically well-circumscribed nodule with a red-brown to yellow cut surface
- May present as localized (giant cell reticulohistiocytoma) or systemic disease (multicentric reticulohistiocytosis)
  - Cutaneous reticulohistiocytoma (localized form)
    - May present as single or multiple skin lesions
    - Clinical features similar to xanthogranuloma
  - Multicentric reticulohistiocytosis (systemic form)
    - Rare condition
    - May involve lymph nodes, heart, bone, and joints in addition to widespread skin involvement

Figure 2-24. Reticulohistiocytic granuloma. The dense dermal infiltrate consists of lymphocytes and histiocytes. The cytoplasm of the histiocytes shows characteristic ground-glass appearance.

◆ Patients may present with progressive erosive arthritis, fever, and weight loss
◆ Association with hyperlipidemia, internal malignancies, and autoimmune diseases

Histopathology

- Essentially similar features in both localized and systemic forms
- Well-defined infiltrate of multinucleated, uniform epithelioid histiocytes with abundant eosinophilic, "glassy" cytoplasm
- Infrequent mitotic activity
- Scattered chronic inflammatory cells

Special Stains and Immunohistochemistry

- Noncontributory

Other Techniques for Diagnosis

- Noncontributory

Differential Diagnosis

▮ Malignant fibrous histiocytoma
- Deep-seated, cellular tumor composed of pleomorphic tumor cells arranged in a storiform pattern
- High mitotic rate often with many atypical forms
- Areas of hemorrhage and necrosis common

▮ Malignant melanoma
- Large, pleomorphic cells with large nuclei and prominent nucleoli
- High mitotic rate often seen
- Melanin pigment may be seen
- Positive for S-100 protein and pan melanocytic marker

Pearls

- Solitary form of reticulohistiocytoma and xanthogranuloma are regarded as part of a spectrum
- Disseminated reticulohistiocytosis is associated with various malignancies (carcinoma of the breast, colon, or lung) or systemic disease (tuberculosis, diabetes, hypothyroidism)
- Polyarthritis seen in the disseminated form is due to infiltrate of similar histiocytic cells found in skin around the joints

Selected References

Miettinen M, Fetsch JF: Reticulohistiocytoma (solitary epithelioid histiocytoma): A clinicopathologic and immunohistochemical study of 44 cases. Am J Surg Pathol 30:521, 2006.

Tajirian AL, Malik MK, Robinson-Bostom L, et al: Multicentric reticulohistiocytosis. Clin Dermatol 24:486, 2006.

Luz FB, Gaspar AP, Ramos-e-Silva M, et al: Immuno-histochemical profile of multicentric reticulohistiocytosis. Skinmed 4:71, 2005.

Snow JL, Muller SA: Malignancy-associated multicentric reticulohistiocytosis: A clinical, histological, and immunophenotypic study. Br J Dermatol 133:71-76, 1995.

Palisading and Necrobiotic Granulomas

Granuloma Annulare

Clinical Features

- Benign granulomatous process of unknown etiology
- Occurs most commonly in children and young adults; females more commonly affected than males
- Predilection for areas of trauma and exposure, typically the dorsal surface of the hands and feet, ankles, knees, and elbows
- Single or multiple annular dermal plaques with central clearing and raised erythematous borders
- Spontaneous regression of the lesions occurs, but they occasionally recur

Histopathology

- Histiocytes in the dermis in an interstitial pattern or as palisades surrounding zones of degenerating collagen with mucin; patterns between the two extremes can occur
- Typically involves upper and middle dermis; occasionally only the upper or deep dermis
- Multinucleated histiocytes, some of which contain elastic fibers in the cytoplasm
- Perivascular infiltrates of lymphocytes; eosinophils in varying numbers may be present
- Occasional neutrophils and nuclear fragmentation in areas of mucinous degeneration

Special Stains and Immunohistochemistry

- Colloidal iron stain highlights mucin

Other Techniques for Diagnosis

- Noncontributory

Figure 2-25. Granuloma annulare. Histologic section shows palisade of histiocytes surrounding zones of myxoid degeneration of collagen. The granulomas are typically located in the upper dermis.

Differential Diagnosis

■ Rheumatoid nodule
  ● Zone of necrobiosis is usually highly eosinophilic, occasionally resembling fibrin and no mucin
  ● Involvement of subcutaneous tissue is typical
■ Necrobiosis lipoidica
  ● Biopsy specimens are usually rectangular
  ● Basophilic degeneration of collagen is stratified between layers of inflammatory cell infiltrate
  ● Plasma cells are frequently present in the inflammatory cell infiltrate
  ● Involvement of deep dermis is typical

Pearls

  ● A subcutaneous variant of granuloma annulare (pseudorheumatoid nodule) typically presents in children with deep-seated nodules in the dermis or subcutaneous fat in which histologic differentiation from rheumatoid nodule can be difficult
  ● A well-known diagnostic pitfall is diagnosing epithelioid sarcoma as granuloma annulare, and vice versa

Selected References

Ko C, Glusac E, Shapiro P: Noninfectious granulomas. In Elder DE, Elenitsas R, Johnson BL Jr, et al (eds): Lever's Histopathology of Skin, 10th ed. Philadelphia, Lippincott Williams & Wilkins, 2008, p 361.

Barren DF, Cootauco MH, Cohen BA: Granuloma annulare: A clinical review. Lippincott Prim Care Pract 1:33-39, 1997.

Magro CM, Crowson AN, Regauer S: Granuloma annulare and necrobiosis lipoidica tissue reactions as a manifestation of systemic disease. Hum Pathol 27:50-56, 1996.

Mullans E, Helm KF: Granuloma annulare: An immuno-histochemical study. J Cutan Pathol 21:135-139, 1994.

Umbert P, Winkelmann RK: Histologic, ultrastructural, and histochemical studies of granuloma annulare. Arch Dermatol 113:1681, 1977.

Necrobiosis Lipoidica

Clinical Features

  ● Degenerative cutaneous disease of unknown etiology, often associated with diabetes
  ● Typically seen in diabetic patients in their fifth and sixth decades and in nondiabetic patients between the ages of 20 and 40 years
  ● Characteristically affects the anterior tibial surface but also has a predilection for the thighs, popliteal areas, and dorsum of the feet and arms
  ● Indurated yellow-brown oval plaques with a violaceous border
  ● Center of the plaque may later become atrophic with a distinctive yellow waxy hue

Figure 2-26. Necrobiosis lipoidica. A, Low-power view shows zones of granulomas alternating with those of fibrosis and extending into deep dermis. **B,** High-power view shows histiocytes, including multinucleated giant cells surrounding zones of collagen degeneration in the deep dermis.

Histopathology

  ● Rectangular contour of biopsy sample
  ● Epidermal atrophy and superficial dermal telangiectasia
  ● Alternating horizontal layers of basophilic degeneration of collagen and palisades consisting of histiocytes, lymphocytes, and plasma cells
  ● Zones of dermal sclerosis

Special Stains and Immunohistochemistry

  ● Noncontributory

Other Techniques for Diagnosis

  ● Noncontributory

Differential Diagnosis

■ Rheumatoid nodule
  ● Areas of fibrinoid degeneration are typically sharply demarcated and involve subcutaneous tissue

Figure 2-27. Rheumatoid nodule. Palisading granulomas surrounding zones of fibrinoid degeneration of collagen are present within the subcutaneous tissue.

■ Granuloma annulare
  ● Demarcated zones of necrobiosis with mucin, typically in the upper half of the dermis
■ Late sclerotic lesions may resemble morphea

Pearls
  ● Less than 1% of the patients with diabetes develop necrobiosis lipoidica
  ● Cases of squamous cell carcinoma (SCC) developing in lesions of necrobiosis are reported

Selected References

Imtiaz KE, Khaleeli AA: Squamous cell carcinoma developing in necrobiosis lipoidica. Diabetic Med 18:325-328, 2001.

O'Toole EA, Kennedy U, Nolan JJ, et al: Necrobiosis lipoidica: Only a minority of patients have diabetes mellitus. Br J Dermatol 140:283-286, 1999.

Magro CM, Crowson AN, Regauer S: Granuloma annulare and necrobiosis lipoidica tissue reactions as a manifestation of systemic disease. Hum Pathol 27:50-56, 1996.

Lowitt MH, Dover JS: Necrobiosis lipoidica. J Am Acad Dermatol 25:735-748, 1991.

Rheumatoid Nodule

Clinical Features
  ● Chronic deeply seated inflammatory nodules that occur in patients with rheumatoid arthritis and occasionally in patients with systemic lupus erythematosus
  ● Rheumatoid nodules are seen in up to 20% of patients with rheumatoid arthritis
  ● Predilection for areas subject to mechanical trauma, typically in para-articular locations, including metacarpophalangeal and proximal interphalangeal joints
  ● Solitary or multiple, firm, nontender, freely mobile, large subcutaneous nodules

Histopathology
  ● Central areas of homogeneous eosinophilic degeneration of collagen surrounded by peripheral palisade of histiocytes and lymphocytes
  ● Located in the subcutaneous tissue and deep dermis
  ● Occasional vascular proliferation associated wtih fibrosis in the surrounding stroma

Special Stains and Immunohistochemistry
  ● Noncontributory

Other Techniques for Diagnosis
  ● Serologic evaluation for rheumatoid factor

Differential Diagnosis
■ Subcutaneous granuloma annulare
  ● Areas of necrobiosis typically contain bluish mucin
■ Necrobiosis lipoidica
  ● Typically seen on the anterior tibial surface
  ● Layers of necrobiosis are stratified with inflammatory cell infiltrates

Pearls
  ● Rheumatoid nodules are almost always associated with high titer of rheumatoid factor

Selected References

Edwards JC, Wilkinson LS, Pitsillides AA: Palisading cells of rheumatoid nodules: Comparison with synovial intimal cells. Ann Rheum Dis 52:801, 1993.

Veys EM, De Keyser F: Rheumatoid nodules: Differential diagnosis and immunohistological findings. Ann Rheum Dis 52:625, 1993.

Dubois EL, Friou GJ, Chandor S: Rheumatoid nodules and rheumatoid granulomas in systemic lupus erythematosus. JAMA 220:515, 1972.

Necrobiotic Xanthogranuloma

Clinical Features
  ● Rare disorder often associated with paraproteinemia
  ● Presents as large, yellow indented plaques with atrophy
  ● Most commonly involves the periorbital region

Histopathology
  ● Granulomatous inflammation in the deep dermis and subcutaneous tissue composed of histiocytes, including many foam cells, Touton giant cells, and lymphoid infiltrate
  ● Intervening broad zones of necrobiosis
  ● Cholesterol clefts
  ● Lymphoid follicles are sometimes present

Figure 2-28. Necrobiotic xanthogranuloma. Histologic section shows a dense dermal infiltrate composed of histiocytes and lymphocytes. Many of the histiocytes have foamy cytoplasm, and some are multinucleated.

Special Stains and Immunohistochemistry

● Noncontributory

Other Techniques for Diagnosis

● Serum protein electrophoresis shows IgG monoclonal gammopathy in most patients

Differential Diagnosis

▌ Necrobiosis lipoidica
  ● Characteristically affects the anterior tibial surface, but also has a predilection for the thighs, popliteal areas, and dorsum of the feet and arms
  ● Alternating horizontal layers of basophilic degeneration of collagen and palisades consisting of histiocytes, lymphocytes, and plasma cells
  ● Less foam cells
▌ Subcutaneous granuloma annulare
  ● May be differentiated by the presence of mucinous degeneration and lack of foam cells
▌ Xanthomas and xanthogranulomas
  ● Do not have areas of necrobiosis

Pearls

● In some patients with necrobiotic xanthogranuloma, an underlying multiple myeloma is present

Selected References

Fernández-Herrera J, Pedraz J: Necrobiotic xanthogranuloma. Semin Cutan Med Surg 26:108-113, 2007.

Cornblath WT, Dotan SA, Trobe JD, Headington JT: Varied clinical spectrum of necrobiotic xanthogranuloma. Ophthalmology 99:103-107, 1992.

Mehregan DA, Winkelmann RK: Necrobiotic xanthogranuloma. Arch Dermatol 128:94-100, 1992.

Finan MC, Winkelmann RK: Histopathology of necrobiotic xanthogranuloma with paraproteinemia. J Cutan Pathol 14:92-99, 1987.

Sarcoidal Granulomas

Sarcoidosis

Clinical Features

● Systemic granulomatous disease of unknown etiology, possibly secondary to activation of an unknown antigen
● Overall, a relatively uncommon disease; usually seen in females living in the north temperature zone (e.g., Scandinavians); in United States, more common in blacks
● Cutaneous involvement is seen in one fourth of patients with systemic sarcoidosis, whereas cutaneous lesions are the only manifestation in about one fourth of patients with sarcoidosis
● Maculopapular eruption with predilection for the face, posterior neck and shoulders, and extensor surfaces of extremities
● Lesions typically appear as small (<1 cm), erythematous to violaceous papules; occasional cutaneous and subcutaneous nodules
● Lesions tend to coalesce into yellow to brown plaques with occasional development of central clearing to form annular lesions

Histopathology

● Superficial and deep coalescent dermal noncaseating granulomas
● Granulomas contain multinucleated eosinophilic epithelioid histiocytes with minimal peripheral lymphocytic infiltrates ("naked" tubercles)
● Multinucleated epithelioid histiocytes may contain asteroid bodies (eosinophilic stellate inclusions)
● Involvement of subcutaneous fat may result in lobular pattern of panniculitis due to noncaseating granulomas

Figure 2-29. Sarcoidosis. Histologic section shows noncaseating granulomas within the dermis. The granulomas are composed of histiocytes with only a sparse lymphocytic component (naked tubercles).

Special Stains and Immunohistochemistry

- Special stains for organisms (GMS, PAS, and acid-fast bacilli) to rule out an infectious etiology

Other Techniques for Diagnosis

- Kveim test has 80% sensitivity
- Chest radiograph: variable bilateral involvement ranging from hilar lymphadenopathy to interstitial pulmonary infiltrates

Differential Diagnosis

- Tuberculoid leprosy
  - Acid-fast stain reveals the presence of bacilli within the histiocytes of granulomas
  - Granulomas follow nerves
- Fungal infection
  - There may be a neutrophilic component to the inflammation
  - PAS and GMS stains reveal the presence of fungal organisms
- Foreign-body granuloma
  - Polarized light reveals the presence of birefringent foreign material in giant cells

Pearls

- Cutaneous lesions of sarcoidosis may localize in previous scars, such as those caused by herpes zoster and tattoos
- Definite diagnosis of systemic sarcoidosis is best made on biopsy

Selected References

Ball NJ, Kho GT, Martinka M: The histologic spectrum of cutaneous sarcoidosis: A study of twenty-eight cases. J Cutan Pathol 31:160-168, 2004.

Newman LS, Rose CS, Maier LA: Sarcoidosis. N Engl J Med 336:1224-1234, 1997.

Sheffield EA: Pathology of sarcoidosis. Clin Chest Med 18:741-754, 1997.

Walsh NM, Hanly JG, Tremaine R, Murray S: Cutaneous sarcoidosis and foreign bodies. Am J Dermatopathol 15:203-207, 1993.

Olive KE, Kataria YP: Cutaneous manifestations of sarcoidosis. Arch Intern Med 145:1811, 1985.

Hanno R, Needelman A, Eiferman RA, et al: Cutaneous sarcoidal granulomas and the development of systemic sarcoidosis. Arch Dermatol 117:203, 1981.

Foreign-Body Granulomas

Clinical Features

- Immune reaction to a foreign body implanted within the viable layers of the skin
- Commonly seen lesion with no age or gender predilection
- Predilection for hands, feet, and other sites subject to trauma

Figure 2-30. Foreign-body granuloma. The granulomas may resemble those of sarcoidosis. However, some of the histiocytes contain foreign-body material.

- Erythematous subcutaneous nodules, typically less than 1 cm

Histopathology

- Early lesions present as a neutrophilic abscess
- Localized granuloma usually surrounding birefringent foreign material or keratin
- Multinucleate histiocytes with centrally located nuclei (foreign-body giant cells)
- Occasional histiocytes filled with cytoplasmic vacuoles of varying diameter (Swiss cheese pattern)

Special Stains and Immunohistochemistry

- Noncontributory

Other Techniques for Diagnosis

- Noncontributory

Differential Diagnosis

- Infectious granuloma
  - Foreign-body giant cells are typically absent
  - Acid-fast, Gram, PAS, and GMS stains highlight causative organisms

Pearls

- Materials capable of producing a foreign-body granuloma include vegetable spines, metals, wooden splinters, silk or nylon sutures, paraffin, silicone, silica, urates, oils, keratinous material, and neoplasms

Selected Reference

Walsh NM, Hanly JG, Tremaine R, Murray S: Cutaneous sarcoidosis and foreign bodies. Am J Dermatopathol 15:203-207, 1993.

Figure 2-31. Leprosy. A, Hematoxylin and eosin–stained section shows poorly formed granulomas within the dermis. Some of the histiocytes have foamy cytoplasm. **B,** Acid-fast bacillus stain demonstrates the presence of acid-fast bacilli within the cytoplasm of some of the histiocytes.

Infectious Granulomas

Leprosy

Clinical Features

- An endemic disease of tropical and subtropical countries including the Indian subcontinent and Southeast Asia
- Caused by *Mycobacterium leprae* and predominantly involves the skin and peripheral nerves
- Shows an immunopathologic spectrum with minimal to marked host response and resulting clinicopathologic spectrum consisting of tuberculoid leprosy with maximal host response at one end to lepromatous leprosy with minimal response at the other end; borderline leprosy shows features intermediate between the two
- Tuberculoid leprosy
  - Lesions are scant and consist of hypopigmented papules and plaques associated with anesthesia

- Lepromatous leprosy
  - Multiple symmetrical macules, papules, or nodules are present
  - Involvement of the face (leonine facies) and ulnar, radial, and common peroneal nerves can occur
- Borderline leprosy
  - Lesions are less numerous and less symmetrical than in lepromatous leprosy

Histopathology

- Tuberculoid leprosy
  - Large, elongated epithelioid granulomas with peripheral lymphocytic infiltrate arranged along neurovascular bundles
- Lepromatous leprosy
  - Dense dermal infiltrate composed predominantly of foam cells, with few lymphocytes and plasma cells
- Borderline leprosy
  - Admixture of foamy macrophages and epithelioid histiocytes but not arranged as well-formed granulomas; lymphocytes in significant numbers

Special Stains and Immunohistochemistry

- Acid-fast bacilli can be demonstrated within the cytoplasm of the histiocytes; maximal numbers are present in lepromatous leprosy and the least in tuberculoid leprosy

Other Techniques for Diagnosis

- PCR techniques for infectious agent

Differential Diagnosis

- Abundant foam cells in lepromatous leprosy may invoke a xanthomatous pattern and require demonstration of the acid-fast bacilli for definite diagnosis
- Tuberculoid granulomas of tuberculoid leprosy may resemble sarcoidosis and occasionally foreign-body granulomas

Pearls

- Histioid leprosy is a variant of lepromatous leprosy that histologically resembles a histiocytoma but shows a high number of bacilli

Selected References

Britton WJ, Lockwood DNJ: Leprosy. Lancet 363:1209-1219, 2004.

Abulafia J, Vignale RA: Leprosy: Pathogenesis updated. Int J Dermatol 38:321-334, 1999.

Jacobson RR, Krahenbuhl JL: Leprosy. Lancet 353:655-660, 1999.

Whitty CJ, Lockwood DN: Leprosy-new perspectives on an old disease. J Infect 38:2-5, 1999.

Choudhuri K: The immunology of leprosy: Unravelling an enigma. Int J Lepr 63:430, 1995.

De Wit MYL, Faber WR, Krieg SR, et al: Application of a polymerase chain reaction for the detection of *Mycobacterium leprae* in skin tissues. J Clin Microbiol 29:906, 1991.

Primary Cutaneous Tuberculosis: Lupus Vulgaris

Clinical Features

- Lupus vulgaris is a form of secondary or reactivation tuberculosis developing in previously infected and sensitized persons
- Usually results from hematogenous spread from an old, reactivated focus in the lung or from lymphatic extension from a tuberculous cervical lymphadenitis
- One or more well-demarcated, reddish-brown patches typically involving the skin of nose and adjacent areas of face
- Chronic course with peripheral extension of the lesions
- Over time, the affected areas become atrophic and occasionally ulcerate

Histopathology

- Most commonly involves the upper half of dermis
- Tuberculoid granulomas characterized by epithelioid and multinucleated histiocytes; scattered lymphocytes in the background
- Giant cells are of both Langerhans and foreign-body type; central caseation is minimal or absent
- In older lesions, extensive fibrosis replaces the granulomas
- Depending on the stage, the overlying epidermis may be atrophic, ulcerated, or hyperplastic; pseudo-epitheliomatous epidermal hyperplasia can be seen at the edge of ulcers

Special Stains and Immunohistochemistry

- Special stains may only rarely demonstrate tubercle bacilli because they are typically present in small numbers

Other Techniques for Diagnosis

- PCR detection of mycobacterial DNA is valuable in confirming the diagnosis

Differential Diagnosis

- Other infectious and noninfectious causes of granulomatous inflammation should be considered

Pearls

- SCC may develop from the edges of the ulcerated lesions of lupus vulgaris

Selected References

Negi SS, Basir SF, Gupta S, et al: Comparative study of PCR, smear examination and culture for diagnosis of cutaneous tuberculosis. J Commun Dis 37:83-92, 2005.

Marcoval J, Servitje O, Moreno A, et al: Lupus vulgaris: Clinical, histopathologic, and bacteriologic study of 10 cases. J Am Acad Dermatol 26:404-407, 1992.

Lao IO, Bronson D, Barsky S: Lupus vulgaris. Cutis 31:177-179, 1993.

Haim S, Friedman-Birnbaum R: Cutaneous tuberculosis and malignancy. Cutis 21:643, 1978.

Deep Fungal Infections

Clinical Features

- Deep mycosis can be primarily a cutaneous fungal infection or be part of systemic infections such as those involving the respiratory system or reticuloendothelial system, especially in immunocompromised hosts
- Primary cutaneous and subcutaneous mycoses are often caused by saprophytic organisms and include sporotrichosis, chromoblastomycosis, histoplasmosis, coccidiomycosis, blastomycosis, and cryptococcosis

Figure 2-32. Blastomycosis. A, Hematoxylin and eosin–stained section shows epidermal hyperplasia associated with suppurative and granulomatous inflammation. **B,** Gomori methenamine silver stain demonstrates yeast forms of blastomycosis, some of which show characteristic broad-based budding.

Histopathology

- Characteristic histologic pattern is pseudoepitheliomatous hyperplasia with extensive suppurative and granulomatous inflammation in the dermis
- Small neurophilic abscesses are surrounded by varying numbers of lymphocytes, plasma cells, epithelioid histiocytes, and multinucleated giant cells
- Involvement of the subcutaneous fat generally results in a lobular pattern of panniculitis that is also suppurative and granulomatous
- Causative fungal organisms can be found in the cytoplasm of the histiocytes or within the abscesses
- Size and morphology of fungal organisms can further help in identification of the specific organisms
  - Blastomycosis: 8- to 15-μm thick-walled spores with single broad-based buds
  - Paracoccidioidomycosis: 6- to 20-μm spores with narrow-necked buds ("mariner's wheels")
  - Chromoblastomycosis: 6- to 12-μm thick-walled dark-brown spores in clusters ("copper pennies")
  - Cryptococcosis: 4- to 12-μm spores with wide capsule in gelatinous background or 2- to 4-μm spores in granulomatous areas; narrow-based buds
  - Histoplasmosis: 2- to 4-μm round or oral spores with clear halo, located in the cytoplasm of histiocytes
  - Sporotrichosis: 4- to 6-μm round to oval spores, intraepidermal abscesses may be present

Special Stains and Immunohistochemistry

- Special stains, PAS, and GMS are invaluable in locating and identifying the causative fungal organisms
- Mucicarmine is used to differentiate *Cryptococcus* species from other fungi such as *Blastomyces* species

Other Techniques for Diagnosis

- Microbiologic cultures to isolate the organisms
- PCR techniques are becoming available for various fungi

Differential Diagnosis

▌ In addition to deep fungal infections, atypical mycobacterial infections, and halogenodermas should be considered in the differential diagnosis of suppurative and granulomatous inflammation with pseudo-epitheliomatous hyperplasia
▌ Subcutaneous phaeohyphomycosis (phaeohyphomycotic cyst)
- Presents as deep coalescing suppurative granulomas surrounded by a fibrous capsule
▌ Suppurative inflammation may also be caused by bacterial and mycobacterial organisms

Pearls

- Necrotizing skin lesions with vasculitis and granulomas can be seen in disseminated aspergillosis, mucormycosis, and *Fusarium* species infections
- Cryptococcosis can present with a xanthomatous pattern, especially in immunocompromised hosts
- Host response may be minimal in immunocompromised hosts and requires high degree of suspicion to evaluate for infectious agents

Selected References

Rivitti EA, Aoki V: Deep fungal infections in tropical countries. Clin Dermatol 17:171-190, 1999.

Ogawa H, Summerbell RC, Clemons KV, et al: Dermatophytes and host defence in cutaneous mycoses. Med Mycol 36(Suppl 1):166-173, 1998.

Body BA: Cutaneous manifestations of systemic mycoses. Dermatol Clin 14:125-135, 1996.

Chapman SW, Daniel CR 3rd: Cutaneous manifestations of fungal infection. Infect Dis Clin N Am 8:879-910, 1994.

Foil CS: Fungal diseases. Clin Dermatol 12:529-542, 1994.

Leishmaniasis

Clinical Features

- Leishmaniasis is a protozoan disease transmitted by the sandfly
- Manifests as localized or diffuse cutaneous, mucocutaneous, and visceral disease
- Two forms of cutaneous leishmaniasis are recognized
  - American cutaneous leishmaniasis
    - Caused by *Leishmania braziliensis* complex or *Leishmania mexicana* complex
    - Occurs in the American continent

Figure 2-33. Leishmaniasis. High-power view shows an infiltrate of plasma cells and histiocytes. Within the cytoplasm of the histiocytes, there are organisms that are 2 to 4 μm in size. A Giemsa stain can also be used to highlight the organisms.

— Oriental cutaneous leishmaniasis
  ◆ Caused by *Leishmania tropica*
  ◆ Occurs in parts of Europe, Middle East, Asia, and Africa
- In both forms, the cutaneous lesions occur as single or multiple erythematous papules on exposed skin several weeks after the bite of infected sandfly
- Papules may enlarge to form nodules that can ulcerate

Histopathology

- Dense diffuse infiltrate of histiocytes with scattered lymphocytes and plasma cells is present in the dermis
- In early lesions, numerous parasites are noted within the cytoplasm of the histiocytes
- A smear from an early lesion can be positive for the parasites
- Late lesions are characterized by tuberculoid-type granulomas and lymphocytes

Special Stains and Immunohistochemistry

- Giemsa stain is helpful in identifying the parasite, which is 2 to 4 μm

Other Techniques for Diagnosis

- Noncontributory

Differential Diagnosis

▌ Rhinoscleroma
  - Histiocytes (Mikulicz cells) are larger than the histiocytes in leishmaniasis
  - Caused by *Klebsiella pneumoniae rhinoscleromatis*, which is 2 to 3 μm
  - Plasma cells and Russell bodies are more prominent
▌ Histoplasmosis
  - Generally associated with necrosis
  - Organisms are 2 to 4 μm, round to oval, and surrounded by a clear halo
  - Best seen with GMS and PAS stains
▌ Granuloma inguinale
  - Histiocytic infiltrate is admixed with neutrophilic abscesses
  - Causative organism is *Calymmatobacterium granulomatis*
  - Histiocytes contain Donovan bodies, which are encapsulated round to oval bodies measuring 1 to 2 μm

Pearls

- Mucocutaneous leishmaniasis may involve upper respiratory tract and nasopharynx and is seen in the American forms
- Visceral leishmaniasis includes kala-azar produced by *Leishmania donovani*, which occurs in Africa, Asia, and parts of Brazil; the Mediterranean kala-azar is seen in parts of Europe and Latin American countries

- Cutaneous leishmaniasis can occur as localized form, mucocutaneous form, chronic or verrucous form, relapse form, or diffuse form
- Localized and diffuse forms are at opposite ends of the spectrum and reflect the strength of immune response of the host to the parasite

Selected References

Choi CM, Lerner EA: Leishmaniasis as an emerging infection. J Invest Dermatol Symp Proc 6:175, 2001.

Dedet JP, Pratlong F, Lanotte G, Ravel C: Cutaneous leishmaniasis: The parasite. Clin Dermatol 17:261-268, 1999.

Herwaldt BL: Leishmaniasis. Lancet 354:1191-1199, 1999.

Mehregan DR, Mehregan AH, Mehregan DA: Histologic diagnosis of cutaneous leishmaniasis. Clin Dermatol 17:297-304, 1999.

Salman SM, Rubeiz NG, Kibbi AG: Cutaneous leishmaniasis: Clinical features and diagnosis. Clin Dermatol 17:291-296, 1999.

Samady JA, Schwartz RA: Old World cutaneous leishmaniasis. Int J Dermatol 36:161-166, 1997.

Vasculitis

Leukocytoclastic Vasculitis

Clinical Features

- Many underlying diseases can manifest clinically as palpable purpuric lesions and histologically as leukocytoclastic vasculitis
- Immune complex–mediated diseases such as Henoch-Schönlein purpura, connective tissue diseases, autoimmune diseases, and drug-induced and infectious etiologies are among the most common causes of leukocytoclastic vasculitis

Figure 2-34. Leukocytoclastic vasculitis. Histologic section shows perivascular infiltrate of neutrophils, neutrophilic nuclear dust, and extravasated red blood cells. Deposits of fibrin are present in and around the damaged blood vessels.

- Microscopic polyangiitis involving skin may show changes of leukocytoclastic vasculitis

Histopathology

- Characteristic pattern is a neutrophilic small-vessel vasculitis involving the dermal vessels
- Leukocytoclasis, or fragmentation of the neutrophilic nuclei into dust; the inflammatory cell infiltrate may also contain eosinophils and lymphocytes
- Damage to the vessel wall (typically postcapillary venules) results in extravasation of red cells
- Deposits of fibrin may be seen around the involved vessels
- In severe cases, luminal occlusion with resulting ischemic necrosis of the epidermis

Special Stains and Immunohistochemistry

- Gram, PAS, and GMS stains are helpful in diagnosing infectious causes
- In leukocytoclastic vasculitis caused by *Neisseria meningitides*, organisms can be demonstrated within the endothelial cells and neutrophils

Other Techniques for Diagnosis

- Immunofluorescence studies demonstrate IgM, C3, and fibrinogen in the dermal vessels; IgA is present in Henoch-Schönlein purpura
- Serologic studies are essential in excluding autoimmune-mediated leukocytoclastic vasculitis

Differential Diagnosis

▮ Other causes of neutrophilic dermatosis such as Sweet syndrome
  - May be considered especially in early lesions, where the vascular damage is not easily seen
▮ Erythema elevatum diutinum
  - Represents a chronic form of leukocytoclastic vasculitis
  - Characterized by red to violaceous papules typically involving extensor surfaces of extremities
▮ Granuloma faciale
  - Another chronic form of leukocytoclastic vasculitis typically presenting as brown-red papules or plaques almost always involving the face
▮ Livedo vasculitis
  - Typically involves lower legs
  - Histologic changes include deposition of fibrinoid material within the vessel walls with resulting luminal occlusion and ulceration of epidermis
  - Inflammatory cell infiltrate is generally sparse
▮ Septic vasculitis
  - Generally associated with thrombi in the vascular lumina, in addition to acute leukocytoclastic vasculitis

Pearls

- A true lymphocytic vasculitis of the small blood vessels is only rarely documented and is reported to occur in collagen vascular disease, pityriasis lichenoides, and lymphomatoid papulosis
- Noninflammatory small-vessel vasculitis histologically characterized by deposits of homogeneous pink material within and around vascular lumina can be seen in monoclonal cryoglobulinemia, thrombotic thrombocytopenic purpura (TTP), and warfarin (Coumadin)- or heparin-induced vasculitis

Selected References

Niiyama S, Amoh Y, Tomita M, et al: Dermatological manifestations associated with microscopic polyangiitis. Rheumatol Int 28:593-595, 2008.

Kawakami T, Kawanabe T, Saito C, et al: Clinical and histopathologic features of 8 patients with microscopic polyangiitis including two with a slowly progressive clinical course. J Am Acad Dermatol 57:840-848, 2007.

Claudy A: Pathogenesis of leukocytoclastic vasculitis. Eur J Dermatol 8:75-79, 1998.

Gibson LE, Su WP: Cutaneous vasculitis. Rheum Dis Clin N Am 21:1097-1113, 1995.

Smith JG Jr: Vasculitis. J Dermatol 22:812-822, 1995.

Szer IS: Henoch-Schönlein purpura. Curr Opin Rheumatol 6:25-31, 1994.

Superficial Migratory Thrombophlebitis

Clinical Features

- Typically presents as multiple, tender erythematous nodules on lower legs
- New lesions erupt as older lesions resolve
- May be a manifestation of Behçet disease and a part of Trousseau syndrome with associated visceral carcinoma

Figure 2-35. Thrombophlebitis. A large blood vessel located in the subcutaneous tissue shows inflammatory cell infiltrate in the wall and an organizing thrombus within the lumen.

Histopathology

- Affected vessel is typically a small or medium-sized vein situated in deep dermis or subcutaneous tissue of lower extremity
- Vascular lumen is completely occluded by thrombus
- An inflammatory cell infiltrate composed of neutrophils, lymphocytes, and histiocytes extends between the muscle bundles of the vein
- Recanalization and resorption of thrombus occurs with granulomatous reaction

Special Stains and Immunohistochemistry

- Elastic tissue stain is helpful to highlight elastic lamina of vessel wall

Other Techniques for Diagnosis

- Noncontributory

Differential Diagnosis

▌ Subcutaneous polyarteritis nodosa
- Can present as nodules on the legs
- Histologic findings are those of a neutrophilic vasculitis of medium-sized arteries with fibrinoid necrosis
- Elastic tissue stain may be helpful in distinguishing the arteries of polyarteritis nodosa from the veins of thrombophlebitis
▌ Nodular vasculitis
- Can resemble thrombophlebitis clinically
- Histologic changes include lymphohistiocytic infiltrates in the vessel wall with intimal thickening and thrombosis
- Small and medium-sized arteries and veins of the subcutaneous fat are typically involved
- An associated lobular panniculitis (erythema induratum) is generally present with granulomatous inflammation surrounding zones of fat necrosis
▌ Wegener granulomatosis
- Although most patients with Wegener granulomatosis typically present with leukocytoclastic vasculitis, true granulomatous inflammation and necrotizing vasculitis can occur in subcutaneous tissue
- Assays for antineutrophil cytoplasmic antibody (ANCA) may be helpful in the diagnosis of Wegener granulomatosis

Pearls

- As a result of stasis and venous hypertension, veins of the legs can show an increase in elastic tissue and smooth muscle in their walls, which can pose a problem in differentiating veins from arteries

Selected References

Luis Rodríguez-Peralto J, Carrillo R, Rosales B, et al: Superficial thrombophlebitis. Semin Cutan Med Surg 26:71-76, 2007.

Pickering MC, Haskard DO: Behçet's syndrome. J R Coll Physicians Lond 34:169-177, 2000.

Sakane T, Takeno M, Suzuki N, Inaba G: Behçet's disease. N Engl J Med 341:1284-1291, 1999.

Samlaska CP, James WD, Simel D: Superficial migratory thrombophlebitis and factor XII deficiency. J Am Acad Dermatol 22:939-943, 1990.

Vesiculobullous Dermatoses

Subcorneal Pustular Dermatosis (Sneddon-Wilkinson Disease)

Clinical Features

- Chronic dermatosis, characterized by sterile pustules typically involving flexural surfaces and axillary and inguinal folds
- Pustules may be arranged in annular or serpiginous patterns

Histopathology

- *Subcorneal* collection of neutrophils and rare eosinophils
- Mild epidermal spongiosis with neutrophils may be present
- Superficial perivascular infiltrate of neutrophils, rare eosinophils, and lymphocytes
- Occasional acantholytic keratinocytes may be seen

Special Stains and Immunohistochemistry

- Noncontributory

Other Techniques for Diagnosis

- Immunofluorescence studies to exclude autoimmune bullous disorders

Figure 2-36. Subcorneal pustular dermatosis. There are neutrophilic aggregates underneath the cornified layer. Acantholytic keratinocytes may be seen in addition to neutrophils.

Differential Diagnosis

▪ Bullous impetigo
  ● Histologic changes in bullous impetigo are identical to those of subcorneal pustular dermatosis
  ● Bullous impetigo is caused in most cases by group A streptococci
  ● Demonstration of bacteria by Gram stain or cultures is diagnostic
▪ Dermatophytosis
  ● Can occasionally present as subcorneal pustules
  ● PAS and GMS stains are useful in demonstrating the fungal organisms
▪ Pemphigus foliaceus and erythematosus
  ● Can present with subcorneal pustules with acantholysis
  ● In general, acantholytic cells are more frequent in pemphigus than in subcorneal pustular dermatosis
  ● For definitive diagnosis, immunofluorescence studies are essential
▪ Psoriasis
  ● Can present with subcorneal pustules
  ● Presence of spongiform pustules in pustular psoriasis helps in the differential diagnosis

Pearls

  ● Subcorneal pustular dermatosis may be associated with monoclonal gammopathy, most commonly IgA paraproteinemia
  ● Acantholysis in subcorneal pustular dermatosis is most likely due to the effect of proteolytic enzymes in the pustules

Selected References

Cheng S, Edmonds E, Ben-Gashir M, Yu RC: Subcorneal pustular dermatosis: 50 Years on. Clin Exp Dermatol 33:229-233, 2008.

Reed J, Wilkinson J: Subcorneal pustular dermatosis. Clin Dermatol 8:301-313, 2000.

Yasuda H, Kobayashi H, Hashimoto T, et al: Subcorneal pustular dermatosis type of IgA pemphigus: Demonstration of autoantibodies to desmocollin-1 and clinical review. Br J Dermatol 143:144-148, 2000.

Pemphigus

Clinical Features

  ● Pemphigus is a group of vesicular dermatoses that includes pemphigus vulgaris and pemphigus vegetans, pemphigus foliaceus and pemphigus erythematosus (superficial forms), IgA pemphigus, and paraneoplastic pemphigus
  ● Generally affects middle-aged and older patients and presents as large, flaccid bullae that break easily
  ● Positive Nikolsky sign is seen when lateral pressure on vesicles causes "sliding off" of the epithelium

Figure 2-37. Pemphigus. Histologic section shows intraepidermal vesicle with prominent suprabasal acantholysis.

  ● Sites of predilection include scalp, periocular region, sternum, middle back, umbilicus, and groin
  ● Oral lesions are present in most cases and may be the presenting symptom in some cases

Histopathology

  ● Characteristic histologic pattern is that of an intraepidermal acantholytic vesicular dermatosis
  ● Acantholysis results in clefts and blisters that are typically suprabasal in location
  ● Basal keratinocytes are attached to the dermis (tombstone-like)
  ● Blister cavity contains acantholytic keratinocytes that appear rounded with condensed cytoplasm and have enlarged nuclei with prominent nucleoli
  ● Acantholysis can extend into epithelium of follicles
  ● Variable amounts of superficial dermal inflammation
  ● Early lesions are characterized only by epidermal spongiosis with eosinophils
  ● Superficial forms of pemphigus show acantholysis in the upper part of the epidermis, close to the granular layer
  ● Concomitant interface dermatitis is present in paraneoplastic pemphigus
  ● IgA pemphigus shows a histologic pattern similar to that of subcorneal pustular dermatosis

Special Stains and Immunohistochemistry

  ● Noncontributory

Other Techniques for Diagnosis

  ● Direct immunofluorescence studies show an intercellular pattern with IgG in pemphigus vulgaris, and IgA in IgA pemphigus; granular deposits of IgG or IgM at the dermoepidermal junction in addition to the characteristic intercellular pattern may be seen in paraneoplastic pemphigus

- Tzanck preparation is helpful in demonstration of acantholytic keratinocytes in the blisters of pemphigus

Differential Diagnosis

- Hailey-Hailey disease (benign familial pemphigus)
  - Inherited as an autosomal dominant trait
  - Characterized histologically by acantholysis and epidermal hyperplasia
  - In contrast to pemphigus, Hailey-Hailey disease shows full-thickness acantholysis (dilapidated brick wall pattern)
  - Involvement of hair follicles is not present
- Grover disease (transient acantholytic dermatosis)
  - Presents clinically as a pruritic, papular, and papulovesicular eruption involving chest, back, and thighs of middle-aged and elderly patients
  - Acantholysis is limited to small foci as opposed to widespread acantholysis seen in pemphigus
  - Acantholysis can also show a histologic pattern similar to that seen in Darier disease and Hailey-Hailey disease; foci of spongiosis may be present
  - Presence of more than one pattern in a single specimen aids in the diagnosis
- Darier disease (keratosis follicularis)
  - Transmitted as an autosomal dominant trait
  - Presents as persistent, slowly progressive hyperkeratotic papules in a follicular distribution
  - Histologic features include suprabasal acantholysis with formation of clefts or lacunae and dyskeratosis resulting in formation of corps ronds and grains
  - Corps ronds and grains are helpful in distinguishing Darier disease from pemphigus
- Herpesvirus infection
  - Acantholytic pattern associated with necrotic keratinocytes
  - Presence of multinucleated cells with characteristic viral changes helps in the differential diagnosis
- Staphylococcal scalded skin syndrome
  - Few acantholytic cells may be present in staphylococcal scalded skin syndrome
  - A cleavage plane in the granular layer is helpful in the diagnosis

Pearls

- Pemphigus vegetans is a variant of pemphigus vulgaris in which the lesions heal with verrucous vegetations
- Immunofluorescence studies are critical in definite diagnosis of pemphigus
- Biopsy of perilesional skin or edge of the blister with surrounding intact skin should be done for best results

Selected References

Benchikhi H, Ghafour S, Disky A, et al: Pemphigus: Analysis of 262 cases. Int J Dermatol 47:973-975, 2008.

Nguyen VT, Ndoye A, Bassler KD, et al: Classification, clinical manifestations, and immunopathological mechanisms of the epithelial variant of paraneoplastic autoimmune multiorgan syndrome: A reappraisal of paraneoplastic pemphigus. Arch Dermatol 137:193-206, 2001.

Nousari HC, Anhalt GJ: Pemphigus and bullous pemphigoid. Lancet 354:667-672, 1999.

Robinson ND, Hashimoto T, Amagai M, Chan LS: The new pemphigus variants. J Am Acad Dermatol 40:649-671; quiz, 672-673, 1999.

Amagai M: Pemphigus: Autoimmunity to epidermal cell adhesion molecules. Adv Dermatol 11:319-352; discussion, 353, 1996.

Calvanico NJ, Robledo MA, Diaz LA: Immunopathology of pemphigus. J Autoimmun 4:3-16, 1991.

Korman NJ: Pemphigus. Dermatol Clin 8:689-700, 1990.

Singer KH, Hashimoto K, Jensen PJ, et al: Pathogenesis of autoimmunity in pemphigus. Ann Rev Immunol 3:87-108, 1985.

Bullous Pemphigoid

Clinical Features

- Bullous pemphigoid affects elderly patients and presents as large, tense bullae involving trunk, extremities, and intertriginous areas
- Nikolsky sign is negative
- Oral lesions are present in about one third of the patients

Histopathology

- *Subepidermal* vesicle often filled with eosinophils is the characteristic feature
- Superficial perivascular mixed inflammatory cell infiltrate rich in eosinophils
- In the cell-poor variant, only scant inflammatory cell infiltrate is present
- Early lesions may present with spongiosis and infiltrate of eosinophils (eosinophilic spongiosis)

Figure 2-38. Bullous pemphigoid. Histologic section shows subepidermal blister containing eosinophils and some neutrophils.

Special Stains and Immunohistochemistry

- Noncontributory

Other Techniques for Diagnosis

- Direct immunofluorescence studies show a linear deposition of C3 and IgG at the dermoepidermal junction
- Salt-split skin immunofluorescence shows that the pemphigoid antibodies are localized to the roof of the blister in most cases

Differential Diagnosis

▌ Herpes gestationis
- Presents as intensely pruritic lesions on the abdomen and extremities of pregnant women in second and third trimesters
- Histologic changes and immunofluorescence findings may be distinguishable from bullous pemphigoid
- However, in herpes gestationis, more neutrophils and basal cell necrosis may be seen
- Clinical information is invaluable

▌ Epidermolysis bullosa acquisita
- Presents as blisters developing on acral areas that heal with scarring
- Histologic and immunofluorescence changes may be identical to that of bullous pemphigoid
- Eosinophils are fewer in number, and lymphocytes and neutrophils may predominate
- Immunofluorescence of salt-split skin shows the localization of IgG antibodies to the floor of the blister

▌ Porphyria cutanea tarda
- Subepidermal blister with minimal inflammatory cell infiltrate
- The dermal papillae extend into the blister cavity with a festooning appearance
- PAS-positive eosinophilic deposits around the blood vessels of the papillary dermis are characteristic

Pearls

- Cicatricial pemphigoid (benign mucosal pemphigoid) typically presents as blisters involving mucous membranes that erode, ulcerate, and heal with scarring
- Mucous membranes of mouth, conjunctiva larynx, nose, and anus can be affected

Selected References

Olasz EB, Yancey KB: Bullous pemphigoid and related subepidermal autoimmune blistering diseases. Curr Dir Autoimmun 10:141-166, 2008.

Engineer L, Bhol K, Ahmed AR: Pemphigoid gestationis: A review. Am J Obstet Gynecol 183:483-491, 2000.

Nousari HC, Anhalt GJ: Pemphigus and bullous pemphigoid. Lancet 354:667-672, 1999.

Dabelsteen E: Molecular biological aspects of acquired bullous diseases. Crit Rev Oral Biol Med 9:162-178, 1998.

Korman NJ: Bullous pemphigoid. Dermatol Clin 11:483-498, 1993.

Gammon WR, Kowalewski C, Chorzelski TP, et al: Direct immunofluorescence studies of sodium chloride-separated skin in the differential diagnosis of bullous pemphigoid and epidermolysis bullosa acquisita. J Am Acad Dermatol 22:664, 1990.

Dermatitis Herpetiformis

Clinical Features

- Young to middle-aged males are usually affected
- Lesions are pruritic, symmetrical, grouped papulovesicles involving elbows, knees, back, buttocks, and scalp

Histopathology

- *Subepidermal* bullae filled with neutrophils and varying numbers of eosinophils characterize a fully evolved vesicle
- Neutrophilic aggregates (microabscesses) are present at the tips of the dermal papillae, at the edge of the blister, and in papular lesions
- Moderate amount of superficial perivascular lymphocytic, neutrophilic, and eosinophilic infiltrate may be present in the dermis

Special Stains and Immunohistochemistry

- Noncontributory

Other Techniques for Diagnosis

- Direct immunofluorescence studies show granular deposits of IgA within the dermal papillae of normal skin and lesional skin

Figure 2-39. Dermatitis herpetiformis. Histologic section shows separation at the dermoepidermal junction associated with aggregates of neutrophils, especially at the tips of the dermal papillae (papillary microabscesses).

- Circulating antibodies against reticulin, smooth muscle endomysium, and dietary antigen gluten may be detected

Differential Diagnosis

▌ Linear IgA dermatosis
- Can be indistinguishable from dermatitis herpetiformis on histology
- However, in linear IgA dermatosis, the neutrophils are often seen in a linear array at the dermoepidermal junction
- Direct immunofluorescence shows a linear pattern of IgA deposition at basement membrane zone

▌ Bullous systemic lupus erythematosus
- Shares histologic features with dermatitis herpetiformis and linear IgA dermatosis
- Immunofluorescence findings of granular bandlike deposits of IgG and C3 at basement membrane zone are characteristic of bullous systemic lupus erythematosus

Pearls

- Dermatitis herpetiformis is associated with gluten-sensitive enteropathy and shows celiac sprue–like changes on jejunal biopsy
- High frequency of HLA-BR, -DR3, and -Dqw2 is seen in patients with dermatitis herpetiformis

Selected References

Scott JE, Ahmed AR: The blistering diseases. Med Clin N Am 82:1239-1283, 1998.

Malmusi M, Manca V, Girolomoni G: Coexistence of dermatitis herpetiformis, gluten-sensitive enteropathy, and ulcerative colitis. J Am Acad Dermatol 31:1050-1051, 1994.

Ahmed AR, Hameed A: Bullous pemphigoid and dermatitis herpetiformis. Clin Dermatol 11:47-52, 1993.

Smith EP, Zone JJ: Dermatitis herpetiformis and linear IgA bullous dermatosis. Dermatol Clin 11:511-526, 1993.

Folliculitis

Acne Vulgaris

Clinical Features

- Common disease of adolescents and young adults
- Manifests as open and closed comedones and inflammatory nodules on the face and anterior and posterior trunk
- Nodulocystic acne and acne conglobata are severe expressions of acne vulgaris

Histopathology

- Comedones show dilated follicular infundibulum that is plugged by keratin, lipid, and microorganisms

Figure 2-40. A, Acne vulgaris. Histologic section shows a disrupted follicle and neutrophilic infiltrate. **B, Majocchi granuloma.** Periodic acid–Schiff stain shows fungal forms in the hair shaft of an inflamed follicle.

- Rupture of the follicular wall results in an intense inflammatory reaction with neutrophils in the early stages and foreign-body–type granulomatous reaction in later stages
- Healing takes place by scarring

Special Stains and Immunohistochemistry

- PAS and GMS stains are helpful in excluding infectious etiology

Other Techniques for Diagnosis

- Noncontributory

Differential Diagnosis

▌ Histologic differential diagnoses of folliculitis and perifolliculitis include various infectious processes such as herpesvirus infection and fungal infection
- Multinucleated cells with viral inclusion are present in the follicular epithelium in herpesvirus folliculitis
- GMS and PAS stains are helpful to rule out fungal infection involving follicles

■ Granulomatous rosacea
  ● Has granulomatous perifollicular inflammation
■ Eosinophilic pustular folliculitis
  ● Generally seen in infants and in association with immunocompromised states
  ● Can be differentiated by the presence of spongiosis with eosinophils, subcorneal pustule with eosinophils, and perifollicular infiltrate rich in eosinophils
■ Majocchi granuloma
  ● Nodular folliculitis and perifolliculitis caused by *Trichophyton rubrum*
  ● PAS stain demonstrates spores and hyphae within hairs and hair follicles and in the dermal inflammatory cell infiltrate

Pearls

  ● Follicular occlusion triad—which includes hidradenitis suppurativa, acne conglobata, and perifolliculitis capitis abscedens et suffodiens—represents a chronic, deep-seated folliculitis resulting in abscesses and sinus tract formation that heals with scarring
  ● Folliculitis barbae, folliculitis decalvans, and folliculitis keloidalis nuchae represent types of chronic deep folliculitis that heal with scarring

Selected References

Brown SK, Shalita AR: Acne vulgaris. Lancet 351:1871-1876, 1998.

Cunliffe WJ, Holland DB, Clark SM, Stables GI: Comedogenesis: Some new aetiological, clinical and therapeutic strategies. Br J Dermatol 142:1084-1091, 2000.

Goodman GJ: Postacne scarring: A review of its pathophysiology and treatment. Dermatol Surg 26:857-871, 2000.

White GM: Recent findings in the epidemiologic evidence, classification, and subtypes of acne vulgaris. J Am Acad Dermatol 39:S34-37, 1998.

Rothman KF, Lucky AW: Acne vulgaris. Adv Dermatol 8:347-374, 1993.

Fibrosing Dermatoses

Morphea and Scleroderma

Clinical Features

  ● Scleroderma is a connective tissue disease of unknown etiology characterized by thickening and sclerosis of skin
  ● Morphea is the cutaneous form of scleroderma without associated systemic involvement; lesions can be plaquelike, linear, segmental, or generalized
  ● Lesions are round to oval, indurated with a smooth surface, and ivory colored; a violaceous border may be present
  ● Morphea presents with generally more circumscribed and well-demarcated lesions than systemic scleroderma

Figure 2-41. Morphea. A, Low-power view shows marked thickening of the dermis with sclerotic bands of collagen extending into the subcutaneous fat. **B,** High-power view shows sclerotic collagen extending into the subcutaneous fat associated with lymphocytic inflammation.

  ● Sites of predilection include face, distal extremities, and trunk

Histopathology

  ● Biopsies of early inflammatory lesions representing the violaceous border of actively enlarging lesions show a perivascular and interstitial infiltrate of lymphocytes and plasma cells associated with thickening of collagen bundles in the reticular dermis
  ● Septa in the subcutaneous fat show marked thickening and inflammatory cell infiltrate; newly formed collagen is seen as fine wavy fibers

- Fully evolved sclerotic lesions show closely packed collagen bundles in the reticular dermis with only minimal inflammatory cell infiltrate
- Eccrine glands appear atrophic and are placed higher in the dermis; there is progressive sclerotic destruction of capillaries and adnexal structures
- Underlying fascia and occasionally skeletal muscle tissue may also show fibrosis and sclerosis

Special Stains and Immunohistochemistry

- Noncontributory

Other Techniques for Diagnosis

- Up to 90% of patients with systemic scleroderma and 50% with localized scleroderma have a positive antinuclear antibody (ANA) test
- More than 90% have anticentromere antibody, which correlates with morphea or CREST (calcinosis cutis, Raynaud phenomenon, esophageal dysfunction, sclerodactyly, and telangiectasia) syndrome (associated with a better prognosis)
- About 20% to 40% have antibodies to Scl 70 (antitopoisomerase), which correlates with systemic sclerosis

Differential Diagnosis

▌ Scleredema
- Presents as diffuse, nonpitting swelling and induration of skin and shows clinical and histologic similarities to scleroderma
- Collagen bundles may be thickened but are not hyalinized
- Widened spaces between collagen bundles are present
- Special stains can be used to demonstrate the presence of hyaluronic acid in these spaces

▌ Lichen sclerosus
- Indistinguishable from lichen sclerosus and perhaps represent a spectrum of the same pathologic process
- Presence of epidermal atrophy, follicular plugging, vacuolar change of basal cell layer, and edema of papillary dermis and absence of elastic fibers in the sclerotic areas favors a diagnosis of lichen sclerosus

▌ Chronic radiation dermatitis
- Dermal collagen bundles are swollen and often hyalinized, showing some similarities to morphea
- Epidermal atrophy, large bizarre fibroblasts with pleomorphic nuclei, inflammation, and telangiectasia in the superficial dermis occur
- Additionally, fibrous thickening of the blood vessels, especially of the deep dermis, is seen

▌ Nephrogenic systemic fibrosis
- Systemic disorder seen in patients with renal impairment and characterized by thickening of skin of trunk and extremities

- Histologic sections show thickened collagen bundles and spindled fibroblasts that extend into subcutaneous septae and subjacent fascia
- Immunohistochemical studies show the spindled cells to be CD34 positive
- Differentiation from scleroderma and other fibrosing dermatitis may require clinical and laboratory evidence of renal impairment

Pearls

- A subset of scleroderma known as *CREST syndrome* presents with Raynaud phenomenon in all affected patients; the manifestations include calcinosis cutis, Raynaud phenomenon, esophageal involvement, sclerodactyly, and telangiectasis
- Eosinophilic fasciitis (Shulman syndrome) is a disorder characterized by involvement of deep fascia by sclerosis and eosinophilic infiltrate and most likely represents a deep form of morphea

Selected References

Morcos SK, Thomsen HS: Nephrogenic systemic fibrosis: More questions and some answers. Nephron Clin Pract 110:c24-31, 2008.

Zulian F: New developments in localized scleroderma. Curr Opin Rheumatol 20:601-607, 2008.

Cowper SE, Boyer PJ: Nephrogenic systemic fibrosis: An update. Curr Rheumatol Rep 8:151-157, 2006.

Mitchell H, Bolster MB, LeRoy EC: Scleroderma and related conditions. Med Clin N Am 81:129-149, 1997.

Uziel Y, Miller ML, Laxer RM: Scleroderma in children. Pediatr Clin N Am 42:1171-1203, 1995.

Wigley FM: Clinical aspects of systemic and localized scleroderma. Curr Opin Rheumatol 6:628-636, 1994.

Uitto J, Santa Cruz DJ, Bauer EA, et al: Morphea and lichen sclerosus et atrophicus: Clinical and histopathologic studies in patients with combined features. J Am Acad Dermatol 3:271, 1980.

Panniculitis

Erythema Nodosum

Clinical Features

- Acute form generally presents with sudden onset of symmetrical, tender, erythematous subcutaneous nodules on the extensor aspects of lower legs
- Associated fever, malaise, and arthropathy may be present
- Chronic form, also known as *erythema nodosum migrans*, presents as unilateral nodules on lower legs

Histopathology

- A granulomatous fibrosing septal panniculitis is the characteristic finding

Figure 2-42. Erythema nodosum. A, Low-power view shows a predominantly septal involvement by a fibrosing process. **B,** High-power view shows broadening of the septa of the subcutaneous fat by fibrosis and granulomatous inflammation.

- Early lesions are characterized by a mixed inflammatory cell infiltrate of lymphocytes, eosinophils, and neutrophils, more intense at the periphery of the lobule
- Later lesions show widening of the septa with increasing number of macrophages in the infiltrate; well-formed granulomas are often in the septa; this feature is more prominent in late stages of acute erythema nodosum and chronic erythema nodosum

Special Stains and Immunohistochemistry

- Special stains and microbiologic cultures to exclude an infectious etiology

Other Techniques for Diagnosis

- Noncontributory

Differential Diagnosis

▪ Erythema induratum and nodular vasculitis
  - A mixed lobular and septal pattern of inflammation
  - Vasculitis and zones of fat necrosis

▪ Subcutaneous sarcoidosis
  - Noncaseating granulomas in the overlying dermis in addition to those in the subcutaneous fat help in differentiating sarcoidosis from erythema nodosum
▪ Infectious panniculitis
  - Presence of neutrophilic infiltrate and granuloma formation should raise the possibility of an underlying infection, in particular subcutaneous tuberculosis
  - Special stains and cultures are necessary

Pearls

- Streptococcal infection is the most common among the known causes of erythema nodosum
- Crohn disease and sarcoidosis are known to be associated with erythema nodosum

Selected References

Requena L, Sanchez Yus E: Panniculitis. Part I. Mostly septal panniculitis. J Am Acad Dermatol 45:163-183, 2001.

White WL, Hitchcock MG: Diagnosis: Erythema nodosum or not? Semin Cutan Med Surg 18:47-55, 1999.

Cribier B, Caille A, Heid E, Grosshans E: Erythema nodosum and associated diseases: A study of 129 cases. Int J Dermatol 37:667-672, 1998.

Meyerson MS: Erythema nodosum leprosum. Int J Dermatol 35:389-392, 1996.

Hannuksela M: Erythema nodosum. Clin Dermatol 4:88-95, 1986.

Subcutaneous Fat Necrosis of the Newborn

Clinical Features

- Uncommon, painless, self-limited disease that affects full-term and post-term infants
- Presents at 1 to 6 weeks of age as asymptomatic, firm nodules on cheeks, shoulders, back, buttocks, and thighs

Histopathology

- Predominantly lobular pattern of inflammation with foci of fat necrosis, surrounded by macrophages and multinucleated giant cells
- Cytoplasm of the macrophages and giant cells contains needle-shaped crystals of lipid arranged in radial array
- Deposits of calcium may be seen

Special Stains and Immunohistochemistry

- Noncontributory

Other Techniques for Diagnosis

- Noncontributory

Figure 2-43. Subcutaneous fat necrosis. A, Low-power view shows a predominantly lobular pattern of inflammation. **B,** High-power view shows the lobules containing areas of fat necrosis and a moderately dense mixed inflammatory cell infiltrate, including lymphocytes and histiocytes. Multinucleated histiocytes containing needle-shaped crystals in radial array are a characteristic finding.

Differential Diagnosis

▌ Sclerema neonatorum
- Usually affects premature, ill newborns
- Presents as rapidly spreading diffuse hardening of subcutaneous tissue of back, shoulders, and buttocks
- Lobular pattern of panniculitis with cells containing needle-shaped crystals arranged in radial array similar to subcutaneous fat necrosis
- Minimal to absent inflammation in the background in sclerema neonatorum is helpful in the differential diagnosis

▌ Poststeroid panniculitis
- May show similar changes with needle-shaped crystals in fat cells
- Clinical history of steroid treatment is essential

▌ Pancreatic fat necrosis
- Can present as lobular panniculitis; however, foci of fat necrosis are associated with ghostlike fat cells with thick borders
- Crystals in radial array are not a feature

▌ Lipodystrophy
- Lobular panniculitis with predominantly histiocytic infiltrate
- No needle-shaped clefts in the histiocytes

Pearls
- Subcutaneous fat necrosis is a self-limited disease of unknown etiology

Selected References

Requena L, Sanchez Yus E: Panniculitis. Part II. Mostly lobular panniculitis. J Am Acad Dermatol 45:325-361, 2001.

Higgins E, Ive FA: Subcutaneous fat necrosis in pancreatic disease. Br J Surg 77:532-533, 1990.

Salas Valien JS, Ribas Arino MT, Egido Romo M, Palau Benavides MT: Subcutaneous fat necrosis of newborn children. Histol Histopathol 5:1-5, 1990.

Friedman SJ, Winkelmann RK: Subcutaneous fat necrosis of the newborn: Light, ultrastructural and histochemical microscopic studies. J Cutan Pathol 16:99-105, 1989.

Katz DA, Huerter C, Bogard P, Braddock SW: Subcutaneous fat necrosis of the newborn. Arch Dermatol 120:1517-1518, 1984.

Horsfield GI, Yardley HJ: Sclerema neonatorum. J Invest Dermatol 44:326-332, 1965.

Cysts, Proliferations, and Neoplasms

Cysts

Epidermal Inclusion Cyst (Infundibular Cyst)

Clinical Features
- Typically results from progressive cystic ectasia of the infundibulum of the hair follicle following mechanical occlusion of the orifice
- Predilection for the head, neck, and trunk
- One or more freely movable, dermal, skin-colored, firm nodules less than 5 cm in diameter

Histopathology
- Rounded dermal cyst filled with laminated keratin that tends to fall out during processing of tissue
- Cyst lining resembles epidermis or infundibular epithelium with prominent granular layer
- Rupture of the cyst into the dermis produces a granulomatous reaction with foreign-body giant cells
- Pseudocarcinomatous hyperplasia may ensue from the remnants of the cyst wall, which can be mistaken for SCC

Special Stains and Immunohistochemistry
- Noncontributory

Other Techniques for Diagnosis
- Noncontributory

Figure 2-44. A, Epidermal inclusion cyst. Histologic section shows a cyst filled with laminated keratin and lined by stratified squamous epithelium with granular layer. **B, Trichilemmal cyst.** The presence of compact keratin in the lumen of this cyst lined by stratified squamous epithelium with no granular layer distinguishes it from an epidermal inclusion cyst. **C, Hidrocystoma.** This cyst, lined by only two layers of cells, an inner luminal row with decapitation secretion and outer myoepithelial cells, is easily differentiated from epidermal inclusion cyst. The cyst lumen contains secretions rather than the laminated keratin seen in epidermal inclusion cyst. **D, Steatocystoma.** The thin epithelial lining of this cyst is covered by an undulating keratin layer.

Differential Diagnosis

▪ Trichilemmal cyst
  - Benign cyst occurring most commonly on the scalp as multiple cystic nodules
  - Cyst contents consist of compact keratin, and the lining resembles the isthmus of hair follicle; abrupt keratinization with absent granular layer is characteristic
  - Calcifications are frequently found
  - Proliferating trichilemmal cystic neoplasm: a low-grade neoplasm characterized by lobules of eosinophilic epithelial cells (isthmic) and infiltrative growth pattern
▪ Steatocystoma
  - Most commonly occurs as multiple nodules on presternal skin, upper arms, axillae, and scrotum; inherited in an autosomal dominant pattern
  - Occasionally may be seen in solitary form
  - Sections show a collapsed cystic space in the dermis lined by squamous epithelium, with the innermost layer composed of homogeneous keratin with an undulating or crenulated appearance
  - Mature sebaceous lobules are present in the vicinity, and hair shafts may be seen in the lumen
▪ Dermoid cyst
  - Usually present at birth
  - Occurs most commonly on the head around the eyes as a result of sequestration of skin along lines of closure
  - Cyst lining is composed of epidermis with associated mature adnexal structures; hair follicles contain hair shafts that project into the lumen

▌ Hidrocystoma
  ● Usually occurs as a translucent nodule with a bluish
    hue on the face
  ● Lining is composed of a row of secretory cells
    surrounded by elongated myoepithelial cells
  ● "Decapitation" secretions when present point
    toward the apocrine nature of the cyst (apocrine
    hidrocystoma)
  ● In contrast, in eccrine hidrocystoma, myoepithelial
    cells and decapitation secretions are not
    apparent
▌ Infectious granuloma
  ● Granulomatous reaction surrounding a ruptured
    epidermal inclusion cyst may raise the possibility of
    an infectious process
  ● Gram and PAS stains may be necessary to
    demonstrate the organisms

Pearls

  ● Incomplete excision often leads to recurrences
  ● Multiple epidermal inclusion cysts occur on
    the face and scalp in patients with Gardner
    syndrome

Selected References

Pariser RJ: Benign neoplasms of the skin. Med Clin N Am
    82:1285-1307, 1998.
Vicente J, Vazquez-Doval FJ: Proliferations of the epidermoid cyst
    wall. Int J Dermatol 37:181-185, 1998.
Perniciaro C: Gardner's syndrome. Dermatol Clin 13:51-56,
    1995.

Epidermal Proliferations and Neoplasms

Seborrheic Keratosis

Clinical Features

  ● Occurs characteristically in middle-aged and elderly
    individuals
  ● Predilection for the trunk with common involvement
    of the extremities, head, and neck
  ● Round, variably sized plaques with stuck-on
    appearance
  ● Plaques are usually tan to dark brown
  ● Small, porelike ostia impacted with keratin

Histopathology

  ● Hyperkeratosis
  ● Proliferation of uniform squamous and basaloid cells
    in the epidermis
  ● Presence of keratin-filled cysts (horn cysts) that
    occasionally communicate with the overlying skin
    (pseudohorn cysts)
  ● Other histologic variants include adenoid, reticulated,
    clonal, and inverted follicular keratosis types

Figure 2-45. Seborrheic keratosis. Histologic section shows an
epidermal proliferation composed of monomorphous keratinocytes.
Laminated hyperkeratosis and pseudohorn cysts are characteristic
features.

Special Stains and Immunohistochemistry

  ● Noncontributory

Other Techniques for Diagnosis

  ● Noncontributory

Differential Diagnosis

▌ Epidermal nevus and acanthosis nigricans
  ● May be indistinguishable from seborrheic keratosis on
    histologic grounds alone
▌ Verruca vulgaris
  ● Papillomatous changes in seborrheic keratosis can
    resemble a verruca vulgaris
  ● In verruca, the tips of the papillae are covered by
    columns of parakeratosis, often with hemorrhages in
    the cornified layer
▌ Clonal pattern of seborrheic keratosis can
  mimic an intraepidermal poroma or even
  Bowen disease; however, cytologic atypia,
  dyskeratosis, and mitotic figures are absent in
  seborrheic keratosis
▌ SCC
  ● Irritated or inverted follicular keratosis variant has
    scattered "squamous eddies" that may resemble
    keratin pearls of SCC; however, squamous eddies are
    simply whorls of keratinocytes and do not contain
    central parakeratosis, which is characteristic of
    keratin pearls

Pearls

  ● Sign of Leser-Trélat: sudden onset of hundreds of
    seborrheic keratoses related to internal malignancy
  ● Dermatosis papulosa nigra: multiple lesions appearing
    on the face of patients of African descent with
    histologic features identical to those of seborrheic
    keratosis

Selected References

Soyer HP, Kenet RO, Wolf IH, et al: Clinicopathological correlation of pigmented skin lesions using dermoscopy. Eur J Dermatol 10:22-28, 2000.

Toussaint S, Salcedo E, Kamino H: Benign epidermal proliferations. Adv Dermatol 14:307-357, 1999.

Eads TJ, Hood AF, Chuang TY, et al: The diagnostic yield of histologic examination of seborrheic keratoses. Arch Dermatol 133:1417-1420, 1997.

Schwartz RA: Sign of Leser-Trélat. J Am Acad Dermatol 35:88-95, 1996.

Clear Cell Acanthoma

Clinical Features

- Commonly affects middle-aged and older individuals
- Predilection for lower extremities
- Lesions grow slowly but frequently ulcerate and have an oozing, erythematous surface
- Small (<2 cm), solitary nodule or plaque that is sharply delineated

Histopathology

- Overlying parakeratotic cornified layer, often containing neutrophils
- Abrupt intraepidermal proliferation of squamoid cells with pale to clear cytoplasm
- Elongated rete ridges with well-vascularized dermal papillae
- Presence of neutrophils within intercellular spaces of the involved epidermis
- Decreased or absent melanin in affected cells

Figure 2-46. **Clear cell acanthoma.** Histologic section shows a sharply demarcated epidermal proliferation composed of keratinocytes with pale cytoplasm. Parakeratosis and neutrophils in the parakeratosis and among the clear cells are typical findings.

Special Stains and Immunohistochemistry

- PAS stain highlights the presence of abundant glycogen in the pale cells

Other Techniques for Diagnosis

- Noncontributory

Differential Diagnosis

- Eccrine poroma
  - Sheetlike down-growth of monomorphous epithelial cells
  - Keratinization and early erosion and ulceration present on the surface of epidermis
  - Richly vascular stroma with dilated, tortuous vessels
  - Small foci of spiraling cuboidal cells lining eccrine ducts may be present in epithelium
- Psoriasis
  - Parakeratosis with neutrophils associated with regular epidermal hyperplasia
  - Cytoplasm of the keratinocytes is not pale or clear

Pearls

- Clinically, clear cell acanthomas appear stuck on like seborrheic keratosis and vascular similar to pyogenic granuloma

Selected References

Toussaint S, Salcedo E, Kamino H: Benign epidermal proliferations. Adv Dermatol 14:307-357, 1999.

Pariser RJ: Benign neoplasms of the skin. Med Clin N Am 82:1285-1307, v-vi, 1998.

Langer K, Wuketich S, Konrad K: Pigmented clear cell acanthoma. Am J Dermatopathol 16:134-139, 1994.

Brownstein MH: The benign acanthomas. J Cutan Pathol 12:172-188, 1985.

Verrucae (Verruca Vulgaris, Plantar Warts, Verruca Plana)

Clinical Features

- Benign epidermal proliferation due to infection with varying strains of human papillomavirus (HPV)
- Verruca vulgaris
  - Associated with HPV-1, -2, -4, -7, -49
  - Most common type of wart
  - Predilection for the dorsal aspect of the hands and feet
  - Circumscribed, papillomatous, flesh-colored nodules
- Palmoplantar warts
  - Associated with HPV-1, -2, -3, -4, -27, -29, -57
  - Predilection for the palms and soles of feet, especially near points of pressure
  - Usually painful and surrounded by a thick reactive callus
  - Hyperkeratotic nodules appearing on the dorsum of the foot surrounded by a thick reactive callus

Figure 2-47. Verruca vulgaris. Histologic section shows papillomatous proliferation of epidermal keratinocytes covered by parakeratosis. Hypergranulosis, presence of vacuolated keratinocytes (koilocytes), and dilated blood vessels in the papillary dermis are additional findings.

▌ Verruca plana
- Associated with HPV-3, -10, -28, -49
- Predilection for the face, larynx, and dorsal aspect of the hands
- Multiple, flesh-colored papules
- Typically distributed in a linear fashion

Histopathology
▌ Verruca vulgaris
- Flame-shaped tongues of epidermis with overlying hyperkeratosis and parakeratosis
- Epithelial cells contain enlarged coarse keratohyalin granules, cytoplasmic pallor, and clearing
- HPV particles cause nuclear pallor and dispersion of chromatin, imparting a steel-gray appearance

▌ Palmoplantar warts
- Endophytic epithelial down-growths covered with dense hyperkeratotic and parakeratotic scale
- Epithelial cells with changes similar to those found in verruca vulgaris
- Uppermost viable epithelial cells also contain irregular eosinophilic cytoplasmic inclusions

▌ Verruca plana
- Multiple blunt epidermal papillae with parakeratosis and minimal hyperkeratosis
- Epithelial cells with changes similar to those found in verruca vulgaris

Special Stains and Immunohistochemistry
- Noncontributory

Other Techniques for Diagnosis
- PCR and ISH techniques may be used to type the HPV

Differential Diagnosis
▌ Molluscum contagiosum
- Cytoplasmic inclusions are typically round to ovoid and eosinophilic
▌ Epidermodysplasia verruciformis
- Shows histologic changes similar to verruca plana
▌ Keratoacanthoma
- Typically has a central crater filled with cornified material
- Large keratinocytes with abundant glassy cytoplasm
- Neutrophilic microabscesses within the epithelial nests

Pearls
- Verrucous carcinoma may be included in the differential diagnosis of single large lesions involving the plantar aspect of foot; a superficial biopsy may show changes indistinguishable from verruca plantaris (clinical suspicion and a deep biopsy are critical in arriving at correct diagnosis)

Selected References
Xu X, Erickson L, Chen L, Elder D: Diseases caused by viruses. In Elder DE, Elenitsas R, Johnson BL Jr, et al (eds): Lever's Histopathology of Skin, 10th ed. Philadelphia, Lippincott Williams & Wilkins, 2008, p 637.

Brentjens MH, Yeung-Yue KA, Lee PC, et al: Human papillomavirus: A review. Dermatol Clin 20:315, 2002.

Beutner KR: Nongenital human papillomavirus infections. Clin Lab Med 20:423-430, 2000.

Carr J, Gyorfi T: Human papillomavirus: Epidemiology, transmission, and pathogenesis. Clin Lab Med 20:235-255, 2000.

Nuovo GJ, Ishag M: The histologic spectrum of epidermodysplasia verruciformis. Am J Surg Pathol 24:1400, 2000.

Tyring SK: Human papillomavirus infections: Epidemiology, pathogenesis, and host immune response. J Am Acad Dermatol 43:S18-26, 2000.

Actinic Keratosis

Clinical Features
- Lesions typically affect middle-aged to older patients
- Predilection for sun-exposed skin of individuals with light skin color
- Lesions are typically multiple and present as small (<1 cm), erythematous papules with adherent scale; occasionally pigmented

Histopathology
- Alternating columns of orthokeratosis and parakeratosis
- Orthokeratotic sparing corresponds to the opening of follicular infundibula
- Budding of basal cell epithelium and keratinocytic atypia

Figure 2-48. Actinic keratosis. Histologic section shows areas of parakeratosis associated with hypogranulosis that spares the openings of the adnexal structures. Budding of the basal cells, keratinocytic atypia, and solar elastosis are present.

Special Stains and Immunohistochemistry

- Noncontributory

Other Techniques for Diagnosis

- Noncontributory

Differential Diagnosis

▮ SCC in situ
- Confluent parakeratosis with no intervening areas of orthokeratosis
- Full-thickness keratinocytic atypia with complete lack of maturation

Pearls

- Actinic cheilitis: actinic keratosis of the vermillion border of the lower lip presenting as zones of discoloration and pallor
- Actinic keratosis can progress into SCC and may represent an incipient SCC

Selected References

Cockerell CJ: Histopathology of incipient intraepidermal squamous cell carcinoma ("actinic keratosis"). J Am Acad Dermatol 42:11-17, 2000.

Cohn BA: From sunlight to actinic keratosis to squamous cell carcinoma. J Am Acad Dermatol 42:143-144, 2000.

Schwartz RA: The actinic keratosis: A perspective and update. Dermatol Surg 23:1009-1019; quiz, 1020-1021, 1997.

Squamous Cell Carcinoma

Clinical Features

- Malignant epithelial tumor of the epidermal keratinocytes
- Commonly affects men older than 60 years old

- Risk factors include solar irradiation, radiation therapy, local carcinogens such as tars and oils, and hereditary diseases such as xeroderma pigmentosa and albinism
- Tumors typically favor sun-exposed areas, including the upper face, ears, lower lip, and dorsum of hands
- Generally presents as solitary, slowly enlarging, indurated nodule that may develop central ulceration
- Variations include verrucous, papillary, and acantholytic forms

Histopathology

- Moderate and confluent parakeratosis
- Epidermal proliferation with full-thickness cytologic atypia, keratin pearl formation, and zones of necrosis
- Neoplastic cells are characterized by moderate amounts of eosinophilic cytoplasm, nuclear enlargement, and hyperchromasia
- Lower part of the neoplasm may show an infiltrative pattern; perineural invasion may be present in deeply invasive neoplasms
- Acantholytic pattern seen in some examples
- Degree of differentiation is generally assessed by the degree of keratin pearl formation

Special Stains and Immunohistochemistry

- Cytokeratin positivity is useful in differentiating poorly differentiated SCC from other neoplasms

Other Techniques for Diagnosis

- Noncontributory

Differential Diagnosis

▮ Bowen disease
- Variant of SCC in situ occurring on sun-exposed and non–sun-exposed skin
- Histologic changes include confluent parakeratosis and marked atypia of the epidermal keratinocytes with frequent mitoses and dyskeratotic cells
- Bowenoid papulosis is a clinical entity characterized by multiple papules in the genital area but histologically indistinguishable from Bowen disease

▮ Keratoacanthoma
- Best regarded as a variant of well-differentiated SCC with a potential for spontaneous regression
- Presents as symmetrical cup-shaped lesions filled with orthokeratotic cornified layer and surrounded by lips of epidermal proliferation
- Epithelial cells typically contain abundant glassy eosinophilic cytoplasm and only mild cytologic atypia
- Neutrophilic microabscesses are a characteristic feature

▮ Verrucous carcinoma
- Plantar verrucous carcinoma can be easily misdiagnosed as verruca if the biopsy is superficial
- Surface shows hyperkeratosis, parakeratosis, and epidermal hyperplasia

Figure 2-49. A, Squamous cell carcinoma. Histologic section shows an irregular proliferation of atypical keratinocytes. Acantholytic pattern is present. Keratin pearls composed of parakeratosis surrounded by atypical keratinocytes are characteristically seen in well-differentiated and moderately differentiated squamous cell carcinoma. **B, Keratoacanthoma.** The characteristic architecture of this exoendophytic neoplasm with a central cup-shaped crater surrounded by proliferation of large keratinocytes with abundant glassy cytoplasm and minimal cytologic atypia differentiates this form of squamous cell carcinoma from the conventional squamous cell carcinoma. Neutrophilic microabscesses may be seen at the base of the neoplasm. **C, Bowen disease.** There is confluent parakeratosis and increased thickness of epidermis. The epidermis contains atypical keratinocytes with pleomorphic nuclei, dyskeratotic cells, and frequent mitotic figures above the basal cell layer. The changes are confined to the epidermis, and therefore this lesion is considered a form of squamous cell carcinoma in situ. **D, Verrucous carcinoma.** The epidermal proliferation shows tunnel-like invaginations filled with parakeratosis. The neoplasm infiltrates as bulbous expansions of the rete.

- Deeper biopsy shows broad bands of epidermal proliferation filled with parakeratotic centers; the bases of the proliferation are large and bulbous and invade the deep dermis in a pushing manner
▪ Spindle cell SCC versus atypical fibroxanthoma
  - Presence of intercellular bridges in SCC
  - Cytokeratin positivity in SCC
▪ Inverted follicular keratosis
  - Shows features of an irritated seborrheic keratosis or verruca with squamous eddies
  - No keratin pearls
▪ Pseudocarcinomatous epidermal hyperplasia
  - Occurs most often at the edges of ulcers, deep fungal infections, pyodermas, and other proliferative inflammatory processes

- Presence of granulomas and neutrophilic microabscesses suggests an inflammatory process

Pearls

- *Marjolin ulcer* refers to SCC arising at the periphery of an ulcer or scar
- SCC arising on sun-damaged skin has low potential for metastasis

Selected References

Brand D, Ackerman AB: Squamous cell carcinoma, not basal cell carcinoma, is the most common cancer in humans. J Am Acad Dermatol 42:523-526, 2000.

Salasche SJ: Epidemiology of actinic keratoses and squamous cell carcinoma. J Am Acad Dermatol 42:4-7, 2000.

Roth JJ, Granick MS: Squamous cell and adnexal carcinomas of the skin. Clin Plast Surg 24:687-703, 1997.

Maguire B, Smith NP: Histopathology of cutaneous squamous cell carcinoma. Clin Dermatol 13:559-568, 1995.

Haydon RC 3rd: Cutaneous squamous carcinoma and related lesions. Otolaryngol Clin N Am 26:57-71, 1993.

Follicular Neoplasms

Trichoepithelioma

Clinical Features

- Trichoepithelioma can occur in either a solitary or multiple form
- Solitary lesions frequently affect adults and have a predilection for the face
- Multiple lesions often present during childhood, with a predilection for the upper trunk, neck, scalp, and face, especially the nasolabial folds and preauricular regions; transmitted as an autosomal dominant trait

Figure 2-50. **Trichoepithelioma. A,** Low-power view shows a well-circumscribed dermal proliferation of basaloid cells embedded in a cellular stroma and containing keratinous cysts. **B,** High-power view shows follicular differentiation in the form of bulbs and papillae.

- Solitary lesions appear as pale, small to medium (<2 cm), skin-colored papules
- Multiple lesions appear as small (<1 cm), flesh-colored papules

Histopathology

- Well-circumscribed, symmetrical lesion composed of basaloid and eosinophilic cells in small or large nodules within a variably cellular stroma; they may also show retiform or cribriform patterns
- Basaloid cells are encircled by fibroblasts resembling follicular germs and bulbs with associated papillae (signs of follicular differentiation)
- Retraction artifacts, if present, are within the fibrotic stroma rather than around the basaloid cells
- Multiple infundibulocystic structures filled with keratin are present within the epithelial islands

Special Stains and Immunohistochemistry

- Noncontributory

Other Techniques for Diagnosis

- Noncontributory

Differential Diagnosis

- Basal cell carcinoma (BCC)
  - Multiple nests of basaloid cells that emanate from the undersurface of the epidermis
  - Nests show peripheral palisading and presence of a mucinous stroma with retraction artifacts
  - Immunohistochemistry: CD10 is positive in the stromal cells but not the epithelial cells in trichoepithelium and is positive in the epithelial cells of BCC
- Syringoma
  - Contains ductal structures filled with proteinaceous material
- Microcystic adnexal carcinoma (sclerosing sweat duct carcinoma)
  - Extends deep into the dermis with neoplastic nests getting smaller toward the base
  - Keratin-filled cysts and ductal structures are present
  - Infiltrative borders and perineural invasion may be present
- Trichoadenoma
  - Characterized by numerous infundibulocystic structures surrounded by eosinophilic cells resembling those of follicular infundibulum; germinative cells are sparse

Pearls

- Desmoplastic trichoepithelioma is a distinct variant of trichoepithelioma that is characterized by narrow strands and columns of germinative epithelial cells, infundibulocystic structures filled with keratin, and a fibrotic stroma

- Giant solitary trichoepithelioma is a variant of trichoepithelioma that measures several centimeters in size and is typically located in the deep dermis and subcutaneous tissue
- Trichoblastoma and trichoepithelioma constitute different morphologic patterns of a benign neoplasm composed of follicular germinative cells

Selected References

Pham TT, Selim MA, Burchette JL Jr, et al: CD10 expression in trichoepithelioma and basal cell carcinoma. J Cutan Pathol 33:123-128, 2006.

Ackerman AB, Reddy VB, Soyer HP: Neoplasms with Follicular Differentiation. New York, Ardor Scribendi, 2001.

Centurion SA, Schwartz RA, Lambert WC: Trichoepithelioma papulosum multiplex. J Dermatol 27:137-143, 2000.

Matt D, Xin H, Vortmeyer AO, et al: Sporadic trichoepithelioma demonstrates deletions at 9q22.3. Arch Dermatol 136:657-660, 2000.

Brownstein MH, Shapiro L: Desmoplastic trichoepithelioma. Cancer 40:2979-2986, 1977.

Pilomatricoma (Pilomatrixoma, Calcifying Epithelioma of Malherbe)

Clinical Features

- Most common in children and adolescents
- Sites of predilection include the face, neck, and upper extremities
- Firm, solitary, deep-seated nodules between 0.5 and 3 cm in diameter

Histopathology

- Sharply demarcated, cystic, well-circumscribed proliferation of dark-staining aggregates of matrical and supramatrical cells
- Pale-staining cells that exhibit a ghost of nucleus ("ghost" or "shadow" cells)
- Granulomatous inflammation with foreign-body giant cells adjacent to shadow cells
- Mitotic figures may be present in the small basophilic cells, but nuclear atypia and infiltrative growth are uncommon
- Early lesions: cystic cavity surrounded by rows of matrical cells
- Older lesions: preponderance of ghost or shadow cells with dystrophic calcification, ossification, and granulomatous inflammation

Special Stains and Immunohistochemistry

- Noncontributory

Other Techniques for Diagnosis

- Noncontributory

Figure 2-51. Pilomatricoma. A, Low-power view shows a well-circumscribed dermal nodule composed of basaloid cells, shadow cells, and areas of calcifications. **B,** High-power view shows basaloid cells and shadow cells with distinct cell borders but only an outline of nucleus. Areas of granulomatous inflammation can be present.

Differential Diagnosis

- Calcified trichilemmal cyst
  - Absence of shadow or ghost cells
  - Cyst lined by epithelial cells with abundant eosinophilic cytoplasm
- Malignant pilomatricoma (matrical carcinoma)
  - Rare entity
  - Infiltrative growth pattern
  - Striking nuclear atypia, frequent abnormal mitoses, and necrosis en masse

Pearls

- Multiple lesions and familial patterns linked to myotonic dystrophy
- Shadow cells represent faulty attempts of the matrical cells to form hair shafts

Selected References

Ackerman AB, Reddy VB, Soyer HP: Neoplasms with Follicular Differentiation. New York, Ardor Scribendi, 2001.

Hardisson D, Linares MD, Cuevas-Santos J, et al: Pilomatrix carcinoma: A clinicopathologic study of six cases and review of the literature. Am J Dermatopathol 23:394-401, 2001.

Nakamura T: A reappraisal on the modes of cell death in pilomatricoma. J Cutan Pathol 26:125-129, 1999.

Berberian BJ, Colonna TM, Battaglia M, Sulica VI: Multiple pilomatricomas in association with myotonic dystrophy and a family history of melanoma. J Am Acad Dermatol 37:268-269, 1997.

Julian CG, Bowers PW: A clinical review of 209 pilomatricomas. J Am Acad Dermatol 39:191-195, 1997.

Kaddu S, Soyer HP, Hodl S, Kerl H: Morphological stages of pilomatricoma. Am J Dermatopathol 18:333-338, 1996.

Trichilemmoma

Clinical Features

- Predilection for the nose, cheek, and upper lip
- Lesions are usually solitary
- Presents as verrucous or smooth, small (<1 cm), flesh-colored papule

Histopathology

- The lesion has the silhouette of a verruca
- Vertically oriented bulbous hyperplasia of infundibular epithelium that contains cells with clear or pale cytoplasm
- The columnar clear cells are arranged in a palisade at the periphery similar to those seen in the outer root sheath of a normal hair follicle
- The epithelial proliferation is surrounded by a thick hyalinized basement membrane

Figure 2-52. Trichilemmoma. Histologic section shows a sharply defined proliferation of cells with clear cytoplasm resembling the outer root sheath of hair follicle.

- Dilated tortuous blood vessels may be present in the papillary dermis
- Desmoplastic trichilemmoma: shows irregular extensions of clear cells into a sclerotic dermis simulating an invasive carcinoma; the upper part of the lesion shows typical features of trichilemmoma

Special Stains and Immunohistochemistry

- PAS stain demonstrates glycogen in the clear cells

Other Techniques for Diagnosis

- Noncontributory

Differential Diagnosis

▌ Verruca
  - Most trichilemmomas have architectural and cytologic features of verruca in the process of involution
  - A typical verruca lacks the epithelial cells with clear cytoplasm (trichilemmal differentiation)
▌ Inverted follicular keratosis
  - Has similar silhouette of verruca and trichilemmoma
  - Additionally, there are squamous eddies within the hyperplastic infundibular epithelium

Pearls

- Cowden disease: autosomal dominant disorder presenting with multiple trichilemmomas associated with a variety of malignancies (breast, gastrointestinal, thyroid, and reproductive organs)

Selected References

Brownstein MH, Shapiro L: Trichilemmoma: Analysis of 40 new cases. Arch Dermatol 107:866-869, 1973.

Lloyd KM, Denis M: Cowden's disease: A possible new symptom complex with multiple system involvement. Ann Intern Med 58:136-142, 1963.

Basal Cell Carcinoma

Clinical Features

- Typically affects older individuals
- Predilection for sun-exposed skin (face, hands)
- Small, well-circumscribed, pearly tan-gray papule devoid of scale
- Lesions enlarge with time and tend to ulcerate (rodent ulcers)

Histopathology

- Nests and islands of basaloid cells attached to the undersurface of epidermis and extending into the dermis
- Peripheral palisading of basaloid cells of the nests
- Basaloid cells are typically uniform with frequent mitotic activity and abundant apoptotic cells

Figure 2-53. A, Basal cell carcinoma, superficial. Histologic section shows small nests of basaloid cells showing peripheral palisading. **B, Basal cell carcinoma, nodular.** Section shows a nodular proliferation of basaloid cells with peripheral palisading.

- Characteristic retraction artifact between the palisading cells and the normal stroma
- Areas of squamous differentiation and perineural invasion are seen in aggressive (infiltrative) forms
- Variants of basal cell carcinoma: pigmented, morphea-like or sclerosing, superficial, nodular, keratotic, adenoid, micronodular, and fibroepithelial types

Special Stains and Immunohistochemistry

- Noncontributory

Other Techniques for Diagnosis

- Noncontributory

Differential Diagnosis

▌ Trichoepithelioma and trichoblastoma
  - Nests of basaloid cells usually without mitotic activity, individual cell necrosis, or separation artifacts
  - Abundant fibrotic stroma
  - Retraction artifacts within a cellular stroma rather than around the epithelial nests
  - Evidence of follicular differentiation in the form of germs, bulbs, and papillae is more common
  - CD10-positive stroma

Pearls

- Basal cell nevus syndrome: multiple basaloid hamartomas on the cutaneous surface associated with palmar keratotic pits, jaw cysts, and basal cell carcinomas in non–sun-exposed locations
- BCCs rarely metastasize; when they do, the primary lesion is usually advanced

Selected References

Ackerman AB, Reddy VB, Soyer HP: Neoplasms with Follicular Differentiation. New York, Ardor Scribendi, 2001.

Rippey JJ: Why classify basal cell carcinomas? Histopathology 32:393-398, 1998.

Strutton GM: Pathological variants of basal cell carcinoma. Aust J Dermatol 38(Suppl 1):S31-35, 1997.

Goldberg DP: Assessment and surgical treatment of basal cell skin cancer. Clin Plast Surg 24:673-686, 1997.

Goldberg LH: Basal cell carcinoma. Lancet 347:663-667, 1996.

Maloney ME: Histology of basal cell carcinoma. Clin Dermatol 13:545-549, 1995.

Mehregan AH: Aggressive basal cell epithelioma on sunlight-protected skin. Am J Dermatopathol 5:221, 1983.

Mason JK, Helwig EB, Graham JH: Pathology of the nevoid basal cell carcinoma syndrome. Arch Pathol 79:401, 1965.

Eccrine and Apocrine Neoplasms

Syringoma

Clinical Features

- Commonly affects females, usually at the onset of puberty
- Predilection for the face, eyelids, neck, and upper anterior chest but can occur at other sites including penis and vulva
- Multiple small (1 to 3 mm), yellowish, firm papules

Histopathology

- Symmetrical, well-circumscribed lesions with an eosinophilic fibrous stroma

Figure 2-54. Syringoma. Histologic section shows nests, strands, and ducts composed of monomorphic epithelial cells. The ductal structures are lined two layers of cells, and some have elongated contours (tadpole-like).

- Confined to the upper half of the dermis
- Elongated aggregates of epithelial cells of varying shapes and tubules in a markedly fibrotic stroma
- Cords and nests of epithelial cells often continuous with tubules (likened to comma shapes or tadpoles)
- Epithelial cells may have scant cytoplasm or abundant pale-staining cytoplasm
- Ductal lumina may contain eosinophilic PAS-positive material
- Clear cell syringoma
  - Contains mostly nests of clear cells with occasional tubules
- Chondroid syringoma (mixed tumor)
  - Composed of syringomatous ductal structures surrounded by a blue-gray mucinous stroma with occasional areas of cartilage formation, similar to mixed tumor of salivary gland

Special Stains and Immunohistochemistry
- PAS: ductal lumina may contain eosinophilic PAS-positive material

Other Techniques for Diagnosis
- Noncontributory

Differential Diagnosis
- BCC (sclerosing and keratotic)
  - Predilection for sun-exposed skin, typically face and hands
  - Multiple nests of basaloid cells with peripheral palisading infiltrating between a sclerotic stroma
- Trichoepithelioma
  - Nests of cells that typically do not show ductal lumina but contain many infundibulocystic structures filled with keratin

- Microcystic adnexal carcinoma (sclerosing sweat duct carcinoma)
  - Clinically presents as a solitary lesion that is typically larger (1 to 3 cm)
  - Deeply infiltrative histologic pattern
  - Perineural invasion

Pearls
- Syringoma is believed to show differentiation toward the intraepidermal portion of the eccrine sweat duct

Selected References
Goyal S, Martins CR: Multiple syringomas on the abdomen, thighs, and groin. Cutis 66:259-262, 2000.
Karam P, Benedetto AV: Syringomas: New approach to an old technique. Int J Dermatol 35:219-220, 1996.
Feibelman CE, Maize JC: Clear-cell syringoma: A study by conventional and electron microscopy. Am J Dermatopathol 6:139-150, 1984.

Poroma

Clinical Features
- Benign adnexal tumor related to the eccrine sweat duct
- Predilection for the palms and soles (60%), trunk, head, and neck
- Lesions have a tendency to crust and ulcerate
- Present as small (2 to 3 cm), firm to rubbery, painless nodules

Histopathology
- Sheetlike down-growth of monomorphous dark (poroid) cells and tubules lined by pale (cuticular) cells
- Intracytoplasmic vacuolization and necrosis en masse may be present
- Cystic spaces and foci of keratinization may be present

Figure 2-55. Poroma. Histologic section shows a sharply demarcated intraepidermal proliferation of monomorphous cuboidal cells with scattered ductal lumina. The stroma is richly vascular.

- Early erosion and ulceration of the superficial epidermis
- Richly vascular stroma with dilated, tortuous vessels
- Variants: intraepidermal poroma (hidroacanthoma simplex), dermal duct tumor, and poroid hidradenoma

Special Stains and Immunohistochemistry
- Noncontributory

Other Techniques for Diagnosis
- Noncontributory

Differential Diagnosis
▍Clear cell acanthoma
- Overlying parakeratotic cornified layer often containing neutrophils
- Abrupt acanthotic proliferation of pale squamoid cells
- Elongated rete ridges with well-vascularized dermal papillae
- Presence of neutrophils within intercellular spaces of the involved epidermis
▍Seborrheic keratosis
- Characteristic horn and pseudohorn cysts
- Stroma is not vascular
▍Porocarcinoma
- Asymmetrical, poorly circumscribed proliferation of cords and lobules of polygonal cells with marked nuclear atypia, frequent mitosis, and necrosis

Pearls
- Poromas display differentiation toward eccrine ducts
- Eccrine poromatosis: multiple lesions affecting the palms and soles

Selected References
Lee NH, Lee SH, Ahn SK: Apocrine poroma with sebaceous differentiation. Am J Dermatopathol 22:261-263, 2000.
Verplancke P, Driessen L, Wynants P, Naeyaert JM: The Schopf-Schulz-Passarge syndrome. Dermatology 196:463-466, 1998.
Hamanaka S, Otsuka F: Multiple malignant eccrine poroma and a linear epidermal nevus. J Dermatol 23:469-471, 1996.
Mousawi A, Kibbi AG: Pigmented eccrine poroma: A simulant of nodular melanoma. Int J Dermatol 34:857-858, 1995.
Pena J, Suster S: Squamous differentiation in malignant eccrine poroma. Am J Dermatopathol 15:492-496, 1993.

Spiradenoma

Clinical Features
- Benign proliferation of eccrine ductal and secretory structures
- Lesions typically occur in children and young to middle-aged adults

Figure 2-56. Spiradenoma. A, Low-power view shows a well-circumscribed dermal nodule with occasional ductal lumina. **B,** High-power view shows sheets of larger cells with pale cytoplasm and smaller cells with scant cytoplasm. Globules of hyaline basement membrane–like material are present within the aggregations.

- Predilection for the trunk and extremities
- Lesions are typically solitary and painful but can occur as multiple lesions infrequently
- Small (1 to 2 cm), dome-shaped, skin-colored nodules

Histopathology
- Relatively well-circumscribed neoplasm with solid and tubular components
- Solid component has up to three types of cells
  — Large cells with ovoid nuclei and pale cytoplasm, located within the centers of the nodules of neoplastic cells
  — Small dark cells with hyperchromatic nuclei and scant cytoplasm, located at the periphery of the aggregations
  — Mature lymphocytes scattered among the small and large neoplastic epithelial cells
- Tubules resembling dilated ducts and lined by large, pale epithelial cells

- Richly vascular stroma
- Evenly distributed globules of eosinophilic basement membrane material within the epithelial aggregates

Special Stains and Immunohistochemistry

- Noncontributory

Other Techniques for Diagnosis

- Noncontributory

Differential Diagnosis

▌ Cylindroma
  - Low magnification reveals multiple nests of basaloid cells that appear to fit together like pieces of a jigsaw puzzle
▌ Benign vascular tumors
  - Lack nodular aggregates of epithelial cells

Pearls

- Painful nature of these lesions is related to the numerous unmyelinated axons in the stroma
- Malignant transformation, although uncommon, has been reported

Selected References

Bedlow AJ, Cook MG, Kurwa A: Extensive naevoid eccrine spiradenoma. Br J Dermatol 140:154-157, 1999.

Argenyi ZB, Nguyen AV, Balogh K, et al: Malignant eccrine spiradenoma: A clinicopathologic study. Am J Dermatopathol 14:381-390, 1992.

Cooper PH, Frierson HF Jr, Morrison AG: Malignant transformation of eccrine spiradenoma. Arch Dermatol 121:1445-1448, 1985.

Mambo NC: Eccrine spiradenoma: Clinical and pathologic study of 49 tumors. J Cutan Pathol 10:312-320, 1983.

Cylindroma

Clinical Features

- Benign adnexal neoplasm with apocrine differentiation
- May occur as a solitary lesion or multiple lesions
- Multiple form is inherited in a dominant pattern and presents in females at an earlier age as multiple dome-shaped nodules on the scalp; other sites of involvement include face and, rarely, trunk and extremities
- Nodules vary in size from a few millimeters to several centimeters
- Over time, the scalp nodules coalesce to larger nodules and may resemble a turban (hatlike growth)

Histopathology

- Well-circumscribed dermal nodules composed of islands of epithelial cells that fit together like pieces of jigsaw puzzle and are separated from each other only by thick hyaline sheaths

Figure 2-57. Cylindroma. Histologic section shows a well-circumscribed dermal nodule composed of epithelial islands that are separated by thick hyaline sheaths and fit together like pieces of a puzzle.

- Two types of cells are present in the epithelial islands
  — Cells with small, dark-staining nuclei at the periphery of the islands
  — Cells with large light-staining nuclei in the center of the islands
- Tubular lumina lined by ductal cells and filled with amorphous material are often present
- Drops of eosinophilic hyaline material can be present within the epithelial islands

Special Stains and Immunohistochemistry

- Hyaline sheaths are PAS positive and diastase resistant
- Human milk-fat globulin (HMFG) positive

Other Techniques for Diagnosis

- Familial cylindromatosis (turban tumor syndrome) is associated with a genetic defect localized to chromosome 16q

Differential Diagnosis

▌ Malignant cylindroma
  - In rare instances, malignant change characterized by cytologic and nuclear pleomorphism, atypical mitotic figures, loss of hyaline sheaths, and infiltrating pattern can be seen
▌ Areas of spiradenoma can coexist within cylindromas

Pearls

- Multiple cylindromas may be associated with multiple trichoepitheliomas and perhaps represent different expressions of same genetic disorder
- Hyaline sheaths are synthesized by the neoplastic cells and are believed to represent basement membrane–like material

Selected References

Meybehm M, Fischer HP: Spiradenoma and dermal cylindroma: Comparative immunohistochemical analysis and histogenetic considerations. Am J Dermatopathol 19:154-161, 1997.

Lee MW, Kelly JW: Dermal cylindroma and eccrine spiradenoma. Aust J Dermatol 37:48-49, 1996.

Biggs PJ, Wooster R, Ford D, et al: Familial cylindromatosis (turban tumour syndrome) gene localized to chromosome 16q12-q13: Evidence for its role as a tumour suppressor gene. Nat Genet 11:441-443, 1995.

Van der Putte SC: The pathogenesis of familial multiple cylindromas, trichoepitheliomas, milia, and spiradenomas. Am J Dermatopathol 17:271-280, 1995.

Clear Cell Hidradenoma (Nodular Hidradenoma)

Clinical Features

- Generally presents as solitary dermal nodule 0.5 to 2 cm in diameter
- May have a cystic component
- Synonyms include *nodular hidradenoma, solid-cystic hidradenoma,* and *eccrine acrospiroma*

Figure 2-58. Clear cell (nodular) hidradenoma. A, Low-power view shows a well-circumscribed, lobulated, and partly cystic dermal nodule. **B,** High-power view shows lobules of cells with clear cytoplasm and ductal lumens lined by cells with decapitation secretions and cystic spaces filled with eosinophilic material.

Histopathology

- Well-circumscribed, lobulated dermal nodule that may extend into the subcutaneous fat
- Lobules contain masses of cells with clear cytoplasm; some cells are polyhedral, and others are fusiform with elongated nuclei
- Occasional lumina lined by cuboidal cells or columnar cells with decapitation secretions
- Cystic spaces filled with eosinophilic homogeneous material, which most likely results from degeneration of neoplastic cells
- Stroma between the nodules is characteristically eosinophilic and hyalinized

Special Stains and Immunohistochemistry

- PAS stain demonstrates glycogen in the clear cells
- Immunohistochemical studies show positivity for cytokeratin, epithelial membrane antigen (EMA), carcinoembryonic antigen (CEA), S-100 protein, and vimentin

Other Techniques for Diagnosis

- Noncontributory

Differential Diagnosis

▌ Trichilemmoma
- Also contains clear cells; however, cystic spaces and tubular lumina characteristic of clear cell hidradenoma are not present

▌ Malignant nodular hidradenoma
- Cytologic pleomorphism and high mitotic rate are suggestive of aggressive behavior
- Zonal or diffuse necrosis in addition to infiltrative, poorly circumscribed borders in an asymmetrical nodular neoplasm should suggest a diagnosis of malignant nodular hidradenoma
- Typically arise de novo rather than in association with preexisting benign lesions

Pearls

- Nodular hidradenomas may occasionally recur; recurrent tumors show frequent mitoses or nuclear pleomorphism and should be completely excised

Selected References

Waxtein L, Vega E, Cortes R, et al: Malignant nodular hidradenoma. Int J Dermatol 37:225-228, 1998.

Touma D, Laporte M, Goossens A, Ledoux M: Malignant clear cell hidradenoma. Dermatology 186:284-286, 1993.

Winkelmann RK, Wolff K: Solid-cystic hidradenoma of the skin: Clinical and histopathologic study. Arch Dermatol 97:651-661, 1968.

Hashimoto K, DiBella RJ, Lever WF: Clear cell hidradenoma: Histological, histochemical, and electron microscopic studies. Arch Dermatol 96:18-38, 1967.

Figure 2-59. A, Syringocystadenoma papilliferum. Histologic section shows cystic epidermal invagination into which papillary structures project. **B, Syringocystadenoma papilliferum.** High-power view shows that the papillae are lined by two rows of cells: the luminal row is composed of columnar cells with decapitation secretions. Plasma cells are present within the stroma. **C, Hidradenoma papilliferum.** In contrast to syringocystadenoma, this is a predominantly dermal nodule with cystic appearance. **D, Hidradenoma papilliferum.** High-power view shows complex papillary fronds lined by columnar cells with decapitation secretions.

Syringocystadenoma Papilliferum

Clinical Features

- Occurs most often on scalp or face, presenting at birth or in early childhood as a single papule or multiple papules or as a solitary plaque
- Occurs near puberty in a preexisting nevus sebaceus on scalp in one third of the cases

Histopathology

- Epidermis shows papillomatous hyperplasia
- One or multiple invaginations extend down from the epidermis

- Upper part of the invaginations is lined by epidermis, whereas lower part is lined by papillary projections extending into the luminal aspect
- Papillary projections are lined by two rows of epithelial cells; the luminal row consists of columnar cells with oval nuclei and occasionally with decapitation secretions; the outer row consists of small cuboidal cells with scant cytoplasm and small, round nuclei
- Within the stroma, a dense plasma cell infiltrate is present
- Apocrine sweat glands are often noted at the base of the lesion

Special Stains and Immunohistochemistry

- Apocrine differentiation is supported by the demonstration of gross cystic disease fluid protein (GCDFP) in some cases

Other Techniques for Diagnosis

- Noncontributory

Differential Diagnosis

❚ Hidradenoma papilliferum
- Occurs on labia majora, perineum, and perianal regions of women
- Presents as a dermal nodule measuring a few millimeters
- Histologically, it is a well-circumscribed nodule that is cystic with no connection to the surface
- Papillary fronds lined by a single row of columnar cells showing decapitation secretions project into the cystic space
- Tubular lumina lined by secretory cells surrounded by myoepithelial cells are also present

❚ Tubular apocrine adenoma
- Generally contains numerous, irregularly shaped tubular structures lined by two rows of cells
- Some may contain papillary projections and resemble syringocystadenoma papilliferum; however, the lesion does not connect to the overlying epidermis

Pearls

- Features of both eccrine and apocrine differentiation can be seen in some examples of syringocystadenoma papilliferum

Figure 2-60. Microcystic adnexal carcinoma. A, Low-power view shows a deeply infiltrative neoplasm composed of ductal structures and keratin-filled cysts. **B,** High-power view shows rather monomorphous epithelial islands infiltrating between the skeletal muscle fibers.

Selected References

de Bliek JP, Starink TM: Multiple linear syringocystadenoma papilliferum [letter]. J Eur Acad Dermatol Venereol 12:74-76, 1999.

Mazoujian G, Margolis R: Immunohistochemistry of gross cystic disease fluid protein (GCDFP-15) in 65 benign sweat gland tumors of the skin. Am J Dermatopathol 10:28-35, 1988.

Toribio J, Zulaica A, Peteiro C: Tubular apocrine adenoma. J Cutan Pathol 14:114-117, 1987.

Numata M, Hosoe S, Itoh N, et al: Syringadenocarcinoma papilliferum. J Cutan Pathol 12:3-7, 1985.

Helwig EB, Hackney VC: Syringocystadenoma papilliferum. Arch Dermatol 71:361, 1955.

Microcystic Adnexal Carcinoma (Sclerosing Sweat Duct Carcinoma)

Clinical Features

- Locally aggressive neoplasm that invades deeply but generally does not metastasize
- Characteristic site of involvement is the upper lip; other sites include chin, nasolabial fold, and cheek

Histopathology

- Poorly circumscribed infiltrating dermal lesion that extends deep into the subcutaneous tissue and skeletal muscle
- Continuity with the epidermis is generally not seen
- Islands of epithelial cells with formation of keratin-filled cysts in a desmoplastic stroma are characteristic; in other areas, ductal structures lined by two cell layers are seen
- Cysts are not detected in all tumors; may be composed entirely of ductlike structures
- Ducts typically become smaller as they infiltrate into deeper tissue
- May have only minimal cytologic atypia, and mitotic figures are often difficult to find
- Perineural invasion is often seen

Special Stains and Immunohistochemistry

- Noncontributory

Other Techniques for Diagnosis

- Noncontributory

Differential Diagnosis

- ▎ Syringoma
  - May be indistinguishable, especially if the deeply infiltrative nature of microcystic adnexal carcinoma cannot be appreciated owing to the superficial nature of the biopsy
  - Lacks infiltrative pattern and perineural invasion
- ▎ Desmoplastic trichoepithelioma
  - Generally confined to the upper half of the dermis
  - May contain cysts but lacks ductal structures
- ▎ Sclerosing basal cell carcinoma
  - Infiltrative pattern of strands and nests of basaloid cells associated with stromal sclerosis
  - No cysts or ductlike structures present

Pearls

- The possibility of microcystic adnexal carcinoma should always be considered in assessment of trichoepitheliomatous and syringomatous neoplasms extending to the base of the specimen

Selected References

Friedman PM, Friedman RH, Jiang SB, et al: Microcystic adnexal carcinoma: Collaborative series review and update. J Am Acad Dermatol 41:225-231, 1999.

Cook TF, Fosko SW: Unusual cutaneous malignancies. Semin Cutan Med Surg 17:114-132, 1998.

Nelson BR, Lowe L, Baker S, et al: Microcystic adnexal carcinoma of the skin: A reappraisal of the differentiation and differential diagnosis of an underrecognized neoplasm. J Am Acad Dermatol 29:840-845, 1993.

Sebastien TS, Nelson BR, Lowe L, et al: Microcystic adnexal carcinoma. J Am Acad Dermatol 29:840-845, 1993.

Goldstein DJ, Barr RJ, Santa Cruz DJ: Microcystic adnexal carcinoma: A distinct clinicopathologic entity. Cancer 50:566-572, 1982.

Sebaceous Proliferations and Neoplasms

Nevus Sebaceus

Clinical Features

- Presents at birth on the scalp or face as a single, yellowish, slightly raised, hairless plaque
- In childhood, it may have a linear configuration; at puberty, the lesions appear verrucous and nodular
- Some patients may present with extensive nevus sebaceous as part of neurocutaneous syndrome

Histopathology

- Sebaceous glands in nevus sebaceus show the same developmental pattern as normal sebaceous glands

Figure 2-61. Nevus sebaceus. Histologic section shows papillomatous epidermal hyperplasia associated with prominent sebaceous lobules and poorly formed follicular units.

- At birth
  - Sebaceous lobules are prominent (result of the effect of maternal hormones)
- After infancy
  - Sebaceous lobules are small and decreased in number
- At puberty
  - Large numbers of mature sebaceous glands are seen
  - Associated epidermal changes include papillomatous hyperplasia
  - Malformed follicular germs resembling basal cell carcinoma can be present
  - Apocrine glands located deep in the dermis are present in most cases
- In adulthood
  - Various adnexal neoplasms, the most common being trichoblastoma and syringocystadenoma papilliferum, can develop in nevus sebaceus

Special Stains and Immunohistochemistry

- Noncontributory

Other Techniques for Diagnosis

- Noncontributory

Differential Diagnosis

- Diagnosis of nevus sebaceus can be missed if the biopsy specimen is taken at a stage at which sebaceous lobules are small and few
- ▎ Epidermal nevus
  - Lacks sebaceous lobules
- ▎ Sebaceous gland hyperplasia
  - Single enlarged sebaceous gland that opens into a dilated duct

Pearls

- BCC and rarely SCC and adnexal carcinomas can develop in nevus sebaceus

- Small biopsy of nevus sebaceus may show only prominent sebaceous lobules and can be misinterpreted as sebaceous gland hyperplasia

Selected References

Miller CJ, Ioffreda MD, Billingsley EM: Sebaceous carcinoma, basal cell carcinoma, trichoadenoma, trichoblastoma, and syringocystadenoma papilliferum arising within a nevus sebaceus. Dermatol Surg 30:1546-1549, 2004.

Cribier B, Scrivener Y, Grosshans E: Tumors arising in nevus sebaceus: A study of 596 cases. J Am Acad Dermatol 42:263-268, 2000.

Jaqueti G, Requena L, Sanchez Yus E: Trichoblastoma is the most common neoplasm developed in nevus sebaceus of Jadassohn: A clinicopathologic study of a series of 155 cases. Am J Dermatopathol 22:108-118, 2000.

Steffen C, Ackerman AB (eds): Nevus Sebaceus. In Steffen C, Ackerman AB (eds): Neoplasms with Sebaceous Differentiation. Philadelphia, Lea & Febiger, 1996, p 89.

Morioka S: The natural history of nevus sebaceus. J Cutan Pathol 12:200, 1985.

Sebaceous Epithelioma (Sebaceoma)

Clinical Features

- Occurs more commonly in middle-aged and older individuals
- Predilection for the facial skin and scalp
- Occasionally bleeds or ulcerates
- Small (<1 cm), solitary, tan-yellow circumscribed papule or ill-defined plaque

Histopathology

- Well-circumscribed lesion
- Preponderance of lipidized (adenoma) or basaloid (epithelioma) cells within an eosinophilic stroma

Figure 2-62. Sebaceous epithelioma (sebaceoma). Well-circumscribed proliferation of an admixture of basaloid cells and cells with abundant vacuolated cytoplasm characteristic of sebaceous differentiation is seen.

- Basaloid cells tend to occur at the periphery of the lesion
- No nuclear atypia; however, mitotic figures may be present
- Rippled pattern sebaceoma: shows a unique arrangement of small, monomorphous, cigar-shaped basaloid cells in linear rows parallel to one another, resembling Verocay bodies; this arrangement of cells produces the rippled pattern; scattered cells and ducts with sebaceous differentiation are seen

Special Stains and Immunohistochemistry

- Oil red O (fresh tissue) highlights the lipid in the sebocytes

Other Techniques for Diagnosis

- Noncontributory

Differential Diagnosis

▌ Sebaceous hyperplasia
- Single enlarged sebaceous gland
- Lobules are composed of mostly mature sebaceous cells and open into a single dilated duct

▌ Sebaceous adenoma
- Sharply demarcated lobules composed of undifferentiated basaloid cells and mature sebaceous cells
- Smaller and more superficial than sebaceoma
- May represent the mature end of the spectrum of sebaceoma

Pearls

- Sebaceous neoplasms may be associated with Muir-Torre syndrome

Selected References

Kiyohara T, Kumakiri M, Kuwahara H, et al: Rippled-pattern sebaceoma: A report of a lesion on the back with a review of the literature. Am J Dermatopathol 28:446-448, 2006.

Dinneen AM, Mehregan DR: Sebaceous epithelioma: A review of twenty-one cases. J Am Acad Dermatol 34:47-50, 1996.

Donati P: Solitary sebaceoma in Muir-Torre syndrome. Int J Dermatol 35:601-602, 1996.

Misago N, Narisawa Y: Sebaceous neoplasms in Muir-Torre syndrome. Am J Dermatopathol 22:155-161, 2000.

Ueda M, Wang Y, Sugimura H, et al: A case of multiple sebaceous epithelioma: Analysis of microsatellite instability. J Dermatol 26:178-182, 1999.

Steffen C, Ackerman AB: Sebaceoma. In Steffen C, Ackerman AB (eds): Neoplasms with Sebaceous Differentiation. Philadelphia, Lea & Febiger, 1994, p 385.

Sebaceous Carcinoma

Clinical Features

- Rare malignant sebaceous gland neoplasm
- Affects women more often than men

Figure 2-63. Sebaceous carcinoma. Histologic section shows irregular lobules of pleomorphic basaloid cells with scattered mature sebocytes. Mitotic figures and individually necrotic cells are present.

- Predilection for the eyelids in association with the meibomian gland and the gland of Zeis
- Related to irradiation and other neoplastic growths, including
  — BCC
  — SCC
  — Keratoacanthoma
  — Visceral carcinomas (Muir-Torre syndrome)
- Presents as asymptomatic, firm, ill-defined nodule, usually less than 1 cm in diameter; may be ulcerated

Histopathology

- Irregular lobules of varying sizes composed of many undifferentiated basaloid cells with some cells showing sebaceous differentiation, usually in the middle of the lobule
- Some lobules may contain squamoid areas resembling SCC
- Sebaceous carcinoma of eyelid typically shows pagetoid spread to the overlying conjunctival epithelium or epidermis

Special Stains and Immunohistochemistry

- Noncontributory

Other Techniques for Diagnosis

- Noncontributory

Differential Diagnosis

▌ Sebaceous epithelioma (sebaceoma)
- Generally circumscribed and symmetrical
- No necrosis or surface ulceration

Pearls

- Sebaceous carcinoma spreads in contiguous fashion, first affecting the regional lymph nodes (periauricular, submaxillary, and cervical chains), then spreading through the viscera
- Sebaceous carcinomas occurring in Muir-Torre syndrome are much less likely to metastasize

Selected References

Nelson BR, Hamlet KR, Gillard M, et al: Sebaceous carcinoma. J Am Acad Dermatol 33:1-15, 1995.

Wick MR, Goellner JR, Wolfe JT 3rd, et al: Adnexal carcinomas of the skin. II. Extraocular sebaceous carcinomas. Cancer 56:1163-1172, 1985.

Rao NA, Hidayat AA, McLean IW, et al: Sebaceous carcinomas of the ocular adnexa: A clinicopathologic study of 104 cases, with five-year follow-up data. Hum Pathol 13:113-122, 1982.

Russell WG, Page DL, Hough AJ, et al: Sebaceous carcinoma of meibomian gland origin: The diagnostic importance of pagetoid spread of neoplastic cells. Am J Clin Pathol 73:504-511, 1980.

Melanocytic Proliferations and Neoplasms

Congenital Melanocytic Nevus

Clinical Features

- Presents at birth or shortly thereafter as variably sized pigmented lesion
- Size varies from 1.5 cm to more than 20 cm (giant congenital nevus)
- Bathing trunk–type congenital nevus is characterized by an uneven verrucous surface, variations of shades of brown and blue, and increased hair growth throughout the lesion
- Large congenital nevi show mild variation in color and epidermal hyperplasia
- Small congenital nevi are seen as solitary light-tan to brown, uniformly pigmented macules

Figure 2-64. Congenital melanocytic nevus. Low-power view shows a broad proliferation of monomorphous melanocytes arranged as nests extending deep into the dermis, where they surround the adnexal structures.

- Congenital nevi change with age and develop darker areas, nodules, and coarse hair
- Giant congenital nevi of head and neck region may be associated with leptomeningeal melanocytosis and neurologic disorders

Histopathology

- Like acquired nevi, congenital nevi may be junctional, compound, or intradermal
- Broad lesions, characterized by nests of monomorphous melanocytes at the dermoepidermal junction and in the dermis
- Dermal nests show marked adnexocentricity and angiocentricity, in addition to infiltrating between the collagen bundles
- Deep infiltration into the reticular dermis and extension along the septa of the subcutaneous fat are seen in giant congenital nevi
- Cellular proliferative nodules with occasional mitotic figures may occur in the dermal component of some congenital nevi

Special Stains and Immunohistochemistry

- Noncontributory

Other Techniques for Diagnosis

- Noncontributory

Differential Diagnosis

- Diagnosis based on clinical and histopathologic findings is generally not problematic
- Small congenital nevi when taken by a shave biopsy may show features similar to Clark dysplastic nevus

Pearls

- Giant congenital nevi when associated with leptomeningeal melanosis may be complicated by development of malignant melanoma and other primitive malignancies such as rhabdomyosarcoma, with an estimated risk of 4% to 12%
- Risk for development of melanoma in giant congenital nevi is reported to be as high as 1000 times greater than in normal population

Selected References

Marghoob AA, Schoenbach SP, Kopf AW, et al: Large congenital melanocytic nevi and the risk for the development of malignant melanoma: A prospective study. Arch Dermatol 132:170-175, 1996.
Sasai S, Kato T, Yoshimura T, et al: Congenital plantar melanocytic nevus with satellite lesions. Dermatology 192:146-148, 1996.
Swerdlow AJ, English JS, Qiao Z: The risk of melanoma in patients with congenital nevi: A cohort study. J Am Acad Dermatol 32:595-599, 1995.
Swerdlow AJ, Green A: Melanocytic naevi and melanoma: An epidemiological perspective. Br J Dermatol 117:137-146, 1987.
Walton RG, Jacobs AH, Cox AJ: Pigmented lesions in newborn infants. Br J Dermatol 95:389-396, 1976.
Mark GJ, Mihm MC Jr, Liteplo MG, et al: Congenital melanocytic nevi of the small and garment type: Clinical, histologic, and ultrastructural studies. Hum Pathol 4:395-418, 1973.

Acquired Melanocytic Nevi

Clinical Features

- Most acquired melanocytic nevi appear within the first two decades of life
- Nevi begin as small, tan-brown macules and progress to become papules
- Acquired melanocytic nevi are characterized by small size, uniform color, and well-defined borders

Histopathology

- Symmetrical, well-circumscribed proliferation of monomorphous melanocytes arranged as well-formed nests at the dermoepidermal junction or in the dermis
- Junctional nests are evenly distributed
- Nests of melanocytes in the dermis show maturation with progressive descent
- Special variants of melanocytic nevi
  — Spitz nevus
    - Presents as solitary, small (<1 cm), pink papule in children younger than 14 years; can occur in older patients and also as a congenital nevus
    - Histologically, Spitz nevi are characterized by a symmetrical, well-circumscribed proliferation of large spindle-shaped and epithelioid melanocytes that are uniform from side to side and mature with progressive descent
    - Pagetoid spread can be seen
    - Eosinophilic hyaline globules (Kamino bodies) located at the dermoepidermal junction
    - Mitotic figures may be present but usually are not atypical and are not present at the base of the lesion
    - Epidermal hyperplasia with hyperkeratosis and parakeratosis, patchy perivascular lymphohistiocytic inflammation, and papillary dermal vascular ectasia are features characteristic of Spitz nevi
    - Some examples of Spitz nevi may be difficult to differentiate from melanomas, especially when they occur in older patients
  — Clark dysplastic nevus
    - Originally described by Clark and others in 1978 in a subgroup of patients with family history of melanoma and multiple clinically atypical nevi (B-K mole syndrome)
    - Histologically, these nevi are broad, with the nests at the dermoepidermal junction extending far beyond the dermal component (shoulders)

Figure 2-65. A, Acquired (compound) melanocytic nevus. Section shows nests of monomorphous melanocytes at the dermoepidermal junction and within the dermis, where they show maturation with progressive descent. **B, Spitz nevus.** Hyperkeratosis and parakeratosis, epidermal hyperplasia, and a proliferation of spindle and epithelioid melanocytes are seen at the dermoepidermal junction and within the dermis. Clefts around the nests and eosinophilic globules are characteristic findings. **C, Compound nevus, Clark dysplastic type.** Section shows junctional nests of melanocytes with bridging between the adjacent rete and associated concentric and lamellar fibroplasia. The melanocytes are slightly large and contain melanin-laden cytoplasm. The dermal nests are surrounded by inflammatory cell infiltrate and melanophages. **D, Halo nevus.** Section shows nests of melanocytes at the dermoepidermal junction and within the dermis, where they are surrounded by a dense infiltrate of lymphocytes. **E, Blue nevus.** Section shows a deep dermal proliferation of spindle-shaped melanocytes containing abundant melanin.

- ◆ Nests at the junction show bridging between adjacent rete and are surrounded by concentric and lamellar fibroplasia
- ◆ Some of the melanocytes at the junction are large with enlarged nuclei and contain dusty melanin-laden cytoplasm; pagetoid spread is not present
- ◆ Mild perivascular lymphocytic infiltrate and increased vascularity may be present in the papillary dermis
  - — Halo nevus
    - ◆ Characterized clinically by the appearance of a zone of depigmentation surrounding a nevus
    - ◆ Most occur on the back of children and young adults
    - ◆ Complete regression can occur, leaving a depigmented macule
    - ◆ Histologically, halo nevus is a compound nevus with a dense lymphocytic inflammation that results in destruction of melanocytes
    - ◆ In the earlier stages, the melanocytes may appear large and atypical; later stages are characterized by complete disappearance of melanocytes
  - — Blue nevus
    - ◆ Clinically presents as blue-gray papule
    - ◆ Histologically, dendritic melanocytes with melanin pigment are present as nests and fascicles within the dermis
    - ◆ In cellular blue nevi, cellular islands of large oval melanocytes with pale cytoplasm extend deep in the dermis
    - ◆ Some blue nevi may be congenital

Special Stains and Immunohistochemistry

- Noncontributory

Other Techniques for Diagnosis

- Noncontributory

Differential Diagnosis

▌ Malignant melanoma
- Acquired melanocytic nevi should be differentiated from malignant melanoma
- In general, the architectural and cytologic features of nevi are distinct from those of melanoma and include small size, symmetry, circumscription, and evenly spaced junctional nests
- Maturation of dermal nests is a helpful histologic feature associated with nevi

Pearls

- Melanocytic nevi on scalp, periauricular area, acral skin, genitalia, breast, and periumbilical location ("nevi on special sites") may simulate malignant melanoma

- Recurrent melanocytic nevus has many histologic features similar to malignant melanoma
- *Spitzoid* melanomas are melanomas that simulate Spitz nevi and pose a challenge to accurate histopathologic diagnosis
- Melanomas simulating Spitz nevi occur in prepubescent children, have architectural and cytopathologic features distinct from those that occur in adults, and require awareness for accurate diagnosis

Selected References

Xu X, Murphy G, Elenitsas R, Elder D: Benign pigmented lesions and malignant melanoma. In Elder DE, Elenitsas R, Johnson BL Jr, et al (eds): Lever's Histopathology of Skin, 10th ed. Philadelphia, Lippincott Williams & Wilkins, 2008, p 699.

Fabrizi G, Pagliarello C, Parente P, et al: Atypical nevi of the scalp in adolescents. J Cutan Pathol 34:365-369, 2007.

Elder DE: Precursors to melanoma and their mimics: nevi of special sites. Mod Pathol 19(Suppl 2):S4-20, 2006.

Mooi WJ, Krausz T: Spitz nevus versus spitzoid melanoma: Diagnostic difficulties, conceptual controversies. Adv Anat Pathol 13:147-156, 2006.

Mones JM, Ackerman AB: Melanomas in prepubescent children: Review comprehensively, critique historically, criteria diagnostically, and course biologically. Am J Dermatopathol 25:223-238, 2003.

Rapini RP: Spitz nevus or melanoma? Semin Cutan Med Surg 18:56-63, 1999.

Spatz A, Calonje E, Handfield-Jones S, Barnhill RL: Spitz tumors in children: A grading system for risk stratification [see comments]. Arch Dermatol 135:282-285, 1999.

Knoell KA, Nelson KC, Patterson JW: Familial multiple blue nevi. J Am Acad Dermatol 39:322-325, 1998.

Clark WH Jr, Reimer RR, Greene M, et al: Origin of familial malignant melanoma from heritable melanocytic lesions. Arch Dermatol 14:732, 1978.

Spitz S: Melanomas of childhood. Am J Pathol 24:591, 1948.

Malignant Melanoma

Clinical Features

- Most melanomas arise de novo and present as asymmetrical, irregularly pigmented lesions with ill-defined borders
- Generally measure more than 4 mm in diameter
- Clinically, melanomas occurring on sun-damaged skin of the face and presenting as large, irregularly pigmented patches have been referred to as *lentigo maligna melanoma*
- Those occurring on acral skin are known as *acral lentiginous melanoma*
- *Superficial spreading melanoma* refers to the histologic pattern of a prominent pagetoid spread
- *Nodular melanoma* refers to a thick, more advanced melanoma

Figure 2-66. A, Malignant melanoma, superficial spreading. Low-power view shows a broad proliferation of large atypical melanocytes arranged in poorly formed nests at the dermoepidermal junction and within the dermis. **B, Malignant melanoma, superficial spreading.** High-power view shows pagetoid melanocytes in a pagetoid pattern involving all levels of epidermis. **C, Malignant melanoma, nodular.** Low-power view shows nodular proliferation of atypical melanocytes arranged as confluent nests and sheets. **D, Malignant melanoma, nodular.** High-power view shows markedly atypical melanocytes with pleomorphic nuclei and prominent nucleoli. Mitotic figures are present.

- Up to 20% of melanomas originate in association with nevi, which include congenital nevi and Clark dysplastic nevi

Histopathology

- Broad, poorly circumscribed, asymmetrical pro-liferation of large atypical melanocytes appearing as single cells and nests at the dermoepidermal junction
- Single melanocytes extend into the overlying epidermis in a pagetoid pattern
- Nests of melanocytes are not distributed evenly at the dermoepidermal junction
- Dermal nests, when present, do not show maturation with progressive descent
- Mitotic figures, including atypical ones and necrosis, may be present
- Clark levels
  — Level 1: melanoma in situ
  — Level 2: extension into papillary dermis
  — Level 3: neoplastic cells fill the papillary dermis and extend up to reticular dermis
  — Level 4: extension into reticular dermis
  — Level 5: extension into subcutaneous fat

Special Stains and Immunohistochemistry

- When a malignant neoplasm is poorly differentiated, melanocytic markers such as S-100 protein and HMB-45 may be useful in confirming the diagnosis of melanoma

Other Techniques for Diagnosis

- Genes believed to be associated with melanoma in a background of multiple dysplastic nevi include (10% of cases)
  — *CMM1* gene on chromosome 1p36
  — Tumor suppressor gene *p16* (chromosome 9p)
  — Cyclin-dependent kinase gene (*CDK4*) located on chromosome 12q
- Comparative genomic hybridization and other molecular techniques are being developed to aid in differentiating nevi from melanoma
- High frequency of *BRAF* mutations are shown to be more common in nevi than melanoma

Differential Diagnosis

- Malignant melanoma can be differentiated from nonmelanocytic neoplasms such as Paget disease and pagetoid Bowen disease by immunohistochemical methods
- Differentiation from melanocytic nevi is best achieved using histologic criteria based on architectural and cytologic features in concert with clinical features; molecular methods hold some promise for the future
- Spitz nevus versus spitzoid melanoma can be a challenge to differentiate and perhaps impossible at times; all Spitz and Spitz-like lesions require complete excision

Pearls

- Desmoplastic and neurotropic malignant melanoma is a variant characterized by the presence of spindle-shaped melanocytes that may be mistaken for fibroblastic proliferation
- Breslow thickness (the thickness of melanoma measured from the granular layer of the epidermis) and presence or absence of ulceration provide useful prognostic information
- Melanoma in situ, when diagnosed and treated early, is associated with 100% cure rate
- About 10% of melanomas are found to run in families and are associated with multiple atypical nevi

Selected References

Xu X, Murphy G, Elenitsas R, Elder D: Benign pigmented lesions and malignant melanoma. In Elder DE, Elenitsas R, Johnson BL Jr, et al (eds): Lever's Histopathology of Skin, 10th ed. Philadelphia, Lippincott Williams & Wilkins, 2008, p 699.

Bauer J, Bastian BC: Distinguishing melanocytic nevi from melanoma by DNA copy number changes: Comparative genomic hybridization as a research and diagnostic tool. Dermatol Ther 19:40-49, 2006.

Harvell JD, Kohler S, Zhu S, et al: High-resolution array-based comparative genomic hybridization for distinguishing paraffin-embedded Spitz nevi and melanomas. Diagn Mol Pathol 13:22-25, 2003.

Pollock PM, Harper UL, Hansen KS, et al: High frequency of BRAF mutations in nevi. Nat Genet 33:19-20, 2003.

Sharpless E, Chin L: The INK4a/ARF locus and melanoma. Oncogene 22:3092-3098, 2003.

Kanzler MH, Mraz-Gernhard S: Primary cutaneous malignant melanoma and its precursor lesions: Diagnostic and therapeutic overview. J Am Acad Dermatol 45:260-276, 2001.

Edwards SL, Blessing K: Problematic pigmented lesions: approach to diagnosis. J Clin Pathol 53:409-418, 2000.

Perniciaro C: Dermatopathologic variants of malignant melanoma. Mayo Clin Proc 72:273-279, 1997.

Greene MH, Clark WH Jr, Tucker MA, et al: The high risk of melanoma in melanoma prone families with dysplastic nevi. Ann Intern Med 102:458, 1985.

Clark WH Jr, Elder DE, Guerry DIV, et al: A study of tumor progression: the precursor lesions of superficial spreading and nodular melanoma. Hum Pathol 15:1147-1165, 1984.

Vascular Proliferations and Neoplasms

Hemangiomas (Capillary Hemangioma and Cavernous Hemangioma, Angiokeratoma)

Clinical Features

- Acquired or congenital lesion consisting of dilated dermal vessels
- Capillary hemangioma
  - Typically affects people in the first decade of life and spontaneously regresses
  - Small (<1 cm), strawberry-red lesions
- Cavernous hemangioma
  - Commonly observed as acquired lesions on the face, neck, and trunk of middle-aged and older individuals
  - Small (<1 cm), bright-red, symmetrical, dome-shaped papules

Histopathology

- Capillary hemangioma
  - Well-circumscribed proliferation of small vessels lined by flattened endothelial cells
  - Congenital lesions are typically lobulated and have numerous vessels
  - Acquired lesions typically develop luminal ectasia with age
- Cavernous hemangioma
  - Poorly circumscribed collections of large ectatic vessels
  - Vessels have thicker walls and occasionally contain intraluminal thrombi
- Angiokeratoma
  - Numerous dilated thin-walled capillaries in the papillary dermis associated with epidermal hyperplasia and hyperkeratosis
  - May be seen in Fabry disease
- Glomus and glomangioma
  - Solitary or multiple painful nodules histologically characterized by vessels surrounded by glomus cells (uniform rounded eosinophilic cells with central nuclei) that show immunohistochemical and ultrastructural features of smooth muscle cells

Special Stains and Immunohistochemistry

- Noncontributory

Other Techniques for Diagnosis

- Noncontributory

Differential Diagnosis

- Pyogenic granuloma
  - Lesions typically show superficial ulceration and a markedly edematous stroma with a mononuclear and neutrophilic infiltrate

Figure 2-67. A, Hemangioma. Histologic section shows well-formed vascular spaces in the dermis filled with red blood cells. **B, Angiokeratoma.** Section shows epidermal hyperplasia, hyperkeratosis, and markedly dilated vascular spaces extending into the epidermis. **C, Glomangioma.** Section shows dilated blood vessels surrounded by a monomorphous population of round to oval cells.

▌ Kaposi sarcoma
  ● Composed of slitlike vascular spaces and surrounding stroma infiltrated with lymphocytes and plasma cells
  ● Extravasated red blood cells

Pearls
  ● Maffucci syndrome: association of cavernous hemangiomas with multiple enchondromas
  ● Kasabach-Merritt syndrome: association of cavernous hemangiomas with a consumptive coagulopathy secondary to intralesional thrombosis
  ● Blue rubber bleb nevus syndrome: association of cavernous hemangiomas with gastrointestinal tract vascular proliferations

Selected References

Mulliken JB, Fishman SJ, Burrows PE: Vascular anomalies. Curr Probl Surg 37:517-584, 2000.

Frieden IJ: Which hemangiomas to treat—and how? Arch Dermatol 133:1593-1595, 1997.

Schiller PI, Itin PH: Angiokeratomas: an update. Dermatology 193:275, 1996.

Esterly NB: Cutaneous hemangiomas, vascular stains and malformations, and associated syndromes. Curr Probl Dermatol 7:6, 1995.

Fishman SJ, Mulliken JB: Hemangiomas and vascular malformations of infancy and childhood. Pediatr Clin N Am 40:1177-1200, 1993.

Pyogenic Granuloma (Lobular Capillary Hemangioma)

Clinical Features
  ● Reactive, proliferating capillary hemangioma usually in response to localized trauma

Figure 2-68. Pyogenic granuloma. Histologic section shows focal epidermal ulceration covered by neutrophilic scale crust and a lobular proliferation of vascular spaces associated with stromal edema and inflammatory cell infiltrate, including neutrophils.

- Commonly affects children
- Predilection for sites of minor trauma, including the face and distal extremities
- Lesions typically enlarge rapidly and have a tendency to bleed with minor trauma
- Friable, small (<1 cm), erythematous papule; often pedunculated
- Lesions are initially finely lobulated and raspberry in color but become yellow, brown, or black with time

Histopathology

- Superficial ulceration typically present in early lesions
- Proliferation of capillary-sized vessels surrounded by an epidermal collarette
- Vessels typically lined by swollen endothelial cells
- Markedly edematous stroma, which fibroses with time
- Inflammatory infiltrate composed of neutrophils and mononuclear cells

Special Stains and Immunohistochemistry

- Noncontributory

Other Techniques for Diagnosis

- Noncontributory

Differential Diagnosis

▌ Capillary or cavernous hemangioma
  - Lesions typically contain dilated vascular channels without significant stromal edema or inflammatory infiltrate
▌ Bacillary angiomatosis
  - Infectious angiomatosis often seen in HIV-infected patients and caused by *Rochalimaea henselae* or *Rochalimaea quintana*, small gram-negative rods belonging to *Bartonella* species
  - Clumps of granular basophilic material that shows bacilli with Warthin-Starry or Giemsa stain are characteristically present in association with neutrophilic infiltrates

Pearls

- Pyogenic granuloma of the gingiva occurring in pregnant women is known as *epulis*

Selected References

Fortna RR, Junkins-Hopkins JM: A case of lobular capillary hemangioma (pyogenic granuloma), localized to the subcutaneous tissue and a review of the literature. Am J Dermatopathol 29:408, 2007.

Chian CA, Arrese JE, Pierard GE: Skin manifestations of Bartonella infections. Int J Dermatol 41:461, 2002.

Plettenberg A, Lorenzen T, Burtsche BT, et al: Bacillary angiomatosis in HIV-infected patients: An epidemiological and clinical study. Dermatology 201:326, 2000.

Requena L, Sangueza OP: Cutaneous vascular proliferation. Part II. Hyperplasias and benign neoplasms. J Am Acad Dermatol 37:887-919, 1997.

Park YH, Houh D, Houh W: Subcutaneous and superficial granuloma pyogenicum. Int J Dermatol 35:205-206, 1996.

Patrice SJ, Wiss K, Mulliken JB: Pyogenic granuloma (lobular capillary hemangioma): A clinicopathologic study of 178 cases. Pediatr Dermatol 8:267, 1994.

Kaposi Sarcoma

Clinical Features

- Slowly progressive multifocal vasoproliferative lesion of low-grade malignancy
- Four forms are recognized
  — Classic Kaposi sarcoma
    ◆ Affects mainly males of Eastern European and Mediterranean descent
    ◆ Presents as slowly developing nodules and plaques primarily affecting lower extremities
  — Endemic Kaposi sarcoma
    ◆ Occurs among native blacks in Central Africa
    ◆ Affects younger patients and children
  — Epidemic Kaposi sarcoma
    ◆ Occurs in immunocompromised states associated with HIV infection
    ◆ Typically involves trunk and mucosal surfaces
  — Kaposi sarcoma associated with iatrogenic immunosuppression
    ◆ Immunosuppressed states, associated with the treatment for transplant rejection, greatly increase the risk for Kaposi sarcoma

Histopathology

- Histopathologic findings are similar in all forms of Kaposi sarcoma
- Early patch stage
  — Characterized by slitlike spaces between the collagen bundles that often follow adnexal structures and preexisting blood vessels that appear to protrude into newly formed blood vessels (promontory sign)
  — Extravasated red blood cells and plasma cells may be present
- Plaque stage
  — Characterized by a proliferation of spindle-shaped cells arranged as short fascicles and a diffuse proliferation of blood vessels
  — Intracytoplasmic hyaline globules may be seen
- Nodular stage
  — Well-defined nodules of vascular spaces and spindle-shaped cells replace the dermis
  — Hemosiderin-laden macrophages are noted in the vicinity
  — Intracellular and extracellular hyaline globules are easily seen
- Late aggressive lesions of Kaposi sarcoma have features of an aggressive sarcoma with greater degree of cytologic atypia and high mitotic rate

Figure 2-69. A, Kaposi sarcoma, patch stage. Histologic section shows slitlike spaces between the collagen bundles and extravasated red blood cells. **B, Kaposi sarcoma, plaque stage.** Histologic section shows a spindle cell proliferation and irregular vascular spaces. **C, Kaposi sarcoma, nodular stage.** Histologic section shows a solid proliferation of spindle-shaped cells associated with extravasated red cells. Nuclear atypia and mitotic figures are present.

Special Stains and Immunohistochemistry

- Hyaline globules are PAS positive and diastase resistant
- Vascular nature of Kaposi sarcoma may be confirmed by immunostains CD31 and CD34

Other Techniques for Diagnosis

- Demonstration of human herpesvirus-8 in lesions of Kaposi sarcoma by ISH and recently by immunohistochemical methods in all clinical subtypes is helpful in differentiating Kaposi sarcoma from other vascular proliferations

Differential Diagnosis

- Early lesions need to be differentiated from benign vascular proliferations such as targetoid hemosiderotic hemangioma and fibrous histiocytoma
- Late aggressive forms need to be differentiated from other aggressive sarcomas and require immunohistochemical stains

▌ Angiosarcoma
- Asymmetrical collection of angulated, irregular vessels infiltrating between collagen bundles
- Vascular lumina lined by endothelial cells that contain hyperchromatic irregular nuclei and prominent nucleoli

Pearls

- Natural course of Kaposi sarcoma varies widely depending on the clinical setting
  — At presentation, the classic form is typically restricted to the surface of the body and has a relatively indolent course (associated with long survival)
  — Endemic and epidemic subsets are typically more widespread at presentation and may have an aggressive clinical course

Selected References

Patel RM, Goldblum JR, His ED: Immunohistochemical detection of human herpes virus-8 latent nuclear antigen-1 is useful in the diagnosis of Kaposi sarcoma. Mod Pathol 17:456, 2004.

Cheuk W, Wong KO, Wong CS, et al: Immunostaining for human herpesvirus 8 latent nuclear antigen-1 helps distinguish Kaposi's sarcoma from its mimics. Am J Clin Pathol 121:335, 2004.

Antman K, Chang Y: Kaposi sarcoma. N Engl J Med 342:1027-1038, 2000.

Iscovich J, Boffetta P, Franceschi S, et al: Classic Kaposi sarcoma: Epidemiology and risk factors. Cancer 88:500-517, 2000.

Friedman-Kien AE, Saltzman BR: Clinical manifestations of classical, endemic African, and epidemic AIDS-associated Kaposi's sarcoma. J Am Acad Dermatol 22:1237, 1990.

Angiosarcoma

Clinical Features

- Malignant proliferation of endothelial cells
- Commonly affects elderly (sixth to seventh decades) males

Figure 2-70. Angiosarcoma. Histologic section shows irregularly shaped vascular spaces lined by highly atypical endothelial cells with marked nuclear pleomorphism.

- Can also occur after lymphedema (postmastectomy) and radiation therapy
- Predilection for the face, scalp, and neck
- Lesions typically progress rapidly, leading to ulceration and hemorrhage
- Present as dusky irregular erythematous plaques, which are often ulcerated

Histopathology

- Asymmetrical collection of angulated, irregular vascular spaces infiltrating between collagen bundles
- Endothelial cells lining the vascular spaces have hyperchromatic irregular nuclei and prominent nucleoli; high mitotic rate
- In epithelioid angiosarcoma, the neoplastic cells are large and pleomorphic with abundant eosinophilic cytoplasm and a large nucleus with a prominent nucleolus
- Adjacent lymphatic spaces are often dilated
- Infiltrate of lymphocytes

Special Stains and Immunohistochemistry

- Factor VIIIR-ag, CD31, and CD34 highlight endothelial cells
- D2-40 staining in tumors of lymphatic origin

Other Techniques for Diagnosis

- Electron microscopy: Weibel-Palade bodies (rod-shaped lysosome-like structures) characteristic of endothelial cells

Differential Diagnosis

- Epithelioid hemangioma
  - Lesions are typically symmetrical and contain plump endothelial cells without nuclear atypia
- Kaposi sarcoma
  - Capillary spaces are typically slitlike
  - Associated inflammatory infiltrate is composed of plasma cells and lymphocytes

- Intravascular papillary endothelial hyperplasia
  - Lesions typically contain papillary fronds with no endothelial cell atypia; most likely represents an organizing thrombus
- Epithelial and melanocytic neoplasms
  - Epithelioid angiosarcoma may lack distinct vascular spaces and simulate epithelial or melanocytic neoplasms
  - Immunohistochemical studies are necessary for accurate diagnosis

Pearls

- Stewart-Treves syndrome: angiosarcoma arising in the upper extremities of patients who have undergone radical mastectomy with axillary lymph node dissection
- A rare variant of angiosarcoma is an entity known as *malignant endovascular papillary angioendothelioma*, or *Dabska tumor*

Selected References

Mendenhall WM, Mendenhall CM, Werning JW, et al: Cutaneous angiosarcoma. Am J Clin Oncol 29:524, 2006.

Billings SD, McKenney JK, Folpe AL, et al: Cutaneous angiosarcoma following breast-conserving surgery and radiation: An analysis of 27 cases. Am J Surg Pathol 28:781, 2004.

Schwartz RA, Dabski C, Dabska M: The Dabska tumor: A thirty-year retrospect. Dermatology 201:1-5, 2000.

Requena L, Sangueza OP: Cutaneous vascular proliferations. Part III. Malignant neoplasms, other cutaneous neoplasms with significant vascular component, and disorders erroneously considered as vascular neoplasms. J Am Acad Dermatol 38:143-175, 1998.

Smooth Muscle Neoplasms

Leiomyomas (Arrector Pili Muscle Type, Angioleiomyoma, Dartoic Leiomyoma)

Clinical Features

- Benign dermal and subcutaneous tumors composed of smooth muscle
- Arrector pili muscle hamartomas are painful lesions commonly affecting persons during the second and third decades of life
- Predilection for the face, anterior aspect of the trunk, and extensor surfaces of the extremities
- Typically present as small (typically <1 cm), smooth, firm, cutaneous nodules
- Nodules are usually pink to yellow or brown and translucent or waxy in appearance
- Angioleiomyomas usually occur as painful solitary subcutaneous lesions affecting the extremities especially the lower extremities

Figure 2-71. A, Leiomyoma, arrector pili muscle type. Fascicles of smooth muscle cells are seen within the upper part of the dermis. **B, Leiomyoma, vascular type.** A deep, dermal, well-circumscribed nodule composed of smooth muscle cells that surround and merge with the vessels walls.

- Dartoic leiomyomas occur as solitary, painless, flesh-colored lesions affecting the genitalia, including the scrotum, labia majora, and areola

Histopathology

▎ Arrector pili muscle type
- Symmetrical proliferation of smooth muscle within the superficial and deep dermis
- Interlacing fascicles of smooth muscle cells containing eosinophilic cytoplasm and cigar-shaped nuclei
▎ Angioleiomyoma
- Well-circumscribed nodule of interlacing bundles of smooth muscle
- Admixture of small branching vessels, typically venules

▎ Dartoic leiomyomas
- Similar in appearance to arrector pili muscle hamartomas

Special Stains and Immunohistochemistry
- Smooth muscle actin (SMA) positive

Other Techniques for Diagnosis
- Noncontributory

Differential Diagnosis

▎ Leiomyosarcoma
- Asymmetrical tumor with infiltrative fascicles of smooth muscle cells with coarse nuclei and numerous mitoses
▎ Neurofibroma
- Well-circumscribed, unencapsulated dermal mass of nerve sheath cells and fibroblasts
- Epidermal atrophy with indistinct rete ridges
- Spindle cells appear as wavy fibers with bland nuclei
- Characteristic presence of mast cells in the background
▎ Dermatofibroma
- Well-circumscribed but unencapsulated proliferation of fibroblasts with entrapped collagen bundles
- Characteristic hyperplasia of the overlying epidermis with basal cell hyperpigmentation
- Thick bundles of collagen are present at the periphery of the lesion

Pearls
- Multiple pilar-type leiomyomas are the commonest type

Selected References

Kawagishi N, Kashiwagi T, Ibe M, et al: Pleomorphic angioleiomyoma. Am J Dermatopathol 22:268-271, 2000.

Sajben FP, Barnette DJ, Barrett TL: Intravascular angioleiomyoma. J Cutan Pathol 26:165-167, 1999.

Heffernan MP, Smoller BR, Kohler S: Cutaneous epithelioid angioleiomyoma. Am J Dermatopathol 20:213-217, 1998.

Spencer JM, Amonette RA: Tumors with smooth muscle differentiation. Dermatol Surg 22:761-768, 1996.

Calonje E, Fletcher CD: New entities in cutaneous soft tissue tumours. Pathologica 85:1-15, 1993.

Cutaneous Leiomyosarcoma

Clinical Features

- Malignant proliferation of smooth muscle cells typically with features of arrector pili muscles
- Lesions commonly affect persons during the second and third decades of life
- Typically widely distributed with no appreciable site predilections
- Bleeding and ulceration of lesions commonly occur
- Firm dermal nodules typically less than 2 cm in diameter with discolored or depressed overlying skin

Figure 2-72. Leiomyosarcoma. Histologic section shows spindle-shaped cells with enlarged and hyperchromatic nuclei. Mitotic figures are present.

Histopathology

- Asymmetrical infiltrative fascicles of smooth muscle
- Intermixed zones of hypercellularity and better-differentiated zones
- Nuclei are hyperchromatic and have coarsely clumped chromatin
- High mitotic rate

Special Stains and Immunohistochemistry

- May be helpful in differentiating leiomyosarcoma from other spindle cell tumors
- Cells of leiomyosarcoma typically show positivity for desmin and SMA

Other Techniques for Diagnosis

- Noncontributory

Differential Diagnosis

▌ Leiomyoma
- Well-circumscribed proliferation of smooth muscle cells that typically form fascicles
- Cells are uniform and lack nuclear atypia
▌ Dermatofibrosarcoma protuberans (DFSP)
- Characterized by a storiform pattern and infiltration into the underlying subcutaneous fat
- Positive for CD34

Pearls

- Leiomyosarcomas typically metastasize through the bloodstream after invasion through the dermis

Selected References

Diaz-Cascajo C, Borghi S, Weyers W: Desmoplastic leiomyosarcoma of the skin. Am J Dermatopathol 22:251-255, 2000.

Lin JY, Tsai RY: Subcutaneous leiomyosarcoma on the face. Dermatol Surg 25:489-491, 1999.

Sidbury R, Heintz PW. Beckstead JH, White CR Jr: Cutaneous malignant epithelioid neoplasms. Adv Dermatol 14:285-306, 1999.

Cook TF, Fosko SW: Unusual cutaneous malignancies. Semin Cutan Med Surg 17:114-132, 1998.

Kaddu S, Beham A, Cerroni L, et al: Cutaneous leiomyosarcoma. Am J Surg Pathol 21:979-987, 1997.

Fish FS: Soft tissue sarcomas in dermatology. Dermatol Surg 22:268-273, 1996.

Spencer JM, Amonette RA: Tumors with smooth muscle differentiation. Dermatol Surg 22:761-768, 1996.

Fibroblastic Proliferations and Neoplasms

Keloid

Clinical Features

- Scar that has grown beyond its initial margins
- Usually presents as a well-defined, round to linear elevation of the skin
- Tends to occur more often in females than males
- Dark-skinned individuals are more commonly affected
- Common sites include the earlobe following ear piercing
- Typically associated with trauma or surgery

Histopathology

- Characterized by accumulation of thick, hyalinized collagen fibers arranged in a haphazard pattern
- Prominent myxoid matrix
- Early lesions are more vascular, whereas older lesions are predominantly fibrous

Figure 2-73. Keloid. Histologic section shows a nodular proliferation of fibroblasts associated with irregularly thickened bundles of collagen.

Special Stains and Immunohistochemistry
- Noncontributory

Other Techniques for Diagnosis
- Noncontributory

Differential Diagnosis
▌ Hypertrophic scar
- Scar is limited to the area of injury
- Also shows thickened collagen fibers, but shows a lesser amount of myxoid matrix

Pearls
- Treated by various modes of therapy ranging from tropical steroid injections to surgical excision
- Unknown etiology; may be familial

Selected References

English RS, Shenefelt PD: Keloids and hypertrophic scars. Dermatol Surg 25:631-638, 1999.

Niessen FB, Spauwen PH, Schalkwijk J, Kon M: On the nature of hypertrophic scars and keloids: a review. Plast Reconstruct Surg 104:1435-1458, 1999.

Sahl WJ Jr, Clever H: Cutaneous scars: Part I. Int J Dermatol 33:681-691, 1994.

Sahl WJ Jr, Clever H: Cutaneous scars: Part II. Int J Dermatol 33:763-769, 1994.

Dermatofibroma

Clinical Features
- Reactive hyperplasia of fibroblasts, histiocytes, and vascular elements
- Common lesion that affects mostly young or middle-aged adults, with slightly higher incidence in females
- Predilection for the arms and legs and other areas exposed to trauma
- Slow-growing, painless, usually single lesions that expand in a symmetrical fashion
- Typically small (<1 cm), freely mobile, and tan to brown colored

Histopathology
- Well-circumscribed but unencapsulated proliferation of fibroblasts with entrapped collagen bundles
- Characteristic hyperplasia of the overlying epidermis with basal cell hyperpigmentation
- Thick bundles of collagen are present at the periphery of the lesion
- Occasional xanthomatous features with admixed histiocytes, foam cells, and multinucleated giant cells
- Occasional vascular proliferation with hemosiderin deposition

Figure 2-74. **Dermatofibroma. A,** Histologic section shows a well-defined dermal nodule of fibroblasts and histiocytes. **B,** High-power view shows fibroblasts and multinucleated histiocytes with foamy cytoplasm and hemosiderin pigment.

Special Stains and Immunohistochemistry
- Negative for CD34
- Positive for factor XIIIa

Other Techniques for Diagnosis
- Noncontributory

Differential Diagnosis
▌ DFSP
- Lesions have a characteristic storiform pattern
- Typically infiltrates the subcutaneous fat in a lacelike pattern
- Foci of hypercellularity and mitoses are usually present
▌ Neurofibroma
- Well-circumscribed, unencapsulated dermal mass of nerve sheath cells and fibers
- Epidermal atrophy with indistinct rete ridges
- Spindle cells appear as wavy fibers with bland nuclei
- Characteristic presence of mast cells in the background

- Basal cell carcinoma
  - Follicular induction seen in dermatofibromas may resemble basal cell carcinoma
  - Predilection for sun-exposed skin, typically face and hands
  - Multiple nests of basaloid cells with peripheral palisading and presence of a mucinous stroma with retraction artifacts
  - Basaloid cells are typically uniform and have frequent mitotic activity and abundant apoptosis

Pearls

- Dermatofibromas rarely present with hyperesthesia and minor pain
- Fitzpatrick sign: application of centripetal compression results in central dimpling of the dermatofibromas due to tethering of the mass to the deep dermis

Selected References

De Unamuno P, Carames Y, Fernandez-Lopez E, et al: Congenital multiple clustered dermatofibroma. Br J Dermatol 142:1040-1043, 2000.

Pariser RJ: Benign neoplasms of the skin. Med Clin N Am 82:1285-1307, v-vi, 1998.

Cohen PR, Rapin RP, Farhood AI: Dermatofibroma and dermatofibrosarcoma protuberans: Differential expression of CD34 and factor XIIIa. Am J Dermatopathol 16:573-574, 1994.

Dermatofibrosarcoma Protuberans

Clinical Features

- Locally invasive fibroblastic tumor
- Uncommon lesion typically seen in males during the third and fourth decades
- Predilection for the trunk and occasionally the proximal extremities
- Initially slow-growing, single lesion that accelerates in growth after a period of quiescence
- Initially presents as firm, freely mobile, tan to brown cutaneous nodule
- With time, lesions enlarge to form a blue-red, multilobular nodules

Histopathology

- Asymmetrical, diffuse, deep dermal to subcutaneous lesion
- Proliferation of bland spindle cells in a typical cartwheel or storiform pattern
- Neoplastic cells infiltrate into the subcutaneous fat in lacelike pattern
- Few mitotic figures; rare atypical mitoses, necrosis, or multinucleated giant cells
- Overlying epidermis is typically thinned

Figure 2-75. Dermatofibrosarcoma protuberans. A, Low-power view shows a deeply infiltrative proliferation of spindle-shaped cells. **B,** High-power view shows the slender spindle-shaped cells infiltrating and replacing the subcutaneous fat.

Special Stains and Immunohistochemistry

- CD34 positive

Other Techniques for Diagnosis

- Noncontributory

Differential Diagnosis

- Dermatofibroma
  - Well-circumscribed but unencapsulated proliferation of fibroblasts with entrapped collagen bundles

- Characteristic hyperplasia of the overlying epidermis with basal cell hyperpigmentation
- Thick bundles of collagen are present at the periphery of the lesion
- Mitotic figures and necrosis are generally absent
▌ Neurofibroma
  - Well-circumscribed, unencapsulated dermal mass of nerve sheath cells and nerve fibers
  - Epidermal atrophy with indistinct rete ridges
  - Spindle cells appear as wavy fibers with bland nuclei
  - Characteristic presence of mast cells in the background

Pearls

- Surgical removal of a DFSP is often followed by a recurrence due to the infiltrative nature of the tumor
- Bednar variant contains spindle-shaped cells with melanin pigment

Selected References

Cohen PR, Rapin RP, Farhood AI: Dermatofibroma and dermatofibrosarcoma protuberans: Differential expression of CD34 and factor XIIIa. Am J Dermatopathol 16:573-574, 1994.

Zelger B, Sidoroff A, Stanzl U, et al: Deep penetrating dermatofibroma versus dermatofibrosarcoma protuberans: A clinicopathologic comparison. Am J Surg Pathol 18:677-686, 1994.

Fletcher CD, Evans BJ, MacArtney, et al: Dermatofibrosarcoma protuberans: A clinicopathologic and immunohistochemical study with a review of the literature. Histopathology 9:921-938, 1985.

Neural Neoplasms

Neurofibroma

Clinical Features

- Benign tumors of perineural supporting cells
- Lesions tend to be solitary and unassociated with any particular age or gender group except when associated with von Recklinghausen neurofibromatosis
- Can involve any site, but lesions tend to avoid palms and soles
- Present as small (<1 cm), soft, tan papules or nodules, occasionally larger or pedunculated

Histopathology

- Well-circumscribed, unencapsulated dermal mass of nerve sheath cells and fibroblasts
- Epidermal atrophy with indistinct rete ridges
- Spindle cells appear as wavy fibers with bland nuclei
- Characteristic presence of mast cells in the background

Figure 2-76. A, Neurofibroma. Histologic section shows a dermal proliferation of spindle-shaped cells with wavy nuclei and a loose myxoid stroma. Mast cells are typically present in the background. **B, Palisaded and encapsulated neuroma.** Histologic section shows a well-circumscribed nodule of spindle-shaped cells with elongated nuclei and a palisaded arrangement.

Special Stains and Immunohistochemistry

- S-100 protein positive

Other Techniques for Diagnosis

- Noncontributory

Differential Diagnosis

▌ Palisaded and encapsulated neuroma
  - Well-circumscribed superficial dermal nodule resembling schwannoma
  - Spindle-shaped cells with elongated nuclei arranged in palisades
▌ Dermatofibroma
  - Well-circumscribed but unencapsulated proliferation of fibroblasts and histiocytes in varying numbers
  - Characteristic hyperplasia of the overlying epidermis with basal cell hyperpigmentation
  - Thick bundles of collagen may be present at the periphery of the lesion

▌ Schwannoma

- Typically consists of an encapsulated spindle cell proliferation with distinct zones
  — Antoni A zones (hypercellular and composed predominantly of spindle cells)
  — Antoni B zones (hypocellular areas composed of spindle cells with abundant mucinous background)
  — Verocay bodies (parallel arrangements of nuclei)

Pearls

- Von Recklinghausen neurofibromatosis is a systemic hereditary disease characterized by café-au-lait spots and multiple neurofibromas composed of cellular and hypertrophied nerve trunks that usually develop after birth but before puberty
- Spindle cell elements of neurofibromas are primarily composed of Schwann cells

Selected References

Argenyi ZB, Santa-Cruz D, Bromley C: Comparative light-microscopic and immunohistochemical study of traumatic and palisaded and encapsulated neuromas of the skin. Am J Dermatopathol 14:504, 1992.

Murphy GF, Elder DE: Atlas of Tumor Pathology: Non-Melanocytic Tumor of the Skin. Third Series, Fascicle 1. Washington, DC, Armed Forces Institute of Pathology, 1990.

Riccardi VM: Von Recklinghausen neurofibromatosis. N Engl J Med 305:1617, 1981.

Merkel Cell Carcinoma (Cutaneous Small Cell Undifferentiated Carcinoma)

Clinical Features

- Uncommon neoplasm with neuroendocrine differentiation
- Most common sites of involvement are head and extremities
- Presents most commonly as a solitary nodule and rarely as multiple nodules
- Lesions are pink, firm, and nodular and typically range in size from 0.8 to 4 cm
- Skin ulceration is uncommon

Histopathology

- Dermal nodule composed of small, round, blue cells with scant cytoplasm and irregular nuclei with uniformly distributed chromatin
- Tumor cells are arranged in sheets or trabeculae and may form pseudorosettes
- Nucleoli are inconspicuous, and nuclear molding may be present
- Frequent mitotic figures and individually necrotic tumor cells are common
- Stroma between the nests of tumor cells is scant

Figure 2-77. Merkel cell carcinoma. A, Low-power view shows a dermal nodule of small blue cells arranged in sheets and trabeculae. **B,** High-power view shows cells with scant cytoplasm and irregular nuclei. Nucleoli are inconspicuous. Mitotic figures and individually necrotic cells are present. **C,** Cytokeratin stain shows perinuclear dotlike positivity of the neoplastic cells.

- Tumor cells may extend into the overlying epidermis in a pagetoid pattern
- Overlying epidermis may show varying degrees of atypia and occasionally SCC

Special Stains and Immunohistochemistry

- Neuron-specific enolase (NSE) and neurofilament positive

- Chromogranin positive
- Cytokeratin 20 positive

Other Techniques for Diagnosis

- Electron microscopy shows membrane-bound dense-core granules and perinuclear bundles or whorls of intermediate filaments

Differential Diagnosis

▮ Metastatic small cell carcinoma
- Immunohistochemical stain for cytokeratin 20 generally negative
▮ Malignant lymphoma
- Immunohistochemical stains leukocyte common antigen (LCA) and T- and B-cell markers are helpful
▮ Other primitive neuroectodermal tumors such as Ewing sarcoma and neuroblastoma should be considered

Pearls

- Divergent differentiation consisting of squamous, adnexal, and melanocytic areas can be seen in neuroendocrine carcinoma of the skin

Selected References

Ratner D, Nelson BR, Brown MD, Johnson TM: Merkel cell carcinoma. J Am Acad Dermatol 29:143, 1993.

Smith KJ, Skelton HG 3rd, Holland TT, et al: Neuroendocrine (Merkel cell) carcinoma with an intraepidermal component. Am J Dermatopathol 15:528, 1993.

Isimbaldi G, Sironi M, Taccagni GL, et al: Tripartite differentiation (squamous, glandular, and melanocytic) of a primary cutaneous neurocrine carcinoma: An immunocytochemical and ultrastructural study. Am J Dermatopathol 15:260, 1993.

Haneke E: Electron microscopy of Merkel cell carcinoma from formalin-fixed tissue. J Am Acad Dermatol 12:487, 1985.

Wick MR, Goellner JR, Scheithauer BW, et al: Primary neuroendocrine carcinomas of the skin (Merkel cell tumors): A clinical, histologic, and ultrastructural study of thirteen cases. Am J Clin Pathol 79:6, 1983.

Hematopoietic Proliferations and Neoplasms

Urticaria Pigmentosa

Clinical Features

- Can present in four forms
  — Arising in infancy and childhood without associated systemic lesions
  — Arising in adolescence or adulthood without associated systemic lesions
  — Systemic mast cell disease
  — Mast cell leukemia

Figure 2-78. Urticaria pigmentosa. A, Hematoxylin and eosin–stained section shows a dense, diffuse dermal infiltrate of mast cells. **B,** Immunohistochemical stain for mast cell tryptase highlights the mast cells.

- Cutaneous lesions can take many forms
  — Maculopapular: can occur in infantile and adult forms
  — Nodular and plaquelike: can occur in infantile and adult forms
  — Solitary nodule: seen in infancy
  — Diffuse erythroderma: always starts in infancy
  — Telangiectasia macularis eruptive perstans: occurs in adults

Histopathology

- Nodules and plaques
  — Dense, diffuse dermal infiltrate composed of mast cells is characteristic
  — Infiltrate may extend into subcutis
  — Mast cells contain metachromatic granules in the cytoplasm
- Maculopapular type and telangiectasia macularis eruptive perstans

— Mast cells are distributed in a perivascular pattern in the upper dermis
- Erythrodermic urticaria pigmentosa
  — Mast cells are arranged in a dense bandlike pattern in the upper dermis
- Eosinophils are present in varying numbers; especially if biopsy is taken after urtication
- Subepidermal bullae may be noted in some cases (bullous mastocytosis)
- Increased pigment in the basal cell layer of epidermis and melanophages in the dermis are responsible for the pigmentation of the lesions clinically

Special Stain and Immunohistochemistry

- Metachromatic granules in mast cells are best seen with Giemsa, toluidine blue, and Leder stains
- Immunohistochemical stain for mast cell tryptase and CD117 positive

Other Techniques for Diagnosis

- Noncontributory

Differential Diagnosis

▮ Langerhans cell histiocytosis
- Can be differentiated by the presence of aggregates of histiocytes in the epidermis that are positive for CD1a and S-100 protein
▮ Inflammatory dermatoses
- In sparsely cellular examples of urticaria pigmentosa, special stains are essential to demonstrate mast cells and differentiate from other dermatitis
- Mast cells have a distinct appearance and are easy to differentiate from other cellular infiltrates in the dermis in most cases

Pearls

- Mast cells stimulate the melanocytes of the epidermis to produce more melanin
- In systemic mast cell disease, mostly seen in adults, massive infiltration of the bones may cause collapse of vertebrae and fractures of large bones
- Systemic mast cell disease can also involve lymph nodes, liver, spleen, gastrointestinal tract, and central nervous system

Selected References

Khanna N, D'Souza P: Urticaria pigmentosa (mastocytosis). Indian Pediatr 35:253-254, 1998.

Topar G, Staudacher C, Geisen F, et al: Urticaria pigmentosa: A clinical, hematopathologic, and serologic study of 30 adults. Am J Clin Pathol 109:279-285, 1998.

Allison MA, Schmidt CP: Urticaria pigmentosa. Int J Dermatol 36:321-325, 1997.

Schneider I, Schwartz RA: Mast cell disease. Cutis 59:63-66, 1997.

Leaf FA, Jaecks EP, Rodriguez DR: Bullous urticaria pigmentosa. Cutis 58:358-360, 1996.

Mihm MC, Clark WH, Reed RJ, et al: Mast cell infiltrates of the skin and the mastocytosis syndrome. Hum Pathol 4:231, 1973.

Langerhans Cell Histiocytosis and Histiocytosis X (Letterer-Siwe Disease, Hand-Schüller-Christian Disease, Eosinophilic Granuloma)

Clinical Features

- A histiocytic proliferative disorder of unknown etiology composed of three separate clinical entities
▮ Letterer-Siwe disease (acute disseminated form)
- Rare disease usually seen in male infants between 3 months and 3 years of age
- Patients commonly present with constitutional signs, extraosseous lesions, hepatosplenomegaly, lymphadenopathy, and cutaneous lesions

Figure 2-79. Langerhans cell histiocytosis. A, Histologic section shows dermal infiltrate of histiocytic cells with abundant cytoplasm and irregular lobulated nuclei; many of the cells extend into the overlying epidermis. B, Immunohistochemical stain for CD1a shows strong positivity of the histiocytic cells.

- Predilection of the cutaneous lesions for the scalp, face, mouth, neck, trunk, and buttocks
- Scaling, yellow-brown, purpuric, papular eruptions

▪ Hand-Schüller-Christian disease (chronic multifocal form)
- Rare disease usually seen in toddlers between 2 and 6 years of age
- Patients commonly present with chronic otitis media and portions of the classical triad of cranial bone defects, exophthalmos, and diabetes insipidus as well as cutaneous lesions
- Predilection of the cutaneous lesions for the chest, axillae, and groin
- Similar to Letterer-Siwe disease with occasional red-brown papulopustular or papulonodular lesions

▪ Eosinophilic granuloma (chronic focal form)
- Rare disease usually seen in toddlers between 2 and 5 years of age
- Patients commonly develop osteolytic, pulmonary, cutaneous, and occasionally cranial lesions
- Predilection of cutaneous lesions for the scalp, face, oral cavity, and groin
- Multiple ulcerative crusted papules or multiple subcutaneous nodules

Histopathology

- The histologic picture is essentially similar in all clinical forms and is characterized by the presence of Langerhans cells in an appropriate context
- Characteristic Langerhans cells are large and rounded with indistinct cell membranes and clearly demarcated lobulated or folded nuclei
- Langerhans cells are variably present throughout the dermis and frequently found in the epidermis
- Prominent infiltrate of eosinophils may be present in the background

Special Stains and Immunohistochemistry

- S-100 protein: Langerhans cells, melanocytes, and activated histiocytes are positive
- CD1a: Langerhans cells are positive

Other Techniques for Diagnosis

- Electron microscopy: presence of tennis racquet–shaped Birbeck granules within Langerhans cells

Differential Diagnosis

▪ Xanthogranuloma
- Lesions contain multinucleated cells with peripheral vacuolization of the cytoplasm

▪ Reticulohistiocytoma
- Lesions contain multinucleated cells with red-purple granular cytoplasm (ground-glass giant cells)

▪ Congenital self-healing reticulohistiocytosis
- Scattered papules and nodules are present at birth or appear shortly after

- Ground-glass giant cells on histology
- Lesions begin to involute in 2 to 3 months and completely regress within 1 year

▪ Cutaneous T-cell lymphoma
- Composed of atypical lymphoid cells
- Positive for LCA and T-cell markers

Pearls

- Langerhans cells may occasionally appear vacuolated and multinucleated, giving a xanthomatous appearance
- Prognosis and clinical course depend on the age of the patient and the extent of organ involvement

Selected References

Kapur P, Erickson C, Rakheja D, et al: Congenital self-healing reticulohistiocytosis (Hashimoto-Pritzker disease): Ten-year experience at Dallas Children's Medical Center. J Am Acad Dermatol 56:290, 2007.

Minkov M, Prosch H, Steiner M, et al: Langerhans cell histiocytosis in neonates. Pediatr Blood Cancer 45:802, 2005.

Howarth DM, Gilchrist GS, Mullan BP, et al: Langerhans cell histiocytosis: Diagnosis, natural history, management, and outcome. Cancer 85:2278, 1999.

Herzog KM, Tubbs RR: Langerhans cell histiocytosis. Adv Anat Pathol 5:347-358, 1998.

Ladisch S: Langerhans cell histiocytosis. Curr Opin Hematol 5:54-58, 1998.

Munn S, Chu AC: Langerhans cell histiocytosis of the skin. Hematol Oncol Clin N Am 12:269-286, 1998.

Favara BE, Jaffe R: The histopathology of Langerhans cell histiocytosis. Br J Cancer 23(Suppl):S17-23, 1994.

Willman CL, Busque L, Griffith BB, et al: Langerhans'-cell histiocytosis (histiocytosis X): A clonal proliferative disease. N Engl J Med 331:154, 1994.

Cutaneous T-Cell Lymphoma (Mycosis Fungoides)

Clinical Features

- Mycosis fungoides is the most common form of primary cutaneous lymphoma
- It may present as a patch, plaque, or nodule or tumor
- Patches of mycosis fungoides are erythematous and scaly and affect trunk and proximal extremities
- Lesions typically vary in size from 1 cm to several centimeters
- Plaques are usually well defined and occasionally annular
- Nodules and tumors represent advanced disease and are indistinguishable from other aggressive cutaneous lymphomas; lesions are reddish-brown and firm and are often ulcerated
- All forms may be seen in the same patient at the same time

Figure 2-80. Mycosis fungoides. A, Psoriasiform epidermal hyperplasia and a bandlike infiltrate of lymphoid cells within a thickened papillary dermis are seen. **B,** Collections of atypical lymphoid cells are seen in the epidermis (epidermotropism, Pautrier microabscesses).

Histopathology

- Patch stage
  - Patchy lichenoid infiltrate of lymphocytes in markedly thickened papillary dermis and in small collections within a minimally spongiotic epidermis
  - Epidermis may show psoriasiform hyperplasia
- Plaque stage
  - Features are similar to those seen in patch stage, but the infiltrate is denser and more bandlike
  - Lymphocytes may be cytologically atypical
- Tumor stage
  - Diffuse dermal infiltrate of atypical lymphocytes with convoluted nuclei
  - Increase in the number of medium to large lymphoid cells

Special Stains and Immunohistochemistry

- Most of the lymphoid cells are CD3, CD4, and CD5 positive and CD8 negative

Other Techniques for Diagnosis

- Gene rearrangement studies for T-cell receptor

Differential Diagnosis

I Spongiotic dermatitis
  - Early lesions of mycosis fungoides may be difficult to differentiate from spongiotic dermatitis
  - Papillary dermal collagen changes and intraepidermal collections of lymphocytes with only minimal spongiosis favor mycosis fungoides
I Nodules of mycosis fungoides need to be differentiated from other cutaneous lymphomas
  - Immunohistochemical studies to confirm T-cell phenotype are helpful in differentiating from B-cell lymphomas and lymphoid hyperplasias
  - CD30 immunostain is useful in distinguishing mycosis fungoides from cutaneous anaplastic large cell lymphoma

Pearls

- Sézary syndrome represents an erythrodermic form of mycosis fungoides with neoplastic cells populating the peripheral blood
- Follicular mucinosis may be a feature in some cases of mycosis fungoides

Selected References

Reddy K, Bhawan J: Histologic mimickers of mycosis fungoides: A review. J Cutan Pathol 34:519-525, 2007.

Willemze R, Jaffe E, Burg G, et al: WHO-EORTC classification for cutaneous lymphomas. Blood 105:3768-3785, 2005.

Siegel RS, Pandolfino T, Guitart J, et al: Primary cutaneous T-cell lymphoma: Review and current concepts. J Clin Oncol 18:2908-2925, 2000.

Dalton JA, Yag-Howard C, Messina JL, Glass LF: Cutaneous T-cell lymphoma. Int J Dermatol 36:801-809, 1997.

Burg G, Dummer R, Dommann S, et al: Pathology of cutaneous T-cell lymphoma. Hematol Oncol Clin North Am 9:961-995, 1995.

Primary Cutaneous CD30-Positive T-Cell Lymphoma (Anaplastic Large Cell Lymphoma)

Clinical Features

- Represents the malignant end in the spectrum of related diseases that include lymphomatoid papulosis
- Characterized by the presence of atypical lymphoid cells expressing CD30 antigen
- Presents as one or multiple large nodules
- Frequently ulcerated

Figure 2-81. Primary cutaneous large cell lymphoma. A, Histologic section shows epidermal ulceration and a dense dermal infiltrate of lymphoid cells. **B,** High-power view shows highly atypical lymphoid cells with irregular vesicular nuclei and coarse chromatin. These cells are typically positive for CD30.

- Patients of any age: systemic involvement more common in children

Histopathology

- Dense dermal infiltrate of large atypical lymphocytes with abundant cytoplasm and irregular vesicular nuclei with coarse chromatin
- Multinucleated cells often seen
- Mitotic figures may be present
- Infiltrate may extend into the subcutaneous tissue

Special Stains and Immunohistochemistry

- Anaplastic lymphoid cells are positive for CD30 (Ki-1)
- Most of the neoplastic cells are CD4 positive

Other Techniques for Diagnosis

- Gene rearrangement studies show clonal rearrangement of the T-cell receptor gene
- Epstein-Barr virus viral genome is identifiable in the neoplastic cells in some cases

Differential Diagnosis

▮ Lymphomatoid papulosis
- Presents clinically as multiple small lesions
- Histologically, the infiltrate is mixed, and fewer atypical lymphoid cells are present

▮ Hodgkin disease
- Cutaneous involvement is secondary to extension from involved lymph nodes
- Characterized by presence of Reed-Sternberg or lacunar cells (positive for CD15 and CD30)

Pearls

- CD30-positive cells can be also found in late-stage mycosis fungoides and pleomorphic T-cell lymphoma
- CD30 expression is also seen in carcinomas such as embryonal carcinoma
- Primary cutaneous anaplastic large cell lymphoma should be differentiated from secondary cutaneous involvement of primary systemic lymphoma and other high-grade lymphomas that are associated with significantly worse prognosis

Selected References

Murphy GF, Hsu M: Cutaneous lymphomas and leukemias. In Elder DE, Elenitsas R, Johnson BL Jr, et al (eds): Lever's Histopathology of Skin, 10th ed. Philadelphia, Lippincott Williams & Wilkins, 2008, p 911.

Bekkenk MW, Geelen FA, van Voorst Vader PC, et al: Primary and secondary cutaneous CD30(+) lymphoproliferative disorders: A report from the Dutch Cutaneous Lymphoma Group on the long-term follow-up data of 219 patients and guidelines for diagnosis and treatment. Blood 95:3653-3661, 2000.

Kummer JA, Vermeer MH, Dukers D, et al: Most primary cutaneous CD30-positive lymphoproliferative disorders have a CD4-positive cytotoxic T-cell phenotype. J Invest Dermatol 109:636-640, 1997.

Leboit PE: Lymphomatoid papulosis and cutaneous CD30+ lymphoma. Am J Dermatopathol 18:221, 1996.

Paulli M, Berti E, Rosso R, et al: CD30/Ki-1-positive lymphoproliferative disorders of the skin: Clinicopathologic correlation and statistical analysis of 86 cases. A multicentric study from the European Organization for Research and Treatment of Cancer. Cutaneous Lymphoma Project Group. J Clin Oncol 13:1343, 1995.

Pallesen G: The diagnostic significance of the CD30 (Ki-1) antigen. Histopathology 16:409, 1990.

Michelle D. Williams and Adel K. El-Naggar

3

Head and Neck

Thyroid Gland

Granulomatous Thyroiditis (de Quervain Thyroiditis)

Clinical Features

- Also called subacute thyroiditis
- Presents with clinically marked tenderness of thyroid, fever, sore throat, malaise most likely related to systemic viral illness
- Most commonly affects middle-aged women
- Majority of cases show complete resolution; initial phase often is hyperthyroid (elevated thyroxine [T_4] and triiodothyronine [T_3] levels); may lead to hypothyroidism, usually euthyroid on resolution
- Rarely comes to surgery; treat with aspirin, steroids

Gross Pathology

- Asymmetrically enlarged, firm thyroid
- Nodular process involving entire gland

Histopathology

- Nodular process, variable fibrosis
- Mixed inflammatory infiltrate: lymphoplasmacytic, giant cells, neutrophils with microabscesses (early), and foamy histiocytes
- Giant cells contain ingested extravasated colloid material
- Centered around follicles, which are lost in later stage

Special Stains and Immunohistochemistry

- May need acid-fast bacillus (AFB) stain and Gomori methenamine silver (GMS) stain to evaluate for infectious etiology

Other Techniques for Diagnosis

- Noncontributory

Differential Diagnosis

▌ Acute thyroiditis
  - Neutrophilic infiltration within thyroid gland parenchyma

Figure 3-1. Subacute thyroiditis (de Quervain thyroiditis). Section shows foreign-body giant cell granulomas. The giant cells contain ingested colloid material.

- Microabscesses and necrosis common, possible vasculitis
- No granuloma formation
- Caused by bacterial, fungal, or viral infections
▌ Granulomatous diseases
- Sarcoidosis: granulomas (noncaseating) in interstitial location
- Tuberculosis: caseating granulomas (AFB stain)
- Fungal: usually acute and necrotizing, less likely granulomatous (GMS stain)
▌ Riedel thyroiditis
- Diffuse fibrotic process involving the thyroid obliterating the thyroid architecture
- Fibrosis extends to soft tissue outside the thyroid
- Giant cells are absent
▌ Hashimoto thyroiditis
- Lymphocytic thyroiditis with germinal center formation and oxyphilic change of the follicular epithelium
- May have extensive fibrosis with follicular loss and architectural distortion
▌ Palpation thyroiditis
- Result of minor trauma to thyroid tissue
- Usually an incidental finding
- Scattered small foci of histiocytes, few lymphocytes, and rare giant cells within thyroid follicles (no neutrophils)

Pearls

- Associated with systemic viral infection, usually self-limited, ending euthyroid
- Neutrophilic inflammation only seen in initial or early stage of disease

Selected References

Benbassat CA, Olchovsky D, Tsvetov G, Shimon I: Subacute thyroiditis: Clinical characteristics and treatment outcome in fifty-six consecutive patients diagnosed between 1999 and 2005. J Endocrinol Invest 30:631-635, 2007.

Duininck TM, van Heerden JA, Fatourechi V, et al: De Quervain's thyroiditis: Surgical experience. Endocrine Pract 8:255-258, 2002.

Kojima M, Nakamura S, Oyama T, et al: Cellular composition of subacute thyroiditis: An immunohistochemical study of six cases. Pathol Res Pract 198:833-837, 2002.

Thompson LD, Heffess CS: Subacute (de Quervain's) thyroiditis. Ear Nose Throat J 81:623, 2002.

Chronic Lymphocytic Thyroiditis (Hashimoto Thyroiditis)

Clinical Features

- Immune-mediated inflammatory disease
- Autoantibodies detected in serum: antithyroglobulin, antithyroid peroxidase, antithyroid microsomal antibodies

Figure 3-2. Hashimoto thyroiditis. A, Gross photograph showing thyroid enlargement with pale lobulated cut surface. **B,** Marked lymphocytic infiltration with germinal center formation; *inset* shows follicular atrophy, marked plasma cell infiltrate, and fibrosis.

- Marked female predominance (5:1); peak in middle-aged women
- Higher incidence in high-iodine areas (United States, Japan)
- Clinically hypothyroid with diffuse, firm, enlarged thyroid
- Familial cases; associations with HLA-DR3 and HLA-DR5
- Higher incidence in Turner and Down syndromes and familial Alzheimer disease
- May coexist with other autoimmune diseases (Sjögren syndrome, diabetes, others)
- Increased risk for primary thyroid lymphoma

Gross Pathology

- Firm, diffusely enlarged thyroid
- Cut surface is pale tan-yellow and nodular

Histopathology

- Marked lymphoplasmacytic infiltration with germinal center formation
- Follicles are small with scant colloid
- Oncocytic metaplasia (Hürthle cell change) with enlarged, hyperchromatic nuclei of follicles may show proliferation (dominant nodules)
- Squamous metaplasia is common
- Fibrosis varies; marked in fibrous variant
- Nodularity of follicles and inflammation may extend into adjacent soft tissue (do not mistake for metastasis in lymph node)
- Optically clear and enlarged follicular nuclei often present

Special Stains and Immunohistochemistry

- Rarely necessary—inflammation is mixed B (CD20) and T (CD3, CD4, CD8) cells, plasma cells polyclonal (κ and λ cells)

Other Techniques for Diagnosis

- Clinical evaluation for antibodies

Differential Diagnosis

- Extranodal marginal zone B-cell lymphoma (mucosa-associated lymphoid tissue [MALT] lymphoma)
  - Rapid enlargement with sheets of lymphocytic infiltrate
  - Increased risk in Hashimoto thyroiditis
- Associated papillary thyroid carcinoma
  - Look for architectural distortion, fibrosis, invasive nests
  - Cellular proliferation with strict nuclear criteria of papillary carcinoma
  - Optically clear and enlarged nuclei may accompany lymphocytic thyroiditis
- Follicular neoplasm
  - Well-circumscribed lesion with capsule
  - Define based on capsular breach and lymphovascular invasion

- Nonspecific lymphocytic thyroiditis
  - Scattered, patchy chronic inflammation, occasional germinal center
  - Lacking oncocytic changes
  - Minimal fibrosis

Pearls

- May coexist with other thyroid neoplasms (especially papillary thyroid carcinoma); follicular nuclear changes may overlap
- Rare malignant transformation into lymphoma (MALT, diffuse large B-cell lymphoma)
- Benign follicles and lymphocytes may form nodules separated from the gland (parasitic nodule) in soft tissue

Selected References

MacDonald L, Yazdi HM: Fine needle aspiration biopsy of Hashimoto's thyroiditis: Sources of diagnostic error. Acta Cytol 43:400-406, 1999.

Nguyen GK, Ginsberg J, Crockford PM, Villanueva RR: Hashimoto's thyroiditis: Cytodiagnostic accuracy and pitfalls. Diagn Cytopathol 16:531-536, 1997.

Mizukami Y, Michigishi T, Kawato M, et al: Chronic thyroiditis: A new clinically relevant classification. Pathol Ann 29:135-158, 1994.

Riedel Thyroiditis

Clinical Features

- Also called Riedel struma, fibrous thyroiditis
- Very rare; predilection for women (5:1) with peak in fifth decade
- Clinically appears as an ill-defined, extremely firm, painless goiter
- May present with dyspnea as a result of tracheal compression

Figure 3-3. Riedel thyroiditis. Diffuse fibrosis is present with scattered inflammatory cells.

- One third of patients will develop a process in other sites: mediastinal or retroperitoneal fibrosis, sclerosing cholangitis (regarded as a manifestation of the idiopathic inflammatory fibrosclerosis disorders)

Gross Pathology
- Diffuse enlargement of thyroid gland, hard, stonelike with adherent soft tissue
- Cut surface white, fibrotic, and "woody"

Histopathology
- Prominent finding is fibrosis extending into soft tissue and muscle (greater than inflammation)
- Scattered mixed chronic inflammatory infiltrate (lymphocytes, plasma cells, neutrophils, monocytes, eosinophils)
- "Occlusive phlebitis" with infiltration of veins by lymphocytes and plasma cells; vessels have thickened wall and myxoid change
- Giant cells or germinal centers are not present

Special Stains and Immunohistochemistry
- Noncontributory

Other Techniques for Diagnosis
- Noncontributory

Differential Diagnosis
▌ Hashimoto thyroiditis (fibrous variant)
- Characterized by lobulated, follicular epithelium with oncocytic change, giant cells, lymphocytes with germinal center formation, and plasma cells
- Eosinophils not identified
▌ Undifferentiated thyroid carcinoma
- Scattered malignant cells (spindle, epithelioid, or pleomorphic) within fibrosis
- Cytokeratin may assist in identification of tumor cells within fibrosis and outside of the thyroid gland
▌ Granulomatous (subacute) thyroiditis
- Asymmetrical enlargement of the thyroid gland
- Granulomas with giant cells involving follicles, neutrophils at early stage

Pearls
- Clinically may be mistaken for malignancy
- Treatment with corticosteroid or tamoxifen therapy; surgery for compression
- Benign: self-limited (almost half develop hypothyroidism)

Selected References

Harigopal M, Sahoo S, Recant WM, DeMay RM: Fine-needle aspiration of Riedel's disease: Report of a case and review of the literature. Diagn Cytopathol 30:193-197, 2004.

Yasmeen T, Khan S, Patel SG, et al: Clinical case seminar. Riedel's thyroiditis: Report of a case complicated by spontaneous hypoparathyroidism, recurrent laryngeal nerve injury, and Horner's syndrome. J Clin Endocrinol Metab 87:3543-3547, 2002.

Schwaegerle SW, Bauer TW, Esselstyn CB: Riedel's thyroiditis. Am J Clin Pathol 90:715-722, 1988.

Graves Disease (Diffuse Toxic Goiter)

Clinical Features
- Autoimmune thyroid disease; thyroid-stimulating immunoglobulin (TSI)
- Peak in third to fourth decade; marked predominance in woman at least 5:1
- Strong association with HLA-DR3 and HLA-B8
- Clinically presents with thyrotoxicosis: muscle weakness, weight loss, exophthalmos, tachycardia, and goiter
- Suppressed thyroid-stimulating hormone (TSH), increased T_4 and T_3

Figure 3-4. Graves disease. A, Gross photograph of a diffusely enlarged pale thyroid. **B,** Low-power view shows scant colloid in hyperplastic follicles with papillary formations and inflammatory infiltrate; *inset* shows bland nuclei, papillary growth pattern, and scalloped colloid.

Gross Pathology

- Diffuse enlargement of the thyroid, usually symmetrical
- Diffusely beefy-red cut surface

Histopathology

- Hyperplastic thyroid follicles with papillary infoldings
- Follicular nuclei remain round and basally located, may be clear
- Colloid is typically decreased; when present, shows prominent peripheral scalloping
- Colloid increases after treatment
- Lymphocytic inflammation patchy in stroma (varies)
- Nuclear atypia and stromal fibrosis may be seen after radioactive iodine therapy

Special Stains and Immunohistochemistry

- Noncontributory

Other Techniques for Diagnosis

- Clinical evaluation for antibodies and thyroid levels

Differential Diagnosis

▌ Adenomatoid nodule, nodular hyperplasia
- Follicles of varying sizes with occasional Sanderson polsters (groups of small, active follicles at one pole)
- Nonencapsulated

▌ Papillary thyroid carcinoma
- Complete nuclear features are absent in Graves disease (overlapping, grooving)
- Invasive pattern when present is helpful

Pearls

- Treatment is drug therapy or radioactive iodine; surgery if uncontrolled
- Morphologic appearance cannot predict the patient's current functional status
- Radioactive iodine causes nuclear atypia in follicular cells of no significance

Selected References

Lloyd RV, Douglas BR, Young WF: Endocrine diseases. In King DW (ed): Atlas of Nontumor Pathology. Washington, ARP Press, 2002, pp 125-133.

LiVolsi VA: The pathology of autoimmune thyroid disease: A review. Thyroid 4:333-339, 1994.

Takamatso J, Takeda K, Katayama S, et al: Epithelial hyperplasia and decreased colloid content of the thyroid gland in tri-iodothyronine predominant Graves disease. J Endocrinol Metab 75:1145-1150, 1992.

Multinodular Goiter

Clinical Features

- Also known as adenomatoid goiter, adenomatous hyperplasia

Figure 3-5. Goiter. A, Gross photograph of an enlarged thyroid with nodularity, fibrosis, and hemorrhage. **B,** Thyroid follicles vary in size and are often dilated with colloid accumulation.

- Incidence of 3% to 5% in general population; endemic in iodine-deficient areas
- Probably caused by impairment of hormone production
- Adult females predominate over adult males (8:1)
- Clinically often asymptomatic; may cause discomfort, compression
- May grow to massive size in neck or mediastinum
- Number and size of nodules varies; dominant nodule leads to workup

Gross Pathology

- Enlarged, nodular thyroid gland, may be asymmetrical
- Cut surface shows various-sized nodules, often with colloid
- Variegated appearance from hemorrhage to cystic degeneration and calcification

Histopathology

- Heterogeneous, unencapsulated, medium to large distended follicles
- May have scattered, solid, microfollicular nodules; papillary hyperplasia; or oncocytic changes
- Surrounding thyroid follicles usually not compressed by nodules
- Background of hemorrhage, fibrosis, calcification
- Parasite nodules (nodules separated from the main gland) are common

Special Stains and Immunohistochemistry

- Noncontributory

Other Techniques for Diagnosis

- Noncontributory

Differential Diagnosis

▌ Follicular adenoma
- Typically solitary
- Composed of uniform small follicles or macrofollicles
- Distinct fibrous capsule surrounds nodular proliferation
- Compression of adjacent thyroid tissue

▌ Graves disease
- Gross examination: diffuse, beefy-red, less nodular than multinodular goiter
- Hyperplastic thyroid follicles with papillary infoldings
- Vacuolated cytoplasm of follicular cells, and colloid with scalloped borders
- Laboratory tests indicate hyperthyroidism

▌ Amyloid goiter
- Diffusely enlarged thyroid; waxy, pale cut surface
- Amyloid deposits around vessels and intercellular between follicles
- Secondary follicle atrophy and squamous metaplasia
- Congo red stain with polarization to detect birefringent apple-green amyloid
- Clinical history, evaluation for cause (e.g., myeloma, rheumatologic diseases)

Pearls

- Cellular hyperplastic nodules can be difficult to distinguish from follicular neoplasms by fine-needle aspiration (FNA)
- Most common cause of sudden increase in size of hyperplastic nodules is hemorrhage and cystic degeneration
- Extensive nodularity and enlargement may extend to mediastinum and cause detached nodules (parasitic thyroid nodules)

Selected References

Kotwal A, Priya R, Qadeer I: Goiter and other iodine deficiency disorders: A systematic review of epidemiological studies to deconstruct the complex web [erratum in: Arch Med Res 38:366, 2007]. Arch Med Res 38:1-14, 2007.

Krohn K, Führer D, Bayer Y, et al. Molecular pathogenesis of euthyroid and toxic multinodular goiter. Endocr Rev 26:504-524, 2005.

Ríos A, Rodríguez JM, Canteras M, et al: Risk factors for malignancy in multinodular goitres. Eur J Surg Oncol 30:58-62, 2004.

Dyshormonogenetic Goiter

Clinical Features

- Rare genetic disorder of defects in thyroid hormone synthesis pathway, most commonly cannot incorporate iodine
- Patients are usually hypothyroid, frequently with enlarged thyroid
- May present with congenital hypothyroidism; mean age, 16 years
- Slight female predominance
- Rare cases of associated carcinoma; predominately follicular carcinomas
- Surgery in children or young adult for dominant nodule or compression

Gross Pathology

- Enlarged for age, frequently nodular, lacking colloid

Histopathology

- Nodular arrangement of small follicles with scant colloid separated by fibrous trabeculae; may show papillary areas
- Often hypercellular with marked cellular pleomorphism (thyroid cancer is not diagnosed by pleomorphism)

Figure 3-6. Dyshormonogenetic goiter. Small thyroid follicles with scant colloid composed of follicular cells with atypical nuclei (*inset*) and surrounded by dense fibrosis.

- Follicles may extend to involve adjacent soft tissue; not a sign of malignancy

Special Stains and Immunohistochemistry

- Noncontributory

Other Techniques for Diagnosis

- Clinical evaluation for underlying genetic defect

Differential Diagnosis

▌ Nodular hyperplasia
  - Bland follicular cells forming nonencapsulated nodules
  - Frequently follicles enlarged with colloid
▌ Follicular adenoma, carcinoma
  - Uniform, small follicles (unlike atypical cytology of background follicles in dyshormonogenetic goiter)
  - Nodule surrounded by fibrous capsule
  - Vascular invasion or capsular invasion must be present to make a diagnosis of follicular carcinoma
▌ Graves disease
  - Hyperplastic thyroid follicles with papillary infoldings
  - Follicular cells with granular cytoplasm
  - Scant colloid; when present, apical vacuolation leads to scalloping of colloid
  - Laboratory tests indicating hyperthyroidism
▌ Post–radioactive iodine therapy
  - Cytologic atypia
  - Various degrees of fibrosis
  - Clinical history of prior therapy
  - Frequently an older patient group

Pearls

- Histology is diagnostic, although clinical history should also be noted; frequently patient is young
- Caution in diagnosing cancer in this setting, requires characteristic nuclear features to diagnosis papillary carcinoma (presence of papillary architecture is not sufficient); diagnosis of follicular carcinoma requires capsular or vascular invasion
- Nuclei of the follicular neoplasm are frequently more uniform than the background dyshormogenetic thyroid

Selected References

Deshpande AH, Bobhate SK: Cytological features of dyshormonogenetic goiter: Case report and review of the literature. Diagn Cytopathol 33:252-254, 2005.

Ghossein RA, Rosai J, Heffess C: Dyshormonogenetic goiter: A clinicopathologic study of 56 cases. Endocr Pathol 8:283-292, 1997.

Kennedy JS. The pathology of dyshormonogenetic goitre. J Pathol 1969;99:251-264.

Thyroglossal Duct Cyst

Clinical Features

- Congenital persistence of the thyroid developmental tract
- Midline, from foramen cecum (tongue) to hyoid bone, to pyramidal lobe or isthmus
- May fistulize to skin
- Moves on swallowing
- Most often detected during childhood or young adulthood
- Associated thyroid tissue may develop well-differentiated thyroid carcinomas

Gross Pathology

- Cystic lesion in soft tissue, middle third of hyoid bone, skin if fistula present

Histopathology

- Cyst is lined by respiratory or squamous epithelium
- Secondary inflammation and granulation tissue if infected; lining may be lost
- Underlying stroma contains mucus glands and thyroid follicles (50% of cases)

Special Stains and Immunohistochemistry

- Thyroid epithelium is positive for thyroid transcription factor-1 (TTF-1) and thyroglobulin

Other Techniques for Diagnosis

- Noncontributory

Figure 3-7. Thyroglossal duct cyst. Respiratory epithelium–lined cyst in the midline, often with thyroid follicles in the wall.

Differential Diagnosis

▌ Branchial cleft cyst
- Located in the lateral neck
- Cyst lined by squamous, columnar, or ciliated epithelium or, if ulcerated, by granulation tissue
- Prominent lymphoid infiltrate in cyst wall
- Cyst may contain anucleated squamous cells, histiocytes, or cholesterol clefts
- Epithelium is thyroglobulin negative (differentiate from metastatic papillary carcinoma)

▌ Adenomatoid, colloid nodule
- May occur in isthmus or pyramidal lobe, leading to midline mass
- Squamous metaplasia can occur, but squamous debris is rare; colloid is typically abundant
- Lacks ciliated cells

Pearls

- Malignancy may occur in the thyroid tissue (majority papillary carcinoma); medullary carcinoma is not seen (different route of embryologic development)
- Ciliated cells are occasionally seen on FNA of thyroid gland nodules near the trachea from "tracheal aspirates" if the needle enters the trachea (patient usually coughs when this occurs)

Selected References

Mondin V, Ferlito A, Muzzi E, et al: Thyroglossal duct cyst: Personal experience and literature review. Auris Nasus Larynx 35:11-25, 2008.

Shahin A, Burroughs FH, Kirby JP, Ali SZ: Thyroglossal duct cyst: A cytopathologic study of 26 cases. Diagn Cytopathol 33:365-369, 2005.

Allard RH: The thyroglossal cyst. Head Neck Surg 5:134-146, 1982.

Branchial Cleft Cyst

Clinical Features

- Anterolateral neck mass, multiple locations based on which pouch is affected
- Derived from first, second, third, or fourth branchial pouches
- Congenital, identified in children and young adults (be wary in older adults)

Gross Pathology

- Mostly unilocular cysts with slightly granular inner surface due to presence of numerous lymphoid follicles
- May be associated with a fistula tract

Histopathology

- Cyst and fistula tracts are lined by squamous, columnar, or ciliated epithelium

Figure 3-8. Branchial cleft cyst. Epithelium-lined cystic space has associated lymphoid stroma; the cyst is often lined by respiratory epithelium but may be squamous, as in this case.

- Subepithelial stroma contains abundant lymphoid tissue
- Lining contains mucinous and serous or even sebaceous glands, particularly when located in lower neck area
- Cyst may contain anucleated squames, histiocytes, and cholesterol clefts

Special Stains and Immunohistochemistry

- Noncontributory

Other Techniques for Diagnosis

- Noncontributory

Differential Diagnosis

▌ Squamous cell carcinoma (SCC) metastatic to lymph node with secondary cystic change
- Must be considered in all adult patients with neck mass
- Aggregates of malignant squamous cells forming cyst in lymph node
- May at times appear cytologically bland
- Squamous pearl formation may be seen
- Sights of primary tumor are frequently in Waldeyer ring (tonsils, base of tongue) and are not apparent at time of presentation (image and biopsy for primary)

▌ Cystic papillary thyroid carcinoma metastatic to lymph node
- Cystic lining may be flattened without overt nuclear changes
- Adequate sections usually show papillary architecture and nuclear features
- Thyroglobulin level on FNA fluid diagnostic
- Lateral neck location of thyroid tissue equals metastasis
- TTF-1 and thyroglobulin will be positive

Pearls

- FNA is a valuable tool in evaluating neck lesions
- Keep cystic papillary thyroid carcinoma in mind for patients of all ages with neck mass
- Use caution in diagnosing branchial cleft cyst in adult patients when metastatic cystic SCC is the overwhelming cause of neck masses

Selected References

Al-Khateeb TH, Al Zoubi F: Congenital neck masses: A descriptive retrospective study of 252 cases. J Oral Maxillofac Surg 65:2242-2247, 2007.

Firat P, Ersoz C, Uguz A, Onder S: Cystic lesions of the head and neck: Cytohistological correlation in 63 cases. Cytopathology 18:184-190, 2007.

Burgess KL, Hartwick RWJ, Bedard YC: Metastatic squamous cell carcinoma presenting as a neck cyst: Differential diagnosis from inflamed branchial cleft cyst in fine-needle aspirates. Acta Cytol 37:494-498, 1993.

Teratoma

Clinical Features

- Very rare primary thyroid neoplasm with trilineage differentiation
- Reported in newborn patients to those in their 50s, males = females
- Teratomas are classified as benign (mature), immature, and malignant
- Teratomas of infants: >90% benign, often contain immature components
- Teratomas in adolescents and adults: 50% malignant

Gross Pathology

- Variable with multiloculated cysts, soft glial tissue, gritty bone or cartilage

Figure 3-9. Thyroid teratoma. Trilineage cellular components are present—mature cartilage, glial tissue, and a malignant epithelial component.

Histopathology

- Mixture of mature or immature tissues (ectoderm, endoderm, and mesoderm)
- Thyroid parenchyma should be identified
- Maturation of neural tissue determines grade
- Frank malignant component may be present (i.e., embryonal carcinoma)

Special Stains and Immunohistochemistry

- Various stains to highlight lineages

Other Techniques for Diagnosis

- Noncontributory

Differential Diagnosis

- ▍ Thyroglossal duct cyst
  - Cyst lined by respiratory or squamous epithelium
  - May be associated with chronic inflammation
  - Clinically correlate with anatomic region (anterior, midline)
- ▍ Lymphoma
  - Single population of atypical small cells
  - Other tissue types are not identified
  - Immunohistochemistry (IHC) to identify cell type
- ▍ Rhabdomyosarcoma
  - Single population of tumor cells without other lineages
  - Rhabdomyoblasts may be found in teratomas

Pearls

- Grading based on percentage of immature component
- Prognosis based on age, size, and proportion of immature component

Selected References

Nishihara E, Miyauchi A, Hirokawa M, et al: Benign thyroid teratomas manifest painful cystic and solid composite nodules: Three case reports and a review of the literature. Endocrine 30:231-236, 2006.

Thompson LD, Rosai J, Heffess CS: Primary thyroid teratomas: A clinicopathologic study of 30 cases. Cancer 88:1149-1158, 2000.

Hyalinizing Trabecular Tumor

Clinical Features

- Follicular neoplasm of debated classification
- Females affected more than males; patients are usually in their 50s and 60s

Gross Pathology

- Solitary, well-circumscribed nodule

Histopathology

- Trabecular and insular growth patterns
- Large elongated cells with oval nuclei

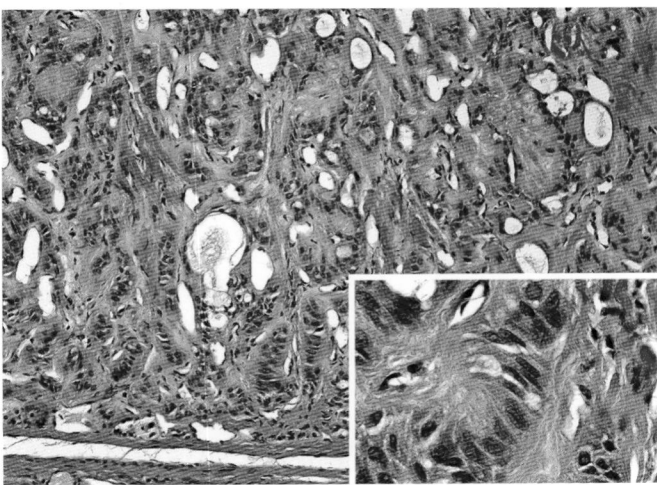

Figure 3-10. Hyalinizing trabecular tumor. Trabeculae and nests of elongated cells with prominent grooves and pseudonuclear inclusions (*inset*).

- Nuclear grooves and intranuclear cytoplasmic inclusions
- Intracytoplasmic bodies and perinuclear halos are common

Special Stains and Immunohistochemistry
- TTF-1 and thyroglobulin positive

Other Techniques for Diagnosis
- *RET/PTC* gene rearrangements in some suggest link to papillary thyroid carcinoma

Differential Diagnosis
▌ Papillary thyroid carcinoma
  - Shares overlapping nuclear features, including clearing and grooves
  - Invasive growth pattern is helpful
  - Lymphovascular invasion is often identified
▌ Follicular adenoma
  - Nuclei in general are bland and round, lacking clearing and grooving
  - Lacks intracytoplasmic bodies
▌ Paraganglioma
  - Rare tumor in thyroid; cells forming nests
  - Nuclear features are bland and round, lacking clearing and grooves
  - Positive for chromogranin, synaptophysin
  - Negative for TTF-1 and thyroglobulin
▌ Medullary thyroid carcinoma
  - Overlapping nuclear features of grooving and elongation
  - Overlapping growth patterns (trabecular)
  - Amyloid helpful when present
  - Thyroglobulin negative
  - Both express TTF-1

Pearls
- Unclear if biologically capable of metastasis
- Suggested relationship to papillary thyroid carcinoma
- Conservative treatment recommended

Selected References
Galgano MT, Mills SE, Stelow EB: Hyalinizing trabecular adenoma of the thyroid revisited: A histologic and immunohistochemical study of thyroid lesions with prominent trabecular architecture and sclerosis. Am J Surg Pathol 30:1269-1273, 2006.

Baloch ZW, LiVolsi VA: Cytologic and architectural mimics of papillary thyroid carcinoma: Diagnostic challenges in fine-needle aspiration and surgical pathology specimens. Am J Clin Pathol 125:S135-144, 2006.

Casey MB, Sebo TJ, Carney JA: Hyalinizing trabecular adenoma of the thyroid gland: Cytologic features in 29 cases. Am J Surg Pathol 28:859-867, 2004.

LiVolsi VA: Hyalinizing trabecular tumor of the thyroid: Adenoma, carcinoma, or neoplasm of uncertain malignant potential? Am J Surg Pathol 24:1683-1684, 2000.

Follicular Adenoma

Clinical Features
- Benign tumor more common (about 5:1) than follicular carcinoma
- Usually solitary lesion; mainly affects lobes of thyroid, rare in isthmus
- Predilection for middle-aged women; clinically euthyroid
- Associated with iodine deficiency and Cowden disease (hamartomas, *PTEN* gene)

Gross Pathology
- Solitary, well-circumscribed, round to oval nodule, thin capsule

Histopathology
- Encapsulated follicular proliferation; variable amount of colloid
- Thin fibrous capsule may contain small blood vessels; thinner than in follicular carcinoma
- Various architectural patterns: trabecular or solid, microfollicular, and macrofollicular, which have no clinical significance
- Central area may be hypocellular with loose and edematous stroma
- Uniform polygonal follicle cells with round or oval nuclei
- Absent or minimal mitotic activity
- Occasionally bizarre nuclei do not indicate malignancy
- Papillary or pseudopapillary structures without nuclear changes

Figure 3-11. Follicular adenoma. A, Gross photograph of a thyroid lobe with a well-defined nodule without a prominent capsule. **B,** The cellular proliferation is well circumscribed with a thin capsule.

- Follicular adenoma variants
  — Adenoma with oncocytic (Hürthle) cells
    ◆ Follicular cells with ample eosinophilic cytoplasm with round nuclei and prominent nucleoli
    ◆ More susceptible to infarction, especially after FNA
    ◆ No clinical significance
  — Atypical adenoma, follicular lesion of uncertain malignant potential
    ◆ May show necrosis, infarction, mitoses
    ◆ Thickened capsule with irregularity and partial capsule invasion
    ◆ Lacks lymphovascular invasion
    ◆ Worrisome features without meeting criteria for carcinoma
  — Toxic adenoma (rare)
    ◆ Also called Plummer adenoma
    ◆ Solitary, hyperfunctioning nodule causing hyperthyroidism
    ◆ Cytologic features within nodule mimics Graves disease

Special Stains and Immunohistochemistry

- Thyroglobulin and TTF-1 positive
- Cytokeratin positive
- Chromogranin and calcitonin negative

Other Techniques for Diagnosis

- One fourth of cases are aneuploid; however, this does not correlate clinically with malignant behavior or recurrence
- Some reports of *Ras* mutations and *PAX/PPARgamma* rearrangements (see "Follicular Carcinoma")

Differential Diagnosis

▮ Hyperplastic nodule
  - Typically multiple; mixture of microfollicles and macrofollicular, marked colloid
  - Incomplete fibrous capsule; does not compress surrounding thyroid tissue
▮ Follicular carcinoma
  - Follicular proliferation with thick capsule and evidence of vascular invasion or full-thickness capsular invasion by neoplastic follicles
▮ Encapsulated follicular variant of papillary carcinoma
  - Characterized by follicular architecture with cytologic features of classic papillary carcinoma, including enlarged, cleared nuclei and intranuclear cytoplasmic pseudoinclusions
  - May have microfollicles or macrofollicles
▮ Medullary thyroid carcinoma, nodular C-cell hyperplasia
  - Not encapsulated
  - Isochromatic cytoplasm versus eosinophilic cytoplasm in follicular cells
  - Calcitonin positive; also frequently expresses TTF-1
▮ Intrathyroidal parathyroid (normal) or parathyroid adenoma
  - Well circumscribed, may or may not have intercellular fat
  - Small, hyperchromatic nuclei in nests which may have cytoplasmic clearing
  - Parathyroid hormone positive
  - Calcitonin and TTF-1 negative

Pearls

- FNA shows follicular lesion or follicular neoplasm
- Treatment is lobectomy or subtotal thyroidectomy
- Frozen sections are of little value and are discouraged
- Thorough examination of the follicular capsule is warranted

Selected References

Baloch ZW, LiVolsi VA: Our approach to follicular-patterned lesions of the thyroid. J Clin Pathol 60:244-250, 2007.

Suster S: Thyroid tumors with a follicular growth pattern: Problems in differential diagnosis. Arch Pathol Lab Med 130:984-988, 2006.

Baloch ZW, Fleisher S, LiVolsi VA, Gupta PK: Diagnosis of "follicular neoplasm": A gray zone in thyroid fine-needle aspiration cytology. Diagn Cytopathol 26:41-44, 2002.

Baloch ZW, Livolsi VA: Follicular-patterned lesions of the thyroid: The bane of the pathologist. Am J Clin Pathol 117:143-150, 2002.

Oertel YC, Oertel JE: Diagnosis of benign thyroid lesions: Fine needle aspiration and histopathologic correlation. Ann Diagn Pathol 2:250-263, 1998.

Follicular Carcinoma

Clinical Features

- Malignant epithelial tumor with follicular cell differentiation and no features of the other distinctive types of thyroid malignancy
- Constitutes about 5% of thyroid cancers
- In iodine-deficient areas comprise between 25% and 40% of thyroid cancers
- Not associated with prior radiation therapy
- Predilection for women
- Patients present with a solitary nodule that is typically "cold" on isotopic scan
- Patients are usually euthyroid

Gross Pathology

- Solid, round tumor with fibrous capsule that is thicker and more irregular than in adenomas, usually larger than 1 cm
- Cut surface is light-tan and solid; secondary changes such as cystic degeneration, hemorrhage, and fibrosis
- Mahogany-colored nodule corresponds to Hürthle cell morphology

Histopathology

- Frequently divided into (1) minimally invasive and (2) widely invasive, although these definitions are variably used
- Cells similar to those of follicular adenoma: round or oval nuclei in follicular cells
- Various architectural patterns: solid, trabecular, microfollicular, macrofollicular (not clinically significant)
- Diagnosis depends on demonstration of full-thickness capsular or vascular invasion
- Capsular invasion
  — Penetration of entire thickness of capsule is required (mere presence of follicular cell clusters within capsule is not regarded as capsular invasion)
  — Caution of FNA defects in capsule with associated hemorrhage and reactive changes

Figure 3-12. Follicular carcinoma. A, Gross photograph of a circumscribed thyroid mass with thickened capsule and gross invasion of the capsule at the superior left aspect of the image. B, Lymphovascular invasion is present within the markedly thickened capsule. C, Widely invasive follicular carcinoma with nodules extending into the adjacent thyroid parenchyma.

- Vascular invasion (also termed *angioinvasive follicular carcinoma*)
  — Vessel should be located within or outside the capsule; frequently of large caliber
  — Tumor cells should be within the vascular lumen and must be at least focally attached to the vessel wall (not pushing beneath the vessel)
  — Some require endothelial growth over a portion of the tumor or fibrin deposition

Special Stains and Immunohistochemistry
- Thyroglobulin positive
- No currently available marker to distinguish adenoma from carcinoma

Other Techniques for Diagnosis
- Translocation of *PAX8/PPARgamma* t(2;3) seen in approximately 35% of follicular carcinomas
- Identification of *Ras* mutations (*K-ras, N-ras,* or *H-ras* in 40% to 50%) (also seen in adenomas and follicular variant of papillary carcinoma)

Differential Diagnosis
▌ Follicular adenoma
  - Thin fibrous capsule without evidence of vascular invasion
▌ Atypical adenoma or follicular lesion of uncertain malignant potential
  - Cellular follicular lesion with thickened capsule
  - Cells may partially invade capsule
  - Lymphovascular invasion is not identified
▌ Dominant nodule of nodular hyperplasia
  - Background of multiple, variably sized nodules
  - No fibrous capsule
▌ Follicular variant of papillary carcinoma
  - Nuclear features of papillary carcinoma present: overlapping and clearing of nuclei, pseudoinclusions, and nuclear grooves, in most of the lesion (not just focally)
▌ Follicular variant of medullary carcinoma
  - Calcitonin positive and thyroglobulin negative
  - Polygonal cells with abundant eosinophilic to clear cytoplasm and coarsely clumped chromatin with inconspicuous nucleoli; may have plasmacytoid appearance

Pearls
- Vascular invasion is a more reliable sign of malignancy than capsular invasion
- FNA cannot distinguish between follicular lesions (i.e., adenoma from carcinoma), requiring surgical excision for diagnosis
- FNA can produce WHAFFT ("worrisome histologic alterations following FNA of the thyroid") (including artifactual capsular invasion)
- Typically metastasize via hematogenous route, most commonly to lung and bone

Selected References
Rosai J, Kuhn E, Carcangiu ML: Pitfalls in thyroid tumour pathology. Histopathology 49:107-120, 2006.

Kroll TG: Molecular events in follicular thyroid tumors. Cancer Treat Res 122:85-105, 2004.

D'Avanzo A, Treseler P, Ituarte PH, et al: Follicular thyroid carcinoma: Histology and prognosis. Cancer 100:1123-1129, 2004.

LiVolsi VA, Baloch ZW: Follicular neoplasms of the thyroid: View, biases, and experiences. Adv Anat Pathol 11:279-287, 2004.

Thompson LD, Wieneke JA, Paal E, et al: A clinicopathologic study of minimally invasive follicular carcinoma of the thyroid gland with a review of the English literature. Cancer 91:505-524, 2001.

Leteurtre E, Leroy X, Pattou F, et al: Why do frozen sections have limited value in encapsulated or minimally invasive follicular carcinoma of the thyroid? Am J Clin Pathol 115:370-374, 2001.

Papillary Thyroid Carcinoma

Clinical Features
- Most common type of thyroid cancer (80%) in the United States
- More common in women (4:1)
- Well-documented association with radiation exposure (after Chernobyl and Hiroshima)
- Relative incidence is higher in areas of high iodine intake compared with follicular carcinoma
- Prognostic features include age and gender (worse when age > 45 years, male)
- Regional lymph node metastasis is common (50% of cases at presentation); does not adversely affect long-term prognosis

Gross Pathology
- Variable, from well circumscribed to diffusely involving lobe or multifocal
- White-gray, firm, granular cut surface; may have small papillary structures
- Calcifications may be present

Histopathology
- Complex branching true papillae (contain fibrovascular stalks)
- Papillae lined by neoplastic epithelial cells with characteristic enlarged optically clear, empty "Orphan Annie eye" nuclei (formalin fixation only), nuclear grooves (usually parallel to long axis), cytoplasmic pseudoinclusions, and overlapping nuclei
- Psammoma bodies seen in up to 50% of cases
- Cystic growth pattern is commonly present in lymph nodes with flattened nuclei
- Solid areas, squamous metaplasia, are not infrequently seen

Figure 3-13. Papillary thyroid carcinoma. A, Gross photograph of a thyroid with a partially calcified tumor. **B,** Papillary architecture with fibrovascular cores. **C,** Papillary thyroid carcinoma growing in microfollicles consistent with the follicular variant. The nuclei are clear, elongated, and grooved.

- Colloid is thick and dark eosinophilic with bubblegum-like quality
- Stroma is often abundant and fibrous
- Lymphatic invasion is common
- Multicentricity is common compared with follicular neoplasms
- Histologic variants
  — Microcarcinoma
    ◆ Microscopic tumor less than 1 cm in diameter
    ◆ Subcapsular region and scar growth pattern is common
    ◆ Common at autopsy
    ◆ Most do not require additional treatment
  — Follicular variant of papillary carcinoma
    ◆ Microfollicular or macrofollicular
    ◆ May mimic adenoma or adenomatous nodule
    ◆ Nuclear features must show enlargement, clearing, and grooves throughout most of lesion
    ◆ Focal papillae may be found if multiple sections are taken
    ◆ Prognosis is similar to that for classic papillary carcinoma
  — Diffuse sclerosing variant
    ◆ Often, diffusely involves both lobes
    ◆ Extensive fibrosis, squamous metaplasia, lymphocytic infiltrate, and psammoma bodies
    ◆ Solid or papillary growth with extensive lymphovascular spread
    ◆ Higher incidence of cervical lymph node and pulmonary metastases
  — Oncocytic variant
    ◆ Distinct Hürthle cell features (abundant eosinophilic cytoplasm) with classic papillary thyroid carcinoma nuclei often with papillary architecture
    ◆ Nuclei frequently do not overlap secondary to ample cytoplasm
    ◆ May be associated with lymphoid stoma in chronic lymphocytic thyroiditis
    ◆ Degenerative changes after FNA are common
  — Tall or columnar cell variant
    ◆ More common in older patients
    ◆ Often greater than 5 cm, extrathyroidal extension and vascular invasion are more frequent
    ◆ Tall cell nuclei at base with cells that are 3 times as tall as wide and have abundant eosinophilic cytoplasm
    ◆ Columnar nuclei are pseudostratified and luminal with basal cytoplasmic vacuoles and squamous metaplasia
    ◆ Stage for stage, similar to conventional papillary thyroid carcinoma

Special Stains and Immunohistochemistry

- Noncontributory—although high-molecular-weight cytokeratins (CK19), galectin-3, and HBME-1 are noted to be expressed in papillary thyroid carcinoma, lack of sensitivity and specificity limits their use

Other Techniques for Diagnosis

- Oncogene alterations
  - Point mutation *BRAF*, exon 15 (up to 60%)
  - Translocations of *RET* proto-oncogene with multiple different genes (*RET/PTC* gene rearrangements, 30%, although higher percentage in children)
  - *N-ras* mutations particularly follicular variant (10%)
  - *TRK* gene rearrangements with multiple genes (10%)
- New tyrosine kinase inhibitors affect the *BRAF* and *RET* pathways and may provide targeted therapy for patients with aggressive disease or distant metastases

Differential Diagnosis

▍ Papillary hyperplasia in Graves disease and adenomatous goiter
  - Classic nuclear features of papillary carcinoma are absent
▍ Follicular adenoma and carcinoma
  - Most commonly microfollicular pattern with fibrous capsule
  - Large-vessel vascular invasion frequently seen in follicular carcinoma
  - Lack characteristic nuclear features such as enlargement and overlapping of cleared-out nuclei
▍ Medullary carcinoma
  - Spindle and plasmacytoid features; may be follicular or papillary growth pattern
  - Amyloid frequently present in stroma (Congo red positive)
  - Calcitonin positive and thyroglobulin negative

Pearls

- All variants of papillary carcinoma, irrespective of architecture, must have characteristic nuclear features (hypochromasia, elongated nucleus with grooves, and intranuclear pseudoinclusions)
- Prognosis correlates with clinical factors (age, sex, stage)
- Clear "Orphan Annie eye" nuclei are an artifact of formalin fixation and are not seen in frozen sections and cytologic preparations
- Psammoma bodies are not pathognomonic

Selected References

Michels JJ, Jacques M, Henry-Amar M, Bardet S: Prevalence and prognostic significance of tall cell variant of papillary thyroid carcinoma. Hum Pathol 38:212-219, 2007.

Sanders EM Jr, LiVolsi VA, Brierley J, et al: An evidence-based review of poorly differentiated thyroid cancer. World J Surg 31:934-945, 2007.

Trovisco V, Soares P, Sobrinho-Simoes M: B-RAF mutations in the etiopathogenesis, diagnosis, and prognosis of thyroid carcinomas. Hum Pathol 37:781-786, 2006.

Al-Brahim N, Asa SL: Papillary thyroid carcinoma: An overview. Arch Pathol Lab Med 130:1057-1062, 2006.

DeLellis RA: Pathology and genetics of thyroid carcinoma. J Surg Oncol 94:662-669, 2006.

Akslen LA, LiVolsi VA: Prognostic significance of histologic grading compared with subclassification of papillary thyroid carcinoma. Cancer 88:1902-1908, 2000.

Medullary Thyroid Carcinoma

Clinical Features

- Malignant tumor composed of neural crest–derived C cells
- Accounts for 5% to 10% of thyroid malignancies
- Can be sporadic (80%) or hereditary (20%); more common in women
- Lymph nodes common at presentation (about 50%)
- Elevated serum calcitonin, can be used to monitor residual, recurrent, or metastatic disease postoperatively; CEA elevation is usually a late finding in progressive disease
- Hereditary types include familial medullary thyroid carcinoma and multiple endocrine neoplasia (MEN) IIA and IIB and are caused by different germline mutations in *RET* proto-oncogene
  - Sporadic type
    - Occurs in middle-aged adults, some show *RET* mutations in the tumors
    - Solitary tumor mass
  - Familial medullary thyroid carcinoma
    - Medullary carcinoma without other endocrine abnormalities, onset in adults
  - MEN IIA
    - Medullary carcinoma, pheochromocytoma, parathyroid adenoma or hyperplasia
    - Mean age at diagnosis in MEN IIA cases is third decade
    - Often multicentric and involve both thyroid lobes
  - MEN IIB
    - All patients develop medullary thyroid carcinoma, onset in childhood or young adult
    - Same possible endocrinopathies as MEN IIA, plus gastrointestinal and ocular ganglioneuromas and skeletal abnormalities

Figure 3-14. Medullary thyroid carcinoma. A, Gross photograph of a pale-tan tumor replacing the thyroid parenchyma. **B,** Nests of neuroendocrine cells are associated with dense amorphous stroma (amyloid). Higher-power magnification (*inset*) of tumor cells shows the amphophilic cytoplasm and the round nuclei with salt-and-pepper chromatin. **C,** Immunohistochemical stain for calcitonin is positive in a medullary thyroid carcinoma with spindled morphology.

Gross Pathology

- Often circumscribed
- Cut section is tan-yellow with soft to firm consistency
- Tumors arise in upper and middle third of lobe, corresponding to the area in which C cells predominate
- May have multifocal nodules in hereditary types

Histopathology

- Wide spectrum of histologic patterns, including solid, lobular, trabecular, insular, and sheetlike
- Tumor cells are round, polygonal, or spindle shaped; frequently mixed cell types
- Polygonal cells have abundant amphophilic to clear cytoplasm, and nuclei often have a plasmacytoid appearance
- Cytoplasmic pseudoinclusions and grooves can be seen
- Nuclear chromatin is coarsely clumped (i.e., salt-and-pepper like) with inconspicuous nucleoli
- Binucleated cells are commonly seen
- Necrosis, hemorrhage, and mitoses are rare features
- Bizarre nuclear atypia can occur
- Variants (have no clinical significance)
  — Follicular or trabecular, papillary, paraganglioma-like, amphicrine, small cell, giant cell, clear cell, encapsulated, oncocytic, melanotic (melanin pigment present), and squamous have been described
- Stromal amyloid is present in up to 80% of cases; amyloid can induce foreign-body giant cell reaction
- Stroma may contain calcifications or rarely psammoma bodies
- Can be diagnosed preoperatively by FNA but should be supported by immunocytochemistry; use caution because nuclear changes include grooving and pseudonuclear inclusions

Special Stains and Immunohistochemistry

- Calcitonin positive
- Chromogranin and synaptophysin positive
- Carcinoembryonic antigen (CEA) positive in tumor cells and serum; may have prognostic value
- Congo red positive in amyloid material (polarizes: birefringence apple-green)
- TTF-1 usually positive
- Thyroglobulin negative

Other Techniques for Diagnosis

- Germline mutations in *RET* proto-oncogene are present in all hereditary forms
- *RET* mutations are identified in some sporadic cases (20% to 80%)
- Genetic testing for germline mutations should be offered to all patients diagnosed with medullary thyroid carcinoma regardless of age at diagnosis

Differential Diagnosis

■ C-cell hyperplasia, reactive
  ● Lacks fibrosis
  ● Proliferations of C cells may surround follicles, mimicking invasion
  ● Scattered cells are often appreciated only by immunostaining
■ C-cell hyperplasia, nodular (preneoplastic)
  ● Greater than 50 cells per cluster
  ● Identified on hematoxylin and eosin stain, confirmed by immunostaining
  ● Lacks fibrosis, infiltration
  ● Nodular proliferation considered preneoplastic
  ● Difficult to separate from or define microscopic medullary thyroid carcinoma
■ Follicular carcinoma
  ● Stroma does not contain amyloid
  ● Thyroglobulin positive and calcitonin negative
■ Papillary carcinoma
  ● Characteristic nuclear features of papillary thyroid carcinoma
  ● Thyroglobulin positive and calcitonin negative
  ● Pseudoinclusions and grooving may be seen in both papillary and medullary carcinoma
■ Poorly differentiated thyroid carcinoma
  ● Islands of tumor cells that typically grow in a solid fashion but may form small follicles
  ● Stroma does not contain amyloid (negative for Congo red)
  ● Thyroglobulin positive and calcitonin negative
■ Plasmacytoma (extramedullary)
  ● Plasmacytoid form of medullary carcinoma can resemble a plasmacytoma
  ● Immunoglobulin light-chain restriction can be demonstrated by kappa and lambda staining, negative for calcitonin
■ Paraganglioma
  ● Lobular, nested growth pattern (Zellenballen)
  ● Nuclei are round with fine granular chromatin
  ● Rare in this location
  ● Negative for calcitonin and TTF-1
■ Hyalinizing trabecular tumor
  ● Well circumscribed
  ● Lacks amyloid
  ● Thyroglobulin positive and calcitonin negative
■ Spindle cell tumor with thymus-like differentiation (SETTLE)
  ● Occurs in young patients (teens to 20s)
  ● Well circumscribed
  ● Biphasic tumor of spindled and epithelial cells in glands, tubules, and sheets
  ● TTF-1, thyroglobulin, and calcitonin negative

Pearls

  ● Medullary carcinoma can mimic a variety of benign and malignant thyroid neoplasms

  ● TTF-1 is positive in most medullary thyroid carcinomas
  ● Presence of C-cell hyperplasia suggests hereditary or germline mutation, as does bilateral and associated endocrine abnormalities (i.e., parathyroid)
  ● Incidental finding of C-cell hyperplasia (>50 cells in aggregate, often seen bilaterally) should be reported
  ● Survival correlates with stage; familial non-MEN related has best overall prognosis of hereditary forms
  ● Radioactive iodine plays no role in treatment

Selected References

Leboulleux S, Baudin E, Travagli JP, Schlumberger M: Medullary thyroid carcinoma. Clin Endocrinol (Oxf) 61:299-310, 2004.

Massoll N, Mazzaferri EL: Diagnosis and management of medullary thyroid carcinoma. Clin Lab Med 24:49-83, 2004.

Guyetant S, Josselin N, Savagner F, et al: C-cell hyperplasia and medullary thyroid carcinoma: Clinicopathological and genetic correlations in 66 consecutive patients. Mod Pathol 16:756-763, 2003.

Simpson NE, Kidd KK, Goodfellow PJ, et al: Assignment of multiple endocrine neoplasia type IIA to chromosome 10 by linkage. Nature 328:528-529, 1987.

Poorly Differentiated Thyroid Carcinoma

Clinical Features

  ● Poorly differentiated carcinoma arising from follicular cells (insular or trabecular pattern)
  ● May arise from follicular carcinoma or papillary carcinoma
  ● Rare in the United States (2% to 3% of thyroid carcinomas)
  ● Mean age at diagnosis is in the fifth and sixth decades
  ● Slightly more common in women

Figure 3-15. Poorly differentiated thyroid carcinoma. Solid nests of follicular cells with scant cytoplasm lacking the nuclear features of papillary thyroid carcinoma.

- Viewed by the World Health Organization (WHO) classification as a morphologic variant of follicular carcinoma
- Intermediate behavior between well-differentiated and anaplastic thyroid carcinomas

Gross Pathology

- Typically greater than 5 cm
- Cut surface is gray-white and solid with areas of necrosis
- Usually extrathyroidal extension with gross invasion into adjacent soft tissue

Histopathology

- Tumor cells with round to oval hyperchromatic nuclei and scant cytoplasm forming a nested pattern (insulae)
- May be defined by the presence of convoluted nuclei; mitotic activity ≥3/10 high-power fields (hpf); or tumor necrosis
- Infiltrative growth pattern with invasion into surrounding tissue

Special Stains and Immunohistochemistry

- Thyroglobulin and TTF-1 often focally or weakly positive
- Cytokeratin positive
- Calcitonin negative (if positive classify as medullary)

Other Techniques for Diagnosis

- See "Papillary Thyroid Carcinoma" and "Follicular Carcinoma" for current expression patterns

Differential Diagnosis

▌ Medullary carcinoma
- Round to oval, spindled, or plasmacytoid
- Amyloid in stroma (Congo red positive)
- Calcitonin positive and thyroglobulin negative

▌ Undifferentiated (anaplastic) carcinoma
- Pleomorphic cellular features may also show giant, spindled, or squamous cells
- Lacks architectural growth pattern (insulae)

▌ Carcinoma showing thymus-like differentiation (CASTLE)
- Occurs in adults, fifth decade
- One third develop metastatic disease
- Invasive growth in sheets and nests with dense fibrosis; moderately pleomorphic cells
- TTF-1, thyroglobulin, and calcitonin negative
- Tumor positive for CD5

Pearls

- May originate from papillary or follicular carcinoma, clinically aggressive
- Not viewed as a distinct tumor but in the spectrum from well-differentiated to anaplastic or undifferentiated thyroid carcinoma

- If calcitonin is positive, classify as medullary thyroid carcinoma

Selected References

Volante M, Collini P, Nikiforov YE, et al: Poorly differentiated thyroid carcinoma: The Turin proposal for the use of uniform diagnostic criteria and an algorithmic diagnostic approach. Am J Surg Pathol 31:1256-1264, 2007.

Sanders EM Jr, LiVolsi VA, Brierley J, et al: An evidence-based review of poorly differentiated thyroid cancer. World J Surg 31:934-945, 2007.

Hiltzik D, Carlson DL, Tuttle RM, et al: Poorly differentiated thyroid carcinomas defined on the basis of mitosis and necrosis: A clinicopathologic study of 58 patients. Cancer 106:1286-1295, 2006.

Volante M, Landolfi S, Chiusa L, et al: Poorly differentiated carcinomas of the thyroid with trabecular, insular, and solid patterns: A clinicopathologic study of 183 patients. Cancer 100:950-957, 2004.

Undifferentiated (Anaplastic) Carcinoma

Clinical Features

- Less than 5% of thyroid neoplasms, also called *pleomorphic carcinoma*
- Highly malignant tumor, totally or partially undifferentiated by microscopy
- Mean age at diagnosis is sixth to seventh decades; slightly more common in women
- Presents as a rapidly enlarging neck mass in the thyroid region associated often with compression signs, including dyspnea, dysphagia, and hoarseness
- High likelihood of cervical lymph node metastases at presentation
- Fatal in most cases within 6 months regardless of treatment
- Most of the anaplastic carcinomas arise from a preexisting tumor, usually a papillary carcinoma

Gross Pathology

- Widely invasive tumor, often with spread beyond the thyroid
- Variegated appearance with necrotic and hemorrhagic areas

Histopathology

- Three patterns may be seen: squamoid, spindle cell, and giant cell (often more than one pattern within a tumor)
  — Squamoid pattern (WHO classifies as SCC)
    ◆ Resembles nonkeratinizing SCC; rarely, squamous pearls are present
    ◆ Exclude direct extension from aerodigestive tract primary
    ◆ Squamous metaplasia in papillary thyroid carcinoma lacks atypia

Figure 3-16. Undifferentiated (anaplastic) carcinoma. A, Gross photograph of the tumor invading trachea and soft tissue. **B,** Anaplastic spindled and giant cells are present. **C,** Papillary thyroid carcinoma (*left side*) merging with an anaplastic thyroid carcinoma with spindled morphology.

— Spindle cell pattern
  ◆ Resembles a sarcoma (fibrosarcoma, malignant fibrous histiocytoma, or angiosarcoma)
  ◆ May have sharply demarcated foci of necrosis, myxoid change, or prominent vascularity
— Giant cell pattern
  ◆ Markedly pleomorphic cellular features, including many tumor giant cells with bizarre nuclei, usually solid growth pattern
- Scattered inflammatory cells, high mitotic activity, necrosis, and infiltrative growth pattern are typically seen in all three patterns
- Rarely heterologous elements are seen, such as neoplastic cartilage and bone (most common in spindle cell type)
- Metastases resemble primary morphology
- Background well-differentiated component (most often papillary) may be identified, confirming thyroid origin of anaplastic carcinoma

Special Stains and Immunohistochemistry

- Cytokeratin (particularly low molecular weight) and epithelial membrane antigen (EMA) patchy positive
- Vimentin positive
- Frequently thyroglobulin and TTF-1 negative; may identify focal weak expression to confirm tumor origin
- If calcitonin is positive, more likely to be an anaplastic variant of medullary carcinoma

Other Techniques for Diagnosis

- Most tumors have complex chromosomal alterations
- Strong association with *TP53* mutations

Differential Diagnosis

▌ Poorly differentiated carcinoma
- Nests of uniform, small, round tumor cells
- Aggressive, but prognosis better than for anaplastic
▌ Medullary carcinoma
- Round to oval, spindled, or plasmacytoid features
- Amyloid stroma (Congo red positive)
- Calcitonin positive and thyroglobulin negative
▌ Papillary carcinoma, solid variant
- Characteristic nuclear features such as cleared-out nuclei, nuclear pseudoinclusions, grooves, and overlapping of nuclei
- Thyroglobulin positive (stronger and more uniform than anaplastic)
▌ True sarcoma of the thyroid
- Rare
- Does not have recognizable foci of epithelial differentiation or various patterns
- Vimentin positive and cytokeratin negative
▌ Metastatic carcinoma to the thyroid
- Well-circumscribed, usually multiple nodules, or intralymphatic
- Does not show as much cytologic pleomorphism
- Clinical history important to rule out metastasis

■ Malignant lymphoma
  ● Source of diagnostic error
  ● Leukocyte common antigen (LCA) positive; cytokeratin negative

Pearls

● Highly aggressive tumor, usually with extrathyroidal extension at the time of diagnosis
● Surgical resection rarely alters tumor progression, which is rapidly fatal even if surgically resected (frequently only a biopsy is performed)
● Coexisting papillary thyroid carcinoma when present aids in confirming thyroid origin

Selected References

Kebebew E, Greenspan FS, Clark OH, et al: Anaplastic thyroid carcinoma: Treatment outcome and prognostic factors. Cancer 103:1330-1335, 2005.
Wiseman SM, Loree TR, Rigual NR, et al: Anaplastic transformation of thyroid cancer: Review of clinical, pathologic, and molecular evidence provides new insights into disease biology and future therapy. Head Neck 25:662-670, 2003.
Venkatesh YS, Ordonez NG, Schultz PN, et al: Anaplastic carcinoma of the thyroid: A clinicopathologic study of 121 cases. Cancer 66:321-330, 1990.

Lymphoma

Clinical Features

● Up to 5% of thyroid tumors; malignant tumor is composed of lymphoid cells
● More common in women; peak incidence is in seventh decade
● Rapidly enlarging, firm, hard thyroid; compression symptoms are common

Figure 3-17. Lymphoma, follicular grade 3. Atypical lymphoid infiltrate surrounds and replaces thyroid follicles. At high power (*inset*), the nuclear atypia and discohesive nature of the lymphoma cells are noted.

● Considered primary when the thyroid gland is the predominant or exclusive site of involvement
● The thyroid is involved in 5% of systemic lymphoma or leukemia
● Primary thyroid lymphoma is rare (about 2% of all thyroid malignancies)
● Primary thyroid lymphoma is often associated with autoimmune thyroiditis (Hashimoto or lymphocytic thyroiditis); causal relationship is widely accepted

Gross Pathology

● Solid, homogeneous, tan mass with a fish-flesh appearance
● Unencapsulated tumor with a poorly defined tumor-gland interface
● No necrosis or hemorrhage

Histopathology

■ Non-Hodgkin lymphoma
  ● Most common
  ● Thyroid is considered to be a MALT site, and low-grade and high-grade lymphomas can occur
  ● Most are of B-cell origin, large cell type
  ● Diffuse pattern of growth with entrapped thyroid follicles
  ● Extends into skeletal muscle and fat
  ● Lymphoma cells may accumulate within follicular lumens
■ T-cell lymphoma
  ● Extranodal involvement by mycosis fungoides can affect the thyroid
■ Hodgkin disease
  ● Rarely involves the thyroid gland
  ● Usually nodular sclerosing type

Special Stains and Immunohistochemistry

● LCA positive
● Cytokeratin and thyroglobulin highlight entrapped follicular structures
● For subtyping, refer to Chapter 14

Other Techniques for Diagnosis

● For subtyping, refer to Chapter 14

Differential Diagnosis

■ Hashimoto thyroiditis, chronic lymphocytic thyroiditis
  ● Infiltrate of mature small lymphocytes without atypia
  ● Lymphoid follicles with germinal centers common
  ● Expansion and effacing of germinal centers not seen

Pearls

● Although patients with chronic lymphocytic thyroiditis are at increased risk, primary lymphomas of the thyroid are still rare
● Accumulation of lymphoid cells is seen within follicular lumens (a histologic feature usually not seen in thyroiditis and Graves disease)

- Prognosis depends on classification and stage of tumor
- Plasmacytomas of the thyroid are believed to represent a variant of MALT with plasma cell differentiation

Selected References

Widder S, Pasieka JL: Primary thyroid lymphomas. Curr Treat Options Oncol 5:307-313, 2004.

Thieblemont C, Mayer A, Dumontet C, et al: Primary thyroid lymphoma is a heterogeneous disease. J Clin Endocrinol Metab 87:105-111, 2002.

Belal AA, Allam A, Kandil A, et al: Primary thyroid lymphoma: A retrospective analysis of prognostic factors and treatment outcome for localized intermediate and high grade lymphoma. Am J Clin Oncol 24:299-305, 2001.

Derringer GA, Thompson LD, Frommelt RA, et al: Malignant lymphoma of the thyroid gland: A clinicopathologic study of 108 cases. Am J Surg Pathol 24:623-639, 2000.

Tumors Metastasizing to the Thyroid Gland

Clinical Features

- Direct extension from carcinomas of the head and neck area (pharynx, larynx, trachea, esophagus); occurs most frequently with SCCs
- Hematogenous metastasis to the thyroid occurs in patients with widespread disease
- Common tumors metastasizing to the thyroid are malignant melanoma and carcinomas of the lung, gastrointestinal tract, breast, kidney, and head and neck area
- Clinically present as thyroid enlargement

Gross Pathology

- Often multiple nodules
- Appearance varies with primary lesion; may be very vascular in the case of renal cell carcinoma

Figure 3-18. Metastasis to thyroid. High-grade adenocarcinoma with comedo necrosis. Tumor nests are present in lymphatic spaces.

Histopathology

- Varies with the histology of the primary tumor
- Metastatic renal cell carcinoma is markedly vascular with clear cytoplasm
- Nuclear atypia may favor metastasis because thyroid carcinomas (well differentiated) have bland nuclear features

Special Stains and Immunohistochemistry

- Thyroglobulin negative in all metastatic tumors
- See "Differential Diagnosis"

Other Techniques for Diagnosis

- Noncontributory

Differential Diagnosis

- Malignant melanoma
  - Variable cytology, often large polygonal cells with prominent nucleoli
  - S-100 protein and HMB-45, melan-A, tyrosinase positive
- Renal cell carcinoma
  - Cells with abundant clear cytoplasm and surrounding delicate vascularity
  - Cytokeratin and vimentin positive (also seen in papillary thyroid carcinomas)
- Carcinoid tumor
  - Typically has a nested architecture
  - Uniform cells with round nuclei and neuroendocrine-type chromatin
  - Chromogranin, synaptophysin, and cytokeratin positive; rarely expresses calcitonin
  - Clinical history required to differentiate from primary medullary carcinoma
- Breast carcinoma
  - Glandular or solid growth pattern typically with marked cytologic atypia and desmoplastic stroma
  - Mucin stains may be positive (mucin may be seen in papillary thyroid carcinomas)

Pearls

- Always obtain a good clinical history so that any previous malignancy is revealed
- If something does not fit into a known primary thyroid tumor, use select immunohistochemical stains and obtain clinical correlation

Selected References

Wood K, Vini L, Harmer C: Metastases to the thyroid gland: The Royal Marsden experience. Eur J Surg Oncol 30:583-588, 2004.

Heffess CS, Wenig BM, Thompson LD: Metastatic renal cell carcinoma to the thyroid gland: A clinicopathologic study of 36 cases. Cancer 95:1869-1878, 2002.

Chen H, Nicol TL, Udelsman R: Clinically significant, isolated metastatic disease to the thyroid gland. World J Surg 23:177-180, 1999.

Parathyroid Glands

Parathyroid Cyst

Clinical Features

- Rare lesions, more common in the neck than mediastinum
- Clinically often mistaken for cystic thyroid nodule, may be palpable
- Can result from degeneration of an adenomatous or hyperplastic parathyroid gland
- Usually nonfunctioning; minority are functioning associated with hyperparathyroidism
- More common in women than men
- Peak incidence in fourth to sixth decades

Gross Pathology

- Can measure up to 10 cm
- Thin-walled, unilocular cyst
- Cyst fluid is thin and watery, occasionally hemorrhagic
- May appear to distend from the surface of the thyroid gland but is loosely attached

Histopathology

- Cyst is lined by flattened to cuboidal epithelium with small, basally located nuclei and clear cytoplasm
- Cyst wall consists of fibrous connective tissue
- Entrapped parathyroid chief cells can be seen in wall in cases resulting from degeneration of adenoma, hyperplasia

Special Stains and Immunohistochemistry

- Parathyroid hormone (PTH) and cytokeratin positive
- Thyroglobulin and TTF-1 negative
- FNA of cyst fluid may be sent for PTH and thyroglobulin levels to confirm diagnosis

Other Techniques for Diagnosis

- Noncontributory

Differential Diagnosis

- Thyroid cyst
  - Fluid on FNA positive for thyroglobulin, negative for PTH
  - Lining cells positive for TTF-1 and thyroglobulin
- Degenerated parathyroid adenoma or hyperplasia
  - Cystic degeneration may occur in either adenoma or hyperplasia
  - Background cells are those of adenomatous or hyperplastic parathyroid tissue
  - Entrapped parathyroid chief cells can be seen in wall in cases resulting from degeneration of adenoma or hyperplasia
- Cystic parathyroid adenoma
  - May be associated with hyperparathyroidism–jaw tumor (HPT-JT) syndrome
  - Higher risk for parathyroid carcinoma

- Third pharyngeal pouch cysts
  - Mediastinal cysts that contain both parathyroid and thymic tissue
- Branchial cleft cyst
  - Located in the lateral neck
  - Cyst lined by squamous, columnar, or ciliated epithelial lining
  - Abundant lymphoid stroma in cyst wall

Pearls

- FNA is the best "first" test to evaluate neck nodules
- When FNA of a neck nodule yields clear fluid, a parathyroid cyst should be in the differential diagnosis, and the fluid should be sent for PTH assay because microscopic examination is nonspecific (histiocytes and few epithelial cells that may be mistaken for follicular thyroid epithelium)

Selected References

Ujiki MB, Nayar R, Sturgeon C, Angelos P: Parathyroid cyst: Often mistaken for a thyroid cyst. World J Surg 31:60-64, 2007.

Ippolito G, Palazzo FF, Sebag F, et al: A single-institution 25-year review of true parathyroid cysts. Langenbecks Arch Surg 391:13-18, 2006.

Layfield LJ: Fine needle aspiration cytology of cystic parathyroid lesions: A cytomorphologic overlap with cystic lesion of the thyroid. Acta Cytol 35:447-450, 1991.

Parathyroid Hyperplasia

Clinical Features

- Hyperplasia of parathyroid tissue that involves more than one gland, usually all four
- *Primary hyperparathyroidism* (result of parathyroid hyperplasia in about 15% of cases)
  - Patients have increased PTH, hypercalcemia, and hypophosphatemia
- Secondary hyperparathyroidism
  - Typically secondary to chronic renal failure, which causes hypocalcemia and hyperphosphatemia leading to increased PTH levels
- Hyperplasia of chief cells may be associated with multiple MEN syndromes (I, IIA, and IIB)

Gross Pathology

- Typically all glands are enlarged, but they may be unequally enlarged (normal glands weigh up to 40 mg)
- Cut section appears homogeneous but may be nodular or have cystic changes

Histopathology

- Proliferation of chief cells, oncocytic cells, transitional cells, or clear cells, which are frequently mixed
- Nodular pattern of cellular growth within the gland

Figure 3-19. A, Normal parathyroid. Note the cellularity of the gland showing nests of chief cells with intercellular adipose tissue. **B, Hyperplastic parathyroid.** Multiple lobulated nests of parathyroid cells show loss of intercellular adipose tissue. **C, Parathyroid adenoma.** Gross photograph shows a smooth, well-circumscribed, enlarged gland. **D, Parathyroid adenoma.** Low-power view shows an expansile nodule (adenoma); note a small, compressed rim of normal parathyroid at top of nodule. **E, Parathyroid carcinoma.** Gross photograph of a parathyroid carcinoma with necrosis. **F, Parathyroid carcinoma.** Low-power view shows infiltrating uniform tumor cells in a dense stromal reaction.

- Cellular growth pattern may be solid, follicular (glandlike), or in cords
- Occasionally mitotic figures may be identified
- Involved glands have decreased intracytoplasmic fat content and decreased intercellular fat

Special Stains and Immunohistochemistry

- Oil red O on frozen section will demonstrate decreased intracytoplasmic fat (also seen in adenomas)

Other Techniques for Diagnosis

- MEN I *menin* gene on chromosome 11q
- MEN II *Ret* proto-oncogene on chromosome 10q

Differential Diagnosis

▍ Parathyroid adenoma
- Typically only one enlarged gland; two adenomas are rare
- Rim of compressed parathyroid tissue, but otherwise normal parathyroidal tissue is often present

Pearls

- Intraparenchymal fat will be reduced in both hyperplasia and adenomas
- Treatment is subtotal parathyroidectomy (i.e., removal of $3\frac{1}{2}$ glands)

Selected References

Elliott DD, Monroe DP, Perrier ND: Parathyroid histopathology: Is it of any value today? J Am Coll Surg 203:758-765, 2006.

Johnson SJ, Sheffield EA, McNicol AM: Best practice no. 183: Examination of parathyroid gland specimens. J Clin Pathol 58:338-342, 2005.

Parathyroid Adenoma

Clinical Features

- Benign neoplasm composed of chief cells
- Most commonly occurs in the fifth and sixth decades, female predominance (3:1)
- Most are single adenomas involving one gland
- May occur in various sites such as within thyroid, mediastinum, or retroesophageal area
- Single most common cause of primary hyperparathyroidism (about 80% of cases)
- Patients may present with signs of hypercalcemia ("stones, moans, psychiatric overtones"), or elevated serum calcium is incidentally found during routine blood tests
- Evaluate by ultrasound, sestamibi scan, or computed tomography
- May be associated with MEN I and II or HPT-JT syndrome (also associated with parathyroid carcinoma)

Gross Pathology

- Single enlarged gland; two adenomas are rare
- Round to oval with thin capsule
- Reddish-brown on cut sectioning, usually homogeneous, may on occasion show cystic changes and hemorrhage
- Typically weigh more than 300 mg and up to several grams

Histopathology

- Well circumscribed; cellular proliferation of chief cells that may have clear or oncocytic changes
- Adjacent rim of compressed normal parathyroid tissue is seen in about half of cases and is not required for diagnosis
- Stromal fat content, although minimal to absent in adenoma, is not reliable in separating adenoma from hyperplasia
- Cells with bizarre nuclei may be seen (endocrine atypia), not a sign of malignancy
- Mitoses are usually absent; high mitotic rate should raise suspicion for malignancy
- Growth pattern is solid, nested, follicular, or pseudopapillary; follicular cystic structures may contain colloid-like periodic acid–Schiff (PAS)–positive material
- Variants
  - Atypical adenoma
    - ◆ Lacks unequivocal evidence of malignancy
    - ◆ May show thickened capsule, dense fibrotic bands without lymphovascular invasion or invasion into adjacent structures (i.e., thyroid, esophagus, larynx)
  - HPT-JT
    - ◆ Familial, autosomal dominant, involving *HRPT2* gene, which encodes parafibromin
    - ◆ Cystic change common
    - ◆ Associated with parathyroid carcinoma in 10% to 15%

Special Stains and Immunohistochemistry

- Cytokeratin, chromogranin, and PTH positive
- Thyroglobulin and TTF-1 negative
- Follicle or cyst contents is PAS positive and thyroglobulin negative

Other Techniques for Diagnosis

- Frequent loss of chromosome 11q (location of MEN I) not seen in carcinomas
- Cyclin D1/*PRAD1* oncogene activated by clonal rearrangement (40%)
- Sestamibi scan can localize most parathyroid adenomas preoperatively, and rapid intraoperative PTH assay allows for a minimally invasive parathyroidectomy (MIP), which is a small incision with removal of only the affected gland,

avoiding neck exploration and identification of all four glands

Differential Diagnosis

▌Parathyroid hyperplasia
  - May be primary or secondary, frequently as a result of renal failure
  - If primary, may be associated with MEN I and II
  - All glands are enlarged, often asymmetrically

▌Parathyroid carcinoma
  - Ill-defined, infiltrative mass with extension into adjacent structures

▌Thyroid nodules
  - Follicular nodules: thyroglobulin and TTF-1 positive and PTH negative
  - Medullary thyroid carcinoma: calcitonin and CEA positive; negative for PTH

▌Oncocytic nodules in parathyroids of elderly patients
  - Oncocytic cells within the parathyroid gland increase with age and may form small nodules

Pearls

  - Most parathyroid adenomas are functionally active
  - Treatment is surgical resection of adenoma—preoperative localization and use of intraoperative PTH assay allows for limited surgical exploration with identification and resection of only the affected gland, resulting in less morbidity
  - Thyroid lesions may coexist

Selected References

Absher KJ, Truong LD, Khurana KK, Ramzy I: Parathyroid cytology: Avoiding diagnostic pitfalls. Head Neck 24:157-164, 2002.

Carling T: Molecular pathology of parathyroid tumors. Trends Endocrinol Metab 12:53-58, 2001.

Grimelius L, Johansson H: Pathology of parathyroid tumors. Semin Surg Oncol 13:142-154, 1997.

Parathyroid Carcinoma

Clinical Features

  - Malignant tumor derived from the chief cells of the parathyroid gland
  - Rare cause of hyperparathyroidism (accounts for <1% of cases)
  - High probability of local recurrence and late metastasis to lymph nodes, distant sites
  - Age range, 45 to 55 years; 10 years younger than adenomas; no sex predilection
  - Usually marked hypercalcemia (higher than in patients with adenomas) at presentation, leading to increased renal and bone disease
  - May be associated with HPT-JT syndrome

Gross Pathology

  - Ill-defined, infiltrative mass with extension into muscle, thyroid, esophagus, or trachea
  - Cut section firm and gray-white
  - Mean size, 3 cm; mean weight, 6 g
  - Lymph nodes usually not involved at time of surgery
  - Surgeons report adherent and difficult-to-remove mass

Histopathology

  - Histology is frequently mild to moderate variation in chief cells resembling adenomas; rarer cases have marked pleomorphism and macronucleoli
  - Various architectural patterns include solid (most often), glandular, and trabecular
  - Thick acellular fibrous bands and thick capsule (60% of cases) are common
  - For diagnosing carcinoma, invasion should extend into adjacent structures (esophagus, larynx, muscle)
  - Necrosis is worrisome for carcinoma
  - Vascular invasion (10% to 15% of cases) is defined as attachment to the wall within a vessel located outside the tumor (diagnostic of carcinoma)
  - Capsule in carcinoma is generally thicker than in adenoma
  - Mitoses are seen in about 50% of cases but can also be seen in adenoma or hyperplasia

Special Stains and Immunohistochemistry

  - Cytokeratin and chromogranin positive
  - TTF-1 and thyroglobulin negative

Other Techniques for Diagnosis

  - Recurrent loss of chromosome 13q (region of retinoblastomas and *BRCA2* tumor suppressor genes)
  - HPT-JT syndrome involving *HRPT2* gene (1q25), which encodes parafibromin

Differential Diagnosis

▌Parathyroid hyperplasia
  - Well-defined growth pattern without extension into adjacent structures
  - Multiple parathyroid glands enlarged

▌Parathyroid adenoma
  - Well-defined mass with a distinct, thin fibrous capsule; lacks infiltrative growth pattern
  - Lacks capsular and vascular invasion

▌Atypical adenoma
  - May have some features associated with parathyroid carcinoma, such as adherence to soft tissue, broad fibrous bands, and capsular invasion
  - The term *atypical adenoma* is used if some of these features are present, but the tumor lacks unequivocal

evidence of malignancy, including vascular invasion or invasion into muscle or adjacent structures
▌ Primary neoplasms of the thyroid
  ● Lack clinical hyperparathyroidism (hypercalcemia)
  ● Papillary and follicular tumors are positive for thyroglobulin and negative for chromogranin; medullary carcinoma is positive for calcitonin and frequently positive for TTF-1

Pearls

  ● Treatment is surgical en bloc resection; if local recurrence happens, it is usually during first 3 years after surgery
  ● Most common sites of metastases are cervical lymph nodes, lung, and liver; metastases typically occur late
  ● No scientific basis for progression from hyperplasia to adenoma to carcinoma

Selected References

DeLellis RA: Parathyroid carcinoma: An overview. Adv Anat Pathol 12:53-61, 2005.

Clayman GL, Gonzalez HE, El-Naggar A, Vassilopoulou-Sellin R: Parathyroid carcinoma: Evaluation and interdisciplinary management. Cancer 100:900-905, 2004.

Evans HL: Criteria for the diagnosis of parathyroid carcinoma: A critical study. Surg Pathol 4:244-265, 1991.

Tumors Metastasizing to the Parathyroid Glands

Clinical Features

  ● Metastases to the parathyroid glands are relatively rare
  ● Most common sites of origin are breast, skin, lung, soft tissue, and involvement by leukemia

Figure 3-20. Metastasis to parathyroid gland. Prostatic adenocarcinoma with large nuclei infiltrating fibrous tissue between parathyroid follicles as seen on frozen section.

  ● Rarely the destruction of parathyroid tissue by the metastases may lead to clinical presentation of hypoparathyroidism

Gross Pathology and Histopathology

  ● Depends on the primary site of malignancy

Special Stains and Immunohistochemistry

  ● Staining for PTH and other epithelial markers may be helpful

Other Techniques for Diagnosis

  ● Depends on primary tumor

Differential Diagnosis

  ● Depends on cell type and pattern
  ● Clinical history is essential

Pearls

  ● Parathyroids may be involved by direct extension of tumors from adjacent structures (thyroid, larynx) or from distant sites (metastatic spread)

Selected References

Venkatraman L, Kalangutkar A, Russell CF: Primary hyperparathyroidism and metastatic carcinoma within parathyroid gland. J Clin Pathol 60:1058-1060, 2007.

De la Monte SM, Hutchins GM, Moore GW: Endocrine organ metastases from breast carcinoma. Am J Pathol 114:131-136, 1984.

Salivary Glands

Sialadenitis

Clinical Features

  ● May present as acute, chronic, and granulomatous forms
  ● Causative agents include viral (paramyxovirus, Epstein-Barr virus [EBV], coxsackievirus, influenza A, parainfluenza virus) and bacterial (*Staphylococcus aureus*, *Streptococcus* species, gram-negative bacteria) organisms
  ● Chronic sialadenitis may be associated with rheumatoid arthritis
  ● Predisposing conditions include dehydration, malnutrition, immunosuppression, and sialolithiasis
  ● Etiology of granulomatous subtype is tuberculosis, mycosis, sarcoidosis, duct obstruction
  ● Male predilection; mean age, 40 years

Gross Pathology

  ● Sialolith (stone) may be present (more common in extraglandular secretory ducts than in gland)

Figure 3-21. Chronic sialadenitis, sialometaplasia. Retained lobular architecture with fibrosis and marked squamous metaplasia of the ducts.

- Firm to hard; gland consistency depends on the extent of fibrosis

Histopathology

- Varies depending on the causative agent (viral versus bacterial), underlying condition (sialolithiasis, obstruction), and age of lesion (acute or chronic)
- Variable atrophic changes, fibrosis, and acute and chronic inflammatory features
- Interlobular variation of the extent of inflammatory and fibrotic changes
- Chronic sclerosing sialadenitis of the submandibular gland is unilateral and characterized by lymphocytic and plasmacytic inflammation encasing ducts

Special Stains and Immunohistochemistry

- Noncontributory

Other Techniques for Diagnosis

- Noncontributory

Differential Diagnosis

▍ Benign lymphoepithelial lesion
- Epimyoepithelial islands within lymphoid stroma
- Parenchymal atrophy

▍ Benign lymphoepithelial cyst
- Almost always in parotid gland
- Often bilateral
- Irregular luminal surface with lymphoid infiltrate in wall of cyst
- Often associated with HIV infection

▍ Necrotizing sialometaplasia
- Reactive inflammatory condition with lobular coagulative necrosis of acini
- Squamous metaplasia and pseudoepitheliomatous hyperplasia of overlying mucosal epithelium

- May resemble neoplasia if unilateral
- Can affect any site (palate is common), probably related to ischemia
- FNA yields mostly ductal elements and some chronic inflammatory cells

Pearls

- Clinically, sialadenitis can be confused with malignancy

Selected References

Richardson MS: Non-neoplastic lesions of the salivary glands. In Thompson LDR, Goldblum JR (eds): Head and Neck Pathology. Philadelphia, Elsevier, 2006, pp 283-286.

O'Brien CJ, Murrant BJ: Surgical management of chronic parotitis. Head Neck 15:445-449, 1993.

Brook I: Diagnosis and management of parotitis. Arch Otolaryngol Head Neck Surg 118:469-471, 1992.

Van der Walt JD, Leake J: Granulomatous sialadenitis of the major salivary glands: A clinicopathological study of 57 cases. Histopathology 11:131-144, 1987.

Benign Lymphoepithelial Lesion (Mikulicz Disease)

Clinical Features

- Most common cause of diffuse bilateral enlargement of salivary and lacrimal glands
- Clinically, slowly increasing bilateral and symmetrical swelling of salivary glands
- One manifestation of Sjögren syndrome
- Systemic autoimmune disease; develop small clonal expansions; can evolve into lymphoma

Gross Pathology

- Multiple small, tan nodules may diffusely replace gland

Figure 3-22. Benign lymphoepithelial lesion. High-power view shows a vaguely defined epimyoepithelial island surrounded by small lymphoid cells.

Histopathology

- Epimyoepithelial islands are solid nests of mainly basal epithelial cells and myoepithelial cells; typically permeated by monocytoid B cells of MALT; they can also be seen in low-grade MALT lymphoma
- Lymphoid infiltrate can contain well-formed germinal centers; polyclonal and composed predominantly of T cells
- Intercellular hyaline material resembling basal lamina is deposited

Special Stains and Immunohistochemistry

- B- and T-cell markers and kappa and lambda stains on paraffin or frozen tissues

Other Techniques for Diagnosis

- Flow cytometry to evaluate clonality
- Gene rearrangement studies to exclude lymphoma, if indicated

Differential Diagnosis

▌ Malignant lymphoepithelial carcinoma
- Undifferentiated carcinoma with lymphoid stroma
- Most in salivary location, EBV associated

Pearls

- Increased risk for developing malignant lymphoma in both salivary and extrasalivary locations
- Lymphomas are mostly B-cell phenotype; large cell lymphoma or MALT type
- Features that indicate development of lymphoma include prominent aggregations of monomorphic medium-sized lymphoid cells with abundant pale cytoplasm and uniform nuclei (monocytoid B cells); involvement of adjacent fat and connective tissue, immunohistochemical evidence of monoclonality

Figure 3-23. Lymphoepithelial cyst. A, Gross photograph of multiple lymphoepithelial cysts within the parotid gland. **B,** Low-power view shows a cyst lined by epithelium and a prominent lymphoid infiltrate in the cyst wall.

Selected References

Peel RL: Diseases of the salivary glands. In Barnes L (ed): Surgical Pathology of the Head and Neck. New York, Marcel Dekker, 2001, pp 635-642.

MacLean H, Ironside JW, Cullen JF, Butt Z: Mikulicz syndrome and disease: 2 case reports highlighting the difference. Acta Ophthalmol 71:136-141, 1993.

McCurley TL, Collins RD, Ball E, Collins RD: Nodal and extranodal lymphoproliferative disorders in Sjögren syndrome: A clinical and immunopathologic study. Hum Pathol 482-492, 1990.

Batsakis JG: Pathology consultation: Carcinoma ex lymphoepithelial lesion. Ann Otol Rhinol Laryngol 92:657-658, 1983.

Lymphoepithelial Cyst

Clinical Features

- Present in the parotid or upper cervical lymph nodes
- Similar to salivary duct cyst

- Etiology
  — Originates from remnant of branchial apparatus and is similar to branchial cleft cyst
  — Cystic formation of salivary gland nests in intraparotid or periparotid lymph node
- Some cases associated with HIV infection, often bilateral

Gross Pathology

- Multiloculated cysts on cut surface
- Solid, tan homogeneous areas in the cyst wall represent lymphoid tissue

Histopathology

- Multilocular cysts covered by glandular or squamous epithelium surrounded by hyperplastic lymphoid follicles with germinal center formation

- HIV-associated cases
  - Multifocal
  - Occur early and associated with florid lymphoid hyperplasia

Special Stains and Immunohistochemistry

- Noncontributory

Other Techniques for Diagnosis

- Noncontributory

Differential Diagnosis

▌ Cystic Warthin tumor
  - Lymphoid follicle formation with oncocytic epithelium
▌ Branchial cleft cyst
  - Lateral location is in neck near sternocleidomastoid muscle
  - Cyst is lined by squamous, columnar, or ciliated epithelium
  - Cyst wall has prominent lymphoid stroma
  - Cyst may contain anucleated keratinized epithelium, histiocytes, or cholesterol clefts

Pearls

- HIV infection show marked increase in dendritic reticular cells and intrafollicular CD8-positive lymphocytes
- FNA can be diagnostic and therapeutic; can be the first indication that the patient should be tested for HIV

Selected References

Richardson MS: Non-neoplastic lesions of the salivary glands. In Thompson LDR, Goldblum JR (eds): Head and Neck Pathology. Philadelphia, Elsevier, 2006, pp 288-290.

Mandel L, Reich R: HIV parotid gland lymphoepithelial cysts: Review and case reports. Oral Surg Oral Med Oral Pathol 74:273-278, 1992.

Terry JH, Loree TR, Thomas MD, Marti JR: Major salivary gland lymphoepithelial lesions and the acquired immunodeficiency syndrome. Am J Surg 162:324-329, 1991.

Cleary KR, Batsakis JG: Lymphoepithelial cysts of the parotid region: A new face on an old lesion. Ann Otol Rhinol Laryngol 99:162-164, 1990.

Salivary Duct Cyst

Clinical Features

- Cystic dilatation of a salivary duct due to ductal obstruction
- Majority occur in parotid

Gross Pathology

- Well-circumscribed, unilocular cyst with smooth lining
- Cyst contains thin, watery to viscous fluid

Figure 3-24. Salivary duct cyst. Low-power view shows a cyst lined by a single layer of epithelium. Notice the adjacent salivary gland tissue and marked fibrosis of the wall.

Histopathology

- Cyst wall consists of dense fibroconnective tissue with mild to moderate infiltrate of chronic inflammatory cells and lined by stratified squamous epithelium
- Goblet-type mucinous or oncocytic cells may be present in the epithelium
- Surrounding parenchyma of parotid is atrophic as a result of compression
- Mild sialadenitis and duct ectasia may be seen

Special Stains and Immunohistochemistry

- Noncontributory

Other Techniques for Diagnosis

- Noncontributory

Differential Diagnosis

▌ Mucus retention cyst (ranula)
  - More common in minor salivary glands, lower lip
  - Lack of cystic wall
  - Pools of mucin in fibrous tissue
▌ Cystic Warthin tumor
  - Cyst wall lined by oncocytic cuboids or columnar epithelium with underlying dense lymphoid stroma

Pearls

- Surgical excision is curative

Selected References

Peel RL: Diseases of the salivary glands. In Barnes L (ed): Surgical Pathology of the Head and Neck. New York, Marcel Dekker, 2001, pp 651-653.

Cohen MN, Rao U, Shedd DP: Benign cysts of the parotid gland. J Surg Oncol 27:85-88, 1984.

Mucocele (Ranula)

Clinical Features

- Most common non-neoplastic lesion of the salivary glands (4% to 9%)
- Two types of mucoceles: extravasation type and retention type
  - Extravasation-type mucocele
    - ◆ Results from extravasation of secreted salivary fluid into surrounding tissue; peak incidence in third decade
    - ◆ Lip most common location
  - Retention-type mucocele (plunging ranula)
    - ◆ Mucus pools within epithelium-lined cysts (partially obstructed excretory ducts with cystic dilatation or congenital or acquired weakness of duct wall)
    - ◆ Occurs in all ages; peak incidence in seventh decade
    - ◆ Clinically may fluctuate in size; can develop within hours to days

Gross Pathology

- Small, dome-shaped swelling of mucosa ranging in size from 0.2 to 1 cm
- Consistency is soft and fluctuant

Histopathology

- Extravasation type
  - Pool of mucin often with scattered inflammation surrounded by granulation tissue
- Retention type
  - Mucin pool surrounded by cuboidal to stratified squamous epithelial lining and fibrotic cyst wall

Special Stains and Immunohistochemistry

- Noncontributory

Figure 3-25. Mucocele (extravasation type). Low-power view shows pools of mucoid material surrounded by inflammation and minor salivary glands.

Other Techniques for Diagnosis

- Noncontributory

Differential Diagnosis

- ▌ Salivary duct cyst
  - True epithelium-lined cyst with chronic inflammation in wall
  - Compression of surrounding parenchyma, which has atrophic changes
- ▌ Lymphoepithelial cyst
  - Multilocular cyst with marked lymphoid tissue in wall

Pearls

- Sublingual mucocele (floor of mouth) is called plunging ranula; can become larger (several centimeters) and dissect through muscles and connective tissue of the neck
- Treatment is local excision

Selected References

Richardson MS: Non-neoplastic lesions of the salivary glands. In Thompson LDR, Goldblum JR (eds): Head and Neck Pathology. Philadelphia, Elsevier, 2006, pp 279-283.

Das S, Das AK: A review of pediatric oral biopsies from a surgical service in a dental school. Pediatr Dent 15:208-211, 1993.

Mixed Tumor (Pleomorphic Adenoma)

Clinical Features

- Benign tumor that manifests both epithelial and mesenchymal elements
- Most common neoplasm of salivary gland origin; constitutes about 30% of all parotid neoplasms and 60% of benign tumors from all salivary gland sites
- Most common salivary gland tumor in children and adolescents; higher incidence in women
- Most common intraoral site is the palate, followed by the upper lip and buccal mucosa
- Usually solitary, most common associated tumor is Warthin tumor
- Peak incidence is in fourth decade
- Typically presents as a slow-growing, asymptomatic, discrete, mobile, often multinodular, firm mass; may become large if untreated
- Often occurs in the lower pole of the superficial lobe; facial paralysis may occur only as result of extrinsic compression of facial nerve, not invasion

Gross Pathology

- Round to ovoid mass with smooth surface
- Most tumors are encapsulated (incomplete fibrous capsule); tumors that originate from minor salivary glands are often unencapsulated

Figure 3-26. Benign mixed tumor (pleomorphic adenoma). A, Gross photograph shows a well-circumscribed, gray-white nodule. **B,** A cellular tumor composed of ducts and myoepithelial cells (*right*) is adjacent to the hypocellular cartilaginous areas (*left*).

- Cut surface is homogeneous or variegated, tan to white, with shiny, translucent zones that represent myxochondroid or cartilaginous areas; often lobulated, especially when larger than 1 cm
- Occasionally, hemorrhage and infarction occur secondary to surgical or FNA biopsy

Histopathology
- Shows both epithelial and mesenchymal differentiation; proportions are variable and heterogeneous cellular composition
  - Epithelial component
    - Well-formed ductal structures formed of inner epithelial and outer myoepithelial cells associated with features of spindle, squamous, basaloid, cuboidal, oncocytoid, mucous, sebaceous, round, plasmacytoid, polygonal, or clear cells
    - Squamous differentiation with keratin pearls can occur

- Cytologic features of epithelial cells are bland; rare, if any, mitotic activity
  - Mesenchymal component
    - Myxoid, hyaline, cartilaginous, or osseous differentiation
- Several variants
  - Cellular type: epithelial element predominates; constitutes more than 80% of tumor in only 12% to 15% of cases
  - Myxoid type: myxochondromatous mesenchymal element predominates (most tumors have a myxoid component that makes up about 30% of tumor)
- Thickness of fibrous capsule varies; often absent in predominantly myxoid tumors and in tumors arising in minor salivary glands

Special Stains and Immunohistochemistry
- Noncontributory

Other Techniques for Diagnosis
- Cytogenetic studies often show clonal chromosomal rearrangements, 8q12 and 12q13-15
- Patients with 8q12 abnormalities are typically younger
- No correlation between cytogenetic findings and prognosis

Differential Diagnosis
▌ Polymorphous low-grade adenocarcinoma (particularly in minor salivary gland)
- Frequently shows perineural growth and is infiltrative into periglandular tissue
- Forms small tubular structures or single-file cords of cells at the periphery
▌ Carcinoma ex pleomorphic adenoma
- Malignant tumor arising in a background of a mixed tumor

Selected References
Das DK, Anim JT: Pleomorphic adenoma of salivary gland: To what extent does fine needle aspiration cytology reflect histopathological features? Cytopathology 16:65-70, 2005.

Brachtel EF, Pilch BZ, Khettry U, et al: Fine-needle aspiration biopsy of a cystic pleomorphic adenoma with extensive adnexa-like differentiation: Differential diagnostic pitfall with mucoepidermoid carcinoma. Diagn Cytopathol 28:100-103, 2003.

Glas AS, Hollema H, Nap RE, Plukker JT: Expression of estrogen receptor, progesterone receptor, and insulin-like growth factor receptor-1 and of MIB-1 in patients with recurrent pleomorphic adenoma of the parotid gland. Cancer 94:2211-2216, 2002.

Lee PS, Sabbath-Solitare M, Redondo TC, Ongcapin EH: Molecular evidence that the stromal and epithelial cells in pleomorphic adenomas of salivary gland arise from the same origin: Clonal analysis using human androgen receptor gene (HUMARA) assay. Hum Pathol 31:498-503, 2000.

Bullerdiek J, Wobst G, Meyer-Bolte K, et al: Cytogenetic subtyping of 220 salivary gland pleomorphic adenomas: Correlation to occurrence, histological subtype, and in vitro cellular behavior. Cancer Genet Cytogenet 65:27-31, 1993.

Myoepithelioma

Clinical Features

- Benign tumor composed entirely of myoepithelial cells
- May represent the end of the pleomorphic adenoma spectrum
- About 2% to 5% of benign salivary gland tumors
- Sites: parotid (50%) and minor salivary glands (40%)
- Men and women affected equally
- Peak incidence in third decade
- Typically presents as an asymptomatic mass

Gross Pathology

- Well circumscribed and may be encapsulated
- Cut surface is solid, tan, or yellow-tan and glistening

Histopathology

- Three characteristic histologic growth patterns
  — Spindle cell variant
    ◆ Composed of interlacing fascicles of uniform spindle cells that have elongated nuclei and eosinophilic cytoplasm
    ◆ May manifest clusters of polygonal or round epithelial or clear cells
    ◆ Minimal formation of myxoid stoma
  — Plasmacytoid cell variant
    ◆ Cells show plasmacytoid features, most common subtype
  — Epithelioid variant
    ◆ Tumors are composed of epithelioid cells with round to oval vesicular nuclei, inconspicuous nucleoli, and eosinophilic cytoplasm
    ◆ Few spindle and plasmacytoid cells may be present
- Occasionally microcystic architecture with mucoid stroma
- Stroma, when present, shows hyaline or myxoid features

Special Stains and Immunohistochemistry

- Cytokeratin, muscle-specific actin (MSA), glial fibrillary acidic protein (GFAP), calponin, and S-100 protein: variable reactivity

Other Techniques for Diagnosis

- Noncontributory

Differential Diagnosis

▮ Myoepithelial-rich mixed tumor (pleomorphic adenoma)
  - Areas of conventional of benign mixed tumor

Figure 3-27. Myoepithelioma. A, Solid sheets of round myoepithelial cells. **B,** Myoepithelial cells are forming trabeculae with a rosette-like pattern. **C,** Marked spindling of the myoepithelial cells.

▮ Myoepithelial carcinoma
  - Mainly spindle cell form but any cellular variants with infiltrative borders with and without cellular features of malignancy
  - Slightly older; mean age, 50 years; males = females

- Most arise in parotid
- Unencapsulated, multinodular
- Morphologic cellular variability (spindled, stellate, epithelioid, plasmacytoid)
- Cytologically, often bland-appearing adenoma but locally invasive
- Also designate carcinoma when perineural or lymphovascular invasion is identified
▌ Spindle cell tumors (rare in the major and minor salivary glands)
- Nerve sheath tumors: schwannoma
  — Cytokeratin negative, S-100 protein positive
- Fibrous histiocytomas: cytokeratin negative
- Nodular fasciitis: cytokeratin negative
- Monophasic spindle cell synovial sarcoma
  — Often has high-grade histology
  — May be positive for cytokeratin, epithelial or mixed forms
▌ Metastatic renal cell carcinoma (differentiate from clear cell myoepithelioma)
- History is important
- Distinct delicate vascularity surrounds tumor cells

Pearls

- Differentiate adenoma from carcinoma by circumscription verses invasion
- Histologically myoepithelial cells are very diverse in appearance

Selected References

Hungermann D, Roeser K, Buerger H, et al: Relative paucity of gross genetic alterations in myoepitheliomas and myoepithelial carcinomas of salivary glands. J Pathol 198:487-494, 2002.

Savera AT, Sloman A, Huvos AG, Klimstra DS: Myoepithelial carcinoma of the salivary glands: A clinicopathologic study of 25 patients. Am J Surg Pathol 24:761-774, 2000.

Nagao T, Sugano I, Ishida Y, et al: Salivary gland malignant myoepithelioma: A clinicopathologic and immuno-histochemical study of ten cases. Cancer 83:1292-1299, 1998.

Simpson RH, Jones H, Beasley P: Benign myoepithelioma of the salivary glands: A true entity? Histopathology 27:1-9, 1995.

Warthin Tumor (Papillary Cystadenoma Lymphomatosum)

Clinical Features

- Second most common benign salivary tumor
- Most occur in parotid gland
- Unusually low frequency in black patients
- More common in males
- Presents as a painless, sometimes fluctuant swelling (usually 2 to 4 cm in diameter)
- May present as multifocal or bilateral lesions

Figure 3-28. Warthin tumor. A, Gross photograph of a parotid mass shows a partially cystic mass with fine nodular, papillary surface. **B,** Section shows a cystic tumor composed of uniform, bland oncocytic epithelium surrounded by lymphoid cells.

Gross Pathology

- Well-circumscribed, fluctuant mass
- Cut surface shows brown mucoid and turbid materials in cystic spaces and small granular tissue excrescences; cystic areas are tan to nodular foci and may be hemorrhagic

Histopathology

- Thin capsule, usually sharply demarcated from surrounding parenchyma
- Epithelial component composed of tall columnar and basaloid oncocytic cells lining cysts and forming prominent papillae
- Cystic spaces lined by papillary proliferation of oncocytic epithelium with lymphoid stroma; can show lymphoid follicles
- Cyst contents include cellular debris and laminated bodies resembling corpora amylacea, and calcifications
- Squamous metaplasia may be present

Special Stains and Immunohistochemistry

- Noncontributory

Other Techniques for Diagnosis

- Noncontributory

Differential Diagnosis

- ❚ Oncocytoma
  - Typically a solid proliferation of oncocytic cells; may occasionally be cystic
  - Lacks lymphoid component
- ❚ Papillary oncocytic cystadenoma
  - Lacks lymphoid component
- ❚ Lymphoepithelial cysts in HIV patients
  - Often bilateral
  - Lacks oncocytes
- ❚ Lymphadenoma
  - Lacks oncocytic cell component
- ❚ Parotid duct cyst
  - Lacks dense lymphoid stroma

Pearls

- Pathogenesis uncertain; possibly two forms: reactive (non-neoplastic) characterized by multifocality and bilaterality, and neoplastic characterized by a single site with rare association with mucoepidermoid carcinoma and oncocytic carcinoma
- May arise in an intraparotid lymph node
- FNA findings (amorphous background, lymphoid cells, oncocytes, and necrosis) can raise differential diagnosis of bronchial cleft cyst, oncocytoma, cystic SCC

Selected References

Webb AJ, Eveson JW: Parotid Warthin's tumour Bristol Royal Infirmary (1985-1995): A study of histopathology in 33 cases. Oral Oncol 38:163-171, 2002.

Maiorano E, Lo Muzio L, Favia G, Piattelli A: Warthin's tumour: A study of 78 cases with emphasis on bilaterality, multifocality and association with other malignancies. Oral Oncol 38:35-40, 2002.

Schwerer MJ, Kraft K, Baczako K, Maier H: Cytokeratin expression and epithelial differentiation in Warthin's tumour and its metaplastic (infarcted) variant. Histopathology 39:347-352, 2001.

Lewis PD, Baxter P, Paul Griffiths A, et al: Detection of damage to the mitochondrial genome in the oncocytic cells of Warthin's tumour. J Pathol 191:274-281, 2000.

Oncocytoma

Clinical Features

- Rare benign epithelial neoplasm composed of oncocytic (mitochondria-rich) cells
- Predominant site is the parotid gland
- Typically occurs in older population

Figure 3-29. **Oncocytoma. A,** Gross photograph shows a lobular mahogany nodule with central scar within the parotid tissue. **B,** Low-power view shows a solid tumor composed of uniform cells with abundant granular eosinophilic cytoplasm and central scar. High-power view (*inset*) shows uniform round nuclei often with prominent nucleoli and granular cytoplasm.

- Presents as swelling, and mass effect may rarely be painful
- Recurrence rate ranges from 0% to 30%

Gross Pathology

- Single, well-defined and encapsulated tan to red-brown mass
- Usually solid, but cysts can be present occasionally

Histopathology

- Sheets of relatively large, oncocytic cells (strongly eosinophilic cells with abundant finely granular cytoplasm) with distinct cell borders that contain centrally placed nuclei with fine chromatin and a single conspicuous nucleolus
- Often arranged in an organoid pattern or in clusters with surrounding thin fibrous bands and capillaries

156 Differential Diagnosis in Surgical Pathology

- Variably sized cystic spaces are present, occasionally with lymphoid infiltrate
- May manifest clear cell features

Special Stains and Immunohistochemistry

- Noncontributory

Other Techniques for Diagnosis

- Noncontributory

Differential Diagnosis

▎ Oncocytic metaplasia in salivary gland
  - Normal salivary gland with focal oncocytic cell overgrowth
  - May be multifocal; occasionally diffuse
  - Oncocytes increase in numbers with increasing age of the patient (most likely due to internal cellular derangement or demand on the respiratory pathway cycle of mitochondria)
▎ Warthin tumor
  - Papillary cystic architecture and lymphoid stroma
  - Squamous metaplasia is a common finding but is rarely seen in oncocytomas
▎ Pleomorphic adenoma with oncocytic metaplasia
  - Varied architectural patterns, chondromyxoid background, and epithelial or myoepithelial cell types
▎ Mucoepidermoid carcinoma
  - May arise or occur within Warthin tumor and show oncocytic features
  - Invasive, multinodular pattern of growth
▎ Metastatic renal cell carcinoma, granular and clear cell types
  - High-grade cellular and nuclear features
  - History of renal cell carcinoma
▎ Clear cell carcinoma, not otherwise specified (NOS)
  - Unencapsulated and infiltrative
  - Nuclei eccentric, often with small nucleoli
▎ Clear cell acinic cell carcinoma
  - Invasive, multilobular pattern
  - Clear cells in this entity will be negative for PAS granules
  - Oncocytic nuclei are not a feature

Pearls

- Neither nuclear atypia nor tumor infiltration correlates with biologic behavior
- Recurrence rates are higher if tumor is multifocal or if incompletely excised
- Excision is the primary treatment because radiation therapy has been linked to malignant transformation

Selected References

Ito K, Tsukuda M, Kawabe R, et al: Benign and malignant oncocytoma of the salivary glands with an immunohistochemical evaluation of Ki-67. ORL J Otorhinolaryngol Relat Spec 62:338-341, 2000.

Paulino AF, Huvos AG: Oncocytic and oncocytoid tumors of the salivary glands. Semin Diagn Pathol 16:98-104, 1999.
Coli A, Bigotti G, Bartolazzi A: Malignant oncocytoma of major salivary glands: Report of a post-irradiation case. J Exp Clin Cancer Res 17:65-70, 1998.
Brandwein MS, Huvos AG: Oncocytic tumors of major salivary glands: A study of 68 cases with follow-up of 44 patients. Am J Surg Pathol 15:514-528, 1991.

Cystadenoma

Clinical Features

- Rare benign cystic epithelial tumor
- Occurs predominantly in parotid and minor salivary glands (lip and buccal mucosa)

Gross Pathology

- Encapsulated, well-circumscribed mass
- Multiple small cystic spaces within salivary gland

Histopathology

- A single cyst or variably sized cysts with variable intraluminal papillary proliferation lined by cuboidal or columnar epithelium
- Lumens contain eosinophilic fluid with epithelial and inflammatory cells; calcifications and crystals rarely seen
- Occasionally, gland formation may be seen
- May display oncocytic cellular and squamous metaplastic features

Special Stains and Immunohistochemistry

- Noncontributory

Other Techniques for Diagnosis

- Noncontributory

Figure 3-30. Cystadenoma. Cystic lesion lined by bland epithelium.

Differential Diagnosis

▌ Warthin tumor
  ● More common in parotid gland
  ● Composed of bilayered oncocytic epithelium and marked lymphoid hyperplasia in surrounding stroma
▌ Congenital polycystic disease
  ● Developmental malformation of ductal system
  ● Multicystic mass with luminal spheroliths and apocrine-like lining epithelium
  ● Mainly in infants and young children
▌ Duct ectasia with focal epithelial proliferation secondary to obstruction
  ● Associated changes include acinar atrophy, chronic inflammation, and fibrosis
  ● No epithelial cell proliferation
▌ Intraductal papilloma
  ● Always unicystic and occur in dilated salivary gland duct
  ● Intraluminal papillary fronds are more numerous and complex
▌ Low-grade papillary cystadenocarcinoma
  ● Must have an invasive growth pattern with infiltration into adjacent tissue
  ● Cytologic atypia can be minimal
  ● Exclude low-grade mucoepidermoid carcinoma

Pearls

  ● Treatment is conservative but complete resection
  ● Differential includes both benign and malignant entities

Selected References

Nakagawa T, Hattori K, Iwata N, Tsujimura T: Papillary cystadenocarcinoma arising from minor salivary glands in the anterior portion of the tongue: A case report. Auris Nasus Larynx 29:87-90, 2002.

Danford M, Eveson JW, Flood TR: Papillary cystadenocarcinoma of the sublingual gland presenting as a ranula. Br J Oral Maxillofac Surg 30:270-272, 1992.

Hemangioma

Clinical Features

  ● May be capillary or cavernous
  ● Occurs in adults and adolescents
  ● About 80% of cases affect females
  ● Juvenile hemangiomas occur in patients younger than 1 year; most occur in parotid gland (previously called *benign infantile hemangioendothelioma*)
  ● Often congenital and present as a bluish discoloration of overlying skin
  ● Can extend into hypopharynx and intracranially
  ● Rapid enlargement suggests malignancy

Figure 3-31. Hemangioma (cavernous). Thin-walled dilated vessels lined by bland endothelial cells.

Gross Pathology

  ● No distinctive mass
  ● Dark red-purple parenchyma

Histopathology

  ● Juvenile hemangioma
    — Closely packed sheets of cells within salivary gland parenchyma
    — Small capillary channels and larger, thin-walled vessels at periphery
    — Variable mitotic rate
  ● Adult-type hemangioma
    — Larger, thin-walled vascular channels lined by plump endothelial cells
    — Variable mitotic rate
    — Minimal cellular features of malignancy

Special Stains and Immunohistochemistry

  ● CD31 positive in endothelial cells

Other Techniques for Diagnosis

  ● Noncontributory

Differential Diagnosis

▌ Lymphangioma
  ● Dilated lymphatic spaces lined by uniform, flattened endothelial cells
  ● Absence of luminal red blood cells
▌ Angiosarcoma
  ● High-grade tumor with irregular vascular spaces lined by pleomorphic, atypical cells
  ● Typically has a high mitotic rate

Pearls

  ● Progressive interstitial fibrosis and infarction of tumors often occur over time

- Treatment may include excision, embolization, alcohol injection, steroid therapy, laser therapy, and radiation; propranolol may also be effective
- By age 7 years, 70% to 90% of hemangiomas will have involuted spontaneously
- Presence of high cellularity and mitotic activity does not make the lesion malignant; be very cautious before making a diagnosis of malignancy in children

Selected References

Peel RL: Diseases of the salivary glands. In Barnes L (ed): Surgical Pathology of the Head and Neck. New York, Marcel Dekker, 2001, pp 684-688.

Mantravadi J, Roth LM, Kafrawy AH: Vascular neoplasms of the parotid gland: Parotid vascular tumors. Oral Surg Oral Med Oral Pathol 75:70-75, 1993.

Livesey JR, Soames JV: Cystic lymphangioma in the adult period. J Laryngol Otol 106:566-568, 1992.

Caldwell RA: A case of congenital capillary hemangioma of the parotid gland. Br J Surg 39:261-263, 1951.

Basal Cell Adenoma

Clinical Features

- A monomorphic adenoma composed of basal cells
- Most commonly involving parotid gland (70%), usually superficial aspect
- Peak incidence in sixth and seventh decades; extremely rare in children; female predominance
- Clinically, presents as a single, well-defined movable nodule; membranous subtype tends to be multifocal

Gross Pathology

- Sharply circumscribed or multinodular mass
- Vary in size

Figure 3-32. Basal cell adenoma. A neoplasm composed of nests of uniform, small basaloid cells with dense basement membrane between nests.

- Cut section shows a homogeneous, gray to tan mass; usually solid, occasionally cystic

Histopathology

- Monotonous cellular growth lacking the myxochondroid stroma of mixed tumors
- Characterized by uniform small cells with round to oval, hyperchromatic nuclei, pale eosinophilic to amphophilic cytoplasm, and indistinct cell borders (basaloid cells)
- Squamous and squamoid features may be seen
- Four recognized subtypes: trabecular, solid, tubular, and membranous (often have mixed patterns)
  — Trabecular type
    ◆ Interlacing narrow bands of basaloid cells
    ◆ May have variable proportion of ductal lumens
    ◆ Loose fibrous stroma surrounding trabeculae
  — Solid type
    ◆ Variably sized aggregates of epithelial tumor cells with scant surrounding dense collagenous stroma
    ◆ Palisading nuclei at border of epithelial cell islands and stroma (stromal interface)
    ◆ Foci of squamous whorls and "eddies" may be seen
  — Tubular type
    ◆ Predominance of ductal differentiation
    ◆ Lumens bordered by cuboidal ductal cells that may show palisading; resembles canalicular adenoma
  — Membranous type
    ◆ Prominent hyaline material or basal lamina forms thick bands surrounding the islands of basal cells

Special Stains and Immunohistochemistry

- Noncontributory

Other Techniques for Diagnosis

- Noncontributory

Differential Diagnosis

▮ Mixed tumor (pleomorphic adenoma)
- Characteristic chondromyxoid stroma is the most helpful distinguishing feature
- Epithelial cells "blend" with mesenchymal (stromal) component (lacks sharp interface)
- Often GFAP positive

▮ Adenoid cystic carcinoma
- Cribriform architecture
- Tumor cells have irregular, hyperchromatic, angulated nuclei
- Infiltrative growth pattern
- Often have perineural invasion

▮ Canalicular adenoma
- Occurs predominantly in the upper lip

- Composed of branching and anastomosing cords two cell layers thick, which are often separate and form small cystic spaces (beads-on-a-string appearance)
- Surrounding loose stroma

▮ Basal cell adenocarcinoma (malignant counterpart to basal cell adenoma)
  - Infiltrative growth pattern
  - Tumor cells have bland cytologic features
  - May have perineural or vascular invasion

▮ Basal cell carcinoma of skin origin
  - Clinical history of locally invasive skin primary
  - May be metastasis from skin of face and scalp
  - Invasive growth pattern
  - May show mitoses and more irregular, hyperchromatic nuclei

Pearls

- Overall excellent prognosis with low recurrence rates following surgical excision, except for membranous subtype, which may recur in up to 25% of cases owing to tendency to be multifocal and unencapsulated
- Membranous basal cell adenomas histologically resemble dermal cylindromas
- Rare reports of malignant transformation; higher rates in membranous subtype

Selected References

Choi HR, Batsakis JG, Callender DL, et al: Molecular analysis of chromosome 16q regions in dermal analogue tumors of salivary glands: A genetic link to dermal cylindroma? Am J Surg Pathol 26:778-783, 2002.

Ferreiro JA: Immunohistochemistry of basal cell adenoma of the major salivary glands. Histopathology 24:539-542, 1994.

Batsakis JG, Luna MA, el-Naggar AK: Basaloid monomorphic adenomas. Ann Otol Rhinol Laryngol 100:687-690, 1991.

Daley TD, Gardner DG, Smout MS: Canalicular adenoma: Not a basal cell adenoma. Oral Surg Oral Med Oral Pathol Oral Radiol Endodontol 57:181-188, 1984.

Sebaceous Lymphadenoma

Clinical Features

- Rare benign tumor (<1% of all adenomas of the major salivary glands)
- Mean age, sixth decade
- Slightly more common in men
- Almost exclusively found in parotid gland
- Presents as a slow-growing, firm mass

Gross Pathology

- Sharply circumscribed and encapsulated
- Usually solid, occasionally cystic
- Gray-white to yellow-gray cut surface
- Usually 1 to 3 cm in diameter

Figure 3-33. Sebaceous adenoma. Nests of cells with various levels of vacuolization of the cytoplasm corresponding to sebaceous differentiation.

Histopathology

- Composed of cells that form solid nests of variable size and cystic areas surrounded by fibrous, often hyalinized stroma and lymphoid stroma
- Sebaceous and squamous differentiation is focal; no or only minimal cytologic atypia
- Foreign-body giant cell reaction and histiocytes may be present

Special Stains and Immunohistochemistry

- Noncontributory

Other Techniques for Diagnosis

- Noncontributory

Differential Diagnosis

▮ Sebaceous carcinoma
  - Infiltrative growth pattern and high-grade cellular features

▮ Metastatic squamous carcinoma with clear cell features
  - May have areas of necrosis
  - Often infiltrates surrounding tissue

Pearls

- Benign behavior; no recurrences or malignant degeneration
- Treatment is typically local excision

Selected References

Peel RL: Diseases of the salivary glands. In Barnes L (ed): Surgical Pathology of the Head and Neck. New York, Marcel Dekker, 2001, pp 728-731.

Merwin WH Jr, Barnes L, Myers EN: Unilocular cystic sebaceous lymphadenoma of the parotid gland. Arch Otolaryngol Head Neck Surg 111:273-275, 1985.

Gnepp DR, Brannon R: Sebaceous neoplasms of salivary gland origin: Report of 21 cases. Cancer 53:2155-2170, 1984.

Cramer SF, Gnepp DR, Kiehn CL, Levitan J: Sebaceous differentiation in adenoid cystic carcinoma of the parotid gland. Cancer 46:1405-1410, 1980.

Adenoid Cystic Carcinoma

Clinical Features

- Constitutes about 10% of all salivary gland tumors
- Most common malignancy of the submandibular gland
- May occur in any site with salivary tissue
- All ages, peak in fourth to sixth decades; slightly more common in females
- Presents as a slow-growing, sometimes painful mass; patients often have a long clinical course
- May present with facial nerve paralysis

Gross Pathology

- May appear well circumscribed, but is deceptively infiltrative; tumor extends well beyond visible and palpable limits of grossly evident tumor
- Solid, gray-white mass with marked propensity to grow along nerves

Histopathology

- Three major growth patterns: cribriform (classic), tubular, and solid; most tumors have mixtures of cytoarchitectural patterns
  — Cribriform pattern (classic)
    ◆ Constitutes about 50% of cases
    ◆ Composed of small cylindrical structures (i.e., sievelike appearance with pseudocystic spaces) that are encased by tumor cells
    ◆ Cylindrical structures contain eosinophilic material (basal lamina) or basophilic substance (glycosaminoglycans)

Figure 3-34. Adenoid cystic carcinoma. A, Maxillectomy specimen with a tan-white tumor of the palate replacing bone. **B,** Proliferation of tumor cells with a cribriform growth pattern. **C,** Tumor cells in a tubular pattern showing marked perineural and intraneural invasion. **D,** High-power view of a solid adenoid cystic carcinoma showing increased pleomorphism and mitotic figures.

◆ Tumor cells are small, pale to clear, and round to oval with angulated, hyperchromatic nuclei, small nucleoli, N/C ratio of 1:1
— Tubular pattern
  ◆ Found in 20% to 30% of cases
  ◆ Tubules lined by cuboidal epithelial cells
— Solid or basaloid pattern
  ◆ Least frequent, 10% to 15% of cases
  ◆ Solid proliferation of monotonous basaloid cells
  ◆ May show necrosis and high-grade malignant cellular features
  ◆ Focal areas, cribriform or tubular patterns must be present
- Stroma is eosinophilic, hyalinized, or collagenous
- Propensity for perineural invasion is found in greater than 50% of cases

Special Stains and Immunohistochemistry

- Noncontributory

Other Techniques for Diagnosis

- Cytogenetics: may have chromosome structural or balanced translocation involving 6q regions
- *C-kit* is expressed in a subset of adenoid cystic carcinomas

Differential Diagnosis

▌ Polymorphous low-grade adenocarcinoma (PLGA)
- Occurs mainly in minor salivary glands
- Wide variety of architectural patterns, but cribriform architecture is typically not prominent
- Perineural invasion is common
▌ Basaloid SCC (solid type)
- Predilection for hypopharynx, base of tongue, and larynx
- Small hyperchromatic cells in lobules and cords
- Squamous component (dysplasia or carcinoma) in mucosal epithelium
▌ Epithelial-myoepithelial carcinoma
- No cribriform pattern
- Both tumors may produce basal lumina and have hyalinized stroma
- Composed of bicellular ductal proliferation
- Outer cell is prominent with clear cytoplasm; inner cell is ductal cells

Pearls

- Characterized by a lengthy clinical course with multiple recurrences and late metastasis
- Adenoid cystic carcinomas with tubular or cribriform growth patterns have better prognosis than solid tumors
- Unlike most other salivary gland carcinomas, distant metastases are far more common than regional lymph node metastases (usually metastasizes by hematogenous route)

- Lung is the most common site for metastases; may remain stable for many years
- Overall has 35% to 60% 5-year survival rate
- Surgical resection with or without radiation is typical treatment; neck dissection if clinically positive

Selected References

Edwards PC, Bhuiya T, Kelsch RD: C-kit expression in the salivary gland neoplasms adenoid cystic carcinoma, polymorphous low-grade adenocarcinoma, and monomorphic adenoma. Oral Surg Oral Med Oral Pathol Oral Radiol Endodontol 95:586-593, 2003.

Stallmach I, Zenklusen P, Komminoth P, et al: Loss of heterozygosity at chromosome 6q23-25 correlates with clinical and histologic parameters in salivary gland adenoid cystic carcinoma. Virchows Arch 440:77-84, 2002.

Martins C, Fonseca I, Roque L, et al: Cytogenetic similarities between two types of salivary gland carcinomas: Adenoid cystic carcinoma and polymorphous low-grade adenocarcinoma. Cancer Genet Cytogenet 128:130-136, 2001.

Chau Y, Hongyo T, Aozasa K, Chan JK: Dedifferentiation of adenoid cystic carcinoma: Report of a case implicating p53 gene mutation. Hum Pathol 32:1403-1407, 2001.

Cheuk W, Chan JK, Ngan RK: Dedifferentiation in adenoid cystic carcinoma of salivary gland: An uncommon complication associated with an accelerated clinical course. Am J Surg Pathol 23:465-472, 1999.

Acinic Cell Carcinoma

Clinical Features

- Constitutes about 2% of all salivary gland tumors and 10% to 15% of malignant tumors
- Up to 90% occur in parotid gland; remainder are found in submandibular and minor salivary glands
- Peak incidence is in fourth and fifth decades; more common in women
- Presents as slow-growing, solitary, mobile mass; may occasionally be painful or fixed to adjacent muscle or skin

Gross Pathology

- Usually single, well-circumscribed nodule; occasionally multiple or bilateral
- Typically 1 to 3 cm
- Cut surface is gray to maroon with lobular and solid-cystic features

Histopathology

- Malignant neoplasm in which neoplastic cells demonstrate acinar differentiation
- Four growth patterns: solid, microcystic, papillary-cystic, and follicular; often have mixed pattern; solid and microcystic are most common and often are intermixed
- Cells may show acinar, intercalated duct, vacuolated, and clear features

Figure 3-35. Acinic cell carcinoma. A, Low-power view shows a basophilic, granular neoplasm with solid growth involving the parotid. **B,** Prominent cystic growth pattern is present with macrocysts and microcysts composed of granular basophilic tumor cells.

- Classic acinic cell carcinoma shows sheets of large, polygonal cells with uniform, round, eccentric nuclei and coarsely granular to vacuolated cytoplasm
- Usually minimal cytologic atypia in all cellular and architectural patterns; mitotic rate is variable
- Most tumors have infiltrative margins (may only be identified at microscopic level)
- Stroma is sparse, may contain marked lymphoid reaction with germinal centers

Special Stains and Immunohistochemistry

- PAS highlights cytoplasmic granularity (diastase resistant)

Other Techniques for Diagnosis

- Noncontributory

Differential Diagnosis

▮ Papillary cystadenocarcinoma of salivary gland
  - Uncommon tumors
  - Presence of mucous cells (mucicarmine positive) favors cystadenocarcinoma
  - Usually does not show microcystic pattern and lacks serous acinar differentiation
▮ Mucoepidermoid carcinoma
  - Lacks serous acinar cell differentiation
  - Clear cell and oncocytic types
▮ Metastatic granular renal carcinoma
  - Lacks serous acinar cell differentiation
  - History of renal cell carcinoma

Pearls

- Difficult to predict biologic behavior based on histology alone
- Aggressive behavior associated with solid pattern, necrosis, large size, hyalinization of stroma, infiltrative borders, high mitotic rate, and cellular atypia; favorable findings include encapsulation and lack of intratumoral vascular permeation
- About 20% of tumors recur locally; may metastasize to regional lymph nodes
- Tumors arising in the minor salivary glands and those with lymphocyte-rich stroma are associated with a favorable clinical outcome
- Papillary-cystic architecture is associated with an aggressive course
- FNA biopsy findings should be distinguished from normal salivary gland acini, which will contain fat and ductal epithelium

Selected References

Hoffman HT, Karnell LH, Robinson RA, et al: National Cancer Data Base report on cancer of the head and neck: Acinic cell carcinoma. Head Neck 21:297-309, 1999.

El-Naggar AK, Abdul-Karim FW, Hurr K, et al: Genetic alterations in acinic cell carcinoma of the parotid gland determined by microsatellite analysis. Cancer Genet Cytogenet 102:19-24, 1998.

Jin C, Jin Y, Hoglund M, et al: Cytogenetic and molecular genetic demonstration of polyclonality in an acinic cell carcinoma. Br J Cancer 78:292-295, 1998.

Laskawi R, Rodel R, Zirk A, Arglebe C: Retrospective analysis of 35 patients with acinic cell carcinoma of the parotid gland. J Oral Maxillofac Surg 56:440-443, 1998.

Ellis GL, Corio RL: Acinic cell adenocarcinoma: A clinicopathologic analysis of 294 cases. Cancer 52:542-549, 1983.

Polymorphous Low-Grade Adenocarcinoma

Clinical Features

- Also called *terminal duct carcinoma* (histogenetic origin)

Figure 3-36. Polymorphous low-grade adenocarcinoma. Histologic section shows a tumor composed of monomorphous tumor cells growing in sheets and nests.

- Occurs predominantly in the intraoral minor salivary glands, especially at the junction of the hard and soft palates
- May occur in the parotid gland
- Wide age range; peaks in fifth and sixth decades
- Female predominance (2:1)
- Frequently presents as a firm, nontender swelling; can erode underlying bone

Gross Pathology

- Polypoid tumor usually with intact mucosal covering; rarely ulcerated
- Circumscribed, unencapsulated, firm mass with tan, homogeneous cut surface
- Typically ranges from 1 to 5 cm

Histopathology

- Well circumscribed, but lacks a capsule and shows peripheral infiltration into surrounding tissue (often infiltrates in single-file pattern)
- Patterns include solid, tubular, trabecular, and ductular (cribriform, cystic, and papillary-cystic may be focally seen); mixed patterns account for the polymorphous appearance
- May show a single-file pattern, narrow ductlike structures; may display a characteristic concentric whirling pattern at the periphery
- Composed of uniform, cytologically bland, cuboidal to columnar to spindle-shaped cells with round to ovoid nuclei and inconspicuous to obvious nucleoli; scant, eosinophilic to clear cytoplasm and indistinct cell borders
- Nuclear clearing that may mimic papillary thyroid carcinoma

- Variable collagenous or hyaline stroma; tyrosine crystals rarely seen
- Mitotic figures and necrosis are rare
- Infiltrative growth pattern; may invade adjacent bone
- Propensity for perineural invasion, vascular invasion is less frequent
- Wide surgical resection is treatment of choice; resection of adjacent bone necessary if bony infiltration is present

Special Stains and Immunohistochemistry

- S-100 often positive

Other Techniques for Diagnosis

- Noncontributory

Differential Diagnosis

- Adenoid cystic carcinoma
  - Occurs mostly in parotid, whereas PLGA occurs mostly in minor salivary glands
  - Characteristic cribriform architecture with nuclei that are hyperchromatic and angulated
- Monomorphic adenoma
  - Well circumscribed without invasion into surrounding tissue
  - Monomorphous architectural pattern
  - No perineural invasion

Pearls

- Most occur in minor salivary glands
- Recognition aided by combination of architectural features and bland cytology
- Mixed growth patterns lead to polymorphous appearance
- Although termed *low grade*, perineural invasion is common and may lead to local recurrences

Selected References

Simpson RH, Pereira EM, Ribeiro AC, et al: Polymorphous low-grade adenocarcinoma of the salivary glands with transformation to high-grade carcinoma. Histopathology 41:250-259, 2002.

Perez-Ordonez B, Linkov I, Huvos AG: Polymorphous low-grade adenocarcinoma of minor salivary glands: A study of 17 cases with emphasis on cell differentiation. Histopathology 32:521-529, 1998.

Kemp BL, Batsakis JG, El-Naggar AK, et al: Terminal duct adenocarcinomas of the parotid gland. J Laryngol Otol 109:466-468, 1995.

Anderson C, Krutchkoff D, Pederson C, et al: Polymorphous low grade carcinoma of minor salivary gland: A clinicopathologic and comparative immunohistochemical study. Mod Pathol 3:76-82, 1990.

Evans HL, Batsakis JG: Polymorphous low-grade adenocarcinoma of minor salivary glands: A study of 14 cases of a distinctive neoplasm. Cancer 53:935-942, 1984.

Mucoepidermoid Carcinoma

Clinical Features

- Constitutes about 5% of all salivary gland tumors; most common malignant tumor of the salivary glands
- Most arise in parotid gland (about 60% of cases); remainder in minor salivary glands
- Slightly more common in women; peak age is in fifth decade
- Wide age distribution, most common malignant salivary gland tumor in children
- Typically presents as solitary, painless mass; variable involvement of facial nerve depending on tumor grade
- Increased risk after exposure to radiation
- May be associated with Warthin tumor

Gross Pathology

- Partially encapsulated and sometimes circumscribed tumors with lobulated, firm, gray-tan cut surface
- On cut sectioning, tumor is variably solid and cystic, with cysts containing viscid mucoid material
- Average size 2 to 5 cm

Histopathology

- Composed of varying proportions of mucous, epidermoid, and intermediate-type cells
  - Mucous cells
    - Neoplastic cells that are columnar and have foamy cytoplasm; may resemble goblet cells or clear cells
    - Found in clusters or interspersed around the epidermoid or intermediate cells
    - Typically line cystic spaces
    - Usually a minor component of the tumor
    - May need mucin stain to identify this component
  - Epidermoid cells
    - Found in clusters; may form a partial lining of the cystic areas

Figure 3-37. Mucoepidermoid carcinoma. A, Gross photograph of a solid, ill-defined mass corresponding to an intermediate-grade tumor. **B,** Low-grade mucoepidermoid carcinoma consisting of prominent mucinous cells surrounding cystic spaces. High-power view (*inset*) shows mucin cells and underlying intermediate cells. **C,** Characteristic features include smaller, basaloid intermediate cells, larger eosinophilic epithelioid cells (central in nests), scattered mucous cells, and cystic spaces. **D,** High-power view showing intermediate, epithelioid, and clear cell changes.

— Intermediate-type cells
  ◆ Most common cell type
  ◆ Variably sized cells ranging from basaloid cells up to larger cells with more abundant cytoplasm
  ◆ Often form islands or grow in sheets
● May also have clear cells, which are usually a minor component; clear cytoplasm is due mainly to glycogen and less often to mucin
● Architecture is cystic or papillary cystic with lumens filled with mucin; often have pools of extravasated mucin in surrounding tissue
● Grading
  — Grade 1 (low): largely cystic with focal cellular proliferation
  — Grade 2 (intermediate): focal cystic areas with intervening cellular proliferation and invasive features
  — Grade 3 (high): solid cellular proliferation with high-grade cellular features
● In general, higher-grade tumors have few cystic spaces and more solid areas, whereas lower-grade tumors are predominantly cystic

Special Stains and Immunohistochemistry

● Mucicarmine: mucous cells are positive
● IHC is noncontributory
● Translocation of (11;19) and resultant fusion gene transcript, *CTRC1/MAML2*

Other Techniques for Diagnosis

● Noncontributory

Differential Diagnosis

▌ Sialometaplasia (from low-grade mucoepidermoid carcinoma)
  ● Reactive condition often secondary to nonspecific inflammation
  ● Proliferation of squamous cells with occasional mucous cells; squamous metaplasia often seen following FNA
  ● Squamous nests are admixed with ductal epithelium
  ● No intermediate-type cells or cystic areas
  ● Squamous carcinoma with clear or dyskeratotic features
▌ Cystadenocarcinoma
  ● Cystic or papillary-cystic architecture
  ● Lacks infiltrative growth pattern
  ● Cysts lined by columnar or cuboidal, monomorphic cells (less variation in cell types)

Pearls

● Prognosis depends on clinical stage and tumor grade
● May rarely be associated with other benign salivary gland tumors (Warthin tumor)
● Local recurrence is common if not completely excised

● Low-grade tumors rarely metastasize; high-grade tumors may metastasize to lung, bone, and brain
● Treatment is typically wide excision with free margins

Selected References

Guzzo M, Andreola S, Sirizzotti G, Cantu G: Mucoepidermoid carcinoma of the salivary glands: Clinicopathologic review of 108 patients treated at the National Cancer Institute of Milan. Ann Surg Oncol 9:688-695, 2002.

Brandwein MS, Ivanov K, Wallace DI, et al: Mucoepidermoid carcinoma: A clinicopathologic study of 80 patients with special reference to histological grading. Am J Surg Pathol 25:835-845, 2001.

Gibbons MD, Manne U, Carroll WR, et al: Molecular differences in mucoepidermoid carcinoma and adenoid cystic carcinoma of the major salivary glands. Laryngoscope 111:1373-1378, 2001.

Auclair PL, Goode RK, Ellis GL: Mucoepidermoid carcinoma of the salivary glands: Evaluation and application of grading criteria in 143 cases. Cancer 69:2021-2030, 1992.

Epithelial-Myoepithelial Carcinoma

Clinical Features

● Rare low-grade malignant tumor
● Constitutes less than 1% of salivary gland tumors
● Most common in major salivary glands, particularly parotid gland
● Peak incidence is in sixth decade; slight female predominance
● Patients typically present with a localized, painful swelling

Gross Pathology

● Typically well circumscribed and multilobular
● Firm, solid, gray-white cut surface
● Occasionally hemorrhage and necrosis are seen
● Typically 2 to 3 cm
● Recurrent tumors often have irregular borders

Histopathology

● Biphasic tumors composed of myoepithelial cells and minor component of ductal cells
  — Myoepithelial cells
    ◆ Relatively large, polygonal to spindle-shaped cells with clear cytoplasm and eccentrically located nuclei
    ◆ Located peripherally and surround the ductal cells
  — Ductal cells
    ◆ Smaller, uniform cuboidal cells with eosinophilic cytoplasm and round nuclei
    ◆ Form the lining of small ducts that contain eosinophilic proteinaceous material
● Cytologic atypia is usually mild; ductal cells are uniform; variable atypia in myoepithelial cells may be seen

Figure 3-38. Epithelial-myoepithelial carcinoma. A, Gross photograph of a large, white-tan mass with focal hemorrhage replacing the parotid. **B,** Histologic section shows nests of ductlike structures (central in nests and more basophilic) surrounded by myoepithelial cells with pale to clear cytoplasm.

- May have clear myoepithelial cells arranged in an organoid pattern, in sheets or in nests; in these cases, ductal cells may be inconspicuous
- Stroma varies from loose and myxoid to collagenous and hyalinized; occasionally, hyaline basement membrane–like material surrounds tumor nests
- Often have distinct fibrous bands of stroma surrounding tumor lobules
- Variably sized cystic spaces are frequently present
- Occasionally has infiltrative growth pattern or perineural invasion

Special Stains and Immunohistochemistry

- Not essential for diagnosis
- Cytokeratin: ductal cells are positive; myoepithelial cells may be positive
- S-100 protein and smooth muscle actin (SMA): myoepithelial cells are positive; ductal cells are negative
- Calponin and p63: myoepithelial cells are positive

Other Techniques for Diagnosis

- Noncontributory

Differential Diagnosis

- ▌ Benign mixed tumor (pleomorphic adenoma)
  - Mesenchymal element (not just myxoid areas)
  - Well circumscribed, noninvasive
- ▌ Myoepithelial carcinoma
  - Most arise in parotid
  - Unencapsulated, multinodular, invasive
  - Cytologically often bland with morphologic cellular variability (spindled, stellate, epithelioid, plasmacytoid)
  - Duct formation is not a component of this tumor
- ▌ Adenoid cystic carcinoma
  - Characteristic ductal and small cribriform architecture
  - Ductal cells often inconspicuous and smaller with more hyperchromatic, angulated nuclei
  - More commonly has infiltrative growth pattern and perineural invasion
- ▌ PLGA
  - Occurs mainly in minor salivary glands
  - Composed of a uniform population of bland-appearing cells
  - Infiltrative growth, often in single-file pattern
  - Myoepithelial component is usually not prominent

Pearls

- Low-grade malignant neoplasm with recurrence rate of about 30%; recurrences may develop many years after initial diagnosis
- May metastasize to regional lymph nodes and occasionally to distant organs; rarely results in death
- No correlation has been established between histology and prognosis

Selected References

Seethala RR, Barnes EL, Hunt JL: Epithelial-myoepithelial carcinoma: A review of the clinicopathologic spectrum and immunophenotypic characteristics in 61 tumors of the salivary glands and upper aerodigestive tract. Am J Surg Pathol 31:44-57, 2007.

Miliauskas JR, Orell SR: Fine-needle aspiration cytological findings in five cases of epithelial-myoepithelial carcinoma of salivary glands. Diagn Cytopathol 28:163-167, 2003.

Lee HM, Kim AR, Lee SH: Epithelial-myoepithelial carcinoma of the nasal cavity. Eur Arch Otorhinolaryngol 257:376-378, 2000.

Batsakis JG, el-Naggar AK, Luna MA: Epithelial-myoepithelial carcinoma of salivary glands. Ann Otol Rhinol Laryngol 101:540-542, 1992.

Simpson RH, Clarke T, Sarsfield PT, Gluckman PG: Epithelial-myoepithelial carcinoma of salivary glands. J Clin Pathol 44:419-423, 1991.

Salivary Duct Carcinoma

Clinical Features

- High-grade ductal carcinoma morphologically resembling breast adenocarcinoma
- About 9% of malignant salivary tumors; more than 90% of cases in major glands
- Wide age distribution (22-91 years), peak in sixth to seventh decades
- Male predominance
- Presents as a rapidly enlarging mass; may ulcerate and cause facial nerve dysfunction
- May arise in long-standing stable lesion with rapid growth (carcinoma ex pleomorphic adenoma)

Gross Pathology

- Solid, white-gray with necrosis; hemorrhage is common

Histopathology

- Glandular or ductal structures with infiltrative growth pattern characteristically seen; variety of other patterns, including solid areas, cords, nests, or small cystic spaces
- Large ducts with "Roman bridges" and comedo necrosis
- Often oncocytic cytoplasm
- Perineural and perivascular invasion common
- Lymph node metastases also common

Special Stains and Immunohistochemistry

- Most express androgen receptor
- *EGFR* expression in half of cases

Figure 3-39. Salivary duct carcinoma. High-grade eosinophilic cells with prominent nucleoli forming glands and nests with comedo necrosis.

- *HER-2* overexpression (secondary to amplification) in a subset

Other Techniques for Diagnosis

- Noncontributory

Differential Diagnosis

▌ SCC
- Poorly differentiated from skin or metastasis; morphologically may overlap
- Keratinization if present is helpful
- Acantholysis may mimic duct formation

▌ Adenocarcinoma, NOS
- A diagnosis of exclusion; tumors must lack morphologic criteria of a more specific salivary gland carcinoma before this diagnosis is made
- Low-grade tumors have minimal pleomorphism and low mitotic rate

▌ Metastatic adenocarcinoma
- Medical history and clinical evaluation provide important data

Pearls

- Salivary duct carcinoma is a high-grade carcinoma with a poor prognosis
- Local recurrence, regional and distant metastases are common
- Rarely may express breast and prostate immunohistochemical markers; clinical history is important to differentiate from metastases

Selected References

Williams MD, Roberts D, Blumenschein GR Jr, et al: Differential expression of hormonal and growth factor receptors in salivary duct carcinomas: Biologic significance and potential role in therapeutic stratification of patients. Am J Surg Pathol 31:1645-1652, 2007.

Jaehne M, Roeser K, Jaekel T, et al: Clinical and immunohistologic typing of salivary duct carcinoma: A report of 50 cases. Cancer 103:2526-2533, 2005.

Valeri RM, Hadjileontis C, Skordalaki A, et al: Salivary duct carcinoma of the parotid gland: Report of a rare case with a comparative study of aspiration cytology and histomorphology. Acta Cytolog 49:61-64, 2005.

Dagrada GP, Negri T, Tamborini E, et al: Expression of HER-2/neu gene and protein in salivary duct carcinomas of parotid gland as revealed by fluorescence in-situ hybridization and immunohistochemistry. Histopathology 44:301-302, 2004.

Nasser SM, Faquin WC, Dayal Y: Expression of androgen, estrogen, and progesterone receptors in salivary gland tumors: Frequent expression of androgen receptor in a subset of malignant salivary gland tumors. Am J Clin Pathol 119:801-806, 2003.

Skalova A, Starek, Kucerova V, et al: Salivary duct carcinoma—a highly aggressive salivary gland tumor with HER-2/neu oncoprotein over-expression. Pathol Res Pract 197:621-626, 2001.

Carcinoma Ex Mixed Tumor (Carcinoma Ex Pleomorphic Adenoma)

Clinical Features

- Malignant transformation of benign mixed tumor occurs in less than 10%
- Most common in the parotid gland (>75% of cases)
- Rare in patients younger than 30 years; more common in women
- Many patients have a long-standing or recurrent parotid mass with recent, rapid growth; typically painless

Gross Pathology

- Poorly circumscribed and often with infiltrative margins
- Cut section is tan-gray with hemorrhage, necrosis, and cystic degeneration
- Variable size

Histopathology

- Diagnosis requires presence of benign mixed tumor areas (either concomitantly or as recurrence from previously excised tumor) in addition to malignant carcinomatous component
- Epithelial component is malignant; most commonly classified as adenocarcinoma NOS and salivary duct carcinoma (e.g., undifferentiated carcinoma, polymorphous low-grade adenocarcinoma, epithelial myoepithelial carcinoma)
- Malignant component often infiltrates capsule and extends into adjacent soft tissue; tumor may be localized without capsular involvement (designated as encapsulated, in situ, or noninvasive carcinoma ex mixed tumor)

- High-grade cellular features; perineural and vascular invasion often seen
- Necrosis and hemorrhage are common but seen more frequently in high-grade tumors

Special Stains and Immunohistochemistry

- Depends on the type of salivary gland carcinoma present; see under specific entities

Other Techniques for Diagnosis

- Noncontributory

Differential Diagnosis

- Salivary duct carcinoma
  - History and thorough sampling of the tumor will identify benign mixed tumor component
- Carcinosarcoma
  - Both epithelial and heterologous mesenchymal malignant components

Pearls

- Local recurrence indicates poorer prognosis and is commonly seen before distant metastases (lung, bone, brain, liver)
- In cases of encapsulated, in situ, or noninvasive carcinoma ex mixed tumor, the prognosis of completely excised tumors equals that of benign mixed tumors

Selected References

Felix A, Rosa-Santos J, Mendonca ME, et al: Intracapsular carcinoma ex pleomorphic adenoma: Report of a case with unusual metastatic behaviour. Oral Oncol 38:107-110, 2002.

Lewis JE, Olsen KD, Sebo TJ: Carcinoma ex pleomorphic adenoma: Pathologic analysis of 73 cases. Hum Pathol 32:596-604, 2001.

El-Naggar AK, Callender D, Coombes MM, et al: Molecular genetic alterations in carcinoma ex-pleomorphic adenoma: A putative progression model? Genes Chromosomes Cancer 27:162-168, 2000.

Duck SW, McConnel FM: Malignant degeneration of pleomorphic adenoma—clinical implications. Am J Otolaryngol 14:175-178, 1993.

LiVolsi VA, Perzin KH: Malignant mixed tumors arising in salivary glands. I. Carcinomas in benign mixed tumors. A clinicopathologic study. Cancer 39:2209-2230, 1977.

Carcinosarcoma

General Features

- Rare
- True malignant mixed tumor with both carcinomatous and sarcomatous components
- Most arise in parotid gland
- Most patients are older than 50 years
- Patients usually present with relatively rapid growth of a parotid mass with pain, facial nerve paralysis, and skin ulceration

Figure 3-40. Carcinoma ex mixed tumor. Low-power view shows a biphasic tumor with a mixed tumor on the left with chondroid matrix and a carcinoma on the right. High-grade ductal carcinoma with eosinophilic cytoplasm and glandular spaces (*inset*).

Figure 3-41. Carcinosarcoma. High-power view shows a neoplasm composed of pleomorphic epithelial cells and malignant mesenchymal elements (osteoid differentiation).

Gross Pathology

- Often large; usually greater than 3 cm
- Unencapsulated with a solid, gray-tan cut surface
- Often have areas of necrosis, hemorrhage, and calcification

Histopathology

- Composed of carcinomatous and sarcomatous components; sarcomatous component usually predominates and usually consists of chondrosarcoma; osteosarcoma, fibrosarcoma, malignant fibrous histiocytoma (MFH), and liposarcoma have been reported
- Carcinomatous component is most commonly high-grade ductal adenocarcinoma, but squamous cell carcinoma, undifferentiated carcinoma, and other salivary gland carcinomas have been reported
- Sarcomatous and carcinomatous components are usually intermixed but may be distinctly separate

Special Stains and Immunohistochemistry

- Carcinomatous component positive for cytokeratin, EMA, and often S-100 protein

Other Techniques for Diagnosis

- Noncontributory

Differential Diagnosis

▋ Sarcomatoid carcinoma (spindle cell carcinoma)
- Presence of cytokeratin in both components would favor this classification
- Spindled and epithelial components are carcinoma (derived from epithelium)

▋ Sarcoma of the salivary glands
- Chondrosarcoma is more likely a component of a carcinosarcoma than a pure chondrosarcoma

- Lack distinct carcinomatous component
- Typically negative for cytokeratin

▋ Synovial sarcoma
- Rare tumor of salivary glands
- Biphasic tumor composed of fascicles of uniform spindle cells admixed with epithelioid cells, often showing focal glandular architecture
- Less cytologic atypia
- Immunostains are typically not helpful because both tumors show variable positivity for cytokeratin and vimentin

Pearls

- Metastases and recurrences may consist of both carcinomatous and sarcomatous components and only sarcomatous component
- High-grade, aggressive neoplasm with predilection for hematogenous spread rather than spread by lymphatics
- Most common metastatic site is the lung

Selected References

Kwon MY, Gu M: True malignant mixed tumor (carcinosarcoma) of parotid gland with unusual mesenchymal component: A case report and review of the literature. Arch Pathol Lab Med 125:812-815, 2001.

Bleiweiss IJ, Huvos AG, Lara J, Strong EW: Carcinosarcoma of the submandibular gland. Immunohistochemical findings. Cancer 69:2031-2035, 1992.

Toynton SC, Wilkins MJ, Cook HT, Stafford ND: True malignant mixed tumor of a minor salivary gland. J Laryngol Otol 108:76-79, 1994.

Undifferentiated Neuroendocrine (Small Cell) Carcinoma

Clinical Features

- Rare tumor (<1% of all salivary gland tumors)
- May involve areas in the head and neck, including the salivary glands, nasal cavity, hypopharynx, larynx, and trachea
- Within the salivary glands, most common in the parotid
- Peak incidence in fifth to seventh decades; much more common in males
- Presents as a rapidly growing, painless mass; patients often have enlarged cervical lymph nodes at the time of presentation

Gross Pathology

- Poorly circumscribed with infiltrative margins
- Often multilobulated with a solid, gray-tan cut surface

Histopathology

- Infiltrative growth pattern with extension into adjacent salivary gland and soft tissue
- Solid sheets, nests, or cords of small, hyperchromatic, uniform cells with inconspicuous to small nucleoli

Figure 3-42. Undifferentiated neuroendocrine carcinoma. High-power view of poorly defined tumor cells with scant cytoplasm and variable nuclear chromatin.

and finely granular chromatin; nuclear molding and marked crush artifact is typical
- High mitotic rate and frequent tumor necrosis
- Nests or sheets of tumors cells surrounded by hyalinized, fibrous stroma
- Some tumors demonstrate focal ductal differentiation or have partially formed glandular spaces
- Vascular invasion often present

Special Stains and Immunohistochemistry
- Cytokeratin positive (characteristic perinuclear staining pattern)
- Synaptophysin, chromogranin, and neuron-specific enolase (NSE) positive
- Vimentin occasionally positive
- S-100 protein and HMB-45 negative

Other Techniques for Diagnosis
- Noncontributory

Differential Diagnosis
▌ Adenoid cystic carcinoma (solid variant)
  - Solid sheets or nests of small cells with hyperchromatic nuclei and a high mitotic rate
  - Lacks nuclear molding
  - Negative for synaptophysin, chromogranin, and NSE
▌ Non-Hodgkin lymphoma
  - More solid growth pattern; does not form nests or cords
  - Often infiltrate around normal salivary gland ducts and acini
  - Positive for LCA
  - Negative for cytokeratin
▌ Metastatic neuroendocrine carcinoma
  - History is important

- Small cell carcinoma of the lung usually TTF-1 positive (not specific)
- Merkel cell carcinoma may metastasize to periparotid lymph node. CK20 positive, dot-like; TTF-1 negative

Pearls
- High-grade malignant neoplasm
- Overall, better prognosis than in patients with small cell carcinomas of the lung
- Less than 50% 5-year survival rate
- Primary treatment is surgical excision followed by radiation or chemotherapy; neck dissection is often performed, especially with clinically positive lymph nodes

Selected References

Nagao T: Small cell carcinoma. In Barnes L, Eveson JW, Reichart P, Sidransky D (eds): World Health Organization Classification of Tumours: Pathology and Genetics: Head and Neck Tumours. Lyon, IARC Press, 2005, pp 247-248.

Cameron WR, Johansson L, Tennvall J: Small cell carcinoma of the parotid: Fine needle aspiration and immunohistochemical findings in a case. Acta Cytolog 34:837-841, 1990.

Gnepp DR, Wick MR: Small cell carcinoma of the major salivary glands: An immunohistochemical study. Cancer 66:185-192, 1990.

Lymphoepithelial Carcinoma

Clinical Features
- Also called *malignant lymphoepithelial lesion* or *undifferentiated carcinoma with lymphoid stroma*
- Rare tumor, making up less than 1% of salivary tumors
- Marked predilection for Eskimos and Arctic inhabitants and Inuits
- Wide age range with a slight female predominance
- Most occur in the parotid gland (>75% of cases)
- May occur in association with or subsequent to a benign lymphoepithelial lesion
- Like nasopharyngeal lymphoepithelial carcinoma, this is also associated with EBV
- Usually presents as a painful mass; patients may have facial nerve paralysis
- Frequently have positive cervical lymph nodes at presentation

Gross Pathology
- Infiltrative margins with involvement of adjacent salivary gland and soft tissue
- Lobulated and firm with a solid, tan cut surface

Histopathology
- Undifferentiated carcinoma associated with abundant lymphoid stroma and often germinal centers

Figure 3-43. Lymphoepithelial carcinoma. High-power view shows a poorly differentiated carcinoma (larger cells, *top half*) surrounded by small uniform lymphoid elements.

— Epithelial component
  ◆ Irregular nests of malignant epithelial cells that are round to polygonal to slightly spindle shaped and have large, atypical, vesicular nuclei, one to many prominent nucleoli, eosinophilic cytoplasm, and indistinct cell borders
  ◆ Epithelial component may consist of small nests, syncytial aggregates, cords, or trabeculae or appear as isolated cells
  ◆ Usually high but variable mitotic rate
— Lymphoid component
  ◆ Surrounding lymphoid stroma is often dense and consists of uniform small lymphocytes admixed with plasma cells and histiocytes
  ◆ Typically have well-formed germinal centers
• Occasional benign epimyoepithelial islands with associated lymphoid stroma admixed with the malignant component
• Marked histologic similarity between salivary gland and nasopharyngeal lymphoepithelial carcinoma

Special Stains and Immunohistochemistry

• Cytokeratin: epithelial cells are positive
• LCA: highlights lymphoid component

Other Techniques for Diagnosis

• EBV genomes can be detected by in situ hybridization in malignant epithelial cells; elevated titers of serum immunoglobulin A (IgA) against EBV capsid antigen or IgG against EBV nuclear antigen

Differential Diagnosis

❚ Metastatic amelanotic melanoma
  • Typically lacks dense lymphoid stroma and germinal centers

  • S-100 protein and HMB-45 positive
  • Cytokeratin negative
❚ Large cell lymphoma
  • Lymphocytic markers positive
❚ Benign lymphoepithelial lesion
  • Well-defined mass without infiltration into adjacent tissue
  • Epithelial component is composed of benign cells with a low mitotic rate
  • Similar-appearing lymphoid component
❚ Large cell undifferentiated carcinoma
  • Malignant component of lymphoepithelial carcinoma has cytologic features similar to those of large cell undifferentiated carcinoma
  • Lacks lymphoid stroma
❚ Metastatic nasopharyngeal lymphoepithelial carcinoma
  • Cannot be reliably distinguished based on histology, IHC, and electron microscopy
  • Careful clinical history and examination are essential
  • Parotid is an uncommon site for metastasis of nasopharyngeal lymphoepithelial carcinoma

Pearls

• Considered an undifferentiated carcinoma but has an overall better prognosis than large cell undifferentiated carcinoma
• Factors indicating a poor prognosis are high mitotic rate, anaplasia, and necrosis
• Most important prognostic factor is clinical stage
• Treatment is typically surgical excision combined with radiation therapy

Selected References

Bialas M, Sinczak A, Choinska-Stefanska A, Zygulska A: EBV-positive lymphoepithelial carcinoma of salivary gland in a woman of a non-endemic area: A case report. Pol J Pathol 53:235-238, 2002.

Leung SY, Chung LP, Yuen ST, et al: Lymphoepithelial carcinoma of the salivary gland: In situ detection of Epstein-Barr virus. J Clin Pathol 48:1022-1027, 1995.

Albeck H, Nielson NH, Hansen HE: Epidemiology of nasopharyngeal and salivary gland carcinoma in Greenland. Arctic Med Res 51:189-195, 1992.

Hamilton-Dutoit SJ, Therkildsen MH, Nielsen NH, et al: Undifferentiated carcinoma of the salivary gland in Greenlandic Eskimos: Demonstration of Epstein-Barr virus DNA by in situ nucleic acid hybridization. Hum Pathol 22:811-815, 1991.

Nagao K, Matsuzaki O, Saiga H: A histopathologic study of benign and malignant lymphoepithelial lesions of the parotid gland. Cancer 52:1044-1052, 1983.

Lymphoma

Clinical Features

• May be primary or secondary; considered secondary if patient has noncontiguous positivity involving multiple sites

Figure 3-44. Lymphoma, B-cell extranodal marginal zone. Fine-needle aspiration shows discohesive lymphoid cells with an immunophenotype of a MALT lymphoma involving the parotid.

- May be nodal or extranodal because parotid gland contains intraparenchymal lymph nodes
- Common tumor of salivary glands; many studies have shown lymphoma to be the fourth or fifth most common tumor involving this location; typically involves the parotid gland
- Most lymphomas are non-Hodgkin lymphomas; Hodgkin disease involving salivary glands is rare
- Increased risk for developing lymphoma in patients with autoimmune disease, particularly Sjögren syndrome
- Most major salivary gland lymphomas arise de novo
- More common in females, especially those with an autoimmune disease
- In young males with salivary gland lymphoma, HIV infection should be ruled out

Gross Pathology

- Firm, solid mass, with a tan, homogeneous cut surface
- May show infiltrative margins with involvement of surrounding tissue

Histopathology

- Most lymphomas are non-Hodgkin lymphomas of B-cell type
- Dense proliferation of lymphoid cells infiltrates and grows around normal salivary gland ducts and acini, resulting in distortion of the normal salivary gland architecture
- Most common lymphomas include follicular small cleaved, follicular mixed, and diffuse large cell lymphomas
- Tumor often infiltrates surrounding soft tissue

- Plasmacytoid lymphocytes, which are common in chronic lymphocytic lymphoma (CLL), may show Dutcher bodies (intranuclear inclusions consisting of immunoglobulin)
- Prominent crush artifact is common
- MALT-type lymphomas show characteristic epimyoepithelial islands and a mixture of small to medium-sized lymphocytes and monocytoid B cells
- Hodgkin lymphoma usually is confined to intraparenchymal lymph node tissue; most frequent histologic types are nodular sclerosing and lymphocyte predominant
- Salivary gland non-MALT, non-Hodgkin lymphomas have similar prognosis as their nodal counterpart

Special Stains and Immunohistochemistry

- LCA positive (CD45)
- Most salivary gland lymphomas are of B-cell type and thus are positive for pan–B-cell markers
- Cytokeratin: epimyoepithelial islands in MALT lymphomas are positive
- See Chapter 14 for immunohistochemical staining patterns of specific lymphomas

Other Techniques for Diagnosis

- Refer to Chapter 14 for specific diagnostic techniques

Differential Diagnosis

▋ Sialadenitis
- Mixture inflammatory infiltrate consisting of lymphocytes, plasma cells, and occasionally neutrophils
- Germinal center formation sometimes seen
- IHC demonstrates a mixed population of T and B cells; often a predominance of T cells

▋ HIV-associated lymphadenopathy
- Lymphoid infiltrate is often atypical, and florid follicular hyperplasia may be seen; tingible body macrophages in germinal centers typically seen
- Commonly have squamous lined cysts and small epithelial nests within lymphoid proliferation
- Often bilateral
- MALT-type salivary gland lymphomas are low-grade, indolent lymphomas; they can transform to more aggressive large cell lymphomas
- Hodgkin disease is rare in salivary glands but occurs most often in the parotid gland; male predominance with a bimodal age distribution

Pearls

- FNA with morphologic and flow-cytometric analysis for diagnosis
- Lymphomas of the salivary glands may involve intraparotid nodes or the parenchyma
- Higher risk in patients with autoimmune disease (Sjögren syndrome)

Selected References

Chan ACL, Chan JKC, Abbondanzo SL: Haematolymphoid tumours. In Barnes EL, Eveson JW, Reichart P, Sidransky D (eds): World Health Organization Classification of Tumours: Pathology and Genetics: Head and Neck Tumours. Lyon, IARC Press, 2005, pp 277-280.

Masaki Y, Sugai S: Lymphoproliferative disorders in Sjögren's syndrome. Autoimmun Rev 3:175-182, 2004.

Royer B, Cazals-Hatem D, Sibilia J, et al: Lymphomas in patients with Sjögren's syndrome are marginal zone B-cell neoplasms, arise in diverse extranodal sites, and are not associated with viruses. Blood 90:766-767, 1997.

Ioachim HL, Ryan JR, Blaugrund SM: Salivary gland lymph nodes. The site of lymphadenopathies and lymphomas associated with human immunodeficiency virus infection. Arch Pathol Lab Med 112:1224-1228, 1988.

Tumors Metastasizing to the Salivary Glands

Clinical Features

- Most metastases to the salivary glands are found in the intraparotid or submandibular lymph nodes
- May mimic a primary tumor of the salivary gland
- Most common metastatic tumors are SCCs of the head and neck or skin, malignant melanoma, or carcinomas from the lung, kidney, and breast; less commonly from the prostate and gastrointestinal tract

Gross Pathology

- Depends on the primary tumor
- Metastatic malignant melanoma may be pigmented

Histopathology

- Histopathologic features resemble those of the primary tumor

Figure 3-45. Metastasis (melanoma) to parotid. Pigmented nodules corresponding to metastatic melanoma to intraparotid lymph nodes are present on gross examination.

Special Stains and Immunohistochemistry

- A battery of epithelial, melanocytic and neuroendocrine markers

Other Techniques for Diagnosis

- Noncontributory

Differential Diagnosis

- Depends on cell type and growth pattern

Pearls

- History is necessary
- Peculiar features for a primary tumor—think possible metastasis
- SCCs in this region are most often metastases from skin

Selected References

Hrebinko R, Taylor SR, Bahnson RR: Carcinoma of prostate metastatic to parotid gland. Urology 41:272-273, 1993.

Seifert G, Hennings K, Caselitz J: Metastatic tumors to the parotid and submandibular glands: Analysis and differential diagnosis of 108 cases. Pathol Res Pract 181:684-692, 1986.

Paranasal Sinuses and Nasopharynx

- See Tables 3-1 and 3-2

Acute and Chronic Sinusitis

Clinical Features

- Common, occurring in 20% of population
- Purulent and nonpurulent types
- Most commonly involves the maxillary sinus
- Acute may be postviral
- Chronic secondary to fungal or bacterial organisms

Gross Pathology

- Edematous, reddish to gray, soft tissue

Histopathology

- Respiratory mucosa with mixed inflammatory infiltrate, edema, glandular hyperplasia, basement membrane thickening, and squamous metaplasia
- Eosinophils may be present
- Underlying bone may show remodeling and thickening

Special Stains and Immunohistochemistry

- Fungal infection should be excluded by GMS and PAS staining

Other Techniques for Diagnosis

- Noncontributory

Table 3-1.　Immunohistochemical Markers Useful in the Differential Diagnosis of Undifferentiated Sinonasal and Skull-Base Neoplasms

Marker	Olfactory Neuroblastoma	Ewing Sarcoma, PNET	RMS	Lymphoma	NEC	Melanoma
Keratin	−, Focal	−	−, Rare	−	+	Rare
Synaptophysin, chromogranin	+++	+	−	−	+++	Rare
HMB-45	−	−	−	−	++	+++
CD99	−	+++	+/−	−	−	−
Desmin	−	−	+++	−	−	−
Myogenin/myoD1	−	−	+++	−	−	−
S-100	Focal	−	−	−	Focal	++
CD45	−	−	−	+++	−	−

NEC, neuroendocrine carcinoma; PNET, peripheral neuroectodermal tumor; RMS, rhabdomyosarcoma.

Table 3-2.　Clinicopathologic Comparisons of Sinonasal and Nasopharyngeal Spindled Lesions

	Nasopharyngeal Angiofibroma	Hemangiopericytoma	Lobular Capillary Hemangioma	Solitary Fibrous Tumor	Kaposi Sarcoma
Age	15-25 yr	50-60 yr most common	Any age; male teens, 30s women	Broad range, 30-60 yr	Non-HIV elderly, HIV+ in 4th decade
Sex	M	M + F	M + F	M + F	M >> F
Location	Nasopharynx	Sinus, nasal cavity	Septum > other	Any	Skin, mucosa
Symptoms	Epistaxis	Congestion, epistaxis	Congestion, epistaxis	Congestion, epistaxis	Asymptomatic
Histology	Stellate stroma	Spindled, epithelioid proliferation	Lobular growth	Variably cellular, spindled cells, ropey collagen	Spindled cells, extravasated red blood cells
Vasculature	Haphazard vessels	Thin, slitlike, irregular branching vessels	Capillary proliferation	Irregular, branching vessels	Irregular, angulated vessels
IHC	Vessels CD34+, SMA partially around vessels	SMA+	Vessels CD34+	Stromal cells CD34+	CD31+, HHV-8+

F, female; HIV, human immunodeficiency virus; HHV-8, human herpesvirus type 8; IHC, immunohistochemistry; M, male; SMA, smooth muscle actin.

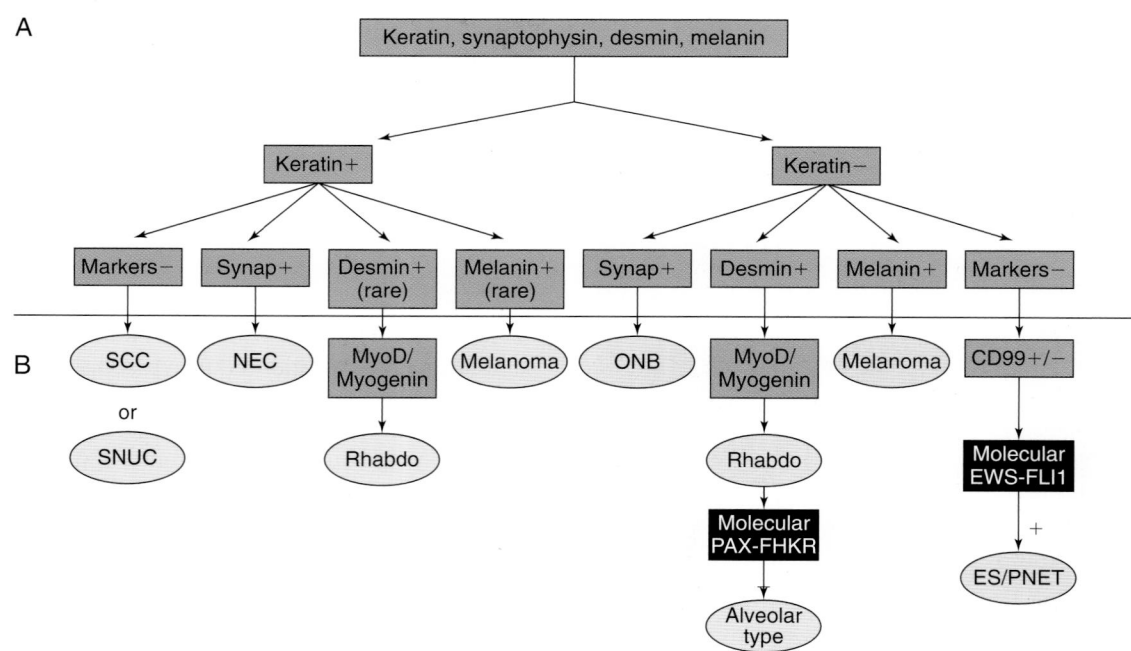

Figure 3-46. Diagnostic algorithm for immunohistochemical evaluation of undifferentiated skull-base tumors. An initial panel (**A**) of keratin, synaptophysin (Synap), desmin, and melanin markers allows for the classification of most neoplasms. Panel **B** includes confirmatory, ancillary markers and molecular studies for rhabdomyosarcoma (Rhabdo), myoD or myogenin, and PAX-FKHR for the alveolar type, and Ewing sarcoma or peripheral neuroectodermal tumor (ES/PNET), CD99, and EWS-FLI1. NEC, neuroendocrine carcinoma; ONB, olfactory neuroblastoma; SCC, squamous cell carcinoma; SNUC, sinonasal undifferentiated carcinoma.

Figure 3-47. A, Chronic sinusitis. A thickened basement layer is present beneath the respiratory epithelium, and chronic inflammation fills the submucosa. **B, Allergic fungal sinusitis.** Thick secretions show layering of mucous and inflammatory cells, a characteristic finding of "tidal waves." **C, Invasive fungal sinusitis.** Marked tissue necrosis and inflammation with fungal hyphae are identified. Gomori methenamine silver stain highlights the fungal wall (*inset*). **D, Rhinoscleroma.** Large vacuolated histocytes (Mikulicz cells) are filled with microorganisms.

Differential Diagnosis

▌ Allergic fungal sinusitis (noninvasive)
- Most common in third to seventh decade; males = females
- Thick, putty-like secretions
- Pools of eosinophilic mucin with abundant eosinophils (layered secretions)
- Charcot-Leyden crystals often present
- Fungal hyphae not associated with tissue (*Aspergillus, Curvularia,* and other species) speciation done by culture

▌ Invasive fungal sinusitis
- Usually associated with diabetes mellitus or immune compromise
- Spreads rapidly; treatment is surgical débridement
- Fungal organisms invade blood vessels and cause thrombosis and necrosis
- Thick, twisted, ribbon-like, nonseptate hyphae (zygomycoses)

▌ Myospherulosis
- Iatrogenically induced by packing the nose with petroleum-based ointments
- Characterized by large spaces (pseudocysts) with brown spherules that represent altered erythrocytes surrounded by a thin membrane

▌ Rhinoscleroma
- Lymphoplasmacytic inflammation with large vacuolated macrophages (Mikulicz cells), may be polypoid
- Caused by *Klebsiella* species; identified on Warthin-Starry stain
- Endemic in Central America, India, and other countries

Pearls

- Complication of chronic sinusitis involving maxillary sinus is mucocele (pseudocyst), which can cause destruction of bone and be clinically mistaken for a malignant process

● Cultures required for speciation if microorganisms are suspected

Selected References

Polzehl D, Moeller P, Riechelmann H, Perner S: Distinct features of chronic rhinosinusitis with and without nasal polyps. Allergy 61:1275-1279, 2006.

Taxy JB: Paranasal fungal sinusitis: Contributions of histopathology to diagnosis. A report of 60 cases and literature review. Am J Surg Pathol 30:713-720, 2006.

Granville L, Chirala M, Cernoch P, et al: Fungal sinusitis: Histologic spectrum and correlation with culture. Hum Pathol 35:474-481, 2004.

Batsakis JG, El-Naggar AK: Rhinoscleroma and rhinosporidiosis. Ann Otol Rhinol Laryngol 101:879-882, 1992.

Nasal Polyp

Clinical Features

● Stromal and epithelial proliferation of uncertain pathogenesis
● Usually bilateral and multiple
● Uncommon under 20 years of age; develops in 10% to 20% of children with cystic fibrosis
● Etiologic factors are inflammation, allergy, and mucoviscidosis (cystic fibrosis)
● May also develop as part of mucopolysaccharidosis (Hurler syndrome)
● Choanal polyps arising from the paranasal sinuses are morphologically similar
● Local recurrence is common

Gross Pathology

● Variably sized, soft, fleshy, gray-pink, polypoid masses
● Cut surface often translucent and edematous
● May fill entire nasal cavity and extend into sinuses

Histopathology

● Loose myxoid stroma and seromucous glands covered by respiratory epithelium with occasional foci of squamous metaplasia
● Thickened basement membrane and submucosal hyalinization
● Mixed acute and chronic inflammatory infiltrate including eosinophils; called *allergic polyp* if eosinophils predominate
● May show a pseudoangiomatous appearance of dilated vascular channels
● May become fibrotic

Special Stains and Immunohistochemistry

● Noncontributory

Other Techniques for Diagnosis

● Noncontributory

Figure 3-48. A, Nasal polyp—inflammatory. Edematous stroma is admixed with inflammatory cells and increased vasculature. **B, Respiratory epithelial adenomatoid hamartoma.** Low-power view shows a polypoid mass with prominent glands within the stroma. At higher power (*inset*), the glands are bilayered and lined by a ciliated epithelium and a surrounding prominent basement membrane.

Differential Diagnosis

▌ Respiratory epithelial adenomatoid hamartoma
 ● Often polypoid mass
 ● Increased glands composed of bland pseudostratified ciliated epithelium surrounded by a thick basement membrane separated by stroma
 ● Glands and ducts often connect to the surface
 ● Rare; males affected more than females, in sixth decade
 ● Differentiate from papillomas and adenocarcinomas
▌ Rhinosporidiosis
 ● Hyperplastic polypoid lesions in nasal cavity
 ● Numerous globular cysts measuring up to 300 μm in diameter containing numerous endospores (2 to 9 μm) of *Rhinosporidium seeberi* highlighted by silver stain, PAS, or mucicarmine
 ● Marked lymphoplasmacytic infiltrate

- Heterotopic glial heterotopia
  - Congenital malformation without connection to the central nervous system
  - Intranasal (30%) or extranasal (60%) manifestations
  - Mature glial elements and fibrosis
  - Astrocytes may show gemistocytic change
  - Encephalocele would connect to the central nervous system and may reveal meninges
- Rhabdomyosarcoma
  - Usually more cellular with small primitive cells
  - Botryoid variant may be polypoid
  - Atypical spindle cells; positive for desmin, myogenin, and MyoD1
- Angiofibroma
  - Almost exclusively found in males aged 10 to 25 years
  - Arise in nasopharynx
  - Haphazardly arranged small, thin-walled blood vessels of varying sizes
  - Stroma frequently collagenous with stellate fibroblasts

Pearls

- Clinical presentation of "polyps" may represent other pathologic diagnoses
- Presence of eosinophils is not restricted to allergic polyps

Selected References

Mortuaire G, Pasquesoone X, Leroy X, Chevalier D: Respiratory epithelial adenomatoid hamartomas of the sinonasal tract. Eur Arch Otorhinolaryngol 264:451-453, 2007.

Garavello W, Gaini RM: Histopathology of routine nasal polypectomy specimens: A review of 2,147 cases. Laryngoscope 115:1866-1868, 2005.

Barnes L: Schneiderian papillomas and nonsalivary glandular neoplasms of the head and neck. Mod Pathol 15:279-297, 2002.

Graeme-Cook F, Pilch BZ: Hamartomas of the nose and nasopharynx. Head Neck 14:321-327, 1992.

Nasopharyngeal Angiofibroma

Clinical Features

- Occurs almost exclusively in young males between the ages of 6 and 29 years (peak, 15 years)
- Arises from fibrovascular stroma in posterolateral wall or roof of the nasopharynx or posterior nasal cavity
- Patients typically present with nasal obstruction and epistaxis
- Locally aggressive, may extend into sinuses or base of skull

Gross Pathology

- Well-circumscribed, unencapsulated, polypoid mass
- Tan-gray and fibrous cut surface may show spongy composition from vasculature

Figure 3-49. Nasopharyngeal angiofibroma. Prominent vessels are surrounded by small, elongated stromal cells in a fibrous background. Embolization material is noted on the *right* with surrounding inflammation.

Histopathology

- Haphazardly arranged blood vessels lined by endothelial cells for various sizes, often thin-walled
- Vessels are various sizes, often slitlike; larger vessels may have incomplete muscular wall
- Stroma varies from loose and edematous to dense, acellular, and collagenous
- May have stellate, spindled, or angulated stromal cells
- Frequent mast cells, rare mitotic activity
- Postembolization inflammation, foreign body giant cells, and foreign material

Special Stains and Immunohistochemistry

- CD31, CD34 positive in endothelial cells lining vascular spaces
- Androgen receptor positive in 75% of cases within endothelial cells
- Stromal cells positive for vimentin; negative for smooth muscle markers and CD34

Other Techniques for Diagnosis

- Noncontributory

Differential Diagnosis

- Lobular capillary hemangioma (pyogenic granuloma)
  - In the respiratory tract, almost always involves the nasal cavity, frequently the septum (60%)
  - Vascular tumor with a lobular arrangement
  - Large central vessel surrounded by tightly packed capillaries
- Hemangiopericytoma (glomangiopericytoma)
  - Rare; has been described in all age groups; slight female predilection
  - Cellular tumor characterized by staghorn-shaped irregular vascular spaces may be hyalinized

Figure 3-50. Hemangiopericytoma. A, Low power shows a marked vascular and spindled proliferation within the submucosa. **B,** High power shows the bland oval to spindled cells and scattered vessels. **C,** Smooth muscle actin immunohistochemical stain is diffusely positive in the spindled cells. **D,** CD34 immunohistochemical stain highlights only the background vessels.

- Spindle, round cells with rare mitotic activity
- Spindle cells positive for SMA and negative for CD34
- Often indolent, without recurrence if completely resected
- Increased mitotic rate and high cytologic atypia associated with aggressive behavior

▌ Solitary fibrous tumor
- Mixture of hyalinized stroma, ropey collagen, spindle cells, and vessels
- Stromal cells are positive for CD34

▌ Kaposi sarcoma
- Typically in immunocompromised patients, most commonly HIV
- Slitlike vascular spaces with extravasated red blood cells and hyaline globules
- Positive for human herpesvirus-8 (HHV-8)

▌ Angiosarcoma
- Rare in nasopharynx
- Characterized by anastomosing, irregularly shaped vascular spaces lined by atypical endothelial cells

- High mitotic rate
- Tumor cells are positive for vascular markers (CD31, CD34, factor VIII-rel antigen)

Pearls
- Clinical correlation is useful regarding age and sex of patient
- As a vascular tumor, presurgical embolization is common, with embolization material frequently seen in resected specimens
- Malignant transformation (rare) is possibly associated with radiation treatment

Selected References

Glad H, Vainer B, Buchwald C, et al: Juvenile nasopharyngeal angiofibromas in Denmark 1981-2003: Diagnosis, incidence, and treatment. Acta Otolaryngol 127:292-299, 2007.

Puxeddu R, Berlucchi M, Ledda GP, et al: Lobular capillary hemangioma of the nasal cavity: A retrospective study on 40 patients. Am J Rhinol 20:480-484, 2006.

Thompson LD, Miettinen M, Wenig BM: Sinonasal-type hemangiopericytoma: A clinicopathologic and immunophenotypic analysis of 104 cases showing perivascular myoid differentiation. Am J Surg Pathol 27:737-749, 2003.

Wyatt ME, Finlayson CJ, Moore-Gillon V: Kaposi's sarcoma masquerading as pyogenic granuloma of the nasal mucosa. J Laryngol Otol 112:280-282, 1998.

Kapadia SB, Heffner DK: Pitfalls in the histopathologic diagnosis of pyogenic granuloma. Eur Arch Otorhinolaryngol 249:195-200, 1992.

Sinonasal Papilloma (Schneiderian Papilloma)

Clinical Features

- Benign neoplasms of the respiratory mucosa subtypes: inverted, fungiform, and cylindrical cell papillomas
- Typically found in the nasal cavity and paranasal sinuses; rare in the nasopharynx
- Most common in adult men (male-to-female ratio, 2:1), occasionally seen in children
- Typically affect patients ages 30 to 50 years
- Clinically present as nasal obstruction or epistaxis
- Unilateral in most cases
- Some studies have demonstrated human papillomavirus (HPV) DNA in certain papillomas (exophytic and inverted)
- Inverted papilloma
  — Most common of the subtypes
  — Arises in the lateral nasal wall and paranasal sinuses
  — Likely to recur if incompletely excised
  — About 10% to 15% of cases may develop malignant transformation
- Exophytic papilloma
  — Also called *fungiform papilloma*
  — Arise on the nasal septum
- Cylindrical cell papilloma (least common)
  — Also called *oncocytic papilloma*
  — Arises in the lateral nasal wall, less often paranasal sinuses
  — May be associated with squamous carcinoma or other carcinomas

Gross Pathology

- Soft tan-white tissue often with small papillae or invaginations

Histopathology

- Most of the nasal cavity is lined by ciliated columnar epithelium (schneiderian), except the nasal vestibule, which is lined by stratified squamous epithelium
- Mixed morphology can occur
- Inverted papilloma
  — Deeply invaginated nests of benign squamous epithelium (5 to 30 cells thick) with intact smooth basement membrane, stroma without desmoplasia

Figure 3-51. Schneiderian papilloma. A, Inverted type. Well-circumscribed nests of transitional epithelium push into the stroma. At high power (*inset*), an intact basement membrane is present with maturation of the epithelium and associated inflammation with intraepithelial cyst formation. **B, Cylindrical cell type.** The surface epithelium is replaced by cells with prominent eosinophilic cytoplasm (oncocytic change) with microcysts filled with neutrophils.

  — Surface epithelium is usually squamous or transitional but may be ciliated, columnar, or mucinous
  — Neutrophils and mixed inflammatory infiltrate are seen
  — Dysplasia may be present and should be reported and graded (low or high grade)
  — May coexist with a frankly invasive carcinoma, most often squamous carcinoma
- Exophytic papilloma
  — Exophytic architecture with well-defined papillae showing fibrovascular cores
  — Surface epithelium is usually squamous, transitional
  — Surface keratinization is absent except in areas of irritation
- Cylindrical cell papilloma
  — Multilayered tall, cytologically bland columnar cells may be oncocytic

— Surface epithelium is often ciliated and typically two to eight cells thick
— Frequently contain mucous cells, inspissated mucin, and mucin pools
— Microabscesses with neutrophils within epithelium
— Inflammatory infiltrate in stroma is common
— May show an exophytic or endophytic growth pattern

Special Stains and Immunohistochemistry

- Cytokeratin positive
- Mucicarmine highlights goblet cells

Other Techniques for Diagnosis

- In situ hybridization or polymerase chain reaction (PCR) detects HPV types 6 and 11 in many cases (some fungiform and inverted papillomas)

Differential Diagnosis

▌ Squamous papilloma
- Arises from the squamous epithelium near the nasal vestibule
- Polypoid mass lined by mature squamous epithelium with keratinization
- Lacks microabscesses, mucin cells

▌ Squamous carcinoma, nonkeratinizing
- Infiltrative growth pattern with stromal invasion and desmoplastic response
- Pleomorphic cells with large, hyperchromatic nuclei and prominent nucleoli; high mitotic rate often with atypical mitoses
- May coexist with or arise from an inverted papilloma

▌ Inflammatory polyp
- Multiple and usually bilateral; involves both the nasal cavity and paranasal sinuses
- Associated with chronic rhinitis and asthma
- Mucous glands within fibroblastic stroma associated with mixed acute and chronic inflammation
- Epithelium lacks histologic features described previously

▌ Respiratory epithelial adenomatoid hamartoma (REAH)
- Increased glands composed of multilayered, columnar cells with cilia surrounded by a thick, prominent basement membrane
- Glands are separated by stroma and often connect to surface
- Rare; males affected more than females, in sixth decade
- Lacks microabscesses

▌ Sinonasal adenocarcinoma (nonenteric type)
- Proliferation of cytologically low-grade, back-to-back glands filling stroma
- In the differential of a cylindrical cell papilloma

▌ Rhinosporidiosis
- Hyperplastic polypoid lesions in nasal cavity

- Numerous globular cysts measuring up to 300 μm in diameter containing numerous endospores (2-9 μm) of *Rhinosporidium seeberi* highlighted by silver stain, PAS, or mucicarmine
- Cysts also present in stroma (cylindrical papilloma "cysts" only in epithelium)

▌ Papillary squamous carcinoma
- Exophytic proliferation with fibrovascular cores
- Epithelium shows full-thickness dysplastic cells
- Invasion may be difficult to identify

Pearls

- Inverted schneiderian papillomas are the most commonly encountered
- Carcinoma may be associated with inverted and cylindrical papillomas
- No current criteria to predict which papillomas will develop carcinoma
- Recurrence is common with incomplete excision

Selected References

Syrjänen KJ: HPV infections in benign and malignant sinonasal lesions. J Clin Pathol 56:174-181, 2003.

Barnes L: Schneiderian papillomas and nonsalivary glandular neoplasms of the head and neck. Mod Pathol 15:279-297, 2002.

Kaufman MR, Brandwein MS, Lawson W: Sinonasal papillomas: Clinicopathologic review of 40 patients with inverted and oncocytic schneiderian papillomas. Laryngoscope 112:1372-1377, 2002.

Batsakis JG, Suarez P: Schneiderian papillomas and carcinomas: A review. Adv Anat Pathol 8:53-64, 2001.

Squamous Cell Carcinoma of the Sinonasal Region

Clinical Features

- SCC of the sinonasal area is rare (about 3% of all head and neck neoplasms)
- More than half of paranasal SCCs occur in the maxillary antrum, about 30% in the nasal cavity, 10% in the ethmoid
- Increased risk related to cigarette smoking and nickel exposure; also related to exposure to chromium, isopropyl alcohol, and radium
- Male predominance (2:1); typically in sixth and seventh decades
- Presenting symptoms include nasal obstruction, epistaxis, pain, and alterations in voice

Gross Pathology

- Cut surface is tan-white with areas of necrosis and hemorrhage
- Infiltrative growth pattern

Histopathology

- Most are easily recognized intermediate- to high-grade tumors with obvious squamous differentiation

Figure 3-52. Squamous cell carcinoma arising in the maxillary sinus. Morphologically similar to squamous cell carcinomas in other head and neck sites, full-thickness pleomorphic cells with hyperchromatic nuclei are seen.

and often focal keratinization; nonkeratinizing carcinomas do occur

- Less common histologic subtypes include verrucous carcinoma, basaloid carcinoma, and spindle cell (sarcomatoid) carcinoma
- Desmoplastic stroma present
- Dysplastic squamous epithelium is seen at the edges of early lesions
- Lymph node involvement in 15%; increases with extension outside of nasal cavity

Special Stains and Immunohistochemistry

- Cytokeratin positive
- Synaptophysin and chromogranin negative

Other Techniques for Diagnosis

- Noncontributory

Differential Diagnosis

▌ Sinonasal undifferentiated carcinoma (SNUC)
- Nests, trabeculae, or sheets of poorly differentiated cells with high mitotic rate and necrosis; lacks squamous differentiation; lacks keratinization
- Moderate-sized cells, frequently with prominent nucleoli

▌ Schneiderian papillomas
- Inverted growth pattern has intact basement membrane without desmoplasia
- Epithelium is uniform; may show dysplasia
- May accompany and give rise to sinonasal squamous carcinoma

Pearls

- Recurrences are common regardless of mode of treatment

- Death typically due to local spread (60% 5-year survival rate)
- High frequency of second primary squamous carcinomas of the oral cavity and larynx and other sites (lung and esophagus)

Selected References

Thompson LDR: Malignant neoplasms of the nasal cavity, paranasal sinuses and nasopharynx. In Thompson LDR, Goldblum JR (eds): Head and Neck Pathology. Philadelphia, Churchill Livingstone, 2006, pp 155-160.

Pilch BZ, Bouqout J, Thompson LDR: Squamous cell carcinoma. In Barnes EL, Evenson JW, Reichart P, Sidransky D (eds): World Health Organization Classification of Tumours: Pathology and Genetics: Head and Neck Tumours. Lyon, IARC Press, 2005, pp 15-17.

Dulguerov P, Jacobsen MS, Allal AS, et al: Nasal and paranasal sinus carcinoma: Are we making progress? A series of 220 patients and a systematic review. Cancer 92:3012-3029, 2001.

Wieneke JA, Thompson LD, Wenig BM: Basaloid squamous cell carcinoma of the sinonasal tract. Cancer 85:841-854, 1999.

Sinonasal Undifferentiated Carcinoma

Clinical Features

- Rare high-grade undifferentiated carcinoma of unclear etiology
- More common in males (3:1); mean age, sixth decade
- Patients present with nasal obstruction, facial pain, proptosis, or epistaxis
- One third develop cervical lymphatic node metastases
- Poor survival; median survival, 18 months

Gross Pathology

- Large irregular mass with bone invasion

Histopathology

- Tumor grows in sheets, trabeculae, or nests
- Moderate-sized hyperchromatic cells with poorly defined cell borders and high N/C ratio
- Prominent single nucleoli
- Frequent mitoses
- Prominent tumor necrosis
- Keratinization not identified
- Lymphocytic infiltrate not identified (differentiates from nasopharyngeal)

Special Stains and Immunohistochemistry

- Positive for pan-cytokeratin, frequently cytokeratin 7
- Negative for cytokeratin 5/6
- Rare, focal synaptophysin, chromogranin

Other Techniques for Diagnosis

- Noncontributory

Figure 3-53. A, Sinonasal undifferentiated carcinoma. Nests of undifferentiated cells with prominent nucleoli and apoptotic figures are seen. **B, Teratocarcinoma.** Mixed cell lineages are identified within the tumor from primitive neuroblastoma (*right*) and cartilage (*left*).

Differential Diagnosis

▌ Nasopharyngeal carcinoma (undifferentiated type)
   ● Site of tumor aids in differential
   ● Accompanying lymphoid infiltrate (absent in SNUC)
   ● EBV frequently positive (negative in SNUC)
▌ SCC
   ● Keratinization usually identified (absent in SNUC)
   ● Grade based on degree of differentiation and keratinization
   ● Basaloid SCC shows focal abrupt keratinization
▌ Adenocarcinoma
   ● Hyperchromatic large cells in glands and nests
   ● Intestinal type shows intracellular mucin
▌ All small, round blue cell tumors in the sinonasal region
   ● Neuroblastoma, rhabdomyosarcoma, Ewing sarcoma, lymphoma, melanoma
   ● IHC panel of markers aids in classification
      — Pan-cytokeratin, CD45, desmin, synaptophysin, chromogranin, S-100, pan-melanin markers

Pearls

● Highly aggressive neoplasm with mean survival less than 2 years
● Strong or diffuse neuroendocrine markers not identified in SNUC
● Differentiation from nasopharyngeal carcinoma difficult in large tumors involving both regions

Selected References

Ejaz A, Wenig BM: Sinonasal undifferentiated carcinoma: Clinical and pathologic features and a discussion on classification, cellular differentiation, and differential diagnosis. Adv Anat Pathol 12:134-143, 2005.

Jeng YM, Sung MT, Fang CL, et al: Sinonasal undifferentiated carcinoma and nasopharyngeal-type undifferentiated carcinoma: Two clinically, biologically, and histopathologically distinct entities. Am J Surg Pathol 26:371-376, 2002.

Franchi A, Moroni M, Massi D, et al: Sinonasal undifferentiated carcinoma, nasopharyngeal-type undifferentiated carcinoma, and keratinizing and nonkeratinizing squamous cell carcinoma express different cytokeratin patterns. Am J Surg Pathol 26:1597-1604, 2002.

Cerilli LA, Holst VA, Brandwein MS, et al: Sinonasal undifferentiated carcinoma: Immunohistochemical profile and lack of EBV association. Am J Surg Pathol 25:156-163, 2001.

Frierson HF Jr, Mills SE, Fechner RE, et al: Sinonasal undifferentiated carcinoma: An aggressive neoplasm derived from Schneiderian epithelium and distinct from olfactory neuroblastoma. Am J Surg Pathol 10:771-779, 1986.

Nasopharyngeal Carcinoma

Clinical Features

● Squamous carcinoma arising in the nasopharynx with features that distinguish it from features of oral cavity and oropharynx SCC by epidemiology
● Adverse prognostic factors: older age, high stage, male sex, bony invasion of skull base, and cranial nerve paralysis
● Divided into keratinizing and nonkeratinizing types (includes undifferentiated carcinoma)
● Nasopharyngeal carcinoma, keratinizing type
   — SCC, graded by degree of differentiation (well, moderately, or poorly differentiated)
   — Keratinization identified
   — Less commonly associated with EBV
   — Occurs in older patients
   — Less radiosensitive, poor outcome
● Nasopharyngeal carcinoma, nonkeratinizing type
   — Recent World Health Organization tumor classification groups nonkeratinizing squamous carcinoma with undifferentiated type because both are strongly associated with EBV

Figure 3-54. Nasopharyngeal carcinoma. A, Undifferentiated type.
Large neoplastic cells are present admixed with a lymphocytic stroma.
B, Epstein-Barr virus. Tumor cell nuclei are positive for EBER (Epstein-
Barr virus–encoded RNA) by in situ hybridization.

— Prevalent in Southeast Asia and Northern Africa,
  rare in United States and Europe
— Peak incidence, 40 to 60 years of age; more
  common in males (3:1)
— Most common presentation is unilateral cervical
  lymphadenopathy; patients also commonly have
  nasal and middle-ear symptoms
— Environmental factors: diet high in nitrosamines-
  salted fish, smoking, formaldehyde, and EBV
  infection
— Etiologic factors include genetic predisposition
  (familial occurrence), associated with specific HLA
  loci, which are prognostic in Chinese patients

Gross Pathology

- Tumor may be difficult to detect clinically; usually
  "blind" biopsies
- Frozen sections used to direct number of biopsies for
  diagnostic material

Histopathology

- Undifferentiated nasopharyngeal carcinoma
  (lymphoepithelial carcinoma)
  — Two growth patterns
    ◆ Regaud type: well-defined tumor nests
      separated by fibrous stroma with inflammatory
      cells
    ◆ Schmincke type: sheets or syncytia of tumor
      cells infiltrated by inflammatory cells (masking
      tumor cells); can mimic malignant lymphoma
  — Nuclei are characteristically vesicular with a
    smooth outline and large eosinophilic nucleolus
  — Spindle cells may be present
  — Mitoses are easily identified; necrosis may be
    extensive
  — In situ component is identified in a minority of
    cases
  — Occasionally, eosinophils can be the predominant
    inflammatory component
  — Desmoplastic stroma is uncommon
  — Stromal amyloid deposition is occasionally seen
- SCC nonkeratinizing
  — Infiltrative growth pattern with stromal invasion
    and desmoplasia
  — Pleomorphic cells with large, hyperchromatic
    nuclei and prominent nuclei; high mitotic rate
    often with atypical mitoses
- Keratinizing nasopharyngeal carcinomas
  — SCC with associated desmoplasia and keratin
    pearls

Special Stains and Immunohistochemistry

- Cytokeratin positive, highlights malignant cells
  within lymphoid stroma
- High-molecular-weight cytokeratins positive (CK 5/6,
  34βE12)
- EBV latent membrane protein-1 (LMP-1) by IHC
  weak and positive in only one third of tumors (in
  situ Epstein-Barr–encoded RNA (EBER) is more
  sensitive)

Other Techniques for Diagnosis

- In situ hybridization demonstrates specific viral
  mRNA of EBV in tumor cell nuclei (EBER)
- Detection of IgG antibody (directed against early EBV
  antigen) and IgA antibody (against capsid viral
  antigen) in serum used in United States for
  presumptive diagnosis of nasopharyngeal
  carcinoma

Differential Diagnosis

▌ Non-Hodgkin (large cell) lymphoma
- Variably large nuclei may morphologically overlap
- Immunohistochemical panel of lymphoid and
  epithelial markers for lineage
▌ Sinus histiocytosis
- Histiocytic cells with small nuclei and low N/C ratio

- Rare or absent mitotic activity
- Positive for CD68; negative for cytokeratin
▌ SNUC
- Tumor bulk should be located in the sinonasal region but may extend to involve nasopharynx
- EBV negative
- No keratinization or lymphocytic infiltrate

Pearls

- Lymphoid tissue is not neoplastic; the term *lymphoepithelial* is a misnomer
- Cervical lymphadenopathy is most common mode of presentation
- Radiation is typical treatment because EBV-positive tumors are sensitive; chemotherapy is frequently added
- Survival is worse for keratinizing SCC, probably secondary to lack of EBV association and radiotherapy resistance

Selected References

Viguer JM, Jimenez-Heffernan JA, Lopez-Ferrer P, et al: Fine-needle aspiration cytology of metastatic nasopharyngeal carcinoma. Diagn Cytopathol 32:233-237, 2005.

Wei WI, Sham JS: Nasopharyngeal carcinoma. Lancet 365:2041-2054, 2005.

Lo KW, To KF, Huang DP: Focus on nasopharyngeal carcinoma. Cancer Cell 5:423-428, 2004.

Shi W, Pataki I, MacMillan C, et al: Molecular pathology parameters in human nasopharyngeal carcinoma. Cancer 94:1997-2006, 2002.

Wenig BM: Nasopharyngeal carcinoma. Ann Diagn Pathol 3:374-385, 1999.

Squamous Cell Carcinoma of the Tonsil or Oropharynx

Clinical Features

- Tonsil is the most common site in the oropharynx for SCC
- More common in men, in fifth and sixth decades, associated with tobacco use
- Also seen in nonsmokers, men and women, usually fourth and fifth decades, associated with high-risk HPV
- Clinically, 30% initially present with neck mass (metastasis)
- Other clinical signs are difficulty swallowing, sore throat, and ear pain

Gross Pathology

- Endophytic tan-pink tumor; may enlarge tonsil
- May be small, poorly visualized in crypts (submit tonsils in entirety for examination in adults)
- Firm white on cut sections

Figure 3-55. A, Tonsil squamous cell carcinoma. Atypical squamous epithelium with invasion into the submucosa is present forming irregular nests with variable keratinization. **B, Tonsil squamous cell carcinoma, human papillomavirus (HPV) positive.** In situ hybridization for HPV-16 is positive within the tumor nuclei. **C, Metastatic cystic squamous cell carcinoma.** A prominent cystic space is present surrounded by a neoplastic lining within a cervical lymph node. At high power (*inset*), the epithelium is hyperchromatic and haphazard (neoplastic).

Histopathology

- Most are easily recognized intermediate- to high-grade tumors with obvious squamous differentiation and at least focal keratinization
- Often, nonkeratinzing/low keratinizing SCC is frequently HPV associated
- Less common histologic subtypes include verrucous carcinoma, basaloid carcinoma, and spindle cell carcinoma

Special Stains and Immunohistochemistry

- Cytokeratin positive

Other Techniques for Diagnosis

- HPV testing for high-risk types (in situ hybridization)
- HPV positivity seen in 30% to 70% of oropharyngeal squamous carcinomas and associated with a better prognosis
- p16 by IHC overexpressed in HPV-positive tumors

Differential Diagnoses

▎ Nasopharyngeal carcinoma, undifferentiated carcinoma
- Composed of groups of undifferentiated large cells with vesicular nuclei associated with prominent lymphoplasmacytic reaction
- EBV often positive (EBER detected by in situ hybridization)

Pearls

- Patients often present with cystic metastasis to neck (not branchial cleft cysts)
- Treatment is often with radiation therapy to primary site and neck (tonsillectomy or biopsy for diagnosis)
- Increased risk for developing a second primary malignancy elsewhere in the head and neck
- HPV positivity often identified in nonsmokers and associates with a better prognosis (more radiosensitive)

Selected References

El-Mofty SK, Patil S: Human papillomavirus (HPV)-related oropharyngeal nonkeratinizing squamous cell carcinoma: Characterization of a distinct phenotype. Oral Surg Oral Med Oral Pathol Oral Radiol Endodont 101:339-345, 2006.

Goldenberg D, Sciubba J, Koch WM: Cystic metastasis from head and neck squamous cell cancer: A distinct disease variant? Head Neck 28:633-638, 2006.

Syrjänen S: HPV infections and tonsillar carcinoma. J Clin Pathol 57:449-455, 2004.

Li W, Thompson CH, O'Brien CJ, et al: Human papillomavirus positivity predicts favourable outcome for squamous carcinoma of the tonsil. Int J Cancer 106:553-558, 2003.

Thompson LD, Heffner DK: The clinical importance of cystic squamous cell carcinomas in the neck: A study of 136 cases. Cancer 82:944-956, 1998.

Sinonasal Adenocarcinoma

Clinical Features

- Arise from either the respiratory epithelium or seromucinous glands
- Tumors may arise in the nasal cavity or sinus region
- Clinical symptoms include obstruction and epistaxis
- Three distinct types of adenocarcinomas: enteric type, nonenteric type, and salivary type
  — Enteric type (intestinal type)
    ◆ Associated with woodworking (hard-wood exposure), leather, some chemical manufacturing
    ◆ Arises from schneiderian surface mucosa involving ethmoids, then nasal, then maxillary
    ◆ Prominent male predominance (9:1), often in the sixth decade
  — Nonenteric type (nonintestinal type)
    ◆ Classified as low- or high-grade nonenteric seromucinous adenocarcinomas
    ◆ Arise from seromucinous glands
    ◆ Wide age range; low-grade median 50 years, high-grade median 60 years
    ◆ No known environmental causes
  — Salivary type
    ◆ Morphologically identical to those in the salivary gland region
    ◆ Adenoid cystic carcinoma is the most frequent type
    ◆ Essentially any salivary histology may be seen

Gross Pathology

- Enteric type (intestinal type)
  — Fungating mass may show ulceration, hemorrhage
  — Friable gray mass with mucoid material
- Nonenteric type (nonintestinal type)
  — Varies based on grade
- Salivary type
  — Submucosal mass with infiltration

Histopathology

- Enteric type (intestinal type)
  — Hyperchromatic, atypical columnar epithelium
  — Invasion with desmoplasia present
  — Mucin and frequently goblet cells present
  — Intestinal metaplasia of schneiderian mucosa without atypia may be present
  — Intermediate- to high-grade tumors
- Nonenteric type (nonintestinal type)
  — Low grade
    ◆ Relatively cytologically bland proliferation of seromucinous glands
    ◆ Small glands are back to back, or papillary growth
    ◆ Can be difficult to distinguish from hyperplastic glands and to identify invasion

Figure 3-56. Sinonasal adenocarcinoma. A, Enteric (intestinal) type. Elongated hyperchromatic nuclei form glandular structures reminiscent of colonic adenocarcinoma. **B, Nonenteric type.** Back-to-back, uniform glands composed of cytologically bland cells fill the stroma (*inset*). **C, Salivary type.** Tubules and cribriform patterns of adenoid cystic carcinoma are invading bone. *Inset*, Higher-power view of the neoplastic cells.

◆ Atypical mitoses and necrosis generally absent
— High grade
  ◆ Solid growth pattern is common
  ◆ Moderate to marked pleomorphism
  ◆ High mitotic rate, prominent necrosis
• Salivary type
— Morphologies include those in the salivary regions (refer to "Salivary Glands" for features)
  ◆ Pleomorphic adenoma
  ◆ Adenoid cystic carcinoma
  ◆ Acinic cell carcinoma
  ◆ Polymorphous low-grade carcinoma
  ◆ Other morphologic entities

Special Stains and Immunohistochemistry

• Enteric type (intestinal type)
— Cytokeratin positive, may express CK7 and CK20
— CDX2 often positive (nuclear)
— As the morphology resembles intestinal-like mucosa, gains marker expression like colon
— Markers cannot be used to distinguish primary from metastasis (clinical correlate required)
• Nonenteric type (nonintestinal type)
— Cytokeratin 7 positive
— May express S-100 protein
• Salivary type
— Cytokeratin 7 positive
— May express S-100 protein

Other Techniques for Diagnosis

• Enteric type (intestinal type)
— *Ras* mutations (15%)
— *TP53* mutations (18% to 44%)

Differential Diagnosis

• Clinical history of exposures is helpful
▌ SNUC
• High-grade tumor with prominent necrosis
• Tumor cells with prominent nucleoli without differentiation
• Mucinous cells and intracellular mucin not identified
▌ Schneiderian papilloma-cylindrical cell type
• Inverted growth pattern has intact basement membrane without desmoplasia
• Epithelium is uniform with cilia identified
• Microabscesses are present within epithelium
▌ Nasopharyngeal papillary adenocarcinoma
• Described in children and adults; males = females
• Papillary growth and nest of uniform tumor cells in nasopharynx
• Nuclei mimic papillary thyroid carcinoma: enlarged, oval, clear, and folds
• TTF-1 is positive in this entity; thyroglobulin is negative
• Low-grade malignancy with resection being curative

- Teratocarcinosarcoma
  - Mixture of several tumor lineages, high-grade carcinoma, neuroblastoma, sarcoma, and occasionally germ cell tumors
  - Large friable mass with extensive necrosis
  - More common in males
  - Poor prognosis

Pearls

- Diverse histologies occur from low- to high-grade tumors
- IHC cannot separate primary from metastatic disease for intestinal-type adenocarcinoma and requires clinical correlation

Selected References

Pineda-Daboin K, Neto A, Ochoa-Perez V, Luna MA: Nasopharyngeal adenocarcinomas: A clinicopathologic study of 44 cases including immunohistochemical features of 18 papillary phenotypes. Ann Diagn Pathol 10:215-221, 2006.

Cathro HP, Mills SE: Immunophenotypic differences between intestinal-type and low-grade papillary sinonasal adenocarcinomas: An immunohistochemical study of 22 cases utilizing CDX2 and MUC2. Am J Surg Pathol 28:1026-1032, 2004.

Neto AG, Pineda-Daboin K, Luna MA: Sinonasal tract seromucous adenocarcinomas: A report of 12 cases. Ann Diagn Pathol 7:154-159, 2003.

Barnes L: Schneiderian papillomas and nonsalivary glandular neoplasms of the head and neck. Mod Pathol 15:279-297, 2002.

Franchi A, Gallo O, Santucci M: Clinical relevance of the histological classification of sinonasal intestinal-type adenocarcinomas. Hum Pathol 30:1140-1145, 1999.

Olfactory Neuroblastoma (Esthesioneuroblastoma)

Clinical Features

- Malignant neuroendocrine neoplasm, 5% of sinonasal tumors
- Wide age range, bimodal peaks around ages 15 and 55 years; no sex predilection
- Most often located at roof of nasal cavity
- Presenting symptoms include nasal obstruction and hemorrhage

Gross Pathology

- Reddish-gray, vascular, polypoid mass with soft consistency

Histopathology

- Lobular nests of uniform, relatively small monomorphic cells with round nuclei, fine and course chromatin, scant cytoplasm, and indistinct cell membrane
- Nests surrounded by fibrovascular cores and sustentacular cells

Figure 3-57. Olfactory neuroblastoma. Neoplastic small blue cells infiltrate into the submucosa as single cells and in nests. Neurofibrillary stroma is present, and rosettes are occasionally identified (*inset*).

- Fibrillary stroma corresponds to neuronal processes seen ultrastructurally
- Ganglion cells are rarely seen but when present are diagnostic
- Homer-Wright pseudorosettes seen in 30% of cases (annular arrays of cells surrounding central aggregates of cytoplasmic fibrils) or Flexner-type rosettes (glandular lumen) seen in 5% of cases
- Higher-grade tumors are less uniform, with more mitoses and pleomorphism

Special Stains and Immunohistochemistry

- Synaptophysin, chromogranin, neuron-specific enolase, neurofilament positive
- S-100 protein positive in sustentacular cells surrounding some nests of tumor
- Cytokeratin occasionally focally positive
- CEA and EMA negative

Other Techniques for Diagnosis

- Electron microscopy: numerous cytoplasmic dense core neurosecretory granules

Differential Diagnosis

- Rhabdomyosarcoma
  - Round to spindled cells, possible rhabdomyoblasts
  - Lacks rosette formation and fibrillary background
  - Positive for muscle differentiation markers; desmin (cytoplasmic) and MyoD1 and myogenin (nuclear)
- SNUC
  - Nests, ribbons, or trabeculae of polygonal cells with round, hyperchromatic nuclei; large, prominent nucleoli; and moderate eosinophilic cytoplasm
  - High mitotic rate and prominent individual cell or central necrosis
  - Vascular or lymphatic invasion often seen

- No rosettes or fibrillar background
- Positive for cytokeratin and may show focal synaptophysin or chromogranin
- Worse prognosis
▌ Sinonasal melanoma
- Primitive, often round tumor cells may show prominent nucleoli
- Discohesive with pseudopapilla
- Express S-100 protein or melan-A, HMB-45, tyrosinase
- Pagetoid spread occasionally seen
- Clinically, nasal obstruction may mimic nasal polyps
▌ Peripheral neuroectodermal tumor (PNET), Ewing sarcoma
- Can resemble SNUC, neuroblastoma, or rhabdomyosarcoma
- Neuroendocrine markers not helpful
- Positive for CD99 (nonspecific)
- Characteristic t(11;22) in 90% of tumors; paraffin sections can be analyzed by fluorescence in situ hybridization (FISH) analysis to confirm diagnosis
▌ Pituitary adenoma
- Ectopic origin or direct extension into paranasal sinuses (sphenoid)
- Positive for cytokeratin and chromogranin; variable positivity for pituitary hormones
▌ Malignant lymphoma
- Diffuse infiltrate of discohesive cells with large nuclei and clumped chromatin
- Lacks rosettes and fibrillary background
- LCA positive
▌ Small cell neuroendocrine carcinoma
- Same histologic features as pulmonary small cell carcinoma
- Small cells with hyperchromatic nuclei, nuclear molding, and scant cytoplasm
- Necrosis and high mitotic rate
- Positive for neuroendocrine markers and cytokeratin

Pearls

- Differential is broad, must consider multiple other tumors in this location
- Local recurrence common secondary to invasion (sinuses, orbit, base of skull)
- Most common sites of metastases are cervical lymph nodes and lung
- Postoperative radiation given to improve local control

Selected References

Mahooti S, Wakely PE Jr: Cytopathologic features of olfactory neuroblastoma. Cancer 108:86-92, 2006.
Diaz EM Jr, Johnigan RH 3rd, Pero C, et al: Olfactory neuroblastoma: The 22-year experience at one comprehensive cancer center. Head Neck 27:138-149, 2005.
Windfuhr JP: Primitive neuroectodermal tumor of the head and neck: Incidence, diagnosis, and management. Ann Otol Rhinol Laryngol 113:533-543, 2004.
Ingeholm P, Theilgaard SA, Buchwald C, et al: Esthesioneuroblastoma: A Danish clinicopathological study of 40 consecutive cases. Acta Pathol Microbiol Immunol Scand 110:639-645, 2002.
Hirose T, Scheithauer BW, Lopes MB, et al: Olfactory neuroblastoma: An immunohistochemical, ultrastructural, and flow cytometric study. Cancer 76:4-19, 1995.

Rhabdomyosarcoma

Clinical Features

- Most common sarcoma arising in the head and neck; accounts for 45% of head and neck sarcomas
- Embryonal type most common in children, alveolar type in adults; pleomorphic variant rare
- Patients present with a soft tissue mass, sinus symptoms, or both
- Nasopharynx more common than sinuses

Gross Pathology

- Poorly circumscribed, fleshy, polypoid (mimicking polyps)
- Cut surface is gray-red with a soft consistency

Histopathology

- Embryonal rhabdomyosarcoma
  — Makes up 80% of rhabdomyosarcoma of the head and neck
  — Hyperchromatic round to spindled cells; rhabdomyoblasts are larger with eosinophilic cytoplasm
  — Cross-striations are rare
  — Stroma may be myxoid
  — Subtypes of embryonal rhabdomyosarcoma include botryoid and spindled
    ◆ Botryoid type
      ◇ Small blue cells in abundant myxoid stroma
      ◇ Cambium layer composed of more compact cells below epithelial surface
    ◆ Spindled type
      ◇ Fairly uniform spindled cells, rare rhabdoid cells, occasional striations
- Alveolar rhabdomyosarcoma
  — Nests of small, discohesive round to oval hyperchromatic tumor cells separated by fibrous tissue
  — Mitotic figures are common
  — Multinucleated giant cells may be present
  — Solid growth and clear cell morphology have been described
- Pleomorphic rhabdomyosarcoma
  — Large, pleomorphic cells rarely showing cross-striations
  — Need immunohistochemical evidence of skeletal muscle differentiation or cytoplasmic cross-striations

Figure 3-58. Rhabdomyosarcoma. A, Embryonal type. Small hyperchromatic neoplastic cells infiltrate the stroma. Desmin, by immunohistochemical analysis, is positive in the cytoplasm of tumor cells (*inset*). **B, Spindled type.** In this variant of embryonal type, the neoplastic cells form elongated fascicles. Myogenin, by immunohistochemical analysis, is positive in the nucleus of tumor cells (*inset*). **C, Alveolar type.** Hyperchromatic tumor cells are discohesive, leaving "alveolar-like" spaces.

Special Stains and Immunohistochemistry

- Positive for desmin, myoglobin, myosin, and MSA (nonspecific)
- Positive for MyoD1 (nuclear expression; regulatory protein in skeletal muscle differentiation)—confirmatory marker
- Myogenin (nuclear expression; regulatory protein in skeletal muscle differentiation)—confirmatory marker
- May rarely express cytokeratin

Other Techniques for Diagnosis

- Embryonal rhabdomyosarcoma has characteristic 11pLOH
- Alveolar rhabdomyosarcoma has characteristic t(2;13); occasionally, t(1;13) *PAX2* or *PAX3* translocated with *FKHR* may have prognostic significance
- FISH can be performed for these translocations on paraffin sections

Differential Diagnosis

- Same as for olfactory neuroblastoma (as listed previously)

Pearls

- Differential diagnosis includes all of the small round blue cell tumors, and evaluation should incorporate morphology and IHC
- A useful initial battery of immunohistochemical stains for differential diagnosis of a small round blue cell tumor in the head and neck includes cytokeratin, LCA, S-100, synaptophysin, desmin, and melanoma marker

Selected References

Nascimento AF, Fletcher CD: Spindle cell rhabdomyosarcoma in adults. Am J Surg Pathol 29:1106-1113, 2005.

Xia SJ, Pressey JG, Barr FG: Molecular pathogenesis of rhabdomyosarcoma. Cancer Biol Therapy 1:97-104, 2002.

Folpe AL: MyoD1 and myogenin expression in human neoplasia: A review and update. Adv Anat Pathol 9:198-203, 2002.

Sorensen PH, Lynch JC, Qualman SJ, et al: PAX3-FKHR and PAX7-FKHR gene fusions are prognostic indicators in alveolar rhabdomyosarcoma: A report from the children's oncology group. J Clin Oncol 20:2672-2679, 2002.

Parham DM: Pathologic classification of rhabdomyosarcomas and correlations with molecular studies. Mod Pathol 14:506-514, 2001.

Sinonasal Melanoma

Clinical Features

- Uncommon (<5%) sinonasal tumor
- Less than 1% of all melanoma cases
- Males = females in fifth to eighth decades
- Higher incidence in Japanese

Figure 3-59. Sinonasal melanoma. Relatively homogeneous tumor cells with prominent nucleoli are present without identifiable pigment.

- Patients present with sinus symptoms, obstruction, or epistaxis
- Generally poor prognosis, less than 50% survival rate at 5 years

Gross Pathology

- Varies from gray to tan, can be pigmented brown or black
- Often polypoid and friable

Histopathology

- Sheets or nests of small to medium-sized epithelioid, rhabdoid, spindled, or pleomorphic cells; may show nucleoli
- Discohesiveness leads to pseudopapillary structure of tumor around vessels
- Mitoses present
- Intracytoplasmic melanin may be present
- Melanocytes at junction of surface respiratory epithelium or pagetoid spread may be noted

Special Stains and Immunohistochemistry

- Positive for S-100 and melanocyte markers (melan-A, HMB-45, tyrosinase)
- No markers to distinguish primary from metastasis (clinical correlate required)

Other Techniques for Diagnosis

- Although rarely performed, electron microscopy will show premelanosomes and melanosomes

Differential Diagnosis

- Olfactory neuroblastoma
  - Growth patterns may be similar
  - Rosette formation and fibrillary background
  - Cells with clumped hyperchromatic chromatin

- Positive for synaptophysin, chromogranin (occasionally in melanoma)
- Rhabdomyosarcoma
  - Hyperchromatic round to spindled cells; rhabdomyoblasts may be seen
  - Striations when present are helpful
  - Positive for muscle differentiation markers; desmin, MyoD1, and myogenin
- SNUC
  - Nests, ribbons, or trabeculae of polygonal cells with round, hyperchromatic nuclei; large, prominent nucleoli; and moderate eosinophilic cytoplasm
  - High mitotic rate and prominent individual cell or central necrosis
  - Vascular or lymphatic invasion often seen
  - Cytokeratin positive
- PNET, Ewing sarcoma
  - High N/C ratio
  - Fine nuclear chromatin and small nucleoli
  - Positive for CD99 (nonspecific)
  - Characteristic t(11;22) in 90% of tumors; paraffin sections can be analyzed by FISH analysis to confirm diagnosis
- Malignant lymphoma
  - Diffuse infiltrate of discohesive lymphoid cells with large nuclei and clumped chromatin
  - LCA positive
  - May be EBV positive depending on type

Pearls

- Morphologically, sinonasal melanoma mimics other primary small round blue cell tumors of this region
- A useful initial battery of immunohistochemical stains for differential diagnosis of a small round blue cell tumor in the head and neck includes cytokeratin, LCA, S-100, synaptophysin, desmin, and a melanoma marker (melan-A)
- Clinical correlation is required to exclude metastasis to sinonasal region (1% of cases); other metastases are usually present with metastatic presentation

Selected References

Thompson LD, Wieneke JA, Miettinen M: Sinonasal tract and nasopharyngeal melanomas: A clinicopathologic study of 115 cases with a proposed staging system. Am J Surg Pathol 27:594-611, 2003.

Prasad ML, Jungbluth AA, Iversen K, et al: Expression of melanocytic differentiation markers in malignant melanomas of the oral and sinonasal mucosa. Am J Surg Pathol 25:782-787, 2001.

O'Sullivan MJ, Perlman EJ, Furman J, et al: Visceral primitive peripheral neuroectodermal tumors: A clinicopathologic and molecular study. Hum Pathol 32:1109-1115, 2001.

Batsakis JG, Suarez P, El-Naggar AK: Mucosal melanomas of the head and neck. Ann Otol Rhinol Laryngol 107:626-630, 1998.

Lymphoma

Clinical Features

- Extranodal natural killer (NK) cell and T-cell lymphoma (angiocentric)
  - Endemic in some Asian countries (Japan, Taiwan), parts of Latin America; less common in Western countries
  - Peaks in sixth decade, more common in males (3:1)
  - Clinical symptoms of obstruction, epistaxis, and septal perforation
  - Most often affecting nasal cavity
  - EBV positive
- Other lymphomas
  - All types of non-Hodgkin lymphomas have been described in this location
  - Most common is diffuse large cell lymphoma involving sinuses
  - B-cell lymphomas, although rare, affect nasopharynx, oropharynx, and sinuses
  - Phenotypically, most Western hemisphere cases are B-cell type (Asian and South American cases are T-cell type)
  - Clinical features are nonspecific and related to obstruction or hemorrhage

Gross Pathology

- Extranodal NK/T-cell lymphoma (angiocentric)
  - Ulcerated lesions often reach large size
- Other lymphomas
  - Typically present as a polypoid mass

Histopathology

- Extranodal NK/T-cell lymphoma (angiocentric)
  - Usually exuberant inflammation
  - Variable cytologic atypia of mostly small to medium-sized lymphocytes; nucleoli are inconspicuous
  - Prominent necrosis and karyorrhexis
  - Vascular invasion and angiocentricity (viable cells seen cuffing a residual blood vessel) may not be demonstrable in all cases
- Other lymphomas
  - Varies with subtype; refer to Chapter 14

Special Stains and Immunohistochemistry

- Extranodal NK/T-cell lymphoma (angiocentric)
  - Lymphocytes are positive for CD2, CD43, and NK cell antigen CD56; negative for CD3, CD57, and CD11
- Other lymphomas
  - LCA positive
  - Cytokeratin negative
  - B-cell (L26/CD20) and T-cell (CD3) markers should be done for phenotyping
  - EMA and CD30 may be positive in anaplastic large cell lymphomas and true histiocytic lymphomas

Other Techniques for Diagnosis

- Extranodal NK/T-cell lymphoma (angiocentric)
  - T-cell receptor rearrangements are usually absent and clonality is difficult to demonstrate
  - EBV positive by in situ hybridization
- Other lymphomas
  - Varies with subtype (refer to Chapter 14)

Differential Diagnosis

▌ Nasopharyngeal carcinoma
- Nuclei are characteristically vesicular with a smooth outline and a single large eosinophilic nucleolus
- Location of nasopharynx
- Cytokeratin-positive tumor in dense lymphocytic infiltrate

Figure 3-60. A, Extranodal NK/T-cell lymphoma. An atypical lymphoid infiltrate shows large pleomorphic cells. **B, Diffuse large B-cell lymphoma.** There is infiltration of tissue by large atypical cells with open chromatin and background of small scattered lymphocytes.

- Often EBV positive (not helpful because EBV is often present in nasal lymphomas)
▌ Olfactory neuroblastoma
  - Rosette formation and fibrillary background may be identified
  - Cells with clumped hyperchromatic chromatin
  - Positive for synaptophysin, chromogranin
▌ Wegener granulomatosis
  - Varying stages of vasculitis involving arterioles, small arteries, and veins can be difficult to find
  - A neutrophilic infiltrate and fibrinoid necrosis
  - Giants cells scattered
  - Areas of geographic necrosis usually predominate
  - Clinical workup shows cytoplasmic antineutrophil cytoplasmic antibodies (c-ANCA) against proteinase-3 (PR3)
▌ Cocaine abuse
  - Shows necrosis and nonspecific inflammation of epithelium and stroma
  - No vasculitis

Pearls

- The term *lethal midline granuloma* is outdated and should not be used as a pathologic diagnosis
- Extranodal NK/T-cell lymphoma is EBV positive and negative for T-cell receptor monoclonal rearrangements
- In Western countries, B-cell lymphomas are more common; T-cell lymphomas are more common in Asia and Latin America

Selected References

Li CC, Tien HF, Tang JL, et al: Treatment outcome and pattern of failure in 77 patients with sinonasal natural killer/T-cell or T-cell lymphoma. Cancer 100:366-375, 2004.

Heffner DK: Wegener's granulomatosis is not a granulomatous disease. Ann Diagn Pathol 6:329-333, 2002.

Seyer BA, Grist W, Muller S: Aggressive destructive midfacial lesion from cocaine abuse. Oral Surg Oral Med Oral Pathol Oral Radiol Endodont 94:465-470, 2002.

Rodriguez J, Romaguera JE, Manning J, et al: Nasal-type T/NK lymphomas: A clinicopathologic study of 13 cases. Leuk Lymphoma 39:139-144, 2000.

Cuadra-Garcia I, Proulx GM, Wu CL, et al: Sinonasal lymphoma: A clinicopathologic analysis of 58 cases from the Massachusetts General Hospital. Am J Surg Pathol 23:1356-1369, 1999.

Jaffe ES, Chan JK, Su IJ, et al: Report of the workshop on nasal and related extranodal angiocentric T/Natural killer cell lymphomas: Definitions, differential diagnosis, and epidemiology. Am J Surg Pathol 20:103-111, 1996.

Tumors Metastasizing to the Paranasal Sinuses and Nasopharynx

Clinical Features

- Metastases to the paranasal sinuses and nasopharynx are rare
- Most common are renal cell carcinoma, melanoma, and breast carcinoma

Gross Pathology

- Depends on location and tumor type

Histopathology

- Renal cell carcinoma
  - Clear cell type mistaken for alveolar rhabdomyosarcoma, clear cell variant
  - Characteristic arborizing vascular pattern surrounds tumor cells
- Malignant melanoma
  - Estimated 1% risk for metastasis to this region
  - Most melanomas encountered are primary sinonasal; however, clinically must exclude metastasis
- Breast carcinoma
  - Infiltrating ductal carcinoma has pleomorphic cells with high mitotic rate
  - Lobular carcinoma can have bland-appearing cells

Special Stains and Immunohistochemistry

- Renal cell carcinoma
  - Cytokeratin and vimentin positive
  - Clear cells contain glycogen
- Malignant melanoma
  - No markers distinguish primary from metastatic
- Breast carcinoma
  - Estrogen receptor and progesterone receptor variably positive
  - *HER-2* may be positive (correlate with primary tumor expression)

Other Techniques for Diagnosis

- Noncontributory

Differential Diagnosis

- Clinical history is essential

Pearls

- Always obtain clinical history when histology is not definitive for primary tumor

Selected References

Lee HM, Kang HJ, Lee SH: Metastatic renal cell carcinoma presenting as epistaxis. Eur Arch Otorhinolaryngol 262:69-71, 2005.

Marchioni D, Monzani D, Rossi G, et al: Breast carcinoma metastases in paranasal sinuses, a rare occurrence mimicking a primary nasal malignancy. Acta Otorhinolaryngol Ital 24:87-91, 2004.

Simo R, Sykes AJ, Hargreaves SP, et al: Metastatic renal cell carcinoma to the nose and paranasal sinuses. Head Neck 22:722-727, 2000.

Wanamaker JR, Kraus DH, Eliacher I, Lavertu P: Manifestations of metastatic breast carcinoma to the head and neck. Head Neck 15:257-262, 1993.

Mickel RA, Zimmerman MC: The sphenoid sinus—a site for metastasis. Otolaryngol Head Neck Surg 102:709-716, 1990.

Oral Cavity

Leukoplakia

Clinical Features

- A clinical term to describe a white patch or plaque that either is localized or has geographic distribution
- Occurs predominantly in older individuals, slightly more common in males
- A subset considered premalignant (4% to 20% may undergo malignant transformation)
- Most common in the buccal mucosa
- Highest incidence of dysplasia in leukoplakia involving the floor of mouth and ventrolateral aspect of the tongue and lip
- Hairy leukoplakia
  — Occurs predominantly in patients with HIV infection
  — Common site, the lateral borders of tongue

Gross Pathology

- White to grayish-yellow plaques on surface epithelium with wrinkled, rough surface

Histopathology

- Hyperkeratosis, parakeratosis, or both
- Acanthosis and hyperplasia of the squamous epithelium
- Mild or moderate (lichenoid) chronic inflammation may be seen in submucosa
- Dysplastic changes may be present (enlarged, hyperchromatic nuclei; loss of maturation); can extend to ducts of minor salivary glands; graded as mild, moderate, or severe
- Often superinfection with *Candida* species

Special Stains and Immunohistochemistry

- Noncontributory

Other Techniques for Diagnosis

- Noncontributory

Differential Diagnosis

▮ Squamous dysplasia (mild to severe)
- May appear grossly white or red-granular (erythroplastic)
- In situ SCC: full-thickness cytologic atypia, disarray of epithelium and intact basement membrane (appears

Figure 3-61. Leukoplakia. A, Clinical photograph shows extensive white patches or plaques of the lower lip and gingiva. **B,** Histologically, the squamous mucosa shows marked hyperkeratosis and parakeratosis and underlying dysplasia.

thinned on staining for type IV collagen and laminin)
▮ Lichen planus
- Less common than leukoplakia
- Bandlike lymphocytic infiltration of the subepithelium, with spongiotic changes in basal cells
- Sawtooth rete ridges
▮ Actinic cheilitis
- Same morphology and pathogenesis as actinic keratosis of the skin
- Biopsy is mandatory because of the lack of reliable clinical signs predicting malignancy; erythematous, granular plaque is worrisome

Pearls

- *Leukoplakia* is a clinical term with variation in pathologic findings

- Leukoplakia may show only hyperkeratosis or be preneoplastic with squamous dysplasia

Selected References

Devaney KO, Rinaldo A, Zeitels SM, et al: Laryngeal dysplasia and other epithelial changes on endoscopic biopsy: What does it all mean to the individual patient? J Otorhinolaryngol Relat Spec 66:1-4, 2004.

Muller S, Waldron CA: Premalignant lesions of the oral cavity. In Barnes L (ed): Surgical Pathology of the Head and Neck. New York, Marcel Dekker, 2001, pp 343-360.

Southam JC, Felix DH, Wray D, Cubie HA: Hairy leukoplakia: A histological study. Histopathology 19:63-67, 1991.

Fernandez JF, Benito MAC, Lizaldez EB, Monatañés MA: Oral hairy leukoplakia: A histopathologic study of 32 cases. Am J Dermatopathol 12:571-578, 1990.

Squamous Papilloma

Clinical Features

- Most common oral neoplasm
- Affects all ages, usually seen in adults
- Etiologic factors are viruses (HPV types 2, 4, 6, 11, 13, 32) and mechanical irritation
- Preferred sites are palate, tongue, gingiva, and lips
- May occur as a component of Cowden syndrome
- Usually single but may be multiple

Gross Pathology

- Painless, exophytic, white to pink mass with warty or papillary surface
- Usually smaller than 1 cm

Figure 3-62. Squamous papilloma. A, Gross evaluation shows exophytic tan-white nodular masses of the oral mucosa. **B,** Low-power view shows papillary fronds covered by stratified squamous epithelium with marked hyperkeratosis.

Histopathology

- Broad papillary projections composed of hyperplastic stratified squamous epithelium around a scant fibrovascular core
- May have varying amounts of parakeratosis, hyperkeratinization, ulceration, inflammation, or superficial *Candida* species infection

Special Stains and Immunohistochemistry

- Noncontributory

Other Techniques for Diagnosis

- In situ hybridization for HPV

Differential Diagnosis

- SCC with papillary growth
  - Marked cytologic atypia, full thickness
  - Infiltrative growth pattern
- Verruca vulgaris (common wart)
  - Uncommonly involves mouth
  - Large basophilic inclusions in epithelial cells

- Condyloma acuminatum
  - Squamous dysplasia with HPV effect (koilocytic atypia)
  - Clusters of coalescing exophytic masses
  - Fronds broader and blunter than papillomas

Pearls

- Squamous atypia and basal cell hyperplasia may occur; dysplasia is rare
- Recurrences are infrequent but may happen after incomplete excision

Selected References

Westra W: Benign neoplasms of the oral cavity and oropharynx. In Thompson LDR, Goldblum JR (eds): Head and Neck Pathology. Philadelphia, Churchill Livingstone, 2006, pp 243-246.

Jenson AB, Lancaster WD, Hartmann DP, Shaffer EL Jr: Frequency and distribution of papillomavirus structural antigens in verrucae, multiple papillomas, and condylomata of the oral cavity. Am J Pathol 107:212-218, 1982.

Abby LJ, Page DG, Sawyer DR: The clinical and histopathologic features of a series of 464 oral squamous cell papillomas. Oral Surg Oral Med Oral Pathol 49:419-428, 1980.

Pyogenic Granuloma (Lobular Capillary Hemangioma)

Clinical Features

- Also called *lobular capillary hemangioma*
- Etiology: infection, trauma, hormonal stimulation (pregnancy)
- May occur at any age; more common in females
- Most common mass of the gingiva

Gross Pathology

- Sharply circumscribed, elevated, dark red, soft nodule
- Often ulcerated
- Sessile or pedunculated, usually friable and hemorrhagic

Histopathology

- Proliferation of small blood vessels arranged in a lobular growth pattern (mass of granulation tissue)
- Fibromyxoid or edematous stroma with acute and chronic inflammation
- Overlying squamous epithelium may be atrophic or ulcerated

Special Stains and Immunohistochemistry

- Noncontributory

Other Techniques for Diagnosis

- Noncontributory

Differential Diagnosis

❚ Hemangioma or lymphangioma
- Occurs mostly in the tongue
- Composed of larger vascular or lymphatic channels

❚ Kaposi sarcoma of oral cavity
- Palate is most common location
- Characterized by slitlike vascular channels with extravasated red blood cells
- Typically associated with HIV-positive patients
- Cells are HHV-8 positive

❚ Peripheral giant cell granuloma
- Nonencapsulated mass of granulation tissue with numerous osteoclast-like giant cells
- Varying degrees of hemorrhage, hemosiderin, and acute and chronic inflammation; metaplastic bone may be seen

Pearls

- May regress completely; can fibrose and resemble fibroepithelial polyp

Figure 3-63. Pyogenic granuloma (lobular capillary hemangioma). **A,** Clinical photograph showing a polypoid mass extending from the gingiva with a ragged erythematous or ulcerated surface. **B,** Low-power view shows a polypoid lesion covered by stratified squamous epithelium and partial ulceration. Note the lobular architecture of the vascular proliferation.

- Recurrence rate after surgical treatment is 16%
- Treatment is local excision

Selected References

Verbin RS, Guggenheimer J, Appel BN: Benign neoplastic and nonneoplastic lesions of the oral cavity and oropharynx. In Barnes L (ed): Surgical Pathology of the Head and Neck. New York, Marcel Dekker, 2001, pp 263-266.

Kapadia SB, Heffner DK: Pitfalls in the histopathologic diagnosis of pyogenic granuloma. Eur Arch Otorhinolaryngol 249:195-200, 1992.

Bodner L, Dayan D: Intravascular papillary endothelial hyperplasia of the mandibular mucosa. Int J Oral Maxillofac Surg 20:263-274, 1991.

Kerr DA: Granuloma pyogenicum. Oral Surg Oral Med Oral Pathol 4:158-176, 1951.

Granular Cell Tumor

Clinical Features

- Can occur anywhere in the oral cavity; most common on the tongue
- Typically presents as a painless submucosal nodule
- No age preference in adults; rare in children; more common in females
- Uncertain etiology

Gross Pathology

- Firm, submucosal nodule
- Typically small, may measure up to 5 cm

Histopathology

- Overlying squamous epithelium shows pseudoepitheliomatous hyperplasia
- Characterized by sheets, nests, or cords of large, polyhedral cells with granular acidophilic cytoplasm and small hyperchromatic nuclei

Special Stains and Immunohistochemistry

- S-100 protein, Leu-7, and myelin basic protein of the granular cell are positive
- Granules are PAS positive and contain lysosomes

Other Techniques for Diagnosis

- Noncontributory

Differential Diagnosis

- Metastatic granular renal cell carcinoma
  - Clinical history helpful
  - Greater cytologic atypia
  - Positive for cytokeratin and vimentin

Figure 3-64. Granular cell tumor. Section shows a hyperplastic pseudoepitheliomatous squamous epithelium with marked irregularity of the nests at the basement membrane. The submucosa is replaced by eosinophilic granular cells with small hyperchromatic nuclei (*inset*).

Pearls

- Pseudoepitheliomatous hyperplasia can be mistaken for SCC
- About 10% of patients have multiple tumors
- Histogenesis believed to be of neural or Schwann cell origin
- Most are benign; rare cases of malignant behavior are seen
- Features of malignancy: high mitotic activity, necrosis, nuclear pleomorphism, and high cellularity; definitive criterion for malignancy is metastasis
- Can occur in nerves (supporting the Schwann cell origin theory)

Selected References

Kapadia SB: Tumors of the nervous system. In Barnes L (ed): Surgical Pathology of the Head and Neck. New York, Marcel Dekker, 2001, pp 813-817.

Muzur MT, Shultz JJ, Myers JL: Granular cell tumor: Immunohistochemical analysis of 21 benign tumors and one malignant tumor. Arch Pathol Lab Med 114:692, 1990.

Radicular Cyst

Clinical Features

- Also called *periapical cyst*
- Accounts for 10% of all inflammatory cysts in the oral mucosa
- Cyst formation caused by infection of the dental pulp by caries or trauma
- Most often involves the root of maxillary incisors and mandibular molars; typically no destruction or displacement of teeth
- Seldom associated with deciduous teeth
- May cause pain or be found incidentally on radiography
- Radiographically shows a round or flask-shaped radiolucency with prominent radiopaque margin

Gross Pathology

- Fragments of glistening or granular soft tissue; rarely is the tooth removed with the cyst intact; cyst lining may or may not be appreciated

Histopathology

- Cyst lined by hyperplastic stratified squamous epithelium with focal keratinization; goblet cells are common
- Hyaline bodies (Rushton bodies) are unique to odontogenic cysts and are seen in about 10% of lesions; helpful in separating odontogenic from fissural cysts
- Cyst wall has chronic inflammation, cholesterol clefts, and foamy histiocytes

Special Stains and Immunohistochemistry

- Noncontributory

Figure 3-65. Radicular cyst. A, Radiograph showing a radiolucent region associated with the tooth root. **B,** Corresponding resection specimen with mass associated with the tooth root. **C,** The mass consists of a cyst with a squamous epithelial lining with marked inflammation. Associated hyaline (Rushton) bodies may be identified (*inset*).

Other Techniques for Diagnosis

- Noncontributory

Differential Diagnosis

▌ Odontogenic keratocyst
  - Radiographically, a unilocular or multilocular radiolucency in posterior mandible or maxilla
  - Keratinizing squamous epithelium with fibrous, noninflammatory cyst wall
  - No Rushton bodies

▌ Dentigerous cyst
  - Atypical cyst of unerupted permanent tooth
  - Lined by stratified squamous epithelium without cyst wall inflammation

Pearls

- Radicular cysts have no potential to differentiate along odontogenic tumor cell lines as do the odontogenic keratocyst and dentigerous cysts
- May rarely undergo neoplastic transformation to SCC, ameloblastoma, or mucoepidermoid carcinoma

Selected References

Verbin RS, Barnes L: Cysts and cyst-like lesions of the oral cavity, jaws and neck. In Barnes L (ed): Surgical Pathology of the Head and Neck. New York, Marcel Dekker, 2001, pp 1464-1468.

High AS, Hirschman PN: Age changes in residual radicular cysts. J Oral Pathol 15:524-528, 1986.

Rushton MA: Hyaline bodies in the epithelium of dental cysts. Proc R Soc Med 48:407-409, 1955.

Dentigerous Cyst

Clinical Features

- Encases the crown of an unerupted permanent tooth
- May clinically present as a missing tooth
- Most often involves third molars
- May be asymptomatic or cause bony expansion and displacement of teeth
- Radiographically, a unilocular radiolucency

Gross Pathology

- Enlarged, swollen soft tissue with cystic formation

Histopathology

- Cyst lined by stratified squamous epithelium in direct continuity with enamel epithelium, which covers the crown of the unerupted tooth
- No inflammation unless superinfected

Special Stains and Immunohistochemistry

- Noncontributory

Other Techniques for Diagnosis

- Noncontributory

Differential Diagnosis

▌ Radicular cyst
  - Associated with root of tooth
  - Cyst wall contains chronic inflammatory cells
  - Hyaline bodies (Rushton bodies) are characteristic but are seen in only about 10% of cases

▌ Odontogenic keratocyst
  - Radiographically, unilocular or multilocular radiolucency in posterior mandible or maxilla
  - Lined by keratinizing squamous epithelium with fibrous, noninflammatory cells

Pearls

- Correlate pathologic findings with radiographic imaging (i.e., Panorex)
- Determine location and association with an unerupted tooth

Selected Reference

Eversole LR, Sabes WR, Rovin S: Aggressive growth and neoplastic potential of odontogenic cysts: With special

Figure 3-66. Dentigerous cyst. A, Radiograph. **B,** Gross photo of the cyst surrounding the crown of an unerupted tooth. **C,** The cyst lining is bland stratified squamous epithelium without inflammation of the cyst wall.

reference to central epidermoid and mucoepidermoid carcinomas. Cancer 35:270-282, 1975.

Odontogenic Keratocyst

Clinical Features

- Radiographically, unilocular or multilocular radiolucency
- Most occur in the posterior mandible or maxilla

Gross Pathology

- Unilocular or more frequently multilocular cyst with creamy fluid representing cytokeratin debris

Histopathology

- Thin keratinizing stratified squamous epithelium with fibrotic cyst wall lacking inflammation

Special Stains and Immunohistochemistry

- Noncontributory

Other Techniques for Diagnosis

- Noncontributory

Differential Diagnosis

- ▌ Radicular cyst
  - Associated with root of tooth
  - Cyst wall contains chronic inflammatory cells
  - Hyaline bodies (Rushton bodies) are characteristic but are seen in only about 10% of cases
- ▌ Dentigerous cyst
  - Atypical cyst of unerupted permanent tooth
  - Lined by stratified squamous epithelium without cyst wall inflammation

Figure 3-67. Odontogenic keratocyst. A, Clinical photograph of a mandibular mass with intact overlying mucosa. **B,** Corresponding radiograph of a translucent, cystic mass extending up the mandibular ramus. **C,** Low-power image shows an epithelial lined cyst with fibrous wall generally without inflammation. **D,** High-power view of the epithelial cyst wall composed of bland stratified squamous epithelium often with a corrugated surface.

Pearls

- Potential for destructive growth and tendency for recurrence
- May be associated with nevoid basal cell carcinoma syndrome (autosomal dominant condition characterized by keratocysts of jaw, multiple basal cell carcinomas of the skin, skeletal anomalies, palmar and plantar dyskeratosis, ectopic soft tissue calcifications, and ovarian fibromas)

Selected References

Verbin RS, Barnes L: Cysts and cyst-like lesions of the oral cavity, jaws and neck. In Barnes L (ed): Surgical Pathology of the Head and Neck. New York, Marcel Dekker, 2001, pp 1452-1460.

Blanas N, Freund B, Schwartz M, Furst IM: Systematic review of the treatment and prognosis of the odontogenic keratocyst. Oral Surg Oral Med Oral Pathol Oral Radiol Endodontol 90:553-558, 2000.

Areen RG, McClatchey KD, Baker HL: Squamous cell carcinoma developing in an odontogenic keratocyst: Report of a case. Arch Otolaryngol Head Neck Surg 107: 568-569, 1981.

Ameloblastoma

Clinical Features

- Most common odontogenic neoplasm
- Males and females equally affected
- Occurs more frequently in whites, followed by blacks and Asians (especially Chinese)
- Average age is 33 years; unicystic lesions occur a decade earlier

Figure 3-68. Ameloblastoma. Low-power view shows epithelial nests with peripheral palisading, loose stellate centers, and microcysts growing in a dense stroma adjacent to thinned bone.

- Location: mandible is affected more than maxilla (ratio 4:1), typically posterior mandible
- Many occur in association with impacted third molars; some arise from the epithelial lining of dentigerous cysts
- Typically grows slowly and is asymptomatic until large; may resorb teeth or infiltrate bone and soft tissue
- Can metastasize (rarely)
- Radiographically, multiloculated, "soap-bubble" radiolucency
- Ameloblastomas of sinonasal region show predilection for older men (more than 80% are infiltrating, solid, or multicystic)
- Clinicopathologic forms: multicystic, unicystic, and peripheral
  - Unicystic and multicystic
    - Occur in younger patients
    - Noninfiltrating form; low recurrence rate after conservative treatment (10% to 15%)
    - May recur as the infiltrating multicystic type
  - Peripheral
    - Least common; more common in older adults
    - Extraosseous location

Gross Pathology

- Cut surface reveals solid and cystic areas
- Solid areas are white to gray with little hemorrhage and no necrosis
- Variably sized cysts that contain clear to yellow fluid

Histopathology

- Follicular and plexiform pattern cellular; other patterns are acanthomatous, granular cell, basaloid, desmoplastic, and keratoameloblastoma-like (exceptionally rare)
  - Follicular pattern (resembles dental follicle)
    - Variably sized islands of odontogenic epithelium whose peripheral palisading tall columnar cells display reverse nuclear polarity and subnuclear vacuoles
    - Fibrous connective tissue stroma surrounds epithelial islands
    - Nuclei are uniform with no mitotic activity
    - Centers of islands have loose-textured stellate epithelial cells, often with microcyst formation
  - Plexiform pattern
    - Broad anastomosing sheets of cells with stellate epithelium at center; peripheral cells are tall columnar with reverse nuclear polarity and subnuclear vacuoles
    - Stroma is looser and can have cyst formation

— Acanthomatous pattern
  ◆ Follicular islands show squamous metaplasia or cytokeratin production
- All ameloblastomas, except for the desmoplastic variant, have mature fibrous stroma; in desmoplastic variant, stromal osteoid production is seen
- Most important prognostic feature is presence or absence of infiltration
- Histologic subtypes do not influence treatment or prognosis

Special Stains and Immunohistochemistry

- Noncontributory

Other Techniques for Diagnosis

- Noncontributory

Differential Diagnosis

❚ Ameloblastic fibroma
- Benign mixed tumor of epithelial-mesenchymal odontogenic neoplasm
- Connective tissue resembles dental papilla
- Epithelial nests of cuboidal to columnar cells with stellate reticulum
- Well-defined basement membrane
- Most in posterior mandible
❚ SCC
- Markedly atypical squamous cells with an infiltrative growth pattern
- Mitoses frequently identified
❚ Basal cell carcinoma
- Desmoplastic stroma
- Often history of prior skin cancer
- Mitoses may be noted
❚ Salivary-type adenocarcinomas
- Rarely primary intraosseous
- Reverse polarization of epithelium not usually seen

Pearls

- Recurrence rate of infiltrating ameloblastomas treated surgically by curettage is high (up to 90%); important to excise with adequate bone margin
- Grows slowly; recurrences may take several years to become radiographically apparent; can recur many years after treatment

Selected References

Chen Y, Wang JM, Li TJ: Ameloblastic fibroma: A review of published studies with special reference to its nature and biological behavior. Oral Oncol 43:960-969, 2007.

Melrose RJ: Benign epithelial odontogenic tumors. Semin Diagn Pathol 16:271-287, 1999.

Feinberg SE, Steinberg B: Surgical management of ameloblastoma: Current status of the literature. Oral Surg Oral Med Oral Pathol 81:383-388, 1996.

Reichart PA, Philopsen HP, Sommer S: Ameloblastoma: Biologic profile of 3677 cases. Eur J Cancer 31B:86-99, 1995.

Calcifying Epithelial Odontogenic Tumor (Pindborg Tumor)

Clinical Features

- Presents as a slow-growing mass with few symptoms; jaw swelling or resorption of teeth may be seen
- Usual age between 30 and 50 years
- No gender predilection
- Most occur in posterior mandible, 25% in the maxilla
- May rarely be extraosseous

Figure 3-69. Calcifying epithelial odontogenic tumor. A, Radiograph of radiolucent mass with fine granular opacifications between two teeth. **B,** Histologic section shows sheets of epithelial cells and calcifications.

- Association with impacted tooth in about 50% of cases
- Radiographically, a poorly demarcated, multilocular radiolucency

Gross Pathology

- Generally a solid mass with variable amount of calcification
- Cortical thinning of bone, but rarely invasion beyond periosteum

Histopathology

- Sheets of large polyhedral epithelial cells often displaying intercellular bridges
- Cells have abundant eosinophilic cytoplasm, pleomorphic nuclei with prominent nucleoli, and intranuclear pseudoinclusions; cells may be binucleated
- No mitosis, necrosis, or inflammation
- Characteristic concentric ring calcifications (Liesegang rings)
- Occasionally pink, amorphous, amyloid-like material present, typically scant stromal fibrosis

Special Stains and Immunohistochemistry

- Congo red positive (amyloid-like material has apple-green birefringence under polarized light)

Other Techniques for Diagnosis

- Noncontributory

Differential Diagnosis

▌ SCC

- Invasive growth pattern
- Cells show cytologic features of malignancy; associated squamous dysplasia in adjacent squamous epithelium is often seen

Pearls

- Even small tumors are infiltrating
- Surgical resection should have adequate bone margin of at least 1 cm
- Recurrence rate is 14%; recurrences are slow growing, and long follow-up is recommended

Selected References

Veness MJ, Morgan G, Collins AP, Walker DM: Calcifying epithelial odontogenic (Pindborg) tumor with malignant transformation and metastatic spread. Head Neck 23:692-696, 2001.

Philipsen HP, Reichart PA: Calcifying epithelial odontogenic tumour: Biological profile based on 181 cases from the literature. Oral Oncol 36:17-26, 2000.

Franlin CD, Pindborg JJ: The calcifying epithelial odontogenic tumor: A review and analysis of 113 cases. Oral Surg Oral Med Oral Pathol 42:753-765, 1976.

Adenomatoid Odontogenic Tumor

Clinical Features

- Uncommon benign lesion
- Typically found in second decade of life
- Female-to-male ratio of 2:1
- Twice as common in maxilla as in mandible
- Predilection for anterior part of both jaws; canine location accounts for about 60% of cases
- Most cases are associated with an impacted tooth; rarely extraosseous
- Radiographically, well-demarcated radiolucency with or without associated impacted tooth

Gross Pathology

- Thick fibrous capsule with abundant gray to white tissue in the center
- Small calcifications give cut surface a gritty feel

Figure 3-70. Adenomatoid odontogenic tumor. A, Radiograph of well-demarcated translucent area of the maxilla with associated impacted tooth. **B,** Microscopic examination shows a neoplasm composed of ductlike spaces in epithelial nests surrounded by solid areas of ameloblast-like fibroblasts.

- May present as a thick-walled cyst with small amount of fluid and a soft, shaggy surface

Histopathology

- Thick fibrous capsule surrounds variably sized nodular areas of epithelium composed of cuboidal or low columnar cells with virtually no connective tissue stroma
- Dystrophic calcification is often associated with the epithelial cell nodules
- Ductlike spaces within epithelial cell nodules contain an amorphous eosinophilic material that does not stain for amyloid but may be an abortive enamel-like product

Special Stains and Immunohistochemistry

- Noncontributory

Other Techniques for Diagnosis

- Noncontributory

Differential Diagnosis

▌ Ameloblastoma
- More commonly found in the posterior mandible (80%)
- Different radiologic appearance
- Typically has a follicular architecture characterized by islands of odontogenic epithelium in a fibrous connective tissue stroma

Pearls

- Prognosis is excellent
- Conservative surgical excision (enucleation) is curative; recurrence is exceptionally rare

Selected References

Rick GM: Adenomatoid odontogenic tumor. Oral Maxillofac Surg Clin N Am 16:333-354, 2004.
Philipsen HP, Reichart PA: Adenomatoid odontogenic tumor: Facts and figures. Oral Oncol 35:125-131, 1998.

Benign Cementoblastoma

Clinical Features

- Rare benign mesenchymal odontogenic tumor
- Slow growing and can reach a large size
- Intimately associated with roots of teeth
- Mostly young adults but may occur in any age
- Most commonly mandibular first molar and premolars
- Typically presents with pain (reminiscent of osteoblastoma)
- Radiographically, well-defined radiopaque mass obliterating the root of the involved tooth and with a peripheral thin radiolucent zone

Gross Pathology

- Calcified mass adherent to the root of affected tooth

Histopathology

- Calcified cemental tissue deposition on a tooth root
- Thick trabeculae of cementum strongly basophilic with numerous irregular reversal lines resembling Paget bone; trabeculae rimmed with active cementoblasts
- Periphery shows radiating columns of cementoid with interspersed fibrovascular tissue
- Dilated vascular spaces and osteoclast-like giant cells are occasionally seen

Special Stains and Immunohistochemistry

- Noncontributory

Other Techniques for Diagnosis

- Noncontributory

Differential Diagnosis

▌ Osteoblastoma of the jaw
- May envelop roots of teeth but does not originate from the cementum of the root surface

Pearls

- Treatment is surgical excision with extraction of affected tooth

Selected References

El-Mofty SK: Cemento-ossifying fibroma and benign cementoblastoma. Semin Diagn Pathol 16:302-307, 1999.
Melrose RJ: Benign epithelial odontogenic tumors. Semin Diagn Pathol 16:271-287, 1999.
Ulmansky M, Hansen EH, Praetorius F: Benign cemento-blastoma: A review and five new cases. Oral Surg Oral Med Oral Pathol 77:48-55, 1994.

Chondrosarcoma

Clinical Features

- Most common site is the pelvis, also in the proximal femur and humerus
- Rarely occurs in the jaw but has predilection for the maxilla and skull base
- Chondrosarcomas may be primary or secondary (arising from enchondromas or osteochondromas)
- Classified into central, peripheral, or juxtacortical tumors depending on location and radiographic characteristics
- More common in men than women (2:1); peak incidence in third to sixth decades, two decades earlier for secondary chondrosarcomas

Figure 3-71. Benign cementoblastoma. A, Radiograph showing a well-defined mass with a peripheral radiolucent zone associated with the tooth root. **B,** Whole-mount section of the corresponding resected specimen with tooth and mass at the root. **C,** Histologic section shows dense bony trabeculae with intervening proliferative fibrovascular tissue.

Gross Pathology

- Central chondrosarcomas grow intramedullarly and may extend into cortical bone
- Peripheral chondrosarcomas grow from the cortex of the bone into soft tissue; may grow into medullary cavity
- Cut surface is white to bluish-gray depending on amount of cartilage
- May be cystic and have myxoid or gelatinous areas; hemorrhage, necrosis, and calcification may be seen

Histopathology

- Composed of conventional, mesenchymal, and dedifferentiated subtypes
- Variable histology depending on amount of chondroid matrix
  - Conventional
    - Irregular lobules of cartilage separated by fibrous strands and invade bone; higher cellularity at the periphery of the lobules

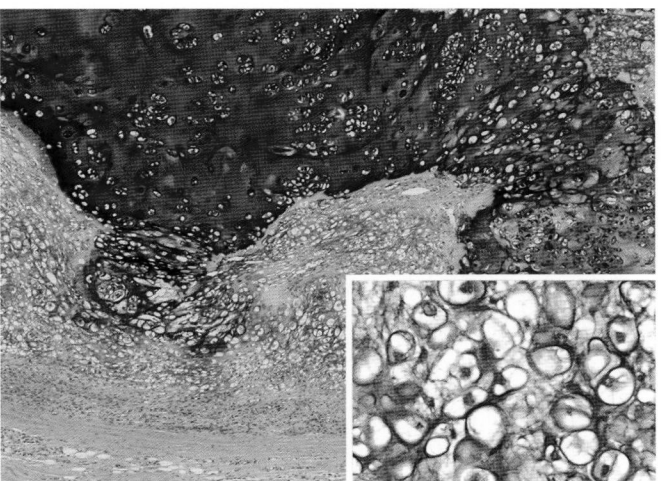

Figure 3-72. Chondrosarcoma. Section shows a lobulated mass composed of variably cellular neoplastic chondrocytes. At high power (*inset*), the chondrocytes have open, large nuclei.

- ◆ Chondrocytes in clusters; atypia varies from slight nuclear enlargement to large, bizarre nuclei
- ◆ Multinucleated chondrocytes may be seen
- ◆ Higher-grade tumors have increased cytologic atypia; grade 3 findings of peripheral spindling or >2 mitoses/10 hpf
- ◆ Mitotic activity is not present in grade I tumors
— Mesenchymal
  - ◆ Spindle cells or small blue cells intermixed with hyaline cartilage
  - ◆ Rare subtype, third decade
  - ◆ Propensity for jawbones
— Dedifferentiated
  - ◆ Two distinct tumor components: chondrosarcoma component (often grade I) and dedifferentiated malignant spindle cell areas that mimic fibrosarcoma or osteosarcoma

Special Stains and Immunohistochemistry

- Noncontributory

Other Techniques for Diagnosis

- Noncontributory

Differential Diagnoses

- ▌ Chondroblastic osteosarcoma
  - May have areas of cartilage but also has atypical osteoblasts and abnormal osteoid formation (irregular, lacelike)
  - May be confused with osseous metaplasia or reactive osteoid within a chondrosarcoma
  - Pure hyaline (without myxoid) frequently in chondrosarcomas, less in osteosarcoma
- ▌ Chondroma
  - Should be distinguished from grade I chondrosarcoma
  - Does not have bony or fibrous trabeculae or islands of bone within cartilage
- ▌ Chordoma
  - Strong predilection for the axial skeleton, particularly the spheno-occipital region
  - Peak incidence in third to fifth decades
  - Radiographically, appears as an expansible, destructive mass, often extending outside of the bone
  - Microscopically, lobules and cords of large cells with low N/C ratio and characteristic vacuolated cytoplasm (physaliferous cells) within myxoid matrix
  - Chondroid type chordoma can be differentiated based on immunohistochemical characteristics: positive for cytokeratin, EMA, Brachyury (notochord) origin marker, and S-100 protein

Pearls

- Metastatic sites are lungs, skin, and soft tissue
- Complete surgical excision should be performed; prognosis depends on stage and histologic grade; metastases are uncommon for grade I chondrosarcomas, but about 70% of grade III chondrosarcomas metastasize; recurrences are often of a higher histologic grade
- Radiologic correlation is crucial

Selected References

Pellitteri PK, Ferlito A, Fagan JJ, et al: Mesenchymal chondrosarcoma of the head and neck. Oral Oncol 43:970-975, 2007.

Thompson LD, Gannon FH: Chondrosarcoma of the larynx: A clinicopathologic study of 111 cases with a review of the literature. Am J Surg Pathol 26:836-851, 2002.

Jeffrey PB, Biava CG, Davis RL: Chondroid chordoma: A hyalinized chordoma without cartilaginous differentiation. Am J Clin Pathol 103:271-279, 1995.

Saito K, Unni KK, Wollan PC, Lund BA: Chondrosarcoma of the jaw and facial bones. Cancer 76:1550-1558, 1995.

Osteosarcoma

Clinical Features

- Rare tumor in the jaw region, constitutes about 5% of all osteosarcomas
- May have predilection for the mandible or equal to maxilla
- Maxillary tumors occur, particularly at alveolar ridge
- Most cases are de novo; may be associated with radiation, Paget disease, and fibrous dysplasia (secondary osteosarcomas)
- Most tumors arise from the medullary cavity or, rarely, periosteum of the jaws (juxtacortical osteosarcomas)

Figure 3-73. Osteosarcoma. Chondroblastic variant with lobules of malignant cartilage. Osteoid is identified within the tumor (*inset*).

- Osteosarcomas of the jaw occur at an older age (third to fourth decades), and swelling, pain, and paresthesias are typical
- Radiographic presentation ranges from radiolucent to radiopaque with classic sunburst pattern
- Jaw osteosarcomas tend to be better differentiated (grade 2-3) than appendicular osteosarcomas
- Genetic predisposition to osteosarcomas in children with familial bilateral retinoblastoma

Gross Pathology

- Cut surface is firm and tan-yellow with bony destruction often into surrounding soft tissue
- Translucent areas (chondroid matrix), hemorrhage, and necrosis may be seen

Histopathology

- Most osteosarcomas of the jaw are chondroblastic
- All osteosarcoma variants in the jaw have histologic features similar to those of osteosarcomas in the appendicular skeleton
  — Chondroblastic (50%-60% of cases)
    ◆ Predominance of malignant-appearing chondroid areas with focal osteoid deposition
    ◆ Chondroid differentiation varies in cellularity and lobulation and may be myxoid
  — Fibroblastic (approximately 25% of cases)
    ◆ Malignant spindle cells, variable cellularity; matrix may be scant
    ◆ May mimic fibrosarcoma
  — Osteoblastic (approximately 20% of cases)
    ◆ Predominance of malignant osteoid, which is irregular with a lacelike filigree pattern
    ◆ Variable mineralization of the osteoid

  — Teleangiectatic (rare)
    ◆ Composed of dilated blood-filled spaces separated by cellular septa containing malignant cells with a high mitotic rate
    ◆ Haphazard distribution of osteoid deposition

Special Stains and Immunohistochemistry

- Noncontributory

Other Techniques for Diagnosis

- Noncontributory

Differential Diagnoses

▪ Chondrosarcoma
  - May be difficult to differentiate from chondroblastic variant
  - Less common in mandible
  - Tumor-forming osteoid is absent
▪ Myxoid and salivary neoplasms
  - Relationship to bone should be considered; radiographic correlation
  - Keep chondroblastic osteosarcoma in differential
  - Search for osteoid is warranted
▪ Ossifying fibroma
  - Often hypercellular, composed of uniform cells lacking nuclear pleomorphism
  - Radiologic features are classic and reliably distinguish these entities
▪ Osteoblastoma
  - Well-defined mass characterized by irregular trabeculae of osteoid and woven bone with vascularized stroma
  - Lacks nuclear pleomorphism
  - Cartilaginous areas are rare

Pearls

- Jaw osteosarcomas are most often chondroblastic
- May mimic myxoid or salivary neoplasms
- Treatment of osteosarcoma of the jaw is surgery; role of chemotherapy is unclear
- Radiologic correlation is of paramount importance in the diagnosis of both cartilaginous and bony lesions

Selected References

Sturgis EM, Potter BO: Sarcomas of the head and neck region. Curr Opin Oncol 15:239-252, 2003.

Kassir RR, Rassekh CH, Kinsella JB, et al: Osteosarcoma of the head and neck: Meta-analysis of nonrandomized studies. Laryngoscope 107:56-61, 1997.

Garrington GE, Scofield HH, Cornyn J, Hooker SP: Osteosarcoma of the jaws: Analysis of 56 cases. Cancer 20:377-391, 1996.

Hadjipavlou A, Lander P, Srolovitz H, Enker IP. Malignant transformation of Paget disease of the bone. Cancer 70:2802-2803, 1992.

Mark RJ, Sercarz JA, Tran L, et al: Osteogenic sarcoma of the head and neck: The UCLA experience. Arch Otolaryngol Head Neck Surg 117:761-766, 1991.

Squamous Cell Carcinoma

Clinical Features

- Predisposing factors are smoking, tobacco, immunosuppression (in organ transplant recipients), mechanical irritation, and sun exposure
- Predominantly affects men older than 50 years, but incidence in younger patients and women is increasing
- Other high-risk areas are floor of mouth and ventrolateral tongue
- Patients have 100-fold increased risk for developing a second primary in the region
- May be multiple; if so, tongue is most commonly affected
- HIV infection: oropharyngeal and tonsillar cancer

Figure 3-74. Squamous cell carcinoma. A, Gross examination of a hemiglossectomy specimen shows a large tumor ulcerating the mucosa of the tongue and deeply invading into skeletal muscle. **B,** An infiltrating neoplasm is present composed of sheets of keratinizing epithelial cells with hyperchromatic nuclei.

Gross Pathology

- Irregular mucosal surface with red granular areas
- Cut surface is tan-white with occasional areas of necrosis or hemorrhage

Histopathology

- Aggressive features: finger-like invasive fronts
- Similar to SCCs in other locations: usually moderately to poorly differentiated
- Epithelium adjacent to invasive tumor often shows carcinoma in situ or varying degrees of squamous dysplasia (field cancerization)
- Perineural invasion

Special Stains and Immunohistochemistry

- Cytokeratin positive: express CK5/6, CK8, and CK19 but are CK20 negative
- Overexpression of *TP53* oncogene in 30% to 50% of cases

Other Techniques for Diagnosis

- Nondiploid tumors are typically more advanced clinically than diploid tumors
- In multiple tumors, TP53 expression is similar, and they are also clonal by karyotypic and FISH analysis
- Loss of heterozygosity (LOH) of TP53 by PCR in 70% of tumors

Differential Diagnosis

▌ Verrucous carcinoma
  - Low-grade variant of SCC
  - Most common in oral cavity (buccal mucosa and lower gingiva)
  - Elderly men more commonly affected
  - Associated with chewing tobacco
  - Grossly large soft papillary tumor
  - Locally aggressive but does not metastasize
  - Characteristically bland cytologic appearance
  - Treatment is surgical because radiation therapy may change the tumor into highly malignant, poorly differentiated, and metastasizing SCC

▌ Nasopharyngeal carcinoma
  - Rare in United States; SCC arising in the nasopharynx, associated with EBV infection
  - Characterized by neoplastic epithelial cells with an intense infiltrate of lymphoid cells

Pearls

- Main prognostic factors are stage, location, depth of invasion, and close margins (<5mm)
- Occasionally, cervical lymph node metastases undergo cystic degeneration or elicit foreign-body giant cell reaction to keratin (can be mistaken for branchial cleft cyst with malignant transformation)

- Lymph nodes with extranodal extension increase recurrence and metastases

Selected References

Cardesa A, Gale N, Nadal A, et al: Squamous cell carcinoma: Verrucous carcinoma. Basaloid squamous cell carcinoma. In Barnes EL, Eveson JW, Reichart P, Sidransky D (eds): World Health Organization Classification of Tumours: Pathology and Genetics: Head and Neck Tumours. Lyon, IARC Press, 2005, pp 118-125.

Wu M, Putti TC, Bhuiya TA: Comparative study in the expression of p53, EGFR, TGF-alpha, and cyclin D1 in verrucous carcinoma, verrucous hyperplasia, and squamous cell carcinoma of head and neck region. Appl Immunohistochem Mol Morphol 10:351-356, 2002.

Koch BB, Trask DK, Hoffman HT, et al: National survey of head and neck verrucous carcinoma: Patterns of presentation, care, and outcome. Cancer 92:110-120, 2001.

Suarez PA, Adler-Storthz K, Luna MA, et al: Papillary squamous cell carcinomas of the upper aerodigestive tract: A clinicopathologic and molecular study. Head Neck 22:360-368, 2000.

Shah JP, Candela FC, Poddar AK: The patterns of cervical lymph node metastases from squamous carcinoma of the oral cavity. Cancer 66:109-113, 1990.

Tumors Metastasizing to the Oral Cavity

Clinical Features

- May present as primary intraoral lesions, most commonly involving the gingiva
- Most common primary tumor site is lung
- Other common primary sites include kidney, breast, skin, prostate, endometrium, and colon

Figure 3-75. Metastasis (renal cell carcinoma) to tongue. Gross photograph shows a submucosal lobulated mass with variable gray translucent to more solid areas.

Gross Pathology

- Gingival nodules
- Cut section varies depending on primary tumor: renal cell carcinoma metastasis may be very hemorrhagic; metastatic colonic tumors may have central areas of necrosis

Histopathology

- Depends on the original tumor cell type and grade

Special Stains and Immunohistochemistry

- Carcinomas: cytokeratin positive
- Renal cell carcinoma: cytokeratin and vimentin positive, contains intracytoplasmic fat but no glycogen (PAS and D-PAS positive)
- Prostate: prostate-specific antigen (PSA) positive (may be lost with treatment)
- Breast: may be positive for *HER-2-neu*, estrogen receptor, progesterone receptor

Other Techniques for Diagnosis

- Noncontributory

Differential Diagnosis

- Metastatic lung, renal cell, colonic, endometrial, breast, prostate carcinoma
- Metastatic melanoma
  - Large polygonal cells with variably pleomorphic nuclei and prominent nucleoli
  - Positive for S-100 protein and HMB-45

Pearls

- Unusual cell type or growth pattern should suggest possibility of a metastasis

Selected References

Hirshberg A, Shnaiderman-Shapiro A, Kaplan I, Berger R: Metastatic tumours to the oral cavity: Pathogenesis and analysis of 673 cases. Oral Oncol 44:743-752, 2008.

Baden E, Duvillard P, Micheau C: Metastatic papillary endometrial carcinoma of the tongue: Case report and review of the literature. Arch Pathol Lab Med 116:965-968, 1992.

Larynx

Laryngeal (Vocal Cord) Nodule or Polyp

Clinical Features

- Also called *singers' nodule*
- Typically develops after prolonged misuse or overuse of voice
- Occurs most commonly in adult men as well as singers and smokers
- Most common on anterior third of vocal cord
- Patients present with hoarseness

Figure 3-76. Vocal cord nodule. Squamous mucosa is present with underlying hyalinized and vascular stroma.

Gross Pathology

- Round, polypoid, often pedunculated whitish nodule on the vocal cord

Histopathology

- Classified as telangiectatic or gelatinous polyps
  — Telangiectatic form
    ◆ Numerous thin-walled vessels in a loose, collagenous stroma
    ◆ Mixed chronic inflammatory exudate in stroma
  — Gelatinous form
    ◆ Nodule composed of scattered fibroblasts, fibrin, and loose, edematous stroma with less obvious thin-walled vessels
- Both are polypoid nodules covered by an intact overlying stratified squamous epithelium
- Hemosiderin deposition is common in long-standing lesions

Special Stains and Immunohistochemistry

- Noncontributory

Other Techniques for Diagnosis

- Noncontributory

Differential Diagnosis

▌Juvenile laryngeal papillomas
- Papillary squamous papillomas with or without koilocytosis
- Immunohistochemical or molecular tests for HPV
- Propensity for recurrence

▌Contact ulcer, granulomatous ulcer
- Typically affects the posterior commissure of vocal cord
- Exuberant granulation tissue and ulceration of overlying squamous epithelium

Pearls

- Florid papillary endothelial hyperplasia can be mistaken for angiosarcoma
- Eosinophilic, proteinaceous material may resemble amyloid but negative staining for Congo red
- Small lesions may regress with voice rest; larger ones often need to be surgically excised
- No association with subsequent development of carcinoma

Selected References

Barnes L: Diseases of the larynx, hypopharynx, and esophagus. In Barnes L (ed): Surgical Pathology of the Head and Neck. New York, Marcel Dekker, 2001, pp 128-132.

McFerran DJ, Abdullah V, Gallimore AP, et al: Vocal process granulomata. J Laryngol Otol 108:216-220, 1994.

Wenig BM, Heffner DK: Contact ulcers of the larynx: A re-acquaintance with the pathology of an often under-diagnosed entity. Arch Pathol Lab Med 114:825-828, 1990.

Kleinsasser O: Pathogenesis of vocal cord polyps. Ann Otol Rhinol Laryngol 91:378-381, 1982.

Laryngeal Papilloma

Clinical Features

- Papillary exophytic squamous epithelial proliferation of the true vocal cords; may also occur in the larynx, oropharynx, and trachea
- Two types: juvenile and adult type
  — Juvenile type
    ◆ Presents in children or adolescents
    ◆ Typically multiple and occurs on true vocal cords
    ◆ Tends to spread to epiglottic and subglottic area, rarely trachea and bronchi
  — Adult type
    ◆ Male predominance
    ◆ Typically solitary
    ◆ Infrequently recurrent
- Etiology: HPV, particularly types 6 and 11

Gross Pathology

- Polypoid soft lesions, variably sized

Histopathology

- Squamous cell papillary proliferation with fibrovascular core, acanthosis, and koilocytosis (HPV effect)
- Mild chronic inflammation and hyperemia of submucosa
- Epithelial atypia may be seen; grade dysplasia if present

Special Stains and Immunohistochemistry

- Noncontributory

Figure 3-77. Respiratory papillomatosis. A, Specimen photograph of extensive exophytic growths (papillomas) covering the laryngeal and tracheal surfaces. **B,** Histologic section shows squamous epithelium with hyperplasia in broad sheets with fibrovascular cords.

Other Techniques for Diagnosis

- In situ and PCR-based techniques for HPV

Differential Diagnosis

▌ SCC

- Invasive growth pattern, desmoplastic stroma
- Cytologic atypia, dyskeratosis

Pearls

- Papillomas with dysplasia or solitary lesions, should be followed closely or surgically excised to rule out invasive carcinoma

- Respiratory papillomas (juvenile and adult) are multiple with propensity for recurrences and a small but definite risk for developing SCC
- Risk for SCC is strongly linked to previous radiation

Selected References

Lele SM, Pou AM, Ventura K, et al: Molecular events in the progression of recurrent respiratory papillomatosis to carcinoma. Arch Pathol Lab Med 126:1184-1188, 2002.

Penaloza-Plascencia M, Montoya-Fuentes H, Flores-Martinez SE, et al: Molecular identification of 7 human papillomavirus types in recurrent respiratory papillomatosis. Arch Otolaryngol Head Neck Surg 126:1119-1123, 2000.

Rimell F, Maisel R, Dayton V: In situ hybridization and laryngeal papillomas. Ann Otol Rhinol Laryngol 101:119-126, 1992.

Lindeberg H, Elbrond O: Laryngeal papillomas: Clinical aspects in a series of 231 patients. Clin Otolaryngol 14:333-342, 1989.

Amyloidosis of the Larynx

Clinical Features

- Uncommon; less than 1% of benign nodules of the larynx
- Most often false cord; may be bilateral or involve true cords
- Usually localized disease; may be familial, secondary, or part of systemic disease
- Laryngeal amyloid in most cases consists of immunoglobulin light chains and is classified as a fibril type similar to primary amyloid
- Hoarseness is often the presenting clinical symptom

Gross Pathology

- Cut surface: firm, translucent, homogeneous tan to red-brown nodule

Figure 3-78. Amyloidosis of larynx. Section shows squamous mucosa with submucosal deposits of amorphous eosinophilic material (amyloid).

Histopathology

- Submucosal amorphous, acellular, eosinophilic material; often perivascular and periglandular
- Chronic inflammatory infiltrate, including plasma cells, histiocytes, and few giant cells

Special Stains and Immunohistochemistry

- Congo red: amyloid displays apple-green birefringence with polarized light

Other Techniques for Diagnosis

- Noncontributory

Differential Diagnosis

▋ Vocal cord nodule
- Amyloid stains are negative

Selected References

Thompson LDR, Derringer GA, Wenig BM: Amyloidosis of the larynx: A clinicopathologic study of 11 cases. Mod Pathol 13:528-535, 2000.

Ferrara G, Boscaino A: Nodular amyloidosis of the larynx. Pathologica 87:94-96, 1995.

Cohen SR: Ligneous conjunctivitis: An ophthalmic disease with potentially fatal tracheobronchial obstruction. Laryngeal and tracheobronchial features. Ann Otol Rhinol Laryngol 90:509-518, 1990.

Richards SH, Bull PD: Lipoid proteinosis of the larynx. J Laryngol Otol 87:187-190, 1973.

Squamous Cell Carcinoma of the Larynx

Clinical Features

- Accounts for 0.4% and 1.3% of carcinomas in women and men, respectively
- Risk factors: smoking and alcohol abuse
- HPV may be associated with a very small number of cases (<5%)
- Locations: supraglottic, glottic, and subglottic sites (different lymphatic drainage)
- Glottic carcinomas (two thirds), most arise anteriorly on the mobile portion of the vocal cord; least common is the subglottic location
- Clinically, hoarseness, mass cause pain, dysphagia, and hemoptysis

Gross Pathology

- Exophytic, fungating lesions of variable sizes, often ulcerated and necrotic

Histopathology

- Premalignant epithelial lesions may border the tumor
- Graded: well, moderately, and poorly differentiated squamous carcinoma based on the degree of cytologic atypia, mitotic activity, and presence of keratin pearl formation
- Most are moderately differentiated

Figure 3-79. Squamous cell carcinoma of larynx. A, Gross photograph of an exophytic and ulcerated glottic tumor. **B,** Histologic section shows an infiltrating neoplasm composed of nests and anastomosing cords of invasive atypical squamous cells with focal keratin pearl formation.

- Subtypes include
  - Nonkeratinizing SCC
    - ◆ Often seen in the supraglottic location
    - ◆ More often has pushing rather than infiltrative margins
  - Verrucous SCC
    - ◆ Markedly keratinized, well-differentiated tumor that is wartlike on low power
    - ◆ Cytologic features are bland, but tumor is locally destructive

Figure 3-80. **Verrucous squamous cell carcinoma. A,** Gross photograph of a broad exophytic epithelial proliferation. **B,** Broad pushing base of squamous epithelium with maturation.

Figure 3-82. **Spindle cell squamous cell carcinoma (sarcomatoid carcinoma). A,** Histologic section showing a cellular spindled neoplasm with cellular atypia and nuclear hyperchromasia. **B,** Cytokeratin immunohistochemical stain highlights some of the tumor cells supporting epithelial origin.

Figure 3-81. **Basaloid squamous cell carcinoma.** Nests of basaloid epithelial cells often with central necrosis and occasional abrupt keratin formation.

- ◆ Parakeratosis is abundant; orthokeratotic squamous cells
- ◆ Broad and sharply demarcated base with bland-appearing squamous epithelium
- ◆ Limited metastatic potential
- — Basaloid SCC
  - ◆ Basaloid cells in nests and cords
  - ◆ Hyaline basement membrane
  - ◆ Often with central necrosis
  - ◆ Minor and localized abrupt keratinization
- — Spindle cell SCC (sarcomatoid carcinoma)
  - ◆ Rare variant
  - ◆ Prominent spindle cell, sarcoma-like with associated minor component of conventional squamous carcinoma
  - ◆ May show metaplastic features and heterologous elements

Special Stains and Immunohistochemistry

- Cytokeratin, for sarcomatoid variant, positive (may be weak or focal in basaloid variant)

Other Techniques for Diagnosis

- Noncontributory

Differential Diagnoses

▎ Verrucous hyperplasia
- Exophytic, noninvasive
- Rete ridges broad
- Stroma may have chronic inflammatory cells
- Cytologic features of squamous epithelium are bland and well differentiated

▎ Squamous papilloma
- Noninvasive, papillary, proliferation of mature squamous cells with or without acanthosis and koilocytosis (HPV effect) overlying thin fibrovascular cores
- Fibrovascular cores are covered by an orderly, stratified squamous epithelium

Pearls

- Prognosis varies with
  - Location: best for glottic, then supraglottic, and worst for subglottic tumors
  - Size: if larger than 2 cm, 40% chance of metastasis
  - Grade: worse prognosis with high-grade tumors
  - Tumor margin: the farther away the surgical margin is from the tumor, the higher the survival rate
- Increased risk for developing other secondary malignancies (often elsewhere in the head and neck or respiratory tract)
- Nonkeratinizing SCC occurs more often in the supraglottic location and spreads along the mucosal surface
- Basaloid SCC typically has poor prognosis; often at an advanced stage when detected

Selected References

Thompson LD, Wieneke JA, Miettinen M, Heffner DK: Spindle cell (sarcomatoid) carcinomas of the larynx: A clinicopathologic study of 187 cases. Am J Surg Pathol 26:153-170, 2002.

Thompson LD, Wenig BM, Heffner DK, Gnepp DR: Exophytic and papillary squamous cell carcinomas of the larynx: A clinicopathologic series of 104 cases. Otolaryngol Head Neck Surg 120:718-724, 1999.

Jovanovic A, van der Tol IG, Schulten EA, et al: Risk of multiple primary tumors following oral squamous cell carcinoma. Int J Cancer 56:320-323, 1994.

Wiernik G, Millard PR, Haybittle JL: The predictive value of histological classification into degrees of differentiation of squamous cell carcinoma of the larynx and hypopharynx

compared with survival of patients. Histopathology 619:411-417, 1991.

Neuroendocrine Carcinoma of the Larynx

Clinical Features

- Classified into carcinoid, atypical carcinoid, and neuroendocrine carcinoma
- Rare (make up less than 1% of all laryngeal malignancies)
- Typically found in men in sixth and seventh decades
- Occurs more often in smokers
- Patients typically present with hoarseness

Figure 3-83. Atypical carcinoid (neuroendocrine carcinoma) of the larynx. An infiltrating cellular mass is present with a trabecular pattern. At higher power (*inset*), nuclei with speckled chromatin is appreciated.

Figure 3-84. Paraganglioma of the larynx. Rare in this location, paragangliomas show classic nested (Zellenballen) growth pattern of neuroendocrine cells (*inset*) surrounded by delicate fibrovascular septae. Focal embolization material is present (*left*).

Gross Pathology

- Submucosal, polypoid mass usually 2 to 4 cm
- Often ulcerated if large

Histopathology

- Carcinoid
  - Tumor cells arranged in nests and cords surrounded by delicate fibrovascular stroma
  - Uniform cytologic features with moderate eosinophilic, finely granular cytoplasm and nuclei with finely granular chromatin
  - Low mitotic rate and no necrosis
- Atypical carcinoid
  - More common in the larynx than typical carcinoid
  - Similar architecture to carcinoid but has higher mitotic activity (2 to 10/10 hpf) and small foci of necrosis
- Neuroendocrine carcinoma
  - Diffuse pattern of growth consisting of small to intermediate-sized cells with hyperchromatic nuclei, inconspicuous nucleoli, scant cytoplasm, and ill-defined cytoplasmic borders; prominent nuclear molding
  - High mitotic rate (more than 10/10 hpf) and often extensive necrosis

Special Stains and Immunohistochemistry

- Neuroendocrine markers (synaptophysin, chromogranin) positive
- Cytokeratin positive

Other Techniques for Diagnosis

- Noncontributory

Differential Diagnosis

▮ Malignant melanoma
  - Other melanoma markers (melan-A, HMB-45) should be used because S-100 protein can be positive in neuroendocrine carcinomas
▮ Metastatic or locally invasive medullary carcinoma
  - History of primary medullary carcinoma
  - Serum calcitonin elevation
  - TTF-1 usually expressed in medullary (thyroid origin)
▮ Paraganglioma
  - S-100 protein positive sustentacular cells
  - Keratin is negative
  - Positive for neuroendocrine markers

Pearls

- Biologic behavior of small cell neuroendocrine tumor is similar to that in the lung
- Poor prognostic features include lymph node metastases, vascular invasion, and positive margins
- Carcinoids are treated surgically
- Neuroendocrine carcinoma multimodality therapy

Selected References

Gillenwater A, Lewin J, Roberts D, El-Naggar AK: Moderately differentiated neuroendocrine carcinoma (atypical carcinoid) of the larynx: A clinically aggressive tumor. Laryngoscope 115:1191-1195, 2005.

Hirsch MS, Faquin WC, Krane JF: Thyroid transcription factor-1, but no p53, is helpful in distinguishing moderately differentiated neuroendocrine carcinoma of the larynx from medullary carcinoma of the thyroid. Mod Pathol 17:631-636, 2004.

Soga J, Osaka M, Yakuwa Y: Laryngeal endocrinomas (carcinoids and relevant neoplasms): Analysis of 278 reported cases. J Exp Clin Cancer Res 21:5-13, 2002.

Ferlito A, Barnes L, Rinaldo A, et al: A review of neuroendocrine neoplasms of the larynx: Update on diagnosis and treatment. J Laryngol Otol 112:827-834, 1998.

Batsakis JG, El-Naggar AK, Luna MA: Neuroendocrine tumors of larynx. Ann Otol Rhinol Laryngol 101:710-714, 1992.

Mills SE, Cooper PH, Garland TA, Johns ME: Small cell undifferentiated carcinoma of the larynx: Report of two patients and review of 13 additional cases. Cancer 51:116-120, 1983.

Trachea

Classification of Tracheal Malignancies

- SCC most common in the lower third; poor prognosis
- Salivary-type carcinoma (adenoid cystic carcinoma) arising in the upper third is second in frequency
- Small cell carcinoma, carcinoid tumor, and adenocarcinoma are rare

Figure 3-85. Squamous cell carcinoma of trachea. Gross photograph of a squamous cell carcinoma filling the tracheal lumen.

Figure 3-86. Adenoid cystic carcinoma of trachea. A, Gross photograph of a polypoid submucosal mass in the trachea. **B,** The tumor cells are growing in tubules beneath the respiratory mucosa.

Squamous Cell Carcinoma

Gross Pathology
- Variably sized, exophytic, ulcerated lesions

Histopathology
- Similar to squamous carcinomas at other sites

Special Stains and Immunohistochemistry
- Noncontributory

Other Techniques for Diagnosis
- Noncontributory

Differential Diagnoses
▌ Papilloma and papillomatosis of the trachea
- Microscopic features are similar to lesions seen in the larynx
- In general, those associated with laryngeal papillomatosis begin in childhood and have lower incidence of malignant transformation than those cases with only bronchial and tracheal involvement

▌ Nonsquamous lesions
- Minor salivary tumors
- Metastases

Pearls
- Tumors involving the larynx may also arise as primary tumors of the trachea
- Predominately SCCs and then salivary gland tumors; other entities are rare

Selected References

Heffner DK: Diseases of the trachea. In Barnes L (ed): Surgical Pathology of the Head and Neck. New York, Marcel Dekker, 2001, pp 601-625.

Allen M: Malignant tracheal tumors. Mayo Clin Proc 68:680-684, 1993.

Horinouchi H, Ishihara T, Kawamura M, et al: Epithelial myoepithelial tumour of the tracheal gland. J Clin Pathol 46:185-187, 1993.

Fechner RE, Fitz-Hugh GS: Invasive tracheal papillomatosis. Am J Surg Pathol 4:79-86, 1980.

Alexander Craig Mackinnon, Jr., and Aliya N. Husain

4

Lung and Pleura

Surgical Complications

Neoplastic Conditions

Benign Epithelial Tumors

Preinvasive Epithelial Lesions

Malignant Epithelial Tumors

Mesenchymal Tumors

Lymphoproliferative Disorders

Other Neoplastic Conditions

Non-neoplastic Conditions

Pediatric and Congenital Diseases

Congenital Pulmonary Airway Malformation (CPAM)

Clinical Features

- Uncommon developmental anomaly predominantly seen in infants that has features of both immaturity and malformation of the airways and distal lung parenchyma (formerly congenital cystic adenomatoid malformation [CCAM])
- Often detected by antenatal ultrasound during the second trimester
- Reported incidence ranges from 1 in 25,000 to 35,000 pregnancies
- About 60% of lesions show variable, spontaneous regression during gestation
- Postnatal diagnosis of CPAM

Figure 4-1. Congenital pulmonary airway malformation. Intermediate-power photomicrograph of H&E-stained section shows cysts lined by a single layer of ciliated columnar epithelial cells. The stroma contains cells with skeletal muscle differentiation (congenital pulmonary airway malformation, type 2).

— About 66% present in the neonatal period either as an infant with respiratory distress (cyanosis, grunting, tachypnea) or as a stillborn infant with anasarca

— The remaining patients present later during childhood with recurrent pneumonia, cough, dyspnea, or cyanosis

Gross Pathology

- Masses of maldeveloped lung tissue composed of cystic or adenomatous overgrowth of terminal bronchioles and air spaces
- CPAM makes direct communication with tracheo-bronchial tree through abnormal connecting bronchi

Histopathology

▌ CPAM type 0
- Small lungs with finely nodular surface in infants who are often less than 50% of expected weight for gestational age; lesions appear solid grossly
- Disorganized proximal airways form the bulk of the lesion; distal components of the normal tracheobronchial tree rarely present
- Mesenchymal cells and collagen, along with thick-walled arteries, large vascular channels, collections of basophilic debris, and foci of extramedullary hematopoiesis, form the prominent intervening tissue

▌ CPAM type 1
- Medium and large interconnecting cysts (1 to 10 cm) usually limited to one lobe
- Cyst walls composed of bronchial epithelium, often with clusters of mucous cells and smooth muscle bands with vascular connective tissue

▌ CPAM type 2
- Back-to-back, dilated bronchiolar-like cysts (0.5 to 2 cm) that blend with normal parenchyma
- Cysts separated by alveolar duct–like structures and small arterioles and venules and sometimes skeletal muscle
- Associated with other severe anomalies in 50% of cases (sirenomelia, renal agenesis or dysgenesis, diaphragmatic hernia, and cardiovascular anomalies)

▌ CPAM type 3
- Original type of CPAM described in 1949 that occurs almost exclusively in males and is associated with maternal polyhydramnios in 80% of cases
- Lesion that forms a solid mass involving the lobe or even entire lung resulting in mediastinal shift and compression with subsequent hypoplasia of adjacent lung
- Composed of randomly arranged glandlike structures resembling bronchioalveolar ducts lined with low cuboidal epithelium

▌ CPAM type 4
- Cysts are distributed peripherally, can be multiple, and involve more than one lobe

- Walls of larger cysts can be thick (0.1 to 0.3 cm) with muscular arteries
- Rare foci of cuboidal epithelium are encountered
- Capillary beds are located beneath epithelial lining

Special Stains and Immunohistochemistry

- Thyroid transcription factor-1 (TTF-1) and surfactant protein A and B label the epithelial lining of CPAM type 4 lesions

Other Techniques for Diagnosis

- Noncontributory

Differential Diagnosis

▌ Pulmonary sequestration
- Pulmonary sequestration has a systemic rather than a pulmonic blood supply and does not communicate with the tracheobronchial tree
- CPAM type 2 is seen in up to 50% of extralobar pulmonary sequestrations
▌ Pleuropulmonary blastoma (PPB)
- CPAM type 1 does not have a subepithelial or septal mesenchymal spindle cell component (with or without cartilage)
- CPAM type 4 is lined by type 2 alveolar cells instead of the cuboidal or columnar cells seen in PPB
▌ Consider congenital diaphragmatic hernia, broncho-genic cyst, congenital lobar emphysema

Pearls

- Diagnosis of CPAM cannot be made in the presence of chronic inflammation
- CPAM is reported to be rarely associated with the development of bronchioloalveolar carcinoma (BAC) and rhabdomyosarcoma (RMS) in adolescent or adult patients
- Presence of mucinous epithelium and completeness of resection should be assessed to assist with follow-up

Selected References

Stocker JT, Husain AN: Cystic lesions of the lung in children: Classification and controversies. Eur Respir Monogr 12:1-20, 2007.

Shimohira M, Hara M, Kitase M, et al: Congenital pulmonary airway malformation: CT-pathologic correlation. J Thorac Imag 22:149-153, 2007.

Ioachimescu OC, Mehta AC: From cystic pulmonary airway malformation, to bronchioloalveolar carcinoma and adenocarcinoma of the lung. Eur Respir J 26:1181-1187, 2005.

Bronchopulmonary Sequestration

Clinical Features

- Rare congenital malformation involving a segment of lung with no connection to the normal tracheo-bronchial tree and with anomalous systemic blood supply

Figure 4-2. Bronchopulmonary sequestration. In this extralobar sequestration, there are too many dilated bronchioles (congenital pulmonary airway malformation) and normal-appearing lung. No cartilage was identified within the lesion.

- Two types: intralobar sequestration (ILS) and extralobar sequestration (ELS)

Gross Pathology

▌ ILS
- Lesions lack pleural covering and are sharply demarcated from adjacent lung parenchyma
- Pedicle or hilus containing vascular structures may be present
- Numerous cysts of variable size within a solid, fibrotic mass

▌ ELS
- Oval or pyramidal, circumscribed, pink to gray-white mass (0.5 to 15 cm)
- Covered with visceral pleura and separate from the normal lung

Histopathology

▌ ILS
- Marked chronic inflammation with mucus accumulation and microcyst formation
- Remnants of bronchi and bronchioles within a dense fibrotic stroma with numerous lymphocytes

▌ ELS
- Irregular, enlarged (2 to 5 times) bronchi, bronchioles, and alveoli
- If present, bronchial structures range from normal to irregular lumens lined with pseudostratified columnar epithelium
- No significant inflammatory or fibrotic component is present
- Dilated subpleural lymphatics may be severe
- Areas of CPAM type 2 are present in up to half the cases

Special Stains and Immunohistochemistry

- Noncontributory

Other Techniques for Diagnosis

- Noncontributory

Differential Diagnosis

▌ CPAM: communicates with tracheobronchial tree and has normal pulmonary arterial supply
▌ Consider bronchogenic cyst, congenital lobar emphysema, primary lung abscess

Pearls

- ELS is frequently associated with CPAM type 2
- ELS is associated with other congenital anomalies, which determine the prognosis
- Ultrasound-detected lesions can partially or completely resolve before delivery

Selected References

Stern R, Berger S, Casaulta C, et al: Bilateral intralobar pulmonary sequestration in a newborn, case report and review of the literature on bilateral pulmonary sequestrations. J Pediatr Surg 42:E19-23, 2007.
Conran RM, Stocker JT: Extralobar sequestration with frequently associated congenital cystic adenomatoid malformation, type 2: Report of 50 cases. Pediatr Dev Pathol 2:454-463, 1999.
Stocker JT, Drake RM, Madewell JE: Cystic and congenital lung disease in the newborn. Perspect Pediatr Pathol 4:93-154, 1978.

Bronchogenic Cyst

Clinical Features

- Cystic lesion arising from anomalous budding of the tracheobronchial anlage of the primitive foregut during development
- Mostly located within the mediastinum, or less frequently at any point along tracheobronchial tree, but does not communicate with it
- Occasionally found peripherally in the lung parenchyma or within the cervical, intrapleural, or suprasternal cutaneous regions or occasionally below the diaphragm or pericardium

Gross Pathology

- Round to oval mass that molds around adjacent structures on radiograph
- Smooth-walled, unilocular or multilocular cystic lesion containing viscous fluid that may form an air-fluid level
- Cysts range from 1 to 10 cm

Histopathology

- Thin-walled cyst lined by ciliated pseudostratified columnar epithelium
- Wall composed of smooth muscle fascicles mixed with cartilage islands and seromucinous glands similar to the normal bronchus, without alveoli
- Squamous metaplasia or chronic inflammation commonly present

Figure 4-3. Bronchogenic cyst. A, Gross picture of bronchogenic cyst that is smooth walled and unilocular. **B,** Microscopic picture of a 6-cm mediastinal cystic mass demonstrates respiratory epithelial lining, seromucinous glands, and cartilage.

Special Stains and Immunohistochemistry

- Noncontributory

Modern Techniques for Diagnosis

- Noncontributory

Differential Diagnosis

▌ CPAM: alveolar tissue can be present
▌ Mediastinal cysts: esophageal cyst (absence of cartilage, double muscular wall layer), enteric cyst (lined by gastric mucosa), thymic cyst, cystic teratoma, pericardial cyst
▌ Consider pulmonary sequestration, abscess, cystic bronchiectasis, postinfarction cyst, interstitial emphysema, pleuropulmonary blastoma

Pearls

- Inflamed cysts may be difficult to definitively diagnose
- Malignant degeneration occurs very rarely in cystic lesions

Selected References

Chang YC, Chang YL, Chen SY, et al: Intrapulmonary bronchogenic cysts: Computed tomography, clinical and histopathologic correlations. J Formos Med Assoc 106:8-15, 2007.

Freedom RM, Yoo SJ, Goo HW, et al: The bronchopulmonary foregut malformation complex. Cardiol Young 16:229-251, 2006.

Congenital Lobar Emphysema (CLE)

Clinical Features

- Hyperinflation of one or more lobes of the lung, often diagnosed on computed tomography (CT)
- Rare, with estimated prevalence of 1 in 20,000 to 30,000
- Males affected more than females (3:1)

- Most patients present within first 6 months of life with tachypnea, cyanosis, wheezing, and increased labor of breathing
- Recurrent pneumonia and failure to thrive can occur

Gross Pathology

- Hyperinflated lobe leads to compression of adjacent normal lung and mediastinal shift
- Upper lobes are involved in virtually all cases, with the left upper lobe being affected more commonly
- Enlarged lobe maintains appropriate shape

Histopathology

- Overinflation of the lobe with alveolar distention without fibrosis

Special Stains and Immunohistochemistry

- Noncontributory

Other Techniques for Diagnosis

- Noncontributory

Differential Diagnosis

▌ Pneumothorax: radiologically lacks the linear bronchovascular and alveolar markings of CLE; treatments aimed at pneumothorax can worsen patient's actual CLE
▌ Consider localized interstitial emphysema, CPAM, pulmonary sequestration, bronchogenic cyst, congenital diaphragmatic hernia

Pearls

- Most cases are idiopathic
- Either intrinsic or extrinsic obstruction of the bronchus supplying the developing lobe is seen in 25% of CLE patients, leading to air trapping within the affected lobe
- Intrinsic obstruction is often secondary to defects in bronchial wall (e.g., decreased bronchial cartilage),

whereas extrinsic obstruction is often caused by vascular malformations or intrathoracic masses (tumor, cyst)
- Cardiovascular anomalies are present in 14% of CLE patients

Selected References

Berrocal T, Madrid C, Novo S, et al: Congenital anomalies of the tracheobronchial tree, lung, and mediastinum: Embryology, radiology, and pathology. Radiographics 24: e17, 2004.

Tander B, Yalçin M, Yilmaz B, et al: Congenital lobar emphysema: A clinicopathologic evaluation of 14 cases. Eur J Pediatr Surg 13:108-111, 2003.

Thakral CL, Maji DC, Sajwani MJ: Congenital lobar emphysema: Experience with 21 cases. Pediatr Surg Int 17:88-91, 2001.

Obstructive Lung Diseases

Large Airway Diseases

Chronic Bronchitis

Clinical Features

- Clinically defined as a productive cough of unknown cause occurring on most days for 3 or more months for at least 2 successive years
- Chronic bronchitis and emphysema share extensive overlap clinically and are often referred to as chronic obstructive pulmonary disease (COPD)
- Most common in cigarette smokers and those exposed to dust or irritating fumes
- Affects 5% of the U.S. population

Gross Pathology

- Increased mucus in the airways due to mucus hypersecretion
- Thickened bronchial wall due to mucous gland enlargement

Histopathology

- Mucus hypersecretion due to increased submucosal glands and goblet cell hyperplasia
- Enlargement and dilation of gland ducts
- Reid index is the ratio of gland thickness to bronchial wall thickness; Reid index greater than 0.5 is consistent with chronic bronchitis
- Chronic inflammation is mild and does not correlate with mucous gland enlargement
- Respiratory bronchiolitis is typically present in cigarette smokers

Special Stains and Immunohistochemistry

- Noncontributory

Other Techniques for Diagnosis

- Noncontributory

Differential Diagnosis

▌ Asthma: associated with eosinophils and sub-basement membrane fibrosis

Pearls

- Diagnosis of chronic bronchitis requires exclusion of other causes of chronic cough, including lung carcinoma, bronchiectasis, cystic fibrosis (CF), congestive heart failure, and tuberculosis

Selected Reference

Travis WD: Non-neoplastic disorders of the lower respiratory tract. In Atlas of Non-tumor Pathology. First Series, Fascicle 2. Washington, DC, American Registry of Pathology: Armed Forces Institute of Pathology; Universities Associated for Research and Education in Pathology, 2002.

Figure 4-4. Asthma. A, This endobronchial biopsy from a treated asthmatic patient shows sub-basement membrane fibrosis and prominent smooth muscle bundles. **B,** High-power photomicrograph shows submucosal eosinophils and chronic inflammation.

Asthma

Clinical Features

- Chronic inflammatory disorder of the airways in which mast cells, eosinophils, T lymphocytes, neutrophils, and epithelial cells play a pathophysiologic role
- Clinical diagnosis: episodic symptoms of airflow obstruction that is at least partially reversible, and alternative diagnoses ruled out
- Status asthmaticus is acute respiratory failure due to refractory bronchospasms with inflammation of the airway, mucus plugging, and edema

Gross Pathology

- Plugging of bronchioles and medium and small bronchi with thick, tenacious mucus
- Hyperinflated lungs and secondary saccular bronchiectasis

Histopathology

- Mucus plugging of bronchi and bronchioles mixed with eosinophils, epithelial cells, and Charcot-Leyden crystals
- Curschmann spirals (mucus plugs) and Creola bodies (whorls of desquamated epithelial cells) seen in sputum cytology
- Sub-basement membrane fibrosis with patchy desquamated or denuded epithelium
- Goblet cell hyperplasia and occasional squamous metaplasia
- Thickened airway walls due to edema, smooth muscle hyperplasia, and submucosal gland hyperplasia
- Eosinophilic infiltration of medium and small bronchi

Special Stains and Immunohistochemistry

- Noncontributory

Other Techniques for Diagnosis

- Noncontributory

Differential Diagnosis

▌ Chronic bronchitis: histologically similar but has few or no eosinophils

Pearls

- Atopy is the strongest predisposing factor to developing asthma
- Inhalation of *Alternaria* species or *Alternaria* species contaminated with endotoxin may be the precipitating factor for patient with sudden fatal asphyxic asthma
- Can be complicated by allergic bronchopulmonary aspergillosis

Selected Reference

Travis WD: Non-neoplastic disorders of the lower respiratory tract. In Atlas of Non-tumor Pathology. First Series, Fascicle 2. Washington, DC, American Registry of Pathology: Armed Forces Institute of Pathology; Universities Associated for Research and Education in Pathology, 2002.

Bronchiectasis

Clinical Features

- Historically, most cases of bronchiectasis were secondary to infection; antibiotic therapy has led to a marked decrease in the incidence of abnormal irreversible bronchial dilation
- Patients present with persistent cough and large amounts of foul-smelling sputum
- High-resolution CT is the procedure of choice for noninvasive diagnosis
- Disease is radiologically classified into cylindrical, varicose, and saccular or cystic bronchiectasis

Gross Pathology

- Slightly less than 50% of cases are bilateral
- Technically, bronchiectasis is present when the diameter of the bronchus exceeds the diameter of the accompanying bronchial artery (corresponds with signet ring sign), ranging from mild to massive dilation
- Dilated bronchi are filled with yellow-green mucopurulent secretions
- Grossly dilated bronchi can extend out to the pleural surface

Histopathology

- Dilated bronchi filled with mucopurulent exudate or necrotic debris
- Mucosa shows varying degrees of necrosis or sloughing, inflammation, and reparative or metaplastic changes
- Chronic inflammation of bronchial wall with fibrosis is seen
- Follicular bronchiectasis describes cases with lymphoid hyperplasia
- Secondary pneumonia and bronchiolitis obliterans are often associated

Special Stains and Immunohistochemistry

- Noncontributory

Other Techniques for Diagnosis

- Screen for known causes of bronchiectasis, such as CF, immotile cilia syndrome

Differential Diagnosis

▌ Postinfectious bronchial damage
- Commonly associated organisms: *Pseudomonas aeruginosa*, *Mycobacterium avium-intracellulare*, gram-negative bacilli, *Haemophilus influenzae*, *Streptococcus pneumoniae*, *Staphylococcus aureus*, β-hemolytic streptococcus

■ Cystic fibrosis
- CF is the most common cause of bronchiectasis in children and is invariably present among bronchiectasis patients older than 6 months
- Widespread bronchiectasis with mucus plugging of large and small airways, pleural adhesions or fibrosis, abscess, and cystic changes

■ Primary cilia dyskinesis
- Immotile cilia, Kartagener syndrome, Young syndrome, secondary cilia dyskinesis
- About 1.5% of patients with bronchiectasis have primary cilia dyskinesia
- Ultrastructural abnormalities affect virtually all cilia and are characterized by loss of dynein arms, absence of radial spokes, microtubule transposition, absence of microtubules, compound cilia, or disorientated cilia

■ Congenital
- α_1-Protease inhibitor deficiency, unilateral hyperlucent lung (Swyer-James syndrome), tracheobronchomegaly, congenital cartilage deficiency, and pulmonary sequestration

■ Middle lobe syndrome
- Recurrent or permanent atelectasis of right middle lobe or lingula, with chronic inflammation
- Strong association with lymphadenopathy and malignancy

Pearls
- Predisposing factors for the development of bronchiectasis include bronchopulmonary infection, bronchopulmonary obstruction, congenital anatomic defect, immunodeficiency states, hereditary abnormalities, and other rare miscellaneous factors
- Antibiotic therapy and prophylaxis for pediatric infections has resulted in a steep decline in the number of cases of bronchiectasis, with many cases in developed countries now due to an underlying disorder
- Can be complicated by allergic bronchopulmonary aspergillosis

Selected References

Ryu JH: Classification and approach to bronchiolar diseases. Curr Opin Pulm Med 12:145-151, 2006.

Rosen MJ: Chronic cough due to bronchiectasis: ACCP evidence-based clinical practice guidelines. Chest 129:122S-131S, 2006.

Takahashi M, Murata K, Takazakura R, et al: Bronchiolar disease: Spectrum and radiological findings. Eur J Radiol 35:15-29, 2000.

Small Airway Diseases and Emphysema

Small Airway Diseases

- See Table 4-1

Emphysema

Clinical Features

- Emphysema is often present in patients with moderate or severe COPD, often with chronic bronchitis; less commonly, some patients have asthma associated with these disorders
- Onset typically occurs during midlife years with slowly progressive shortness of breath in patients with a long smoking history

Gross Pathology

- Proximal acinar or centrilobular emphysema is most often seen in cigarette smokers
- Panacinar or panlobular emphysema is seen in patients with α_1-antitrypsin deficiency
- Distal acinar or paraseptal emphysema is characteristically found in the subpleural areas of the upper lobes and posterior aspects of the lower lobes, and it may be related to bullous disease or idiopathic spontaneous pneumothorax
- Irregular or scar emphysema is found at the periphery of scars, adjacent to healed granulomas, or in association with interstitial lung disease

Figure 4-5. Cystic fibrosis. A, Gross picture of the cut surface of the explanted lung shows dilated bronchi throughout. **B,** The dilated bronchi are thick walled and filled with green-yellow mucoid material.

Table 4-1. Clinical and Pathologic Features of Small Airway Diseases

	Constrictive Bronchiolitis	Acute Bronchiolitis	Diffuse Bronchiolitis	Respiratory Bronchiolitis	Mineral Dust Bronchiolitis	Follicular Bronchiolitis
General features	Mainly involves terminal conducting airway Associated with obstructive airway disease	Children and infants with wheezing and associated viral infection	Rare form affecting Asian adults, particularly Japanese	Common in cigarette smokers	Restrictive lung disease due to parenchymal fibrosis (pneumoconiosis)	Obstructive lesions due to external compression of the bronchioles
Histopathology	Peribronchiolar and submucosal fibrosis Incomplete or complete luminal obliteration Chronic inflammation Epithelial metaplasia Smooth muscle hyperplasia	Intense acute and chronic inflammation of small bronchioles Associated epithelial necrosis and sloughing Edema Inflammatory exudate in bronchiole lumen	Infiltration of lymphocytes, plasma cells, and foamy macrophages Prominent intraluminal neutrophils Organization of exudate with polypoid plugs	Inflammatory infiltrate within respiratory bronchiole interstitium and adjacent alveoli Smooth muscle hypertrophy Mild fibrosis Prominent pigmented alveolar macrophages	Deposits of inhaled dust primarily around respiratory bronchioles Increased fibrosis Luminal narrowing	1- to 2-mm peribronchial nodules Lymphoid hyperplasia and reactive germinal centers Hyperplasia of bronchus-associated lymphoid tissue (BALT)
Associated conditions	CVD Infection (viral) Inhalation injury CHP Drugs Organ transplantation IBD Neuroendocrine cell hyperplasia Multiple carcinoid tumorlets	Viral infection Bacterial infection	Associated with human leukocyte antigen Bw54 Increased cold agglutinins, ESR, and leukocytosis	Inhalation of asbestos, iron oxide, aluminum oxide, talc, mica, silica, silicate, coal	N/A	CVD (rheumatoid arthritis, Sjögren syndrome) Immunodeficiency (AIDS) Infection (mycoplasma, tuberculosis) Hypersensitivity reaction Cystic fibrosis Bronchiectasis Chronic aspiration

CHP, chronic hypersensitivity pneumonia; CVD, collagen vascular disease; ESR, erythrocyte sedimentation rate; IBD, inflammatory bowel disease.

Figure 4-6. Emphysema. The alveolar spaces are markedly enlarged without any interstitial fibrosis. Note the club-shaped alveolar walls projecting into the spaces.

Histopathology

- *Emphysema* is a pathologic term used to describe abnormal, permanent enlargement of air spaces distal to the terminal bronchioles due to destruction of the walls without fibrosis
- All forms of emphysema have a similar underlying histologic pattern of large, dilated alveoli, many with club-shaped septa projecting into the air spaces
- No interstitial fibrosis is present, except for some peribronchial fibrosis associated with pigmented macrophages and chronic inflammation seen in smokers
- Secondary hypertensive changes are commonly present

Special Stains and Immunohistochemistry

- Noncontributory

Other Techniques for Diagnosis

● Noncontributory

Differential Diagnosis

▮ Interstitial emphysema
● Air dissects out of the alveolar spaces and into the loose connective tissue of the interlobular septa, the subpleural region, and around bronchovascular bundles forming clear cystic spaces

Pearls

● There is too much air for the amount of lung parenchyma, even in atelectatic areas
● Inflating emphysematous lungs with formalin before taking histologic sections is recommended

Selected Reference

Travis WD: Non-neoplastic disorders of the lower respiratory tract. In Atlas of Non-tumor Pathology. First Series, Fascicle 2. Washington, DC, American Registry of Pathology: Armed Forces Institute of Pathology; Universities Associated for Research and Education in Pathology, 2002.

Restrictive and Interstitial Lung Diseases

Interstitial Pneumonias

Diffuse Alveolar Damage (DAD), Acute Respiratory Distress Syndrome (ARDS), and Acute Interstitial Pneumonia (AIP)

Clinical Features

● ARDS: severe fulminant form of lung injury caused by sepsis, shock, hypoxia, direct damage by inhalants often with multiorgan involvement
● Acute lung injury (ALI): less severe form of lung injury, same causes as ARDS, other organs not involved
● AIP: lung injury with no known etiology,
● DAD: pathologic correlate of ARDS, ALI, and AIP (Table 4-2)

Gross Pathology

● Rigid, heavy, hemorrhagic lungs in exudative phase
● Firm, consolidated, pale-gray lungs in proliferative phase
● Spongy, cystic, pale-gray lungs in fibrotic phase

Histopathology

● DAD is bilateral and patchy (*diffuse* refers to the whole alveolus, not the whole lung) with an early or exudative phase followed by a proliferative or organizing phase (but combinations can be seen) and a late fibrotic phase (in a minority of patients)
● Exudative phase (first week after injury)
● Type 1 pneumocyte necrosis, inflammatory exudate, hyaline membranes, partial alveolar collapse with interstitial edema

Figure 4-7. Acute interstitial pneumonia. This photomicrograph of the exudative phase shows patchy widening of interstitium due to hyaline membranes, edema, and a sparse inflammatory infiltrate in the lobule seen in the lower part of the picture, whereas the upper lobule is spared.

● Endothelial injury with congestion, neutrophil aggregates, and minimal microthrombi
● Proliferative phase (second week after injury)
● Florid fibroblastic and myofibroblastic proliferation within interstitium and alveolar air spaces with type 2 pneumocyte proliferation
● Remnants of hyaline membranes occasionally seen within air spaces or incorporated into the interstitium
● Occasional squamous metaplasia with atypia
● Intimal proliferation, medial hypertrophy, and thrombi in small pulmonary arteries
● Fibrotic phase (late)
● Thick interstitial fibrosis and microcyst formation

Special Stains and Immunohistochemistry

● Noncontributory

Other Techniques for Diagnosis

● Noncontributory

Differential Diagnosis

▮ Infection
● Granulomas, viral inclusions (e.g., cytomegalovirus [CMV]), foci of necrosis, neutrophil aggregates or microabscess formation
▮ Usual interstitial pneumonia (UIP) or accelerated UIP
● Fibrotic areas shows temporal heterogeneity in UIP, whereas histopathologic changes in DAD are relatively uniform from field to field
● Fibrosis encountered in DAD contains more fibroblasts and myofibroblasts, more edematous stroma, and less collagen deposition
▮ DAD in patients with collagen vascular disease
● Dermatomyositis, polymyositis, scleroderma, and rheumatoid arthritis may present with DAD pattern

Table 4-2. Clinical, Radiologic, and Prognostic Features of Idiopathic Interstitial Pneumonias

Clinical Diagnosis	Histologic Pattern	Duration of Illness	Distribution and Typical Computed Tomography Findings	Prognosis
IPF	UIP	Chronic (>12 mo)	Subpleural predominance Honeycombing Reticular opacities Traction bronchiectasis Ground-glass opacities	5-yr survival, 20% (2-3 yr mean)
NSIP	NSIP	Subacute to chronic (months to years)	Subpleural, basal, symmetrical peribronchovascular ground-glass opacities Reticular opacities Lower lobe volume loss Rare honeycombing	Cellular NSIP: 10-yr survival, >90% Fibrotic NSIP: 5-yr survival, 90%; 10-yr survival, 35%
COP	OP	Subacute (<3 mo)	Subpleural, peribronchial patchy consolidation, nodularity	5-yr survival, >95%
ARDS, ALI, AIP	DAD	Acute (1-2 wk)	Lower zone, peripheral consolidation Ground-glass opacities with lobular sparing	40%-60% mortality rate in <6 mo
DIP	DIP	Subacute (weeks to months)	Subpleural predominance Ground-glass opacities Thin-walled cysts Reticular opacities Rare honeycombing	5-yr survival, >95%
RB-ILD	RB	Subacute (weeks to months)	Diffuse bronchial wall thickening Centrilobular nodules Patchy ground-glass opacity	No deaths reported

AIP, acute interstitial pneumonia; ALI, acute lung injury; ARDS, acute respiratory distress syndrome; COP, cryptogenic organizing pneumonia; DAD, diffuse alveolar damage; DIP, desquamative interstitial pneumonia; IPF, idiopathic pulmonary fibrosis; NSIP, nonspecific interstitial pneumonia; OP, organizing pneumonia; RB, respiratory bronchiolitis; RB-ILD, respiratory bronchiolitis–associated interstitial lung disease; UIP, usual interstitial pneumonia.

- Acute lupus pneumonitis, Takayasu arteritis, polyarteritis nodosa, Behçet syndrome, and microscopic polyarteritis can present with an AIP-like clinical picture

Pearls

- Hyaline membranes are a histologic hallmark of DAD and are seen in ARDS/ALI/AIP but are not present in UIP, nonspecific interstitial pneumonia (NSIP), or cryptogenic organizing pneumonia (COP)
- Diagnosis of AIP is considered in patients presenting with severe community-acquired pneumonia who fail to respond to appropriate antibiotic therapy and in whom no other causative etiology is identified
- The clinical course of AIP is rapidly progressive, with more than 78% (range, 60% to 100%) of patients dying within 6 months due to respiratory failure and right heart failure
- Most patients who recover from ALI/ARDS have near-normal lung function

Selected References

Thannickal VJ: Idiopathic interstitial pneumonia: A clinico-pathological perspective. Semin Respir Crit Care Med 27:569-573, 2006.

Swigris JJ, Brown KK: Acute interstitial pneumonia and acute exacerbations of idiopathic pulmonary fibrosis. Semin Respir Crit Care Med 27:659-667, 2006.

Visscher DW, Myers J: Histologic spectrum of idiopathic interstitial pneumonias. Proc Am Thorac Soc 3:322-329, 2006.

Cryptogenic Organizing Pneumonia (COP)

Clinical Features

- Mean age of onset is 55 years
- No known etiology; cigarette exposure is not a predisposing factor
- Patients present with subacute illness (median, 3 months) consisting of cough and dyspnea, often associated with weight loss, sweats, chills, fever, and myalgia
- Most patients recover after steroid therapy; however, there is a significant relapse rate 1 to 3 months after cessation of therapy

Gross Pathology

- See Table 4-2

Histopathology

- Intraluminal plugs (Masson bodies) composed of fibroblasts and myofibroblasts embedded in loose connective tissue that invariably occlude alveoli, alveolar ducts, and less frequently the bronchioles (bronchiolar component may be minor or absent)

Figure 4-8. Cryptogenic organizing pneumonia. A, Lower-power photomicrograph shows nodules of myxoid loose fibrous tissue filling alveolar spaces and streaming from one space to another. **B,** Nodules of young fibrous tissue (Masson bodies) are seen distending some alveolar spaces. The interstitium is relatively normal.

- Patchy, bronchiolocentric distribution of Masson bodies, with extension into adjacent alveoli through the intra-alveolar pores of Kohn, giving a butterfly pattern
- Within the intraluminal plugs are small clusters of lymphocytes, plasma cells, histiocytes, and endothelial proliferation, resembling granulation tissue
- Mild chronic interstitial inflammation with foci of foamy macrophages
- Pertinent negatives: honeycombing, dense interstitial fibrosis, granulomas, neutrophils or abscess formation, necrosis, hyaline membranes or air space fibrin, predominant eosinophilic infiltrates, and vasculitis

Special Stains and Immunohistochemistry

- Loose connective tissue stains green with the Movat stain compared with the yellow staining pattern characteristic of dense fibrosis

Other Techniques for Diagnosis

- Noncontributory

Differential Diagnosis

❚ UIP
- Chronic clinical course
- Extensive, temporally heterogeneous pattern of fibrosis with dense scarring, honeycombing, and architectural destruction
- Fibroblastic foci of UIP adjacent to areas of dense fibrosis, in contrast to the polypoid intraluminal location of connective tissue seen in COP

❚ NSIP
- Mild to moderate chronic interstitial inflammation or fibrosis without Masson bodies

❚ Desquamative interstitial pneumonia (DIP)
- Intra-alveolar finely pigmented smoker's macrophages without Masson bodies

❚ DAD
- Patients are acutely ill
- Depending on time of biopsy, there is interstitial edema, hyaline membranes, type 2 pneumocyte hyperplasia, and organized fibrosis within alveolar walls and, occasionally, alveolar spaces

Pearls

- COP is a distinct clinicopathologic diagnosis of exclusion employed when all other underlying causes of organizing pneumonia are excluded

Selected References

Cordier JF: Cryptogenic organizing pneumonia. Eur Respir J 28:422-446, 2006.

Schlesinger C, Koss MN: The organizing pneumonias: An update and review. Curr Opin Pulm Med 11:422-430, 2005.

Usual Interstitial Pneumonia (UIP)

Clinical Features

- UIP is a histologic pattern of lung disease that occurs in a variety of clinical settings; when no underlying disease is identified, the clinical diagnosis of idiopathic pulmonary fibrosis (IPF) is made
- Patients present with progressive, chronic exertional dyspnea associated with nonproductive cough
- Incidence of 7.4 to 10.7 cases per 100,000 and prevalence of 13 to 20 per 100,000 make UIP the most common type of idiopathic interstitial pneumonia (47% to 62%)
- Average age of onset is 67 years, with median survival of 3 years
- More common in males and smokers
- Associated clinical conditions include IPF, collagen vascular disease, drug toxicity, chronic hypersensitivity pneumonia, asbestosis, familial IPF, Hermansky-Pudlak syndrome

Figure 4-9. Usual interstitial pneumonia. A, Patchy fibrosis is seen in the subpleural region, which is extending into deeper lung parenchyma, whereas some alveolar walls are not involved (variation in intensity). **B,** Fibroblastic foci can often be seen, even in areas of honeycombing (fibrosis causing destruction of alveolar architecture with remaining air spaces lined by bronchiolar epithelium). **C,** Fibroblastic focus is a subepithelial area of young fibrosis with abundant myxoid intercellular matrix and fibroblasts running parallel to the airspace. Older (*pink*) collagen is seen immediately under the focus (variation in time).

Gross Pathology
- See Table 4-2

Histopathology
- Patchy fibrosis with subpleural and paraseptal distribution
- Areas of fibrosis adjacent to normal-appearing lung parenchyma creating a variegated appearance on low power (variation in intensity)
- Dense, pink fibrosis, which represents chronic scarring adjacent to pale, light blue, myxoid fibroblastic foci, which represent acute or active wound repair (temporal heterogeneity)
- Fibroblastic foci composed of parallel palisades of fibroblasts and connective tissue beneath hyperplastic type 2 pneumocytes or bronchiolar epithelium
- Little to no interstitial inflammation away from areas of fibrosis
- Honeycomb change is often present and is an important diagnostic feature

- Cystically dilated bronchioles lined by ciliated columnar respiratory epithelium within areas of fibrosis that replace normal alveoli
- Secondary traction bronchiectasis and peribronchiolar fibrosis with associated epithelial hyperplasia (peribronchiolar metaplasia) can also occur
- Lower lobes are most severely affected

Special Stains and Immunohistochemistry
- Noncontributory

Other Techniques for Diagnosis
- High-resolution CT scan is often diagnostic in the appropriate clinical setting

Differential Diagnosis
- Chronic hypersensitivity pneumonia with fibrosis
  - Predominantly bronchocentric and mostly involves upper lobes

- Poorly formed granulomas or scattered giant cells
- More cellular, less subpleural fibrosis and less honeycomb change
▌ Langerhans cell histiocytosis
  - Stellate configuration and bronchiolocentric distribution of nodules
  - Emphysematous changes prominent in long-standing cases
  - Fibroblastic foci are rare
▌ Organizing pneumonia
  - Lack of fibrosis or interstitial pneumonia away from intraluminal fibrosis
  - Little or no architectural distortion

Pearls

- Diagnosis of UIP is confounded by inadequate sampling, microscopic findings resembling other conditions (e.g., DIP-like areas), and the fact that UIP-like fibrosis occurs in other conditions
- American Thoracic Society/European Respiratory Society (ATS/ERS) guidelines define IPF as a distinct type of chronic fibrosing interstitial pneumonia of unknown cause limited to the lungs and associated with a surgical specimen showing a histologic UIP pattern
- If in addition to UIP, other histologic patterns of other interstitial lung disease are present (e.g., NSIP), the final diagnosis is based on the worst area seen and hence remains UIP
- Clinician should identify cases of UIP associated with an underlying collagen vascular disease because of the markedly better clinical course
- Cigarette smoking confers a 1.6- to 2.3-fold increased risk for developing UIP
- Fibroblastic foci are not specific to UIP but are always present in UIP and are a key feature for diagnosis
- Combined findings of UIP and DAD, capillaritis, infection, or organizing pneumonia with extensive fibroblastic proliferation are associated with an accelerated or acute phase of IPF and often represent the terminal phase of the illness

Selected References

Dempsey OJ, Kerr KM, Gomersall L, et al: Idiopathic pulmonary fibrosis: An update. Q J Med 99:643-654, 2006.

Kim D, Collard HR, King TE Jr: Classification and natural history of the idiopathic interstitial pneumonias. Proc Am Thorac Soc 3:285-292, 2006.

Khalil N, O'Connor R: Idiopathic pulmonary fibrosis: Current understanding of the pathogenesis and the status of treatment. CMAJ 171:153-160, 2004.

Flaherty KR, Colby TV, Travis WD, et al: Fibroblastic foci in usual interstitial pneumonia: Idiopathic versus collagen vascular disease. Am J Respir Crit Care Med 167:1410-1415, 2003.

Nonspecific Interstitial Pneumonia (NSIP)

Clinical Features

- Characterized by varying degrees of fibrosis and inflammation (cellular and fibrotic subtypes) and does not meet the criteria for other forms of idiopathic interstitial pneumonia
- Second most common subtype of idiopathic interstitial pneumonia that accounts for 14% to 36% of all idiopathic interstitial pneumonia
- Commonly recognized pattern in patients with collagen vascular diseases, hypersensitivity pneumonia, drug toxicity, and immunodeficiency
- Patients present with a subacute illness with dyspnea, cough, or fever and typically have a history of cigarette smoking
- Cellular NSIP: average age of diagnosis is 39 years; 5- and 10-year survival rates approach 100%
- Fibrotic NSIP: average age of diagnosis is 51 years; 5- and 10-year survival rates are 90% and 35%, respectively

Gross Pathology

- See Table 4-2

Histopathology

▌ Cellular NSIP
  - Diffuse interstitial lymphoplasmacytic infiltrate with no significant fibrosis and preservation of lung architecture
  - Type 2 pneumocyte hyperplasia
  - Minor features: focal organizing pneumonia, lymphoid aggregates, alveolar macrophages
  - Pertinent negatives: dense fibrosis, honeycombing, fibroblastic foci, granulomas, eosinophils, neutrophils, organisms, necrosis

Figure 4-10. Nonspecific interstitial pneumonia. The alveolar walls are uniformly thickened by small lymphocytes and mild fibrosis.

- Fibrotic NSIP
  - Loose to dense interstitial fibrosis causing uniform thickening of alveolar walls with preservation of lung architecture
  - Fibrosis lacks temporal heterogeneity of UIP (fibroblastic foci are inconspicuous or insignificant in number) and no honeycombing
  - Mild to moderate chronic inflammation
  - Minor features: organizing pneumonia, lymphoid aggregates, alveolar macrophages, bronchial metaplasia, metaplastic calcifications or bone formation
  - Pertinent negatives: inconspicuous to rare granulomas, no eosinophils or organisms

Special Stains and Immunohistochemistry
- Noncontributory

Other Techniques for Diagnosis
- Noncontributory

Differential Diagnosis
- UIP versus NSIP
  - Underlying lung architecture is preserved in NSIP
  - Fibrosis is heterogenous in UIP and homogeneous in NSIP (fibrotic type)
  - Fibroblastic foci and honeycomb fibrosis are rare or inconspicuous in NSIP
  - Inflammation is relatively more abundant in NSIP (cellular type)
- Hypersensitivity pneumonitis
  - Scattered, poorly formed granulomas and intraluminal fibrosis in hypersensitivity pneumonitis
  - Slightly more diffuse pattern in NSIP
- Lymphoid interstitial pneumonia
  - Extensive, chronic alveolar septal inflammation with architectural distortion in lymphoid interstitial pneumonia versus mild, patchy inflammation in NSIP (cellular type)
- Organizing pneumonia
  - Intraluminal plugs of fibrotic tissue within distal airways and alveoli

Pearls
- NSIP is a diagnosis of exclusion; it lacks the features of UIP, DIP, COP, and DAD
- NSIP is the most common histologic pattern of lung damage observed in patients with collagen vascular disease
- Extensive lymphoid follicles or plasmacytic differentiation within interstitial infiltrates is suggestive of associated collagen vascular disease
- Efforts to identify a causative etiology (e.g., infection, collagen vascular disease) should be exhaustive when NSIP pattern is encountered on biopsy material due to prognostic implications

- An accumulation of S-100–positive, HLA-DR–positive, CD1a-negative dendritic cells is present in NSIP but not in idiopathic UIP and may be a marker of an underlying, immune-mediated etiology or process unique to NSIP

Selected References

Churg A, Muller NL, Flint J, Wright JL: Chronic hypersensitivity pneumonitis. Am J Surg Pathol 30:201-208, 2006.

Collard HR, King TE Jr: Demystifying idiopathic interstitial pneumonia. Arch Intern Med 163:17-29, 2003.

Katzenstein AL, Fiorelli RF: Nonspecific interstitial pneumonia/fibrosis: Histologic features and clinical significance. Am J Surg Pathol 18:136-147, 1994.

Desquamative Interstitial Pneumonia (DIP)

Clinical Features
- Clusters of pigmented macrophages within the distal air spaces that were thought to be desquamated pneumocytes when first described
- Uncommon disease, which along with respiratory bronchiolitis–associated interstitial lung disease (RB-ILD), accounts for 10% to 17% of all interstitial pneumonias
- About 90% of patients report current or past history of cigarette smoking
- Shares many histologic and epidemiologic features with RB-ILD
- DIP and RB-ILD likely represent different spectra of a single smoking-related interstitial lung disease
- Average age of onset is 46 years, with a male-to-female ratio of 2:1
- Subacute illness lasting weeks to months with dyspnea, cough, or chest pain

Figure 4-11. Desquamative interstitial pneumonitis. The alveolar spaces contain clusters of macrophages. There is only minimal interstitial fibrosis and rare lymphocytes.

Gross Pathology

- See Table 4-2

Histopathology

- Even, uniform filling of distal air spaces by cohesive clusters of pigmented alveolar macrophages with finely granular brown pigment within abundant cytoplasm
- Subtle to mild uniform interstitial fibrosis with hyperplasia of type 2 pneumocytes
- Scattered lymphoid aggregates, often with germinal centers
- Blue bodies (intra-alveolar laminated basophilic concretions) sometimes present
- Medial and intimal thickening of vascular structures
- Mild bronchiolar fibrosis with minimal inflammation
- Pleural inflammation and fibrosis sometimes present along with dilated pleural lymphatics
- Negative findings: architectural remodeling, dense fibrosis, honeycombing, fibroblastic foci

Special Stains and Immunohistochemistry

- Prussian blue stain for iron demonstrates finely granular pigment within macrophages that contrasts with coarse brown hemosiderin granules associated with pulmonary hemorrhage

Other Techniques for Diagnosis

- Noncontributory

Differential Diagnosis

▌ RB-ILD
- Bronchiolocentric accumulation of macrophages with sparing of distal air spaces in RB-ILD, whereas DIP has more extensive and diffuse changes
- RB-ILD associated with more benign clinical course

▌ UIP
- DIP lacks the architectural distortion and honeycombing seen in UIP
- Fibrous component of DIP (if present) is mild and without fibroblastic foci

▌ NSIP
- Cellular NSIP: increased interstitial inflammation, few alveolar macrophages
- Fibrosing NSIP: interstitial fibrosis, few alveolar macrophages

▌ Focal, nonspecific DIP-like reactions
- Likely represent RB-ILD and often seen around scar, tumor, or infarction

Pearls

- ATS/ERS Panel for Classification of Idiopathic Interstitial Pneumonia recommends using the term *DIP* for both the histologic pattern and the clinical diagnosis
- DIP-like condition described in infants with mutations in the *SP-C* gene coding for surfactant protein C
- DIP and RB-ILD lesions can persist for long periods of time after smoking cessation
- Reported association of DIP with sirolimus therapy

Selected References

Flores-Franco RA, Luevano-Flores E, Gaston-Ramirez C: Sirolimus-associated desquamative interstitial pneumonia. Respiration 74:237-238, 2007.

Ryu JH, Myers JL, Capizzi SA, et al: Desquamative interstitial pneumonia and respiratory bronchiolitis-associated interstitial lung disease. Chest 127:178-184, 2005.

Nogee LM, Dunbar AE 3rd, Wert SE, et al: A mutation in the surfactant protein C gene associated with familial interstitial lung disease. N Engl J Med 344:573-579, 2001.

Liebow AA, Steer A, Billingsley JG: Desquamative interstitial pneumonia. Am J Med 39:369-404, 1965.

Lymphoid Interstitial Pneumonia (LIP)

Clinical Features

- True idiopathic LIP is extremely rare
- Historically, most cases previously diagnosed as LIP were actually low-grade B-cell lymphomas, typically marginal zone B-cell lymphoma of the mucosa-associated lymphoid tissue (MALT) type (discussed later)
- In children, LIP is a common manifestation of HIV infection and establishes the diagnosis of AIDS
- In adults, LIP can be associated with HIV, AIDS, or other immunocompromised states
- Clinical presentation in children includes recurrent bacterial and viral infections, failure to thrive, parotiditis, and occasionally respiratory failure
- Chest radiograph
  — In children, bilateral miliary reticulonodular infiltrates
  — In adults, patchy areas of alveolar consolidation as well as miliary-type infiltrates

Figure 4-12. Lymphoid interstitial pneumonia. There is a marked mononuclear cell infiltrate in the alveolar septa and around blood vessels and airways partially obliterating lung architecture.

Gross Pathology

- Scattered nodular solid areas

Histopathology

- Early lesions: aggregates of lymphocytes and plasma cells around airways and blood vessels with extension along the alveolar septa in more advanced lesions
- Later stages: formation of confluent solid nodules, resembling intraparenchymal lymph nodes

Special Stains and Immunohistochemistry

- Not monoclonal, stains for fungi and bacteria are negative

Other Techniques for Diagnosis

- Epstein-Barr virus (EBV) can be detected in most cases by in situ hybridization

Differential Diagnosis

▌ Viral pneumonitis: may need to be determined by serologic testing

Pearls

- Pathogenesis of LIP is unknown and presumably caused by the direct effects of HIV on the lung tissue
- EBV plays a cofactor in triggering the lymphoproliferative response; however, EBV is not isolated from all patients with the disease
- LIP does not progress to interstitial fibrosis of the lung in children or adults

Selected References

Kaan PM, Hegele RG, Hayashi S, Hogg JC: Expression of bcl-2 and Epstein-Barr virus LMP1 in lymphocytic interstitial pneumonia. Thorax 52:12-16, 1997.

Angritt P, Mones JM: Pulmonary pathology in acquired immunodeficiency syndrome. In Saldana MJ (ed): Pathology of Pulmonary Disease. Philadelphia, JB Lippincott, 1994, pp 503-520.

Chayt KJ, Harper ME, Marselle LM, et al: Detection of HTLV-III RNA in lungs of patients with AIDS and pulmonary involvement. JAMA 256:2356-2359, 1986.

Hypersensitivity Pneumonitis (HP)

Clinical Features

- Bilateral, interstitial granulomatous lung disease representing an immune-mediated reaction to inhaled organic antigens or chemicals, with upper lobe predominance
- More than 200 different organic antigens are associated with HP, with thermophilic actinomycetes and avian proteins responsible for most cases
- Prevalence ranges from 5% to 15% of the population exposed to known inciting antigens
- Acute HP: onset within 4 to 8 hours of exposure to high levels of antigen and resolves within 24 to 48 hours

Figure 4-13. Hypersensitivity pneumonitis. Poorly formed granuloma with a multinucleated giant cell is seen together with histiocytes, eosinophils, and focal organizing pneumonia (to the left of the granuloma).

- Subacute HP: continuous or intermittent exposure to low levels of antigen; symptoms can resolve following steroid treatment and removal of offending antigen
- Chronic HP: similar to subacute HP, but fibrosis is present, and long-term prognosis is worse

Gross Pathology

- Patchy to diffuse ground-glass opacities on CT
- Poorly defined centrilobular nodules corresponding to cellular bronchiolitis, organizing pneumonia, or peribronchiolar interstitial pneumonitis

Histopathology

- Acute phase: biopsy rarely done
- Subacute phase
  - Small, poorly formed, noncaseating granulomas with occasional multinucleated giant cells and a patchy mononuclear cell infiltration consisting of lymphocytes and plasma cells adjacent to respiratory or terminal bronchioles
  - Large histiocytes with foamy cytoplasm present in the alveoli and the interstitium
- Chronic phase: HP has three distinct histologic patterns
  - UIP-like pattern: subpleural, patchy, pauci-cellular fibrosis and architectural distortion; fibroblastic foci; focal areas of subacute HP pattern
  - Fibrotic NSIP-like pattern: homogeneous, linear fibrosis with preservation of lung architecture
  - Irregular peribronchiolar pattern: peribronchiolar fibrosis; additional UIP-like pattern of subpleural fibrosis

Special Stains and Immunohistochemistry

- Negative fungal and acid-fast bacilli (AFB) stains

Other Techniques for Diagnosis

- Noncontributory

Differential Diagnosis

▌ NSIP

- Granulomas and giant cells are not features of NSIP
- NSIP may be the sole histologic lesion of HP, and careful exposure history potentially is the best method to distinguish NSIP from HP in these cases

▌ UIP

- Giant cells and granulomas are not features of UIP
- Peribronchiolar fibrosis and upper lobe predominance favor HP
- UIP is most severe in lower lobes with subpleural distribution

▌ LIP

- More prominent interstitial lymphoid infiltrate with extensive alveolar septal involvement
- Granulomas and intraluminal fibrosis are less common in LIP (5% in LIP versus 67% in HP)

▌ Sarcoidosis

- Granulomas are well formed, tightly packed, and sharply delineated with a hyalinized rim and are distributed along bronchovascular bundles and pleura
- Intraluminal fibrosis and UIP-like or NSIP-like component absent in sarcoidosis

Pearls

- Best diagnosed by wedge biopsy
- The chronic form of HP is the type that will eventually be presented to the pathologist
- Chronic hypersensitivity pneumonitis has a fibrotic component that can resemble UIP
- Presence of fibrosis on lung biopsy is an important prognostic factor
- If a known history of exposure exists, but the biopsy shows only NSIP-like or UIP-like fibrosis, the possibility of chronic HP should be considered
- About 95% of HP cases occur in nonsmokers

Selected References

Silva CI, Churg A, Muller NL: Hypersensitivity pneumonitis: Spectrum of high-resolution CT and pathologic findings. AJR Am J Roentgenol 188:334-344, 2007.

Churg A, Muller NL, Flint J, Wright JL, et al: Chronic hypersensitivity pneumonitis. Am J Surg Pathol 30:201-208, 2006.

Mohr LC: Hypersensitivity pneumonitis. Curr Opin Pulm Med 10:401-411, 2004.

Vourlekis JS, Schwarz MI, Cool CD, et al: Nonspecific interstitial pneumonitis as the sole histologic expression of hypersensitivity pneumonitis. Am J Med 112:490-493, 2002.

Eosinophilic Lung Diseases

Clinical Features

- Eosinophilic lung diseases are classified into three major categories
  - Eosinophilic lung disease of unknown etiology
    - Simple pulmonary eosinophilia/Löffler syndrome (SEP)

Figure 4-14. Eosinophilic pneumonia. Marked eosinophilic infiltration is seen both in the interstitium and in the alveolar spaces with organizing pneumonia.

- Acute eosinophilic pneumonia (AEP)
- Chronic eosinophilic pneumonia (CEP)
- Idiopathic hypereosinophilic syndrome (HIS)
  - Eosinophilic lung disease of determined cause
    - Allergic bronchopulmonary aspergillosis (ABPA)
    - Bronchocentric granulomatosis (BG)
    - Parasitic infections
    - Drug reaction
  - Eosinophilic vasculitis
    - Allergic angiitis
    - Churg-Strauss syndrome

▌ Acute eosinophilic pneumonia

- Diagnostic criteria include high eosinophil percentage on bronchoalveolar lavage (BAL) (>25%), but peripheral blood eosinophil percentages usually normal
- Associated with cigarette smoke and dust exposure
- Bilateral patchy areas of ground-glass opacities with interstitial thickening on CT
- Histologic appearance similar to acute phase of diffuse alveolar damage but with alveolar and interstitial eosinophilic infiltrates
- Hypertrophic, detached type 2 pneumocytes without disruption of the basal lamina
- Prompt and complete clinical response to corticosteroid therapy

▌ Chronic eosinophilic pneumonia

- Peripheral eosinophilia ranging from mild to severe
- Elevated IgE in 7% of patients
- Peripheral consolidation, most commonly involving the middle and lower zones (reversed pulmonary edema pattern on CT)
- Eosinophils, lymphocytes, and deeply eosinophilic macrophages (forming pseudogranulomas) in the intra-alveolar air spaces and interstitium; eosinophilic microabscesses

- Damage to the basal lamina with subsequent interstitial and intra-alveolar fibrosis in 50% of patients

Special Stains and Immunohistochemistry
- Noncontributory

Other Techniques for Diagnosis
- Noncontributory

Differential Diagnosis
▮ Asthma, drug reaction, Churg-Strauss syndrome
▮ Some fungal infections (e.g., coccidioidomycosis)
▮ Parasite infestation
- Allergic reaction: *Entamoeba, Toxocara* species; *Clonorchis sinensis*
- Direct invasion: *Ascaris lumbricoides* infection (strong association with SEP), schistosomiasis, *Paragonimus westermani, Ancylostoma duodenale* infection
- Others: dirofilariasis, *Strongyloides stercoralis, Wuchereria bancrofti,* and *Brugia malayi* infection

Pearls
- The diagnosis of eosinophilic lung disease can be made if any of the following are present: pulmonary opacities with peripheral eosinophilia, biopsy-proved tissue eosinophilia, or increased eosinophils in BAL
- CEP can be histologically differentiated from AEP based on the greater extent of basal lamina disruption and greater amount of intraluminal fibrosis
- White blood cell differential count is a crucial aspect of the evaluation because most eosinophilic lung diseases manifest with peripheral eosinophilia
- Charcot-Leyden crystals are bipyramidal crystals that may be present in sputum or tissue and are a hallmark of eosinophil-related disease

Selected References

Jeong YJ, Kim KI, Seo IJ, et al: Eosinophilic lung diseases: A clinical, radiologic, and pathologic overview. Radiographics 27:617-637; discussion, 637-639, 2007.

Leslie KO, Gruden JF, Parish JM, Scholand MB: Transbronchial biopsy interpretation in the patient with diffuse parenchymal lung disease. Arch Pathol Lab Med 131:407-423, 2007.

Cottin V, Cordier JF: Eosinophilic pneumonias. Allergy 60:841-857, 2005.

Mochimaru H, Kawamoto M, Fukuda Y, Kudoh S: Clinico-pathological differences between acute and chronic eosinophilic pneumonia. Respirology 10:76-85, 2005.

Alberts WM: Eosinophilic interstitial lung disease. Curr Opin Pulm Med 10:419-424, 2004.

Sarcoidosis

Clinical Features
- Chronic, multisystem granulomatous disorder of unknown etiology

- Occurs most commonly in young adults (20 to 40 years old) with slight female predominance
- In United States, higher incidence in African Americans; also common in Scandinavians and Irish
- The lung is involved in 90% to 95% of patients
- Patients present with either an abrupt, acute illness showing a better prognosis or with a chronic, insidious illness and a persistent, progressive disease course
- Angiotensin-converting enzyme (ACE) serum levels can be elevated during active phases

Gross Pathology
- Irregular, well-circumscribed nodules (2 to 5 mm) have a perilymphatic distribution and are most numerous along the bronchi and pulmonary vessels
- Late-stage sarcoidosis shows interstitial fibrosis and cavitary lesions
- About 5% of cases have a single or multiple large nodules (nodular sarcoidosis)

Histopathology
- Interstitial noncaseating granulomas distributed along lymphatic routes: pleura, interlobular septa, and bronchovascular bundles
- Granulomas composed of epithelioid histiocytes with or without multinucleated giant cells
- Granulomas are tightly clustered, well formed, and often surrounded by concentric fibrosis, which over time becomes hyalinized with a lamellar appearance
- Necrosis is usually absent; however, a minority of cases demonstrate small, punctate foci of necrosis
- Granulomas directly involve vessels (67% of cases) and pleura (10% of cases)
- Variety of inclusions, some of which may be confused for microorganisms
  — Asteroid bodies (2% to 9%)
  — Schaumann bodies, conchoidal bodies (70%)
  — Hamazaki-Wesenberg bodies (GMS stain positive, Ziehl-Neelsen acid fast, misinterpreted for fungi)
  — Microcalcifications, birefringent calcium oxalate, and calcium carbonate (mistaken for fungi or *Pneumocystis jiroveci*)
- Small number of patients progress to end-stage fibrosis and honeycombing, with an associated risk for cavitation, *Aspergillus* species infection, and subsequent hemoptysis

Special Stains and Immunohistochemistry
- GMS, periodic acid–Schiff (PAS), AFB stains negative for microorganisms

Other Techniques for Diagnosis
- Noncontributory

Figure 4-15. Sarcoidosis. A, Low-power photomicrograph shows non-necrotizing granulomas in the bronchovascular bundle. **B,** The sarcoid granuloma is well defined and is formed by histiocytes and lymphocytes. Langerhans-type giant cells, with peripheral horseshoe arrangement of nuclei, are present. **C,** Various inclusions (asteroid body in the lower left and Schumann body in the upper right) can be seen within the cytoplasm of the giant cells, which are characteristic, but not diagnostic, for sarcoidosis.

Differential Diagnosis

▌ Infection
- Special stains to exclude fungal (e.g., histoplasmosis) and mycobacterial infection
- *Mycobacterium avium-intracellulare*: granulomas are distributed around airways (bronchocentric) and may fill bronchiolar lumen, along with a granulomatous vasculitis component

▌ Hypersensitivity pneumonitis
- Granulomas are not as well formed or as sharply delineated
- More prominent interstitial chronic inflammation

▌ Reaction to inhaled substances (e.g., talc, aluminum, beryllium)
- Consider exposure history and beryllium lymphocyte stimulation test

▌ Conditions associated with sarcoid-like disorders
- Malignancies (lymphoma, lung carcinoma, carcinoid tumors, testicular germ cell tumors)
- Collagen vascular disease (systemic lupus erythematosus [SLE], Sjögren syndrome, primary biliary cirrhosis)

Pearls

- Sarcoidosis is a clinical diagnosis, and the pathologic diagnosis of non-necrotizing (or noncaseating) granulomatous inflammation, etiology undetermined, with comments regarding the negative results of special stains for microorganisms is appropriate
- Hemoptysis suggests the presence of mycetoma

Selected References

El-Zammar OA, Katzenstein AL: Pathological diagnosis of granulomatous lung disease: A review. Histopathology 50:289-310, 2007.

Leslie KO, Gruden JF, Parish JM, Scholand MB: Transbronchial biopsy interpretation in the patient with diffuse parenchymal lung disease. Arch Pathol Lab Med 131:407-423, 2007.

Hemorrhagic Diseases

Idiopathic Pulmonary Hemosiderosis

Clinical Features

- Recurrent, diffuse alveolar hemorrhage with no known etiology
- Occurs almost exclusively in children and adolescents with an equal sex distribution
- Patients present with an insidious onset of productive cough, hemoptysis, iron deficiency anemia, and weight loss
- Spontaneous remissions and exacerbations are common
- Coexists with several other diseases: IgA nephropathy, celiac disease, and dermatitis herpetiformis
- Radiographic studies reveal bilateral alveolar and reticulonodular infiltrates

Gross Pathology

- Marked increase in lung weight with areas of red-brown consolidation

Histopathology

- Dense aggregates of hemosiderin-laden macrophages with mild septal fibrosis to severe intra-alveolar hemorrhage
- Degeneration, sloughing, and hyperplasia of alveolar epithelial cells

Special Stains and Immunohistochemistry

- Noncontributory

Other Techniques for Diagnosis

- Noncontributory

Figure 4-16. Idiopathic pulmonary hemosiderosis. Prussian blue staining is positive for iron, within intra-alveolar macrophages containing hemosiderin.

Differential Diagnosis

▌ Other pulmonary hemorrhagic syndromes
  - Goodpasture syndrome: circulating anti–basement membrane antibodies
  - Vasculitis-associated angiitis, Wegener granulomatosis, and SLE

Pearls

- Biopsy specimens should be assessed for immune complex or immunoglobulin deposition using immunofluorescence or immunohistochemistry because these findings are inconsistent with IPH
- Biopsies should not demonstrate any specific pathologic findings such as granulomas, vasculitis or capillaritis, pulmonary infarction, or infection
- Outcome has improved dramatically after implementation of immunosuppressive therapy, leading to the presumption that this is an immune-mediated disease

Selected References

Nuesslein TG, Teig N, Rieger CH: Pulmonary haemosiderosis in infants and children. Paediatr Respir Rev 7:45-48, 2006.

Collard HR, Schwarz MI: Diffuse alveolar hemorrhage. Clin Chest Med 25:583-592, vii, 2004

Ioachimescu OC, Sieber S, Kotch A: Idiopathic pulmonary haemosiderosis revisited. Eur Respir J 24:162-170, 2004.

Goodpasture Syndrome and Anti–Basement Membrane Antibody Disease (ABMABD)

Clinical Features

- Autoimmune disorder caused by antibodies that react with glomerular and pulmonary basement membranes
- Rare disease with an incidence of 0.9 per million persons per year
- Typically affects young white males or elderly women with renal disease
- Younger patients frequently present with pulmonary symptoms (e.g., hemoptysis) before manifesting renal symptoms, whereas older patients develop glomerulonephritis and renal failure before the onset of pulmonary problems
- Hemoptysis ranges from mild to life threatening

Gross Pathology

- Diffusely consolidated lungs with areas of red-brown consolidation

Histopathology

- Lung biopsy is useful in cases with limited renal involvement
- Extensive intra-alveolar hemorrhage and numerous hemosiderin-laden macrophages

Figure 4-17. Goodpasture syndrome. H&E-stained section shows recent hemorrhage and hemosiderin-laden intra-alveolar macrophages, indicating old hemorrhage, as well as a mild interstitial chronic inflammation.

- Fibrous thickening of alveolar septa with pneumocyte hyperplasia

Special Stains and Immunohistochemistry

- Immunofluorescence studies: linear staining of basement membrane along alveolar septa for IgG, IgM, or IgA and complement
- Circulating autoantibodies can be detected by serology

Other Techniques for Diagnosis

- Electron microscopy: widened gaps between endothelial cells and fragmentation of capillary basement membranes

Differential Diagnosis

▌ Idiopathic pulmonary hemosiderosis
- No renal involvement
- Anti–basement membrane antibodies are not identified

▌ Wegener granulomatosis
- PR3-ANCA (c-ANCA) in serum
- Necrotizing capillaritis and granulomas are prominent features

▌ SLE
- Antinuclear antibody (ANA) positive
- Necrotizing capillaritis is a prominent feature

Pearls

- One third of patients have positive serum c-ANCA or p-ANCA in addition to ABMABD
- Antibodies of ABMABD target the noncollagenous domain of the α_3 chain of type IV collagen, and antibody titer correlates with disease severity
- About 90% of patients have HLA-DR2
- Diagnosis is often established from kidney biopsy specimens

Selected References

Frankel SK, Cosgrove GO, Fischer A, et al: Update in the diagnosis and management of pulmonary vasculitis. Chest 129:452-465, 2006.

Collard HR, Schwarz MI: Diffuse alveolar hemorrhage. Clin Chest Med 25:583-592, vii, 2004.

Pneumoconioses

Silicosis

Clinical Features

- Chronic lung disease is distinguished by parenchymal nodules and interstitial fibrosis due to inhalation of dust containing crystalline silicon dioxide
- Roughly 1500 cases are diagnosed annually in the United States
- Acute silicosis: patients develop symptoms within 3 years of exposure
- Classic or chronic silicosis: disease develops at least 20 years after exposure
- Accelerated silicosis: similar to acute silicosis, but symptoms develop later, typically within 3 to 10 years of exposure
- Simple silicosis: nodules 10 mm or less
- Progressive massive fibrosis: nodules are greater than 1 cm

Gross Pathology

- Firm, spherical, slate-gray to tan hyalinized nodules
- Nodules may coalesce to form irregular masses predominantly in the upper lobes

Histopathology

▌ Acute silicosis
- Pulmonary edema and interstitial inflammation
- Alveoli become filled by a granular, eosinophilic, PAS-positive lipoproteinaceous substance with prominent cholesterol clefts (pulmonary alveolar proteinosis)

▌ Classic silicosis
- Firm, rounded, sharply demarcated nodules, from a few millimeters to several centimeters in diameter, predominantly localized to upper lobes and subpleural regions
- Nodules are composed of an amorphous center surrounded by whorls of mature, dense, lamellar collagen showing varying degrees of calcification and necrosis
- A peripheral zone of particle-laden macrophages, lymphocytes, and fibroblasts cuffs the nodule
- Weakly birefringent silicate crystals can be identified with polarized light

▌ Silicotuberculosis
- Tuberculosis is a common complication of silicosis and occurs in 25% of patients with acute or classic silicosis
- Silicotic nodules demonstrate central necrosis and epithelioid granulomatous reaction

Special Stains and Immunohistochemistry
- Elastic stain can facilitate the identification of obliterated vessels within the lesions

Other Techniques for Diagnosis
- Noncontributory

Differential Diagnosis
▌ Pulmonary alveolar proteinosis (PAP)
- Resembles acute silicosis
- Eosinophilic material is present within alveolar spaces, alveolar ducts, and bronchioles
- The intra-alveolar material stains with surfactant apoprotein antibodies
- Little inflammation or fibrosis is present
- Secondary infection with *Nocardia* infection, fungi, viruses, mycobacteria, or *Pneumocystis jiroveci* pneumonia (PCP) can occur

- PAP can be associated with hematologic malignancy, inorganic dust exposure, or immunodeficiency

Pearls
- Silicosis, coal worker pneumoconiosis, asbestosis are the most common types of pneumoconioses
- Pneumoconiosis can be clinicopathologically classified as
  — Fibrotic: focal nodularity or diffuse fibrosis
    ◆ Silicosis, coal worker pneumoconiosis, asbestosis, berylliosis, and talcosis
  — Nonfibrotic: particle-laden macrophages with minimal or no fibrosis
    ◆ Siderosis (iron oxide), stannosis (tin oxide), baritosis (barium sulfate)
- A small but definite association between silicosis and lung cancer has been described in the literature

Selected References
Pelucchi C, Pira E, Piolatto G, et al: Occupational silica exposure and lung cancer risk: A review of epidemiological studies 1996-2005. Ann Oncol 17:1039-1050, 2006.

Chong S, Lee KS, Chung MJ, et al: Pneumoconiosis: Comparison of imaging and pathologic findings. Radiographics 26:59-77, 2006.

Castranova V, Vallyathan V: Silicosis and coal workers' pneumoconiosis. Environ Health Perspect 108(Suppl 4): 675-684, 2000.

Asbestosis

Clinical Features
- Asbestosis is primarily associated with four settings in developed countries
  — Older workers exposed to asbestos years ago
  — Workers managing existing sources (building or facility managers)
  — Asbestos abatement procedures
  — Renovation or demolition of asbestos-containing structures

Figure 4-18. Pulmonary alveolar proteinosis. Pink granular proteinaceous material is seen filling the alveolar spaces with only minimal inflammation.

Figure 4-19. Asbestosis. A, Asbestos bodies appear brown on H&E stain because they are covered with protein containing hemosiderin. **B,** This high-power photomicrograph of a Prussian blue reaction shows an asbestos body with a bulbous end and beads along its length. The other bulbous end is not present, presumably because of the plane of sectioning.

- Asbestosis typically occurs 15 to 20 years after exposure
- Inhaled asbestos fibers are deposited deep in the lungs and reach the pleura through lymphatic channels in macrophages or through direct penetration
- Patients present with dyspnea, clubbing, and restrictive lung disease

Gross Pathology

- Fibrosis is predominantly distributed in the lower lobes
- Pleural fibrosis, calcifications, and honeycombing are common findings

Histopathology

- Asbestos fibers or asbestos bodies accompanied by interstitial fibrosis
- Diffuse interstitial fibrosis with chronic inflammation and type 2 pneumocyte hyperplasia
- Alveolar epithelial cells often contain eosinophilic material that resembles Mallory hyaline
- Asbestos bodies are straight or curved, 10- to 100-μm fibers with a central clear core and diffusely beaded pattern surrounded by a gold to yellow coating with terminal bulbs or knobs
- Ferruginous bodies: similar to asbestos bodies but lack a clear central core

Special Studies and Immunohistochemistry

- Electron microscopy: facilitates the identification and characterization of asbestos fibers

Other Techniques for Diagnosis

- Amount of asbestos can be quantified in tissue by mass spectrometry

Differential Diagnosis

▌ NSIP
- Lacks asbestos fibers

▌ UIP
- Patchy fibrosis with temporal heterogeneity that is more pronounced in the lower lobes
- Lacks asbestos bodies

Pearls

- Transbronchial biopsy specimens are usually too small for analysis for asbestos bodies; BAL can be more useful to identify asbestos bodies
- Asbestos is a heterogenous group of hydrated magnesium silicate materials that typically separate into fibers when crushed
- An important implication for significant asbestos exposure is the associated increased risk for malignancy (e.g., lung cancer or mesothelioma)
- Asbestos exposure is the largest single cause of occupational cancer in the United States; it is also a significant cause of morbidity from nonmalignant disease
- However, most patients with asbestosis (lung fibrosis) do not develop cancer

Selected Reference

Smith DD: Diagnosis and initial management of nonmalignant diseases related to asbestos. Am J Respir Crit Care Med 170:691-715, 2004.

Iatrogenic Diseases

Radiation Pneumonitis

Clinical Features

- Clinical symptoms of acute radiation pneumonitis (dyspnea on exertion and nonproductive cough) usually develop 6 weeks to 6 months after completion of therapy
- The likelihood of a patient's developing an adverse response to radiation therapy depends on (1) individual susceptibility; (2) amount of radiation; (3) dose rate; (4) duration of therapy; (5) and the volume of lung irradiated
- Several factors add to the toxic effects of radiation, including (1) concomitant chemotherapy; (2) prior history of irradiation; and (3) infection

Gross Pathology

- Noncontributory

Histopathology

- Acute pneumonitis: similar to acute or organizing DAD with hyaline membranes, type 2 pneumocyte hyperplasia, and interstitial fibroblast proliferation
- Fibrotic stage: may follow clinically apparent acute radiation pneumonitis or may develop insidiously

Figure 4-20. Radiation pneumonitis. High-power photomicrograph shows reactive atypical fibroblasts with enlarged nuclei in a background of young fibrosis.

without a previous acute illness and is similar to nonspecific fibrosis with hyperplasia and cytologic atypia of type 2 pneumocytes
- Regardless of the process, the presence of foam cells and interstitial atypical stromal cells (radiation fibroblasts) is relatively distinctive for radiation injury
- Foam cells are lipid-rich modified macrophages and smooth muscle cells similar to the cells that accumulate in fatty streaks and atheromatous plaques and may be found in the intima of arterioles of any irradiated organ
- Atypical stromal cells have abundant, usually basophilic cytoplasm and enlarged hyperchromatic nuclei with or without prominent nucleoli; mitotic figures are rare

Special Stains and Immunohistochemistry
- CT scanning is sensitive in detecting radiographic evidence of pneumonitis

Other Techniques for Diagnosis
- Noncontributory

Differential Diagnosis
▌ Consider other causes of DAD

Pearls
- Foam cells and atypical stromal cells are distinctive features of radiation injury
- The injury is largely confined to the radiation field; however, it has been reported in contralateral nonirradiated lung
- Acute radiation pneumonitis is usually responsive to corticosteroid therapy
- Radiation-induced carcinomas usually have an induction period of more than 10 years

Selected References
Prakash UB: Radiation-induced injury in the "nonirradiated" lung. Eur Respir J 13:715-717, 1999.
Dail DH, Hammar SP: Iatrogenic injury: Radiation and drug effects. In Dail DH, Hammar SP (eds): Pulmonary Pathology, 2nd ed. New York, Springer-Verlag, 1994, pp 779-805.
Fajardo LF, Berthrong M: Radiation injury in surgical pathology: Part 1. Am J Surg Pathol 2:159-199, 1978.

Bleomycin Toxicity

Clinical Features
- Bleomycin is an antitumor antibiotic isolated from *Streptomyces verticillus*
- Incidence of bleomycin toxicity is less than 5%
- The sensitivity of lungs to bleomycin is attributed to hydrolase, an enzyme that inactivates the drug; bleomycin is concentrated in the lung, which is relatively deficient in the enzyme

Figure 4-21. Bleomycin toxicity. There is interstitial fibrosis with mild chronic inflammation. The pneumocytes are hyperplastic with reactive atypia.

- Patients present with insidious onset of dry cough, dyspnea, and fever

Gross Pathology
- Noncontributory

Histopathology
- DAD is present, usually in acute or organizing phase, with hyperplasia of type II pneumocytes
- Pneumocyte atypia is a characteristic feature but is not specific
- Some cases progress to fibrotic phase with interstitial scarring; the fibrosis tends to be nonuniform, focal, or nodular

Special Stains and Immunohistochemistry
- Noncontributory

Other Techniques for Diagnosis
- Noncontributory

Differential Diagnosis
▌ DAD, acute interstitial pneumonia
▌ Amiodarone toxicity
- Amiodarone causes DAD, possibly through direct toxic effect, in about one third of patients
- In addition to interstitial inflammation and hyperplasia of type II pneumocytes, there is an accumulation of foamy histiocytes in air spaces
- Electron microscopy shows lamellar inclusions in alveolar macrophages
▌ Methotrexate toxicity

Pearls
- Toxicity of bleomycin is dose related; toxicity tends to increase by concomitant use of oxygen, drugs (e.g., cyclophosphamide), and radiation therapy

Figure 4-22. Amiodarone toxicity. Finely vacuolated cytoplasm is seen both in the alveolar macrophages and in the reactive pneumocytes.

Figure 4-23. Methotrexate pneumonitis. Poorly formed granulomas and a mixed inflammatory infiltrate, including eosinophils, are seen.

- Bleomycin is one of the drugs suggested to elicit the radio-recall phenomenon, that is, a phenomenon in which previous irradiation appears to cause latent damage that may be unmasked later (e.g., by use of bleomycin)

Selected References

Cohen MB, Austin JHM, Smith-Vaniz A, et al: Nodular bleomycin toxicity. Am J Clin Pathol 92:101-104, 1989.

Kennedy J, Myers J, Plum V, Fulmer J: Amiodarone pulmonary toxicity: Clinical, radiologic and pathologic correlations. Arch Intern Med 147:50-55, 1987.

Cooper JA Jr, White DA, Matthay RA: Drug induced pulmonary disease: Part 1: Cytoxic drugs. Am Rev Respir Dis 133:321-340, 1986.

Einhorn L, Krause M, Hornback N, Furnas B: Enhanced pulmonary toxicity with bleomycin and radiotherapy in oat cell lung cancer. Cancer 37:2414-2426, 1976.

Vascular Conditions

Vasculitides

- See Table 4-3

Selected References

Chernick V: Pulmonary vasculitides in children. Paediatr Respir Rev 7(Suppl 1):S243-244, 2006.

Frankel SK, Cosgrave GP, Fischer A, et al: Update in the diagnosis and management of pulmonary vasculitis. Chest 129:452-465, 2006.

Collins CE, Quismorio FP Jr: Pulmonary involvement in microscopic polyangiitis. Curr Opin Pulm Med 11:447-451, 2005.

Pulmonary Hypertension

Clinical Features

- See Table 4-4 for the Revised Clinical Classification of Pulmonary Hypertension (Venice 2003)

Figure 4-24. Wegener granulomatosis. A, Low-power photomicrograph shows a granuloma with geographic basophilic necrosis, which is characteristic of Wegener granulomatosis. **B,** High-power photomicrograph shows granulomatous vasculitis.

Table 4-3. Clinical and Pathologic Features of Wegener Granulomatosis and Churg-Strauss Syndrome

	Wegener Granulomatosis	Churg-Strauss Syndrome
General	Triad of upper airway involvement (e.g., sinusitis), lower respiratory tract involvement, and glomerulonephritis	Multisystem disorder with asthma, rhinitis, peripheral eosinophilia, and systemic vasculitis
Target organs	Head and neck, lungs, renal	Lungs, skin, heart, central nervous system, joints, gastrointestinal system, kidneys
ANCA	c-ANCA (>90%) Usually PR3-ANCA	p-ANCA (40%-60%) Usually MPO-ANCA Occasionally PR3-ANCA
Gross findings	Multiple nodules (0.5-10 cm) 50% demonstrate cavitation Lower lobe predominance	Multifocal parenchymal consolidations Eosinophilic pleural effusions (30%) Stellate-shaped peripheral pulmonary arteries Rare cavitations
Histologic findings	Parenchymal necrosis (microscopic or geographic) Small vessel vasculitis (arteritis, venulitis, capillaritis) Elastic lamina destruction Granulomatous inflammation Microabscess Palisading histiocytes Scattered giant cells Poorly formed granulomas	Asthmatic bronchitis Eosinophilic pneumonia Occasional pleural and septal inflammation Extravascular granuloma with palisading histiocytes and MNGC surrounding central necrosis ("allergic granuloma") Vasculitis with chronic inflammatory cells, eosinophils, epithelioid cells, MNGC, or neutrophils Diffuse hemorrhage
Differential diagnosis	Lymphoma Churg-Strauss syndrome Sarcoidosis Necrotizing sarcoid granulomatosis Granulomatous infection Rheumatoid nodules DPHS	Wegener granulomatosis EP (no systemic vasculitis) ABPFD (no systemic vasculitis) Parasites (*Strongyloides stercoralis, Toxocara canis*) Fungal infection Hodgkin disease Drug-induced vasculitis (carbamazepine)
Pearls	Tissue and peripheral eosinophilia, <10% Asthma is rare Cardiac disease is rare Severe renal disease Severe, destructive sinus disease	Tissue and peripheral eosinophilia typical Asthma is typical Cardiac disease is common Mild renal disease Mild sinus involvement, typically allergic rhinitis Consider in patients with difficult-to-control asthma who develop significant cardiac, gastrointestinal, or neurologic disease

ABPFD, allergic bronchopulmonary fungal disease; ANCA, antineutrophil cytoplasmic antibody; DPHS, diffuse pulmonary hemorrhage syndrome; EP, eosinophilic pneumonia; MNGC, multinucleated giant cells.

Figure 4-25. Pulmonary hypertension. H&E-stained section shows a plexiform lesion within a pulmonary artery branch.

- Idiopathic pulmonary arterial hypertension (IPAH) is a rare disease with an incidence of 2 to 3 cases per 1 million persons per year and a prevalence of 15 cases per 1 million persons
- IPAH is 3 times more common in women than men
- Other forms of PAH are much more common
  - About 8% to 60% of all patients with scleroderma
  - Up to 20% of patients with rheumatoid arthritis, 5% to 15% of patients with SLE
  - About 20% to 40% of patients with sickle cell disease
- Most patients with pulmonary hypertension present with dyspnea, fatigue, anginal chest pain, syncope, nonproductive cough, peripheral edema, and rarely hemoptysis
- The most common cause of pulmonary hypertension is left heart failure
- Pulmonary systolic pressure is greater than 40 mm Hg owing to a decrease in the cross-sectional area of the pulmonary vascular bed

Table 4-4. Revised Clinical Classification of Pulmonary Hypertension (Venice 2003)

Pulmonary Arterial Hypertension (PAH)

- Idiopathic (IPAH)
- Familial (FPAH)
- Associated with (APAH)
  Collagen vascular disease
  Congenital systemic-to-pulmonary shunts
  Portal hypertension
  HIV infection
  Drugs and toxins
  Other (thyroid disorders, glycogen storage disease, Gaucher disease, hereditary hemorrhagic telangiectasia, hemoglobinopathies, myeloproliferative disorders, splenectomy)
- Associated with significant venous or capillary involvement
- Pulmonary veno-occlusive disease (PVOD)
- Pulmonary capillary hemangiomatosis (PCH)

Pulmonary Hypertension with Left Heart Disease

- Left-sided atrial or ventricular heart disease
- Left-sided valvular heart disease

Pulmonary Hypertension Associated with Lung Disease and Hypoxemia

- Chronic obstructive pulmonary disease
- Interstitial lung disease
- Sleep-disordered breathing and alveolar hypoventilation disorders
- Chronic exposure to high altitude
- Developmental abnormalities

Pulmonary Hypertension Due to Chronic Thrombotic or Embolic Disease

- Thromboembolic obstruction of proximal pulmonary arteries
- Thromboembolic obstruction of distal pulmonary arteries
- Nonthrombotic pulmonary embolism (tumor, parasites, foreign material)

Miscellaneous

- Sarcoidosis, histiocytosis X, lymphangiomatosis, compression of pulmonary vessels (adenopathy, tumor, fibrosing mediastinitis)

From Simonneau G, Galie N, Rubin LJ, et al: Clinical classification of pulmonary hypertension. J Am Coll Cardiol 43(Suppl S):5S-12S, 2004.

Gross Pathology

- Atherosclerotic plaques, usually small, develop in large pulmonary arteries

Histopathology

- See Table 4-5
- Grading scheme applies only to IPAH and APAH (associated with pulmonary arterial hypertension) secondary to congenital heart disease and some drugs (e.g., phenytoin)
- Only grades I, II, and III are seen in secondary pulmonary hypertension
- Plexiform lesions (present in severe disease)
- Areas of dilation due to thinning of arterial walls
- Within dilated vessels, glomeruloid plexus of slitlike vascular channels

Special Stains and Immunohistochemistry

- Trichrome and elastic von Gieson stains highlight the vascular lesions

Table 4-5. Grading Scheme for Idiopathic Pulmonary Arterial Hypertension and Disease Associated with Pulmonary Arterial Hypertension

Grade	Reversible	Histologic Features
I	Yes	Medial hypertrophy of pulmonary arteries Extension of muscle into the wall of pulmonary arterioles
II	Yes	Muscle hypertrophy plus proliferation of intimal cells in arterioles and small muscular arteries
III	Yes	Muscle hypertrophy plus subendothelial fibrosis Concentric masses of fibrous tissue and reduplicated internal elastic lamina with vascular lumen occlusion of small arteries and arterioles Large elastic arteries show atherosclerosis
IV	No	Muscle hypertrophy is less apparent Progressive dilation of small arteries, particularly vessels with intimal fibrous occlusion Plexiform lesions occur
V	No	Plexiform and angiomatoid lesions Intra-alveolar hemosiderin-filled macrophages
VI	No	Necrotizing arteritis with thrombosis Fibrinoid necrosis of the arterial wall with transmural neutrophilic and eosinophilic infiltrates

Other Techniques for Diagnosis

- Noncontributory

Differential Diagnosis

▮ Pulmonary veno-occlusive disease (PVOD)
  - Rare cause of pulmonary hypertension, with estimated annual incidence of 0.1 cases per million persons and occurring more commonly in children and young adults
  - Extensive and diffuse occlusion of pulmonary venules and small veins in lobular septa by intimal fibrosis; involvement of larger veins is rare
  - Media of the veins may become arterialized with increased elastic fibers
  - Pulmonary arterioles demonstrate moderate to severe medial hypertrophy in about half of cases
  - Alveolar capillaries may become dilated and tortuous such that PVOD can be confused with pulmonary capillary hemangiomatosis
  - Hemosiderin may be prominent and confused with idiopathic pulmonary hemosiderosis
  - Arteritis and plexiform lesions are usually absent

▮ Pulmonary hypertension due to chronic thrombotic or embolic disease
  - Little or no medial hypertrophy in pulmonary arteries and arterioles
  - Recent organizing and organized thrombi possible
  - Eccentric intimal fibrosis that focally obliterates the lumen
  - Recanalization of thrombi common

■ Pulmonary capillary hemangiomatosis (PCH)
  ● Extremely rare disorder with dense proliferation of capillaries within the alveolar septa causing thickening of the alveolar walls

Pearls

● The terms *primary* and *secondary* pulmonary hypertension are no longer used in the clinical medicine literature
● Familial pulmonary arterial hypertension (FPAH) is linked to mutations in the *BMPR2* gene on 2q33-q34

Selected References

Frazier AA, Franks TJ, Mohammed TL, et al: From the Archives of the AFIP: Pulmonary veno-occlusive disease and pulmonary capillary hemangiomatosis. Radiographics 27:867-882, 2007.

Galambos C, deMello DE: Molecular mechanisms of pulmonary vascular development. Pediatr Dev Pathol 10(1):1-17, 2007.

Taichman DB, Mandel J: Epidemiology of pulmonary arterial hypertension. Clin Chest Med 28:1-22, vii, 2007.

Tuder RM, Marecki JC, Richter A, et al: Pathology of pulmonary hypertension. Clin Chest Med 28:23-42, vii, 2007.

Simonneau G, Galiè N, Rubin LJ, et al: Clinical classification of pulmonary hypertension. J Am Coll Cardiol 43(12 Suppl S):5S-12S, 2004.

Infectious Diseases

Viral

Cytomegalovirus (CMV) Pneumonia

Clinical Features

● CMV infects healthy individuals in whom it remains dormant in white cells; it reactivates in immunocompromised hosts

● In addition to pneumonia, CMV causes hepatitis, esophagitis, colitis, meningoencephalitis, chorioretinitis, and congenital and neonatal infections

Gross Pathology

● High-resolution CT demonstrates micronodules, consolidations, ground-glass opacities, and irregular reticular opacities in transplant recipients
● One- to 3-cm nodular masses in AIDS patients

Histopathology

● Based on its characteristic cytopathic changes in lung tissue specimens (Table 4-6), CMV is the most commonly recognized pneumonia-causing virus by pathologists
● CMV infects endothelial cells, respiratory epithelial cells, fibroblasts, and macrophages
● Infected cells with CMV inclusions vary in number from few to numerous

Special Stains and Immunohistochemistry

● Immunohistochemistry usually highlights more viral inclusions than seen on H&E

Other Techniques for Diagnosis

● Noncontributory

Differential Diagnosis

● See Table 4-6

Pearls

● In the nonimmunocompromised host, with little or no histopathologic reaction, rare CMV inclusions may represent an incidental finding

Figure 4-26. Cytomegalovirus (CMV) pneumonia. A, In the center of the picture there is an enlarged cell, with a single large intranuclear inclusion, perinuclear halo or clearing, and multiple small intracytoplasmic inclusions, diagnostic for CMV. **B,** Immunoperoxidase stain using antibody mixture against immediate-early and early nuclear antigens demonstrates infected normal-sized nuclei that are not yet showing the cytopathic effect of CMV as well as classically enlarged nuclei. This allows for early diagnosis of CMV when diagnostic inclusions are not present in the biopsy.

Table 4-6. Diagnostic Features of Viral Pneumonias

Virus	Inclusions		Cytologic Features	Histopathologic Features
	Nuclear	*Cytoplasmic*		
Cytomegalovirus (CMV)	Yes	Yes	**Nuclear features:** Single 20-μm inclusion with halo, thickened nuclear membrane, rounded clump of chromatin extending into halo **Cytoplasmic features:** multiple, 1- to 3-μm inclusions	Miliary pattern, inflammation, and necrosis Diffuse interstitial pneumonitis Hemorrhagic pneumonia CMV inclusions with minimal inflammation
Herpes simplex virus	Yes	No	Squamous cells with dense, eosinophilic inclusions surrounded by clear halo and marginated, bead chromatin at the periphery; best found at interface between viable and necrotic lung Rare multinucleated cells with nuclear inclusions	Necrotizing tracheobronchitis with ulceration Necrotizing bronchiolocentric pneumonia Interstitial pneumonitis resembling diffuse alveolar damage
Measles	Yes	Yes	Very large (100-μm diameter), multinucleated giant cells with nuclear and large eosinophilic cytoplasmic inclusions	Necrotizing bronchiolitis Giant cell pneumonia
Adenovirus	Yes	No	Smudge cells with basophilic inclusion with smudgy nuclear membrane often filling entire nucleus *or* Densely eosinophilic nuclear inclusions	Necrotizing bronchitis, bronchiolitis Interstitial pneumonia with necrosis, hemorrhage, and diffuse alveolar damage–like features
Influenza	No	No	N/A	Squamous metaplasia
Respiratory syncytial virus	No	Yes	Multinucleated syncytial cells in airway walls Eosinophilic cytoplasmic inclusions	Bronchiolitis with focal epithelial ulceration Interstitial pneumonia
Parainfluenza virus	No	Yes	Multinucleated giant cells with small cytoplasmic inclusions	Giant cell pneumonia with genotypes 2 and 3
Hantavirus	No	No	Virus is identified by immunohistochemistry or polymerase chain reaction	Marked alveolar edema Immature leukocytes within alveolar capillaries

Data from Travis WD: Non-neoplastic Disorders of the Lower Respiratory Tract. Atlas of Non-tumor Pathology. First Series, Fascicle 2. Washington, DC, American Registry of Pathology: Armed Forces Institute of Pathology; Universities Associated for Research and Education in Pathology, 2002.

- Ganciclovir therapy induces morphologic changes to the intranuclear inclusions such that they become globular and eosinophilic
- CMV immunohistochemistry or in situ hybridization is helpful for identifying rare, occult inclusions as well as early infection before cytopathic changes develop
- Additional infectious agents may be present in immunocompromised patients, particularly *Pneumocystis jiroveci* in AIDS patients
- If the clinical, histologic, and radiologic findings are inconsistent with pneumonia, positive CMV BAL cultures and serum polymerase chain reaction (PCR) should be interpreted conservatively

Bacterial

Legionella Pneumonia

Clinical Features

- The gram-negative bacteria *Legionella* species are believed to cause 1% of all pulmonary infections and 15% of pneumonia in hospitalized patients
- *Legionella* causes two diseases: *Legionella* pneumonia and the milder Pontiac fever

Gross Pathology

- Focal and nodular pattern of lung involvement
- Rounded lesions occasionally seen

Histopathology

- A neutrophilic infiltrate, a monocyte and macrophage infiltrate, or a combined neutrophil, monocyte, and macrophage infiltrate is present
- Intra-alveolar fibrin and hemorrhage are common
- Prominent nuclear debris creates a dusty or dirty appearance
- Occasional vasculitic component is present

Special Stains and Immunohistochemistry

- Tissue silver stains (Warthin-Starry, Steiner, and Dieterle stains) demonstrate the bacteria
- Immunofluorescence methods on tissue sections are available

Other Techniques for Diagnosis

- Electron microscopy demonstrates bacteria within macrophages and neutrophils

Differential Diagnosis

▌ Bronchopneumonia and lobar pneumonia due to other bacterial infections

Pearls

- *Legionella* is a relatively common cause of both community-acquired and hospital-acquired pneumonia
- The major disadvantage of the urinary antigen test is that it is specific for *Legionella pneumophila*, serogroup 1 only

Nocardiosis

Clinical Features

- Rare lung infection caused by the gram-positive bacilli *Nocardia* species (*Nocardia asteroides* accounts for more than 80% of cases), with an incidence of 500 to 1000 cases per year in the United States
- Inhalation of the saprophytic organisms in decaying organic matter and soil is the main route of infection
- Chronic immunosuppression is secondary to AIDS, Cushing disease, corticosteroid therapy, lymphoma, and chronic granulomatous disease
- At the time of diagnosis, 50% of cases of pulmonary nocardiosis have disseminated to other organs (e.g., skin, bone, kidney, and brain)

Gross Pathology

- Numerous, often coalescent abscesses that may contain think, green pus

Histopathology

- *Nocardia* species are long, thin, beaded bacterial filaments 1 μm in thickness that branch at right angles (Chinese character pattern)
- Neutrophils form microabscesses, leading to necrotizing pneumonia in acute nocardiosis
- Organisms are best seen in areas of necrosis or suppuration
- *Nocardia* species form a ball-like mass within cavitary spaces in rare instances

Figure 4-27. Nocardiosis. Branching thin filamentous bacteria are best visualized on GMS stain.

- In immunocompromised patients, there are small, poorly formed granulomas with few neutrophils

Special Stains and Immunohistochemistry

- *Nocardia* species are difficult to identify, so a high index of suspicion and knowledge of the morphology increase the chances of positive identification
- GMS, Brown and Brenn, and Brown and Hopps stains demonstrate the organisms
- Coates-Fite, Kinyoun, and Fite-Faraco stains show the weakly acid-fast organisms

Other Techniques for Diagnosis

- PCR methods are available to identify *Nocardia* species from BAL or tissue biopsy specimens

Differential Diagnosis

▌ Actinomycosis
- Uncommon pulmonary infection caused by the anaerobic filamentous *Actinomyces* species
- Gram-positive, beaded, branching, filamentous bacteria that branch at right angles
- Sulfur granule formation often accompanied by the Splendore-Hoeppli phenomenon is a feature of *Actinomyces* but not *Nocardia* species

Pearls

- Organisms are difficult to recognize; silver stains are most helpful, but molecular or immunohistochemical methods may be needed to establish the diagnosis

Mycobacterium tuberculosis

Clinical Features

- Tuberculosis is a chronic infection caused by the bacillus *Mycobacterium tuberculosis*
- In the United States, tuberculosis most often occurs in homeless, incarcerated, impoverished, elderly, and immunosuppressed individuals
- Primary tuberculosis is transmitted through the inhalation of 1- to 5-μm airborne droplets containing the bacillus
- Secondary tuberculosis is due to reactivation of primary infection or, less likely, reinfection
- Miliary tuberculosis reflects hematogenous spread of the organism, causing systemic tuberculosis

Gross Pathology

- Ghon lesion: round, 1- to 2-cm, gray-white pulmonary parenchymal nodule with a necrotic center, usually close to the pleura in the lower upper lobe or upper lower lobe
- Ghon complex: Ghon lesion associated with enlarged hilar lymph nodal involvement
- Ranke complex: in 95% of cases, cell-mediated immunity controls the infection, and the Ghon complex undergoes progressive fibrosis and calcification

Figure 4-28. Tuberculosis. A, Gross picture of the cut surface of a lung shows caseating granulomas (cheesy white appearance). **B,** H&E-stained section shows a granuloma with central necrosis (*left side*) and Langerhans-type giant cells (peripherally arranged nuclei). **C,** Acid-fast bacillus stain shows few acid-fast bacilli (pink rods) in this nonimmunocompromised patient.

Histopathology

- Necrotizing granulomas containing mycobacterial organisms (4-µm, slim, beaded rods) are present within the lung parenchyma and mediastinal lymph nodes
- Granulomas are bordered by palisading histiocytes and contain epithelioid cells, which often fuse to form Langerhans-type multinucleated giant cells
- Severe pulmonary complications include
  - Enlargement of necrotizing granuloma into cavitary lesion
  - Rupture of necrotizing granuloma into pleura, vascular structure, or bronchus with subsequent empyema, embolization, and bronchopneumonia, respectively

Special Stains and Immunohistochemistry

- Ziehl-Neelsen acid-fast stain is the optimal staining method for identification
- Other staining methods are auramine-rhodamine fluorescent, Fite, and Kinyoun stains

Other Techniques for Diagnosis

- PCR-based identification is faster than culture and is useful in cases in which specimen was not obtained for culture

Differential Diagnosis

❚ Nontuberculosis mycobacterial pneumonia, fungal pneumonia, Wegener granulomatosis, sarcoidosis, *Nocardia* species

Pearls

- About 1×10^4 to 10^6 organisms/mL are needed for a positive Ziehl-Neelsen acid-fast stain
- The diagnosis of most cases of *Mycobacterium tuberculosis* pneumonia is based on clinical presentation, history, physical signs and symptoms, and sputum culture
- Virulence is attributed to particular cell envelope components (peptidoglycan, arabin galactan, and mycolic acids), the lipopolysaccharide lipoarabinomannan (LAM), and mycobacterial cell entry protein (Mcep) encoded by *mce1A*

Atypical Mycobacterial Pneumonia

Clinical Features

- Atypical mycobacterial infection is important in AIDS and other immunosuppressed patients, older persons with or without underlying lung disease, and patients with CF
- The most common atypical mycobacterial agent of human infection is *Mycobacterium avium* complex (MAC)
- MAC infections tend to occur late in the course of AIDS
- The portal of entry is most likely the gastrointestinal tract
- MAC can be cultured from lungs, lymph nodes, spleen, liver, bone marrow, and gastrointestinal tract

Gross Pathology

- Cavitary lesions in the upper lobes, similar to pulmonary tuberculosis, are seen in about 90% of HIV patients with *Mycobacterium kansasii* infection and in perhaps 50% of HIV patients with MAC infection
- About 50% patients with MAC lung disease have nodules associated with bronchiectasis, which occur most frequently in the right middle lobe and lingula

Histopathology

- Similar to that seen in ordinary tuberculosis, necrotizing granulomatous inflammation is the most common feature
- Non-necrotizing granulomas are often present as well
- In AIDS and other immunocompromised patients, there may be a nonspecific inflammatory reaction composed of poorly organized histiocytic infiltrates, acute and chronic inflammation, fibrosis, and organizing pneumonia

Figure 4-29. Atypical mycobacterial pneumonia. Acid-fast stain demonstrates numerous bright pink intracellular organisms, which can be easily seen in this biopsy specimen from an AIDS patient.

Special Stains and Immunohistochemistry

- Organisms appear as long, thin, beaded, red bacilli on acid-fast stains
- Immunohistochemical methods using antibody to *Mycobacterium tuberculosis* is sensitive and specific

Other Techniques for Diagnosis

- Auramine-rhodamine fluorescent stain outlines the organisms in sputum and tissue

Differential Diagnosis

- Other granulomatous infections, sarcoidosis

Pearls

- The ATS diagnostic criteria for nontuberculous mycobacterial infections include both imaging studies consistent with pulmonary disease and recurrent isolation of mycobacteria from sputum or bronchial wash in a symptomatic patient
- Other *Mycobacterium* species that cause lung disease include *M. abscessus, M. fortuitum, M. xenopi, M. malmoense, M. szulgai, M. simiae,* and *M. asiatica*
- Pulmonary disease due to rapidly growing mycobacteria (RGM) is predominantly due to *M. abscessus* (80% of cases) and *M. fortuitum* (15% of cases)

Selected References (Bacterial Pneumonia)

Sutcliffe IC, Harrington DJ: Lipoproteins of *Mycobacterium tuberculosis*: An abundant and functionally diverse class of cell envelope components. FEMS Microbiol Rev 28:645-659, 2004.

Collins DM: Virulence factors of *Mycobacterium bovis.* Tuberculosis (Edinb) 81(1-2):97-102, 2001.

Fungal

Aspergillosis

- See Table 4-7

Clinical Features

- Pulmonary aspergillosis is usually caused by *Aspergillus fumigatus, Aspergillus niger,* or *Aspergillus flavus*
- Hemoptysis is frequently reported and can be so massive as to be life threatening
- Patterns of pulmonary aspergillosis
  — Colonization of preexisting cavities in the lung (fungus ball)
  — Hypersensitivity reaction: allergic broncho-pulmonary aspergillosis, eosinophilic pneumonia, bronchocentric granulomatosis, and hypersensitivity pneumonia
  — Invasive: acute invasive aspergillosis, necrotizing pseudomembranous tracheobronchitis, chronic necrotizing aspergillosis, bronchopleural fistula

Figure 4-30. Aspergillosis. A, Radiating arrangement of fungal hyphae invading through arterial wall can be easily seen on H&E stain. **B,** GMS stain shows characteristic septate hyphae with parallel walls and acute angle branching.

Gross Pathology

- Areas of hemorrhage and necrosis with consolidation or cavitation
- Fungal balls are friable, brown to red lesions ranging in size from 1 to 7 cm that are loosely associated with the cavity wall
- Target lesion: nodular pulmonary infarct with central pale necrotic zone surrounded by a hemorrhagic rim or infarct

Histopathology

- Usual form is hyphae; conidial heads form rarely where organism is exposed to air
- Splendore-Hoeppli phenomenon: radiating eosinophilic material at edges of fungal masses
- Classic tissue reaction is in the form of a hemorrhagic infarct with sparse inflammatory infiltrate that evolves into necrotizing pneumonia
- Fungal hyphae are found invading blood vessel walls and permeating alveolar septae
- Fungal emboli can completely occlude vessels, causing the so-called target lesion

Special Stains and Immunohistochemistry

- GMS and PAS highlight fungal structures

Other Techniques for Diagnosis

- PCR methods available in reference labs for identification

Differential Diagnosis

- Other fungal infections: zygomycosis and *Candida*, *Fusarium*, *Penicillium* species
- Allergic bronchopulmonary aspergillosis
  - Hypersensitivity reaction that occurs mostly in patients with CF or asthma due to colonization with *Aspergillus* species
  - Mucoid impaction of the bronchi and eosinophilic pneumonia
- Bronchocentric granulomatosis (BCG)
  - BCG represents a histopathologic pattern of injury secondary to infectious or noninfectious etiology (e.g., allergy)
  - Necrotizing granulomatous inflammation destroys the walls of small bronchi and bronchioles
  - Palisading histiocytic reaction replaces the airway wall

Pearls

- Definitive diagnosis requires culture, molecular, or immunohistochemical methods
- Pattern of infection depends on the patient's immune status and underlying lung disease

Table 4-7. Differential Diagnosis of Hyphal Fungi

	Aspergillus Species	*Zygomycetes* Species	*Fusarium* Species	*Pseudallescheria boydii*
Width	3-6 μm	5-25 μm	3-8 μm	2-5 μm
Outline	Parallel	Irregular	Parallel	Parallel
Branching pattern	Dichotomous* Acute angle	Haphazard, >90-degree angle	Right angle, occasionally 45 degrees	Haphazard
Septation	Frequent	Inconspicuous	Frequent	Frequent

*Dichotomous indicates that the daughter branch is same width as the parental branch.

Zygomycosis

Clinical Features

- Uncommon opportunistic fungal infection is most commonly due to *Rhizopus* species acquired through spore inhalation
- Patients present with fever, cough, chest pain, dyspnea, and hemoptysis, which can be massive
- Infection begins in the nasal turbinates and then spreads to the orbits, brain, or lungs
- Mortality rate due to infection or hemoptysis usually exceeds 50%
- Almost all cases of zygomycosis occur in the presence of some underlying condition: diabetes mellitus, hematologic malignancies (neutropenia), organ transplantation (immunosuppressive therapy), broad-spectrum antibiotic therapy, severe malnutrition, and skin or mucosal lesions secondary to burns, trauma, or surgical incisions

Gross Pathology

- Diffuse pneumonia with infarction and necrosis
- Direct extension to the mediastinum, pericardium, and heart

Histopathology

- Cross-sectioned hyphae are round or oval with clear centers
- Rare chlamydoconidium forms when the organism is exposed to air
- Zygomycetes are angioinvasive, and infarcts are a hallmark of infection
- Granulomatous vasculitis is occasionally present

Special Stains and Immunohistochemistry

- Organisms can be identified with GMS and PAS stains

Other Techniques for Diagnosis

- PCR methods available in reference laboratories for identification

Figure 4-31. Zygomycosis. GMS stain shows broad wavy ribbon-like hyphae, some with 90-degree branching.

Differential Diagnosis

- See Table 4-7

Pearls

- The term *zygomycosis* is more precise than the commonly used term *mucormycosis* because other members of this class of fungi cause infection
- Ketone reductase is produced by the organism and allows it to survive in high-glucose, acidic conditions (e.g., diabetic ketoacidosis)
- Iron availability is crucial for the growth of *Zygomycetes* species, and paradoxically, deferoxamine increases susceptibility to zygomycosis—perhaps by functioning as a siderophore for the fungi
- Rhinocerebral and pulmonary zygomycosis is acquired through spore inhalation

Histoplasmosis

- See Table 4-8

Clinical Features

- Dimorphic, soil-dwelling fungus
- Most infected persons show few or no symptoms
- Acute pulmonary histoplasmosis
  - Self-limited illness in young children exposed to the fungus for the first time
  - Acute, severe pulmonary infection following exposure to a large inoculum of *Histoplasma capsulatum* with clinical manifestations similar to ARDS
- Disseminated histoplasmosis
  - Frequently occurs in patients with underlying immune dysfunction (infants; patients with AIDS, hematologic malignancy, immunosuppressive therapy, congenital T-cell deficiency)
- Chronic pulmonary histoplasmosis
  - Most patients are adults with some form of underlying lung disease (e.g., emphysema)
  - Patients can develop chronic, cavitary lesions

Gross Pathology

- Pathology varies from chronic fibrocavitary lesions with hilar lymphadenopathy to circumscribed, solitary fibrocaseous nodules with concentric, calcified lamellae (tree-barking) to miliary nodules (buckshot appearance)

Histopathology

- Narrow-based budding yeast with one blunt end and one pointed end (i.e., pear shaped), often found in clusters
- Budding forms are relatively difficult to find, and hyphal forms are incredibly rare
- Necrotizing granulomatous inflammation occurs in the setting of chronic infection

Figure 4-33. Histoplasmosis. A. Low-power photomicrograph of an H&E-stained section shows circular deposits of calcium in the granuloma (tree-bark appearance). **B,** GMS stain shows small pear-shaped yeasts that are pointed at one end and rounded at the other. Occasional budding yeasts can also be seen.

Table 4-8. Differential Diagnosis of Yeastlike Fungi

	Coccidioides immitis	*Histoplasma capsulatum*	*Cryptococcus neoformans*	*Blastomyces dermatitidis*	*Candida* Species	*Torulopsis glabrata*
Size	Spherules: 30-100 μm Endospores: 2-5 μm	2-4 μm	2-20 μm	8-15 μm	2-6 μm	2-5 μm
Shape	Round to oval	Round to oval, pear shaped	Round to oval	Round to oval	Round to oval	Round to oval
Budding	Endosporulation	Single, narrow based	Single to multiple, narrow based	Single, broad based	Single, chains, narrow based	Single, narrow based
Cell wall	Thin	Thin	Thick mucinous capsule	Thick, refractile	Thin	Thin
Hyphae, pseudohyphae	Rare	Rare	Rare	Rare	Pseudohyphae and rare true hyphae	None
Nuclei	Single	Single	Single	Multiple	Single	Single
Mucicarmine staining	Negative	Negative	Positive	Negative	Negative	Negative

- Granulomas are well circumscribed with a thick fibrous capsule, are not infrequently calcified, and have necrotic central areas, which are the best place to find organisms
- Clusters of organisms are found within foamy macrophages in the immunocompromised

Special Stains and Immunohistochemistry

- GMS is the best stain to identify *Histoplasma* species

Other Techniques for Diagnosis

- Direct immunofluorescence on histologic sections can assist with the diagnosis

Differential Diagnosis

- See Table 4-8

Pearls

- In the United States, histoplasmosis is most common in the Midwest within the Ohio and Mississippi River

Figure 4-32. Candidiasis. GMS stain shows budding yeasts and pseudohyphae. Note sausage-link appearance caused by pinching in of the wall.

valleys, where more than 80% of young adults have been previously infected

- Histoplasmosis has a predilection for elderly patients, likely because of the association of histoplasmosis with emphysema
- Granulomatous mediastinitis is a complication of pulmonary infection with massive enlargement of multiple nodes that are often matted and undergo caseous necrosis
- Mediastinal fibrosis is a rare, frequently lethal complication of pulmonary histoplasmosis affecting younger patients 20 to 40 years old
- Pericarditis, pleural disease, and broncholithiasis are additional rare complications

Coccidioidomycosis

Clinical Features

- Dimorphic fungus is endemic to the southwestern United States and Central America and causes granulomatous disease in humans
- Primary pulmonary coccidioidomycosis is usually asymptomatic, subclinical, and self-limited
- Patients who develop clinically apparent pulmonary disease show a range of pathologic findings: acute pneumonia; eosinophilic pneumonia; solitary pulmonary nodule; chronic progressive infection with fibrocavitary lesions, bronchopleural fistula, or empyema
- Disseminated disease shows miliary or extrapulmonary dissemination

Gross Pathology

▌ Acute coccidioidomycosis
- Patchy, unilateral parenchymal consolidations that are often perihilar or in lower lobes
- Multifocal, peripheral, subpleural nodules or masses

▌ Persistent pulmonary coccidioidomycosis
- Pulmonary nodules typically develop in areas of previous consolidation
  — Single, peripheral, spherical, and well delineated
- Single, thin-walled cavitary lesions occur in a subset of patients
  — Upper lobe predominance
  — May rupture into pleural cavity, resulting in bronchopleural fistula or pneumothorax

▌ Chronic progressive coccidioidomycosis
- Unilateral or bilateral apical consolidations with occasional cavitation

Figure 4-34. Coccidioidomycosis. A, A necrotizing granuloma with multiple organisms (*right side*) is seen in this medium-power photomicrograph of an H&E-stained section. **B,** On periodic acid–Schiff stain, large spherules and hyphae are stained pink. **C,** On GMS stain, large spherules and numerous endospores are stained black.

Histopathology

- Grossly apparent pulmonary nodules typically correspond with necrotizing granulomas
- Organisms likely to be found within neutrophilic infiltrates or necrotic zones
- Immature spherules, mature spherules, and endospores are present in the biopsy tissue
- Immature spherules lack endospores and are PAS positive
- Mature spherules possess a thick, refractile wall that is either lined or filled with endospores (diagnostic feature)
- Endospores are mononuclear with punctate, PAS positive, cytoplasmic inclusions
- Mycelia can be observed in aerated cavitary lesions or bronchopleural fistulas

Special Stains and Immunohistochemistry

- PAS and GMS stains help identify the organisms

Other Techniques for Diagnosis

- Noncontributory

Differential Diagnosis

- See Table 4-8

Pearls

- Cutaneous manifestations of pulmonary coccidioidomycosis include erythema nodosum and erythema multiforme and occur in about 20% of patients, typically young white women

Blastomycosis

Clinical Features

- Blastomycosis occurs predominantly in the Mississippi, Missouri, and Ohio River valleys, as well as the Great Lakes region and the southeastern United States
- Patients present with no history of antecedent infection, or blastomycosis can develop months to years after an episode of acute pulmonary blastomycosis
- Patients present with cough, high temperature, arthralgias, and myalgias
- Extrapulmonary spread to bone and skin can occur
- It is much more common in immunosuppressed patients

Gross Pathology

- Pleural involvement is common and often associated with pleural effusions
- Bilateral, patchy parenchymal consolidations have predilection for posterior lower lobes

Histopathology

- Intense neutrophilic infiltrates with abscess formation is the initial response
- Necrotizing granulomatous inflammation ensues
- Organisms can be identified in necrotic areas, between the inflammation, and in multinucleated giant cells
- Large aggregates of organisms form in cases of disseminated infection, forming so-called yeast lakes, with minimal associated inflammation

Special Stains and Immunohistochemistry

- GMS and PAS stains adequately demonstrate the organisms

Other Techniques for Diagnosis

- Noncontributory

Differential Diagnosis

- See Table 4-8

Figure 4-35. Blastomycosis. A, Within the mixed inflammatory infiltrate (granulomatous and neutrophilic), large budding yeasts can be seen on H&E. **B,** GMS stain shows broad-based budding yeasts.

Pearls

- Pulmonary blastomycosis can present virtually identically to bacterial pneumonia, tuberculosis, histoplasmosis, ARDS, or lung carcinoma
- Blastomycosis can form nodules or masses that are radiographically indistinguishable from primary pulmonary malignancy, particularly if hilar or mediastinal lymphadenopathy is present
- *Blastomycoses dermatitidis* can take 4 to 5 weeks to culture, so prompt histologic diagnosis can have a big effect on patient management

Cryptococcosis

Clinical Features

- Pulmonary lesions of cryptococcosis are usually clinically and radiographically silent
- Severe disease occurs only in immunosuppressed patients
- Diagnosis is established by culture or histologic examination of tissue or BAL fluid

Gross Pathology

- Focal parenchymal consolidation with a gelatinous cut surface

Histopathology

- Capsule-deficient forms are typically encountered in immunocompetent hosts
- Histologic reaction can be minimal with organisms filling in alveolar spaces
- Fibrohistiocytic reaction accompanies numerous, densely packed organisms, mimicking lipoid pneumonia
- Granulomatous inflammation with fibrosis occurs in immunocompetent patients with organisms found within giant cells and macrophages

Special Stains and Immunohistochemistry

- GMS stain identifies all forms of the organism
- Mucicarmine, Alcian blue, and DPAS stain the mucinous capsule

Other Techniques for Diagnosis

- PCR methods available in reference laboratories for identification

Differential Diagnosis

- See Table 4-8

Pearls

- Although the lung is the most likely initial portal of entry and infection, disseminated foci with a normal chest radiograph can be seen

Pneumocystis jiroveci Pneumonia (PCP)

Clinical Features

- Pneumocystis is one of the major causes of opportunistic fungal pneumonia in immunocompromised patients
- Four clinical forms: asymptomatic infections, infantile pneumonia, pneumonia in immunocompromised hosts, and extrapulmonary infections
- Infantile pneumonia typically presents as an epidemic in malnourished or premature children
- Extrapulmonary infections result from dissemination from lungs to other organs, such as lymph nodes, spleen, bone marrow, liver, kidneys, heart, brain, pancreas, and skin

Gross Pathology

- Bilateral alveolar and interstitial infiltrates radiating out from the hilum on CT

Histopathology

- Alveoli are filled with frothy, acellular, eosinophilic, proteinaceous material

Figure 4-36. Cryptococcosis. A, H&E stain of this endobronchial biopsy shows numerous yeasts with no inflammatory response. **B,** Mucicarmine stain demonstrates thick mucinous capsules, which stain bright red.

Figure 4-37. *Pneumocystis jiroveci* **pneumonia. A,** H&E-stained section shows eosinophilic frothy acellular intra-alveolar exudate characteristic of *Pneumocystis* pneumonia. **B,** GMS stains the cysts black. Some cysts are round to oval with dotlike structures, and some are helmet shaped.

- The material is composed of masses of cysts and trophozoites, desquamated alveolar cells, alveolar macrophages, and few inflammatory cells
- Multiple morphologic forms of *Pneumocystic jiroveci*
  — Trophozoites are pleomorphic, measure 2 to 4 μm, and conjugate to produce a diploid zygote that develops into a cyst
  — Cysts are spherical when they contain sporozoites; empty cysts are indented or cup shaped
  — Up to eight intracystic sporozoites measuring 1 to 2 μm develop within the cysts and are subsequently released and go on to develop into trophic forms
- Less common reactions to *Pneumocystis* species include granulomas, infarcts, giant cells, interstitial fibrosis, and interstitial plasma cell infiltrates

Special Stains and Immunohistochemistry

- GMS stain is most useful to demonstrate the cyst forms, which stain black or brown; cysts often contain dark bodies or dots, which correspond to focal thickening of cyst wall and should not be confused with sporozoites
- Toluidine blue stains the cyst wall blue and also stains fungal elements
- Giemsa, Wright, and Wright-Giemsa (Diff-Quik) dyes stain the trophozoites and intracystic sporozoites pale blue with a punctate red nucleus; these dyes do not stain the cyst forms

Other Techniques for Diagnosis

- Monoclonal immunofluorescent antibodies recognize the cyst wall and have increased specificity compared with other staining methods
- PCR targets include mitochondrial 23S rRNA (mtLSUrRNA) and internal transcribed spacers (ITS), which have higher sensitivity than methods targeting cytoplasmic 5S rRNA and dihydrofolate reductase (DHFR) regions

Differential Diagnosis

▮ DAD, histoplasmosis

Pearls

- Coinfection with other organisms (e.g., CMV) occurs, particularly in immunosuppressed patients
- *Pneumocystis* microbes are classified as fungi on the basis of rRNA and mitochondrial sequence homologies
- *Pneumocystis jiroveci* is the organism that infects humans and causes PCP, whereas *Pneumocystis carinii* is found in rats
- PCP is the most common cause of pneumothorax in patients with HIV
- Highest incidence of PCP in HIV-infected children is in the first year of life, with peak incidence at ages 3 to 6 months and is often accompanied with a significant lymphoplasmacytic interstitial infiltrate

Selected References (Fungal Pneumonia)

Jeong YJ, Kim KI, Seo IJ, et al: Eosinophilic lung diseases: A clinical, radiologic, and pathologic overview. Radiographics 27:617-637; discussion, 637-639, 2007.

Almyroudis NG, Sutton DA, Linden P, et al: Zygomycosis in solid organ transplant recipients in a tertiary transplant center and review of the literature. Am J Transplant 6:2365-2374, 2006.

Kauffman CA: Endemic mycoses: Blastomycosis, histoplasmosis, and sporotrichosis. Infect Dis Clin North Am 20:645-662, vii, 2006.

Chong S, Lee KS, Yi CA, et al: Pulmonary fungal infection: Imaging findings in immunocompetent and immuno-compromised patients. Eur J Radiol 59:371-383, 2006.

Subramanian S, Mathai D: Clinical manifestations and management of cryptococcal infection. J Postgrad Med 51(Suppl 1):S21-26, 2005.

Galgiani JN, Ampel NM, Blair JE, et al: Coccidioidomycosis. Clin Infect Dis 41:1217-1223, 2005.

Roden MM, Zaoutis TE, Buchanan WL, et al: Epidemiology and outcome of zygomycosis: A review of 929 reported cases. Clin Infect Dis 41:634-653, 2005.

Robinson C, Singh N, Addis B: Eosinophilic pneumonia and *Aspergillus* colonization of rheumatoid nodules. Histopathology 46:709-710, 2005.

Wazir JF, Ansari NA: *Pneumocystis carinii* infection: Update and review. Arch Pathol Lab Med 128:1023-1027, 2004.

Franquet T, Müller NL, Giménez A, et al: Spectrum of pulmonary aspergillosis: Histologic, clinical, and radiologic findings. Radiographics 21:825-837, 2001.

Surgical Complications

Lung Transplantation

Clinical Features

- Early complications include acute rejection, bacterial infection, pulmonary edema, acute respiratory distress syndrome (ARDS), diffuse alveolar hemorrhage
- Patients are evaluated for these complications with transbronchial biopsy and BAL
- Acute cellular rejection typically occurs within the first 3 to 6 months; however, the earliest manifestations of rejection can occur within the first week
- More than 80% of lung transplant recipients experience an episode of acute cellular rejection
- It can be difficult to differentiate acute cellular rejection from infection owing to overlapping clinical findings; reduction of forced expiratory volume in 1 second (FEV_1) is the most sensitive clinical finding for rejection

Gross Pathology

- Radiologic findings range from normal to interstitial pulmonary edema and are nonspecific

Histopathology

- See Table 4-9
- Transbronchial biopsy should yield at least 3 to 5 tissue fragments, and ideally more than 100 alveoli and 1 bronchiole should be present
- Acute rejection
  - Lymphoid infiltration of the airways often accompanies acute rejection in the form of lymphocytic bronchitis and bronchiolitis
  - However, lymphocytic bronchitis or bronchiolitis can occur in the absence of parenchymal acute rejection
- Airway inflammation
- Bronchiolitis obliterans (BO, chronic rejection): deposition of bland fibrous tissue within the submucosa of bronchioles in either a concentric or eccentric fashion, consequently, the airway lumen becomes narrowed
- Usually develops at the end of the first year or later; 50% of patients show evidence of bronchiolitis obliterans at 5 years

Special Stains and Immunohistochemistry

- CMV stain is most helpful; GMS and AFB stains are used when histology indicates infection
- Elastic or trichrome stains may be helpful in the workup of chronic rejection

Other Techniques for Diagnosis

- Noncontributory

Differential Diagnosis

▮ Infection
  - Perivascular lymphoid infiltrates also occur in the setting of CMV and *Pneumocystis* species infection

▮ Post-transplantation lymphoproliferative disorder

Figure 4-38. A, Acute rejection in lung transplantation. There is a complete cuff of inflammatory cells (predominantly lymphocytes) more than three layers thick around the pulmonary arteriole (grade A2). **B, Chronic rejection in lung transplantation.** There is near-total occlusion of the bronchiole by submucosal fibrosis. Note the residual discontinuous smooth muscle of the bronchiole in contrast to the adjacent artery.

Table 4-9. Grading Scheme for Transplant Rejection

Rejection Grade	Histologic Findings
A0	No evidence of mononuclear leukocyte infiltration, hemorrhage, or necrosis
A1	Perivascular or perivenular lymphoid cuffing Difficult to observe at low-power microscopy Density of lymphoid cells should be at least two cell layers thick
A2	Perivascular infiltrate expands and becomes easier to detect at low-power microscopy (more than three cell layers) Rare eosinophils, but not neutrophils, may be seen
A3	Expansion of the mononuclear infiltrate into perivascular and peribronchiolar alveolar interstitium Neutrophils may be apparent Endothelialitis, a subendothelial infiltration along with reactive or hyperplastic endothelial changes, is occasionally present
A4	Diffuse infiltrates extending from the perivascular areas to the pulmonary interstitium Diffuse alveolar damage with hyaline membranes, parenchymal necrosis, and hemorrhage Neutrophils may be seen in small numbers
B0	No airway inflammation
B1	Minimal airway inflammation
B2	Circumferential band of mononuclear cells with occasional eosinophils within the submucosa of bronchi or bronchioles
B3	Expansion of the infiltrate into a dense, bandlike process composed of mononuclear leukocytes, activated lymphocytes, and eosinophils Satellitosis of lymphocytes and epithelial cell necrosis
B4	Severe airway inflammation composed of dense bands of mononuclear leukocytes with ulceration of the airway epithelium Fibropurulent exudates containing neutrophils and necrotic debris

Pearls

- Minimal acute rejection is treated only when patient is symptomatic, whereas mild rejection is treated regardless of symptoms
- BO is the hallmark of chronic rejection; however, biopsy is not required for diagnosis of bronchiolitis obliterans syndrome, which is based on irreversible deterioration of lung function tests

Selected Reference

Leslie KO, Wick MR: Practical pulmonary pathology: A diagnostic approach. Philadelphia, Churchill Livingstone, 2005.

Neoplastic Conditions

Benign Epithelial Tumors

- See Table 4-10

Preinvasive Epithelial Lesions

Squamous Dysplasia (SD) and Carcinoma In Situ (CIS)

Clinical Features

- Relatively common, centrally localized lesion occurs in large airways of patients with history of cigarette smoke exposure
- SD/CIS is almost always asymptomatic
- Most patients have a previous high-grade preinvasive lesion, a history of lung or head and neck cancer, or synchronous lung cancer

Gross Pathology

- Difficult to detect grossly or bronchoscopically
- Detection is facilitated by autofluorescence bronchoscopy (AFB)
- About 75% of lesions are flat or superficial; 25% are nodular or polypoid
- CIS usually arises near bifurcations in segmental bronchi

Histopathology

- Often multifocal lesions ranging from 1 to 3 mm (SD) to 4 to 12 mm (CIS)
- Four histologic grades: mild, moderate, and severe dysplasia, and CIS
- Severe dysplasia shows cytologic atypia (increased cell size and pleomorphism) and mitoses extending to the upper third of the epithelium
- CIS shows extreme atypia without maturation extending to the surface and replacing the entire thickness of the of the epithelium

Special Stains and Immunohistochemistry

- Noncontributory

Other Techniques for Diagnosis

- Noncontributory

Differential Diagnosis

▌ Basal cell hyperplasia (BCH)
- BCH shows more than three layers of basal cells in otherwise normal pseudostratified columnar respiratory-type epithelium

Figure 4-39. **Squamous papilloma. A,** Low-power photomicrograph shows a papillary lesion composed of acanthotic squamous epithelium with fibrovascular cores. **B,** At higher power, human papillomavirus–related changes (koilocytes) are seen in the upper layers of the squamous epithelium (*right side*).

Table 4-10. Diagnostic Features of Benign Epithelial Neoplasms

	Juvenile Laryngotracheal Papillomatosis and Squamous Cell Papilloma	Alveolar Adenoma	Papillary Adenoma	Mucous Gland Adenoma	Mucinous Cystadenoma
Clinical features	Rare primary lung tumor (<0.5%) Associated with human papillomavirus- 6 and -11 Obstructive symptoms	Rare Most cases are asymptomatic	Rare Most cases are asymptomatic	Extremely rare Patients complain of obstructive symptoms	Extraordinarily rare
Gross findings	Arise from main bronchus Exophytic, cauliflower-like papillary projection into lumina, 0.7 to 9 cm (mean, 1.5 cm)	Most tumors are peripheral or subpleural, 0.7 to 6 cm Well-demarcated, smooth, lobulated, multicystic, yellow-tan lesions	Well-defined, soft, spongy to firm, gray-white to brown lesion, 1 to 4 cm	White-pink to tan, smooth, gelatinous, mucoid, solid or cystic, cut surface, 0.7 to 7.5 cm	Unilocular, mucus-filled cyst, 1 to 5 cm Thin cyst walls (0.1 cm)
Histology	Loose fibrovascular cores covered by stratified squamous epithelium 20% show koilocyte-like cytologic atypia	Unencapsulated, multicystic lesions Lined by bland, flattened, cuboidal, and hobnailed cells Cystic spaces are larger centrally and filled with eosinophilic fluid and periodic acid–Schiff–positive granular debris Squamous metaplasia	Well circumscribed Papillary growth with fibrovascular cores lined by cuboidal or columnar cells Ciliated or oxyphilic cells can also be found Intracellular mucin, atypia, and mitoses are rare to absent	Circumscribed, exophytic nodules Mucin-filled cystic spaces, microacini, glands, tubules, and papillae Cysts lined by bland flat, cuboidal or columnar mucus-producing cells	Mucinous cystic lesion lined by discontinuous layer of cuboidal or columnar mucinous cells Basal, hyperchromatic nuclei Multinucleated giant cell associated with extravasated mucin
Differential diagnosis	Squamous cell carcinoma shows invasion and malignant cytology Juvenile laryngotracheal papillomatosis rarely involves the lower respiratory tract	Lymphangioma Sclerosing hemangioma Adenocarcinoma Bronchioloalveolar carcinoma Primary or metastatic spindle cell tumor	Sclerosing hemangioma Alveolar adenoma Papillary adenocarcinoma Primary lung Metastatic thyroid	Low-grade mucoepidermoid carcinoma Mucinous cystadenoma Adenocarcinoma	Mucinous cystadenocarcinoma, adenocarcinoma, colloid bronchioloalveolar carcinoma, Mucinous congenital pulmonary airway malformation Bronchogenic cyst

▌ Squamous metaplasia (SM)
  ● SM likely arises from BCH
  ● Found in chronic inflammatory conditions
▌ Reactive atypia of inflammation, infection, and chemoradiation
  ● Reactive lesions show hypercellularity but lack the cytologic dysplasia
▌ Invasive carcinoma in transbronchial biopsy specimens
  ● Free, detached fragments of CIS are difficult to distinguish from invasive carcinoma, and helpful clues favoring CIS include straight to curvilinear fragment edges, a flat superficial epithelial surface, and a straight to undulating basement membrane
  ● Endobronchial papillary squamous cell carcinoma can be difficult to diagnose

Pearls

● The progression is thought to be from basal cell hyperplasia to squamous metaplasia to SD to CIS and finally to invasive SCC
● The follow-up behavior of severe SD/CIS lesions varies by study: some authors show invariable progression to invasive cancer, others show that only a minority of high-grade SD/CIS progresses
● The risk for low-grade SD progressing to invasive cancer is minimal
● Two additional subtypes of bronchial epithelial dysplasia have recently been described: columnar cell dysplasia (CCD) and bronchial epithelial dysplasia with transitional differentiation (TD type)

Selected Reference

Wistuba II, Gazdar AF: Lung cancer preneoplasia. Annu Rev Pathol 1:331-348, 2006.

Atypical Adenomatous Hyperplasia (AAH)

Clinical Features

● A peripheral lesion found in the centriacinar region close to respiratory bronchioles that arises from bronchioloalveolar epithelium
● Almost always found as an incidental histologic finding in lungs with existing bronchioloalveolar carcinoma (BAC) or primary carcinoma
● About 50% of cases show between two and six lesions

Gross Pathology

● AAH appears as a gray to yellow discrete nodule ranging from 1 to 5 mm, with most smaller than 3 mm

Histopathology

● Lesions stand out at scanning-power magnification
● Alveolar walls are thickened by fibrosis and lined by a heterogeneous population of cells including cuboidal cells, peg cells, and flat type 1 pneumocytes
● Large gaps can exist between cells conferring an interrupted appearance
● Occasional large or multinucleated cells are present
● Intranuclear inclusions that stain positive for surfactant apoprotein A (PE10) are present in up to 25% of the cells
● Ciliated and mucous cells are virtually absent, and mitoses are rare
● Cellularity and cytologic atypia are variable

Special Stains and Immunohistochemistry

● Noncontributory

Other Techniques for Diagnosis

● Noncontributory

Figure 4-40. Atypical adenomatous hyperplasia. A, Low-power photomicrograph shows a distinct small lesion with atypical pneumocytes lining alveolar septa with mild fibrosis. **B,** High power shows atypical pneumocytes with a hobnail appearance.

Differential Diagnosis

- Localized nonmucinous BAC
  - Alveolar architecture is preserved in both AAH and BAC
  - BACs are usually more than 10 mm in diameter, with a more homogeneous cell population; large BACs show central collapse with fibrosis or scar (an important area to look for evidence of invasion)
  - BACs show three or more of the following: marked cell stratification, high cell density with nuclear overlap, coarse nuclear chromatin with prominent nucleoli, true papillae, and increased cell height; AAH rarely displays more than one of those features
- Diffuse interstitial lung disease
  - AAH occurs in the absence of underlying interstitial inflammation or fibrosis
- Peribronchiolar metaplasia
  - Centriacinar lesion composed of ciliated bronchiolar-type cells with fibrosis
- Papillary adenoma
  - About 1- to 4-cm, well-demarcated tumor with papillary architecture
  - True papillae are not a feature of AAH
- Alveolar adenoma
  - Peripheral, well-circumscribed tumor smaller than 6 cm
  - Composed of variably sized spaces lined with cuboidal cells overlying a spindle cell–rich stroma with focal myxoid changes
- Micronodular pneumocyte hyperplasia
  - Extremely rare lesion associated with tuberous sclerosis or lymphangioleiomyomatosis (LAM)
  - Well-demarcated lesion several millimeters in diameter composed of uniform cuboidal cells arranged in a more solid pattern than AAH

Pearls

- AAH is thought to be the precursor of nonmucinous BAC and invasive adenocarcinoma; it is also seen in patients with squamous cell carcinoma (field effect)
- Similar to invasive adenocarcinoma, AAH show mutations in the *Kras* and *EGFR* genes, but the invasive potential of *Kras* mutations is not clearly demonstrated

Selected Reference

Wistuba II, Gazdar AF: Lung cancer preneoplasia. Annu Rev Pathol 1:331-348, 2006.

Diffuse Idiopathic Pulmonary Neuroendocrine Cell Hyperplasia (DIPNECH)

Clinical Features

- Extremely rare lesion that gives rise to low-grade, peripheral carcinoid tumor

Gross Pathology

- As lesions progress to carcinoid tumorlets and carcinoid tumors they appear as small, well-demarcated, gray-white nodules resembling miliary bodies

Histopathology

- Widespread proliferation of pulmonary neuroendocrine cells manifesting as increased numbers of individual cells, small groups, or nodular aggregates or nests in the bronchial or bronchiolar epithelium
- Nodules of neuroendocrine cells can protrude into airway lumens and occasionally cause an occlusion
- As lesions advance, pulmonary neuroendocrine cells break through the basement membrane and form 2- to 5-mm carcinoid tumorlets
- Marked fibrosis is often associated with carcinoid tumorlets and carcinoid tumor (lesions larger than 5 mm are classified as carcinoids)

Special Stains and Immunohistochemistry

- Positive for chromogranin, synaptophysin, and cytokeratin 8/18

Other Techniques for Diagnosis

- Noncontributory

Differential Diagnosis for DIPNECH

- Pulmonary neuroendocrine cell (PNEC) hyperplasia in fibroinflammatory disease (e.g., bronchiectasis), incidental PNEC hyperplasia, minute meningothelial nodules

Pearls

- DIPNECH may be a precursor lesion of a subset of carcinoid tumors that are invariably low grade and peripheral; the precursor to centrally localized, high-grade carcinoid tumors has not yet been clearly identified

Selected References

Kerr KM, Popper HH: The differential diagnosis of pulmonary pre-invasive lesions. Eur Respir Monogr 12:37-62, 2007.
Kerr KM: Pulmonary preinvasive neoplasia. J Clin Pathol 54:257-271, 2001.

Malignant Epithelial Tumors

Adenocarcinoma

Clinical Features

- Most common type of lung cancer, accounting for about 40% of all cases of invasive lung cancer in the United States; increasing incidence in the past decade
- Roughly 75% of lung adenocarcinomas are peripheral
- The most common variant of lung cancer in women and nonsmokers; its association with cigarette smoking is weaker than with other types of lung carcinoma

Figure 4-41. Adenocarcinoma. This photomicrograph shows a mixed pattern with solid areas and gland formation in this moderately to poorly differentiated adenocarcinoma.

Gross Pathology

- Disease classically arises as a single mass or as multiple nodular tumors of variable size; also arises centrally in the hilum or perihilar bronchus
- Tumors are gray-tan and firm with variable amounts of necrosis
- Tumors demonstrate one of six growth patterns
  - Peripheral tumor with desmoplastic retraction of overlying pleura creating a puckered appearance with or without scarring
  - Endobronchial adenocarcinoma
  - Pneumonia-like consolidation associated with bronchioloalveolar or papillary growth patterns
  - Visceral pleural-based, pseudomesotheliomatous carcinoma
  - Adenocarcinoma arising in the background of underlying fibrosis
  - Diffuse bilateral lung disease
- Penetration of the pleura leads to dissemination within the pleural cavity, pleural effusions, and occasionally chest wall invasion

Histopathology

- Tumor is characterized by gland formation or mucin production
- Intracytoplasmic mucin or mucin within glandular lumina is a key feature
- Glands are usually surrounded by desmoplastic stroma
- A spectrum of morphology is seen, with varying amounts of differentiation and atypia
- Major histologic subtypes
  - Acinar pattern
    - Acini and tubules formed by cuboidal or columnar cells resembling bronchial glands with mucin production
  - Papillary pattern
    - Usually a solitary tumor formed by papillae lined by large, atypical cells with enlarged, hyperchromatic nuclei, prominent nucleoli, and frequent mitoses (in contrast to BAC)
    - Papillae often show secondary and tertiary branching patterns
    - Psammoma bodies can be present
    - Foci of conventional adenocarcinoma or BAC are often present
    - Pure papillary growth pattern must be distinguished from metastatic tumor
  - Bronchioloalveolar pattern
    - Composed of mature, well-differentiated tumor cells growing along preexisting alveolar walls demonstrating no stromal, vascular, or pleural invasion
    - Often seen at the periphery of an otherwise invasive adenocarcinoma, which should be classified as adenocarcinoma mixed-type with predominant bronchioloalveolar pattern
  - Solid pattern
    - Lacks papillae, tubules, and acini and is composed sheets of polygonal cells with at least five mucin-positive cells in each of 2 high-power fields (hpf)
  - Well-differentiated fetal adenocarcinoma (WDFA)
    - Endometrioid appearance composed of complex, back-to-back glands and occasional desmoplastic stromal reaction resembling the stroma of secretory endometrium
    - Glands lined by nonciliated columnar cells with clear cytoplasm and basally orientated nuclei
    - Pleomorphism and atypia are inconspicuous
    - Resembles monophasic pulmonary blastoma and fetal-type adenocarcinoma
    - Tumor cells show weak, multifocal staining for chromogranin or synaptophysin in roughly 70% of cases
  - Mucinous or colloid adenocarcinoma
    - Dissecting pools of mucin with islands of neoplasia
  - Mucinous cystadenocarcinoma
    - Lower-grade variant of adenocarcinoma
  - Signet ring adenocarcinoma: rule out metastasis from gastric primary
    - Acinar or diffuse histologic pattern composed of tumor cells with large cytoplasmic mucin vacuoles and peripherally displaced nuclei
  - Clear cell adenocarcinoma: rule out metastatic renal cell carcinoma

Special Stains and Immunohistochemistry

- Mucin production can be demonstrated with mucicarmine, PAS, or Alcian blue stains
- Tumor cells are positive for the epithelial markers: CAM5.2, pancytokeratin AE1/AE3, epithelial

membrane antigen (EMA), carcinoembryonic antigen (CEA), Leu-M1, Ber-Ep4, and B72.3/BRST-3/TAG-72
- Adenocarcinomas usually express CK7 more often than CK20
- TTF-1 (nuclear) is expressed in roughly 75% to 95% of lung adenocarcinomas

Other Techniques for Diagnosis
- *EGFR* mutations seen in less than 10% of patients allow for targeted therapy

Differential Diagnosis
▪ Metastatic adenocarcinoma
- Presentation with multiple lung masses favors metastasis
- Metastatic colonic adenocarcinoma is typically CK7 negative and CK20 positive
- CDX2 is positive in mucinous BAC and gastrointestinal lesions
- Estrogen and progesterone receptors and gross cystic disease fluid protein-15 are often positive in breast carcinomas
- Prostate-specific antigen, prostatic acid phosphatase are positive in metastatic prostate carcinoma
- TTF-1 is positive in primary lung and metastatic thyroid carcinoma; thyroglobulin is positive in the latter, and mucin staining is positive in the former
▪ Mesothelioma
- IHC panel should include TTF-1, two epithelial markers (CEA, BG8, or MOC 31), and two mesothelial markers (calretinin, CK5/6, WT-1, or D2-40)
▪ Bronchiolar metaplasia
- Bronchiolar metaplasia often occurs in fibrotic processes such as UIP
- Papillary or invasive growth patterns or intracytoplasmic mucin production favors adenocarcinoma

Pearls
- The pathologic diagnosis should include the histologic subtypes, for example, "adenocarcinoma, with acinar, papillary, and bronchioloalveolar patterns"
- Small, peripheral adenocarcinomas with minimal invasion (5 mm or less) within lepidic growth areas have the same excellent clinical prognosis as BAC
- Micropapillary pattern is associated with poorer prognosis
- WDFA can occur in the setting of familial adenomatous polyposis (FAP) and is correlated with abnormally elevated β-catenin signaling
- Incidence of intrapulmonary metastasis is most common in adenocarcinoma
- Molecular analysis of adenocarcinoma suggests two differing pathways involving either the *K-ras* gene or the *EGFR* gene
- *K-ras* mutations in codons 12, 13, or 61 are present in 30% of adenocarcinomas, are particularly common in smokers, and are occasionally present in SCC
- Activating mutations in *EGFR* are clustered in exons 18 to 21 and associated with female sex, never-smoked status, adenocarcinoma histology, and Asian ethnicity
- Optimal patient selection for *EGFR*-directed therapies is currently being defined, and the highest response rates appear to occur in tumors with activating *EGFR* mutations or a prominent nonmucinous BAC component
- Inactivation of p16Ink4 occurs often in adenocarcinoma and is associated with cigarette smoking
- Overexpression of p27 correlates with increased tumor differentiation and better prognosis

Selected References
Weydert JA, Cohen MB: Small peripheral pulmonary adenocarcinoma: Morphologic and molecular update. Adv Anat Pathol 14:120-128, 2007.
Travis WD, Garg K, Franklin WA, et al: Bronchioloalveolar carcinoma and lung adenocarcinoma: The clinical importance and research relevance of the 2004 World Health Organization pathologic criteria. J Thorac Oncol 1(9 Suppl):S13-139, 2006.
Moran CA: Pulmonary adenocarcinoma: The expanding spectrum of histologic variants. Arch Pathol Lab Med 130:958-962, 2006.
Dennis JL, Hvidsten TR, Wit EC, et al: Markers of adenocarcinoma characteristic of the site of origin: development of a diagnostic algorithm. Clin Cancer Res 11:3766-3772, 2005.
Meyerson M, Franklin WA, Kelley MJ: Molecular classification and molecular genetics of human lung cancers. Semin Oncol 31(1 Suppl 1):4-19, 2004.

Bronchioloalveolar Carcinoma (BAC)

Clinical Features
- Wide age distribution ranging from 20 years to old age, with equal distribution between men and women and no association with smoking

Gross Pathology
- Mostly occurs in the peripheral portions of the lung as either single or multiple subpleural nodules
- Solitary nodules are usually associated with nonmucinous BAC
- Tumors are soft, are poorly circumscribed, and may be mucinous

Histopathology
- Neoplastic cells grow along preexisting alveolar septa with no evidence of stromal, vascular, or pleural invasion
  — Nonmucinous variant of BAC
    ◆ Accounts for roughly 75% of BAC and likely arises from AAH
    ◆ Tumor cells display either Clara cell or type 2 pneumocyte differentiation

Figure 4-42. Bronchioloalveolar carcinoma. A, Gross picture of explanted lung shows one large irregular tan-white tumor and innumerable smaller areas of pneumonic consolidation, which is due to the intrapulmonary spread of tumor. **B,** Columnar tumor cells are growing along preexisting alveolar septa with no desmoplastic reaction.

◇ Clara cell differentiation: columnar cells with pale, eosinophilic cytoplasm and cytoplasmic snouts

◇ Type 2 pneumocyte differentiation: cuboidal with fine cytoplasmic vacuoles or clear to foamy cytoplasm; eosinophilic intranuclear inclusions may be present

— Mucinous variant of BAC

♦ About 25% of BAC, frequently associated with significant bronchorrhea

♦ Tumor cells are tall columnar with basal nuclei, amphophilic cytoplasm, and varying amounts of mucin production; minimal cytologic atypia

♦ Transition from tumor cells to uninvolved alveoli is often abrupt

♦ Mucin accumulation within surrounding alveolar spaces can occur

Special Stains and Immunohistochemistry

- Nonmucinous BAC has an immunophenotype similar to adenocarcinoma, i.e., CK7 positive, TTF-1 positive, CK20 negative
- Mucinous BAC is often positive for CK7 and CK20 but negative for TTF-1, which is important to be aware of to avoid misinterpreting mucinous BAC for a metastasis from gastrointestinal tract primary
- PAS positive granules may be identified in nonmucinous BAC with Clara cell differentiation

Other Techniques for Diagnosis

- Mucinous BACs have frequent mutations at codon 12 of the *K-ras* gene
- Loss of heterozygosity within the fragile histidine triad gene (*FHIT*) is commonly observed in all BAC subtypes
- Nonmucinous BACs often have *p53* mutations and are associated with more aggressive tumors

Differential Diagnosis

▐ Invasive adenocarcinoma
- Invasive adenocarcinoma displays significant atypia, fibroblastic stromal response, and glandular differentiation

▐ Type 2 pneumocyte hyperplasia
- Occurs in the setting of underlying fibrosis (i.e., UIP)
- Additional cell types, including low cuboidal, flattened epithelial, and nonmucinous columnar bronchial cells, are unusual in BAC

▐ Mucinous BAC versus metastatic gastrointestinal adenocarcinoma
- Gastrointestinal adenocarcinomas also express COX2, which is usually negative in mucinous BAC

Pearls

- Mucinous and nonmucinous BACs are likely two entirely separate clinical entities in which patients with mucinous BAC present with higher-stage disease or more extensive, multifocal, pneumonic spread of the tumor cells
- Features favoring true invasion versus stromal collapse: angulated glands, increased cytologic, desmoplastic stromal reaction, complex acinar or cribriform growth, individual cell infiltration, necrosis, and destruction of the elastica or normal parenchyma (laminin stain may be helpful here)
- Tumors with the bronchioloalveolar pattern that are smaller than 2 cm need to be completely sampled and submitted to search for foci of invasion
- The diagnosis of BAC requires that no pleural, vascular, or stromal invasion is present, and the diagnosis of BAC should not be made on a small biopsy or cytology specimen
- Some pathologists consider BACs measuring less than 0.5 cm to be AAH; however, this is not a recognized World Health Organization (WHO) criterion or classification

- Many conventional adenocarcinomas show a component of lepidic growth, particularly at their periphery, and these should not be diagnosed as BAC
  — WHO classification recommends such tumors be termed *adenocarcinoma with prominent bronchioloalveolar pattern* or *mixed subtype adenocarcinoma*
- Aerogenous spread is common, leading to numerous satellite lesions adjacent to main tumor mass or manifesting as extensive consolidation
- Cathepsin K is a proteinase that is involved in extracellular matrix remodeling and has been reported to be expressed in areas of invasive growth but not in areas of lepidic growth or alveolar collapse

Selected References

Yousem SA, Beasley MB: Bronchioloalveolar carcinoma: A review of current concepts and evolving issues. Arch Pathol Lab Med 131:1027-1032, 2007.

Weydert JA, Cohen MB: Small peripheral pulmonary adenocarcinoma: Morphologic and molecular update. Adv Anat Pathol 14:120-128, 2007.

Travis WD, Garg K, Franklin WA, et al: Bronchioloalveolar carcinoma and lung adenocarcinoma: The clinical importance and research relevance of the 2004 World Health Organization pathologic criteria. J Thorac Oncol 1(9 Suppl):S13-19, 2006.

Squamous Cell Carcinoma (SCC)

Clinical Features

- Accounts for roughly 20% of all invasive lung cancer
- Strong association with cigarette smoking
- Small minority of patients presenting with signs of obstruction (e.g., recurrent infection, hemoptysis, cough)

Figure 4-43. Squamous cell carcinoma. This moderately well-differentiated squamous cell carcinoma shows focal keratinization with formation of keratin pearls. Marked desmoplastic reaction is present.

Gross Pathology

- About 75% of cases are centrally located, arising from proximal bronchi
- Tumor forms a firm gray-white mass with desmoplastic stromal reaction
- Areas of necrosis and cavitation can be present
- Endobronchial growth may occlude the airway lumen, leading to bronchiectasis, infection, or bronchopneumonia

Histopathology

- Tumor cells display squamous cell differentiation in the form of keratinization, pearl formation, and intercellular bridges
- ▌ Papillary variant
  - Exophytic, papillary, and endobronchial growth pattern
  - Most patients present with low-stage disease and a relatively good prognosis with greater than 60% 5-year survival
- ▌ Clear cell variant
  - This variant is rare (<0.3% of all lung cancer)
  - Tumor is composed almost entirely of large, polygonal cells with clear cytoplasm; note, clear cell change is common, and up to one third of all primary lung cancers have foci of clear cell change composing 10% to 20% of the tumor
  - Resembles metastatic renal clear cell carcinoma, metastatic thyroid carcinoma, adenocarcinoma with clear cell change, and large cell carcinoma
- ▌ Small cell variant
  - Poorly differentiated carcinoma with small cells, hyperchromatic, irregular nuclei, prominent nucleoli, moderate cytoplasm, and distinct cell-cell boundaries
  - Focal squamous differentiation
  - Lacks the even, homogeneous, salt-and-pepper chromatin pattern and nuclear molding seen in small cell lung carcinoma (SCLC) and stains negative for chromogranin and synaptophysin
- ▌ Basaloid variant
  - Nests of poorly differentiated tumor cells with prominent palisading peripheral nuclei
  - Differential diagnosis of this variant of SCC includes adenoid cystic carcinoma, which occurs in younger patients and has a better prognosis
- ▌ Nonkeratinizing variant
  - Resembles urothelial carcinoma

Special Stains and Immunohistochemistry

- SCC express high-molecular-weight keratin 34βE12, CK5/6, CEA, p63, and low-molecular-weight keratin (35βH11)
- SCC rarely expresses CK7 or TTF-1

Other Techniques for Diagnosis

- Gain of the chromosomal locus 3q26 through either 3q26 amplification or polysomy is the most common genomic abnormalities in SCC

- Expression of *p53* gradually increases in dysplastic squamous epithelium

Differential Diagnosis

▌ SCC versus SCLC
  - SCLC is p63 negative and TTF-1 positive, whereas SCC is generally p63 positive and TTF-1 negative

Pearls

- Five-year survival rate for SCC is generally better than that of adenocarcinoma
- In addition to 3q26 amplification, other cytogenetic features of SCC include loss on 3p, 9p, and 8p, and *p53* mutation
- Loss of p16INK4A correlates with significantly worse survival in NSCLC, particularly for SCC

Selected References

Meyerson M, Franklin WA, Kelley MJ:. Molecular classification and molecular genetics of human lung cancers. Semin Oncol 31(Suppl 1):4-19, 2004.

Massion PP, Taflan P, Jamshedur Rahman SM, et al: Significance of p63 amplification and overexpression in lung cancer development and prognosis. Cancer Res 63:7113-7121, 2003.

Small Cell Lung Carcinoma (SCLC)

Clinical Features

- SCLC occurs almost exclusively in smokers
- It accounts for about 13% of lung cancer cases in the United States
- The proportion of women with SCLC has increased and accounts for roughly half of all cases
- In general, SCLC initially responds to chemotherapy and therefore needs to be separated from non–small cell lung carcinoma (NSCLC)
- Combined small cell carcinoma variant displays classic SCLC features, with an additional component consisting of any histologic subtype of NSCLC
- Because SCLC is a high-grade tumor with widespread dissemination at presentation, it is staged as limited disease versus extensive disease rather than using the TNM system, although there are emerging data to support use of the TNM system
- Limited disease (30% to 40% of patients): disease confined to the ipsilateral hemithorax and within a single radiotherapy port (corresponding in part to TNM stages I through IIIB)
- Extensive disease (60% to 70% of patients): evident metastatic disease outside the ipsilateral hemithorax

Gross Pathology

- White-tan, soft, friable perihilar mass with extensive necrosis and frequent nodal metastases
- Tumor spreads along bronchi in a submucosal and circumferential pattern with usual lymphatic invasion

- About 5% of cases present as peripheral coin-shaped lesions

Histopathology

- Tumor cells are generally smaller than the size of three resting lymphocytes
- Tumor cells have round, oval, or spindle-shaped nuclei and scanty cytoplasm
- Cell borders are indistinct, and molding is a common feature
- An important diagnostic feature is the absence of nucleoli; however, larger tumor cells can occasionally display a few inconspicuous nucleoli
- Mitotic rates are high, averaging more than 60 mitoses/10 hpf, and necrosis is often extensive
- Growth patterns include nesting, trabeculated, peripheral palisading, and rosette formation—similar to other neuroendocrine tumors; sheetlike growth without a neuroendocrine pattern is also common
- Combined SCLC represents less than 3% of SCLC cases and is the only variant of SCLC recognized by the 2004 WHO Classification
  - Non–small cell component is usually squamous cell, adenocarcinoma, or large cell carcinoma; less commonly, spindle cell or giant cell carcinoma
  - The non–small cell component needs to be specified in the diagnosis

Special Stains and Immunohistochemistry

- Virtually all SCLC stain with cytokeratin (including CK7) and EMA
- About 90% of SCLC cells express TTF-1
- About 90% of SCLC cells stain positive for one or more of the neuroendocrine markers; less than 10% of SCLC cases are negative for all neuroendocrine markers

Other Techniques for Diagnosis

- Deletion of chromosome 3p is a consistent finding in SCLC, and this region may include the fragile histidine triad gene (*FHIT*) located at 3p14.2
- About 20% of SCLCs show mutations in the *Rb* gene
- About 70% to 95% of SCLCs show *Bcl-2* expression
- SCLC shows the highest rate of *p53* mutation of all lung carcinomas, and consequently a strong nuclear p53 staining pattern in greater than 10% to 20% percent of cells is strongly suggestive of a *p53* mutation

Differential Diagnosis

▌ Lymphocytic infiltrate
  - In a small biopsy sample, crushed lymphocytes can be difficult to distinguish from SCLC without IHC analysis (LCA, keratin AE1/AE3, and CAM5.2)
▌ Atypical carcinoid
  - SCLC displays relatively more necrosis, karyorrhexis, and mitoses than atypical carcinoid
  - Carcinoid tumors generally show more extensive and robust staining for chromogranin

Figure 4-44. Small cell carcinoma. A, Grossly, all lung carcinomas tend to have a similar appearance. In this resection specimen, a large irregular tan-white tumor mass is seen in the lung. **B,** Low-power photomicrograph shows nests of crushed cells and large areas of necrosis, typical of transbronchial biopsies. **C,** This photomicrograph of a resected tumor shows well-preserved intermediate-sized tumor cells forming pseudorosettes with mitoses, salt-and-pepper chromatin, and rare inconspicuous nucleoli. **D,** Azzopardi effect is seen with crushed DNA around a blood vessel in this largely necrotic tumor. **E,** Immunoperoxidase stain for keratin CAM5.2 can be helpful in distinguishing carcinoma from lymphocytes. **F,** Thyroid transcription factor-1 (TTF-1) shows nuclear staining in the tumor as well as in adjacent normal pneumocytes.

Pearls

- The diagnosis of SCLC is made by light microscopy, and negative staining for neuroendocrine markers does not exclude the diagnosis
- SCLC shows a tendency to crush in forceps and bronchial biopsies
- DNA from necrotic tumor cells can get deposited in the walls of vessels and connective tissue (the Azzopardi phenomenon)

- Infrequently, patients produce autoantibodies that bind to SCLC cells and non-neoplastic cells of the central nervous system or neuromuscular junction, resulting in cerebellar degenerative syndromes or Lambert-Eaton myasthenic syndrome
- SCLC cells can also produce a number of polypeptide hormones, including adrenocorticotropic hormone and vasopressin, resulting in various paraneoplastic and ectopic hormonal syndromes

- The *Rb* gene has been reported to be deleted in more than 90% of SCLCs and in 15% of NSCLCs

Selected References

Chong S, Lee KS, Chung MJ, et al: Neuroendocrine tumors of the lung: Clinical, pathologic, and imaging findings. Radiographics 26:41-57; discussion, 57-58, 2006.

Meyerson M, Franklin WA, Kelley MJ: Molecular classification and molecular genetics of human lung cancers. Semin Oncol 31(Suppl 1):4-19, 2004.

Large Cell Carcinoma and Large Cell Neuroendocrine Carcinoma (LCNEC)

Clinical Features

- Undifferentiated tumor lacks the diagnostic features of squamous cell carcinoma, adenocarcinoma, or small cell carcinoma by light microscopy
- Represents 9% of all lung cancers

Gross Pathology

- Usually is a large central or peripheral tumor with a fleshy, pink-tan cut surface
- Foci of tumor necrosis are common
- Invasion through the pleura into the chest wall or adjacent structures frequently occurs

Histopathology

- A diagnosis of exclusion after adenocarcinoma, squamous cell carcinoma, and small cell carcinoma have been ruled out
- Tumor cells possess large vesicular nuclei with prominent nucleoli, moderate amounts of cytoplasm, and well-defined cell-cell borders
- Tumor cells are arranged in sheets or nests

Figure 4-45. Large cell carcinoma. Clusters of highly atypical large cells (compare size to normal lymphocytes) are seen within fibrous tissue. Nucleoli are prominent.

- Variants
  — Large cell neuroendocrine carcinoma variant (LCNEC)
    ◆ LCNEC represents 3% of lung cancers
    ◆ Has organoid nesting, trabecular growth, rosette formation, and perilobular palisading patterns of growth
    ◆ Tumor cells are large with abundant cytoplasm
    ◆ Prominent nucleoli help differentiate from small cell carcinoma
    ◆ Mitotic activity is robust (>10 mitoses/10 hpf; average, 66 mitoses/10 hpf), and large zones of necrosis are common
  — Combined large cell neuroendocrine variant
    ◆ Component of adenocarcinoma, squamous cells carcinoma, giant cell carcinoma, or spindle cell carcinoma is present
  — Basaloid carcinoma
    ◆ Conspicuous palisading at the periphery of tumor nests
  — Lymphoepithelioma-like carcinoma
    ◆ Large tumor cells intermixed with a lymphoid infiltrate
  — Clear cell carcinoma
  — Large cell carcinoma with rhabdoid phenotype
    ◆ More than 10% of the tumor cells must be rhabdoid, with eosinophilic cytoplasmic inclusions composed of intermediate filaments

Special Stains and Immunohistochemistry

▌ LCNEC
- Staining with neuroendocrine markers is often patchy and relatively weak, similar to SCLC and in stark contrast to the robust, diffuse staining seen in carcinoids
- Diffusely positive for keratin and CEA; 50% of LCNEC tumors express TTF-1

▌ Basaloid carcinoma
- Neuroendocrine markers and TTF-1 are usually negative
- High-molecular-weight cytokeratin (34βE12) is positive

Other Techniques for Diagnosis

▌ Lymphoepithelioma-like carcinoma
- EBV-encoded small RNA (EBER RNA) expression is present in the nuclei of tumor cells but not in the surrounding lymphocytic infiltrate

Differential Diagnosis

▌ Poorly differentiated squamous cell carcinoma
- Foci of intercellular bridges and keratin formation are present in SCC

▌ Basaloid carcinoma versus basaloid variant of squamous cell carcinoma
- Presence of squamous differentiation, even if focal, favors the basaloid variant of squamous cell carcinoma

- ▌ Solid type of adenocarcinoma
  - ● Minimum of 5 mucin droplets/2 hpf
- ▌ Atypical carcinoid
  - ● 2 to 10 mitoses/10 hpf and punctate necrosis

Pearls

- ● Diagnosis of large cell carcinoma should not be made on a small transbronchial biopsy because adenocarcinoma, squamous cell carcinoma, and other types of carcinoma may have foci with features of large cell carcinoma
- ● LCNEC is an aggressive, rare tumor with dismal prognosis that is difficult to diagnose because the neuroendocrine component (organoid pattern) must first be identified by light microscopy, and at least one specific neuroendocrine marker must be demonstrated by immunohistochemistry

Selected References

Chong S, Lee KS, Chung MJ, et al: Neuroendocrine tumors of the lung: Clinical, pathologic, and imaging findings. Radiographics 26:41-57; discussion, 57-58, 2006.

Hage R, Seldenrijk K, de Bruin P, et al: Pulmonary large-cell neuroendocrine carcinoma (LCNEC). Eur J Cardiothorac Surg 23:457-460, 2003.

Carcinoid Tumor

Clinical Features

- ● Carcinoid tumors are low-grade malignancies that make up 1% to 2% of all primary lung cancers
- ● Mean age of diagnosis for typical and atypical carcinoid tumors is 45 and 55 years, respectively
- ● Atypical carcinoid is associated with cigarette smoking
- ● Young adults, adolescents, and children can get carcinoid tumors
- ● Carcinoid tumors arise at numerous sites in the body, with lung being the second most common site after the gastrointestinal tract
- ● Bronchial carcinoid may present with obstructive symptoms due to mass effect: cough, wheezing, dyspnea, chest pain, hemoptysis, and recurrent pneumonia; peripheral carcinoid tumors are usually asymptomatic

Gross Pathology

- ● Most tumors (70%) arise centrally in the main or major bronchi and are frequently endobronchial; 30% are peripheral, arising in segmental bronchi or beyond
- ● Tumors are firm, well-demarcated, yellow-tan, nodular masses with a glistening cut surface and usually measure less than 2 cm
- ● The overlying mucosa may be intact or ulcerated

Histopathology

- ● Carcinoid tumors are part of the spectrum of neuroendocrine lung tumors that includes large cell neuroendocrine carcinoma, small cell carcinoma, and typical and atypical carcinoid tumors
- ● Carcinoid tumors are composed of a uniform population of polygonal cells with fine, granular cytoplasm, inconspicuous nucleoli, and scanty cytoplasm
- ● Nuclear atypia and pleomorphism may be marked, but these features do not distinguish between typical and atypical carcinoid
- ● Growth patterns suggestive of neuroendocrine differentiation include organoid, trabecular, spindle cell, papillary, pseudoglandular, rosette, and follicular
- ● True gland formation is rare, and spindling of tumor cells can be significant—particularly in peripherally localized carcinoid tumors

Figure 4-46. Carcinoid tumor. A, A polypoid lesion with a uniform appearance is seen protruding into the lumen of the bronchus. **B,** At high power, an organoid pattern is seen. The cells are uniform, with abundant cytoplasm, round to oval nuclei, and salt-and-pepper chromatin.

- The stroma is typically vascular, or less often, hyalinized with cartilage or metaplastic bone formation
- Typical carcinoid (80% to 90% of pulmonary carcinoids): greater than 0.5 cm in diameter, 1 mitosis/10 hpf, and no evidence of necrosis
- Atypical carcinoid (10% to 20% of pulmonary carcinoids): focal necrosis or 2 to 10 mitoses/10 hpf

Special Stains and Immunohistochemistry

- About 80% of carcinoid tumors stain with cytokeratin antibodies
- Typical carcinoid tumors are strongly positive for neuroendocrine markers
- Atypical carcinoid tumors show modestly reduced staining for neuroendocrine markers; however, the difference does not distinguish atypical from typical carcinoid
- Sustentacular cells express S-100
- Most carcinoid tumors express CD99

Other Techniques for Diagnosis

- Noncontributory

Differential Diagnosis

- Other neuroendocrine tumors
  - SCLC and LCNEC show fewer positive cells with less intense staining for neuroendocrine markers
  - Carcinoid and large cell neuroendocrine tumors make up less than 3% of all lung cancers, whereas small cell lung cancer is more common, accounting for 13% of all lung cancers
  - Carcinoid tumorlets resemble typical carcinoid and are less than 5 mm in diameter
- Large cell neuroendocrine carcinoma (LCNEC)
  - Greater than 10 mitoses/10 hpf (median, 70/10 hpf)
  - Relatively more necrosis
  - Larger cell size with vesicular, coarse, or fine chromatin, visible nucleoli, and lower nuclear-to-cytoplasmic ratio than atypical carcinoid
- Small cell lung carcinoma (SCLC)
  - High mitotic rates (median, 80/10 hpf)
  - Frequent, extensive necrosis
  - Fine granular chromatin, absent or faint nucleoli, scanty cytoplasm, and nuclear molding
- Pulmonary carcinoid versus intestinal or pancreatic carcinoid tumors
  - About 80% to 95% of pulmonary carcinoid tumors are TTF-1 positive, whereas intestinal and pancreatic carcinoids do not express TTF-1
- Adenocarcinoma and other carcinomas
  - Pseudoglandular growth patterns may mimic adenocarcinoma, mucoepidermoid, or acinic cell carcinoma
  - Adenocarcinoma displays more atypia, more mucin production, and less expression of neuroendocrine markers than carcinoid tumors

Pearls

- Typical carcinoid tumors rarely metastasize and have a good prognosis (about 90% 5-year survival rate after complete resection)
- Atypical carcinoid tumors show a greater propensity for metastasis, and 5-year survival rate is about 50%
- Typical and atypical carcinoid tumors can occur in patients with multiple endocrine neoplasia type I syndrome (MEN I)
- Gene mutations in *p53*, *Rb*, and *cyclin D1* are much more common in LCNEC and SCLC than in carcinoid tumors
- Carcinoid syndrome, Cushing syndrome, and synthesis of ectopic growth hormone–releasing hormone is rare in pulmonary carcinoid tumors

Selected References

Kloppel G: Tumour biology and histopathology of neuroendocrine tumours. Best Pract Res Clin Endocrinol Metab 21:15-31, 2007.

Chong S, Lee KS, Chung MJ, et al: Neuroendocrine tumors of the lung: Clinical, pathologic, and imaging findings. Radiographics 26:41-57; discussion, 57-58, 2006.

Hage R, Seldenrijk K, de Bruin P, et al: Pulmonary large-cell neuroendocrine carcinoma (LCNEC). Eur J Cardiothorac Surg 23:457-460, 2003.

Flieder DB: Neuroendocrine tumors of the lung: Recent developments in histopathology. Curr Opin Pulm Med 8:275-280, 2002.

Mesenchymal Tumors

Pulmonary Hamartoma

Clinical Features

- About 5% to 8% of all solitary pulmonary nodules and 75% of all benign lung tumors

Figure 4-47. Hamartoma. Benign cartilage, fat, and bronchial epithelium are seen in this low-power photomicrograph.

- Most hamartomas are discovered between the ages of 50 and 60 years, and men are affected 2 to 3 times more frequently than women
- Most patients have a history of cigarette smoke exposure
- Most peripheral lesions are clinically silent, whereas endobronchial lesions may cause obstructive symptoms

Gross Pathology

- About 90% of tumors are located in the lung periphery, whereas 10% are located centrally
- Gray-white, sharply demarcated, firm, lobulated nodule ranging in size from 1 to 9 cm with mean diameter of 1.5 cm

Histopathology

- Benign neoplasm containing a mixture of epithelial and mesenchymal tissues
- The tumor is composed of a haphazard arrangement of cartilage, fibromyxoid tissue, fat, smooth muscle, or bone
- Nodules are separated by clefts lined with non-neoplastic, ciliated, or nonciliated respiratory epithelium
- All components are well differentiated, and fat is present in more than half of all specimens

Special Stains and Immunohistochemistry

- Noncontributory

Other Techniques for Diagnosis

- Noncontributory

Differential Diagnosis

▌ Carney triad
- Rare disorder that predominantly affects women and often presents during teenage years, with epithelioid gastrointestinal stromal tumors (GISTs) and extra-adrenal paragangliomas
- Pulmonary chondromas, often multiple and lacking cleftlike spaces, lined by respiratory epithelium
▌ Leiomyoma
- Leiomyomas do not contain fat or cartilage
▌ Lipoma
- Typically found in central bronchi, more often left-sided, and can present with obstructive symptoms (wheezing, recurrent pneumonia, or bronchiectasis)
- Smooth-walled polypoid lesion projecting into bronchus lumen
- Mature adipose tissue with occasional giant cells
- Lacks other mesenchymal elements

Pearls

- Cartilage is the most common type of tissue in pulmonary hamartomas
- Chromosomal regions 12q15 and 6p21, corresponding to high mobility group (HMG) loci, are often involved in many benign tumors, including pulmonary hamartoma and lipoma
- The presence of both fat and calcification on high-resolution CT is a specific combination for hamartomas, particularly in tumors smaller than 2.5 cm in diameter
- Malignant transformation is very rare

Selected References

Trahan S, Erickson-Johnsons MR, Rodriguez F, et al: Formation of the 12q14-q15 amplicon precedes the development of a well-differentiated liposarcoma arising from a nonchondroid pulmonary hamartoma. Am J Surg Pathol 30:1326-1329, 2006.

Kayser K, Dünnewald D, Kazmierczak B, et al: Chromosomal aberrations, profiles of expression of growth-related markers including galectins and environmental hazards in relation to the incidence of chondroid pulmonary hamartomas. Pathol Res Pract 199:589-598, 2003.

Lemke I, Rogalla P, Grundmann F, et al: Expression of the HMGA2-LPP fusion transcript in only 1 of 61 karyotypically normal pulmonary chondroid hamartomas. Cancer Genet Cytogenet 138:160-164, 2002.

Tallini G, Vanni R, Manfioletti G, et al: HMGI-C and HMGI(Y) immunoreactivity correlates with cytogenetic abnormalities in lipomas, pulmonary chondroid hamartomas, endometrial polyps, and uterine leiomyomas and is compatible with rearrangement of the HMGI-C and HMGI(Y) genes. Lab Invest 80:359-369, 2000.

Lymphangioleiomyomatosis (LAM)

Clinical Features

- Diffuse, extensive proliferation of smooth muscle–like spindle cells (LAM cells) frequently associated with cystic changes occurring almost exclusively in women during their reproductive years
- Rare disease; estimated incidence of 1 case per 100,000 persons per year

Figure 4-48. Lymphangioleiomyomatosis. There is an abnormal proliferation of bland uniform spindle cells with eosinophilic cytoplasm (smooth muscle cells).

- LAM is a multisystem disease involving the lungs; axillary, thoracic, and retroperitoneal lymph nodes (where it manifests as fluid-filled cystic structures known as *lymphangioleiomyomas*); renal angiomyolipomas; hamartomas; and uterine leiomyomas
- Patients typically present with progressive dyspnea, cough, chylous pleural effusions, recurrent pneumothoraces, and hemoptysis
- Ten-year survival rate is more than 90%

Gross Pathology

- High-resolution CT shows numerous bilateral, 2- to 5-mm thin-walled cysts, which in the clinical context of pneumothorax or chylothorax, as well as obstructive pulmonary function tests and impaired diffusion capacity, is diagnostic for LAM
- Hyperaerated lungs with extensive, diffuse cysts measuring 0.5 to 2 cm in diameter affecting both lungs and distorting the pleural surfaces

Histopathology

- Two major lesions in LAM
  - Disorderly proliferation of benign-appearing smooth muscle cells in peribronchial, perivascular, and perilymphatic regions throughout the lung
  - Variably sized, air-filled cysts lined by plaquelike or nodular aggregates of smooth muscle bundles
- Two types of LAM cells
  - Small spindle cells that react with proliferating cell nuclear antigen (PCNA; see later) and likely represent a more proliferative state
  - Larger epithelioid cells that react with HMB-45 and likely represent a more differentiated state
- LAM cells have no significant atypia or mitotic activity; however, over time, these cells proliferate and destroy lung parenchyma
- Secondary to hemorrhage, hemosiderin-laden macrophages or a foreign-body granulomatous reaction may be present
- LAM histology score (LHS) corresponds with prognosis and may be quantified by the extent of replacement of normal lung tissue with cystic lesions and LAM cell nodules
  - LHS-1: <25%
  - LHS-2: 25% to 50%
  - LHS-3: >50%

Special Stains and Immunohistochemistry

- Desmin, smooth muscle actin, and vimentin expression is present, consistent with smooth muscle differentiation
- Smooth muscle bundles stain positive for HMB-45, estrogen receptor, and bcl-2

Other Techniques for Diagnosis

- Molecular analysis demonstrates the loss of heterozygosity and somatic mutations in the gene

TSC2 (16p13), a tumor suppressor gene that codes for tuberin

Differential Diagnosis

- Benign metastasizing leiomyoma
  - Lacks the delicate, thin-walled cysts seen in LAM
  - Patient history of uterine leiomyoma
  - Smooth muscle bundles typically form nodular arrangements
  - HMB-45 negative
- Leiomyosarcoma
  - No diffuse cystic changes
  - Cellular atypia, mitoses, and necrosis
  - Negative for HMB-45
- Peribronchiolar smooth muscle hyperplasia in honeycomb fibrosing lesions
  - Reactive smooth muscle hyperplasia and cystic changes are common findings in pulmonary fibrosis; however, extensive, diffuse interstitial fibrosis and remodeled lung architecture with some inflammation are absent in LAM
  - HMB-45 negative

Pearls

- A spectrum of mutations in the *TSC2* gene have been identified in patients with LAM
- Some studies suggest that LAM cells migrate or metastasize to the lung from angiomyolipomas or lymph nodes
- Women with LAM appear to have a high prevalence of meningiomas
- An inverse relationship exists in LAM smooth muscle cells between immunoreactivity for HMB-45 and for PCNA, suggesting that LAM cells represent a population of smooth muscle cells in variable states of differentiation

Selected References

Taveira-DaSilva AM, Steagall WK, Moss J: Lymphangioleiomyomatosis. Cancer Control 13:276-285, 2006.

Ryu JH, Moss J, Beck GJ, et al: The NHLBI lymphangioleiomyomatosis registry: Characteristics of 230 patients at enrollment. Am J Respir Crit Care Med 173:105-111, 2006.

Zhe X, Schuger L: Combined smooth muscle and melanocytic differentiation in lymphangioleiomyomatosis. J Histochem Cytochem 52:1537-1542, 2004.

Finlay G: The LAM cell: What is it, where does it come from, and why does it grow? Am J Physiol Lung Cell Mol Physiol 286: L690-693, 2004.

Inflammatory Myofibroblastic Tumor (IMT)

Clinical Features

- IMT is most common in lung, but it can be found in most major organs, the retroperitoneum, the mesentery, the mediastinum, the dura, and the abdominal cavity

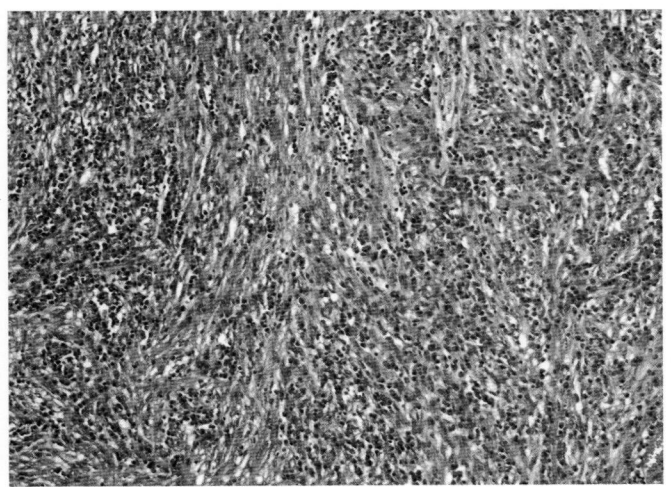

Figure 4-49. Inflammatory myofibroblastic tumor. This photomicrograph shows a cellular lesion composed of bland spindle cells admixed with inflammatory cells (plasma cells and lymphocytes).

- IMT can affect individuals of any age (range, 0 to 87 years), but most patients are children or young adults (mean age, 30 years) with an equal male-to-female ratio
- IMT accounts for more than 50% of pulmonary tumors in children
- Some cases are associated with human herpesvirus-8 (HHV-8); EBV is associated with splenic and nodal-based but not pulmonary IMT
- Reported rates of recurrence range from 25% to 40% and are more common with extrapulmonary IMT

Gross Pathology

- Generally solitary, unencapsulated, round, rubbery masses sharply demarcated from the adjacent lung parenchyma
- Cut surface varies from yellow-grey, to tan, to white
- Size ranges from 1 to 6 cm (mean, 3 cm); they can become as large as 36 cm
- Penetration of the pleura is common, and polypoid endobronchial protrusions occasionally occur

Histopathology

- Composed of spindle cells with fibroblastic and myofibroblastic differentiation arranged in a fascicular or storiform pattern mixed with inflammatory cells in a myxoid, fibrotic, or hyalinized stroma
- Lesions often obliterate the underlying lung architecture
- Variable proportions of cellular elements from predominantly myofibroblastic to predominantly plasmacytic
- Spindle cells have oval nuclei, fine chromatin, inconspicuous nucleoli, and abundant eosinophilic cytoplasm
- Nuclear atypia is minimal to none, but occasional spindle cells have large vesicular nuclei with

prominent nucleoli resembling ganglion cells or Reed-Sternberg cells
  — These rare atypical cells often display granular, cytoplasmic overexpression of the ALK protein
- Mitoses are generally scanty (0 to 2/10 hpf) but can be as numerous as 15/10 hpf
- A robust inflammatory component composed of plasma cells, lymphocytes, macrophages, foamy histiocytes, occasional Touton-type giant cells, and small numbers of eosinophils or neutrophils is present and may be so prominent as to obscure the spindle cells
- Invasion of small vessels, the chest wall, or hilar soft tissue occasionally occurs

Special Stains and Immunohistochemistry

- Spindle cells express vimentin (>95%), smooth muscle actin (86%), muscle-specific actin (82%), and focally desmin (41%)
- ALK-1 and p80 expression occurs in about 45% of cases
- Cytokeratin immunoreactivity likely represents entrapped epithelial elements
- The spindle cells are negative for CD117/c-KIT, S-100, myogenin, and myoglobin

Other Techniques for Diagnosis

- Noncontributory

Differential Diagnosis

- Fibrous histiocytoma of soft tissue
  - Shares a similar storiform histologic pattern with IMT
- Plasmacytoma
  - Rarely involves the lungs
  - Composed of atypical, monoclonal plasma cells with numerous mitotic figures and little to no fibrosis
- Pulmonary amyloidosis
  - Waxy, hard irregular nodules
  - Congo red stain is useful to differentiate amyloid tumor from IMT
- Pulmonary hyalinizing granuloma
  - Multiple lesions with extensive hyalinization and mild lymphocytic infiltrate
  - Lamellar collagen arranged in storiform or whorled arrays
- Inflammatory fibrosarcoma
  - Low-grade sarcoma composed of fascicles or whorls of fibroblastic or myofibroblastic cells mixed with plasma cells and collagen
  - Spindle cells show prominent nuclear atypia and can invade large vessels or the pleura

Pearls

- The current consensus is that the spindle cell component is neoplastic in most cases of IMT

- Recent work suggests that the spindle cells are derived from fibroblastic reticulum cells (FBRCs), which are a subtype of accessory immune cells that interact with lymphocytes and their progeny during immune responses
- The presence of chromosomal abnormalities is consistent with a clonal origin and can help to explain, in part, the spectrum of aggressive behavior of these lesions
- A subset of IMT occurring in the lung or abdomen during the first decade of life has been shown to possess a chromosomal rearrangement involving the ALK locus at 2p23; these tumors may show more aggressive behavior and increased recurrence rates
- Complete excision is recommended if possible to minimize the rate of recurrence

Selected References

Kovach SJ, Fischer AC, Katzman PJ, et al: Inflammatory myofibroblastic tumors. J Surg Oncol 94:385-391, 2006.

Nonaka D, Birbe R, Rosai J: So-called inflammatory myofibroblastic tumour: A proliferative lesion of fibroblastic reticulum cells? Histopathology 46:604-613, 2005.

Dehner LP: Inflammatory myofibroblastic tumor: The continued definition of one type of so-called inflammatory pseudotumor. Am J Surg Pathol 28:1652-1654, 2004.

Janik JS, Janik JP, Lovell MA, et al: Recurrent inflammatory pseudotumors in children. J Pediatr Surg 38:1491-1495, 2003.

Pleuropulmonary Blastoma (PPB)

Clinical Features

- Rare childhood tumor arising in the lung parenchyma in association with the pleura or in the mediastinum

- Mean age of patients is 2.5 years, but occasionally older children and adolescents are affected
- Three morphologic subtypes represent a continuum of histologic and biologic progression
  — Type I is the least common, accounting for less than 15% of PPB cases, and affects the youngest group of patients (median, 10 months)
  — Type II accounts for 40% to 50% of all PPB and affects somewhat older children than type I (median, 34 months)
  — Type III accounts for 40% of PPB cases and occurs in older patients (median, 44 months)

Gross Pathology

- The neoplasms appear cystic, solid, or mixed and are subtyped accordingly
  — Type I: purely cystic
  — Type II: combined cystic and solid pattern
  — Type III: well-circumscribed, solid, mucoid, tan-white, partially friable or necrotic mass with pleural attachments, involving either one lobe or entire lung

Histopathology

- Malignant cells are a biphasic mixture of
  — Primitive, small, elliptical, undifferentiated blastemal cells with scanty cytoplasm and solitary, spherical hyperchromatic nuclei with occasional distinct nucleoli
  — Larger, spindle-shaped, often rhabdomyoblastic cells
- Epithelial cells are not a component of the neoplasm and when present represent entrapped mesothelial or epithelial elements
- Focal rhabdomyosarcomatous differentiation, either as individual or groups of strap cells with cross striations, is present in most cases

Figure 4-50. Pleuropulmonary blastoma. A, Epithelial lining is present in the *upper right-hand corner*. The solid portion of the tumor is composed of solid and loose sarcomatous tissue and nodules of malignant cartilage. **B,** High-power photomicrograph shows high-grade undifferentiated blastomatous and chondrosarcomatous components.

Special Stains and Immunohistochemistry

- Blastemal cells and proliferating spindle cells react with vimentin; they are negative for cytokeratin and epithelial membrane antigen
- Neoplastic cells displaying differentiation often react with desmin, smooth muscle actin, and muscle specific actin
- Cartilaginous nodules express S-100

Other Techniques for Diagnosis

- Trisomy 8 is a common cytogenetic abnormality in PPB

Differential Diagnosis

▌ CPAM
  - CPAM and type I PPB affect infants and young children
  - Type I PPB shows the presence of dense subepithelial or septal spindle cells with or without foci of immature cartilage
▌ Metastatic Wilms tumor
  - PPB is negative for cytokeratin, whereas epithelial component of Wilms tumor is positive
  - Wilms tumor is positive for WT-1 (nuclear)
▌ Primary pulmonary sarcomas of children
  - Rhabdomyosarcoma and leiomyosarcoma show monophasic myogenous differentiation
▌ Adult pulmonary blastoma (APB)
  - Despite its similar nomenclature, APB is an altogether separate entity considered to be a sarcomatoid carcinoma
  - Relative to other rare lung tumors, APB is relatively common and usually presents as a well-defined peripheral lung mass in adults with a female predominance
  - APB is a biphasic tumor composed of malignant, fetal-type tubular epithelial structures and an immature mesenchymal stroma, whereas the epithelial structures in PPB are entrapped, nonmalignant components
  - The tubules and stroma of APB resemble fetal lung between 10 and 16 weeks' gestation (the pseudoglandular stage of lung development)
  - Tubules in APB contain nonciliated, pseudostratified columnar cells with an endometrioid appearance and PAS-positive subnuclear or supranuclear vacuoles
  - The stroma in APB has a blastema-like morphology composed of small, oval to spindle-shaped cells in a myxoid matrix with occasional foci of differentiated sarcomatous elements (i.e., rhabdomyosarcoma, chondrosarcoma, and osteosarcoma)
  - The stroma shows a tendency to condense around the malignant glands in APB
  - Morulas are seen at the bases of glands in close to half of APB

Pearls

- Roughly 25% of PPB cases are associated with familial cancer syndrome: thyroid tumors, cystic nephroma, ovarian teratoma, multiple intestinal polyps, and other tumors
- It is believed that PPB progresses from type I to type III over time, and definitive surgery before progression from type I to either type II or type III is the key to successful management of PPB

Selected References

Hill DA: USCAP Specialty Conference: Case 1-type I pleuropulmonary blastoma. Pediatr Dev Pathol 8:77-84, 2005.

Wright JR Jr: Pleuropulmonary blastoma: A case report documenting transition from type I (cystic) to type III (solid). Cancer 88:2853-2858, 2000.

Nicol KK, Geisinger KR: The cytomorphology of pleuropulmonary blastoma. Arch Pathol Lab Med 124:416-418, 2000.

Baraniya J, Desai S, Kane S, et al: Pleuropulmonary blastoma. Med Pediatr Oncol 32:52-56, 1999.

Priest JR, McDermott MB, Bhatia S, et al: Pleuropulmonary blastoma: A clinicopathologic study of 50 cases. Cancer 80:147-161, 1997.

Lymphoproliferative Disorders

Marginal Zone B-Cell Lymphoma of the Mucosa-Associated Lymphoid Tissue (MALT) Type

Clinical Features

- Primary pulmonary lymphoma is rare, representing 0.5% to 1% of primary pulmonary malignancies
- Pulmonary MALT lymphoma accounts for 70% to 90% of primary lung lymphoma, making it a "common rare tumor"
- Presentation in patients younger than 50 years is rare unless some underlying immunosuppression is present (i.e., autoimmune disease, HIV)
- An associated monoclonal gammopathy is present in 30% of cases
- Pleural effusions are rare to absent

Gross Pathology

- Consolidated, yellow-tan mass

Histopathology

- Lymphoid infiltrates composed of a monomorphic population of malignant cells with centrocyte-like morphology consisting of slightly irregular nuclei with scanty cytoplasm surrounding reactive follicles
- Follicles may be obscured by an exuberant lymphoma infiltrate (follicular colonization or mantle zone colonization)
- There is lymphangitic pattern of growth along interlobular septa and bronchovascular bundles creating a nodular interstitial infiltrate

Figure 4-51. Mucosa-associated lymphoid tissue (MALT) lymphoma. A, The malignant cells form nodules and infiltrate alveolar septa. **B,** High-power photomicrograph shows the malignant lymphoid cells infiltrating a blood vessel wall.

- Expansion of the nodules into solid masses effaces and obliterates the underlying lung architecture
- Lymphoepithelial lesions are formed as lymphoma cells infiltrate the bronchial epithelium and are a common finding
- Plasmacytoid lymphocytes, plasma cells with intranuclear Dutcher bodies, small normal lymphocytes, and large transformed cells may be present
- Central necrosis and giant lamellar bodies are occasional features

Special Stains and Immunohistochemistry

- Tumor cells express CD20, CD43, bcl-2, PAX5, and CD79
- Tumor cells are negative for CD5, CD10, CD21, CD23, bcl-6, and cyclin D1
- Follicular dendritic cells can be identified with CD21, CD23, and CD35

Other Techniques for Diagnosis

- About 60% to 70% of tumors show clonal rearrangements of the JH region of the immunoglobulin heavy chain
- Roughly two thirds of MALT lymphomas display trisomy 3
- About 20% to 50% of MALT lymphomas show t(11;18)(q21;q21)
- Translocations t(14;18)(q32;q21) and t(1;14)(p22;q32) are also present in some MALT lymphomas and may function by up-regulating NF-κB signaling

Differential Diagnosis

▌ Follicular bronchitis or bronchiolitis
- Lymphoepithelial lesions can occur in reactive conditions and lymphoma

- MALT lymphoma displays an expanded B-cell infiltrate beyond the follicles
- Reactive lymphocytic infiltrates form small aggregates of B-cells
- Clonality can be demonstrated by light-chain restriction in MALT lymphoma cells

▌ Lymphoid interstitial pneumonia (LIP)
- Seen in immunocompromised patients, especially pediatric AIDS patients
- Not monoclonal

▌ Chronic lymphocytic lymphoma (CLL)
- CLL infiltrates are limited to the bronchovascular bundles without infiltration and destruction of the lung architecture
- CLL is positive for CD20, PAX5, CD79a, CD5, CD43, and bcl-2; and negative for CD10, CD23, and bcl-6

Pearls

- MALT is absent from the lung in physiologic conditions and becomes apparent during chronic antigenic stimulation
- No antigens have been identified, but certain autoimmune disorders (e.g., SLE, multiple sclerosis, Hashimoto thyroiditis, and Sjögren syndrome) may play a role in MALT lymphoma

Selected References

Bacon CM, Du MQ, Dogan A: Mucosa-associated lymphoid tissue (MALT) lymphoma: A practical guide for pathologists. J Clin Pathol 60:361-372, 2007.

Do KH, Lee JS, Seo JB, et al: Pulmonary parenchymal involvement of low-grade lymphoproliferative disorders. J Comput Assist Tomogr 29:825-830, 2005.

Chilosi M, Zinzani PL, Poletti V: Lymphoproliferative lung disorders. Semin Respir Crit Care Med 26:490-501, 2005.

Pulmonary Langerhans Cell Histiocytosis (PLCH)

Clinical Features

- Occurs in young adults, most commonly between the ages of 30 and 50 years
- Strong association with cigarette smoking
- Uncommon in African Americans and Asians
- Patients present with dyspnea, cough, and occasionally pneumothorax (10% to 15%)
- Can involve extrapulmonary sites, especially bone, pituitary, skin, and lymph nodes (10% to 15%)

Gross Pathology

- Early stages: multiple small nodules (1 to 5 mm) in a centrilobular distribution with middle and upper zone predominance
- Later stages: larger, irregular, tan-gray nodules with central lucency due to cavitation or bronchiolar dilation
- Disease becomes progressively cystic with irregular, bizarre shapes

Histopathology

- Characteristic low-magnification pattern of multiple nodular infiltrates with stellate borders centered around small airways
- Nodules can have a Medusa-head appearance due to tendrils of cellular infiltrates extending into the surrounding alveolar interstitium
- A distinctive form of cicatricial change occurs as nodules interconnect with adjacent nodules
- Infiltrate is composed of uniform sheets of Langerhans cells with varying numbers of eosinophils, lymphocytes, and plasma cells

Figure 4-52. Pulmonary Langerhans cell histiocytosis. High-power photomicrograph shows histiocytes with characteristic grooved nuclei. The same nuclei are present in the multinucleated giant cell. Eosinophils are also present, although not required for diagnosis.

- Langerhans cells have moderate amounts of eosinophilic cytoplasm and pale nuclei with prominent nuclear grooves
- PLCH lesions progress from cellular nodules to intermediate cellular-fibrotic nodules to fibrotic scars, and biopsy specimens often show a spectrum of these changes
- End-stage nodules are pauci-cellular, are fibrotic, and lack Langerhans cells yet retain the stellate pattern facilitating the diagnosis of PLCH
- Nodular lesions can invade vascular structures, causing vasculopathy and abnormal pulmonary hemodynamics
- Smoking associated respiratory bronchiolitis is invariably present in adjacent lung tissue

Special Stains and Immunohistochemistry

- Langerhans cells stain positive for S-100 and CD1a and are negative for CD68
- Various studies examining clonality favor the notion that Langerhans cells are a reactive, polyclonal proliferation secondary to chronic antigenic stimulation due to cigarette smoking

Other Techniques for Diagnosis

- Electron microscopy: Birbeck granules within the Langerhans cells

Differential Diagnosis

▌ Respiratory bronchiolitis
- Weakly brown pigmented alveolar macrophages adjacent to respiratory bronchioles
- Lacks the cellular and nodular interstitial lesions

▌ Chronic eosinophilic pneumonia (CEP)
- Intra-alveolar eosinophils in CEP without Langerhans cells

▌ UIP
- Fibrotic scars in PLCH retain a stellate shape with a bronchiolocentric distribution and lack UIP-like temporal heterogeneity

▌ Reactive eosinophilic pleuritis
- Nonspecific pleural reaction occurring in the setting of pneumothorax
- Restricted to the pleura
- Prominent eosinophils mixed with proliferating mesothelial cells and chronic inflammation

Pearls

- Histology of PLCH in children is essentially identical to that in adults
- High-resolution CT studies demonstrate that PLCH lesions evolve in the following sequence: nodules, cavitated nodules, cysts, and eventually confluent cysts
- PLCH is regarded as a reactive proliferative disease of Langerhans cells, in contrast to the extrapulmonary forms of Langerhans cell histiocytosis, which are neoplastic processes

- Pulmonary lesions show abundant expression of transforming growth factor-β_1 and granulocyte-macrophage colony-stimulating factor

Selected References

Leslie KO, Gruden JF, Parish JM, Scholand MB: Transbronchial biopsy interpretation in the patient with diffuse parenchymal lung disease. Arch Pathol Lab Med 131:407-423, 2007.

Vassallo R Ryu JR: Pulmonary Langerhans' cell histiocytosis. Clin Chest Med 25:561-571, 2004.

Post-transplantation Lymphoproliferative Disorder (PTLD)

Clinical Features

- A morphologically heterogeneous group of EBV-driven lymphoid proliferations
- Occurs more frequently with solid organ transplantation (3% to 5% of heart and lung transplantations)
- A localized or multifocal lymphoproliferative process in which the transplanted lung is often involved
- Proliferations are composed of polyclonal to monoclonal populations of cells

Gross Pathology

- Single or multifocal well-defined solid nodules or diffuse consolidations of lung parenchyma

Histopathology

- Abnormal lymphocytic proliferation occurring in the setting of chronic immunosuppression for organ transplantation that is associated with EBV
- Lymphoid cell populations range from a mixed lymphocytic hyperplasia composed of polyclonal B cells and other polymorphic cell types to monomorphic, monoclonal lymphoplasmacytoid, immunoblastic, or large B-cell lymphomas

- Hence, PTLD encompasses a spectrum of lesions that range from histologically benign lymphoid proliferations to frankly malignant lymphoma, as follows
  - Plasmacytic hyperplasia
    - ◆ Underlying lung architecture is maintained
    - ◆ Small polyclonal T and B lymphocytes, plasma cells, and occasional immunoblasts are present
    - ◆ EBV can be detected in most cases
    - ◆ Most common pattern to occur in children and young adults
  - Polymorphic lymphoproliferative disorder
    - ◆ Lymphoid infiltrate distorts the underlying lung architecture
    - ◆ Mixture of lymphocytes, plasmacytoid cells, and occasional immunoblasts, which may resemble Reed-Sternberg cells
    - ◆ The lymphoid cells are generally clonal and contain EBV
  - Malignant lymphoma or multiple myeloma
    - ◆ Monotonous population of lymphocytes or plasma cells that resemble lymphoma or multiple myeloma
    - ◆ Most tumors are diffuse large B-cell lymphomas and contain EBV

Special Stains and Immunohistochemistry

- EBV, CD45, B-cell markers, and T-cell markers permit further characterization
- Flow cytometry is useful for phenotype analysis of the proliferating lymphocytes

Other Techniques for Diagnosis

- Gene rearrangement studies useful in establishing clonality

Differential Diagnosis

▐ Lymphoid interstitial pneumonia (LIP)

Figure 4-53. Post-transplantation lymphoproliferative disorder. A, Gross picture of cut surface of lung at autopsy in this lung transplant recipient shows tan-white nodules. **B,** Highly atypical lymphocytes are seen infiltrating the lung parenchyma and blood vessel wall.

Pearls

- In bone marrow transplantations, PTLD is usually of donor origin, whereas in solid organ transplantation, it is usually of recipient origin
- Interval between transplantation and development of PTLD is 1 month to 4 years
- Regression or resolution commonly occurs after reduction in immunosuppressive therapy on PTLD occurring in the first year after transplantation

Other Neoplastic Conditions

Malignant Mesothelioma

Clinical Features

- Rare tumor showing a male predominance and an association with asbestos exposure
- Most patients are between 50 and 70 years old
- Associated with a poor prognosis, with average survival of less than 1 year

- Smoking does not increase the risk for malignant mesothelioma; however, the combination of smoking and asbestos exposure greatly increases the risk for lung carcinoma

Gross Pathology

- Malignant mesothelioma encases the lungs and extends diffusely through the pleural space

Histopathology

- A malignant tumor of mesothelial cells with a diffuse growth pattern involving the visceral and parietal pleura and, less commonly, the peritoneum
- Three histologic categories: epithelioid, sarcomatoid, and biphasic
  — Epithelioid variant
    ◆ Represents 65% to 70% of malignant mesothelioma
    ◆ Growth patterns are tubulopapillary, glandular or acinar, sheets, or mixed

Figure 4-54. Malignant mesothelioma. A, Gross photograph of the pneumonectomy specimen shows tumor encasing the lung. **B,** Gross photograph of cut surface shows malignant mesothelioma growing along the pleura and encasing the dark-red lung parenchyma. **C,** H&E-stained section shows glandular and papillary patterns of epithelioid malignant mesothelioma. **D,** Calretinin stain shows both nuclear and cytoplasmic staining in most epithelioid tumors.

- ◆ Neoplastic cells are usually bland and cytologically homogeneous with round nuclei, vesicular chromatin with prominent nucleoli, and a moderate amount of eosinophilic cytoplasm
  - — Sarcomatoid variant
    - ◆ Pleomorphic spindle cells growing in short fascicles, typically with a storiform pattern, within a fibrous stroma
    - ◆ Desmoplastic mesothelioma, a subtype of the sarcomatoid variant representing roughly 10% of all cases of mesothelioma, shows a dense, collagenous stroma separating the neoplastic cells
  - — Biphasic variant
    - ◆ Tumors contain both epithelioid and sarcomatous components in which the minor component exceeds 10% of the tumor

Special Stains and Immunohistochemistry

- Positive for keratin AE1/AE3, CAM5.2, and CK7; specific markers include calretinin, CK5/6, WT-1, D2-40

Other Techniques for Diagnosis

- Inactivation of the CDKN2A/ARF locus at 9p21, which codes for the tumor suppressor genes p16INK4a and p14ARF, is a common finding

Differential Diagnosis

- Adenocarcinoma
  - A panel of immunohistochemical stains that includes at least two mesothelial markers and at least two markers for adenocarcinoma
  - Adenocarcinoma markers include MOC-31, BG8, CEA, Leu-M1 (CD15), Ber-Ep4, B72.3, TTF-1, and estrogen and progesterone receptors for breast and gynecologic carcinomas
  - Calretinin is the most useful mesothelial marker for this and demonstrates strong and diffuse staining of the cytoplasm and nuclei of both benign and malignant mesothelial cells; nuclear staining must be present to make the diagnosis of malignant mesothelioma
  - CK5/6 is expressed in the cytoplasm of mesothelial and squamous cells; it is rarely expressed by adenocarcinoma
  - WT-1 shows a nuclear expression pattern in mesothelioma as well as in serous carcinomas of the ovary

- Reactive mesothelial hyperplasia
  - Invasion of mesothelioma cells into the adipose tissue of the parietal pleura is evidence of malignancy
  - Cytoplasmic desmin staining is more consistent with reactive mesothelial hyperplasia, whereas diffuse, linear membranous EMA, strong p53, and GLUT1 staining supports malignant epithelioid mesothelioma
- Desmoplastic mesothelioma versus chronic fibrosing pleuritis
  - Mesothelial markers are not helpful, and both desmoplastic mesothelioma and reactive mesothelial cells express cytokeratins and vimentin
  - Cytokeratin antibody cocktails help to identify invasion into adjacent adipose tissue
  - Cytokeratin cocktails also demonstrate the disordered growth pattern of desmoplastic mesothelioma
  - In contrast, reactive mesothelial cells in chronic fibrosing pleuritis are arranged in a more orderly manner parallel to the pleural surface
- Solitary fibrous tumor
  - Most commonly involves pleura as a slow-growing, localized mass
  - Grossly, firm with white cut surface; focal necrosis, cystic degeneration may be present
  - Proliferation of uniform spindle-shaped cells in a collagenous background
  - Hemangiopericytoma-like vascular pattern with alternating hypocellular and hypercellular areas
  - CD34, CD99, and bcl-2 positivity in most cases, negative for cytokeratins

Pearls

- Calretinin stains both nucleus and cytoplasm with stronger nuclear staining, which is a helpful feature of mesothelial cells
- Invasion is the best indication of malignant mesothelioma
- Patients with purely epithelioid mesothelioma show the longest survival, whereas the shortest survival occurs with sarcomatoid histology—yet the difference between the two survival rates is only a matter of months

Selected Reference

Travis WD, Brambilla E, Muller-Hermelink H, Harris CC (eds): World Health Organization Classification of Tumours: Pathology and genetics: Tumours of the Lung, Pleura, Thymus, and Heart. Lyon, IARC Press, 2004.

Jose A. Plaza, Cesar A. Moran, and Saul Suster

5 Thymus and Mediastinum

Thymic Cyst

Clinical Features

- Uncommon; constitutes less than 10% of mediastinal cysts
- May be congenital or acquired
- Found in the anterior mediastinum, but may occur in ectopic locations such as neck, pleura, and posterior mediastinum
- Invariably benign
- Age range: 20 to 50 years, often asymptomatic; larger cysts can present with cough, dyspnea, and chest pain
- Acquired thymic cysts are associated with inflammatory processes and have been found in association with mediastinal Hodgkin lymphoma or its treatment, occasionally non-Hodgkin lymphoma, germinoma, yolk sac tumor, thymoma, thymic

carcinoma, Langerhans cell granulomatosis, congenital syphilis, or prior thoracotomy for other diseases
- Radiologic findings: well-circumscribed mass in the anterior mediastinum measuring up to 18 cm in diameter

Gross Pathology

- Typically presents as a large encapsulated mass attached directly to thymic remnant or attached by a pedicle
- Calcifications may be present in the cyst wall
- Two types
  - Unilocular (congenital): thin-walled cyst filled with serous fluid
  - Multilocular (acquired): thick-walled cyst filled with thick, turbid hemorrhagic fluid

Histopathology

- Unilocular cysts usually have a flat or cuboidal lining; thymic remnants are not usually appreciated in their walls
- Multilocular cysts have a lining that is usually flattened but may be stratified squamous, cuboidal, columnar, or ciliated
- Cyst lining is often in continuity with thymic remnants in the wall of the cyst and may be traced to dilated Hassall corpuscles
- Inflammatory infiltrate present in the walls of the cysts, often with hyperplastic follicles with prominent germinal centers
- Cholesterol cleft granulomas
- No cartilage, smooth muscle, or other differentiated mesenchymal tissue

Figure 5-1. Thymic cyst. Cyst wall lined by simple cuboidal epithelium. The cyst wall contains lymphocytic infiltrate and cholesterol cleft granulomas.

Special Stains and Immunohistochemistry

- Cytokeratin may highlight the epithelium and demonstrate thymic tissue in the wall

Other Techniques for Diagnosis

- Noncontributory

Differential Diagnosis

▌ Parathyroid cyst
- Typically found in anterior-superior mediastinum
- Thin-walled cyst lined by attenuated parathyroid endocrine cells and filled with clear fluid

▌ Cystic hygroma (lymphangioma)
- Most common in childhood
- Composed of nonencapsulated complex cavernous spaces lined by flattened endothelium and filled with clear fluid and occasional small lymphocytes
- Embedded in collagenous fibroblastic tissue with sparse lymphoid infiltrate
- No epithelial elements present

▌ Esophageal cyst
- Usually in continuity with the esophagus in the middle mediastinum
- Cyst wall shows alternating layers of smooth muscle
- No thymic tissue identifiable in the wall, usually with few or no lymphocytes

▌ Bronchial cyst
- Attached to trachea or major bronchi
- Lined by ciliated columnar (respiratory) epithelium but may occasionally undergo metaplastic changes
- Smooth muscle and cartilage in cyst wall
- No thymic tissue in wall

▌ Cystic teratoma
- Cysts are lined by any type of epithelium and may contain sebaceous glands and hair follicles
- Other common components include neural tissue, gastrointestinal tract elements, cartilage, and respiratory structures
- Monodermal teratoma may show only epithelial elements and prominent granulomatous foreign body–type response

▌ Cystic thymoma
- May present as a discrete area of thickening or nodularity in the wall of a multilocular cyst
- Expansile nodule showing biphasic population of small T lymphocytes and thymic epithelial cells devoid of normal thymic architecture

▌ Cystic degeneration in Hodgkin lymphoma
- Represents cystic degeneration of thymic tissue within or adjacent to the tumor
- Solid foci showing a mixed population of lymphocytes with atypical lymphoid cells
- Demonstration of Reed-Sternberg cells by immunohistochemical staining with appropriate markers (e.g., Ber-H2, CD30)

Selected References

Suster S, Rosai J: Multilocular thymic cyst: An acquired reactive process. Study of 18 cases. Am J Surg Pathol 15:388-398, 1991.

Suster S, Barbuto D, Carlson G, Rosai J: Multilocular thymic cysts with pseudoepitheliomatous hyperplasia. Hum Pathol 22:455-460, 1991.

Foregut Cysts of the Mediastinum: Bronchial (Bronchogenic) Cyst, Esophageal Cyst, Enteric Duplication Cyst*

Clinical Features

- These foregut cysts of the mediastinum are believed to represent congenital developmental anomalies
- Bronchial and esophageal cysts may be asymptomatic or present with cough, dyspnea, pain, or dysphagia due to compression

❚ Bronchial cyst
  - Usually in adults
  - Moves with respiration

❚ Esophageal cyst (esophageal duplication)
  - Presents in childhood or adolescence
  - Male predominance

❚ Enteric duplication cyst
  - Also known as *foregut duplication cyst* or *enterogenous cyst*
  - Usually presents in infancy or childhood
  - Strong male predominance
  - Patients may have cough, pain, dysphagia, dyspnea, failure to thrive; rarely presents with massive hemoptysis

*Cystic neoplasms are discussed with the corresponding tumor types.

Figure 5-2. Foregut cyst. The lining is composed of tall, pseudostratified columnar ciliated epithelium.

- May be associated with other congenital malformations, including vertebral abnormalities, intestinal atresia or malrotation, and congenital cardiac malformations

Gross Pathology

- Round and usually unilocular
- Size varies from a few millimeters up to 15 cm

❚ Bronchial cyst
  - Attached to trachea or major bronchus
  - Mucinous contents

❚ Esophageal cyst
  - Typically located at the level of the mid-esophagus; may be attached to or within wall of esophagus
  - Mucinous contents

❚ Enteric cyst
  - Mostly confined to posterior mediastinum
  - Predilection for children and adolescents
  - Usually attached to the vertebral column
  - Thin wall
  - May present with dysphagia if there is compression of the esophagus

Histopathology

❚ Bronchial cyst
  - Epithelium is typically respiratory columnar but may undergo squamous metaplasia
  - Cartilage and smooth muscle are present in the cyst wall

❚ Esophageal cyst
  - Epithelium is typically squamous but may be columnar
  - Two discrete layers of smooth muscle are present at least focally in the cyst wall
  - No cartilage

❚ Enteric cyst
  - Epithelium may be of gastric type (including parietal cells), intestinal, colonic, or squamous
  - Cyst lining has a lamina propria, muscularis mucosae, and muscularis propria
  - Cyst wall may contain ganglion cells
  - Particularly with gastric mucosa, ulceration and hemorrhage may be present because of the effects of acid production

Special Stains and Immunohistochemistry

- Noncontributory

Other Techniques for Diagnosis

- Noncontributory

Differential Diagnosis

❚ Thymic cyst
  - Lining epithelium is usually squamous
  - Lymphocytes and true thymic tissue in the wall
  - No well-defined smooth muscle layers
  - No cartilage

▌ Mesothelial cyst
  ● Distinctive mesothelial lining
  ● Filled with clear thin fluid
  ● Lacks well-developed muscle bundles and lamina propria
▌ Cystic teratoma
  ● Generally located in the anterior mediastinum
  ● Typically has focal solid areas
  ● Additional tissue types foreign to the site of origin are common and often consist of neural elements, cartilage, and pancreatic islets
  ● Not attached to bronchus, esophagus, or vertebral column
▌ Foregut cysts
  ● Some cysts show overlap features between different types of cysts in this section; these represent partial duplication of structures derived from the foregut but cannot be subclassified into one of the three types described here and are generically termed foregut cysts

Pearls

  ● Computed tomography (CT) and magnetic resonance imaging can define the anatomic relationships and the cystic nature of the lesion
  ● Surgical resection is curative

Selected References

Wick MR: Cystic lesions of the mediastinum. Semin Diagn Pathol 22:241-253, 2005.
Strollo DC, Rosado-de-Christenson ML, Jett JR: Primary mediastinal tumors: Part II. Tumors of the middle and posterior mediastinum. Chest 112:1344-1357, 1997.

Mesothelial Cyst

Clinical Features

  ● Typically found at the costophrenic angle; may occur in the mediastinum
  ● Affects men and women of all ages; more common in adults than children
  ● When attached to pericardium, are designated as pericardial cyst

Gross Pathology

  ● Thin-walled cyst filled with clear serous fluid
  ● Typically unilocular
  ● Pericardial cysts may have mucoid contents

Histopathology

  ● Typically has an attenuated mesothelial lining with fibrous tissue within the cyst wall
  ● Lacks smooth muscle, specialized epithelium, or cholesterol granulomas

Special Stains and Immunohistochemistry

  ● Noncontributory

Other Techniques for Diagnosis

  ● Noncontributory

Differential Diagnosis

▌ Thymic cyst
  ● Located in the anterior mediastinum; more superior than pericardial and mesothelial cysts
  ● Residual thymic tissue is found in the wall on careful examination
  ● Epithelium is sometimes hyperplastic
▌ Lymphangioma
  ● Typically found in anterior mediastinum
  ● More common in childhood
  ● Usually multiloculated with fibrous walls lined by attenuated cells
  ● Cyst lining cells are cytokeratin negative, but may express one or more antigens of endothelial cells (CD31 or CD34)

Pearls

  ● Mesothelial cysts are most often asymptomatic and found as incidental radiologic findings
  ● Differentiation between mesothelial and pericardial cysts is based on anatomic location
    — Cysts attached to the pericardium are pericardial cysts
    — Mesothelial-lined cysts elsewhere in the mediastinum are mesothelial cysts
    — Careful gross and histologic examination may be necessary to exclude thymic tissue or elements of a foregut cyst
    — Always benign
    — Drainage under radiologic guidance may be an alternative to surgical resection

Selected References

Wick MR: Cystic lesions of the mediastinum. Semin Diagn Pathol 22:241-253, 2005.
Strollo DC, Rosado-de-Christenson ML, Jett JR: Primary mediastinal tumors: Part II. Tumors of the middle and posterior mediastinum. Chest 112:1344-1357, 1997.

True Thymic Hyperplasia

Clinical Features

  ● Seen in children and occasionally in adults after chemotherapy for malignancy
  ● May be associated with hyperthyroidism, myasthenia gravis, or other autoimmune disease

Gross Pathology

  ● Thymic enlargement with increase in volume and normal weight of the gland

Histopathology

- Normal lobular architecture with normal distribution of lymphocytes and epithelial cells
- Preservation of corticomedullary differentiation

Special Stains and Immunohistochemistry

- Noncontributory

Other Techniques for Diagnosis

- Noncontributory

Differential Diagnosis

▌ Thymoma
- Differentiation into cortex and medulla is usually absent
- If areas resembling cortex and medulla are present, they are not arranged normally and do not display the normal lobulation

▌ Thymic follicular hyperplasia
- Well-formed lymphoid follicles with germinal centers
- CD20-positive B lymphocytes are present within germinal centers

Pearls

- Tables of normal thymic weights are derived from autopsy data; most of the specimens were therefore obtained from ill patients; data on normal thymic weights in previously healthy persons, especially infants and children, are relatively scant
- Thymic hyperplasia after chemotherapy, especially when given for Hodgkin disease, may mimic recurrent tumor radiologically

Selected References

Suster S, Rosai J: The thymus. In Mill SE (ed): Histology for Pathologists, 3rd ed. Philadelphia, Lippincott Williams & Wilkins, Philadelphia, 2006, pp 505-526.

Steinmann GG: Changes in the human thymus during aging. In Müller-Hermelink HK (ed): The Human Thymus: Histophysiology and Pathology. Berlin, Springer-Verlag, 1986, pp 43-88.

Carmosino L, Di Benedetto A, Feffer S: Thymic hyperplasia following successful chemotherapy: A report of two cases and review of the literature. Cancer 56:1526-1528, 1985.

Thymic Follicular Hyperplasia

Clinical Features

- Associated with myasthenia gravis, rheumatoid arthritis, systemic lupus erythematosus, and other autoimmune disorders

Gross Pathology

- Thymus is of normal size and weight in most cases

Histopathology

- Thymic hyperplasia characterized by numerous follicles with germinal centers

Special Stains and Immunohistochemistry

- Follicles are composed of normal B cells and will show reactivity with CD20

Other Techniques for Diagnosis

- Flow cytometry or molecular diagnostic techniques, that is, gene rearrangement; can rule out clonality if lymphoma is in the differential

Differential Diagnosis

▌ Follicular lymphoma
- Patients usually have widespread systemic disease
- Uncommon in young adults
- More uniform population of lymphoid cells
- Few or no tingible body macrophages
- Flow cytometry and molecular diagnostic techniques demonstrate monoclonal population of B cells
- B cells in follicles strongly express bcl-2 protein

▌ Normal thymus with prominent corticomedullary differentiation
- Normal thymic lobules show sharp angles; follicles are round
- Hassall corpuscles are seen in thymic medulla, not in germinal centers
- Thymic medulla contains cytokeratin-positive epithelial cells, which are not seen in germinal centers

Pearls

- Thymic gland usually is of normal size and weight
- Follicular lymphoid hyperplasia is usually present in non-neoplastic thymic tissue of patients with myasthenia gravis
- About 10% of patients with myasthenia gravis have thymoma
- About 25% to 50% of patients with thymoma have myasthenia gravis
- About 25% of patients with myasthenia gravis have normal thymic histology

Selected References

Moran C, Suster S, Gil J, Jagirdaar J: Morphometric analysis of germinal centers in the thymuses of nonthymomatous patients with myasthenia gravis. Arch Pathol Lab Med 114:689-691, 1990.

Kornstein MJ, Brooks JJ, Anderson AO, et al: The immuno-histology of the thymus in myasthenia gravis. Am J Pathol 117:184-194, 1984.

Loning T, Caselitz, Otto HF: The epithelial framework of the thymus in normal and pathological conditions. Virchows Archiv 329:7-20, 1981.

Okabe H: Thymic lymph follicles: A histopathological study of 1,356 autopsy cases. Acta Pathol Japonica 16:109-130, 1966.

Thymolipoma

Clinical Features

- Rare tumor
- Peak incidence in young adults
- Often large, and patients are symptomatic (dyspnea, cough) as a result of compression of adjacent structures

Gross Pathology

- Thymus gland is enlarged but soft, with preserved lobulation
- Yellow cut surface with whitish fibrous strands

Histopathology

- Mature adipose tissue interspersed with strands of unremarkable thymic tissue
- Thymic component may be well populated with lymphocytes

Special Stains and Immunohistochemistry

- Noncontributory

Other Techniques for Diagnosis

- Noncontributory

Differential Diagnosis

❚ Involution of thymus gland
- Involuted thymus is normal size or smaller than normal for age
❚ Thymoma
- Contain little or no fat
❚ Lipoma
- Occurs mostly in middle-aged to older adults
- Occurs anywhere in mediastinum but rarely within the thymus
- Does not contain thymic tissue

Pearls

- Appearance on CT may suggest a cyst
- Probably a hamartoma
- Rare associations include Graves disease, Hodgkin lymphoma, and myasthenia gravis

Selected References

Moran CA, Rosado-de-Christenson ML, Suster S: Thymolipoma: Clinicopathologic review of 33 cases. Mod Pathol 8:741-744, 1995.

Rosado-de-Christenson ML, Pugatch RD, Moran CA, Galobardes J: Thymolipoma: Analysis of 27 cases. Radiology 193:121-126, 1994.

Thymoma

Clinical Features

- Most commonly found in adults; peak incidence in the fifth decade
- Most common solid primary neoplasm of the mediastinum
- Typically in anterior-superior mediastinum; may also occur in thymic tissue rests: pleura, pulmonary hilum, pericardium, and thyroid
- Radiograph shows a lobulated mass that is occasionally calcified
- Clinical associations
  — Myasthenia gravis (thymic follicular hyperplasia and thymoma)
  — Acquired hypogammaglobulinemia
  — Pure red cell aplasia
  — Hypogammaglobulinemia
- Other associations
  — Systemic lupus erythematosus
  — Rheumatoid arthritis
  — Scleroderma
  — Polymyositis
  — Prognosis and staging: thymomas exhibit a range of biologic behavior from noninvasive, encapsulated tumors to aggressive infiltrative tumors
  — Most noninvasive tumors are cured by surgical resection

Figure 5-3. Thymoma type A. The tumor cells are elongated and spindled with scant cytoplasm.

Figure 5-4. Thymoma type B. The tumor is composed predominantly of lymphocytes with a background containing round epithelial cells with vesicular nuclei and abundant cytoplasm.

Figure 5-6. Thymoma type B3. The tumor is composed predominantly of large epithelioid cells with enlarged and hyperchromatic nuclei and sharp cell borders. Rare mitotic figures can be seen (*center*).

Figure 5-5. Thymoma type B1. Scanning magnification shows a predominant population of small lymphocytes with scant epithelial cells separated by broad bands of fibrous connective tissue.

— Most important predictor of clinical course is the presence and extent of invasion into other mediastinal structures
• Staging system used for thymomas reflects this range of behavior (Masaoka et al, 1981)

— Stage I: completely encapsulated
— Stage IIa: microscopic invasion into capsule, completely resected
— Stage IIb: macroscopic invasion into adjacent fatty tissue or pleura
— Stage III: invades pericardium, great vessels, or lung
— Stage IV: multifocal pericardial or pleural invasion, or distant metastases
— Careful examination of the margins of a resected thymoma is critical for assessing completeness of resection and guiding possible adjuvant therapy

Gross Pathology

• Most are lobulated and encapsulated with a solid, gray-white cut surface
• Larger tumors may show extensive cystic changes

Histopathology

• Thymomas exhibit a range of histologic features
• Generally encapsulated with a distinct fibrous capsule
• Dual cell population composed of neoplastic proliferation of thymic epithelial cells admixed with variable numbers of non-neoplastic T lymphocytes
• T lymphocytes may be cortical (immature), medullary, or peripheral (mature)

- Most thymomas display organotypic morphology, meaning that the tumors will display features that are distinctive of the normal thymus, including
  — Fibrous bands forming angulated tumor lobules
  — Variable numbers of immature T lymphocytes
  — Proliferation of bland-appearing thymic epithelial cells
  — Perivascular spaces
  — Foci of so-called medullary differentiation (rounded areas with lower lymphocyte density)
  — No significant cytologic atypia or pleomorphism
- Neoplastic epithelial cells may be of two types
  — Oval or spindled cells with bland nuclei and dispersed chromatin and occasional small chromocenters
  — Round or polygonal (epithelioid) cells with abundant lightly eosinophilic or amphophilic cytoplasm and distinct round eosinophilic nucleolus
- Histologic classification is still a matter of debate; most commonly accepted scheme is the one proposed by the World Health Organization (Travis, 2004)
  — WHO thymoma type A: composed primarily of benign-appearing spindle cells
  — WHO thymoma type AB (mixed): composed of a combination of spindle cells (type A) and round epithelioid cells (type B)
  — WHO thymoma type B: composed of round or polygonal epithelial cells with varying amounts of immature and mature T lymphocytes; this group is subdivided into three types (B1 to B3) based on progressive decrease in the proportion of lymphocytes to epithelial cells and progressive increase in cytologic atypia of neoplastic epithelial cells
    ◆ Type B1: large number of T lymphocytes containing few, isolated, scattered round or polygonal thymic epithelial cells with minimal cytologic atypia
    ◆ Type B2: about equal number of T lymphocytes and thymic epithelial cells showing mild to minimal cytologic atypia
    ◆ Type B3: large number of polygonal epithelial cells admixed with few lymphocytes; the epithelial cells show enlarged nuclei with increased chromatin pattern, occasional prominent nucleoli, and rare mitotic figures and contain abundant eosinophilic cytoplasm with sharp cell borders
  — WHO thymomas of special types, including micronodular thymoma, metaplastic thymoma, microscopic thymoma, thymoma with anaplasia, and thymic carcinoma
- Limitations of above scheme include difficulties in interobserver reproducibility, overlap in cytologic features for the various categories due to tumor heterogeneity, conflicting results of clinical survival studies for the various categories, lack of a biologic substrate for the classification, and the existence of numerous morphologic variants that do not fit into any of the standard categories
- Unusual morphologic variants include thymomas with clear cells, glandlike structures, cribriform areas, macrocystic and microcystic structures, papillary structures, rhabdomyomatous cells, heavy plasma cell stromal infiltration, extensive areas of infarction and necrosis, starry-sky pattern, storiform pattern (in spindle cell thymoma), hemangiopericytic pattern (in spindle cell thymoma), rosette-like structures (in spindle cell thymoma), desmoplastic pseudosarcomatous stroma, massive stromal sclerosis, and others
- Classification of thymomas
  — There has been considerable controversy in recent years regarding which (if any) of these histologic features predict clinical behavior or reflect the differentiation of the tumor cells
  — Table 5-1 shows the numerous classification schemes for thymoma
- Features used for classification
  — Type of epithelial cell (spindle versus round or polygonal)
  — Organotypic organization
  — Relative proportion of epithelial cells and lymphocytes
  — Degree of epithelial atypia
- Features predictive of invasion or metastatic potential seem to include
  — Predominance of polygonal epithelial cells
  — Epithelial pleomorphism and atypia
  — Loss of organotypic features
- Thymic tumors with overtly malignant epithelium are called *thymic carcinomas* (see under "Thymic Carcinoma")

Special Stains and Immunohistochemistry

- Have limited role in diagnosis
- Cytokeratin: highlights epithelial cells, particularly in lymphocyte-rich tumors
- CD3: highlights T-cell population
- CD1a/CD99: highlight immature T lymphocytes
- CD20: may be positive in epithelial cells of some thymomas

Other Techniques for Diagnosis

- Electron microscopy: very limited role; can demonstrate tonofilaments, tight intercellular junctions, desmosomes, elongated cytoplasmic processes, and basal lamina of epithelial cells; high potential for sampling error
- Flow cytometry: can be misleading in cases of lymphocyte-rich thymoma by showing an immature terminal deoxynucleotidyl transferase (TdT)-positive lymphoblastic population that can lead to an erroneous diagnosis of lymphoblastic lymphoma

Table 5-1. Comparison of Classifications of Thymoma

World Health Organization (Travis, 2004)	Traditional (Bernatz et al, 1961)	Histogenetic (Marino and Müller-Hermelink, 1969)	Suster and Moran (1999)
Type A	Spindle cell thymoma	Medullary thymoma	Thymoma, well differentiated
Type AB	—	Mixed thymoma	Thymoma, well differentiated
Type B1	Lymphocyte-rich thymoma	Cortical thymoma	Thymoma, well differentiated
Type B2	Lymphoepithelial thymoma	Predominantly cortical	Thymoma, well differentiated
Type B3	Epithelial-rich thymoma	Well-differentiated thymic carcinoma	Atypical thymoma (moderately differentiated)
Thymic carcinoma (formerly thymoma type C)	Thymic carcinoma	Thymic carcinoma	Thymic carcinoma (poorly differentiated thymic epithelial neoplasm)

- Ras p21 protein: increased expression reported in aggressive tumors
- Gene rearrangement studies: no clonality is found in the lymphocytes of thymoma
- Other molecular studies: no role identified yet for diagnosis

Differential Diagnosis

▌ Thymic hyperplasia versus lymphocyte-rich thymoma
- Thymic tissue maintains normal thymic architecture in hyperplasia; architecture and cortical or medullary proportions are distorted in thymoma
- Cases with lymphoid follicular hyperplasia contain follicles with active germinal centers

▌ Lymphoma versus lymphocyte-rich thymoma
- Most likely lymphoid neoplasms to be confused for thymoma are lymphoblastic, Burkitt, and Hodgkin lymphoma

▌ Lymphoblastic lymphoma
- Most often seen in children and adolescents
- Patients often have leukemia with blasts in peripheral blood
- Medium-sized lymphoid cells with fine blastic chromatin; mitoses typically numerous
- Most often of T-cell lineage; expresses TdT and other early T-cell antigens
- May reflect the pattern of antigen expression seen on normal and mature cortical or medullary thymocytes; therefore, flow cytometry must be interpreted with caution
- Molecular diagnostics, that is, gene rearrangement studies, may be needed to rule out a clonal T-cell process
- Most important stain for diagnosis is cytokeratin; shows scattered keratin-positive thymic epithelial cells admixed with the immature lymphoid cell population in lymphocyte-rich thymoma

▌ Burkitt lymphoma
- Clonal B-cell process that can be demonstrated by flow cytometry
- Can be confused with lymphocyte-rich thymoma owing to starry-sky pattern

- Cytokeratin demonstrates no epithelial cell component
- Ki-67 shows virtually 100% positivity of the lymphoid cells

▌ Nodular sclerosing Hodgkin lymphoma
- Reed-Sternberg and lacunar cells may be identified immunohistochemically (positive for CD15 and CD30, negative for CD3, CD45, and CD20), whereas the atypical epithelial cells of thymoma demonstrate cytokeratin staining
- Hodgkin lymphoma is often associated with cystic changes of the thymus

▌ Castleman disease
- Characteristic follicles with hyalinized vessels and sclerotic germinal centers surrounded by concentrically arranged layers of lymphocytes in the mantle zone (onion-skinning)

▌ Spindle cell sarcoma versus spindle cell thymoma
- Both can show a storiform pattern
- Spindle cells in spindle cell sarcomas are reactive for vimentin and negative for cytokeratin
- Spindle cell thymoma can resemble solitary fibrous tumors due to prominent hemangiopericytic growth pattern; cells are positive for cytokeratin in thymoma

Pearls

- Thymomas are tumors of the epithelial component of the thymus; associated lymphocytes in the background are benign
- Thymomas have a strong association with myasthenia gravis
- Primary treatment is surgical excision
- Classification is still controversial
- Invasion of adjacent mediastinal structures remains the most widely accepted predictor of aggressive behavior

Selected References

Suster S, Moran CA: Thymoma classification: Current status and future trends. Am J Clin Pathol 125:542-554, 2006.

Suster S, Moran CA: Problem areas and inconsistencies in the WHO classification of thymoma. Semin Diagn Pathol 22:188-197, 2005.

Travis WD, Brambilla E, Muller-Hermelink HK, Harris CC: Pathology and genetics of tumors of the lung, pleura, thymus and heart. In World Health Organization Classification of Tumours, Lyon, IARC Press, 2004.

Suster S, Moran CA: Thymoma, atypical thymoma and thymic carcinoma: A novel conceptual approach to the classification of thymic epithelial neoplasms. Am J Surg Pathol 111:826-833, 1999.

Suster S, Moran CA: Primary thymic epithelial neoplasms: Spectrum of differentiation and histological features. Semin Diagn Pathol 16:2-17, 1999.

Pan CC, Wu HP, Yang CF, et al: The clinicopathological correlation of epithelial subtyping in thymoma: a study of 112 consecutive cases. Hum Pathol 25:893-899, 1994.

Koga K, Matsuno Y, Noguchi M, et al: A review of 79 thymomas: Modification of staging system and reappraisal of conventional division into invasive and non-invasive thymoma. Pathol Int 44:359-367, 1994.

Kornstein MJ, Curran WJ Jr, Turrisi AT III, Brooks JJ: Cortical versus medullary thymomas: A useful morphologic distinction? Hum Pathol 19:1335-1339, 1988.

Marino M, Müller-Hermelink HK: Thymoma and thymic carcinoma: Relation of thymoma epithelial cells to the cortical and medullary differentiation of the thymus. Virch Arch 407:119-149, 1985.

Masaoka A, Monden Y, Nakahara K, et al: Follow-up study of thymomas with special reference to their clinical stages. Cancer 48:2485-2492, 1981.

Bernatz PE, Harrison EG, Claggett OT: Thymoma. A clinicopathologic study. J Thorac Cardiovasc Surg 42:424-444, 1961.

Thymic Carcinoma

Clinical Features

- Thymic epithelial neoplasm with cellular atypia and aggressive clinical course
- No association with paraneoplastic syndromes of thymoma such as myasthenia gravis or pure red cell aplasia
- May arise from malignant progression in a long-standing, preexisting thymoma
- Predominantly found in middle age to late adulthood
- Patients may present with chest pain, dyspnea, or superior vena cava syndrome
- Primary thymic carcinomas are rare; secondary invasion of the thymus by primary carcinoma of the lung or metastatic tumor in mediastinal lymph nodes is more common
- Thymic carcinoma is a diagnosis of exclusion; extensive clinical and radiologic studies must be undertaken to rule out the possibility of an occult or late metastasis from another organ before rendering this diagnosis

Figure 5-7. Thymic carcinoma, poorly differentiated, nonkeratinizing squamous cell type (lymphoepithelioma-like carcinoma). The tumor is composed of sheets of large cells with vesicular nuclei and prominent eosinophilic nucleoli with a scant and indistinct rim of cytoplasm. Notice the adjacent dense lymphoid stroma.

Figure 5-8. Thymic carcinoma, mucoepidermoid type. The tumor is composed of sheets of squamoid intermediate cells admixed with mucocytes and cystic spaces filled with mucin.

Gross Pathology

- Usually not encapsulated
- Gray-white tumor with a hard, gritty cut surface often showing hemorrhage and necrosis
- Stroma may be desmoplastic, but these tumors do not have the broad fibrous septa seen in thymoma
- Some variants may have prominent cystic changes

Histopathology

- Differs from thymoma by having overt histologic features of a malignancy and complete loss of organotypic features of thymic differentiation
- Lymphocytes are of B-cell type instead of immature T lymphocytes

Figure 5-9. Thymic carcinoma, basaloid type. The tumor is composed of a monotonous proliferation of hyperchromatic cells showing striking peripheral palisading of nuclei.

- Numerous microscopic subtypes; they essentially resemble a variety of other carcinomas in other organs
- Can be divided into histologically low-grade and high-grade tumors (Table 5-2)
▌ Keratinizing squamous cell carcinoma of the thymus
- Resembles invasive squamous cell carcinoma seen elsewhere; must rule out early massive mediastinal spread from an occult bronchial primary by bronchoscopy
▌ Poorly differentiated (lymphoepithelioma-like) non-keratinizing squamous cell carcinoma
- Histologic features similar to lymphoepithelioma-like carcinoma of the nasopharynx
- Comedo-like central areas of necrosis are a distinctive and constant feature
- Lymphocytes in the stroma may or may not be present
- Rarely related to Epstein-Barr virus (EBV) as seen in nasopharyngeal carcinomas
▌ Mucoepidermoid carcinoma
- Resembles that seen in salivary glands; may be low grade (well differentiated) and high grade (moderately and poorly differentiated)

Table 5-2. Comparison of Low-Grade and High-Grade Thymic Carcinomas

Low-Grade	High-Grade
Well-differentiated squamous cell carcinoma	Moderate to poorly differentiated (lymphoepithelioma-like) nonkeratinizing squamous cell carcinoma
Well-differentiated mucoepidermoid carcinoma	
Basaloid carcinoma	Moderate to poorly differentiated mucoepidermoid carcinoma
Papillary carcinoma	
Well-differentiated mucinous adenocarcinoma	Spindle cell carcinoma and thymic carcinosarcoma
	Clear cell carcinoma
	Anaplastic carcinoma

- Can be associated with prominent cystic changes
- Mucicarmine stain is helpful for highlighting cytoplasmic mucin in the tumor cells
▌ Clear cell carcinoma
- Composed of clear cells containing abundant glycogen with surrounding delicate stroma
- May resemble clear cell carcinoma of the kidney, or may result from clear cell changes in well-differentiated squamous cell carcinoma
▌ Basaloid carcinoma
- Composed of nests of basaloid cells that may show peripheral palisading
- Can present in association with prominent cystic changes
▌ Spindle cell (sarcomatoid) carcinoma
- Extremely rare
- Spindle and pleomorphic cells with hyperchromatic nuclei, prominent nucleoli, and eosinophilic cytoplasm
- Spindle cells are cytokeratin positive
- Often associated with preexisting spindle cell thymoma
- When associated with clear-cut sarcomatous elements, is designated thymic carcinosarcoma

Special Stains and Immunohistochemistry

- Periodic acid–Schiff (PAS) and mucicarmine stains may be useful in clear cell carcinoma and mucoepidermoid carcinoma to identify intracytoplasmic glycogen and mucin, respectively
- Universally express cytokeratin intermediate filaments and may react with other epithelial markers such as CEA, EMA, and MOC31
- May express CD5

Other Techniques for Diagnosis

- Noncontributory

Differential Diagnosis

▌ Metastatic carcinoma
- Clinical history is important; possibility of metastasis from occult primary elsewhere must first be ruled out
▌ Epithelioid hemangioendothelioma
- May closely resemble carcinoma
- Cells contain abundant cytoplasm with prominent cytoplasmic vacuoles
- Cells are positive for FVIII-RA and CD31 in epithelioid hemangioendothelioma
- Caveat: some cases of epithelioid hemangioendothelioma can be keratin positive; must always add vascular markers to distinguish from carcinoma
▌ Germ cell tumors
- Positive for placental alkaline phosphatase (PLAP), human chorionic gonadotropin (HCG), or α-fetoprotein (AFP)
- Serum AFP or HCG is often elevated

❚ Lymphoma
- Positive for leukocyte common antigen (LCA) and other lymphoid markers (e.g., CD3, CD20, CD30) and negative for cytokeratin
- Flow cytometry and gene rearrangement studies helpful to document monoclonality

Pearls

- Careful history and clinical and radiologic evaluation are needed to diagnose a carcinoma in the thymus as a primary thymic carcinoma
- Variants that may be cured by surgical excision include well-differentiated squamous cell, mucoepidermoid, and basaloid carcinoma; other variants have poor prognosis and are fatal

Selected References

Suster S: Thymic carcinoma: Update of current diagnostic criteria and histologic types. Semin Diagn Pathol 22:188-197, 2005.

Suster S, Moran CA: Spindle cell carcinoma of the thymus: Clinicopathologic and immunohistochemical study of 15 cases of a novel form of thymic carcinoma. Am J Surg Pathol 23:691-700, 1999.

Suster S, Moran CA: Thymic carcinoma: Spectrum of differentiation and histologic types. Pathology 30:111-122, 1998.

Suster S, Moran CA: Primary thymic epithelial neoplasms showing combined features of thymoma and thymic carcinoma: Clinic pathologic study of 22 cases. Am J Surg Pathol 20:1469-1480, 1996.

Moran CA, Suster S: Mucoepidermoid carcinoma of the thymus: Clinicopathologic study of six cases. Am J Surg Pathol 19:826-834, 1995.

Suster S, Rosai J: Thymic carcinoma: Clinicopathologic study of 60 cases. Cancer 67:1025-1032, 1991.

Wick MR, Scheithauer BW, Weiland LH, Bernatz PE: Primary thymic carcinomas. Am J Surg Pathol 6:613-630, 1982.

Neuroendocrine Neoplasms of the Thymus

Clinical Features

- Most common in middle-aged adults
- Strong male predominance
- Histologic spectrum from well-differentiated tumors (carcinoid) to poorly differentiated carcinomas histologically similar to oat cell carcinoma of the lung; histologic features and clinical behavior correlate
- Carcinoids arising in the mediastinum are most often of thymic origin
- Thymic carcinoid
  - Typically more aggressive than bronchial carcinoid; biologically they are low-grade neuroendocrine carcinomas
  - May be locally invasive or can metastasize
  - May recur after a long disease-free interval
  - Paraneoplastic syndromes are found in one third of these patients and include Cushing syndrome,

Figure 5-10. Well-differentiated neuroendocrine carcinoma of the thymus (thymic carcinoid). The tumor shows a monotonous population of tumor cells with small nuclei and dispersed chromatin pattern (salt-and-pepper). Some of the tumor cells form balls with central, comedo-like areas of necrosis and artifactual retraction from the surrounding stroma.

syndrome of inappropriate antidiuretic hormone (SIADH), and Eaton-Lambert syndrome
  - No expression of the full carcinoid syndrome
- Up to one third of low-grade tumors occur in association with multiple endocrine neoplasia (MEN) types I or II and tend to follow a more aggressive course
  - MEN I: pituitary adenoma, parathyroid adenoma, pancreatic islet cell tumor
  - MEN II: medullary carcinoma of thyroid, pheochromocytoma, parathyroid hyperplasia, mucocutaneous ganglioneuromas

Gross Pathology

- Unencapsulated, firm mass with a gray-pink, gritty texture due to fine calcifications
- Focal hemorrhage and necrosis are common
- No fibrous septa or lobulation (in contrast to thymoma)

Histopathology

- Classification based on histologic grade
  - Well differentiated
    - Fewer than 3 mitoses/10 high-power fields (hpf)
    - Minimal atypia
    - Classic organoid pattern
    - No more than small foci of necrosis
  - Moderately differentiated
    - Intermediate features between well-differentiated and poorly differentiated tumors
    - Organoid architecture is generally not present

- ◆ Moderate cytologic atypia with prominent nucleoli
- ◆ Moderate mitotic activity (3 to 10 mitoses/10 hpf)
  - — Poorly differentiated (high-grade) neuroendocrine carcinoma
    - ◆ More than 10 mitoses/10 hpf
    - ◆ Marked atypia or areas of small cell carcinoma
    - ◆ Extensive necrosis
    - ◆ Total loss of organoid architecture
    - ◆ Some tumors may show admixtures of differing histologic grades
- • Histologic features
  - — Low-grade tumors
    - ◆ Uniform polygonal cells with oval nucleus, stippled chromatin, and granular cytoplasm
    - ◆ Cells arranged in nests, trabeculae, ribbons, and cords; may have pseudorosette formation
    - ◆ Nests may show focal central areas of comedo-like necrosis and calcification
    - ◆ Artifactual clefts between nests of tumor cells and surrounding stroma
  - — Variant morphologic findings
    - ◆ Amyloid-like stroma associated occasionally with calcitonin production
    - ◆ Spindle cell morphology
    - ◆ Oncocytic cytoplasmic features
    - ◆ Pigmentation: melanin, lipofuscin
  - — Moderate- to high-grade tumors
    - ◆ Diffuse, lymphoma-like architecture
    - ◆ Histology similar to small cell (oat cell) neuroendocrine carcinoma of the lung
    - ◆ Pulmonary neuroendocrine carcinomas can have widespread metastases from a small primary lesion; thorough clinical and radiologic evaluation is necessary to prove that such a tumor in the thymus is a primary thymic carcinoma
    - ◆ Small cells with nuclear moulding and scant cytoplasm
    - ◆ Fine salt-and-pepper, stippled chromatin
    - ◆ A large cell variant of poorly differentiated neuroendocrine carcinoma has also been described
    - ◆ Prominent crush artefact
    - ◆ Cases showing transitions between low-grade (well-differentiated) and high-grade (poorly differentiated) neuroendocrine carcinoma have also been described

Special Stains and Immunohistochemistry

- • Neoplastic cells are reactive for cytokeratin, chromogranin, synaptophysin, and CD57
- • May express neuropeptides: adrenocorticotropic hormone (ACTH), serotonin, somatostatin, gastrin, and others

Other Techniques for Diagnosis

- • Electron microscopy: cells contain cytoplasmic dense core neurosecretory granules

Differential Diagnosis

- ▌ Large cell lymphoma
  - • Diffuse growth pattern; no ribbons, festoons, or trabecular pattern
  - • Tumor cells have vesicular nuclei
  - • Mitotic and apoptotic figures are numerous
  - • Positive for LCA and CD20
- ▌ Metastatic malignant melanoma
  - • Cells are generally more pleomorphic and have more abundant cytoplasm and prominent macronucleoli
  - • Positive for S-100 protein and HMB-45
  - • Cytokeratin negative
- ▌ Medullary carcinoma of thyroid gland
  - • Neuroendocrine carcinoma of the thymus can also have scattered cells reactive for calcitonin
  - • Neoplastic C cells are reactive for carcinoembryonic antigen (CEA) and calcitonin
- ▌ Paraganglioma
  - • Prominent atypia (nucleomegaly) in the absence of mitotic activity
  - • Negative for cytokeratin
- ▌ Metastatic carcinoid or neuroendocrine carcinoma
  - • Careful clinical and radiologic evaluation are the only tools to differentiate primary from secondary thymic involvement

Pearls

- • Neuroendocrine neoplasms of the thymus are best considered as a spectrum from low-grade tumors (carcinoid) to high-grade carcinomas similar to small cell carcinoma of the lung
- • Metastasis or extension from the lung to the thymus of small cell carcinoma of pulmonary origin is more common than a thymic primary
- • Low-grade tumors (carcinoid)
  - — Any thymic carcinoid has the potential for metastasis
  - — Poorer prognosis when associated with MEN syndromes or with ACTH production
  - — Treated with surgical excision; tumor is resistant to chemotherapy and radiation
  - — May recur after long intervals (e.g., 10 years)
- • High-grade neuroendocrine carcinoma
  - — Treatment approach is generally the same as for a pulmonary tumor of similar histology

Selected References

Moran CA: Primary neuroendocrine carcinomas of the mediastinum: Review of current criteria for histopathologic diagnosis and classification. Semin Diagn Pathol 22:223-229, 2005.

Suster S, Moran CA: Neuroendocrine neoplasms of the mediastinum. Am J Clin Pathol 115(S1):17-27, 2001.

Moran CA, Suster S: Neuroendocrine carcinomas (carcinoid tumor) of the thymus: A clinicopathologic analysis of 80 cases. Am J Clin Pathol 114:100-110, 2000.

Moran CA, Suster S: Thymic neuroendocrine carcinomas with combined features ranging from well-differentiated (carcinoid) to small cell carcinoma: A clinicopathologic and immunohistochemical study of 11 cases. Am J Clin Pathol 113:345-350, 2000.

Klemm KM, Moran CA: Primary neuroendocrine carcinomas of the thymus. Semin Diagn Pathol 16:32-41, 1999.

Wick MR, Scheithauer BW: Thymic carcinoid: A histologic, immunohistochemical, and ultrastructural study of 12 cases. Cancer 53:475-484, 1984.

Wick MR, Danney JA, Bernatz PE, Brown LR: Primary mediastinal carcinoid tumors. Am J Surg Pathol 6:195-205, 1982.

Rosai J, Higa E: Mediastinal endocrine neoplasm, of probable thymic origin, related to carcinoid tumor. Clinicopathologic study of 8 cases. Cancer 29:1061-1074, 1972.

Chronic Mediastinitis

Clinical Features

- Generally affects anterior-superior mediastinum; often just anterior to the carina
- Occurs at any age; most common in young adult years
- Female predominance is seen
- About half the cases are associated with fungal infection (commonly histoplasmosis), also *Aspergillus* and *Nocardia* species and mycobacteria; also following methysergide treatment
- About half the cases are idiopathic
- Delayed cell-mediated hypersensitivity response is the postulated mechanism in the infectious cases
- Radiologic appearance is an asymmetrical widening of the mediastinum
- Is the most common non-neoplastic cause of superior vena cava syndrome
- Can cause pulmonary vein compression and thrombosis

Gross Pathology

- Firm, white, densely fibrotic tissue
- Generally compresses rather than invades mediastinal structures

Histopathology

- Dense, hypocellular, hypovascular fibrohyaline tissue
- Entrapped lymphocytes
- Granulomas (caseating or noncaseating)
- May see infectious organisms

Special Stains and Immunohistochemistry

- PAS and Grocott methenamine silver (GMS): help identify fungal organisms
- Acid-fast stain for mycobacteria

Other Techniques for Diagnosis

- Microbiology: Gram stain, cultures, and serology
- Polymerase chain reaction (PCR) may be useful for rapid detection of mycobacteria or fungi

Differential Diagnosis

- Solitary fibrous tumor
  - Well-defined neoplasm composed of haphazardly arranged bland spindle cells in a dense, well-vascularized collagenous stroma
  - Positive for CD34 and bcl-2
- Hodgkin lymphoma, nodular sclerosing
  - Relatively acellular fibrous bands separate highly cellular nodules containing a mixed infiltrate
  - Characterized by scattered atypical cells consisting of Hodgkin cells, Reed-Sternberg cells, or lacunar cells
  - Inflammatory infiltrate includes lymphocytes, plasma cells, and eosinophils
  - Granulomas may be present
- Large cell lymphoma with sclerosis
  - Numerous atypical large lymphoid cells in a fibrous tissue background
  - Highly proliferative tumor with mitoses and apoptotic bodies
  - Large cells are CD20 positive

Pearls

- Special stains should be performed to rule out microorganisms
- Some authors consider sclerosing mediastinitis and chronic mediastinitis as separate entities; others believe this process is a reaction pattern that may occur in response to infection or drugs, or as an autoimmune-type reaction
- Sclerosing mediastinitis is reportedly more cellular than chronic mediastinitis and is composed of fibroblasts, lymphocytes, plasma cells, and eosinophils
- At later stages, the lesion becomes hypocellular and hypovascular with dense collagenous fibrosis
- Treated with excision and corticosteroids

Selected Reference

Flieder DB, Moran C, Suster S: Idiopathic fibroinflammatory (fibrosing/sclerosing) lesions of the mediastinum: A study of 30 cases with emphasis on morphologic heterogeneity. Mod Pathol 12:257-264, 1999.

Hodgkin Lymphoma

Clinical Features

- Most common malignant tumor of the mediastinum
- Occurs predominantly in the anterior compartment
- Lymph nodes and thymus may be involved
- Young women in their 20s and 30s are most commonly affected
- Often presents with B symptoms, including fever, night sweats, weight loss, and fatigue

Figure 5-11. Hodgkin lymphoma with cystic changes. A, Low magnification shows cystically dilated thymic epithelium infiltrated by dense lymphoid cell population. **B,** Higher magnification shows large binucleated and mononuclear forms of Hodgkin cells.

Gross Pathology

- Fleshy mass with sclerotic bands
- With thymic involvement, cystic degeneration is common

Histopathology

- Nodular sclerosing variant is the most common type
- Type is best determined by lymph node analysis, as the diagnostic features may not be represented in extranodal sites
- When extranodal, such as in the thymus, Hodgkin disease generally forms a discrete mass
  — Collagenous fibrosis and the typical background cells (small lymphocytes, plasma cells, and eosinophils) are present
  — Classic Reed-Sternberg cells in a background consistent with Hodgkin lymphoma are needed to establish a new diagnosis of Hodgkin lymphoma in an extranodal site
  — In a patient with an established diagnosis of Hodgkin lymphoma, mononuclear cells with the other features of Reed-Sternberg cells (Hodgkin cells) in the background of collagen and cells typical of Hodgkin lymphoma are sufficient to diagnose involvement of an extranodal site

Special Stains and Immunohistochemistry

- Immunohistochemical confirmation is often desirable even if the histology is characteristic
- Reed-Sternberg cells and their lacunar variants are reactive with CD15 and CD30 antibodies
- Hodgkin and Reed-Sternberg cells are usually negative with CD45
- Occasionally Reed-Sternberg cells and their variants are positive for CD20 (L26) or T-cell marker CD45RO (UCHL 1) antibody

Other Techniques for Diagnosis

- Negative for T- or B-cell gene rearrangements

Differential Diagnosis

▍ Thymoma
  - Low-power view can mimic Hodgkin disease because of sclerosis' forming well-defined nodules composed of large and small cells
  - No atypical lymphoid cells (Hodgkin cells)
  - Eosinophils and plasma cells are rare
  - Thymoma cells are positive for epithelial markers (cytokeratin)
▍ Thymic cyst
  - Cyst has an epithelial cell lining
  - No atypical lymphoid cells are seen
  - Adequate and extensive sampling is required in thymic cysts to rule out Hodgkin disease
▍ Sclerosing large cell non-Hodgkin lymphoma
  - Monotonous population of large, atypical lymphoid cells without distinctive milieu of Hodgkin lymphoma (i.e., small lymphocytes, plasma cells, and eosinophils)
  - Tumor cells are almost always of B-cell lineage and express CD19, CD20, and CD22
  - Negative for CD15, but many cases can be CD30 positive

Pearls

- Nodular sclerosing is the most common type of Hodgkin lymphoma seen in the mediastinum
- Young women most commonly affected
- Can be often cystic—thorough sampling is necessary to identify diagnostic areas

Selected References

Kim HC, Nosher J, Haas A, et al: Cystic degeneration of thymic Hodgkin's disease following radiation therapy. Cancer 55:354-356, 1985.

Katz A, Lattes R: Granulomatous thymoma or Hodgkin's disease of thymus? A clinical and histologic study and a re-evaluation. Cancer 23:1-15, 1969.

Fechner RE: Hodgkin's disease of the thymus. Cancer 23:16-23, 1969.

Burke WA, Burford TH, Dorfman RF: Hodgkin's disease in the mediastinum. J Thorac Cardiovasc Surg 3:287-296, 1967.

Diffuse Large Cell Lymphoma, B-Cell Type

Clinical Features

- Second most common type of lymphoid malignancy of the mediastinum after Hodgkin lymphoma
- Predominantly affects females; peak incidence between 20 and 40 years of age
- Typically found in anterior mediastinum
- Almost always of B-cell lineage
- Usually involves the thymus with or without lymph node involvement
- Signs and symptoms may include superior vena cava syndrome and pleural effusions

Gross Pathology

- Firm mass with foci of necrosis
- Typically shows extensive infiltration into surrounding tissue

Histopathology

- Diffuse growth pattern composed of large atypical lymphoid cells with reniform or multilobated nuclei, vesicular chromatin, and distinct nucleoli
- Large amounts of pale or clear cytoplasm
- Often shows a pattern of stromal sclerosis characterized by compartmentalization of the tumor into discrete nests and islands simulating epithelial malignancy

Figure 5-12. Diffuse large cell lymphoma with sclerosis. The tumor is composed of large atypical lymphoid cells showing a compartmentalized appearance owing to fine bands of sclerosis that separate them into small islands.

- Entrapment of thymic and extrathymic fat often seen

Special Stains and Immunohistochemistry

- CD19, CD20, CD22, and CD45 positive
- CD10, CD5, CD43, CD21, and immunoglobulin negative (resembling the phenotype of normal thymic B cells)
- Negative for CD15
- Significant percentage of these cases can be CD30 positive

Other Techniques for Diagnosis

- Flow cytometric or gene rearrangement studies to verify lymphoid B- or T-cell lineage

Differential Diagnosis

- Germinoma
  - Almost all cases occur in males
  - Composed of diffuse population of large cells with abundant cytoplasm and large nuclei with irregular (spiked) nucleoli
  - Small lymphocytes are concentrated along delicate fibrovascular septa rather than scattered throughout the tumor
  - Presence of glycogen in the clear cytoplasm favors the diagnosis of germinoma
  - Positive for PLAP by immunohistochemistry
  - Negative for CD20 and CD45
  - Can show striking dotlike paranuclear positivity for cytokeratin and positive staining for C-kit (CD117)
- Hodgkin lymphoma, syncytial variant
  - Sclerosis is present in broad bands rather than diffusely
  - Characterized by large multinucleated tumor cells (Reed-Sternberg cells)
  - Large cells are CD15 and CD30 positive
  - Large cells usually negative for CD20 and CD45
- Lymphoblastic lymphoma
  - Male predominance
  - Patients may have frank leukemia, which is exceptional in mediastinal large cell lymphoma
  - Cells have very scant cytoplasm and blastic chromatin
  - Cells express CD1, CD3, CD43, TdT
  - Negative for CD20
- Metastatic carcinoma
  - Sheets or nests of cohesive neoplastic cells
  - May form glands or show obvious keratinization
  - Tumor cells express cytokeratin; negative for CD20 and CD45

Pearls

- Generally affects young women (second to fourth decades)
- May involve the thymus
- Sclerosis and necrosis are common findings
- Almost always B-cell lineage

- Good response to multiagent chemotherapy with consolidation radiation therapy

Selected References

Suster S: Primary large-cell lymphomas of the mediastinum. Semin Diagn Pathol 16:51-64, 1999.

Davis RE, Dorfman RF, Warnke RA: Primary large cell lymphoma of the thymus: A diffuse B-cell neoplasm presenting as primary mediastinal lymphoma. Hum Pathol 21:1262-1268, 1990.

Jacobson JO, Aisenberg AC, Lamarre L, et al: Mediastinal large cell lymphoma: An uncommon subset of adult lymphoma curable with combined modality therapy. Cancer 62:1893-1898, 1988.

Menestrina F, Chelosi M, Bonetti F, et al: Mediastinal large cell lymphoma of B-cell type with sclerosis: Histopathological and immunohistochemical study of 8 cases. Histopathology 10:589-600, 1986.

Perrone T, Frizzera G, Rosai J: Mediastinal diffuse large cell lymphoma with sclerosis: A clinicopathological study of 60 cases. Am J Surg Pathol 10:176-191, 1986.

Lymphoblastic Lymphoma

Clinical Features

- Predominantly seen in older children and adolescents but can also occur in older adult patients
- Disease shows male predominance (2:1)
- Patients may have a concomitant leukemic phase
- Almost all cases with a mediastinal mass at presentation are of T-cell lineage (see Chapter 14 for discussion on B-lineage lymphoblastic lymphoma)

Figure 5-13. Lymphoblastic lymphoma. Atypical lymphoid cells with fine chromatin, inconspicuous nucleoli, and frequent nuclear membrane infoldings are seen.

- Mediastinum is most common location, and thymus is usually involved; with thymic involvement, residual lobules and infiltrated Hassall corpuscles may be seen
- Patients often present with acute onset of respiratory distress owing to the rapidly growing nature of the tumor
- Patients may have central nervous system and gonadal involvement at presentation

Gross Pathology

- Usually solid, infiltrative, and lacks a capsule

Histopathology

- Diffuse growth pattern composed of atypical lymphoid cells with fine (blastic) chromatin pattern
- Medium-sized cells with high nuclear-to-cytoplasmic ratio
- Cells may have nuclear convolutions with finely dispersed chromatin and inconspicuous nucleoli (at high power, nuclear outline suggests outline of a brain as seen on CT) or may be of nonconvoluted type
- Numerous mitotic figures
- Necrosis can be extensive
- Blood vessel invasion and extension into perithymic fibroadipose tissue may be prominent features
- Neoplastic cells can infiltrate the thymus
- May have scattered tingible body macrophages, creating a starry-sky pattern

Special Stains and Immunohistochemistry

- TdT positive in almost all cases
- LCA positive in 80% of cases
- CD99 positive in most cases
- Tumor cells usually express CD1, CD43, and CD3
- Tumor cells may be positive or negative for CD4 and CD8
- CD45RO expressed in 50% of cases; CD20 is negative

Other Techniques for Diagnosis

- Flow cytometry
  - May be misleading because lymphocytes in lymphocyte-rich thymomas show similar immunophenotype (i.e., immature, blastic T cells)
  - May not always differentiate clonal immature T cells from benign prethymic cells that may be found in thymoma
- Molecular studies: useful to detect gene rearrangement in lymphoblasts to verify clonality
  - Cytogenetics: helps with diagnosis and is related to prognosis; particularly for B-lineage lymphoblastic lymphoma

Differential Diagnosis

▌ Thymoma
- Rare in children; however, adults can develop either disease

- Lymphocytic component may be phenotypically indistinguishable from lymphoblastic lymphoma
- Apoptotic lymphocytes may simulate a starry-sky pattern
- Cytokeratin highlights network of epithelial cells throughout the tumor
- Lymphocytes are not clonal

▌ Large B-cell lymphoma
- Tumor cells are larger and have clear cytoplasm, vesicular nuclei, and usually prominent nucleoli; convoluted nuclei are uncommon
- Phenotype is that of a B-cell neoplasm
- Positive for CD20; negative for TdT, CD99, CD1a

▌ Other small round blue cell tumors of childhood

▌ Granulocytic sarcoma
- Extremely uncommon
- Search carefully for cells with granular cytoplasm
- Tumor cells positive for myeloperoxidase; negative for TdT
- CD43 and CD45 may be positive and are not helpful in this differential diagnosis

▌ Neuroblastoma
- Typically found in posterior mediastinum
- More commonly seen in younger children
- Composed of smaller round cells with scant cytoplasm forming characteristic rosettes; look for neuropil in the background
- Positive for neuron-specific enolase (NSE), negative for lymphoid markers

▌ Embryonal rhabdomyosarcoma
- Mixture of haphazardly arranged rhabdomyoblasts and undifferentiated primitive cells
- Positive for MyoD1, myogenin, and other markers of muscle differentiation (desmin, actin, and myosin)
- Negative for TdT and lymphoid markers

▌ Primitive neuroectodermal tumor (PNET)
- Rare in this location
- May have limited neural differentiation (usually positive for synaptophysin and chromogranin)
- Positive for CD99
- Intracytoplasmic glycogen (PAS positive)
- Negative for TdT and lymphoid markers
- Characteristic translocation t(11;22)

▌ Small cell carcinoma (neuroendocrine carcinoma, oat cell carcinoma)
- Mostly in older adults
- May be primary or metastatic
- Small cells with nuclear molding and scant cytoplasm
- Nuclei have fine salt-and-pepper stippled chromatin or smudged chromatin pattern
- Prominent crush artefact and extensive necrosis
- Tumor cells express cytokeratin, chromogranin, and synaptophysin
- Negative for TdT, CD45, and CD3

Pearls

- This rapidly growing tumor is seen predominantly in children and adolescents; male predominance

- Leukemia and bone marrow involvement is common
- Almost all cases presenting with a mediastinal mass are of T-cell lineage
- Always include a cytokeratin stain in your panel to make sure you do not miss a lymphocyte-rich thymoma

Selected References

Devoe K, Weidner N: Immunohistochemistry of small round cell tumors. Semin Diagn Pathol 17:216-225, 2000.

Ha K, Minded M, Hozumi N, Gelfano EW: Phenotypic heterogeneity at the DNA level in childhood leukemia with a mediastinal mass. Cancer 56:509-513, 1985.

Benerjee D, Silva E: Mediastinal mass with acute leukemia: Myeloblastoma masquerading as lymphoblastic lymphoma. Arch Pathol 105:126-129, 1981.

Nathwani BN, Kim H, Rappaport H: Malignant lymphoma, lymphoblastic. Cancer 38:966-983, 1976.

Castleman Disease

Clinical Features

- Reactive condition; also known as *angiofollicular lymph node hyperplasia*
- Found predominantly involving lymph nodes; occasionally may involve the thymus
- Both sexes may be affected
- Wide age range
- Three types: hyaline vascular, plasma cell, and mixed
  — Hyaline vascular type (about 80% of cases)
    ◆ Usually asymptomatic except for effects of compression by mass
  — Plasma cell type
    ◆ Patients may have anemia, hypergammaglobulinemia, and fever
    ◆ Typically solitary, but multicentric variant does exist

Figure 5-14. Castleman disease. This histologic section shows a germinal center with hyalinized blood vessels and distinct concentric layering.

— Multicentric variant: multiple lymph nodes at multiple sites are involved
- Hepatosplenomegaly
- Hematologic and immunologic abnormalities (pancytopenia, increased erythrocyte sedimentation rate, proteinuria)
- One third of patients develop other malignancies (non-Hodgkin lymphoma [NHL], carcinoma, or Kaposi sarcoma)
- More frequent in patients with human immunodeficiency virus (HIV) infection
- Associated with infection with Kaposi sarcoma–associated herpesvirus (KSHV, human herpesvirus-8 [HHV-8]), especially in HIV-positive patients

Gross Pathology
- Hyaline vascular type
  - Large single mass
  - Well-circumscribed round nodule usually located in the anterior-superior aspect of the mediastinum
- Plasma cell type
  - Forms a mass and more commonly affects multiple lymph nodes

Histopathology
- Hyaline vascular type (about 80% of cases)
  - Multiple follicles with small germinal centers
  - Hyalinized blood vessels penetrate the germinal centers (lollipop sign)
  - Germinal centers may show concentric foci of hyalinization resembling Hassall corpuscles
  - Small cells of the mantle zone may show distinct concentric layering (onion-skinning)
  - Abnormal follicles may contain multiple small germinal centers
  - Rich network of capillaries in the interfollicular zone
  - Perivascular fibrosis may be seen around interfollicular vessels
  - Interfollicular regions are composed primarily of lymphocytes but also contain plasma cells, immunoblasts, and eosinophils
- Plasma cell type (10% to 20%)
  - Interfollicular areas contain sheets of plasma cells (diagnostic feature)
  - Germinal centers are large and reactive
- Mixed (rare)
  - Combination of features from hyaline vascular and plasma cell variants
  - Generally asymptomatic unless mass causes compression

Special Stains and Immunohistochemistry
- CD5-positive lymphoid cells are seen at the periphery of the abnormal follicles (suggesting that Castleman disease is a proliferation of CD5-positive lymphocytes stimulated by specific lymphokines)
- Polyclonal population of B-lymphocytes and plasma cells

Other Techniques for Diagnosis
- Flow cytometry and gene rearrangement studies: polyclonal

Differential Diagnosis
- Follicular lymphoma
  - Monotonous follicles composed of atypical lymphocytes
  - Cytologically abnormal cells, most of which have cleaved nuclei (centrocytes)
  - Monoclonal B cells
  - Positive for CD20 and bcl-2
- Plasmacytoma
  - Pure plasmacytic population composed of clonal plasma cells
  - Generally lacks hyalinized germinal centers and onion-skinning of mantle zone
  - Must be careful with clonality because several reports have demonstrated a monoclonal plasma cell component in the interfollicular area in Castleman disease

Pearls
- Mediastinum is the most common location and most commonly involves lymph nodes
- Multicentric type is more common in HIV-positive patients
- Multicentric type in HIV-positive patients is associated with HHV-8 infection

Selected References
O'Reilly PE Jr, Joshi V, Holbrook CT, Weisenburger DD: Multicentric Castleman's disease in a child with prominent thymic involvement: A case report and brief review of the literature. Mod Pathol 6:776-780, 1993.

Frizzera G: Atypical lymphoproliferative disorders. In Knowles DM (ed): Neoplastic Hematopathology. Baltimore, Williams & Wilkins, 1992, pp 459-495.

Keller AR, Hochholzer L, Castleman B: Hyaline-vascular and plasma-cell types of giant lymph node hyperplasia of mediastinum and other locations. Cancer 29:670-683, 1972.

Thymic Histology in Immune Deficiencies

Clinical Features
- Thymic histology can be abnormal in a variety of congenital and acquired immune deficiency diseases, particularly in T-lymphocyte deficiencies
- Generally a clinical diagnosis, with patients having characteristic clinical presentations and features of an immune deficiency

Gross Pathology
- DiGeorge syndrome: thymic hypoplasia or aplasia with reduced to absent normal thymic tissue
- Other congenital immune defects: atrophic thymic tissue

Histopathology

- ▐ DiGeorge syndrome
  - Whatever thymic tissue is present is histologically normal or shows variable stress involution
- ▐ B-cell immune defects
  - Features of exaggerated stress involution
  - Decreased corticomedullary differentiation
  - Decreased number of lymphocytes
  - Variable number of Hassall corpuscles
- ▐ Severe combined immune deficiency (SCID)
  - Pattern is called *thymic dysplasia*
  - Small round to oval lobules of spindle to polygonal epithelial cells
  - Few or no lymphocytes and absence of Hassall corpuscles
  - Patients with less severe forms of deficiency may have a few lymphocytes and Hassall corpuscles
- ▐ Severe acquired immune damage (AIDS and graft-versus-host disease [GVHD])
  - Severe lymphocyte depletion
  - Hassall corpuscles may disappear
  - Apoptotic bodies can be seen
  - Apoptosis of thymic epithelial cells has been reported in GVHD

Special Stains and Immunohistochemistry

- Noncontributory

Other Techniques for Diagnosis

- Immunologic studies and lymphocyte function tests used to classify the defect are usually performed on the peripheral blood lymphocytes

Differential Diagnosis

- ▐ Stress involution
  - Clinically important in infants
  - Stress involution and immune deficiencies create an overlapping range of histologic and functional alterations in the thymus (differences are those of degree)
  - Hassall corpuscles are more often present than in severe thymic dysplasia
  - Lobules tend to be triangular rather than rounded
  - Apoptotic cells are usually lymphoid

Pearls

- Thymus may be a target of attack in GVHD
- There may be overlap of histologic features between stress involution and milder forms of thymic dysplasia in congenital immune deficiencies

Selected Reference

Nezelof C: Pathology of the thymus in immunodeficiency states. In Müller-Hermelink HK (ed): The Human Thymus: Histophysiology and Pathology. Berlin, Springer-Verlag, 1986, pp 151-177.

Teratoma

Clinical Features

- Generally found in early adulthood
- Males and females are affected
- Most common type of mediastinal germ cell tumor

Gross Pathology

- Large, uniloculated or multiloculated cystic mass, often with calcification in the wall
- Greasy or fatty material, hair, and degenerated debris in cysts
- May erode into adjacent structures, including the trachea

Histopathology

- Microscopic appearance is similar to that of cystic teratoma of the ovary
- Cysts are lined by any type of epithelium and may contain sebaceous glands and hair follicles
- Other common components include neural tissue, gastrointestinal tract elements, cartilage, and respiratory structures
- Pancreatic acini are a frequent finding in teratomas in mediastinal location
- Immature teratoma
  - In addition to the components of mature teratoma, immature fetal type epithelial, neural, or mesenchymal elements are present
  - See Chapter 12 for more detailed information

Special Stains and Immunohistochemistry

- Noncontributory

Modern Techniques for Diagnosis

- Noncontributory

Figure 5-15. Mature teratoma. The tumor shows mature pancreatic tissue in the wall of a cyst.

Figure 5-16. Immature teratoma. Histologic section demonstrates immature neural tubules surrounded by immature mesenchymal tissue.

Differential Diagnosis

▌ Teratomas with additional malignant components
  ● Malignant mixed germ cell tumor composed of carcinoma and teratoma, teratoma plus another type of malignant germ cell tumor (such as embryonal carcinoma), and teratoma with a sarcoma
▌ Bronchial cyst
  ● Connected to bronchus or trachea
  ● Cyst with epithelial lining, smooth muscle, and cartilage
  ● Neural or other ectopic elements are absent
▌ Foregut cysts
  ● Connected to esophagus or stomach
  ● Cyst with smooth muscle in wall
  ● No ectopic elements

Pearls

● Benign tumor
● Generous sampling of solid areas is advised to rule out immature components and malignant components
● Residual mediastinal masses removed after treatment for a malignant germ cell tumor may contain only mature or immature teratoma; thorough sampling is needed to exclude residual malignant components

Selected References

Suster S, Moran CA, Dominguez-Malagon H, Quevedo-Blanco P: Germ cell tumors of the mediastinum and testis: A comparative immunohistochemical study of 120 cases. Hum Pathol 29:737-742, 1998.

Moran CA, Suster S: Primary germ cell tumors of the mediastinum. I. Analysis of 322 cases with special emphasis on teratomatous lesions and a proposal for histopathologic classification and clinical staging. Cancer 80:681-690, 1997.

Carter D, Bibro MC, Touloukian RJ: Benign clinical behavior of immature mediastinal teratoma in infancy and childhood: Report of two cases and review of the literature. Cancer 49:398-402, 1982.

Gonzalez-Crussi F: Extragonadal teratoma. Atlas of Tumor Pathology, 2nd series, Fascicle 18. Washington, DC, Armed Forces Institute of Pathology, 1982.

Teratoma with Additional Malignant Components

Clinical Features

● Usually present as large, bulky, and invasive anterior mediastinal masses
● May have elevated levels of HCG or AFP

Gross Features

● Large, fleshy tumors with extensive areas of hemorrhage and necrosis

Histologic Features

▌ Type I: teratoma with malignant epithelial component (e.g., adenocarcinoma, squamous cell carcinoma)
▌ Type II: teratoma with additional nonteratomatous germ cell tumor component (e.g., seminoma, choriocarcinoma, yolk sac tumor, embryonal carcinoma)
▌ Type III: teratoma with sarcomatous components (e.g., liposarcoma, leiomyosarcoma, rhabdomyosarcoma)
▌ Type IV: teratoma with a combination of any of the above

Special Stains and Immunohistochemistry

● Epithelial markers (e.g., keratin, EMA, CEA): useful for identifying malignant epithelial components
● Specific markers for mesenchymal neoplasms (e.g., smooth muscle actin [SMA], desmin, S-100 protein, myogenin): useful for identifying specific lines of differentiation in sarcomatous components

Other Techniques for Diagnosis

● Noncontributory

Selected References

Dominguez-Malagon H, Cano-Valdez AM, Moran CA, Suster S: Germ cell tumors with sarcomatous components: A clinicopathologic and immunohistochemical study of 46 cases. Am J Surg Pathol 31:1356-1362, 2007.

Moran CA, Suster S: Germ cell tumors of the mediastinum. Adv Anat Pathol 5:1-15, 1998.

Moran CA, Suster S: Primary germ cell tumors of the mediastinum. I. Analysis of 322 cases with special emphasis on teratomatous lesions and a new proposal for histopathologic classification and clinical staging. Cancer 80:681-690, 1997.

Germinoma (Mediastinal Seminoma)

Clinical Features

● Mediastinum is the most common extragonadal site for germ cell tumors

Figure 5-17. Mediastinal seminoma. The tumor is composed of cells with abundant clear cytoplasm, round nuclei, and prominent nucleoli admixed with epithelioid granulomas.

- Usually arises in the thymus
- Marked male predominance, rare in females
- Most commonly found in second through fourth decades
- Patients may present with superior vena cava syndrome and cervical lymphadenopathy

Gross Pathology
- Lobulated, large, soft, solid yellow tumor
- May be cystic in 10% of cases

Histopathology
- Fibrous septa divide tumor into lobules containing nests of neoplastic tumor cells
- Tumor cells have abundant pale cytoplasm, central round nuclei with irregular, spiked nucleoli, and distinct cell borders
- Lymphocytes are mostly located in the fibrous septa
- Tumor cells may be obscured by extensive granulomatous reaction, florid lymphoid follicular hyperplasia, or extensive sclerosis and hyalinization of the stroma
- Spermatocytic and anaplastic variants of seminoma do not occur in the mediastinum

Special Stains and Immunohistochemistry
- Germ cells
  — PLAP positive
  — C-kit (CD117) positive
  — Cytokeratin positive in 80% of cases with a distinct dotlike, paranuclear pattern
  — PAS: cytoplasmic positivity due to intra-cytoplasmic glycogen

  — Vimentin occasionally positive
  — CD30 may be positive in up to 4% of cases
  — LCA negative

Other Techniques for Diagnosis
- Noncontributory

Differential Diagnosis
▌ Diffuse large cell lymphoma with sclerosis
- Diffuse large cell population with monotonous compartmentalization due to thin sclerotic bands
- LCA, CD20 positive
- PLAP, CD117 negative
▌ Nodular sclerosing Hodgkin lymphoma, syncytial variant
- Relatively acellular fibrous bands separate cellular nodules containing a mixed infiltrate
- Characterized by scattered atypical cells consisting of Hodgkin cells, Reed-Sternberg cells, or lacunar cells
- Inflammatory infiltrate includes lymphocytes, plasma cells, and eosinophils
- Hodgkin cells are positive for CD15 and CD30
- Negative for PLAP

Pearls
- Mediastinal seminomas are reportedly more often positive for cytokeratin and vimentin than testicular seminomas
- Germinoma is highly sensitive to radiation therapy
- Predominantly a male disease
- Careful clinical evaluation for a gonadal primary is essential
- Thorough sampling and examination for other germ cell elements is necessary

Selected References
Suster S, Moran CA, Dominguez-Malagon H, Quevedo-Blanco P: Germ cell tumors of the mediastinum and testis: A comparative immunohistochemical study of 120 cases. Hum Pathol 29:737-742, 1998.

Moran CA, Suster S, Przygodzki RM, Koss MN: Primary germ cell tumors of the mediastinum: II. Mediastinal seminomas—a clinicopathologic and immunohistochemical study of 120 cases. Cancer 80:691-698, 1997.

Moran CA, Suster S: Mediastinal seminomas with prominent cystic changes: A clinicopathological study of 10 cases. Am J Surg Pathol 19:1047-1053, 1995.

Burns BF, McCaughey WTE: Unusual thymic seminomas. Arch Pathol Lab Med 110:539-541, 1986.

Hunt RD, Bruckman JE, Farrow GM, et al: Primary anterior mediastinal seminoma. Cancer 49:1658-1663, 1982.

Schantz A, Sewall W, Castleman B: Mediastinal germinoma. A study of 21 cases with an excellent prognosis. Cancer 30:1189-1194, 1972.

Nonseminomatous Germ Cell Tumors (NSGCTs): Embryonal Carcinoma, Yolk Sac Tumor (Endodermal Sinus Tumor), Choriocarcinoma, Mixed Germ Cell Tumor

Clinical Features

- These tumors occur almost entirely in males
- Tumors can occur at any age, peak in 20s through 40s
- Patients may present with cough, dyspnea, chest pain, or fatigue
- Gynecomastia at presentation generally indicates a choriocarcinoma component
- Mediastinum is the most common site for extragonadal germ cell tumors
- About 75% or more of mediastinal germ cell tumors are teratomas or seminoma; others are extremely rare
- Tumors have 30 to 40 times greater frequency in patients with Klinefelter syndrome
- At the time of diagnosis, tumors are usually large with invasion into surrounding organs or structures
- Elevated serum AFP in a patient with a germ cell tumor is diagnostic of a nonseminomatous component, usually yolk sac tumor
- Serum HCG may be elevated in any type; HCG above 500 IU is indicative of a choriocarcinoma component
- Response to therapy and overall survival is worse than for testicular germ cell tumors

Gross Pathology

- Large infiltrative tumors often with hemorrhage and necrosis
- Usually solid but may have cystic areas because of necrosis
- Extensive hemorrhage is characteristic of choriocarcinoma
- Classic rule of thumb for sectioning is to take one block per centimeter of greatest tumor dimension

Histopathology

- Embryonal carcinoma
  - Cohesive clusters of primitive, anaplastic cells arranged in solid or abortive glandular structures
  - Large polygonal cells with pleomorphic, round to oval nuclei, prominent nucleoli, and abundant, pale-staining cytoplasm
  - High mitotic rate
  - Necrosis and hemorrhage are common
- Yolk sac tumor
  - Variable tumor cytomorphology, ranging from small, round to polygonal monotonous tumor cells with minimal atypia to large, pleomorphic tumor cells
  - Reticular or microcystic pattern is characterized by various-sized cystic spaces lined by flattened cells (most common pattern)

Figure 5-18. Embryonal carcinoma. The tumor shows a solid proliferation of primitive-appearing large cells with oval to round nuclei, prominent nucleoli, and large amounts of pale-staining cytoplasm.

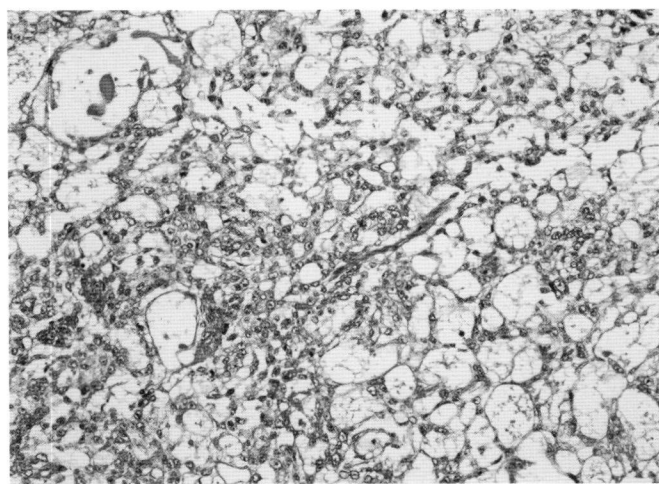

Figure 5-19. Yolk sac tumor (endodermal sinus tumor), reticular pattern. Low-power view shows a reticular pattern with variably sized spaces.

- May form tubules and papillary structures
- Polyvesicular vitelline pattern is characterized by saclike structures in a background of myxoid or fibrous stroma
- Rarely, hepatoid pattern resembling liver cells in thick plates
- Schiller-Duval bodies (papillary structures with central vascular core covered by neoplastic epithelium) characteristic but are not always present
- Intracellular or extracellular eosinophilic hyaline globules often seen regardless of which pattern predominates
- Sarcomatoid foci may be seen

Figure 5-20. Yolk sac tumor with myxoid background. The tumor is characterized by cords of hyperchromatic cells set against a prominent myxoid background.

Figure 5-21. Mixed nonteratomatous germ cell tumor. The tumor shows an admixture of seminomatous (*left*) and yolk sac tumor (*right*) components within the same lesion.

▌ Choriocarcinoma
  ● Neoplasm composed of cytotrophoblastic cells admixed with giant syncytiotrophoblastic cells
  ● Extensive necrosis and hemorrhage common
▌ Mixed nonteratomatous germ cell tumors
  ● Foci with features of different types of germ cell tumor, often including seminoma
  ● Those with choriocarcinoma and yolk sac components usually show elevated serum levels of both β-HCG and AFP

Special Stains and Immunohistochemistry

  ● Immunohistochemistry useful in differentiating germ cell tumors from other malignancies in the mediastinum but not for subclassifying NSGCT
  ● Cytokeratin positive in all nonseminomatous germ cell tumors

  ● PLAP positive in about 50% of NSGCTs
  ● AFP positive in about 30% of cases of embryonal carcinoma and in most cases of yolk sac tumor
  ● HCG positive in giant cells and cytotrophoblastic cells in any germ cell tumor
  ● Embryonal carcinoma
    — CD30 (Ki-1) often positive
    — CD57 often positive
  ● Yolk sac tumor
    — Positive for AFP
    — α_1-Antitrypsin positive in hyaline droplets
  ● Choriocarcinoma
    — β-HCG positive in syncytiotrophoblastic cells and focally in cytotrophoblastic cells
    — Epithelial membrane antigen (EMA) positive in about 50% of cases

Other Techniques for Diagnosis

  ● Cytogenetics: isochromosome 12p is characteristic

Differential Diagnosis

  ● Subclassification depends on thorough sampling and meticulous microscopic examination
▌ Metastatic adenocarcinoma
  ● Thorough history and clinical-radiologic evaluation is necessary
  ● Usually negative for AFP (serum and immunohistochemically)
  ● HCG negative
▌ Thymic carcinoma
  ● Usually occurs in patients older than 40 years
  ● May have squamous or neuroendocrine differentiation
  ● HCG, AFP, and PLAP negative
▌ Metastatic melanoma
  ● Detailed history is important
  ● S-100 protein, vimentin, and HMB-45 are generally positive
  ● Negative for PLAP, HCG, or AFP

Pearls

  ● Almost all cases occur in males
  ● AFP positivity virtually excludes a metastatic adenocarcinoma
  ● Residual mediastinal mass after chemotherapy for a germ cell tumor may be mature teratoma or scar tissue; thorough sampling is necessary to exclude residual malignancy
  ● Most patients have invasion of other organs or distant metastases at time of presentation, and most of these patients die of their disease
  ● Sarcomatous transformation
  ● May have foci of cartilaginous matrix (chondrosarcoma) or skeletal muscle (rhabdomyosarcoma)
  ● Prognosis is extremely poor

- Association with hematologic malignancy
- Seen with yolk sac tumor
- Believed to be due to differentiation of tumor into hematopoietic cells, which migrate to liver, spleen, and bone marrow
- Most are acute myelomonocytic or acute megakaryocytic leukemia

Selected References

Moran CA, Suster S: Hepatoid yolk sac tumors of the mediastinum: A clinicopathological and immuno-histochemical study of four cases. Am J Surg Pathol 21:1210-1214, 1997.

Moran CA, Suster S: Yolk sac tumors of the mediastinum with prominent spindle cell features: A clinicopathologic study of three cases. Am J Surg Pathol 21:1173-1177, 1997.

Moran CA, Suster S: Primary mediastinal choriocarcinomas. A clinicopathologic and immunohistochemical study of 8 cases. Am J Surg Pathol 21:1007-1012, 1997.

Moran CA, Suster S, Koss MN: Primary germ cell tumors of the mediastinum. III. Yolk sac tumor, embryonal carcinoma, choriocarcinoma, and combined nonteratomatous germ cell tumors of the mediastinum—a clinicopathologic and immunohistochemical study of 64 cases. Cancer 80:699-707, 1997.

Moran CA, Suster S: Mediastinal yolk sac tumors associated with prominent multilocular cystic changes of thymic epithelium: A clinicopathologic and immunohistochemical study of five cases. Mod Pathol 10:800-803, 1997.

Truong LD, Harris L, Mattioli C, et al: Endodermal sinus tumor of the mediastinum: A report of 7 cases and review of the literature. Cancer 58:730-739, 1986.

Grego FA, Oldham RK, Fez MF: The extragonadal germ cell cancer syndrome. Semin Oncol 9:448-455, 1982.

McNeil MM, Leong AS, Sage RE: Primary mediastinal embryonal carcinoma in association with Klinefelter's syndrome. Cancer 47:343-345, 1981.

Sickels EA, Belliveau RE, Wiernik PH: Primary mediastinal choriocarcinoma in the male. Cancer 33:1196-1203, 1974.

Neurogenic Tumors: Neuroblastoma, Ganglioneuroblastoma, Ganglioneuroma

Clinical Features

- Tumors are associated with the sympathetic chain and may be found in the neck, mediastinum, retroperitoneum, and adrenal medulla
- Tumors are categorized as neuroblastoma (NB), ganglioneuroblastoma (GNB), and ganglioneuroma (GN) based on the maturation of the neurons and accompanying Schwann cells
- Tumors in the mediastinum are more likely to show maturation than those in the retroperitoneum or adrenal medulla
- Neuroblastoma is the most common solid tumor of young children
- Ganglioneuroma is the most common in the mediastinum

Figure 5-22. Neuroblastoma. The tumor is composed of small round blue cells with scant cytoplasm. Notice the fibrillary background.

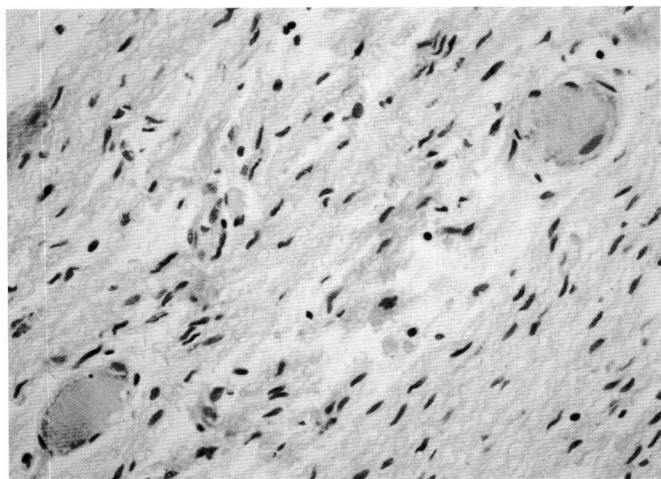

Figure 5-23. Ganglioneuroma. Histologic section shows a tumor composed of spindle cells with wavy nuclei and scattered mature ganglion cells.

- Presents with mass effects, including compression of nerve roots and erosion of vertebral bone
- Serum or urine shows elevated catecholamine metabolites homovanillic acid (HMV) and vanillylmandelic acid (VMA)

Gross Pathology

❚ Neuroblastoma
- Large, well-circumscribed mass with a gray, soft cut surface; often has hemorrhage, necrosis, and calcification

❚ Ganglioneuroblastoma
- Large, well-circumscribed, firm mass with tan-white areas and hemorrhagic areas; focal calcification often seen

❚ Ganglioneuroma
- Large, encapsulated tumor with a firm, gray-white, homogeneous cut surface

Histopathology

- See Chapter 9 for more detailed histologic features
- See Table 5-3
▌ Neuroblastoma
- Cellular tumor composed of nodular aggregates of small round blue cells (neuroblasts) separated by delicate fibrovascular septa
- Characterized by Homer-Wright pseudorosettes (round spaces surrounded by palisading peripheral nuclei and filled with a faintly eosinophilic fibrillary matrix)
▌ Ganglioneuroblastoma
- Similar histology to neuroblastoma except ganglion cell differentiation is seen (admixture of ganglion cells and undifferentiated cells)
- Developing or mature ganglion cells make up more than half the cell population
- Small undifferentiated cells make up a minority of the tumor
▌ Ganglioneuroma
- Spindle cell tumor resembling neurofibroma but with numerous ganglion cells
- Maturing tumors are composed of differentiating neuroblasts, ganglion cells, and neuropil
- Mature tumors are composed of sheets of Schwann cells admixed with clusters of mature ganglion cells in a loose myxoid background

Special Stains and Immunohistochemistry

- Neuroblastoma and ganglion cells are reactive for
  — Neurofilament
  — Synaptophysin
  — Chromogranin
  — NSE (caution: NSE has broad cross-reactivity with other cell types)
- Stromal cells (Schwann cells) are reactive for
  — S-100 protein
  — Glial fibrillary acidic protein (GFAP)
  — Myelin basic protein

Other Techniques for Diagnosis

- Electron microscopy: neuroblastoma is composed of undifferentiated small cells with round nuclei and scant cytoplasm; neurofilaments, neurosecretory granules, or both may be present

- Cytogenetics (neuroblastoma): may be associated with deletion of chromosome 1p

Differential Diagnosis

▌ Neuroblastoma
▌ Ewing sarcoma, PNET
- Generally found in long bones or occasionally in soft tissue; rare in mediastinum
- Tumor cells may have clear cytoplasm containing glycogen (positive for PAS)
- Positive for CD99
- Characteristic translocation t(11;22)
▌ Embryonal rhabdomyosarcoma
- Admixture of small primitive blue cells and scattered larger cells with abundant eosinophilic cytoplasm (rhabdomyoblasts)
- Positive for muscle markers such as desmin, myogenin, MyoD1, and muscle-specific actin (MSA)
- Negative for neural markers
▌ Lymphoblastic lymphoma
- Positive for TdT, CD3, and CD45
- Usually clonal T-cell population; rarely clonal B-cell population
- *Caution:* also positive for CD99
▌ Small cell carcinoma
- Typically found in older adults
- Lung primary far more common than mediastinal primary
- Positive for low-molecular-weight cytokeratins; negative for NSE
▌ Ganglioneuroblastoma and ganglioneuroma
- Malignant melanoma
  — Positive for HMB-45, melan-A, and S-100 protein
- Paraganglioma
  — Zellballen pattern with surrounding sustentacular cells
  — Sustentacular cells positive for S-100 protein
  — Positive for chromogranin and synaptophysin
- Schwannoma and malignant schwannoma
  — Typically show Antoni A and B areas and Verocay bodies
  — Absent ganglion cells
- Neurofibroma
  — Spindle cell tumor with no ganglion cells

Table 5-3. Comparison of Features of Neurogenic Tumors

	Neuroblastoma	**Ganglioneuroblastoma**	**Ganglioneuroma**
Age	Young children; 90% <5 years old	Older children	Older children to adults
Maturation	Minimal to none	Mixed	Mixed to fully mature
Location	Adrenal gland, rarely posterior mediastinum	Posterior mediastinum or retroperitoneum	Posterior mediastinum or retroperitoneum
Behavior	Dismal to excellent depending on stage; average 3-year survival rate of 30%	Overall better prognosis than neuroblastoma	Maturing: favorable Mature: benign

Table 5-4. Prognostic Factors for Neurogenic Tumors

Good Prognosis	Poor Prognosis
Near triploid or hyperdiploid (aneuploid)	Tetraploid or near diploid
Presence of 1p36 tumor suppressor gene	Loss of heterozygosity
No amplification of *N-myc*	Amplification of *N-myc* (>10 copies)
No expression of TRKA factor receptor	

Pearls

- Neuroblastoma: prognosis is related to disease stage, which is a complex scheme based on age at diagnosis and cytogenetic and histologic findings
- Stages I and II (good prognosis) are associated with specific cytogenetic findings (chromosome 1 deletion), no amplification of *N-myc* gene, and greater than 95% 3-year survival rate
- Stages III and IV (poor prognosis) have from less than 5% to about 50% survival rate (Table 5-4)

Selected References

Devoe K, Weidner N: Immunohistochemistry of small round cell tumors. Semin Diagn Pathol 17:216-224, 2000.

Joshi VV: Peripheral neuroblastic tumors: Pathologic classification based on recommendations of international neuroblastoma pathology committee (modification of Shimada classification). Pediatr Dev Pathol 3:184-199, 2000.

Ambros PF, Ambros IM, Strehl S, et al: Regression and progression in neuroblastoma. Does genetics predict tumor behavior? Eur J Cancer 31A:510-515, 1995.

Brodeur GM: Molecular basis for heterogeneity in human neuroblastomas. Eur J Cancer 31A:505-510, 1995.

Young DG: Thoracic neuroblastoma/ganglioneuroma. J Pediatr Surg 18:37-41, 1983.

Adam A, Hochholzer L: Ganglioneuroblastoma of the posterior mediastinum: A clinicopathologic review of 80 cases. Cancer 47:373-381, 1981.

Schwannoma

Clinical Features

- Most common tumor in the posterior mediastinum
- Generally a single mass; multiple schwannomas may be associated with von Recklinghausen disease (neurofibromatosis type I)
- May be asymptomatic or present with pain, cough, or symptoms related to nerve involvement or compression
- No sex predilection
- Peak incidence in third and fourth decades

Gross Pathology

- Round to oval encapsulated tumor
- Usually attached to a nerve trunk
- About 10% have an intravertebral tumor and are dumbbell shaped
- Firm, solid tumor with a tan to yellow cut surface
- Cystic changes and myxoid areas may be seen

Histopathology

- Well-formed fibrous capsule
- Spindle cell tumor composed of Antoni A and B patterns (hypercellular and hypocellular areas, respectively)
- Verocay bodies are characteristic and consist of palisading nuclei with central hypocellular area
- Blood vessels are hyalinized and thick walled
- Focal collections of foamy histiocytes
- Osseous and cartilaginous metaplasia can be seen
- Cystic changes may be seen
- Ancient schwannoma
  — Atypical nuclei
  — Stromal sclerosis
  — Little or no mitotic activity
- Cellular schwannoma
  — Encapsulated, but can erode adjacent structures
  — Highly cellular spindle cell proliferation with predominance of Antoni A areas and no Antoni B areas
  — Variable nuclear atypia
  — Low mitotic activity
  — Strong S-100 protein positivity

Special Stains and Immunohistochemistry

- S-100 protein positive (more often in benign tumors)
- CD57 positive
- GFAP: some schwannomas may be positive

Other Techniques for Diagnosis

- Electron microscopy: spindle cells show numerous long-spaced (130-nm periodicity) collagen fibrils referred to as *Luse bodies* and reduplication of the basal lamina; pigment, if present, is neuromelanin, and is not in melanosomes; long, slender cytoplasmic prolongations are characteristic

Differential Diagnosis

▌ Neurofibroma
- Stronger association with neurofibromatosis
- Lacks thick fibrous capsule
- Grows within and enlarges nerve
- Hypocellular, myxoid areas without hypercellular areas
- Absence of Antoni A and B areas and Verocay bodies
- Silver stain may reveal nerve fibers within the tumor

▌ Leiomyoma
- Less common in this location
- Negative for S-100 protein
- Positive for SMA

Pearls

- Multiple schwannomas may be associated with von Recklinghausen disease
- Well-formed fibrous capsule with typical histologic features, including Verocay bodies and Antoni A and Antoni B areas
- Excellent prognosis; surgical excision of solitary tumors is curative

Selected References

Marchevsky AM: Mediastinal tumors of peripheral nervous system origin. Semin Diagn Pathol 16:65-78, 1999.

Dickersin GR: The electron microscopic spectrum of nerve sheath tumors. Ultrastruct Pathol 11:103-146, 1987.

Weiss SW, Langloss JM, Enzinger FM: Value of S-100 protein in the diagnosis of soft tissue tumors with particular reference to benign and malignant Schwann cell tumors. Lab Invest 49:299-308, 1983.

Ackerman LV, Taylor FH: Neurogenous tumors within the thorax: A clinical pathologic evaluation of 48 cases. Cancer 4:669-691, 1951.

Metastatic Tumors

Clinical Features

- Both small cell and non–small cell carcinomas of the lung can metastasize early to the mediastinum
- Large mediastinal mass and small lung primary may be seen
- Other tumors arising in neighboring structures, including esophagus, trachea, chest wall, pleura, and vertebrae, may also appear to be arising in the mediastinum
- Tumors metastasizing to mediastinal lymph nodes may expand and appear as thymic primary tumors on gross and microscopic examination (particularly breast, thyroid, kidney, prostate, testis, and malignant melanoma)
- Clinical history and radiologic findings are important

Gross Pathology

- Noncontributory

Histopathology

- Histologic features are those seen in primary malignancies

Special Stains and Immunohistochemistry

- Often not helpful because many metastatic carcinomas are cytokeratin positive but have no other specific staining characteristics

- S-100 protein and HMB-45 are useful in the diagnosis of malignant melanoma
- Prostatic-specific antigen (PSA) and prostatic acid phosphatase (PSAP) may be useful in diagnosing a metastasis from a prostatic primary
- BRST2 or GCDFP15 positive in breast carcinoma
- Thyroid transcription factor-1 (TTF-1) positive in lung and thyroid gland tumors
- Synaptophysin and chromogranin positive in small cell carcinomas from lung or other primary site
- LCA positive in lymphoma

Other Techniques for Diagnosis

- As per suspected primary tumor

Differential Diagnosis

- Clinical history is essential when evaluating malignant mediastinal neoplasms
▌ Thymic carcinoma
  - Diagnosis of exclusion
▌ Germinoma
  - Positive for PLAP
▌ Yolk sac tumor
  - Positive for AFP; may be positive for PLAP
▌ Embryonal carcinoma
  - Positive for PLAP and CD30 (Ki-1); may be positive for AFP
▌ Lymphoma
  - Positive for CD45
  - Anaplastic lymphoma positive for CD30 (Ki-1)
  - Flow cytometry or gene rearrangements to demonstrate clonal lymphoid population

Pearls

- Metastatic tumors account for most epithelial malignancies in the mediastinum
- Most common primary sites include trachea, bronchi, lung parenchyma, and esophagus
- Immunohistochemical staining is important when evaluating metastatic tumors in this location

Selected References

McLoud TC, Meyer JE: Mediastinal metastasis. Radiol Clin North Am 20:453-468, 1982.

McLoud TC, Kalisher L, Stark P, Green R: Intrathoracic lymph node metastases from extrathoracic neoplasms. Am J Radiol 131:403-407, 1978.

Middleton G: Involvement of the thymus by metastatic neoplasms. Br J Cancer 20:41-46, 1966.

Jean E. Blair and Robert E. Petras

6 Gastrointestinal System

Esophagus

Congenital and Acquired Esophageal Abnormalities

Clinical Features

▌ Esophageal ectopias
  • Gastric
    — Affects up to 20% of population
    — Found in cervical esophagus; referred to as *inlet patch*
    — May produce peptic symptoms in older patients
    — Rare examples of dysplasia or carcinoma reported complicating inlet patches

Figure 6-1. Endoscopic photograph of inlet patch in the cervical esophagus. Areas of erythematous gastric-type mucosa are surrounded by gray-white glistening squamous mucosa.

  • Sebaceous: so-called Fordyce granules
  • Pancreatic
    — Rare in esophagus
    — Can be seen with trisomy 18 or trisomy 13
    — More often seen as a metaplasia in reflux
▌ Esophageal atresia
  • Complete atresia is found in about 1 in 3000 live births
  • Associated with tracheoesophageal fistula in about 1 in 1000 live births
  • Risk factors include male sex, low birth weight, premature birth, and twin gestation (monozygotic)
  • Classic presentation includes choking in a newborn infant and excessive drooling; affected patients have a propensity to aspirate or develop respiratory distress
  • Atresia is associated with Down syndrome (10% of atresias), single umbilical artery, and other syndromes involving the heart, urogenital tract, and skeleton
  • May be associated with VATER syndrome (vertebral anomalies, anal atresia, tracheoesophageal fistula, renal defects)
▌ Congenital esophageal duplication
  • Manifests as cysts, diverticula, or tubular malformations
  • Most common form: cysts
  • Cysts occur as a result of partial arrest during early development (<8 weeks), when esophagus is lined by columnar epithelium; lined by gastric epithelium if lesion persists into adulthood
  • Symptoms include dysphagia, anorexia, dyspnea, and pain
▌ Esophageal diverticula
  • Saccular protrusions of the esophagus
  • Zenker diverticulum is most common (70%); located immediately above the upper esophageal sphincter (associated with cricopharyngeal motor dysfunction)
  • Less commonly, diverticula develop at the midpoint of the esophagus or immediately proximal to the lower

esophageal sphincter (epiphrenic) (so-called traction diverticulum)
- Typically present in elderly patients
- Produce a repository for swallowed food; complicated by dysphagia and halitosis

▋ Esophageal webs and rings
- Webs
  — Congenital and acquired constrictions caused by diaphragm-like sleeve of mucosa (at right angle to long axis of esophagus)
  — Often symptomatic and typically cause dysphagia
  — Upper esophageal webbing associated with iron deficiency anemia, glossitis, and cheilosis is called *Plummer-Vinson syndrome* and in many patients also includes autoimmune disorders (thyroid disorders, Sjögren syndrome, and inflammatory bowel disease); predisposes to squamous cell carcinoma of the upper esophagus
  — Webs associated with Plummer-Vinson syndrome are proximal, arise anteriorly, and are up to 0.2 cm thick; may occasionally be circumferential
- Rings
  — Developmental constrictions secondary to chronic disease states, which may include reflux or scleroderma
  — May be mucosal or muscular; muscular rings are almost always associated with hiatal hernia
  — Called *Schatzki rings* if located at or immediately above the gastroesophageal junction
  — Rings and corrugations (so-called feline esophagus) can be a manifestation of eosinophilic esophagitis (see "Eosinophilic Esophagitis")

▋ Esophageal hernia (diaphragmatic hernia)
- Generally an acquired condition
- Displacement of the distal esophagus from normal (subdiaphragm) intra-abdominal location into thoracic cavity
- May move caudad to cephalad (sliding) or incarcerate in the anterior mediastinum (paraesophageal)

Gross and Endoscopic Pathology

▋ Esophageal ectopias
- Gastric
  — Discrete pink to red area in cervical esophagus surrounded by gray-white squamous mucosa
  — Variable sizes (several millimeters to large enough to encircle esophagus)
- Sebaceous
  — Small, light-yellow plaques
- Pancreatic
  — Smooth, well-defined submucosal mass resembling leiomyoma or lipoma, sometimes with central dimple

▋ Esophageal atresia (tracheoesophageal fistula)
- Type I: blind proximal esophagus with no fistula
- Type II: proximal fistula with completely interrupted distal esophagus

- Type III: blind proximal esophagus with distal tracheoesophageal fistula arising at tracheal bifurcation (most common)
- Type IV: esophagus with both proximal and distal communications with trachea

▋ Esophageal duplication
- Commonly see posterior cysts
- May be within esophageal wall or extramural

▋ Esophageal diverticula
- Zenker diverticulum
  — Saccular protrusion immediately above the upper esophageal sphincter
  — May be several centimeters

▋ Esophageal webs and rings
- Webs
  — Often produce strictures
- Rings
  — Encircle esophagus and generally occur at the esophagogastric junction (Schatzki ring)
  — Muscular rings arise at the phrenoesophageal membrane attachment

▋ Esophageal hernia (diaphragmatic hernia)
- Intrathoracic portion tends to dilate and undergo ischemic changes
- May lead to ischemic necrosis (rare)

Histopathology

▋ Esophageal ectopias
- Gastric
  — Foveolar mucosa with specialized glands, complete with parietal, chief, and endocrine cells
  — May resemble specialized columnar epithelium of Barrett esophagus with mucin-producing goblet cells
  — May contain *Helicobacter pylori* (rare)
- Sebaceous
  — Mucosal and submucosal sebaceous glands
- Pancreatic
  — Typically pancreatic acinar tissue; may also contain islet cells

▋ Esophageal duplication
- Intramural or extramural cysts lined by respiratory, gastric, intestinal, or squamous mucosa
- May contain hyaline cartilage or duplicated muscularis externa

▋ Esophageal diverticula
- Zenker diverticulum
  — Squamous-lined sac displaying variable acanthosis, chronic inflammation, and ulceration
  — May have thin muscular layer

▋ Esophageal webs and rings
- Webs
  — Thin sleeve of fibrovascular connective tissue covered by squamous mucosa on both sides
  — Gastric mucosa may line distal side
  — Inflammation often present
  — Muscle layer is absent

- Rings
  — Mucosal rings are similar to webs except they have a few fibers of muscularis mucosae (squamous epithelium covering a thin sleeve of connective tissue) and are often covered by gastric mucosa distally
  — Muscular rings have a prominent muscle component
  — Those associated with eosinophilic esophagitis show an increase in the squamous basal cell layer with papillomatosis and increased (>20 per high-power field [hpf]) intraepithelial eosinophils (see "Eosinophilic Esophagitis")
- Esophageal hernia (diaphragmatic hernia)
  - Variable degrees of chronic inflammation, fibromuscular proliferation in the lamina propria, and regenerative epithelial changes

Special Stains and Immunohistochemistry

- Noncontributory

Other Techniques for Diagnosis

- Noncontributory

Differential Diagnosis

- Esophageal ectopias
  - Generally must be differentiated from benign and malignant esophageal tumors; requires biopsy
  - Rare examples of proximal esophageal adenocarcinoma arising in gastric heterotopia are described
- Esophageal atresia
  - Relatively straightforward clinical diagnosis
  - May overlap clinically with respiratory conditions, particularly if associated with tracheoesophageal fistula
- Bronchogenic cysts and esophageal duplication
  - May be difficult to distinguish
  - Bronchogenic cysts are typically anterior, contain cartilage, and are lined by respiratory mucosa

Pearls

- A posterior cyst with two muscular layers, no cartilage, and attachment to esophagus is most likely an esophageal duplication but must be differentiated from a bronchogenic cyst
- Ectopias, atresia, and duplication are congenital conditions; diverticula, rings, webs, and diaphragmatic hernias are acquired conditions

Selected References

Tang P, McKinley MJ, Sporrer M, Kahn E: Inlet patch: Prevalence, histologic type and association with esophagitis, Barrett esophagus and antritis. Arch Pathol Lab Med 128:444-447, 2004.

Dantas RO, Villanova MG: Esophageal motility impairment in Plummer-Vinson syndrome: Correction by iron treatment. Dig Dis Sci 38:968-971, 1993.

Borhan-Manesh F, Farnum JB: Incidence of heterotopic gastric mucosa in the upper oesophagus. Gut 32:968-972, 1991.

Hocking M, Young DG: Duplication of the alimentary tract. Br J Surg 68:92-96, 1981.

Quan L, Smith DW: The VATER association: Vertebral defects, anal atresia, tracheoesophageal fistulas with esophageal atresia, radial and renal dysplasia. A spectrum of associated defects. J Pediatr 82:104-107, 1973.

Infectious Esophagitis

Clinical Features

- Consists primarily of opportunistic viral and fungal infections in immunocompromised patients, including
  — Patients with acquired immunodeficiency syndrome (AIDS)
  — Patients on steroids or immune modulators (after transplantation)
  — Diabetic patients
  — Debilitated or elderly patients

Gross and Endoscopic Pathology

- Herpesvirus infection: punched-out ulcers
- Cytomegalovirus (CMV): nonspecific ulcer
- *Candida* species: pseudomembranous, gray-white patches
- Pathogenic bacteria: superficial necrosis

Histopathology

- Herpes simplex virus (HSV)
  - Biopsies taken from the ulcer edge show acantholysis with multinucleated squamous cells with steel-blue nuclei or Cowdry type A inclusions

Figure 6-2. Endoscopic photograph of herpes esophagitis demonstrating well-circumscribed ulcers.

Figure 6-3. Herpes esophagitis. Squamous mucosa adjacent to an ulcer shows multinucleate giant cells with intranuclear inclusions intermingled with fibrinopurulent exudate.

Figure 6-4. Candida esophagitis (Alcian blue and periodic acid–Schiff stains) with budding yeast forms and pseudohyphae among acantholytic squamous cells.

▌ CMV
 ● Deep biopsies from the ulcer base show classic Cowdry type A inclusions
 ● Cellular enlargement with granular basophilic intracytoplasmic inclusions and intranuclear inclusions, which are sometimes eosinophilic, large, and targetoid
 ● Preferentially involves endothelial cells, fibroblasts, or glandular epithelium (rarely infects squamous cells)
▌ Fungi
 ● Nonspecific mixed inflammation, ulceration, and granulation tissue with admixed fungal structures
 ● *Candida*: blastoconidia and pseudohyphae

 ● *Histoplasma*: small, 1- to 2-μm organisms within histiocyte cytoplasm (rare)
 ● *Aspergillus*: true hyphae demonstrating dichotomous branching at 45-degree angles (extremely rare in biopsy or surgical specimens)
 ● *Mucor*: aseptate, folded, ribbon-like hyphae often in an infarcted background (extremely rare in biopsy or surgical specimens)
▌ Bacterial
 ● Bacteria present in esophageal biopsy are generally nonpathogenic
 ● True bacterial infection is characterized by bacteria present in deeper levels of tissue associated with neutrophilic exudate and necrosis

Special Stains and Immunohistochemistry

 ● Fungal structures are Grocott methenamine silver (GMS) and periodic acid–Schiff (PAS) stain positive
 ● Alcian blue and PAS stain with hematoxylin counterstain is recommended for esophageal tissues because it can also be a useful screen for signet ring cell adenocarcinoma and for Barrett esophagus

Other Techniques for Diagnosis

 ● Immunohistochemistry for HSV and CMV
 ● Polymerase chain reaction (PCR) for HSV and CMV (rarely, if ever, needed)

Differential Diagnosis

▌ Corrosive esophagitis
 ● Acute lesions are similar to infections and are best distinguished by clinical history and by the lack of pathologic organisms
▌ Reflux esophagitis
 ● Can have areas of giant cell change within squamous epithelium in reflux: distinguished from hepatic infection by its lack of characteristic viral inclusions
 ● Reflux typically causes the characteristic histologic triad involving squamous mucosa
  — Hyperplasia: elongated lamina propria papillae (more than two thirds of thickness of epithelium)
  — Thickened basal layer (more than 15% of epithelial thickness)
  — Increased intraepithelial lymphocytes (with characteristic compressed, irregular nuclear contours and eosinophils); neutrophils may also be present—although fairly specific for reflux, they occur only in some cases and are therefore not sensitive
 ● Consistent clinical history
 ● No organisms identified

Pearls

 ● Look for cytopathic changes of CMV in the stromal cells at the base of ulcer
 ● Look for HSV inclusions in squamous cells at the edge of ulcer

Selected References

McBane RD, Gross JB Jr: Herpes esophagitis: Clinical symptoms, endoscopic appearance and diagnosis in 23 patients. Gastrointest Endosc 37:600-603, 1991.

Haulk AA, Sugar AM: Candida esophagitis. Adv Intern Med 36:307-318, 1991.

Myerson D, Hackman RC, Nelson JA, et al: Widespread presence of histologically occult cytomegalovirus. Hum Pathol 15:430-439, 1984.

Knoke M, Bernhardt H: Endoscopic aspects of mycosis in the upper digestive tract. Endoscopy 12:295-298, 1980.

Injurious Esophagitis

Clinical Features

- Chemical esophagitis
  - Most severe injury follows suicide attempts (acid, alkali) in adults and accidental ingestion in children
- Drug esophagitis
  - "Pill" esophagitis: patients report feeling a lump in the throat; can occur after ingestion of any oral medication without adequate hydration
  - Some oral medications are particularly corrosive (e.g., alendronate, iron-containing compounds)
  - Chemotherapeutic agents are generally directly toxic (rather than by allergic mechanisms)
- Radiation esophagitis
  - Produces dysphagia and odynophagia
  - Location depends on area exposed to the radiation
  - Large superficial ulcers occur with more than 6000-cGy exposure
  - May be combined with chemical (chemotherapy) injury

Gross and Endoscopic Pathology

- Chemical esophagitis
  - Affects narrowest esophageal segments (proximal and distal ends and mid-esophagus where esophagus is compressed by aorta and main-stem bronchus)
  - Acute corrosive chemical injury varies from mild erythema to mucosal sloughing, ulceration, or frank necrosis with perforation
  - Chronic injury can cause stricture due to fibrosis
- Drug esophagitis
  - Direct caustic effect of pill produces a localized lesion
  - Chemotherapeutic agents may produce diffuse lesions
- Radiation esophagitis
  - Location depends on area exposed to the radiation
  - Typically causes large superficial ulcers

Histopathology

- Chemical esophagitis
  - Variable histologic features range from mild congestion to severe acute inflammation, erosion, ulceration, and granulation tissue reaction
  - Lesions heal with submucosal fibrosis

- Drug esophagitis
  - Pill esophagitis produces discrete, superficial ulceration that is nonspecific
    - Vascular endothelial proliferation can be prominent
  - Allergic drug reactions produce eosinophilia
  - Chemotherapeutic agents interfere with cell replication, producing basal cell hyperplasia, cytologic atypia
- Radiation esophagitis
  - Radiation injury is recognized by acanthosis, parakeratosis, necrosis, and stromal cell atypia, including enlarged, stellate fibroblasts and hyalinized blood vessels with enlarged, vesicular endothelial cell nuclei
  - All lesions may heal with lamina propria and submucosal fibrosis, leading to stricture

Special Stains and Immunohistochemistry

- Noncontributory

Other Techniques for Diagnosis

- Noncontributory

Differential Diagnosis

- Reflux esophagitis
  - Location, histologic appearance, and clinical history are usually diagnostic
- Infectious esophagitis
  - Diagnosed by detection of organisms, sometimes using special stains and immunohistochemical reactions and recognition of cytopathic viral changes
- Acute esophageal necrosis (so-called black esophagus)
  - Biopsy specimen contains necrotic tissue
  - Appears black on endoscopy; patients present with upper gastrointestinal bleeding
  - Usually associated with comorbid conditions such as severe cardiovascular disease with hemodynamic compromise
  - High mortality rate (about 30%)

Pearls

- Important to have a complete patient clinical history
- Consider radiation exposure when bizarre epithelial and stromal cells are encountered

Selected References

Gurvits GE, Shapsis A, Lau N, et al: Acute esophageal necrosis: a rare syndrome. J Gastroenterol 42:29-38, 2007.

Misra SP, Dwivedi M: Pill-induced esophagitis. Gastrointest Endosc 55:81, 2002.

Kikendall JW: Pill esophagitis. J Clin Gastroenterol 28:298-305, 1999.

Abraham SC, Yardley JH, Wu TT: Erosive injury in the upper gastrointestinal tract in patients receiving iron medication: An underrecognized entity. Am J Surg Pathol 23:1241-1247, 1999.

DeGroen PC, Lubbe DF, Hirsch LJ, et al: Esophagitis associated with the use of alendronate. N Engl J Med 335:1016-1021, 1996.

Oren R, Fich A: Oral contraceptive-induced esophageal ulcer: Two cases and literature review. Dig Dis Sci 36:1489-1490, 1991.

Inflammatory Esophagitis

Clinical Features

▌ Dermatologic conditions
- Pemphigus vulgaris
  — Antibody-mediated, blistering skin disorder that may affect skin or squamous mucosa
  — May be induced by drugs
  — May be fatal
  — Peak ages: 40 to 60 years
- Bullous pemphigoid
  — Bullous skin disease affecting mainly elderly patients (fifth to ninth decades)
  — Rarely affects the esophagus
  — Increased incidence in men
- Erythema multiforme
  — Acute eruption of skin and mucosal surfaces
  — Mucosal involvement is termed *Stevens-Johnson syndrome*
- Lichen planus
  — Common inflammatory disorder usually affecting skin and mucosal surfaces but rarely involving the esophagus

▌ Graft-versus-host disease (GVHD)
- Necrotizing inflammation of mucosa, skin, or glandular epithelia after bone marrow transplantation
- Transplanted T cells attack host

Gross and Endoscopic Pathology

▌ Dermatologic conditions
- Pemphigus vulgaris
  — Bleeding and esophageal strictures
- Bullous pemphigoid
  — Esophageal blisters
- Erythema multiforme (Stevens-Johnson syndrome)
  — Resembles reflux or peptic esophagitis
  — Pseudomembranes may form
- Lichen planus
  — Esophageal papules, plaques, or stricture

▌ GVHD
- Typically involves the upper third of the esophagus
- May be focal or diffuse
- Desquamative lesion can cause web formation

Histopathology

▌ Dermatologic conditions
- All conditions tend to mirror cutaneous histology
- Pemphigus vulgaris
  — Acantholysis
  — Suprabasal blister formation
  — Conspicuous eosinophilic infiltrate
- Bullous pemphigoid
  — Subepithelial blister formation
  — Conspicuous eosinophilic infiltrate
- Erythema multiforme (Stevens-Johnson syndrome)
  — Focal to diffuse keratinocyte necrosis (forming rounded, eosinophilic bodies)
  — Mixed acute and chronic inflammation
- Lichen planus
  — Submucosal, bandlike lymphocytic infiltrate
  — Civatte bodies

▌ GVHD
- Karyorrhexis and apoptosis of epithelial cells
- Variable T-cell infiltrates
- Epithelial atrophy
- Fibrosis of lamina propria

Special Stains and Immunohistochemistry

▌ Dermatologic conditions
- Pemphigus vulgaris
  — Immunofluorescence studies for antibodies (immunoglobulin G [IgG]) localized to intercellular region of acantholytic cells (requires fresh-frozen tissue)
- Bullous pemphigus
  — Immunofluorescence studies for IgG or IgA localized along basement membranes (requires fresh-frozen tissue)
- GVHD
  — Immunostains can be used to confirm intraepithelial T lymphocytes but are rarely useful

Modern Techniques for Diagnosis

- Noncontributory

Differential Diagnosis

▌ Infectious esophagitis
- HSV or CMV infection
  — Typically found in immunocompromised hosts
  — Characterized by typical cytopathic changes (viral inclusions)
  — May coexist with GVHD
- Candidiasis
  — "Cheesy" exudates present in immunosuppressed, diabetic, or long-term antibiotic-treated patients
  — Characteristic fungal structures are present
  — May coexist with GVHD

▌ Reflux esophagitis
- Much more common
- Characterized by involvement of lower esophagus near gastroesophageal junction
- Absent history of coexistent skin disorders or bone marrow transplantation

Pearls

- Primary dermatologic conditions may involve esophagus because both are composed of squamous epithelium; thus, skin and esophageal histology and immunology are similar

Selected References

McKee P, Calonje J, Granter S (eds): Pathology of the Skin with Clinical Correlations. St Louis, Mosby, 2005.

Goldman H, Antonioli DA: Mucosal biopsy of the esophagus, stomach, and proximal duodenum. Hum Pathol 13:423-448, 1982.

McDonald GB, Sullivan KM, Schuffler MD, et al: Esophageal abnormalities in chronic graft-versus-host disease in humans. Gastroenterology 80:914-921, 1981.

Eosinophilic Esophagitis

Clinical Features

- Can be isolated to esophagus or can be part of a multifocal or diffuse process involving various areas of the gastrointestinal tract (eosinophilic gastroenteritis)
- Can occur in atopic children and young men (male-to-female ratio of 3:1)
- Synchronous eosinophilic gastritis or enteritis is more common in pediatric cases
- Patients may also have peripheral eosinophilia, food sensitivity, asthma, or allergies
- Patients often present with dysphagia

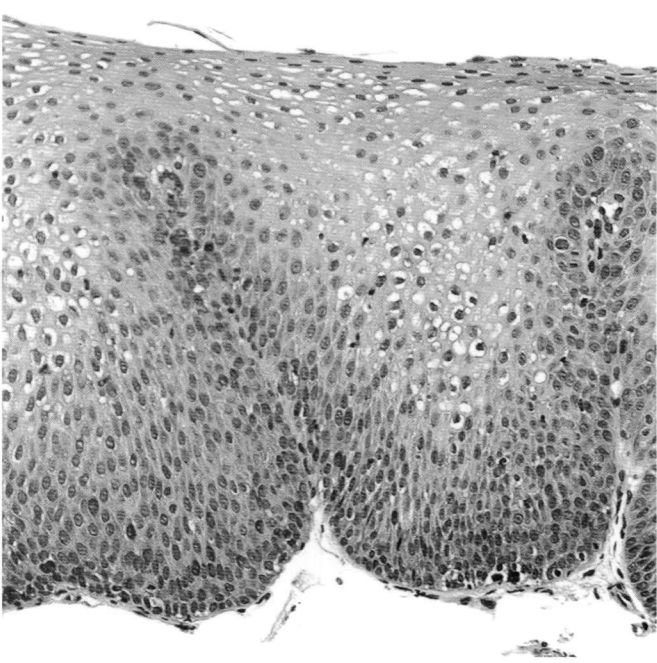

Figure 6-5. Squamous mucosal changes in reflux esophagitis include elongated lamina propria papillae, an increase in the basal cell layer, and scattered intraepithelial eosinophils.

Figure 6-6. Allergic (eosinophilic) esophagitis. Histologic section shows full-thickness squamous basal cells with numerous (>20 per high-power field) intraepithelial eosinophils.

Gross and Endoscopic Pathology

- Patients may develop esophageal strictures or webs usually in the mid- and upper esophagus
- Linear mucosal ulceration may be seen
- White pustules or exudates are also common

Histopathology

- Marked eosinophilic infiltrate (>20 eosinophils/hpf); also within the squamous mucosa; intraepithelial eosinophilic abscesses may also develop
- Eosinophils in muscularis mucosae, submucosa, and muscularis propria are less commonly seen
- Elongated rete pegs and marked squamous basal cell hyperplasia are typical

Special Stains and Immunohistochemistry

- Noncontributory

Other Techniques for Diagnosis

- Serum test for eotaxin-3

Differential Diagnosis

▮ Reflux esophagitis
- Closely simulates eosinophilic gastroenteritis in some cases; however, reflux generally occurs in the distal esophagus and causes pyrosis and acid regurgitation
- Reflux generally shows less than 5 eosinophils/hpf

Pearls

- Esophagus with webs or corrugation with numerous (>20 eosinophils/hpf) usually indicates eosinophilic esophagitis
- Eosinophilic esophagitis often responds to asthma therapy (steroid treatment, fluticasone), with or without mast cell stabilizers, and tends not to respond to proton pump inhibitors

Selected References

Vanderheyden AD, Petras RE, DeYoung BR, Mitros FA: Emerging eosinophilic (allergic) esophagitis: Increased incidence or increased recognition? Arch Pathol Lab Med 131:777-779, 2007.

Teitelbaum JE, Fox VL, Twarog FJ, et al: Eosinophilic esophagitis in children: Immunopathological analysis and response to fluticasone propionate. Gastroenterology 122:1216-1225, 2002.

Walsh SV, Antonioli DA, Goldman H, et al: Allergic esophagitis in children: A clinicopathologic entity. Am J Surg Pathol 23:390-396, 1999.

Mahajau L, Wyllie R, Petras R, et al: Idiopathic eosinophilic esophagitis with stricture formation in a patient with longstanding eosinophilic gastroenteritis. Gastrointest Endosc 46:557-560, 1997.

Reflux Esophagitis and Gastroesophageal Reflux Disease (GERD)

Clinical Features

- Occurs in all ages, including children; most common in adult men older than 40 years
- Patients typically present with dysphagia, heartburn, and acid regurgitation
- Symptoms may be rarely mistaken for angina or myocardial infarction
- Complications include stricture, hemorrhage, and Barrett esophagus (see "Barrett Esophagus")

Gross and Endoscopic Pathology

- One third of patients have normal or slightly erythematous mucosa on endoscopy
- Subset of patients has glandular metaplasia, erosions, or ulcers
- About 30% of patients with documented abnormal histology have no endoscopic lesion

Histopathology

- Characteristic histologic triad involving squamous mucosa
  — Hyperplasia with elongated or lengthened lamina propria papillae (more than two thirds of thickness of epithelium)
  — Thickened basal layer (more than 15% of epithelial thickness)
  — Increased intraepithelial lymphocytes and eosinophils; neutrophils may also be present but occur only in severe reflux
- Erosive and ulcerated lesions show neutrophilic and eosinophilic exudate over a granulation tissue base
- Barrett esophagus with intestinal metaplasia (goblet cell metaplasia) may be present
- Inflammation of gastric cardia–type mucosa with or without intestinal metaplasia may also be present

Special Stains and Immunohistochemistry

- Combined Alcian blue and PAS staining: serves four purposes
  — Defines the relatively PAS-negative, glycogen-free basal layer of the esophagus
  — Detects dark-blue intestinal mucus in goblet cells when intestinal metaplasia is present
  — Identifies fungi, if present
  — Good screening stain for signet cell adenocarcinoma
- Stains for *Helicobacter pylori* (Warthin-Starry, Diff-Quik, Giemsa): may be helpful when differential includes chronic gastritis and probably should be done routinely in specimens obtained from the distal esophagus and gastroesophageal junction

Other Techniques for Diagnosis

- Noncontributory

Differential Diagnosis

▎ Infectious esophagitis
- May resemble reflux esophagitis endoscopically, but usually more focal
- Differentiated by the presence of characteristic organisms or cytopathic changes
- Most common organisms are
  — HSV
  — CMV
  — *Candida* species

▎ *Helicobacter pylori* gastritis of cardia (carditis) with or without intestinal metaplasia
- Histologically indistinguishable from reflux-related inflammation of gastric cardia type mucosa; *H. pylori* infection typically causes more chronic and active inflammatory cells; *H. pylori* seen on hematoxylin and eosin (H&E) or special stain
- Most cases of chronic inflammation of gastric cardia–type mucosa at the gastroesophageal junction or in lower esophagus are examples of reflux

▎ Allergic and eosinophilic esophagitis
- Typically in children or young men with an allergic history
- Characterized by numerous intraepithelial eosinophils (usually >20 eosinophils/hpf)
- Many cases cannot be reliably separated from reflux esophagitis without clinical history and response to therapy

▎ Pill esophagitis
- Typically associated with odynophagia (painful swallowing), lump in the throat sensation, and history of consuming oral medications with inadequate amounts of water
- Occurs more proximally in esophagus than do changes caused by reflux
- Nonspecific histology with ulcer

■ Squamous dysplasia, squamous cell carcinoma
  ● Less likely than reflux-associated regenerative changes because incidence of esophageal squamous cell carcinoma is declining in the United States
  ● Dysplasia and carcinoma show
    — Overlapping, pleomorphic nuclei with high nuclear-to-cytoplasmic ratio
    — Atypical mitoses
    — Single-cell necrosis
    — Paradoxical maturation
    — Squamous pearl formation

Pearls

  ● GERD: classic histologic triad
    — Thickened basal layer
    — Elongated papillae
    — Intraepithelial inflammatory cells, including eosinophils
  ● Always evaluate for presence of intestinal metaplasia when glandular mucosa is present; routine use of Alcian blue and PAS combination stain, with hematoxylin counterstain recommended

Selected References

Haggitt RC: Histopathology of reflux-induced esophageal and supra esophageal injuries. Am J Med 108:109S-111S, 2000.

Black DD, Haggitt RC, Orenstein SR, Whitington PF: Esophagitis in infants: Morphometric histological diagnosis and correlation with measures of gastroesophageal reflux. Gastroenterology 98:1408-1414, 1990.

Wienbeck M, Barnert J: Epidemiology of reflux disease and reflux esophagitis. Scand J Gastroenterol Suppl 156:7-13, 1989.

Barrett Esophagus

Clinical Features

  ● Defined by the American College of Gastroenterology as an endoscopic abnormality (red, velvety mucosa) in the esophagus proved by biopsy to contain intestinal metaplasia
  ● Occurs in up to 45% of patients with chronic gastroesophageal reflux
  ● Affected patients tend to be white men with reflux symptoms; often have hiatal hernia
  ● Disease occurs at two age peaks: younger than 15 years and older than 40 years
  ● Increased risk for adenocarcinoma

Gross and Endoscopic Pathology

  ● Seen on endoscopy as tongues or islands of flat, red, velvety mucosa or as a circumferential zone of red, velvety mucosa against a pale gray-white esophageal squamous mucosal background

Histopathology

  ● Esophageal squamous epithelium is replaced by specialized columnar epithelium; columnar

Figure 6-7. Endoscopic photograph of Barrett esophagus. Note the erythematous mucosa that resembles gastric mucosa, which contrasts to the gray-white glistening squamous esophageal mucosa (*foreground*).

Figure 6-8. Specialized columnar epithelium (intestinal metaplasia) of Barrett esophagus composed of goblet cells interspersed between cells resembling gastric foveolar epithelium.

epithelium containing goblet cells usually interspersed between cells resembling gastric foveolar epithelium
  ● To qualify, the goblet cells must have distinct globoid clear cytoplasm on H&E stain; verification of goblet cells by positive staining with Alcian blue stain (pH 2.5) is desirable and recommended
  ● Neither foveolar cells with Alcian blue–negative cytoplasmic vacuoles nor diffuse, "blush" positivity in

the regenerative zone of foveolar cells qualifies as intestinal metaplasia
- Careful search must be made for dysplastic glandular epithelium
- Dysplastic glandular cells contain enlarged hyperchromatic, stratified nuclei involving luminal surface
- Dysplasia is categorized as low grade, high grade, or indefinite for dysplasia (see section on dysplasia under "Barrett Esophagus")

Special Stains and Immunohistochemistry

- Combined Alcian blue and PAS: serves four purposes
  — Defines the PAS-negative, glycogen-free basal layer of the esophagus
  — Detects dark-blue, globoid goblet cells when intestinal metaplasia is present
  — Highlights fungal structures
  — Is a useful screening stain for signet cell adenocarcinoma
- Cytokeratin 7 and 20 profiles can help differentiate gastric cardia intestinal metaplasia from esophageal (Barrett) intestinal metaplasia but are rarely indicated clinically
  — The "Barrett pattern" shows diffuse (superficial and deep) cytokeratin 7 positivity and bandlike superficial cytokeratin 20 positivity; other patterns usually correlate with gastric-type intestinal metaplasia

Other Techniques for Diagnosis

- Use of p53 and Ki-67 staining can improve interobserver agreement on diagnosis of dysplasia
- DNA ploidy studies and use of other markers of cancer risk are reported but are not used clinically

Differential Diagnosis

- Chronic gastritis involving cardia-type mucosa with intestinal metaplasia
  - Indistinguishable from Barrett esophagus unless seen by the endoscopist in the esophagus
  - May be caused by *Helicobacter pylori* infection rather than reflux in some patients
- Ectopic gastric mucosa
  - Small foci of gastric mucosa, usually in the cervical esophagus (so-called inlet patch) unassociated with gastroesophageal reflux
- Adenocarcinoma
  - Prevalence is estimated to be as high as 10% at time of diagnosis of Barrett esophagus
  - Risk estimates vary widely (30- to 125-fold) in patients with Barrett esophagus
  - May be difficult to distinguish intramucosal adenocarcinoma from high-grade dysplasia

Pearls

- Generally high-grade dysplasia in a background of Barrett esophagus; prompts surgical or endoscopic intervention

Selected References

Sampliner RE: Updated guidelines for the diagnosis, surveillance and therapy of Barrett's esophagus. Am J Gastroenterol 97:1888-1895, 2002.

Ormsby AH, Goldblum JR, Rice TW, et al: Cytokeratin subsets can reliably distinguish Barrett's esophagus from intestinal metaplasia of the stomach. Hum Pathol 30:288-294, 1999.

Antonioli DA, Wang HH: Morphology of Barrett's esophagus and Barrett's-associated dysplasia and adenocarcinoma. Gastroenterol Clin North Am 26:495-506, 1997.

Dysplastic Lesions Associated with Barrett Esophagus

Clinical Features

- Dysplasia is defined as a proliferation of neoplastic cells that are cytologically abnormal yet are still confined within their original basement membrane
- Periodic endoscopic surveillance of patients with Barrett esophagus increases survival (62% versus 20%) over patients without surveillance

Figure 6-9. High-grade glandular dysplasia arising in Barrett esophagus. There is altered mucosal architecture. The cells demonstrate a high nuclear-to-cytoplasmic size ratio, irregular nuclear crowding, and nuclear stratification.

- Studies indicate that dysplasia may progress to carcinoma, but estimates of exact pace vary widely (from less than 2 years to up to 10 years)
- Patients harboring low-grade dysplasia are usually treated with antireflux therapy and should be followed closely
- Patients with high-grade dysplasia who are physically fit and have a life expectancy of at least 10 years are generally advised to undergo esophagectomy once dysplasia is confirmed; other therapies (e.g., endoscopic mucosal resection, photodynamic therapy, cryoablation, laser ablation) are usually palliative

Gross and Endoscopic Pathology

- Dysplasia usually cannot be grossly or endoscopically distinguished from surrounding Barrett esophagus

Histopathology

▮ Dysplasia
- Histologically consists of a continuous spectrum of architectural and cytologic abnormalities
- Divided into low-grade dysplasia, high-grade dysplasia, and indefinite for dysplasia
- Changes rarely resemble those of an adenoma
- Low-grade dysplasia
  — Slight increase in gland complexity, which consists of branching glands with irregular contours
  — Cytologic atypia consisting of enlarged, pleomorphic, stratified nuclei with surface involvement; abnormal nuclei are generally confined to the basal half of each cell
- High-grade dysplasia
  — Further increase in gland complexity characterized by lateral branching and often back-to-back glands
  — Progressive increase in cytologic atypia
    ◆ Greater nuclear enlargement and pleomorphism
    ◆ Stratified nuclei involving luminal surface haphazardly scattered with nuclei located in apical portion of many cells
    ◆ Atypical cells often with prominent nucleoli and a high nuclear-to-cytoplasmic ratio, high mitotic rate with atypical mitotic figures, and progressive loss of goblet cells
    ◆ Similar cytologic changes to those seen in adenocarcinoma
  — Changes involve surface mucosa as well as crypts
  — Complexity and atypia may be so marked that intramucosal carcinoma (infiltration of carcinoma cells beyond basement membrane into the muscularis mucosae or lamina propria alone, but not into submucosa) cannot be ruled out

- Indefinite for dysplasia
  — Designates changes that have features of dysplasia and regenerative mucosa, usually in an inflamed background, making precise distinction impossible

Special Stains and Immunohistochemistry

- Use of p53 and Ki-67 staining may aid in difficult cases (e.g., indefinite versus low-grade dysplasia only)
- Several "markers" have been studied (DCC, *C-myc*, and others), but none is of clinical value

Other Techniques for Diagnosis

- Flow cytometry
  — DNA aneuploidy and elevated S-phase fractions may correlate with progression to carcinoma; experimental only

Differential Diagnosis

▮ Regenerative atypia
- Generally involves areas adjacent to erosions and ulcerations with active inflammation
- Glands may have villiform surface but show normal maturation at surface
- Cells characteristically have equally enlarged cytoplasm and nuclei
- Cytoplasm is typically eosinophilic rather than basophilic
- May be difficult to distinguish from dysplasia

▮ Adenocarcinoma
- Characterized by individual cell infiltration or desmoplastic reaction
- Intramucosal carcinoma may be difficult to differentiate reliably from high-grade dysplasia

Pearls

- Variability of individual nuclei is greater in dysplasia (regenerative atypia is composed of a more uniform population of glands and nuclei)
- Regenerative glands generally show mature cells (basal nuclei and abundant mucin) at mucosal surface
- Uncertain cases may be legitimately diagnosed as indefinite for dysplasia, followed by antireflux therapy and rebiopsy
- Villiform architecture is seen in both regenerative glands and dysplasia

Selected References

Flejou JF, Svrcek M: Barrett's oesophagus: A pathologist's view. Histopathology 50:3-14, 2007.

Lorinc E, Jakobsson B, Landberg G, Veress B: Ki67 and p53 immunohistochemistry reduces interobserver variation in assessment of Barrett's oesophagus. Histopathology 46:642-648, 2005.

Skacel M, Petras RE, Rybicki LA, et al: P53 expression in low-grade dysplasia in Barrett's esophagus: Correlation with interobserver agreement and disease progression. Am J Gastroenterol 97:2508-2513, 2002.

Ormsby AH, Petras RE, Henricks WH, et al: Observer variation in the diagnosis of superficial oesophageal adenocarcinoma. Gut 51:671-676, 2002

Adenocarcinoma Associated with Barrett Esophagus

Clinical Features

- Most esophageal adenocarcinomas are associated with Barrett esophagus
- Exact increase in risk posed by Barrett esophagus is unknown; estimates range from 30- to 125-fold increase in risk
- Occurs in 800 per 100,000 Barrett patients per year
- Is present in 10% of patients at initial diagnosis of Barrett esophagus
- Occurs with higher rate in white males
- Risk factors include hiatal hernia, stricture, and chronic reflux
- Most common symptom is dysphagia, but can be asymptomatic

Gross and Endoscopic Pathology

- Tends to occur near gastroesophageal junction
- May form an exophytic mass or can be flat with an infiltrative architecture
- Only 50% are grossly visible endoscopically

Histopathology

- Resembles gastric adenocarcinoma, with both intestinal and diffuse (signet ring cell) types

Figure 6-10. Endoscopic photograph of carcinoma complicating Barrett esophagus showing complex intraluminal mass with superficial exudate.

- Barrett esophagus with dysplasia of varying degree is present in adjacent mucosa

Special Stains and Immunohistochemistry

- Mucin stain positive in signet ring cells; may be helpful in identifying infiltrating carcinoma cells

Other Techniques for Diagnosis

- Noncontributory

Differential Diagnosis

▮ Barrett esophagus–associated dysplasia
- Characterized by glandular and cytologic atypia without infiltration pattern
▮ Gastric cardia adenocarcinoma
- May be identical to Barrett esophagus–associated adenocarcinoma
- Staining for CK7 and CK20 can help distinguish Barrett esophagus–related adenocarcinoma (CK7 positive; CK20 negative) from gastric adenocarcinoma

Pearls

- A search for goblet cells in glandular epithelium adjacent to any gastroesophageal junction adenocarcinoma helps to identify preexisting Barrett esophagus
- Documentation of a squamous proximal mucosal margin is desirable in cases of surgically resected Barrett esophagus–associated adenocarcinoma
- Overall prognosis is dismal for invasive adenocarcinoma (75% 5-year survival); prognosis is better for small, well-differentiated adenocarcinoma with fewer than four positive nodes

Selected References

Ormsby AH, Goldblum JR, Rice TW, et al: The utility of cytokeratin subsets in distinguishing Barrett's-related oesophageal adenocarcinoma from gastric adenocarcinoma. Histopathology 38:307-311, 2001.

Bollschweiler E, Wolfgarten E, Gutschow C, et al: Demographic variations and the rising incidence of esophageal adenocarcinoma in white males. Cancer 92:549-555, 2001.

Drewitz DJ, Sampliner RE, Garewell HS: The incidence of adenocarcinoma in Barrett's esophagus: A prospective study of 170 patients followed 4.8 years. Am J Gastroenterol 92:212-215, 1997.

Cameron AJ, Lomboy CT, Pera M, Carpenter HA: Adenocarcinoma of the esophagogastric junction and Barrett's esophagus. Gastroenterology 109:1541-1546, 1995.

Benign Esophageal Lesions

Clinical Features

▮ Glycogen acanthosis
- Asymptomatic

Figure 6-11. Resection specimen of giant fibrovascular polyp of the esophagus. The lobulated intraluminal mass is covered by intact squamous mucosa.

Figure 6-12. Glycogen acanthosis. Note the marked thickening of the squamous mucosa composed of squamous cells with increased intracellular glycogen.

▌ Inflammatory fibroid polyp
  ● Usually occurs in the stomach and small intestine but may arise in the esophagus
  ● May produce mild obstructive symptoms
▌ Fibrovascular polyp
  ● Rare, slow-growing polyp
  ● Mild obstructive symptoms may occur
  ● May rarely prolapse into oral cavity

Figure 6-13. Inflammatory fibroid polyp of the esophagus demonstrates edema and inflammatory cells including plasma cells and eosinophils interspersed between elongate spindle cells and dilated blood vessels.

Gross and Endoscopic Pathology

▌ Glycogen acanthosis
  ● Raised, white plaques
  ● Usually less than 0.3 cm in diameter
▌ Inflammatory fibroid polyp
  ● Raised, pedunculated, polypoid mass, often with surface ulceration
▌ Fibrovascular polyp
  ● Usually attached in upper esophagus
  ● Polypoid mass; can be extremely large (e.g., 25 cm)
  ● Smooth surface that may be ulcerated

Histopathology

▌ Glycogen acanthosis
  ● Discrete focus of hyperplastic squamous epithelium containing abundant glycogen (squamous cells with prominent clear cytoplasm)
▌ Inflammatory fibroid polyp
  ● Polypoid mass covered by benign squamous mucosa that may be focally ulcerated
  ● Stromal component varies in cellularity, edema, and inflammation that is often rich in eosinophils and plasma cells
  ● Stromal component typically has prominent vascularity with perivascular onion-skinning composed of fibroblasts, myofibroblasts, and macrophages
  ● Occasionally stroma has a pseudosarcomatous appearance
▌ Fibrovascular polyps
  ● Dense or myxoid fibrovascular core sometimes with adipose tissue covered by benign squamous epithelium

Special Stains and Immunohistochemistry

▌ Inflammatory fibroid polyp and fibrovascular polyp
- Stromal cells are positive for vimentin and negative for cytokeratin
- CD34 immunostain highlights blood vessels and may stain stromal cells; CD117 is negative

▌ Glycogen acanthosis
- PAS-positive epithelium

Other Techniques for Diagnosis
- Noncontributory

Differential Diagnosis
- Inflammatory fibroid polyp should be differentiated from sarcomatoid carcinoma, sarcoma, and stromal tumors

▌ Sarcomatoid carcinoma
- Biphasic histology with both carcinomatous and spindle cell components
- Typically greater cellularity with increased nuclear pleomorphism
- Usually positive for cytokeratin, but staining may be focal

▌ Sarcoma
- Typically a highly cellular malignant spindle cell neoplasm resembling leiomyosarcoma, fibrosarcoma, or malignant fibrous histiocytoma

▌ Gastrointestinal stromal tumor
- Rare in the esophagus
- Spindle cell or epithelioid neoplasm; CD117 positive
- Glycogen acanthosis should be differentiated from squamous papilloma, condyloma, and fungal esophagitis

▌ Squamous papilloma
- Characterized by a greater degree of squamous hyperplasia, papillary structure with a fibrovascular core, and less prominent cytoplasmic glycogenization

▌ Condyloma
- Characteristic viral cytopathic changes (koilocytosis), squamous atypia, and hyperkeratosis

▌ Fungal esophagitis
- Recognized by detection of fungal organisms; may require use of special stains

Pearls
- Careful attention to cytologic characteristics and to the makeup of the inflammatory component and background is important to avoid misdiagnosis of sarcoma and sarcomatous carcinoma

Selected References
Avezzano EA, Fleischer DE, Merida MA, et al: Giant fibrovascular polyps of the esophagus. Am J Gastroenterol 85:299-302, 1990.

Nash S: Benign lesions of the gastrointestinal tract that may be misdiagnosed as malignant tumors. Semin Diagn Pathol 7:102-114, 1990.

Granular Cell Tumor

Clinical Features
- Usually a solitary nodule in the lower esophagus; can be multiple (10% of cases)
- Typically slow growing and generally does not produce symptoms (incidental finding)

Gross and Endoscopic Pathology
- Can be seen throughout the gastrointestinal tract; the esophagus is the preferred site, followed by the large intestine
- Generally small, yellow-white, subepithelial mass
- Typically less than 2 cm; tumors larger than 4 cm may indicate malignancy

Histopathology
- Similar to granular tumors of other sites
- Aggregates of rounded and spindle-shaped cells that resemble smooth muscle with small, round to oval nuclei and granular eosinophilic cytoplasm
- May appear to be arising from nerve or muscle
- Pseudoepitheliomatous hyperplasia of the overlying squamous epithelium is common and can be misinterpreted as squamous carcinoma
  — Malignant granular cell tumor
    ◆ May be suspected by the presence of increased cellularity, nuclear atypia, and increased

Figure 6-14. Granular cell tumor of the esophagus. Squamous mucosa overlies the uniform population of cells with variably shaped small nuclei, abundant eosinophilic granular cytoplasm, and poorly defined cell borders.

mitotic activity; however, the only definite criterion is metastasis

Special Stains and Immunohistochemistry

- Cytoplasmic positivity for PAS and immunostain positive for S-100 protein

Other Techniques for Diagnosis

- Noncontributory

Differential Diagnosis

▌ Squamous cell carcinoma
- Especially on small biopsies, granular cell tumors have many times been misdiagnosed as squamous cell carcinoma because of the pseudoepitheliomatous hyperplasia that accompanies the tumor

Pearls

- Typically slow growing and cured by local surgical excision; malignant granular cell tumors with metastases have been reported

Selected References

Goldblum JR, Rice TW, Zuccaro G, et al: Granular cell tumor of the esophagus: A clinical and pathologic study of 13 cases. Ann Thorac Surg 62:860-865, 1996.

Brady PG, Nord HJ, Connar RG: Granular cell tumor of the esophagus: Natural history, diagnosis and therapy. Dig Dis Sci 33:1329-1333, 1988.

Squamous Papilloma and Carcinoma

Clinical Features

- Most symptomatic esophageal tumors are malignant
▌ Squamous papilloma
- More common in males (male-to-female ratio is 2.5:1)
- Occur throughout life
- Two types of squamous papilloma
  — Human papillomavirus (HPV) associated
    ◆ About 30% of esophageal papillomas
    ◆ May coexist with laryngeal papillomatosis; associated with HPV-6 and HPV-11 infections
  — Not HPV associated
    ◆ May be related to reflux esophagitis or trauma
- Patients typically present with dysphagia and heartburn
▌ Squamous cell carcinoma
- About 1% of all cancers in the United States
- Risk factors include
  — Male gender (male-to-female ratio is 5:1)
  — Black race
  — Tobacco and ethanol use
  — Low socioeconomic status
  — Diet low in trace elements, minerals, and vitamins or high in hot liquids

Figure 6-15. Resection specimen of esophageal squamous carcinoma with an ulcerated mass lesion.

Figure 6-16. Squamous carcinoma of the esophagus characterized by an infiltrative growth pattern and marked cellular atypia.

- Premalignant conditions include chronic esophagitis and squamous dysplasia or carcinoma in situ and are typically asymptomatic
- Dysphagia is the most common symptom associated with invasive carcinoma; cancer is often advanced at presentation
- Complications of invasive carcinoma include
  — Invasion into adjacent structures (major blood vessel, trachea, laryngeal nerve), causing hemorrhage, aspiration, and hiccups
  — More than half of all patients have positive lymph nodes at diagnosis; many are unresectable

- Most common metastatic sites are liver and lung
- Carcinomas that are considered variants of squamous cell carcinoma include
  — Undifferentiated carcinoma
  — Verrucous carcinoma
  — Spindle cell (sarcomatoid) carcinoma
- Other rare esophageal carcinomas
  — Adenosquamous carcinoma (mucoepidermoid carcinoma)
    ◆ May arise from submucosal glands
  — Adenoid cystic carcinoma (sometimes called *basaloid carcinoma*)
    ◆ May arise from submucosal glands

Gross and Endoscopic Pathology

❚ Squamous papilloma
- Exophytic, partially pedunculated, soft, pink-tan mass
- About 95% occur in mid- or lower esophagus
- Typically smaller than 1 cm
❚ Squamous cell dysplasia and carcinoma
- Dysplasia
  — Often multifocal
  — Dysplastic lesions vary widely in size and may be extensive
  — Most are at least focally erosive
  — Most involve mid- to lower esophagus
- Invasive carcinoma
  — Most (90%) occur in mid- and lower esophagus
  — Most tumors are large, discrete masses projecting into the lumen with variable intramural extension
  — Ulcerating tumors are less common and are typically erosive with infiltration and expansion of esophageal wall
  — Least common is an infiltrating tumor with similar intramural invasion but little or no ulceration
  — Prognosis is generally poor
  — Polypoid tumors have better survival than ulcerative and infiltrative tumors
  — Early lesions (T1) may be multifocal and combined with dysplasia of varying degrees and carcinoma in situ over a wide area

Histopathology

❚ Squamous papilloma
- Exophytic and endophytic proliferations of benign squamous epithelium
- Papillary proliferation with fibromuscular core; koilocytosis, hyperkeratosis, and hypergranulosis may occur
- Patterns are often mixed
❚ Squamous cell dysplasia and carcinoma
- Dysplasia and carcinoma in situ
  — Variable combination of nuclear anaplasia (hyperchromasia, pleomorphism) and disordered maturation

  — As in the cervix, dysplastic lesions are defined as those showing some evidence of maturation and are graded in three or two tiers: mild, moderate, and severe; or low grade and high grade
  — Full-thickness atypia without superficial maturation is termed *carcinoma in situ*
  — Dysplastic cells may extend into metaplastic submucosal glands
- Invasive squamous carcinoma
  — Low-grade carcinomas are characterized by obvious recapitulation of benign counterpart and are composed of syncytial nests of cells with abundant pink cytoplasm, intercellular bridges, and keratin pearls
  — High-grade carcinomas may show only solid nests of cells with pleomorphic nuclei and vague pink cytoplasm
  — Necrosis is often seen in high-grade carcinomas
  — Infiltration is often marked by paradoxical maturation of invading cells with squamous pearl formation and stromal desmoplasia
  — Effects of preoperative radiation include
    ◆ Marked atypia of stromal, endothelial, and squamous metaplasia in the submucosal glandular cells with atypia
    ◆ Postradiation changes include foci of calcified keratinized cells and foreign-body giant cell reaction

Special Stains and Immunohistochemistry

❚ Squamous papilloma
- Noncontributory
❚ Squamous cell carcinoma
- Cytokeratin immunostain is positive in virtually all squamous cell carcinomas; exceptions include a minority of high-grade carcinomas; positive in less than 50% of sarcomatoid carcinomas (sarcomatoid areas may react focally with cytokeratin and generally are reactive with vimentin antibodies; antibodies to desmin and muscle-specific actin may be positive)

Other Techniques for Diagnosis

❚ Squamous papilloma
- In situ hybridization and PCR to detect and classify HPV
❚ Squamous cell carcinoma
- Proliferative index (Mib-1 and Ki-67) and ploidy status may correlate with prognosis; usually not routinely performed

Differential Diagnosis

❚ Ulcerative esophagitis
- Usually recognizable endoscopically and usually covers a wide area of distal esophagus
- Biopsies demonstrate regenerative squamous epithelium characterized by basal cell hyperplasia and

orderly superficial maturation without significant nuclear pleomorphism
  - Keratinization is usually absent
- Infectious esophagitis
  - Similar histology to ulcerative esophagitis with detection of responsible organism
- Barrett esophagus
  - Many show inflamed, regenerating squamous epithelium adjacent to diagnostic columnar glands with intestinal metaplasia (goblet cells)

Pearls

- Extensive, diffusely ulcerated, flat lesions by endoscopy are most likely benign esophagitis with regenerative atypia
- Most squamous cell carcinomas form an exophytic mass with ulceration
- Keratinization or keratin pearls, particularly those containing hyperchromatic and atypical cells, are highly suggestive of infiltrating squamous carcinoma
- Five-year survival is dictated largely by depth of invasion and lymph node status
  — T1 lesions (mucosa and submucosa involved) and negative nodes: 90%
  — T2 lesion (into muscularis propria) and negative nodes: 47%
  — Overall 5-year survival with positive lymph nodes: 34%
- Tylosis is an autosomal dominant condition consisting of hyperkeratosis of the palms and soles and oral leukoplakia and is associated with squamous cell carcinoma of the esophagus

Selected References

Blot W: Esophageal cancer trends and risk factors. Semin Oncol 21:403-410, 1994.

Gabbert HE, Nakamura Y, Shimoda T, et al: Squamous cell carcinoma of the oesophagus. In Hamilton SR, Aaltonen LA (eds): World Health Organization Classification of Tumours. Pathology and Genetics: Tumours of the Digestive System. Lyon, IARC Press, 2000, pp 11-19.

Iezzoni JC, Mills SE: Sarcomatoid carcinomas (carcinosarcomas) of the gastrointestinal tract: A review. Semin Diagn Pathol 10:176-187, 1993.

Lewin KJ, Appelman HD: Tumors of the esophagus and stomach. In Atlas of Tumor Pathology, 3rd series, vol 18. Washington, DC, Armed Forces Institute of Pathology, 1996.

Odze R, Antonioli D, Shocket D, et al: Esophageal squamous papillomas: A clinicopathologic study of 38 lesions and analysis for human papillomavirus by the polymerase chain reaction. Am J Surg Pathol 17:803-812, 1993.

Torres CM, Wang HH, Turner JR, et al: Pathologic prognostic factors in esophageal squamous cell carcinoma: A follow-up study of 74 patients with or without preoperative chemoradiation therapy. Mod Pathol 12:961-968, 1999.

Squamous Cell Carcinoma Variants

Clinical Features

- Undifferentiated carcinoma
  - About 20% of esophageal malignancies
  - Highly aggressive
- Verrucous carcinoma
  - Considered a well-differentiated variant of squamous cell carcinoma
  - Slow growing but often recurs; low metastatic risk
  - Some cases reported after acid ingestion or with achalasia
- Sarcomatoid carcinoma
  - Represents a carcinoma with mesenchymal differentiation
  - Rare (<2% of esophageal malignances)
  - Affects mainly older men (mean age, 62 years)
  - Male-to-female ratio is 9:1
  - Patients often present with dysphagia and weight loss
  - Occasionally arises against a background of Barrett esophagus

Gross and Endoscopic Pathology

- Undifferentiated carcinoma
  - Typically large tumor with no distinctive gross features
- Verrucous carcinoma
  - Distinctive warty, exophytic mass
- Sarcomatoid carcinoma
  - Lobulated, large mass (1.5 to 15 cm)
  - May be polypoid or pedunculated and usually has a broad attachment to the underlying mucosa
  - Minority are flat with an ulcerated surface
  - Cut surface is gray and fleshy

Histopathology

- Undifferentiated carcinoma
  - As the name implies, the tumor is composed of large, anaplastic cells growing in a nonorganoid pattern
  - Tumor cells have pleomorphic, vesicular nuclei with prominent nucleoli and often have prominent eosinophilic cytoplasm (may impart a squamoid appearance)
- Verrucous carcinoma
  - Papillary fronds composed of well-differentiated squamous cells with little cytologic atypia
  - Parakeratosis and hyperkeratosis
  - Characteristic feature is the "pushing" deep tumor margin (rather than irregular areas of invasion)
- Sarcomatoid carcinoma
  - Although a recognizable invasive or in situ squamous carcinoma is usually present, most of the mass is composed of sarcomatous tissue showing variable cellularity
  - Biphasic histology has both carcinomatous and spindle cell components

- Spindle cell component is generally hypercellular and composed of malignant-appearing sarcomatous cells; may resemble malignant fibrous histiocytoma (MFH) or fibrosarcoma
- Chondroid, osseous, and rhabdomyoblastic differentiation may be present
- Epithelial component may be sharply demarcated or admixed and may show squamous, glandular, or undifferentiated morphology
- Metastases may contain any or all components

Special Stains and Immunohistochemistry

▌ Undifferentiated carcinoma
- Cytokeratin typically positive
- Vimentin negative

▌ Verrucous carcinoma
- Noncontributory

▌ Sarcomatoid carcinoma
- Carcinomatous elements are generally positive for cytokeratin and may show vimentin positivity
- Sarcomatous elements are strongly positive for vimentin and may show patchy positivity for cytokeratin

Other Techniques for Diagnosis

- Noncontributory

Differential Diagnosis

▌ Undifferentiated carcinoma versus lymphoma, melanoma, and sarcoma
- Presents a diagnostic challenge requiring a thorough immunohistochemical workup to demonstrate epithelial differentiation and to rule out anaplastic lymphoma, melanoma, and sarcoma

▌ Verrucous carcinoma versus papilloma and condyloma
- Generally have similar histologic features; however, they are best differentiated clinically and with a biopsy specimen large enough to demonstrate the broad pushing deep margin characteristic of verrucous carcinoma

▌ Sarcomatoid carcinoma versus sarcoma, melanoma, and inflammatory myofibroblastic tumor
- Diffuse, strong positivity for smooth muscle actin (SMA) supports diagnosis of leiomyosarcoma (although some leiomyosarcomas are cytokeratin positive, and some sarcomatoid carcinomas are SMA positive)
- Positive staining for cytokeratin, negative S-100 protein, HMB-45, and melan-A immunostaining essentially rule out melanoma
- Tumor composed of stromal cells with a low mitotic rate, no abnormal mitoses, and no significant cytologic anaplasia is typically a benign tumor, and in combination with inflammation, an inflammatory myofibroblastic tumor should be considered

Pearls

- Undifferentiated carcinoma is a highly aggressive neoplasm with a poor prognosis
- Verrucous carcinoma is a low-grade neoplasm that frequently recurs locally and only rarely metastasizes

Selected References

Gabbert HE, Nakamura Y, Shimoda T, et al: Squamous cell carcinoma of the oesophagus. In Hamilton SR, Aaltonen LA (ed): World Health Organization Classification of Tumours. Pathology and Genetics: Tumours of the Digestive System. Lyon, IARC Press, 2000, pp 11-19.

Lewin KJ, Appelman HD: Tumors of the esophagus and stomach. In Atlas of Tumor Pathology, 3rd series, vol 18. Washington, DC, Armed Forces Institute of Pathology, 1996.

Iezzoni JC, Mills SE: Sarcomatoid carcinomas (carcinosarcomas) of the gastrointestinal tract: A review. Semin Diagn Pathol 10:176-187, 1993.

Rare Esophageal Neoplasms

Clinical Features

- Most esophageal malignancies are squamous cell carcinomas (and variants) and adenocarcinomas; uncommon primary esophageal malignancies include small cell carcinoma and melanoma

▌ Small cell carcinoma
- Rare esophageal neoplasm
- Few cases have been studied; incidence varies depending on country reporting (<1%, up to 7%)
- Symptoms include dysphagia, weight loss, and chest pain
- Typically presents in older patients (65 years)
- Tumors reported to secrete adrenocorticotropic hormone (ACTH), calcitonin, vasoactive intestinal polyprotein (VIP), gastrin, and antidiuretic hormone (ADH)
- Associated conditions include Cushing syndrome, hypercalcemia, watery diarrhea, hypokalemia, and achlorhydria

▌ Malignant melanoma
- Rare in esophagus (<1% of esophageal malignancies)
- A primary tumor is less common than metastases from cutaneous melanoma
- Slightly more common in males
- Wide age range, 7 to 80 years (mean, 60 years)
- Symptoms include dysphagia and weight loss

Gross and Endoscopic Pathology

▌ Small cell carcinoma
- May be exophytic, flat, or ulcerative
- May occur in any part of the esophagus
- May erode into tracheobronchial tree, making it difficult to determine the primary site

▌ Malignant melanoma
- Often polypoid with a black or gray cut surface

- May arise in any part of the esophagus
- Average size is 7 cm

Histopathology

▌ Small cell carcinoma
- Similar to small cell carcinomas elsewhere
  — Composed of small to medium-sized, round to oval cells arranged in sheets, nests, rosettes, or ribbons
  — Tumor cells have densely hyperchromatic nuclei with scant cytoplasm
  — Crush artifact is characteristic (smeared chromatin)
  — High mitotic rate
  — Tumor cell necrosis is typical
  — May occasionally coexist with squamous carcinoma in situ, invasive squamous carcinoma, adenocarcinoma, or carcinoid tumors
▌ Malignant melanoma
- Similar to melanomas elsewhere
  — May have epithelioid, spindle, or anaplastic cell morphology
  — Unusual variants include small cell, signet ring cell, and balloon cell types
  — Adjacent squamous mucosa may demonstrate in situ lentiginous melanoma growth pattern, melanosis (increased pigmentation), melanocytosis (proliferation of benign melanocytes), or junctional activity

Special Stains and Immunohistochemistry

▌ Small cell carcinoma
- Variable positivity with chromogranin and synaptophysin antibodies
- Immunostain for thyroid transcription factor-1 (TTF-1) may help identify primary site
▌ Malignant melanoma
- Immunoreactivity with S-100 protein, HMB-45, and melan-A supports the diagnosis

Other Techniques for Diagnosis

- Noncontributory

Differential Diagnosis

▌ Small cell carcinoma and malignant melanoma (metastatic versus primary)
- Both tumors are more common outside the esophagus; therefore, the possibility of a metastasis to the esophagus must be considered
- Other than a careful history, differentiation from metastatic small cell carcinoma may be impossible; however, this may be irrelevant clinically because small cell carcinoma from any site usually presents as a widely disseminated process
- TTF-1 immunohistochemistry may help identify a pulmonary primary
- Diagnostic criteria for primary esophageal melanoma
  — Melanocytosis (proliferation of benign melanocytes) in adjacent squamous mucosa
  — Premalignant melanocytic lesions and melanoma in situ in adjacent epithelium is generally proof of a primary neoplasm
▌ Lymphoma
- May be distinguished from small cell carcinoma with leukocyte common antigen (LCA) immunostain and by recognizing the discohesive character of the lymphoid cells

Pearls

- Always consider metastases when diagnosing an uncommon esophageal malignancy
- If the melanoma has overgrown the premalignant changes, it may be impossible to determine whether the neoplasm is a primary tumor or a metastasis
- Both tumors have an extremely poor prognosis
  — Small cell carcinoma: average of 3 months' median survival
  — Melanoma: worse prognosis than cutaneous counterpart

Selected References

Li B, Lei W, Shao K, et al: Characteristics and prognosis of primary malignant melanoma of the esophagus. Melanoma Res 17:239-242, 2007.

Law S, Fok M, Lam K, et al: Small cell carcinoma of the esophagus. Cancer 73:2894-2899, 1994.

Caldwell CB, Bains MS, Burt M: Unusual malignant neoplasms of the esophagus: Oat cell carcinoma, melanoma, and sarcoma. J Thorac Cardiovasc Surg 101:100-107, 1991.

Stomach

Congenital and Acquired Gastric Abnormalities

Clinical Features

▌ Gastric duplication
- More common in females
- Clinically apparent in first year of life; rarely seen in adults
- One third of patients have other anomalies
- Typically presents as an intrathoracic or intra-abdominal mass
- Complications include ulceration, hemorrhage, rupture, fistula, and rarely malignancy
- Typically fails to be visualized on barium swallow
▌ Congenital pyloric stenosis
- Incidence is about 3 to 4 per 100 live births
- Typically male neonates and more common in first-born child (3 to 4 times more common in males)
- Presentation
  — Neonatal period
  — Projectile vomiting (nonbilious, postprandial)
  — Abdominal pain

- Abdominal examination classically reveals "pyloric olive"
- Heterotopia
  - Pancreatic
    - Normal pancreatic tissue entrapped during morphogenesis
    - Represents accessory pancreatic bud

Gross and Endoscopic Pathology

- Gastric duplication
  - Typically a cystic mass of variable size (<1 cm to >10 cm)
  - Generally intramural and on the greater curvature of the stomach
  - Usually does not communicate with the gastric lumen; if it does, it can be referred to as a *congenital diverticulum*
- Congenital pyloric stenosis
  - Progressive hypertrophy and hyperplasia of pyloric sphincter musculature
  - Thickness of the pyloric sphincter may be more than 1 cm (2 times normal), which results in narrowing of the pyloric channel
- Heterotopia
  - Pancreatic
    - Presents as a small (<4 cm), dome-shaped, umbilicated, submucosal mass
    - Central, nipple-like duct
    - Cut surface contains typical lobulated pancreatic parenchyma

Histopathology

- Gastric duplication
  - May contain normal gastric mucosa; occasionally see small intestinal, respiratory, or pancreas tissue
  - Organized muscular wall
- Heterotopia
  - Pancreatic
    - Most cases contain normal lobulated pancreatic tissue with ducts, acini, and islet cells and variable superimposed inflammation; other changes include
      - Cystic duct dilation
      - Pancreatitis
      - Ductal dysplasia
      - Tumors (islet cell, adenocarcinoma)
      - Cases without pancreatic acinar elements or islet cells are classified as adenomyoma

Special Stains and Immunohistochemistry

- Noncontributory

Modern Techniques for Diagnosis

- Pyloric stenosis: may be associated with chromosome 9q duplications

- Pancreatic heterotopia versus adenocarcinoma
  - Heterotopic pancreas and adenomyoma may occasionally produce benign, dilated ducts containing exfoliated cell clusters mimicking carcinoma; however, a benign process is recognized by its orderly lobular arrangement, lack of epithelial anaplasia, and absence of desmoplasia

Pearls

- Pancreatic heterotopia: carefully note the normal relationship of ducts, smooth muscle, and lobulated acini to avoid misinterpretation of heterotopia as carcinoma

Selected References

Mills SE: The stomach. In Sternberg S (ed): Diagnostic Surgical Pathology. Philadelphia, Lippincott Williams & Wilkins, 2004, pp 1435-1474.

Batcup G, Spitz L: A histopathological study of gastric mucosal biopsies in infantile hypertrophic pyloric stenosis. J Clin Pathol 32:625-628, 1979.

Xanthelasma

Clinical Features

- No association with hyperlipidemia
- Strong association with duodenal reflux, gastritis, or previous gastric surgery

Gross and Endoscopic Pathology

- Single or multiple, flat, discrete, tan-yellow plaques on the gastric mucosa
- Usually 0.1 to 0.2 cm (almost always <0.5 cm)

Figure 6-17. Endoscopic view of gastric xanthelasma appearing as two cream-colored to yellow papules.

Figure 6-18. Gastric xanthelasma showing aggregates of foamy histiocytes in the lamina propria.

Histopathology

- Characterized by sheets of foamy histiocytes (lipid filled) within superficial lamina propria
- Cells have a central, small, benign nucleus and finely vacuolated cytoplasm

Special Stains and Immunohistochemistry

- KP1 and CD68 positive
- PAS and mucin negative
- Cytokeratin negative

Other Techniques for Diagnosis

- Noncontributory

Differential Diagnosis

❚ Signet ring cell carcinoma versus xanthelasma
  - Signet ring cell carcinoma may contain seemingly bland cells with clear cytoplasm but is also composed of cells with atypical nuclei
  - Mucin stains and cytokeratin immunostains are positive in signet ring cell adenocarcinoma

Pearls

- Common incidental finding in autopsy studies and occasionally seen in endoscopic biopsy specimens

Selected References

Gencosmanoglu R, Sen-Oran E, Kurtkaya-Yapicier O, Tozun N: Xanthelasmas of the upper gastrointestinal tract. J Gastroenterol 39:215-219, 2004.

Kaiserling E, Heinle H, Itabe H, et al: Lipid islands in human gastric mucosa: Morphological and immunohistochemical findings. Gastroenterology 110:369-374, 1996.

Acute Erosive Gastritis

Clinical Features

- Variable symptoms; may be asymptomatic or cause epigastric pain, nausea, vomiting, mild gastrointestinal hemorrhage, or massive hematemesis
- May occasionally cause fatal hematemesis, particularly in alcoholics
- Occurs in significant percentage of patients taking anti-inflammatory medication
- Frequently associated with use of nonsteroidal anti-inflammatory drugs (NSAIDs), particularly aspirin (typically more than 8 aspirin tablets/day)
- Also associated with alcohol, heavy smoking, chemotherapy, stress (trauma, burns), and nasogastric intubation

Gross and Endoscopic Pathology

- Varies from mild mucosal hyperemia to mucosal erosion, ulcer, and hemorrhage (acute erosive gastritis)

Figure 6-19. Acute erosive gastritis. Note the absence of gastric foveolar epithelium along with the surface eosinophilic change with fibrin, debris, and capillary ectasia.

Histopathology

- Mild: edematous mucosa with scattered neutrophils among superficial epithelial cells or within glands above basement membrane ("active" gastritis)
- Moderate: mucosal erosion characterized by loss of epithelium and superficial exudate containing hemorrhage, fibrin, and neutrophils
- Severe: confluent erosions with similar morphology sometimes with ulcer
- All grades are usually accompanied by reactive gastropathy changes (see "Reactive Gastropathy")

Special Stains and Immunohistochemistry

- Noncontributory (most causes are noninfectious)

Other Techniques for Diagnosis

- Noncontributory

Differential Diagnosis

▌ Chronic gastritis
- Characterized by a dense chronic inflammatory infiltrate consisting of both lymphocytes and plasma cells
- Usually lacks mucosal erosions, hemorrhage, and ulceration

Pearls

- In fragmented biopsy specimens, look for subtle mix of fibrin, blood, and neutrophils within superficial epithelium
- Stain for *Helicobacter pylori* should be performed (Giemsa, Diff-Quik, immunohistochemistry or silver stain)

Selected References

Parfitt JR, Driman DK: Pathological effects of drugs on the gastrointestinal tract: A review. Hum Pathol 38:527-536, 2007.

Haber MM, Lopez I: Gastric histologic findings in patients with nonsteroidal anti-inflammatory drug-associated gastric ulcer. Mod Pathol 12:592-596, 1999.

Dixon MF, Genta RM, Yardley JH, et al: Classification and grading of gastritis. The updated Sydney system. Am J Surg Pathol 20:1161-1181, 1996.

Reactive Gastropathy

Clinical Features

- Incompletely understood adaptive response to more chronic exposure to many of the factors that are associated with erosive acute gastritis
- Often seen with chronic exposures to ethanol, NSAIDs, steroids, other medicines, stress, and reflux of duodenal contents

Figure 6-20. Endoscopic photograph of reactive gastropathy with diffusely erythematous gastric antrum.

Figure 6-21. Reactive gastropathy with lamina propria edema, fibromuscular proliferation within the superficial mucosa, capillary ectasia, and marked tortuous gastric foveolar hyperplasia. The foveolar epithelium demonstrates reduced intracellular mucus.

Gross and Endoscopic Pathology

- Usually seen as diffuse antral erythema with linear erosions
- Focal mucosal erosion and ulcers can be seen

Histopathology

- Regenerative epithelial changes, including foveolar hyperplasia (elongated, sometimes tortuous gastric pits with serrated luminal border), cytologic atypia (enlarged, mildly hyperchromatic nuclei with prominent nucleoli), and decreased foveolar mucin

- Lamina propria may be congested and have thin strands of connective tissue or smooth muscle
- Inflammation is typically sparse, but scattered chronic inflammatory cells are not uncommon
- Can be associated with mucosal capillary ectasia

Special Stains and Immunohistochemistry

- Noncontributory

Other Techniques for Diagnosis

- Noncontributory

Differential Diagnosis

▌ Chronic gastritis and *Helicobacter pylori* gastritis
- Diffuse lymphoplasmacytic infiltrate separating gastric pits sometimes containing neutrophils is highly specific for *H. pylori* infection
- Lymphoid aggregates with germinal centers are common
- If numerous, *H. pylori* organisms may be seen on routine stains; organisms are best highlighted with special stains (Giemsa, Diff-Quik, immunohistochemistry or silver stains)

▌ Gastric antral vascular ectasia ("watermelon stomach")
- Endoscopy shows nearly parallel erythematous stripes traversing the gastric antrum that resemble the stripes on a watermelon
- Accentuation of reactive gastropathy is seen in patients with atrophic gastritis
- Dilated mucosal capillaries containing fibrin thrombi are present

Pearls

- Conceptually, reactive gastropathy represents a mucosal response to injury
- Sometimes referred to as *chemical gastritis* or *chemical gastropathy*

Selected References

Parfitt JR, Driman DK: Pathological effects of drugs on the gastrointestinal tract: A review. Hum Pathol 38:527-536, 2007.

Laine L: Nonsteroidal anti-inflammatory drug gastropathy. [Review] Gastroenterol Endosc Clin North Am 6:489-504, 1996.

Suit P, Petras R, Bauer T, Petrini J: Gastric antral vascular ectasia: A histologic and morphometric study of "the watermelon stomach." Am J Surg Pathol 11:750-757, 1987.

Helicobacter pylori–Associated Gastritis (Chronic Gastritis)

Clinical Features

- Generally asymptomatic; can have symptoms related to peptic ulcer
- Relationship to nonulcer dyspepsia controversial

Figure 6-22. Chronic superficial gastritis associated with *Helicobacter pylori* infection.

Figure 6-23. *Helicobacter pylori* on Warthin-Starry stain.

- Affects all populations worldwide; affects nearly 100% of persons in developing countries
- Diffuse antral gastritis commonly affects whites in the United States
- Multifocal atrophic gastritis more common in blacks, Asians, Hispanics, and Scandinavians
- Affects 10% of children and up to half of the adults in the United States
- Affects lower socioeconomic and institutionalized groups at higher rates in all geographic areas
- *H. pylori* is clearly established as the cause of diffuse antral gastritis and is strongly associated with duodenal and gastric ulcers; predisposes certain

Figure 6-24. *Helicobacter heilmannii* on Giemsa stain. These organisms are larger than *Helicobacter pylori* and are tightly spiraled.

patients to mucosa-associated lymphoid tissue (MALT) lymphoma or gastric adenocarcinoma
- Most patients with *H. pylori* have chronic gastritis but are generally asymptomatic

Gross and Endoscopic Pathology

- Classic *H. pylori*–associated chronic gastritis primarily involves the antrum and causes diffuse antral gastritis (DAG)
- Multifocal atrophic gastritis (MAG) typically affects the antral-body junction
- Active lesions may have a reddened, boggy mucosa with thickened rugae and may mimic an infiltrative disease; chronic lesions may produce a thinned, flat mucosa
- Several studies report no characteristic endoscopic or gross finding; most appear unremarkable at endoscopy
- Correlation between endoscopic impression and histologic findings of gastritis is poor

Histopathology

▌Diffuse antral gastritis
- DAG is characterized by a diffuse lymphoplasmacytic infiltrate that appears to widen the intercryptal and interglandular area and is often accompanied by a neutrophilic component that permeates the epithelium; this chronic active gastritis pattern is associated with *H. pylori* organisms in more than 90% of cases
- Lymphoid aggregates with germinal centers are common with *H. pylori* infection
- May be associated with intestinal metaplasia
- Strong association with duodenal and pyloric ulcers

- *H. pylori* organisms may be seen on H&E staining in most cases; identification is enhanced with special stains
- Gastric body may show chronic superficial gastritis

▌Multifocal atrophic gastritis
- Thought to occur as sequela of *H. pylori* infection
- Minimal, focal chronic superficial and deep gastritis with islands of pseudopyloric and intestinal metaplasia
- Active inflammation (neutrophilic) is minimal
- Lymphoid follicles with germinal centers may persist
- Prevalence of *H. pylori* organisms in the lesion is lower
- Association with high gastric ulcers and adenocarcinoma (risk parallels degree of intestinal metaplasia)
  — Intestinal metaplasia may be
    ◆ Complete (type I): recapitulates true small bowel with goblet cells separated by enterocyte-type absorptive cells
    ◆ Incomplete (type II): "hybrid" mucosa containing goblet cells separated by gastric foveolar cells
  — Other changes include glandular atrophy, pseudopyloric metaplasia, regenerative epithelial changes, and glandular dysplasia

Special Stains and Immunohistochemistry

- Giemsa, Diff-Quik, immunostain and silver stains (e.g., Warthin-Starry): all visualize *H. pylori* along the luminal surface of gastric foveolar epithelium; sometimes organisms can be detected in the gastric glands
- Combined Alcian blue and PAS stain best separates intestinal metaplasia (Alcian blue positive) from foveolar gastric cells with prominent vacuoles (PAS positive)

Other Techniques for Diagnosis

- Antigen can be detected in stool
- Breath test and *Campylobacter*-like organism (CLO) test exploit urease production by *H. pylori* and can be useful to diagnose or follow up patients

Differential Diagnosis

▌Autoimmune gastritis (diffuse corporal atrophic gastritis)
- Affects body and fundus glands including parietal cells, producing atrophy and pyloric metaplasia and areas of intestinal metaplasia
- Autoantibodies to parietal cells or intrinsic factor are present
- Enterochromaffin-like cell hyperplasia and dysplasia and carcinoid tumors may develop as a consequence of hypergastrinemia

■ Acute erosive gastritis and reactive gastropathy
- Superficial erosion, hemorrhage, and neutrophilic infiltrate are accentuated over the chronic inflammation of the *H. pylori* gastritis
- Clinical history often detects inciting agent (ethanol, medication, radiation)

■ *Helicobacter heilmannii* gastritis
- Can cause gastritis; is associated with carcinoma and MALT-type lymphoma
- Organism is larger (7 μm) than *H. pylori* and tightly spiraled, resembling a corkscrew

Pearls
- In general, a diffuse lymphoplasmacytic infiltrate separating glands containing neutrophils is highly specific for *H. pylori* infection
- *H. pylori* is a gram-negative spiral rod about 3.5 μm in size with a flagellum
- Diagnosis may be based on breath test and CLO test; however, the gold standard is histologic identification either by H&E alone or by use of special stains to detect the organism
- *H. pylori*–like inflammation without identifiable organisms can sometimes be explained on the basis of prior antibiotic exposure or migration of *H. pylori* organisms in the setting of proton pump inhibitors; remember to look for organisms in the deep glands

Selected References
Fallone CA, Chiba N, Buchan A, et al: Two decades of *Helicobacter pylori*: A review of the fourth western *Helicobacter* congress. Can J Gastroenterol 16:559-563, 2002.

Dixon MF, Genta RM, Yardley J, et al: Classification and grading of gastritis: The updated Sydney system. Am J Surg Pathol 20:1161-1181, 1996.

Goldman H, Pronjansky R: Allergic proctitis and gastroenteritis in children: Clinical and mucosal biopsy features of 53 cases. Am J Surg Pathol 10:75-86, 1986.

Special Types of Gastritis

■ Lymphocytic gastritis
- Surface epithelial lymphocytosis (>25 lymphocytes per 100 gastric foveolar cells) on a background of superficial and deep chronic gastritis
- Associations include past or present *Helicobacter pylori* infection, celiac sprue, lymphocytic colitis, Ménétrier disease–like protein-losing gastropathy, and varioliform gastritis

■ Collagenous gastritis
- Increased (>15 μm) subepithelial collagen plate, sometimes associated with lymphocytic gastritis
- In children and young adults, may present with anemia and gastric nodules
- In adults, collagenous gastritis can be associated with collagenous colitis and collagenous sprue

■ Granulomatous gastritis
- Can be seen with infection (e.g., tuberculosis), Crohn disease, and sarcoidosis, and as a foreign-body giant cell reaction (e.g., so-called cereal granuloma, mucin granuloma)
- In some patients, granulomatous gastritis is considered idiopathic

■ Eosinophilic gastritis
- Usually seen in children and adolescents
- Presents with abdominal pain, nausea, vomiting, diarrhea, anemia, and protein loss
- Occasionally linked to food allergy

Selected References
Haot J, Jouret A, Willette M, et al: Lymphocytic gastritis: perspective study of its interrelationship to varioliform gastritis. Gut 31:283-285, 1990.

Lagorce-Pages C, Fabiani B, Bouvier R: Collagenous gastritis: A report of six cases. Am J Surg Pathol 25:1174-1179, 2001.

Shapiro JL, Goldblum JR, Petras RE: A clinicopathologic study of 42 patients with granulomatous gastritis: Is there really "idiopathic" granulomatous gastritis? Am J Surg Pathol 20:462-470, 1996.

Singhal AV, Sepulveda AR: *Helicobacter heilmannii* gastritis: A case study with review of literature. Am J Surg Pathol 29:1537-1539, 2005.

Suerbaum S, Michetti P: *Helicobacter pylori* infection. N Eng J Med 347:1175-1186, 2002.

Peptic Ulcer Disease

Clinical Features
- Affects 4 million people in the United States; 350,000 new cases/year
- Lifetime risk: 10% of men and 4% of women
- Typically occurs in middle-aged or older adults
- Gastric *Helicobacter pylori* is present in 100% of patients with duodenal ulcers and in 80% of patients with gastric ulcers
- Only 10% of patients with *H. pylori* infection develop peptic ulcers
- Symptoms
  — Most patients have epigastric pain
  — Hemorrhage, anemia, or perforation occurs in a minority of patients
  — Pain is worse at night and several hours postprandially; classically relieved by food or antacids
  — Without treatment, ulcers often require years to heal
  — Malignant transformation is rare
  — Complications include bleeding and perforation; bleeding may be massive

Gross and Endoscopic Pathology
- Most occur near pyloric ring (4:1 duodenal)
- Generally smaller than 2 cm; 10% are larger than 4 cm

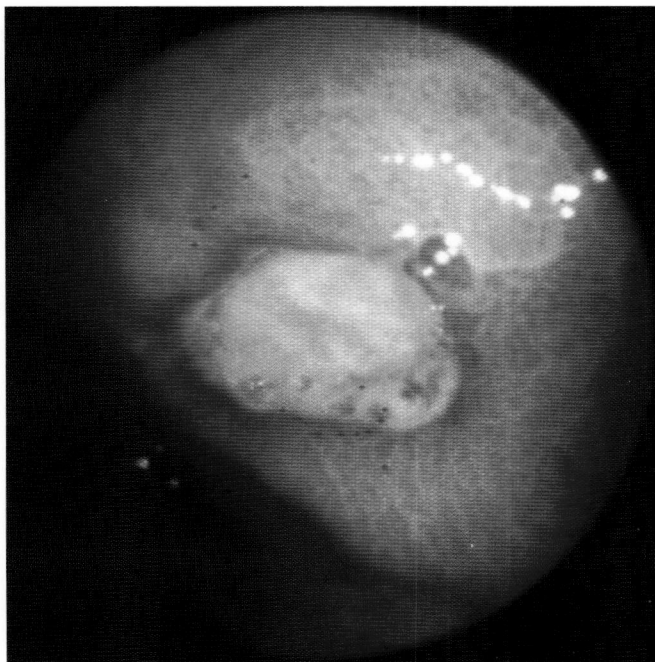

Figure 6-25. Endoscopic view of peptic ulcer of the stomach showing sharply demarcated margins and a clear base.

- Classically discrete, single ulcer with flat margins and a clean base
- No gross or endoscopic feature can reliably distinguish benign from malignant ulcers

Histopathology

- One can often observe four levels in well-developed ulcer
  — Overlying layer of neutrophils and debris
  — Layer of fibrin and necrotic material
  — Superficial zone of active granulation tissue
  — Fibrous scar that by definition interrupts the muscularis mucosae
- Chronic gastritis is present in most patients (unlike with stress ulcers or acute erosive gastritis and reactive gastropathy)

Special Stains and Immunohistochemistry

- Noncontributory

Other Techniques for Diagnosis

- Noncontributory

Differential Diagnosis

▌ Gastric carcinoma with ulcer
- Classically has raised, irregular margins and a necrotic base, but in many cases it is impossible to distinguish based solely on gross and endoscopic appearance
- Histologic features are confirmatory

▌ Acute erosive gastritis and reactive gastropathy

- Similar histology to the ulcer; however, surrounding gastric tissue does not show chronic gastritis and usually demonstrates reactive gastropathy

Pearls

- Always consider carcinoma when evaluating biopsies or resections with a clinical diagnosis of peptic ulcer by carefully examining ulcer margins and base for malignant cells; Alcian blue and PAS stain is helpful by showing abnormal mucin pattern in malignant cells or by highlighting signet ring cells

Selected References

Makola D, Peura DA, Crowe SE: *Helicobacter pylori* infection and related gastrointestinal diseases. J Clin Gastroenterol 41:548-558, 2007.

Dekigai H, Murakami M, Kita T: Mechanism of *H. pylori*-associated gastric mucosal injury. Dig Dis Sci 40:1332-1339, 1995.

Hersey SJ, Sachs G: Gastric acid secretion. Physiol Rev 75:155-189, 1995.

Soll AH: Pathogenesis of peptic ulcer and implications for therapy. N Engl J Med 322:909-916, 1990.

Hypertrophic Gastropathy

Clinical Features

- Expansion of gastric mucosa results in large rugae
- Either the superficial or the deep gastric epithelial zones may be involved
  — Superficial zone: top half of the mucosa that contains the surface foveolar cells and the "pits" (the upper portion of the tubular epithelium with the mucus neck region)
  — Deep zone: lower portion of the mucosa that contains the glands composed of the differentiated

Figure 6-26. Resection specimen of Ménétrier disease with large cerebriform gastric rugae.

Figure 6-27. Lymphocytic gastritis associated with Ménétrier disease–like gastropathy. Note the foveolar hyperplasia with numerous (>25 per 100 gastric foveolar cells) intraepithelial lymphocytes.

functional cells (parietal, zymogenic, and endocrine)
- Greater than 1- to 1.5-mm-thick mucosa is hypertrophic, which is usually due to epithelial hyperplasia
- Specific syndromes are defined by clinical features (gastrin level and presence of ulcers or protein loss) and gastric architecture (which component is hyperplastic)
- Many gastropathies are described, but two are well characterized: Ménétrier disease and Zollinger-Ellison syndrome
  — Both conditions may mimic an infiltrating carcinoma on radiologic or endoscopic examination
  — High risk for duodenal and jejunal ulcers owing to excessive gastrin secretion and increased acid production in Zollinger-Ellison syndrome
▌ Ménétrier disease
- Idiopathic condition
- Typically affects males ages 30 to 50 years
- Patients often have abdominal pain, diarrhea, weight loss, and peripheral edema
- Hypersecretion of gastric epithelium leads to hypoproteinemia and edema (protein-losing enteropathy); deep glandular atrophy is associated with hypochlorhydria

- Associations include eosinophilia, pulmonary infections, and thromboses
- Pediatric cases and some cases seen in immunosuppressed patients can occur and are associated with cytomegalovirus infection; in this setting, the hypertrophic gastropathy is often self-limited
▌ Zollinger-Ellison syndrome
- Mucosal hypertrophy due to gastrinoma-driven parietal cell hyperplasia
- Rare disease, fewer than 1 case per 1 million population
- Affects any age from childhood to elderly
- Peak incidence between ages 20 and 50 years
- Affects both genders equally
- Common symptoms include abdominal pain and diarrhea
▌ *Helicobacter pylori*–associated gastropathy
- Increased mucosal thickness is due to edema and inflammation; mucosa is not hyperplastic

Gross and Endoscopic Pathology
▌ Ménétrier disease
- Thick gastric wall with enlarged, cerebriform rugae
- Tends to spare antrum (in adults)
▌ Zollinger-Ellison syndrome
- Similar to Ménétrier disease; giant rugae
- Spares antrum

Histopathology
▌ Ménétrier disease
- Hyperplasia of superficial foveolar epithelium
- Atrophy of fundic glands
- Superficial pits are elongated and tortuous but are lined by cytologically normal cells
- Hyperplastic foveolar cells secrete excess mucus
- Evolving lesions include
  — Dilated pits producing cysts, which may extend through the muscularis mucosae
  — Expanding pits induce glandular atrophy and hypochlorhydria
  — Mixed inflammatory infiltrate
  — Hyperplasia of muscularis mucosae with extension upward between glands
▌ Zollinger-Ellison syndrome
- Specialized glands are hyperplastic
- Parietal cells occupy most of the deep portions of the glands and extend high up the neck
- Surface foveolar cells are atrophic
- Most easily identified by recognizing the abnormal pit-to-gland ratio (normal, 1:5)

Special Stains and Immunohistochemistry
- Enterochromaffin-like cell hyperplasia, endocrine cell dysplasia, and carcinoid tumors can arise in the setting of Zollinger-Ellison syndrome and are best

seen with immunostain for chromogranin or synaptophysin

Other Techniques for Diagnosis

- Noncontributory

Differential Diagnosis

- ❚ Ménétrier disease–like hypertrophic gastropathy associated with lymphocytic gastritis
  - Associated with giant gastric folds, hypoalbuminemia, and hypochlorhydria
  - Background gastritis characterized by large numbers of intraepithelial lymphocytes (>25 per 100 gastric foveolar cells)
- ❚ Ménétrier disease
  - Can be histologically indistinguishable from gastric hyperplastic polyp, juvenile polyp, Cronkhite-Canada polyp, or reactive gastropathy in small biopsy specimens
  - Careful attention to exact clinical setting and status of adjacent mucosa is critical to accurate diagnosis
- ❚ Gastritis glandularis et cystica profunda
  - Synonyms include diffuse cystic glandular malformation and diffuse cystic malformation
  - Mucosal and submucosal cyst lined by mucus cells, pyloric or Brunner-type glands, or rarely gastric body–type glands enveloped by smooth muscle
  - Rare but may be associated with increased risk for gastric carcinoma
- ❚ Zollinger-Ellison syndrome versus peptic ulcer disease
  - Peptic ulcer disease may have surface foveolar hyperplasia but no parietal cell hyperplasia

Pearls

- Hypertrophic gastropathy is characterized by giant cerebriform enlargement of the gastric rugae
- Ménétrier disease and Zollinger-Ellison syndrome are the most common causes; large folds are less commonly seen with *H. pylori* infection
- Most common complication is peptic ulcer, which may cause gastrointestinal hemorrhage; rarely, the hyperplastic mucosa becomes metaplastic and may subsequently undergo malignant transformation

Selected References

Qualman SJ, Hamoudi AB: Pediatric hypertrophic gastropathy (Ménétrier's disease). Pediatr Pathol 12:263-268, 1992.

Haot J, Bogomoletz WV, Jouret A, Manquet P: Ménétrier's disease with lymphocytic gastritis: An unusual association with possible pathogenic implications. Human Pathol 22:379-386, 1991.

Komorowski RA, Caya JG: Hyperplastic gastropathy: Clinicopathologic correlation. Am J Surg Pathol 15:577-585, 1991.

Honore LH, Lewis AS, O'Hara KE: Gastric glandularis et cystica profunda: A report of 3 cases with discussion of etiology and pathogenesis. Dig Dis Sci 24:48-52, 1979.

Non-neoplastic Gastric Polyps

Clinical Features

- ❚ Hyperplastic polyp
  - A common polyp in the stomach (accounts for 85% to 90% of gastric polyps in some series); ratio depends on prevalence of familial adenomatous polyposis syndrome patients and the use of proton pump inhibitors in the study group
  - Most common in older adults
  - Generally occurs in body or antrum

Figure 6-28. Endoscopic photograph of fundic gland polyposis in a patient with familial adenomatous polyposis. Note the small hemispheric polyps on the summit of rugae.

Figure 6-29. Hyperplastic polyp of the stomach showing edematous and inflammatory expansion of the lamina propria associated with mucosal microcyst formation.

Figure 6-30. Fundic gland polyp associated with familial adenomatous polyposis. In addition to the dilated gastric glands, the surface epithelium shows atypia, a phenotypic marker for familial adenomatous polyposis syndrome–associated fundic gland polyps.

- Associated mainly with chronic gastritis, but also occurs in reactive gastropathy adjacent to ulcers, surgical anastomosis, or gastrostomy sites
- Low malignant potential, but hyperplastic polyps may coexist with adenomas and carcinoma

▌ Fundic gland polyp
- May occur sporadically, can be part of familial adenomatous polyposis (FAP) syndromes (FAP, attenuated FAP, and [*mutY* homologue] MYH-associated polyposis syndrome), and is a common polyp type seen in patients taking proton pump inhibitors
- Adenomatous polyposis coli (APC)-associated fundic gland polyps affect one third to one half of all FAP patients and typically occur at a young age (10 to 30 years)
- Sporadic fundic gland polyps are typically found in older women
- Similar polyps seen in patients taking proton pump inhibitors

▌ Inflammatory fibroid polyp
- Occurs throughout gastrointestinal tract
- Identical to those described in esophagus
- Typically occurs in adults between 50 and 60 years of age
- Often asymptomatic (incidental finding); large polyps may cause abdominal pain or obstructive symptoms

Gross and Endoscopic Pathology

▌ Hyperplastic polyp
- Typically small and sessile with a smooth, bosselated surface
- Generally less than 2 cm
- About one third of affected patients have multiple polyps

- Most occur in patients with chronic gastritis or reactive gastropathy

▌ Fundic gland polyp
- Small (0.1 to 0.5 cm), nonpedunculated mucosal nodules
- Most involve the fundic mucosa
- Sporadic polyps
  — May be multiple but generally fewer than 20
- Fundic gland polyposis associated with FAP syndrome
  — Characterized by hundreds of polyps covering the gastric mucosa; often many more polyps than in non-FAP–associated fundic gland polyposis; concentrate on greater curvature and usually spares the antrum

▌ Inflammatory fibroid polyp
- Most occur in the antrum
- Most are small (<2 cm) and usually sessile
- May be single or multiple
- Circumscribed, firm nodules of gray tissue
- Overlying mucosa is often eroded or ulcerated
- Sometimes referred to as *Vanek polyp*

Histopathology

▌ Hyperplastic polyp
- Elongated, distorted, and branched foveolar pits in a background of edematous and inflamed lamina propria
- Often areas of surface ulceration, granulation tissue, and adjacent regenerative glands
- Glandular lining cells may show intestinal metaplasia; epithelial dysplasia can occur in this setting

▌ Fundic gland polyp
- Proliferation of small and dilated (cystic) glands lined by cytologically bland parietal and chief cells
- Occasional polyps show surface atypia; more commonly seen in FAP syndrome–associated polyps; essentially no malignant potential

▌ Inflammatory fibroid polyp
- Appear to arise in the submucosa as a granulation tissue–like reactive phenomenon
- Variable mixture of fibroblasts, myofibroblasts, thin-walled dilated blood vessels, and scattered mixed inflammation (lymphocytes, eosinophils, plasma cells), sometimes with giant cells
- Typically have a hypocellular stroma, but some polyps may be hypercellular
- Predictable evolution
  — Nodular stage: "tissue-culture" fibroblasts and myxoid stroma
  — Fibrovascular stage: vessels within concentric arrays of stromal spindle cells and eosinophils
  — Sclerotic: collagenization as final stage

Special Stains and Immunohistochemistry

▌ Inflammatory fibroid polyp
- Vimentin and CD34 positive
- Cytokeratin and CD117 negative

Other Techniques for Diagnosis

- Inflammatory fibroid polyps harbor mutations in *PDGFRA* gene (platelet-derived growth factor receptor alpha)

Differential Diagnosis

▌ Adenomatous polyp versus hyperplastic polyp
- Adenomatous polyps are characterized by dysplastic epithelium and typically do not contain as much inflamed stroma or gland dilatation

▌ Gastrointestinal stromal tumor (GIST) and sarcoma versus inflammatory fibroid polyp
- GIST
  — Composed of interlacing fascicles and whorls of spindle cells with elongated, cigar-shaped nuclei and epithelioid cells
  — Can usually be distinguished based on immuno-histochemistry for CD117
- Sarcoma
  — Hypercellular tumors composed of spindle or round cells with nuclear pleomorphism and high mitotic rate

Pearls

- Pathogenesis of fundic gland polyps related to mutations of APC and β-catenin genes
- Fundic gland polyps essentially occur in three settings (sporadic polyps, non-FAP–associated fundic gland polyps, and FAP-associated polyposis); best distinguished clinically
- On small biopsy specimens, the combination of non-neoplastic, irregular, dilated glands and inflamed stroma is a clue to hyperplastic polyp

Selected References

Abraham SC, Park SJ, Mugartegui L, et al: Sporadic fundic gland polyps with epithelial dysplasia: Evidence for preferential targeting for mutations in the adenomatous polyposis coli gene. Am J Pathol 161:1735-1742, 2002.

Abraham SC, Nobukawa B, Giardiello FM, et al: Fundic gland polyps in familial adenomatous polyposis: Neoplasms with frequent somatic adenomatous polyposis coli gene alterations. Am J Pathol 157:747-754, 2002.

Oberhuber G, Stolte M: Gastric polyps: An update on their pathology and biological significance. Virchows Arch 437:581-590, 2000.

Sarre R, Frost A, Jagelman D, et al: Gastric and duodenal polyps in familial adenomatous polyposis: A prospective study of the nature and prevalence of upper gastrointestinal polyps. Gut 28:306-314, 1987.

Gastric Carcinoma and Precursor Lesions

Clinical Features

- Two distinct clinicopathologic presentations of gastric adenocarcinoma

Figure 6-31. Endoscopic photograph of gastric adenocarcinoma demonstrating an irregularly shaped ulcer with undermining infiltrative edges.

Figure 6-32. Gastric adenoma. The histology is similar to a tubular adenoma seen in the intestines and is arising in intestinal metaplasia.

  — Intestinal-type tumors: an exophytic neoplasm similar to colorectal carcinoma
  — Diffuse-type tumors: an infiltrative process causing a thickening of the gastric wall
  — Each type has separate epidemiologic and predisposing factors

Figure 6-33. Infiltrating gastric adenocarcinoma, mixed intestinal and diffuse type of Lauren with an infiltrative pattern composed of carcinoma cells showing a high nuclear-to-cytoplasmic ratio and some gland formation.

Figure 6-34. Infiltrating poorly differentiated adenocarcinoma, diffuse type of Lauren with signet ring cell differentiation.

— In the United States, the overall incidence of gastric carcinoma is decreasing (particularly the intestinal type); however, carcinoma of the proximal stomach is increasing
— Certain countries, such as China and Latin America, have a much higher incidence of gastric carcinoma, usually the intestinal type
● Male-to-female ratio is about 2:1, particularly in older patients

● Risk factors include
— Diet
◆ High intake of complex carbohydrates and nitrates
◆ Low intake of leafy vegetables, salads, and fresh fruits
◆ Consumption of nitrates (or environmental exposure from fertilizer) is deleterious because they are reduced in the stomach to nitrites, which are strong mutagens
◆ Salt (used in food preservation) potentiates the carcinogenic effects of nitrites by causing increased cell turnover
— *Helicobacter pylori*
◆ Colonization by *H. pylori* in childhood leads to chronic gastritis, oxidative effects on DNA, and cell proliferation
▌ Precursor lesions
● Protracted chronic gastritis
— Produces intestinal metaplasia, which epidemiologically correlates with gastric carcinoma of intestinal type
● Dysplasia: as in Barrett esophagus and ulcerative colitis, the gastric dysplasias include flat dysplasia and adenomas
— Flat dysplasia: classified as low grade or high grade
◆ Low-grade dysplasia
◇ Slight increase in glandular complexity and cytologic aberrations, including loss of mucinous cells and hyperchromatic, mildly stratified nuclei
◆ High-grade dysplasia
◇ Marked glandular complexity and frank cytologic anaplasia including regular nuclear stratification, hyperchromasia, and pleomorphism with abnormal mitotic figures and loss of mucinous cells
◇ At times the glandular complexity is such that distinction from carcinoma is impossible
◇ Progression from dysplasia is thought to be slow and may remain stable for years
— Adenomas
◆ Polypoid proliferations; considered to be a localized area of dysplasia
◆ Less common than hyperplastic polyps
◆ Develop in areas of intestinal metaplasia
◆ Epidemiology is similar to intestinal-type gastric adenocarcinoma
◆ Estimates of coexistent gastric carcinoma range from 8% to 59%, as do estimates of carcinoma arising in the adenoma (11% to 69%)
◆ Gastric carcinoma more commonly complicates larger adenomas (>2 cm)
◆ Numerous subtypes
◇ Tubular, villous, tubulovillous
◇ Antral-foveolar type

- Ulcers
  - Although one fourth of all gastric carcinomas contain a discrete ulcer, less than 1% arise in a preceding, documented benign ulcer
  - In most cases, it is difficult to determine whether the cancer arose in an ulcer or whether a cancer ulcerated
  - About 5% of clinically and endoscopically presumed benign ulcers are eventually proved to be carcinoma

▌ Gastric carcinoma
- Common symptoms include early satiety, anorexia, and weight loss
- Like the epithelium from which it arises, gastric carcinoma is a heterogeneous tumor
- Fundamental differences in characteristics of two types of gastric carcinoma
  - Intestinal type
    - More common in elderly men
    - Seen in countries with high gastric cancer risk
    - Associated with dietary and environmental substances
    - Associated with *H. pylori* infection and intestinal metaplasia
    - Arises in a dysplastic precursor
    - Expands centripetally into gastric lumen and wall
    - Better prognosis than diffuse type carcinoma
  - Diffuse type
    - Younger patients and more common in women
    - No identifiable nutritional risk factor
    - May also be associated with *H. pylori* infection
    - Thought to arise from undifferentiated neck cells
    - Subtle precursor lesion seen in familial cases associated with germline E-cadherin mutations
    - Infiltrates into and expands gastric wall
    - Poor prognosis

▌ Early gastric carcinoma
- Superficial malignant tumor that invades the muscularis mucosae and submucosa but has not invaded the muscularis propria
- In large-scale screening programs in countries with a high incidence of gastric carcinoma (Japan), early gastric carcinoma is frequently diagnosed
- Distinct from other entities, such as
  - High-grade dysplasia
    - An incipient malignancy still confined within its original glandular basement membrane

Gross and Endoscopic Pathology

▌ Precursor lesions
- Flat dysplasia
  - Often associated with chronic gastritis, which is endoscopically diffuse

  - Mucosa may be hyperemic or eroded
  - Dysplasia is not endoscopically discernible
- Adenoma
  - Sessile or pedunculated polyp; may be endoscopically indistinguishable from a hyperplastic polyp
- Ulcer
  - Benign form characteristically has discrete, smooth, flat margins and a clean base

▌ Gastric carcinoma
- May be raised, flat, or ulcerated
- Some tumors are minute (<0.5 cm)
- Earliest classification (Borrman, 1926) divided tumors into two exophytic and two endophytic lesions
  - Polypoid (Borrman type I): protruding, bosselated tumor covered by intact mucosa
  - Fungating (Borrman type II): generally large, protruding tumor with ulcerated overlying mucosa
  - Ulcerated (Borrman type III): classic malignant ulcer characterized by irregular, raised, overhanging margins and a necrotic base
  - Infiltrative (Borrman type IV): flat plaques with shallow irregular ulcers and erosions that flatten and fix mucosa to underlying tissue; diffuse infiltration produces a thick gastric wall (linitis plastica or "leather-bottle stomach")
- Excluding association with types of carcinoma (e.g., Borrman type IV and carcinoma of diffuse type), classification of gross or endoscopic features is of little value clinically

Histopathology

▌ Precursor lesions
- Dysplasia (low and high grade)
  - A spectrum of changes involving increased architectural complexity and cytologic atypia (increased nuclear size, hyperchromasia, pleomorphism, and nuclear stratification)
  - Low-grade lesions resemble adenomas similar to those seen in the colon and small bowel
  - High-grade lesions show increased complexity and cellular atypia
- Adenoma
  - Essentially the same as colorectal adenomas
  - Characterized by variable loss of mucinous cells, nuclear enlargement, pleomorphism, and stratification
  - Can be classified as tubular, villous, and tubulovillous

▌ Gastric carcinoma
- Expresses a wide variety of histologic phenotypes
- Many histologic classification schemes have been proposed, but none is universally followed or accepted
- Many carcinomas are reminiscent of colorectal malignancies, whereas some retain mucinous features resembling foveolar cells

- World Health Organization classification includes four types
  — Papillary: exophytic, frondlike projections covered by cuboidal to columnar cells with variable amounts of mucin production
  — Tubular: tumors with prominent gland formation and variable degrees of differentiation; may be solid and usually have prominent desmoplastic stroma
  — Mucinous: gland formations are accompanied by excessive mucin production forming mucus cysts and pools that may contain floating fragments of malignant epithelium
  — Signet ring cell: population of single malignant cells with eccentric nuclei and a single, large, cytoplasmic mucin vacuole
  — Most prefer separation into diffuse and intestinal type of Lauren
- Other rare gastric carcinomas
  — Small cell carcinoma, parietal cell carcinoma, hepatoid adenocarcinoma, endodermal sinus tumor and embryonal carcinoma, choriocarcinoma, adenosquamous carcinoma, carcinosarcoma, and spindle cell carcinoma have been described
  — Lymphoepithelioma-like
    ◆ Uncommon undifferentiated carcinoma with dense lymphoid infiltrate
    ◆ Can often find evidence of Epstein-Barr virus infection

Special Stains and Immunohistochemistry

- Cytokeratin: useful stain to confirm poorly differentiated or signet ring cell carcinoma, which may be present within an ulcer base or at ulcer margins or infiltrate between benign glands; requires experience to accurately interpret
- Mucin stains (PAS, Alcian blue, mucicarmine): serve similar role as cytokeratin, but not all carcinomas are strongly positive; histiocytes may engulf mucin (mucinophages), causing confusion with signet ring cells
- Combined Alcian blue and PAS stain with a hematoxylin counterstain: detects intestinal metaplasia (dark blue, globoid goblet cells against magenta foveolar cells); the Alcian blue and PAS stain helps to detect carcinoma cells with abnormal mucin pattern in the lamina propria

Other Techniques for Diagnosis

- Noncontributory

Differential Diagnosis

▌ Chemotherapy or radiation effect
- Accentuated atypia mimicking cancer and dysplasia can be seen with regional chemotherapy (e.g., hepatic arteriole infusion chemotherapy) and radiation therapy (e.g., SIR-Spheres)
- Radiation and chemotherapy effect is usually associated with preserved mucosa architecture, marked cellular enlargement, bizarre atypia, a low nuclear-to-cytoplasmic ratio, and cytoplasmic eosinophilia with vacuolization

▌ Chronic gastritis with erosion and glandular regeneration
- Characterized by maintained architecture, hyperplastic glands containing normal mitotic figures, and enlarged but uniform nuclei (compared with carcinoma or dysplasia)
- Glands mature superficially, and the gland nuclei are not pleomorphic or stratified

▌ Ulcer
- Glandular epithelium at ulcer margin demonstrates regeneration
- Foamy histiocytes may be present, but infiltrating single malignant cells, malignant glands, and desmoplasia are absent
- Stroma may contain atypical but reactive fibroblasts, particularly following radiation

▌ Intestinal metaplasia with dysplasia
- Characterized by a background of goblet cells and atypical glands containing cells with stratified, pleomorphic, hyperchromatic nuclei
- Distinction from carcinoma may be difficult but is best made by absence of an infiltrating pattern, frankly malignant cytology, and desmoplasia

Pearls

- Overall 5-year survival rate for gastric carcinoma following gastrectomy is 10% to 20%
  — Most carcinomas present as stage IV (53%)
  — Tumor type, size, and grade all have prognostic value
  — Single best predictor of survival is depth of invasion; survival is 95% for tumors confined to the submucosa but drops to 50% with involvement through the muscularis propria to the subserosa (T3); T2 lesions have intermediate survival
- In gastric biopsies
  — If intestinal metaplasia is present, always look for dysplasia and carcinoma
  — If the glands appear farther apart than normal, be certain to determine what is separating them; it could be
    ◆ Signet ring cell carcinoma, lymphoma, benign lymphoplasmacytic infiltrate, foamy histiocytes, infected histiocytes (fungal or mycobacteria), or atrophy
- Surgical reports for resections should include enough information to determine tumor, node, metastisis (TNM) stage, tumor location, histologic type, degree of differentiation, and presence or absence of tumor at the resection margins

Selected References

Abraham SC, Montgomery EA, Singh VK, et al: Gastric adenomas: Intestinal-type and gastric-type adenomas differ in the risk of adenocarcinoma and presence of background mucosal pathology. Am J Surg Pathol 26:1276-1285, 2002.

Fenoglio-Preiser C, Carneiro F, Correa P, et al: Gastric carcinoma. In Hamilton SR, Aaltonen LA (eds): World Health Organization Classification of Tumours. Pathology and Genetics of Tumours of the Digestive System. Lyon, France, ARC Press, 2000, pp 38-52.

Petras R, Hart W, Bukowski R: Gastric epithelial atypia associated with hepatic arterial infusion chemotherapy: Its distinction from early gastric carcinoma. Cancer 56:745-750, 1985.

Lauren T: The two histologic main types of gastric carcinoma. Acta Pathol Microbiol Scand 64:34, 1965.

Gastric Carcinoid Tumor

Clinical Features

- Two types
  - Sporadic tumors
    - Typically solitary
    - Can secrete gastrin, serotonin, somatostatin, histamine, or bradykinin
    - Can behave in an aggressive manner, especially those larger than 2 cm; can be associated with invasion into the gastric wall and metastases to regional lymph nodes and the liver
    - Not associated with endocrine cell hyperplasia in adjacent mucosa
    - No response to antral resection or induction of hypogastrinemia

Figure 6-36. Intramucosal gastric carcinoid tumor arising in association with atrophic gastritis and intestinal metaplasia.

  - Tumors arising in a background of hypergastrinemia (usually resulting from chronic atrophic gastritis with pernicious anemia)
    - More common type
    - Associated with achlorhydria and hypergastrinemia
    - Arise following progression from simple hyperplasia of enterochromaffin-like cells to nodular hyperplasia to dysplasia to neoplasia
    - Multiple small mucosal or submucosal nodules, typically smaller than 1 cm
    - Indolent tumors that rarely metastasize
    - May regress following antrectomy (reduction of gastrin secretion)
    - May be seen in patients with Zollinger-Ellison syndrome as part of multiple endocrine neoplasia (MEN) syndrome type I, or rarely in patients with a primary defect of the proton pump

Gross and Endoscopic Pathology

- Small tumors (several micrometers up to 2 cm); sporadic tumors are usually larger (mean 2 cm)
- Larger lesions are often centrally umbilicated
- Hypergastrinemia related tumors are typically multiple and small (0.1 to 0.3 cm)

Histopathology

- Monomorphic nests, trabeculae, festoons, or glandlike formations

Figure 6-35. Endoscopic photograph of sporadic gastric carcinoid tumor with ulcer (foreground).

- Tumor cells have central, uniform, rounded nuclei with coarse chromatin pattern and sharply demarcated nuclear membrane and a low mitotic rate
- Typically arise in the deep mucosa and are covered by intact superficial epithelium; can invade the gastric wall and produce desmoplastic reaction
- Hypergastrinemia-associated and sporadic carcinoids can be histologically indistinguishable
- High mitotic rate, nuclear anaplasia, and necrosis are components of intermediate or high-grade neuroendocrine carcinoma and predict aggressive behavior

Special Stains and Immunohistochemistry

- Immunoreactive with antibodies to chromogranin and synaptophysin help verify neuroendocrine differentiation and help classify tumors as sporadic (no hyperplasia or dysplasia of enterochromaffin-like cells) or hypergastrinemia related
- Adjacent mucosa in hypergastrinemia-related carcinoids can show linear hyperplasia (5 or more endocrine cells in a line), nodular hyperplasia (clusters of 5 or more endocrine cells smaller than 150 μm), endocrine cell dysplasia (growths larger than 150 μm but smaller than 0.5 mm), or carcinoid tumors (growths larger than 0.5 mm)

Other Techniques for Diagnosis

- Noncontributory

Differential Diagnosis

▌ Gastric adenocarcinoma
- Typically forms recognizable glandular proliferation with a destructive and invasive growth pattern

▌ Lymphoma
- Particularly in small biopsies, the small, monomorphic lymphoid cells may superficially resemble those of carcinoid
- Lymphocytic infiltrate is positive for LCA and other lymphoid markers

Pearls

- In tumors associated with chronic atrophic (autoimmune) gastritis, lymph node metastases are extremely rare and generally occur only in tumors larger than 1 cm
- Sporadic carcinoids typically behave in a more aggressive manner and may prompt more aggressive surgery (complete or partial gastrectomy with lymph node resection)

Selected References

Williams GT: Endocrine tumours of the gastrointestinal tract: Selected topics. Histopathology 50:30-41, 2007.

Modlin IM, Kidd M, Latich I, et al: Current status of gastrointestinal carcinoids. Gastroenterology 128:1717-1751, 2005.

Solcia E, Fiocca R, Villani L: Hyperplastic, dysplastic, and neoplastic enterochromaffin-like-cell proliferations of the gastric mucosa: Classification and histogenesis. Am J Surg Pathol 19:S1-7, 1995.

Thomas RM, Baybick JH, Elsayed AM, Sobin LH: Gastric carcinoids: An immunohistochemical and clinicopathologic study of 104 patients. Cancer 73:2053-2058, 1994.

Gastric Lymphoma

Clinical Features

- Gastric lymphoma accounts for 60% to 65% of all gastrointestinal lymphomas
- Diffuse large B-cell lymphoma is most common
- Many gastric lymphomas are derived from MALT
- Generally affects patients in their fifth and sixth decades of life
- May be asymptomatic or present with an abdominal mass, abdominal pain (related to gastritis or ulcer), weight loss, or less commonly, bleeding
- Clear association between gastric marginal zone B-cell lymphoma of MALT type and *Helicobacter pylori* infection (92% to 100% of cases); treatment of *H. pylori* induces regression in 77% of early lesions
- Indolent behavior and generally an excellent prognosis with marginal zone B-cell lymphoma of MALT type

Gross and Endoscopic Pathology

- Most arise in the antrum
- Early lesions typically form a plaque or small mucosal erosions
- Advanced lesions cause ulcers, diffuse thickening of mucosal folds, or obvious masses

Figure 6-37. Extranodal marginal zone B-cell lymphoma of the mucosa-associated lymphoid tissue involving the stomach. A destructive lymphoepithelial lesion is associated with a proliferation of marginal zone lymphoma cells within the lamina propria.

Histopathology

- Marginal zone B-cell lymphoma of MALT type
  - Expansive proliferation of marginal zone lymphocytes at least 150 μm in size with neoplastic lymphocytes can have cytologic diversity ranging from small lymphocytes with round, dark nuclei to small lymphocytes with irregular nuclear contours and pale cytoplasm (small cleaved follicular center cells) to medium-sized lymphocytes with indented nuclei and abundant clear cytoplasm (resemble monocytoid B cells) to plasma cells with Dutcher bodies and rarely large blastic cells (large noncleaved follicular center cells)
  - Three additional characteristic features
    - Classic feature is the lymphoepithelial lesion (caused by invasion and destruction of gland or cyst by aggregates of neoplastic lymphocytes)
    - Lymphoid follicles often with germinal centers
    - Neoplastic plasma cells
- Diffuse large B-cell lymphoma
  - More than 20% of the tumor is composed of cells that have a blastic appearance (large noncleaved lymphocytes or bizarre, multinucleated lymphocytes)
  - Some of these could represent transformation from marginal zone B-cell lymphoma of MALT type; this is suggested by a mixture of low- and high-grade histology in the same tumor and presence of same immunophenotype and genotype

Special Stains and Immunohistochemistry

- Large cell lymphoma; confirm B-cell lineage with CD20 immunostain
  - Differentiate germinal center (better prognosis) from nongerminal center type using immunostains for CD10, BCL-6, and MUM-1
- Gastric marginal zone B-cell lymphoma of MALT type
  - Workup includes immunostains for pan B-cell marker such as CD19, CD20, and CD79A as well as negative staining for CD3, CD5, CD10, CD23, and cyclin D1

Other Techniques for Diagnosis

- PCR for B-cell clonality is supportive (with appropriate histology) but may be positive in some cases of gastritis
- Cytogenetics: t(11;18), t(14;18), trisomy 3, and 18q21 rearrangements may be seen
- Translocation of t(11;18) predicts resistance to *H. pylori* therapy
- Flow cytometry positive for CD19, CD20, CD21, and bcl-2; negative for CD5, CD10, and CD23

Differential Diagnosis

- ▌ Lymphocytic gastritis versus MALT lymphoma
  - Gastritis lacks lymphoepithelial lesion (cluster of three or more B-cell lymphocytes within gastric glands), which is characteristic of MALT lymphoma
  - Intraepithelial lymphocytes are T cells rather than B cells
  - Lacks characteristic immunophenotype of MALT lymphoma

Pearls

- MALT lymphomas have an excellent prognosis and typically remain confined to the stomach for many years; early lesions often improve with treatment for *H. pylori*
- Biopsy fragments showing diffuse sheets of lymphoplasmacytic cells with lymphoepithelial lesions, particularly in an older patient, are suggestive of MALT lymphoma

Selected References

Banks PM: Gastrointestinal lymphoproliferative disorders. Histopathology 50:42-54, 2007.

Isaacson PG: Gastric lymphoma and *Helicobacter pylori*. N Engl J Med 330:1310-1311, 1994.

Chan JK, Ng CS, Isaacson PG: Relationship between high-grade lymphoma and low-grade B-cell mucosa-associated lymphoid tissue (MALToma) of the stomach. Am J Pathol 126:1153-1165, 1990.

Isaacson PG: Lymphomas of mucosa-associated lymphoid tissue (MALT). Histopathology 16:617-619, 1990.

Lower Gastrointestinal Tract (Small and Large Intestine)

Congenital Anomalies

Clinical Features

- ▌ Malrotation
  - Results from disturbance of normal counterclockwise rotation of bowel around the superior mesenteric artery
  - Occurs in 1 in 6000 live births
  - Presenting symptoms are obstruction, bilious vomiting, abdominal distention, steatorrhea, and failure to thrive
- ▌ Omphalocele
  - Affects about 1 in 6000 to 1 in 10,000 births
  - Results from failure of the intestines to return to the abdominal cavity during the 10th week of development (essentially herniation of all or part of the small intestine)
  - May occur as a result of incomplete closure of the abdominal wall during the fourth week of development, which produces a large defect in the

Figure 6-38. Meckel diverticulum (autopsy photograph).

anterior abdominal wall (as a result, most of the abdominal viscera remain outside the embryo)
- In both situations, the herniated intestines are contained within a thin membranous sac (composed of peritoneal lining and amnion)
- Up to 50% of affected infants have additional anomalies, including malrotation, Meckel diverticulum, imperforate anus, and cardiovascular defects

▌ Gastroschisis
- Literally means split or open stomach (misnomer because it is the abdominal wall that is split, not the stomach)
- Uncommon, but more common in males
- Incidence is estimated at 1 to 2 cases per 100,000 births
- Presumed to be due to a vascular accident in early embryogenesis (before 12 weeks)
- Results from a defect in the anterior abdominal wall that permits extrusion of the abdominal viscera
- No membranous sac surrounds the extruded viscera

▌ Atresia and stenosis
- Rare conditions; found in 1 in 2000 to 1 in 6000 live births
- Duodenal atresia is most common and is associated with other anomalies in 35% of cases
- Higher incidence in twin gestations and in infants of mothers using cocaine
- Colonic atresia virtually never occurs
- Atresia presents in early neonatal period with bilious vomiting

▌ Meckel diverticulum
- Failure of the vitelline duct (connects the lumen of the bowel to the yolk sac) to involute produces a Meckel diverticulum
- Generally found within 85 to 100 cm of the ileocecal valve in adults
- About 1% to 4% prevalence
- No gender predilection
- Complications include hemorrhage, peptic ulceration, intussusception, and diverticulitis

▌ Intussusception
- Telescoping of one intestinal segment into another
- Affects about 2 to 4 per 1000 live births
- Twice as common in males
- Symptoms include abdominal pain, bloody diarrhea, and obstruction
- Complications include bowel infarction and peritonitis
- Children usually have no underlying anatomic abnormalities; intussusception in adults is typically associated with an intraluminal mass

▌ Volvulus
- Twisting of a bowel segment around mesentery
- Thought to cause about 10% of all bowel obstructions
- Occurs with or without predisposing causes, including
  — Congenitally long mesentery
  — Meckel diverticulum
  — Congenital band
- Most commonly occurs with redundant loops of sigmoid colon; less common in small intestine, and rarely involves the stomach or transverse colon
- Patients generally present with abdominal pain and obstruction
- Occurs acutely and may produce bowel infarction and peritonitis

Gross and Endoscopic Pathology

▌ Malrotation
- Intestines occupy abnormal positions
- Generally small bowel appears as a coiled mass of intestine pushed to one side of the abdomen
- Cecum may be on left side of the abdomen
- Fixation band may cause intestinal torsion and infarction

▌ Omphalocele
- Extra-abdominal viscera are covered by a thin membranous sac composed of peritoneum and amnion
- Herniated viscera typically includes intestines; may involve stomach and liver
- Umbilical cord arises from the center of the overlying sac

▌ Gastroschisis
- Abdominal viscera herniate through a defect in the abdominal wall

- Extruded viscera do not have an overlying thin membranous sac
- No involvement of the umbilical cord

❚ Atresia and stenosis
- Multiple types of atresias exist and may coexist
    — Imperforate septum across intestinal lumen
    — Bowel segment replaced by a fibrotic cord
    — Bowel segment and associated mesentery completely absent
    — Atretic bowel of variable length
- Intestinal stenosis is similar to atresia; has a variable reduction of the lumen diameter over a long segment or contains a septum with a central communication

❚ Meckel diverticulum
- Antimesenteric ileum is most common location
- Located 30 cm from ileocecal valve in infants and 85 to 100 cm from ileocecal valve in adults
- Usually 2 to 15 cm in length

❚ Intussusception
- Invagination or telescoping of proximal small or large bowel (intussusceptum) into the adjacent distal bowel that encircles it

❚ Volvulus
- Segment of bowel may twist around its mesentery
- Involved bowel is ischemic or frankly infarcted (35% to 40% of cases)
- Associated fibrous band or adhesion may be found

Histopathology

❚ Malrotation, omphalocele, and gastroschisis
- Normal bowel histology unless complicated by ischemia or peritonitis

❚ Atresia and stenosis
- Bowel proximal to the atretic or stenotic area may show ischemic or gangrenous changes (due to dilation of bowel)
- Villous blunting, ulceration, and granulation tissue can be seen; with time, marked submucosal fibrosis and muscularis propria hypertrophy occur
- Blind segment contains meconium, lanugo hair, and mucin

❚ Meckel diverticulum
- Usually lined by normal small intestinal mucosa
- May contain ectopic pancreatic or gastric tissue

❚ Intussusception
- Ischemic changes are common
- Vascular proliferation in lamina propria and deeper bowel layers develops in recurrent cases and can mimic vascular tumors

❚ Volvulus
- Variable degrees of ischemia

Special Stains and Immunohistochemistry
- Noncontributory

Other Techniques for Diagnosis
- Noncontributory

Differential Diagnosis
- Malrotation, atresia, Meckel diverticulum, intussusception, and volvulus all are considered in the differential diagnosis in patients with bowel obstruction symptoms
- Combination of clinical, radiographic, and surgical findings is usually diagnostic

Pearls
- Meckel diverticulum may contain heterotopic rests of gastric or pancreatic tissue (80% of cases); complications include peptic ulceration, hemorrhage, and diverticulitis
- Omphalocele is characterized by a central protrusion of abdominal contents, directly beneath (and with attachment to) the umbilical cord; protruding abdominal organs are covered by a membrane
- Omphalocele is typically due to failure of abdominal wall to form rather than to a focal abdominal wall defect, as in gastroschisis

Selected References

Dillon PW, Cilley RE: Newborn surgical emergencies: Gastrointestinal anomalies, abdominal wall defects. Pediatr Surg 40:1289-1314, 1993.

Dimmick JE, Kalousek DK: Developmental Pathology of the Embryonal Fetus. Philadelphia, JB Lippincott, 1992, p 526.

Rescorla FJ, Shedd FK, Grosfeld JL, et al: Anomalies of intestinal rotation in childhood: Analysis of 447 cases. Surgery 108:710-715, 1990.

Enteric Infections in Immunocompetent Hosts

Clinical Features
- Populations affected are generally those from underdeveloped countries and immunologically naive travelers to these areas
- Associated with poor sanitation in industrialized nations
- Food- and water-borne illnesses also occur after ingestion of large amounts of bacteria owing to contamination by food handlers or improper preparation or refrigeration and in institutionalized settings

❚ *Escherichia coli* infection
- Pathologic subtypes cannot be routinely differentiated from nonpathogenic forms
- May cause prolonged diarrhea; some *E. coli* elaborate an enterotoxin after the bacteria colonize the intestinal epithelium, leading to watery diarrhea and dehydration
- Enterohemorrhagic *E. coli* (e.g., *E. coli* O157:H7) produces a Shiga toxin. This infection is becoming increasingly prevalent in the United States (8% of routine stool cultures); generally occurs in the summer months; severe infection occurs in very

Figure 6-39. Endoscopic photograph of the transverse colon in a patient with enterohemorrhagic *Escherichia coli* infection. A linear shallow ulcer is surrounded by patchy erythematous mucosa.

Figure 6-41. Acute ischemic colitis pattern of injury in a patient with enterohemorrhagic *Escherichia coli* infection. There is superficial coagulative necrosis and hemorrhage of the colonic mucosa associated with inflammatory pseudomembrane formation. There is preservation of the deep colonic crypts.

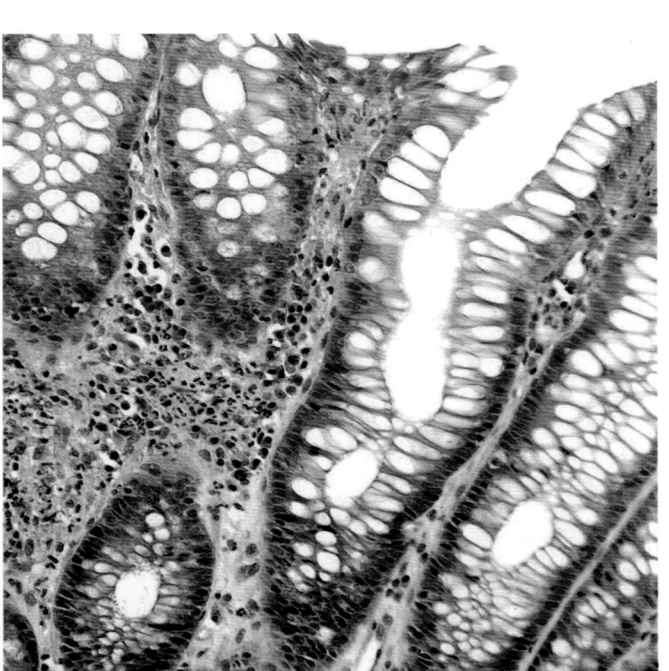

Figure 6-40. Enterohemorrhagic *Escherichia coli* infection showing the infectious pattern of injury with neutrophils loose within the lamina propria.

Figure 6-42. Endoscopic photograph of cytomegalovirus-associated colitis showing three well-circumscribed "punched-out" ulcers.

young or very old patients who eat contaminated food
- Most infections are mild and self-limited, but hemolytic-uremic syndrome and thrombocytopenic purpura may occur

- At least five other categories of *E. coli* pathogens recognized
  — Enteroinvasive *E. coli* are associated with a dysentery-like clinical picture
  — Enterotoxigenic, enteropathogenic, enteroaggregative, and diffusely adherent *E. coli* may cause traveler's diarrhea and diarrhea in children

- Shigellosis
  - *Shigella* species are virulent invasive gram-negative bacilli that cause bloody diarrhea
  - *Shigella dysenteriae* is most common, but infections with *Shigella sonnei* and *Shigella flexneri* are reported
  - Associated with fecal contamination of water supply
  - Most severe infection seen in infants and children, homosexual men, and malnourished and debilitated individuals
- Salmonellosis
  - Produces several distinct disease states; the two with primary gastrointestinal involvement are typhoid fever and salmonella gastroenteritis
  - Organisms replicate within intracellular vacuoles in enterocytes and macrophages and disseminate systemically
  - Typhoid fever
    — Caused by consumption of contaminated food or water
    — Fecal-oral transmission occurs
    — One case per 500,000 people in United States
    — Causes a systemic febrile and diarrheal illness following a 1-week incubation period
    — Complications include massive hemorrhage, peritonitis, and perforation
    — About 15% mortality rate in untreated patients
  - *Salmonella* gastroenteritis
    — Produces febrile diarrheal illness within hours of consumption of food contaminated by one of several types of *Salmonella* (other than *Salmonella typhi*)
    — Can mimic appendicitis
    — Causes 80% of food poisoning incidents
    — Strains resistant to multiple antibiotics have arisen as a result of agricultural practices (feed with antibiotic-supplemented grains)
- Campylobacteriosis
  - Causes both enteritis and colitis
  - Common stool pathogen in infants, teens, and young adults
  - Common cause of traveler's diarrhea and illness in hikers who consume untreated mountain water; 3 times more common than giardiasis in the Rocky Mountains
  - *Campylobacter fetus* is a cause of severe systemic illness
  - Produces bloody diarrhea up to 1 week after infection
  - Complications include meningitis, pseudomembranous colitis, arthropathy, and Guillain-Barré syndrome
- Cholera
  - Produces massive watery diarrhea due to antiabsorptive effect of endotoxin on small intestinal villi
  - Incubation period ranges from a few hours to 2 days
  - Recovery takes up to 1 week
  - Untreated mortality rate of 50% to 75%

- Losses of 15 to 20 L of fluid per day reported (when fluid replacement provided)
- Yersiniosis
  - Can clinically mimic Crohn disease
  - Aerobic bacteria present in contaminated food or blood products
  - Enterocolitis is the most common clinical manifestation and usually affects young children
  - Often associated with mesenteric lymphadenitis
  - Fatal infections occur in immunosuppressed patients and patients with iron overload

Gross and Endoscopic Pathology

- *Escherichia coli* O157:H7 (enterohemorrhagic *E. coli*)
  - Hemorrhagic, oozing mucosa
  - Pseudomembranes may be present but are rare
  - Generally affects the right side of the colon
  - Other *E. coli* pathogens may cause edema or patchy erythema of colon
- Shigellosis
  - Typically affects large bowel
  - Can see mucosal hemorrhage, ulcer, and occasionally pseudomembranes
  - Typical cases show patchy erythema of colonic mucosa
- Salmonellosis
  - Typhoid fever or *Salmonella* enteritis
    — Longitudinal oval ulcers with elevated edges
    — Ulcers are typically on top of Peyer patches in the terminal ileum
  - Nontyphoidal species may cause edema or patchy erythema of colon
- Campylobacteriosis
  - Diffuse, hemorrhagic, and focally ulcerative enterocolitis
  - Often near ileocecal valve with involvement of Peyer patches
- Cholera
  - Edematous small bowel mucosa
- Yersiniosis
  - Diffuse and focal ulcerations and edema in the ileum and colon
  - Enlarged mesenteric lymph nodes with foci of necrosis
  - Hyperplastic lymphoid follicles in epithelium often with overlying aphthous ulcers

Histopathology

- *Escherichia coli* infection including *E. coli* O157:H7 (enterohemorrhagic *E. coli*)
  - Enterohemorrhagic *E. coli* produces both ischemic and infectious colitis (toxin interferes with protein synthesis, causing epithelial and endothelial cell damage)
  - Mucosal hemorrhage, infarct, and pseudomembranes can occur
  - Focal neutrophilic infiltrates, cryptitis, and crypt abscesses may be present

- Adherent bacteria can be seen in some cases of infection with adherent *E. coli* pathogens
- Shigellosis
  - Infective-type pattern of colitis (focal active colitis) characterized by
    - Limited areas of increased inflammatory cells; sometimes seen with focal architectural changes
    - Some areas of biopsy specimen maintain an essentially normal appearance
    - Inflammation is typically acute with patchy cryptitis and neutrophils within the lamina propria without lamina propria plasmacytosis
- Salmonellosis
  - Typhoid fever or salmonella enteritis
    - Hyperplastic lymphoid follicles with adjacent mucosal hemorrhage, neutrophilic infiltrates, and atrophy and regeneration
    - Progressive hemorrhage and inflammation may produce perforation
    - Can cause focal active colitis pattern of injury
- Campylobacteriosis
  - Focal active colitis with neutrophilic infiltrates with cryptitis, hemorrhage, and necrosis
- Cholera
  - Intact mucosa with minimal changes
- Yersiniosis
  - Hyperplastic lymphoid follicles with large germinal centers
  - Punctate ulcers with neutrophilic fissures over hyperplastic lymphoid follicles (similar to Crohn disease)
  - Suppurative epithelioid granulomas in bowel wall and regional lymph nodes
  - Acute cryptitis occurs in colon

Special Stains and Immunohistochemistry

- Organisms are not reliably detected with histologic stains

Other Techniques for Diagnosis

- Pathogenic *Escherichia coli*
  - Requires sophisticated techniques such as a serotyping, PCR, or DNA hybridization for diagnosis, although *E. coli* O157:H7 can be detected from stool culture using specific growth media
- Most pathogenic bacteria are best characterized using microbiologic techniques, serum antibody assays, or occasionally PCR in biopsy specimens

Differential Diagnosis

- Enterohemorrhagic *Escherichia coli*, *Campylobacter* species, and *Salmonella* species infection versus inflammatory bowel disease, ischemic colitis, and pseudomembranous colitis
  - Inflammatory bowel disease

- Characterized by a similar neutrophilic infiltrate but distinguished by a more diffuse involvement, less mucosal hemorrhage, basal plasmacytosis, and greater glandular changes (mucin depletion, gland distortion)
    - Giant cells may be present in any infection, but not the well-formed noncaseating granulomas seen in Crohn disease
    - Suppurative granulomas may be seen with *Campylobacter* species infection
  - Ischemic colitis
    - Characterized by superficial necrosis and less acute inflammation than infectious enterocolitis
    - Clinical history and symptoms are often suggestive of ischemia
  - Pseudomembranous colitis (*Clostridium difficile*–associated colitis)
    - May be histologically indistinguishable from other causes of infectious colitis
    - Pseudomembrane is composed of desquamated epithelial cells, inflammatory cells, and fibrin material
    - Requires clinical history (i.e., previous antibiotic use) and diagnostic tests for identification
    - Diagnosis is based on detection of toxins (toxin A and toxin B); culture is not helpful
- *Yersinia* species infection versus Crohn disease
  - Similar clinical involvement of the terminal ileum with aphthous ulcers
  - Crohn disease typically does not produce the extensive suppurative granulomas seen with *Yersinia* species

Pearls

- *Campylobacter* species infection may be complicated by meningitis, Guillain-Barré syndrome, and pseudomembranous colitis
- *Yersinia* species infection is generally associated with mesenteric lymphadenitis

Selected References

Lamps LW: Infective disorders of the gastrointestinal tract. Histopathology 50:55-63, 2007.

Nataro JP, Kaper JB: Diarrheogenic *Escherichia coli*. Clin Microbiol Rev 11:142-210, 1998.

Griffin P, Olmstead L, Petras R: *Escherichia coli* O157:H7-associated colitis: A clinical and histologic study of 11 cases. Gastroenterology 99:142-149, 1990.

Norstrant TT, Kumar NB, Appelman HD: Histopathology differentiates acute self-limited colitis from ulcerative colitis. Gastroenterology 92:318-328, 1987.

Infections in Immunocompromised Patients

Clinical Features

- Enteric infections are common in immunocompromised patients, particularly patients with AIDS; other causes include

Figure 6-45. Cryptosporidiosis showing developmental forms attached to cell surfaces.

Figure 6-43. Cytomegalovirus-associated colitis showing infected stromal cells with cytomegaly, cytoplasmic inclusions, and prominent intranuclear inclusions with surrounding halo.

Figure 6-46. Intestinal spirochetosis showing numerous organisms attached to the brushed border.

Figure 6-44. Giardiasis. *Giardia lamblia* organisms en face appear pear shaped with paired nuclei.

— Hemodialysis
— Postoperative complications
— Indwelling vascular devices
• Infection may occur at any level of the gastrointestinal tract, and symptoms depend on level infected
— Esophageal infections: dysphagia, odynophagia, chest pain
— Gastric infections: nausea, vomiting, abdominal pain
— Intestinal infections: diarrhea
• Complications include bleeding, obstruction, and perforation

— Transplantation (solid organ and bone marrow)
— Cancer chemotherapy
— Autoimmune diseases (treated with steroids)
— Advanced age
— Diabetes
— Long-term antibiotic use

Figure 6-47. *Mycobacterium avium-intracellulare* **complex** infection involving proximal small intestine. The lamina propria is variably expanded with foamy macrophages.

Figure 6-48. *Mycobacterium avium-intracellulare* **complex infection** (acid-fast stain).

- In AIDS patients, about one half of all diarrheal episodes are due to infections; some of the remainder are due to AIDS enteropathy (syndrome characterized by chronic diarrhea, malnutrition, and wasting without evidence of gastrointestinal infection)
  — Fungal, parasitic, bacterial, and viral infections are all common in untreated AIDS and immunocompromised patients

Gross and Endoscopic Pathology

▌ Viral infections
  - CMV: variable, often discrete, ulcers affecting the esophagus, stomach, or intestines
  - HSV: painful ulcers or vesicles, often in esophagus, low rectum and anus and perianal skin
  - Adenovirus: nonspecific appearance
▌ Parasitic infections
  - Giardiasis (*Giardia intestinalis*): nonspecific changes
  - Coccidiosis (*Cryptosporidium parvum, Isospora belli*, and *Cyclospora* species)
    — *Cryptosporidium* and *Isospora* species are most commonly found in patients with AIDS
    — Cyclosporidiosis is more commonly traveler's diarrhea or associated with contaminated food
    — All show mild, nonspecific features
  - Microsporidiosis (*Enterocytozoon bieneusi* and *Encephalitozoon intestinalis*): mild, nonspecific abnormalities in small bowel
▌ Fungal infections
  - Candidiasis
    — Most common cause of esophagitis in AIDS patients
    — Esophagus is most common site (affects small bowel in disseminated disease)
    — Forms adherent, white-brown plaques with mucosal hyperemia and ulceration
    — May completely denude esophagus
  - Aspergillosis
    — Typically involves esophagus, although rare in gastrointestinal tract
    — Often produces necrotic ulcers (due to angioinvasive properties resulting in ischemia)
  - Mucormycosis
    — Often produces extensive necrosis (due to angioinvasive properties resulting in ischemia); rarely in gastrointestinal tract
  - Histoplasmosis
    — May spread to esophagus and elsewhere from lung
    — Rarely causes esophageal perforation or esophagobronchial fistula
▌ Bacterial infections
  - Bacterial pathogens common to the immunocompromised host include *Salmonella, Shigella*, and *Campylobacter* species (may be difficult to eradicate in AIDS patients)
  - Intestinal spirochetosis typically involves the colon diffusely, usually with no endoscopic abnormality; more often seen in immune competent individuals in whom it may be considered a commensal
  - Tuberculosis causes shallow ulcers with confluent granulomas; most commonly involves ileocecal region (90%)

- *Mycobacterium avium-intracellulare* (MAI): causes poorly delineated, often plaquelike lesions anywhere in gastrointestinal tract
▌ Noninfectious AIDS-related enteropathy
  - Often has minimal disease

Histopathology

▌ Viral infections
  - CMV
    — Variable, but often mild mixed inflammation with ulceration and characteristic nuclear or cytoplasmic inclusions typically in endothelial or mesenchymal cells
    — Rarely causes severe disease with vasculitis and intestinal perforation
  - HSV
    — In esophageal and perianal lesions, acute inflammation and necrosis predominate; classic multinucleated cells, acantholysis, and nuclear inclusions in squamous epithelium may be observed
  - Adenovirus
    — Mild, nonspecific chronic inflammation in colon with dystrophic goblet cells containing amorphic nuclei and rarely containing diagnostic inclusion bodies
▌ Parasite infections
  - Giardiasis
    — Pear-shaped organism similar in size to an enterocyte nucleus
    — Trophozoite has two symmetrical nuclei ("monkey face")
    — Organisms are generally found along the luminal border and induce a variable mucosal inflammatory infiltrate
  - Coccidial infections
    — *Cryptosporidium parvum*
      ◆ Basophilic dotlike organisms (1 to 3 μm) attached to luminal border (brush border) of small intestinal or colonic epithelial cells
      ◆ Usually minimal associated chronic inflammation and variable villous abnormalities; mild villous shortening may be seen
    — *Isospora belli*
      ◆ Coccidia are tiny ovoid structures within the epithelial cells of the intestinal villi (may be difficult to detect); merozoites are banana shaped
    — *Cyclospora cayetanensis*
      ◆ Tiny ovoid structures in enterocytes (similar to *Isospora* species)
  - Microsporidiosis
    — Two forms
      ◆ Mature spores appear as a cluster of dotlike structures (1.5 μm) in the apical cytoplasm of

epithelial cell in the small bowel or colon (often difficult to detect)
      ◆ Larger nucleated sporont (3 to 5 μm) is a basophilic structure in epithelial cells near the villus tips; may cause nuclear indentation
▌ Fungal infections
  - Candidiasis
    — Acantholysis with superficial neutrophils within squamous epithelium; can be associated with focal squamous epithelial lymphocytosis
    — Mucosal ulceration with neutrophilic infiltrates in severe cases
    — Yeast and pseudohyphae form within necrotic debris
    — Invasion of submucosa verifies significant disease
    — Invasive disease is characterized by mixture of dimorphic forms, including the 3- to 5-μm blastoconidia (budding oval yeasts) and pseudohyphae (elongated blastoconidia with indentation at pseudosepta representing several separate yeast organisms)
    — True hyphae may form (one elongated organism with parallel walls and no indentation at true septa); branching is absent
  - Aspergillosis
    — Often admixed with necrotic or infarcted debris owing to ischemia caused by the angioinvasive properties of the fungus
    — Dichotomous branching at 45-degree angles; 2- to 4-μm-wide hyphae with parallel walls and true septa
    — Rarely seen in surgical or biopsy specimens
  - Mucormycosis
    — Wide (10 to 20 μm) aseptate hyphae that are irregularly branched and often create folded, ribbon-like structures
    — Rarely seen in surgical or biopsy specimens
  - Histoplasmosis
    — May cause granuloma formation or diffuse collections of histiocytes in the lamina propria
    — Intracellular organisms are 2 to 3 μm
    — Granulomatous inflammation can mimic Crohn disease
▌ Bacterial infections
  - Spirochetosis
    — Organisms form a basophilic haze on the luminal surface
    — Can be verified with silver stains (e.g., Warthin-Starry) or immunostains for *Treponema* species
  - Tuberculosis
    — Ulceration and necrotizing granulomas with Langhans giant cells
  - MAI
    — Lamina propria contains foamy histiocytes stuffed with acid-fast bacilli (AFB; modified AFB)

■ AIDS-related enteropathy
- Nonspecific apoptosis, chronic inflammation, and villous atrophy due to HIV infections of enterocytes and other cells
- Regenerating immature cells have no microvilli
- Noninfectious esophageal ulcers
- Range of histologic features, including focal edema, apoptotic cells, and dense neutrophilic inflammation with erosion
- Erosion may produce large ulcers that are potentially life threatening
- Electron microscopy reveals viral particles, presumed to be HIV, in mononuclear cells
- Rarely seen since advent of aggressive antiretroviral therapy

Special Stains and Immunohistochemistry
- PAS and GMS: fungal structures are highlighted (best used to detect fungi within ulcerated or necrotic tissue in esophageal and gastric biopsy specimens)
- Giemsa: highlights *Cryptosporidium*, *Isospora*, and *Microsporidium* species
- Trichrome: helps differentiate *Giardia* species from mucus
- Modified AFB: detects MAI infection
- Warthin-Starry or Dieterle: highlights spirochetes
- Immunostains available for CMV (useful), HSV, *Cryptosporidium* and *Microsporidia* species (immunofluorescence), adenovirus, and *Cyclospora* species

Other Techniques for Diagnosis
- PCR available for numerous microorganisms, including CMV and *Microsporidia* species; may work in paraffin blocks
- Diagnosis of parasitic infections is readily made by detecting oocytes or cyst forms in stool specimens; AFB stain detects oocyst of *Cryptosporidia* species in stool samples (not in histologic sections)
- Electron microscopy: may be helpful to identify and speciate some microorganisms (e.g., *Microsporidium* species)

Differential Diagnosis
- Gastrointestinal infection is the foremost consideration in immunocompromised hosts
■ Kaposi sarcoma
- Prevalent in AIDS patients; relatively common in gastrointestinal tract
- Characterized by macular red lesions, composed of a spindle cell proliferation in the lamina propria containing extravasated red blood cells in slitlike spaces
■ Whipple disease
- Closely simulates MAI with PAS-positive foamy histiocytes

- Lacks fat vacuoles and AFB positivity characteristic of MAI infection

Pearls
- Even though the patient is immunocompromised, there is usually some inflammation
- Consider an opportunistic infection when you see inflammation that you are unable otherwise to account for (even if the patient is not known to be immunocompromised)
- Small blue dots in a row *on* the surface of enterocytes: think of cryptosporidiosis
- Small blue dots *in* the enterocyte: think of microsporidiosis
- Blue haze on surface of colonic cells: think of spirochetosis
- When mesenchymal cells look too big or there are subtle erosions or inflammation, check mesenchymal cells—particularly endothelial cells—for CMV inclusions
- Do not confuse luminal mucin globules for *Cryptosporidium* species (*C. parvum* are deeper blue on H&E stain, and generally there are many organisms of equal size along the luminal surface) or for *Giardia* species (trichrome stain can help)
- Giardiasis is also associated with selective IgA immunodeficiency and common variable immunodeficiency disease (CVID)
- Mentally rule out infection in *every* small bowel biopsy specimen
- Consider immunostain for CMV, AFB, and PAS or GMS for gastrointestinal biopsies (unless the tissue is perfectly normal and the endoscopy detected no lesions) in immunocompromised patients

Selected References

Calderaro A, Bommezzadri S, Gorrini C, et al: Infective colitis associated with human intestinal spirochetosis. J Gastroenterol Hepatol 22:1772-1779, 2007.

Varma M, Hester JD, Schaefer FW 3rd, et al: Detection of *Cyclospora cayetanensis* using a quantitative real-time PCR assay. J Microbiol Methods 53:27-36, 2003.

Greenberg PD, Koch J, Cello JP: Diagnosis of *Cryptosporidium parvum* in patients with severe diarrhea and AIDS. Dig Dis Sci 41:2286-2290, 1996.

Greenson JK, Belitos PC, Yardley JH, Bartlett JG: AIDS enteropathy: Occult enteric infections and duodenal mucosal alterations in chronic diarrhea. Ann Intern Med 114:366-372, 1991.

Gutierrez Y: Diagnostic Pathology of Parasitic Infections with Clinical Correlations. Philadelphia, Lea & Febiger, 1990.

Orenstein JM, Chlang J, Steinberg W, et al: Intestinal microsporidiosis as a cause of diarrhea in human immunodeficiency virus-infected patients. Hum Pathol 21:475-481, 1990.

Strom RL, Gruninger RP: AIDS with *Mycobacterium avium-intracellulare* lesions resembling those of Whipple's disease. N Engl J Med 309:1324, 1983.

Whipple Disease

Clinical Features

- Rare, chronic systemic illness with prominent gastrointestinal symptoms
- Commonly affects white adults between 30 and 50 years of age; strong male predominance

Figure 6-49. Whipple disease within duodenum biopsy specimen. Histologic section shows flattening of the villi and an expansion of the lamina propria by foamy macrophages with fat vacuoles.

Figure 6-50. Whipple disease. Periodic acid–Schiff stain shows brightly staining, coarsely granular intracytoplasmic inclusions.

- More common in people of North American and European ancestry
- May involve any organ of the body, most commonly the gastrointestinal tract, joints, and central nervous system
- Common associations
  - Malabsorption and diarrhea
  - Abdominal pain
  - Weight loss
  - Polyarthralgia
  - Peripheral lymphadenopathy
  - Cardiac dysfunction
  - Central nervous system disease (10%)
- Characteristically responsive to antibiotics; often fatal without treatment

Gross and Endoscopic Pathology

- Widespread infiltration of organs by mixed infiltrate consisting of foamy histiocytes, causing
  - Yellowish mucosal plaques in small bowel
  - Occasional shallow ulcers and hemorrhage
  - Thickened bowel wall
  - Enlarged mesenteric and retroperitoneal lymph nodes
  - Hepatosplenomegaly
  - Mesenteric fat and peritoneal plaques

Histopathology

- Lamina propria, muscularis mucosae, and superficial submucosa infiltrated by PAS, diastase-resistant–positive, foamy histiocytes, which contain the Whipple bacillus
- Intestinal villi are blunted by histiocytic infiltrate other than the histiocytes
- Typically minimal or no associated inflammatory infiltrate
- Characteristic large open round spaces in mucosa and submucosa (so-called fat vacuoles), although some represent dilated lymphatics
- Regional lymph nodes may contain foamy histiocytes
- Foreign-body epithelioid granulomas and lipogranulomas are sometimes seen in gastrointestinal mucosa, lymph nodes, spleen, muscles, lung, kidney, and brain

Special Stains and Immunohistochemistry

- Diastase-resistant PAS stain: Whipple bacilli within histiocytes are strongly positive; stain is coarsely granular, and bacillary structure cannot be seen
- AFB stain negative

Other Techniques for Diagnosis

- PCR: used to sequence the bacterial *16s* ribosomal gene
- Electron microscopy: demonstrates bacterial rods in macrophage cytoplasm

Differential Diagnosis

▌ MAI infection

- Similar histologic profile with sheets of foamy histiocyte-like cells in the lamina propria
- Differs in the conspicuous absence of fat vacuoles and dilated lymphatics
- Is faintly PAS positive; bacillary shape can still be seen
- More commonly seen in immunocompromised patients

▌ Histoplasmosis

- Characterized by presence of well-formed granulomas and infiltrates of histiocytes with less "foamy" cytoplasm
- Intracellular, 2- to 3-μm organisms seen with PAS or silver stain

Pearls

- Whipple disease is caused by an uncultured gram-positive bacillus called *Tropheryma whippelii*

Selected References

Baisden BL, Lepidi H, Raoult D, et al: Diagnosis of Whipple disease by immunohistochemical analysis. Am J Clin Pathol 118:742-748, 2002.

Dobbins WO III: Whipple's Disease. Springfield, IL, Charles C. Thomas, 1987.

Relman DA, Schmidt TM, MacDermott RP, Falkow S: Identification of the uncultured bacillus of Whipple's disease. N Engl J Med 327:293-301, 1992.

Figure 6-51. Endoscopic photograph of duodenum showing scalloped valvulae conniventes of celiac sprue.

Celiac Sprue

Clinical Features

- Also called gluten-sensitive enteropathy or celiac disease
- Malabsorptive disorder related to immunologic reaction to the toxic component of cereal grains, the gliadin-related proteins in wheat, rye, and barley
- Genetic predisposition in people of Irish and Northern European descent; much more common in whites; prevalence in the United States could be as high as 1%
- Classic presentation includes diarrhea, steatorrhea, flatulence, weight loss, and fatigue; failure to thrive may be seen in infants
- Can also present with iron or folate deficiency, anorexia, bone pain related to osteoporosis, and infertility
- Serologic testing includes IgA antiendomysial and anti–tissue transglutaminase antibody test; both are sensitive and specific
- Strong association with HLA-DQ2 (more than 98% of cases) and HLA-DQ8

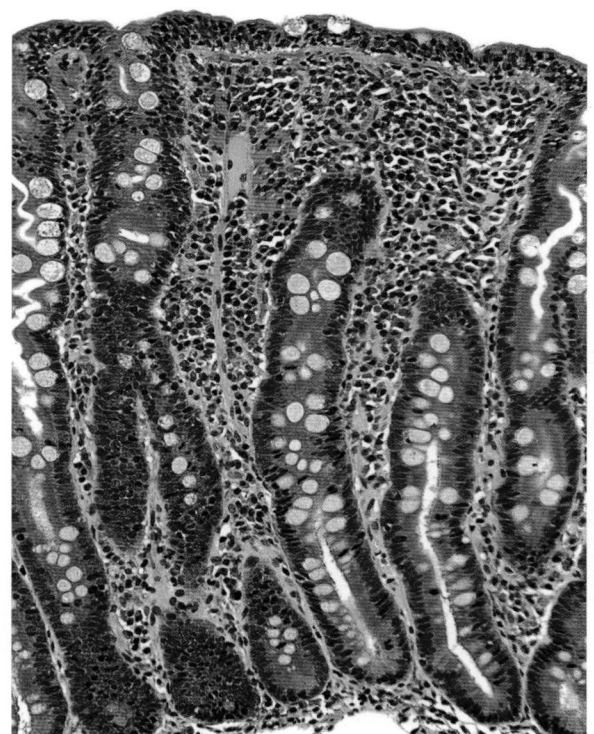

Figure 6-52. Celiac sprue. Histologic section shows a diffuse severe villous abnormality with crypt hyperplasia and epithelial lymphocytosis. The lamina propria is expanded by chronic inflammatory cells including plasma cells.

Figure 6-53. Celiac sprue at high magnification emphasizing the intraepithelial lymphocytosis.

Gross and Endoscopic Pathology

- Flattened mucosa typically most prominent in the proximal small intestine; may show scalloping of the valvulae conniventes

Histopathology

- Characteristic features include shortening of villi and transformation of tall, absorptive enterocytes interspersed with goblet cells and occasional intraepithelial lymphocytes into nonabsorptive low-cuboidal epithelium with nuclear stratification, few goblet cells, and many (>40 per 100 enterocytes) intraepithelial lymphocytes
- Surface epithelium shows loss of brush border, and crypts typically show increased mitotic activity
- Secondary features include crypt elongation and hyperplasia
- Lamina propria contains mixed inflammatory infiltrate (T and B lymphocytes, plasma cells, and eosinophils)

Special Stains and Immunohistochemistry

- Immunostains for LCA or CD3 can be used to evaluate intraepithelial component and may be helpful in recognizing epithelial lymphocytosis; immunostaining is not recommended
- PAS reveals loss of brush border

Other Techniques for Diagnosis

- Molecular evaluation should be considered in patients with refractory sprue or in celiac sprue patients developing small intestinal ulcer

Differential Diagnosis

- ▌ Normal mucosa
  - Malabsorption can be seen with normal small bowel histology (e.g., disaccharidase deficiency)
  - Normal villous to crypt ratio of 3:1 to 5:1
  - Up to 20 intraepithelial lymphocytes are considered normal
- ▌ Lymphocytic enterocolitis
  - Coexisting lymphocytic colitis and celiac sprue–like lesion of the proximal small bowel that is not responsive to gluten withdrawal
- ▌ Refractory or unclassified sprue
  - Refractory to gluten withdrawal
    - Refractory sprue type I
      - ◆ No atypical lymphocytes
      - ◆ Normal surface CD3 and CD8 intraepithelial lymphocytes
      - ◆ Polyclonal T-cell receptor
      - ◆ Responds to azathioprine and prednisone
      - ◆ Low rate of progression to enteropathy-associated T-cell lymphoma
    - Refractory sprue type II
      - ◆ May have scattered atypical lymphocytes
      - ◆ Loss of surface CD3 or CD8
      - ◆ Monoclonal T-cell receptor gene rearrangement (cryptic T-cell lymphoma)
      - ◆ Not responsive to azathioprine, prednisone, or interleukin-10 (IL-10)
      - ◆ About 50% case fatality rate, with most cases developing enteropathy-associated T-cell lymphoma
  - Allergic reaction to protein other than gluten
- ▌ Entities associated with variable villous abnormality with intraepithelial lymphocytosis (>30 lymphocytes per 100 enterocytes)
  - Latent or partially treated celiac sprue (about 10% of patients)
  - Tropical sprue (2% of patients)
    - Occurs in natives and naive visitors to specific tropical locations (e.g., India, Africa, Southeast Asia, Central America, West Indies)
    - Treated with broad-spectrum antibiotics (believed to be infectious etiology) and vitamins
  - Dermatitis herpetiformis
  - Infectious gastroenteritis and stasis
  - Peptic ulceration
  - Autoimmune diseases (e.g., rheumatoid arthritis, Graves disease, Crohn disease)
  - NSAID-related lesions
  - Autoimmune enteritis
- ▌ Entities associated with severe villous abnormality and crypt hypoplasia
  - Kwashiorkor, marasmus
  - Megaloblastic anemia
  - Radiation and chemotherapy effect
  - Microvillus inclusion disease

❚ Entities associated with variable villous abnormality that contain specific diagnostic changes
  ● Collagenous sprue
    — Increased subepithelial collagen plate
  ● Common variable immune deficiency and selective IgA immunodeficiency
    — Nodular lymphoid hyperplasia with reduced numbers of plasma cells within the lamina propria
    — Increased apoptotic bodies
    — May have comorbid giardiasis
  ● Eosinophilic gastroenteritis
  ● Parasitic infestation
  ● Waldenström macroglobulinemia
    — Lymphangiectasia with intralymphatic amorphous eosinophilic material
    — Foamy macrophages in lamina propria
  ● Lymphangiectasia
  ● Abetalipoproteinemia
    — Enterocytes with intracytoplasmic vacuoles

Pearls

● Diagnosis is best made by correlation of clinical history with serology and histologic features (documentation of malabsorption, characteristic histologic features, and improvement of symptoms and resolution of histologic abnormalities on removal of gluten from the diet)
● Removal of gluten from the diet is typically curative
● Withdrawal of gluten causes a return to normal that progresses from distal to proximal (i.e., duodenum is the last to recover); must consider where biopsy is taken from when evaluating recovery
● Fundamental pathology is derived from an immunologic attack on surface enterocytes (transformation to nonabsorptive, low-cuboidal cells with stratified nuclei and numerous interspersed lymphocytes)
● Always consider T-cell lymphoma in patients who present with refractory sprue or in celiac sprue patients who have developed small intestinal ulcers (perform immunohistochemistry or PCR)

Selected References

Hadithi M, vonBlomberg BM, Crusius JB, et al: Accuracy of serologic tests and HLA-DQ typing for diagnosing celiac disease. Ann Intern Med 147:294-302, 2007.

Cellier C, Cerf-Bensussan N: Treatment of clonal refractory celiac disease or cryptic intraepithelial lymphoma: A long road from bench to bedside. Clin Gastroenterol Hepatol 4:1320-1321, 2006.

Gramlich T, Petras R: The small intestine. In Sternberg SS (ed): Histology for Pathologists, 3rd ed. Philadelphia, Lippincott Williams & Wilkins, 2006, pp 603-626.

Kagnoff MF: AGA Institute Medical Position Statement on the Diagnosis and Management of Celiac Disease. Gastroenterology 131:1977-1980, 2006.

Rostom A, Murray JA, Kagnoff MF: American Gastroenterological Association (AGA) Institute Technical Review on the Diagnosis and Management of Celiac Disease. Gastroenterology 131:1981-2002, 2006.

Petras R: Non-Neoplastic Intestinal Diseases. In Mills SE (ed): Sternberg's Diagnostic Surgical Pathology, 4th ed. New York, Lippincott Williams & Wilkins, 2004, pp 1475-1541.

Kakar S, Nehra V, Murray JA, et al: Significance of intraepithelial lymphocytosis in small bowel biopsy samples with normal mucosal architecture. Am J Gastroenterol 98:2027-2033, 2003.

Small Intestinal Adenoma and Adenocarcinoma

Clinical Features

● Primary adenomas and adenocarcinomas that occur in the small intestine are often associated with underlying conditions such as the FAP syndromes (FAP, attenuated FAP, and MYH-associated polyposis syndrome) and Lynch syndrome
● More common small bowel malignancies are metastases, lymphoma, and carcinoid tumor
❚ Adenoma
  ● Small intestinal adenomas are extremely rare (<0.05% of all intestinal adenomas)
  ● Often admixed with adenocarcinoma (65% of all small bowel adenomas)

Figure 6-54. Duodenal intraepithelial lymphocytosis. This variable villous abnormality shows villi of near-normal length with increased (>30 per 100 enterocytes) intraepithelial lymphocytes.

Figure 6-55. Small bowel adenoma in familial adenomatous polyposis. The adenoma resembles colonic tubular adenomas.

Figure 6-56. Gastric heterotopia. This histologic section shows specialized gastric glands beneath surface duodenal mucosa.

- Most arise around the major duodenal papilla and present with biliary colic, cholangitis, jaundice, and pancreatitis
- Patients with the familial adenomatous polyposis syndromes have up to a 300 times greater risk for developing carcinoma than nonpolyposis patients

- Adenocarcinoma
  - Far less common than colonic adenocarcinoma
  - Risk factors include Lynch syndrome, Peutz-Jeghers syndrome, and Crohn disease
  - More common in black men; mean age at diagnosis is 55 years
  - Most cases occur in duodenum near major duodenal papilla; Crohn disease–associated adenocarcinoma tends to involve the ileum
  - Symptoms include obstruction or bleeding as well as jaundice and pancreatitis

Gross and Endoscopic Pathology

- Adenoma
  - Typically multilobulated and soft
  - May be pedunculated or sessile
  - Tubular adenomas tend to be small (<3 cm)
  - Villous adenomas are more common and are larger (mean, 5 cm)
  - Adenomas in patients with FAP are often multiple
- Adenocarcinoma
  - About 25% of lesions are polypoid
  - About 75% are ulcerated
  - Range in size from less than 2 cm up to 15 cm
  - Those described with Crohn disease are often strictured

Histopathology

- Adenoma
  - Recapitulates histology of colonic adenomas with tubular, tubulovillous, and villous morphology
  - Tubular adenoma
    - Tubelike glands lined by epithelial cells containing hyperchromatic stratified nuclei with mitotic figures at all crypt levels, and few goblet cells
    - About 20% of tubular adenomas contain cancer
  - Villous adenoma
    - Papillary fronds containing central lamina propria cores lined by similar epithelium to that seen in tubular adenomas
    - Nearly 30% to 60% of villous lesions harbor invasive cancer
  - Glandular complexity with complete loss of polarity indicates high-grade dysplasia and carcinoma in situ; glandular fusion or an infiltrative pattern indicates at least intramucosal carcinoma; an infiltration pattern to atypical glands and desmoplasia indicates invasion of at least the submucosa
- Adenocarcinoma
  - Typically arises in association with an adenoma; adenocarcinoma in the setting of Crohn disease often demonstrates glandular dysplasia
  - Malignant histology includes mucinous differentiation, cribriform glands, fused glands, marked stratification, cytologic anaplasia, and, most important, desmoplasia; atypical glands adjacent to

large blood vessels, fat, or ganglion cells often accompany submucosal invasion
- Uncommon histology includes papillary adenosquamous carcinoma, signet ring cell carcinoma, and small cell carcinoma

Special Stains and Immunohistochemistry
- Noncontributory

Other Techniques for Diagnosis
- Noncontributory

Differential Diagnosis
▌ Brunner gland nodules
- Most cases of Brunner gland enlargement are probably hyperplasia because they maintain a normal lobular architecture, demonstrate little mitotic activity, and are histologically mature
- Brunner gland nodules may produce a mass lesion, but the histology is usually not adenomatous and can be readily distinguished from adenoma and adenocarcinoma
- True Brunner gland adenoma and adenocarcinoma are thought to be rare but typically demonstrate transition from normal Brunner glands to adenomatous or adenocarcinomatous tissue

▌ Heterotopic gastric mucosa
- Generally small mucosal lesions that are polypoid and are composed of recognizable gastric mucosa with specialized glands (heterotopia) or foveolar epithelium (metaplasia)
- Hyperplastic polyp of gastric type can develop from either; probably the most common proximal small bowel polyp

Pearls
- Many adenomas are complicated by invasive malignancy; specimens require careful examination
- When high-grade dysplasia or intramucosal carcinoma is identified in an adenoma, endoscopic mucosal resection or operative resection should be considered because of the high risk for coexisting invasive carcinoma
- Carcinoma in the small bowel away from the major duodenal papilla is more likely to be metastatic than primary; get the patient's full clinical history
- Ileal small bowel adenocarcinoma can be seen in patients with Crohn disease

Selected References
Riddell RH, Petras RE, Williams GT, Sobin LH: Tumors of the intestines. Atlas of Tumor Pathology Third Series, Fascicle #32. Washington, DC, Armed Forces Institute of Pathology, 2003.

Bjork J, Akerbant H, Iselius L, et al: Periampullary adenomas and adenocarcinomas in familial adenomatous polyposis: cumulative risks and APC gene mutations. Gastroenterology 121:1127-1135, 2001.

Sigel JE, Petras RE, Lashner BA, et al: Intestinal adenocarcinoma in Crohn's disease: A report of 30 cases with a focus on coexisting dysplasia. Am J Surg Pathol 23:651-655, 1999.

Lein GS, Mori M, Enjoji M: Primary carcinoma of the small intestine: A clinicopathologic and immunohistochemical study. Cancer 61:316-323, 1988.

Petras R, Mir-Madjlessi S, Farmer R: Crohn's disease and intestinal carcinoma: A report of 11 cases with emphasis on epithelial dysplasia. Gastroenterology 93:1307-1314, 1987.

Sarre R, Frost A, Jagelman D, et al: Gastric and duodenal polyps in familial adenomatous polyposis: A prospective study of the nature and prevalence of upper gastrointestinal polyps. Gut 28:306-314, 1987.

Zollinger RM Jr: Primary neoplasms of the small intestine. Am J Surg 151:654-658, 1986.

Reddy RR, Schuman BM, Priest RJ: Duodenal polyps: diagnosis and management. J Clin Gastroenterol 3:139-147, 1981.

Carcinoid Tumor of the Small and Large Intestine

Clinical Features
- Carcinoid tumors may be found in any organ in which neuroendocrine cells occur
- About 85% of carcinoid tumors arise in the gastrointestinal tract (constitute about 50% of small intestinal malignancies and less than 2% of colorectal malignancies)
- Most gastrointestinal carcinoid tumors occur in the vermiform appendix, followed by the small intestine (typically ileum), rectum, stomach, and colon
- Most patients are 50 to 70 years old
- May be found incidentally, or patients may present with weight loss, obstruction, or carcinoid syndrome
- Possible secretory products include serotonin, gastrin, somatostatin, VIP, ACTH, and insulin

Figure 6-57. Ileal carcinoid in a resection specimen presenting as a polypoid intraluminal lesion.

Figure 6-58. Carcinoid tumor of the terminal ileum infiltrating the lamina propria. Note the insular arrangement of carcinoid tumor cells showing pseudoglandular formation.

— Carcinoid syndrome
  ◆ Occurs in 10% of patients; more common in patients with an ileal carcinoid tumor
  ◆ Usually indicates hepatic metastasis (precluding hepatic degradation of vasoactive amines)
  ◆ Symptoms include flushing, sweating, cardiac symptoms, and diarrhea
  ◆ About 50% of patients have endocardial right heart lesion
  ◆ Symptoms arise because of increased levels of 5-HT and 5-HIAA

Gross and Endoscopic Pathology

- Location of small and large intestinal carcinoid tumors is as follows: 1% duodenal, 7% jejunal, 80% ileal, and 10% rectal
- Typically small, firm, tan-yellow mucosal or mural nodules that are covered by intact mucosa; sometimes present with mural thickening and stricture
- Rarely larger than 3 cm (often smaller than 1 cm, making them difficult to locate clinically)

Histopathology

- Composed of uniform cells with round, central, monomorphic nuclei showing finely stippled chromatin and scant cytoplasm; faint red cytoplasmic granules can often be seen

- Mitotic rate is low
- Classic architectural patterns include
  — Solid or insular arrangement of cells
  — Ribbons (festoons) or trabeculae
  — Tubules or glands (rosette-like)
- Some tumors may show glandular differentiation
- Typically well circumscribed but may have an infiltrative growth pattern at the periphery
- Cytologic features and evidence of vascular, lymphatic, or perineural invasion do not predict behavior
- Atypical carcinoid (intermediate-grade neuroendocrine carcinoma)
  — Occasionally tumors show neuroendocrine cellular morphology but are composed of pleomorphic cells with large, irregular hyperchromatic nuclei and prominent nucleoli
  — Increased mitotic activity and necrosis are common in these tumors
- Small cell carcinoma, similar to pulmonary primary

Special Stains and Immunohistochemistry

- Chromogranin, synaptophysin positive
- Virtually all carcinoid tumors contain varying numbers of cells that can be identified with hormonal antibodies, including
  — Serotonin
  — Somatostatin
  — Gastrin
  — VIP
  — ACTH
  — Insulin
- Cytokeratin positive in 65% to 70% of cases

Other Techniques for Diagnosis

- Proliferative index and DNA content reportedly correlate with survival (not routinely performed)

Differential Diagnosis

▌ Mixed carcinoid-adenocarcinoma
- Tends to be larger infiltrating tumors
- Mixed histology, including areas of typical carcinoid admixed with carcinomatous areas; carcinoma typically constitutes greater than 50% of the tumor
- Must be distinguished from benign epithelial differentiation within typical carcinoid tumors
- More aggressive behavior; will act like adenocarcinoma

▌ Adenocarcinoma
- Invasive growth pattern with glandular differentiation
- Increased cytologic atypia
- Generally lacks neuroendocrine differentiation (i.e., only scattered cells)
- Lacks the monomorphic nuclear characteristics of carcinoid tumor

Pearls

- Risk for metastasis increases with tumor size
  — Less than 1 cm: 2%
  — One to 2 cm: 50% (ileal); 15% (rectal)
  — More than 2 cm: 80%
- All carcinoids are potentially malignant
- Clinical evidence of metastases is best method to determine malignant potential; histologic features are unreliable
- Deep local mural penetration by tumor correlates with decreased survival, as does presence of hepatic and nodal metastasis
- Overall (5-year) survival rate for small bowel carcinoid tumors is 90%
- Gastrinoma
  — Often multiple, but typically small
  — Associated with Zollinger-Ellison syndrome and MEN-I syndrome
  — Usually malignant behavior
- Insulinoma
  — May also be associated with MEN-I syndrome and hypoglycemia
  — Usually benign behavior

Selected References

Williams GT: Endocrine tumours of the gastrointestinal tract: Selected topics. Histopathology 50:30-41, 2007.

Nikou GC, Lygidakis NJ, Toubanakis C, et al: Current diagnosis and treatment of gastrointestinal carcinoids in a series of 101 patients: The significance of serum chromogranin-A, somatostatin receptor scintigraphy and somatostatin analogues. Hepatogastroenterology 52:731-741, 2005.

Riddell RH, Petras RE, Williams GT, Sobin LH: Tumors of the intestines. Atlas of Tumor Pathology Third Series, Fascicle #32. Washington, DC, Armed Forces Institute of Pathology, 2003.

Capella C, Heitz PU, Hofler H, et al: Revised classification of neuroendocrine tumors of the lung, pancreas and gut. Virchows Arch 425:547-560, 1995.

Dayal Y, O'Brian DS, Wolfe HJ, et al: Carcinoid tumors: a comparison of their immunocytochemical hormonal profile with morphologic and histochemical characteristics. Lab Invest 42:1111, 1980.

Hirschsprung Disease (HD)

Clinical Features

- Uncommon disease affecting 1 in 5000 to 30,000 live births
- About 80% of patients are male
- Small percentage of patients have other congenital anomalies
- Presenting features include constipation, abdominal obstruction, meconium plug
- Patients with Down syndrome are at increased risk for HD

Gross and Endoscopic Pathology

- Classic resected colon consists of a dilated (neurologically normal) proximal segment that narrows (hypoganglionated area) into a contracted (aganglionic) distal segment
- May produce toxic megacolon
- Multiple forms exist
  — Short-segment HD: as little as 3 cm of distal rectum affected (most common form)
  — Long-segment HD: extends beyond sigmoid colon, can involve entire colon and a variable length of small intestine (about 10% of patients)

Histopathology

- Absence of ganglion cells from the submucosal and myenteric plexuses
- Hypertrophy of the mural nerves
- Long-segment HD may have normal caliber nerves and false-negative acetylcholinesterase stain (see later)

Special Stains and Immunohistochemistry

- Acetylcholinesterase reactions (on frozen tissue): patients with HD demonstrate coarse, irregular nerve fibers extending from the muscularis mucosae up into the lamina propria (normal tissue contains only thin fibers, which are only in muscularis mucosae)
- Neuron-specific enolase (NSE) positive in ganglion cells; other immunostains (e.g., Cathepsin D, PGP9.5, bcl-2) can decorate ganglion cells
- S-100 protein: Schwann cells show perinuclear positivity

Other Techniques for Diagnosis

- Gene mutations detected in 50% of patients include inactivation mutation of *RET* oncogene, mutations in endothelin receptor B; at least nine other gene mutations have been implicated

Differential Diagnosis

▌ Hypoganglionosis
- Can cause HD-like syndrome with megacolon
- No accepted definition, but should be diagnosed in patients with a substantial reduction in ganglion cell numbers compared with normal (40 to 80 myenteric neurons per 1 cm of bowel); can be zonal
- Some examples of hypoganglionosis could be similar to idiopathic constipation

▌ Intestinal neuronal dysplasia
- Clinically mimics HD, and patients typically present with constipation
- Differentiated by presence of hyperplastic plexuses and giant ganglia containing more than seven neurons

- Diagnostic criteria and even the existence of intestinal neuronal dysplasia debated
- Diagnosis should be reserved for florid cases

▌ Idiopathic constipation

- Occurs more often in females and produces intestinal pseudo-obstruction
- Ganglion cells are present; distinctive abnormalities of the myenteric plexus (e.g., loss of argyrophilic neurons) described
- Reduced volume of interstitial cells of Cajal reported in some cases

Pearls

- Biopsy specimens in actual cases of HD usually contain hypertrophic nerves, but their presence is not diagnostic
- There can be overlap in the histologic changes described in intestinal neuronal dysplasia and neurofibromatosis

Selected References

Kapur RP: Can we stop looking? Immunohistochemistry and the diagnosis of Hirschsprung's disease. Am J Clin Pathol 126:9-12, 2006.

Toman J, Turina M, Ray M, et al: Slow transit colon constipation is not related to the number of interstitial cells of Cajal. Int J Colorectal Dis 21:527-532, 2006.

Meier-Ruge WA, Ammann K, Bruder E, et al: Updated results on intestinal neuronal dysplasia. Eur J Pediatr Surg 14:384-391, 2004.

Streutker CJ, Huizinga JD, Campbell F, et al: Loss of CD117 (c-kit) and CD34-positive ICC and associated CD34-positive fibroblasts defines a subpopulation of chronic intestinal pseudo-obstruction. Am J Surg Pathol 27:228-235, 2003.

Maia DM: The reliability of frozen-section diagnosis in the pathologic evaluation of Hirschsprung's disease. Am J Surg Pathol 24:1675-1677, 2000.

Robertson K, Mason I, Hall S: Hirschsprung's disease: Genetic mutation in mice and men. Gut 41:436-441, 1997.

Lake BD: Intestinal neuronal dysplasia: Why does it only occur in parts of Europe? Virchows Arch 426:537-539, 1995.

Yunis EJ, Dobbins EW, Sherman FE: Rectal suction biopsy in the diagnosis of Hirschsprung's disease in infants. Arch Pathol Lab Med 100:329-333, 1976.

Diverticular Disease

Clinical Features

- Most common in societies consuming a Western-style diet (high fat, low fiber)
- In the United States, 50% of adults older than 40 years are affected
- Only 20% of patients have symptoms; particularly obese individuals
- Formation of diverticula is related to weakness in the colonic wall and increased intraluminal pressure
- Symptoms may be related to diverticulitis, which includes lower abdominal pain, rebound tenderness, and fever; symptoms can occur without inflammation
- Patients may have symptoms related to anemia from chronic hemorrhage or have massive acute lower gastrointestinal bleeding
- Complications include obstruction, perforation, peritonitis, hemorrhage, abscess formation, and fistula
- Mucosal prolapse is common in patients with diverticular disease

Gross and Endoscopic Pathology

- Small oval or spherical outpouchings along the large intestine
- About 90% involve the sigmoid colon
- Typically form adjacent to penetrating mural arteries and alongside taeniae coli
- Adjacent muscularis propria may be thickened

Histopathology

- Classic lesion is a protrusion of the mucosa and submucosa through the muscularis propria
- Diverticula may have a flattened or atrophic mucosa and compressed submucosa
- Adjacent tissue, including the muscular propria, is hypertrophied, fibrotic, and chronically inflamed
- Acute inflammation indicates acute diverticulitis; may form peridiverticular abscesses

Special Stains and Immunohistochemistry

- Noncontributory

Other Techniques for Diagnosis

- Noncontributory

Differential Diagnosis

▌ Inflammatory bowel disease (particularly Crohn disease)

- Both conditions may cause focal mucosal inflammation and thickening of the bowel wall with stricture and fistula; conditions may coexist
- Crohn disease is distinguished by fissural ulcers, ulcers and mucosal inflammation outside of the areas of diverticulitis, transmural inflammation, serosal lymphoid aggregates, superficial aphthous ulcers, and granulomas

Pearls

- Comprehensive gross examination may be necessary to detect subtle luminal openings of the diverticula in the resected colon
- Clinical, radiographic, and even, to some extent, gross features of diverticulosis may mimic carcinoma; however, a mucosal mass is absent
- Colovesical and colovaginal fistula can complicate diverticular disease; other fistulas must increase index of suspicion for coexisting Crohn disease

Selected References

Goldstein NS, Leon-Armin C, Mani A: Crohn's colitis-like changes in sigmoid diverticulitis specimens is usually an idiosyncratic inflammatory response to the diverticulosis rather than Crohn's colitis. Am J Surg Pathol 24:668-675, 2000.

Imperiali G, Meucci G, Alvisi C, et al: Segmental colitis associated with diverticula: A prospective study. Gruppo di Studio per le Malattie Infiammatorie Intestinali (GSMII). Am J Gastroenterol 95:1014-1016, 2000.

Makapugay LM, Dean PJ: Diverticular disease-associated chronic colitis. Am J Surg Pathol 20:94-102, 1996.

Shepherd NA: Diverticular disease and chronic idiopathic inflammatory bowel disease: Associations and masquerades. Gut 38:801-802, 1996.

Eosinophilic Gastroenteritis

Clinical Features

- Syndrome characterized by gastrointestinal symptoms combined with eosinophilic infiltration of the gastrointestinal tract in the absence of a specific allergen or parasitic infestation, usually seen in children and young adults
- Most patients have peripheral blood eosinophilia (70% of cases)
- Most patients have a history of allergies
- Patients present with variable symptoms ranging from mild nausea and vomiting to an acute abdomen
- Other symptoms include diarrhea, malabsorption, obstruction, or ascites (often depends on level of the bowel wall involved)
- Often have elevation of serum IL-5 levels

Gross and Endoscopic Pathology

- Affects any level of gastrointestinal tract; stomach and small bowel are most common sites; less commonly affects the colon
- Radiographic studies often disclose widened mucosal folds and mural thickening
- Diffuse involvement may occur, producing bowel rigidity and edema

Histopathology

- Three patterns of eosinophilic gastroenteritis described
  — Mucosal involvement typically causing diarrhea and malabsorption
  — Submucosal involvement associated with intestinal obstruction
  — Mural and serosal involvement leading to ascites and eosinophilic peritonitis
- Diffuse, sheetlike infiltrate of eosinophils typically involving the lamina propria, crypts, or villi
- Often associated with mucosal edema, crypt hyperplasia, or villous atrophy
- Mural fibrosis or muscular hypertrophy can occur
- Serosal involvement may induce subserosal fibrosis

Special Stains and Immunohistochemistry

- Noncontributory

Other Techniques for Diagnosis

- Noncontributory

Differential Diagnosis

- Numerous diseases present with eosinophilic infiltrates; rule out allergies, lymphoma, foreign bodies, systemic vasculitis, drug reaction, and parasitic infestation
- ▌Cow's milk allergy
  - Typically affects neonatal or young infants with sensitivity to milk protein; generally responds to prompt switch to soy-based or hydrolysate formula
  - Infants present with severe diarrhea, dehydration, and failure to thrive
  - Characterized by villous atrophy, neutrophilic infiltrates, and eosinophilic infiltrate
  - Overall prognosis is excellent
- ▌Other food allergies
  - Affects 45% of the population and nearly 10% of children
  - Histologically similar to eosinophilic gastroenteritis
  - Requires correlation of symptoms with exposure to a specific food

Pearls

- Resist temptation to suggest eosinophilic gastroenteritis at the sight of eosinophils, which are a normal component of the gastrointestinal mucosa
  — Collections of eosinophils not associated with other inflammatory cells, groupings of eosinophils associated with mucosal architectural change or injury (e.g., crypt abscesses), and infiltration of the muscularis mucosae and deeper bowel layers are all considered abnormal and in a corroborative clinical setting should be considered diagnostic of eosinophilic gastroenteritis
- Whenever collections of eosinophils are seen, it makes sense to check for parasites

Selected References

Orenstein SR, Shalaby TM, DiLorenzo C, et al: The spectrum of pediatric eosinophilic esophagitis beyond infancy: A clinical series of 30 children. Am J Gastroenterol 95:1422-1430, 2000.

Walsh SV, Antonioli DA, Goldman H, et al: Allergic esophagitis in children: A clinicopathologic entity. Am J Surg Pathol 23:390-396, 1999.

Lee M, Hodges WG, Huggins TL: Eosinophilic gastroenteritis. South Med J 89:189-194, 1996.

Steffen RM, Wyllie R, Petras RE, et al: The spectrum of eosinophilic gastroenteritis: Report of six pediatric cases and review of the literature. Clin Pediatr 30:404-411, 1991.

McNabb PC, Fleming CR, Higgins JA, Davis GL: Transmural
eosinophilic gastroenteritis with ascites. Mayo Clin Proc
54:119-122, 1979.

Graft-versus-Host Disease (GVHD)

Clinical Features

- Characterized by immunologic reaction between
  (engrafted) donor T lymphocytes and epithelial cells
  of recipient (host)
- Skin, biliary tract, and gastrointestinal epithelium
  may be involved
- Most commonly occurs after bone marrow
  transplantation
- Clinical severity is determined partially by degree of
  histocompatibility mismatch; however, may also
  occur in exact major histocompatibility matches,
  owing to minor histocompatibility antigen mismatch
- Acute GVHD
  — Usually occurs within first 100 days of
    transplantation
  — Typical gastrointestinal symptoms include
    diarrhea and abdominal pain
- Recalcitrant cases may progress to chronic GVHD
- Most episodes initially involve skin
- Gastrointestinal tract is involved in 70% of cases

Gross and Endoscopic Pathology

- Variable appearance
- Mucosal erythema and ulcers can be seen
  endoscopically
- Gross and endoscopic features generally do not
  correlate well with clinical severity

Histopathology

- Base of crypts shows single epithelial cell necrosis
  creating a lacuna containing nuclear debris (known
  as apoptosis)

Figure 6-59. Graft-versus-host disease demonstrating numerous
apoptotic bodies.

- May progressively worsen to include many crypts or
  entire epithelium; may produce crypt abscess and
  large areas of ulceration and fungal secondary
  infection
- Chronic or unresolved episodes may contain
  atrophic, fibrotic, or regenerating epithelium and
  mucosa

Special Stains and Immunohistochemistry

- Generally unnecessary in the diagnosis of GVHD, but
  stains for fungi, parasites, and viruses (particularly
  CMV) may be indicated

Other Techniques for Diagnosis

- Noncontributory

Differential Diagnosis

▌ Chemotherapy and radiation effect
  - Causes apoptosis; these changes last up to 100 days
▌ Opportunistic infection
  - Must always be considered along with GVHD in the
    post-transplantation setting
  - Characteristic organisms or cytopathic changes must
    be recognized for diagnosis

Pearls

- Apoptotic cells are present in the skin, bile duct
  epithelium, and gastrointestinal tract in GVHD
- Cytotoxic T cell is the perpetrator
- Steroids given for GVHD treatment may predispose to
  reactivation of CMV infection

Selected References

Asplund S, Gramlich TL: Chronic mucosal changes of the colon
in graft-versus-host disease. Mod Pathol 11:513-515, 1998.
Cox G, Matsui S, Lo R, et al: Etiology and outcome of diarrhea
after marrow transplantation: A prospective study.
Gastroenterology 107:1398-1407, 1994.
McGregor GI, Shepherd JD, Phillips G: Acute graft-versus-host
disease of the intestine: A surgical perspective. Am J Surg
155:680-682, 1988.
McDonal GB, Shulman HM, Sullivan KM, Spencer GD: Intestinal
and hepatic complications of human bone marrow
transplantation. Parts I and II. Gastroenterology 90:460–477,
770-784, 1986.
Sale GE, Shulman HM: The pathology of bone marrow
transplantation. New York, Masson, 1984.
Sale GE, Shulman HM, McDonald GB, Thomas ED:
Gastrointestinal graft-versus-host disease in man: A clinical
pathologic study of the rectal biopsy. Am J Surg Pathol 3:291-
299, 1979.

Inflammatory Bowel Disease (IBD)

Clinical Features

- Chronic, recurrent gastrointestinal inflammatory
  disease of unknown etiology

Figure 6-60. Resection specimen of small intestinal Crohn disease with areas of stricture and fat wrapping.

Figure 6-62. Resection specimen of ulcerative colitis. The distalmost margin is involved by the inflammatory process. More proximal involvement is in continuity with the involved rectum.

Figure 6-61. Colonic resection specimen of Crohn disease showing cobblestoning. Cobblestoning is created by the combination of two ulcer patterns, longitudinally oriented linear ulcers and small horizontal crevices, which isolate small islands of relatively intact colonic mucosa.

Figure 6-63. Crohn disease of the colon showing transmural lymphoid aggregates in an area not deeply ulcerated.

- Familial predisposition; 10-fold increased risk for first-degree relatives
- Peak incidence in young adults
- Whites are more commonly affected than nonwhites
- Slight female predominance
▌Crohn disease
- Incidence of 3 per 100,000 people in United States
- Small bowel Crohn disease is associated with IBD-1 gene (*NOD2/CARD15*)

- Usually begins with intermittent episodes of mild diarrhea, fever, and abdominal pain over weeks to months
- About 20% of patients present with severe, acute onset of abdominal pain
- Intestinal complications include strictures, fistula, and malabsorption

Figure 6-64. Ulcerative colitis in a resection specimen showing architectural and inflammatory changes limited to the mucosa.

Figure 6-65. Gross photograph of fulminant primary inflammatory bowel disease of an indeterminate type, probably Crohn disease, showing areas of deep ulceration and involvement of the terminal ileum.

- Extraintestinal complications include polyarthritis, ankylosing spondylitis, primary sclerosing cholangitis (uncommon), and uveitis
- Increased risk for small bowel and colonic adenocarcinoma
▍ Ulcerative colitis
  - Incidence of 4 to 12 per 100,000 people in the United States

- Presents with episodic attacks of lower abdominal pain and bloody diarrhea over months, years, or decades
- About 30% require colectomy within 3 years
- Intestinal complications include toxic megacolon and perforation; both can occur during severe episodes
- Extraintestinal complications include polyarthritis, sacroiliitis, ankylosing spondylitis, uveitis, and primary sclerosing cholangitis
- Risk for carcinoma: previous reports have estimated 30% at 35 years after onset; however, recent estimates now indicate that progression may actually be lower

Gross and Endoscopic Pathology

▍ Crohn disease
  - Involves any level of gastrointestinal tract from mouth to anus; classically affects the small bowel
  - Mesenteric fat of the involved segment wraps around the bowel surface ("creeping fat" or "fat wrapping")
  - Thickened, stiff intestinal wall (stovepipe) with normal-appearing intervening segments (skip lesions)
  - Early disease is characterized by aphthous ulcers that progress to discrete ulceration, serpiginous ulcers, linear ulcers, or cobblestoning
  - Cobblestoning results from two different ulceration patterns: linear ulcers and small horizontal crevices. The sharp demarcation between edematous but otherwise normal mucosa and surrounding ulcers gives the mucosa a cobblestone appearance
  - Ulcers deepen into fissures and can ultimately produce fistulas
  - Luminal narrowing often causes characteristic string sign on x-ray
▍ Ulcerative colitis
  - Classically demonstrates involvement of the rectum and variable length of large intestine (without skip lesions)
  - Often involves the entire colon (pan-colitis) and occasionally spills into ileum (so-called backwash ileitis); in some classification schemes, ileal involvement is a criterion for inflammatory bowel disease of indeterminate type
  - Irregular areas of ulceration, which may be widespread, can surround islands of preserved mucosa (pseudopolyps and inflammatory polyps)
  - Deep ulcers extending to the muscularis externa usually correlate with fulminant clinical disease and are a pathologic criterion for inflammatory bowel disease of an indeterminate type in some schemes
  - Normal serosa unless complicated by fulminant disease

Histopathology

■ Crohn disease
- Classic features include patchy, transmural chronic inflammation with intervening normal areas (skip lesions)
- Acute inflammatory fissures penetrate the muscularis externa
- Associated lymphoid aggregates occur throughout the bowel wall but often along the serosa (rosary bead pattern)
- Granulomas occur in up to 50% cases, both in actively involved and uninvolved tissue
- In chronic disease, Paneth cell and pyloric metaplasia occur
- Neutrophilic infiltrates and crypt abscesses may occur
- Hypertrophied muscularis mucosae, submucosal neural hyperplasia, and mural fibrosis may evolve into strictures

■ Ulcerative colitis
- Characterized by a dense lymphoplasmacytic and neutrophilic infiltrate generally limited to the mucosa and superficial submucosa
- Inflammatory infiltrate is between widely spaced, regenerating, architecturally distorted glands containing intraepithelial and luminal neutrophils (cryptitis and crypt abscess)
- Inflammation may extend into muscularis propria beneath areas of ulceration in fulminant disease; in some classification schemes, this feature would indicate fulminant primary inflammatory bowel disease of an indeterminate type
- In chronic disease, regenerated glands are distorted and may be branched or shortened (above muscularis mucosae); may contain decreased numbers of goblet cells
- Some patients develop epithelial dysplasia in both flat and elevated lesions (see "Dysplasia in Inflammatory Bowel Disease")

Special Stains and Immunohistochemistry

- Noncontributory

Other Techniques for Diagnosis

- Serologic tests such as pANCA (for ulcerative colitis) and ASCA (for Crohn disease) can be helpful but are positive in only 50% of patients
- Genetic test for *NOD2/CARD15* mutation associated with small bowel Crohn disease is commercially available

Differential Diagnosis

■ Acute self-limited colitis
- A self-limited, short-lived (<6 months) disease presumably due to pathogenic organisms
- Characterized clinically by sudden onset of diarrhea and abdominal pain
- Shows the focal colitis pattern of injury with acute inflammation that predominates over chronic lymphoplasmacytic infiltrates
- Gland alterations are not seen
- Active inflammation associated with little or no mucin depletion
- Neutrophils in the lamina propria

■ Lymphocytic colitis
- Characterized by a moderate mixed inflammatory infiltrate in the lamina propria but lacking architectural distortion and crypt abscesses
- By definition, lymphocytic colitis demonstrates increased intraepithelial lymphocytes (>15 per 100 surface epithelial cells)
- Unlike that in IBD, the clinical setting includes profuse, watery diarrhea and normal colonoscopy

■ Collagenous colitis
- Histologically similar to lymphocytic colitis, but distinguished by presence of a thickened collagen layer beneath the surface basement membrane (>15 μm)
- Feathery strands of collagen extend between glands and displace the inflammatory cells downward
- Presence of Paneth cell metaplasia in collagenous colitis correlates with more severe diarrhea and can cause confusion with IBD
- IBD typically shows greater inflammation, lacks the subepithelial collagen layer, includes more neutrophils, crypt abscesses, architectural distortion (bifid and widely spaced glands), minimal intraepithelial lymphocytes (<6 per 100 colonic epithelial cells), and abnormal endoscopy

■ Diversion colitis
- Occurs in a segment of colon excluded from the fecal stream; most often a Hartmann pouch constructed at the time of resection of a proximal segment of colon
- About one third of patients are symptomatic with passage of mucous discharge or blood
- Histologic features include prominent lymphoid aggregates and follicles and a dense lymphoid infiltrate in lamina propria
- Scattered neutrophilic infiltrate with foci of cryptitis and rare crypt abscesses may be seen
- Crypt architecture is usually normal
- Often superimposed on changes of ulcerative colitis or Crohn disease in the rectum following colectomy in patients with primary inflammatory bowel disease
- Cured by resumption of fecal stream; can be treated with short-chain fatty acid enemas

■ Indeterminate colitis
- Diagnosed when clinical, endoscopic, and biopsy findings have features of both Crohn disease and ulcerative colitis or when resected specimen shows deep ulceration, pseudopolyps, and glandular alterations with ambiguous gross and histologic features

Pearls

- IBD is characterized by increased mixed inflammation of the lamina propria, increased basal plasma cells reaching the muscularis mucosae, glandular alterations (mucin depletion, branching, shortening, and atrophy) with scattered cryptitis, crypt abscess formation
- When acute inflammation predominates without glandular architectural changes, consider acute self-limited colitis
- In cases of suspected IBD, it is difficult to confirm a diagnosis of Crohn disease on biopsy; diagnosis may be suggested when granulomas are present, particularly when both normal and inflamed mucosa are identified in biopsies taken during the same colonoscopy
- Dysplasia generally recapitulates adenomatous changes

Selected References

Martland GT, Shepherd NA: Indeterminate colitis: Definition, diagnostic implication and a plea for nosological sanity. Histopathology 50:83-96, 2007.

Wehkamp J, Harder J, Weichenthal M, et al: NOD2 (CARD15) mutations in Crohn's disease are associated with diminished alpha-defensin expression. Gut 53:1658-1664, 2004.

Bonner GF, Petras RE, Cheong DMO, et al: Short- and long-term follow-up of treatment for lymphocytic and collagenous colitis. Inflamm Bowel Dis 6:85-91, 2000.

Farmer M, Petras RE, Hunt LE, et al: The importance of diagnostic accuracy in colonic inflammatory bowel disease. Am J Gastroenterol 95:3184-3188, 2000.

Wang N, Dumot JA, Achkar E, et al: Colonic epithelial lymphocytosis without a thickened subepithelial collagen table: A clinicopathologic study of forty cases supporting a heterogeneous entity. Am J Surg Pathol 23:1068-1074, 1999.

Kleer CG, Appleman HD: Ulcerative colitis: Patterns of involvement in colorectal biopsies and changes with time. Am J Surg Pathol 22:983–989, 1998.

Jenkins D, Balsitis M, Gallivan S, et al: Guidelines for the initial biopsy diagnosis of suspected chronic idiopathic inflammatory bowel disease. British Society of Gastroenterology Initiative. J Clin Pathol 50:93-105, 1997.

Bernstein CN, Shanahan F, Anton PA, Weinstein WM: Patchiness of mucosal inflammation in treated ulcerative colitis: A prospective study. Gastrointest Endosc 42:232-237, 1995.

LeBerre N, Heresbach D, Kerbaol M, et al: Histologic discrimination of idiopathic inflammatory bowel disease from other types of colitis. J Clin Pathol 48:749-753, 1995.

Lazenby AJ, Yardley JH, Giardiello FM, et al: Lymphocytic ("microscopic") colitis: A comparative histopathologic study with particular reference to collagenous colitis. Hum Pathol 20:18-28, 1989.

Norstrant TT, Kumar NB, Appelman HD: Histopathology differentiates acute self-limited colitis from ulcerative colitis. Gastroenterology 92:318-328, 1987.

Biopsy of Ileum and Pouches

- Lymphoid aggregates, pigment, and fibromuscular proliferation within the lamina propria are normally seen in the ileum and should not be misinterpreted as pathologic
  - The pigment is environmental or dietary in origin and deposits in macrophages; it has no clinical significance
  - Pathologic changes in the ileum include inflammation, parasitic infestation, and epithelial lymphocytosis
  - Minimal focal active enteritis can be related to bowel preparation or trauma and prolapse
  - Increased amounts of inflammation with architectural change and pyloric gland metaplasia usually are caused by Crohn disease or can be associated with NSAIDs
  - Giardiasis can be seen in terminal ileal biopsy specimens
  - Epithelial lymphocytosis can be a manifestation of celiac sprue or lymphocytic enterocolitis
- Ileal reservoirs (pouches)
  - The term *pouch* is the colloquialism given to the postcolectomy continence restoring operations (continent ileostomy, ileal pouch–anal anastomosis), which are surgical treatments of choice for ulcerative colitis and FAP
  - These operations have in common the creation of a pouch or reservoir formed by interconnecting loops of the terminal ileum
  - Pouch procedures are not usually done on patients with Crohn disease
  - A common late complication of pouch construction is the development of primary inflammation in the pouch, termed *pouchitis*
    - Patients present with increased effluent that can be bloody and foul smelling; patients often have fever and malaise
    - Pouch biopsy is typically done to confirm inflammation and to rule out Crohn disease
      - Pouchitis typically shows ulcers, granulation tissue, architectural change, and depletion or absence of normal lymphoid follicles
      - Afferent limb ulcers and non-necrotizing granulomas should suggest Crohn disease
      - Pyloric gland metaplasia is not usually seen in classic pouchitis and when present suggests Crohn disease, an NSAID-related lesion, or primary refractory pouchitis, a lesion that can be related to colonic change within the pouch

Selected References

McHugh JB, Appelman HD, McKenna BJ: The diagnostic value of terminal ileum biopsies. Am J Gastroenterol 102:1090-1092, 2007.

Goldstein NS: Isolated ileal erosion in patients with mildly altered bowel habits: A follow-up study of 28 patients. Am J Clin Pathol 125:838-846, 2006.

Wolf JM, Achkar JP, Lashner BA, et al: Afferent limb ulcers predict Crohn's disease in patients with ileal pouch-anal anastomosis. Gastroenterology 126:1686-1691, 2004.

Lengeling RW, Mitros FA, Brennan JA, Schulze KS: Ulcerative ileitis encountered at ileo-colonoscopy: Likely role of nonsteroidal agents. Clin Gastroenterol Hepatol 1:160-169, 2003.

Petras R: Role of the pathologist in evaluating chronic pouches. In Hanauer SB, Bayless TM (eds): Advanced Therapy of Inflammatory Bowel Disease, 2nd ed. Hamilton, Ontario, BC Decker, 2001, pp 229-232.

Shen B, Achkar J, Lashner BA, et al: Endoscopic and histologic evaluation together with symptom assessment are required to diagnose pouchitis. Gastroenterology 121:216-267, 2001.

Sarigol S, Wyllie R, Gramlich T, et al: Incidence of dysplasia in pelvic pouches in pediatric patients after ileal pouch-anal anastomosis for ulcerative colitis. J Pediatr Gastroenterol Nutr 28:429-434, 1999.

Sandborn WJ: Pouchitis following ileal pouch anal anastomosis: Definition, pathogenesis, and treatment. Gastroenterology 107:1856-1860, 1994.

Madden MV, Farthing MJ, Nicholls RJ: Inflammation in ileal reservoirs: "Pouchitis." Gut 31:247-249, 1990.

Dysplasia in Inflammatory Bowel Disease

Clinical Features

- Dysplasia and carcinoma may occur in both long-standing ulcerative colitis and Crohn disease
- Cancer risk in ulcerative colitis is estimated at up to 20% at 30 years
- Cancer risk in Crohn disease is estimated at 3% at 20 years
- Proctocolectomy is advised when dysplasia, especially high-grade dysplasia, is found

Figure 6-66. Endoscopic photograph of a dysplasia-associated lesion or mass.

Figure 6-67. High-grade glandular dysplasia in ulcerative colitis. This biopsy specimen from the lesion illustrated in Figure 6-66 shows adenoma-like dysplasia.

- Dysplasia is by nature patchy in distribution and requires multiple biopsy specimens to detect

Gross and Endoscopic Pathology

- Some areas of dysplasia are not grossly distinguishable from adjacent nondysplastic normal or inflamed mucosa (so-called flat dysplasia)
- Many cases are associated with mucosal polyps or plaques (so-called dysplasia-associated lesion or mass [DALM])
  — DALM is the term used to describe a dysplastic area in long-standing ulcerative colitis associated with a raised or mass lesion (any lesion grossly discernible—a mass, a plaquelike region, a polyp, or a group of polyps)
  — Identifies increased risk for carcinoma, whether high- or low-grade dysplasia is present
  — Often is impossible to distinguish from a sporadic adenoma

Histopathology

- Tissue specimens in IBD are categorized as negative for dysplasia, indefinite for dysplasia, positive low-grade dysplasia, or positive high-grade dysplasia
  — Negative for dysplasia
    ◆ Affected mucosa, although at times inflamed or regenerating, demonstrates normal maturation of the glandular epithelium
    ◆ Mitotic figures and histologic features of regeneration are generally confined to the lower half of the glands
  — Indefinite for dysplasia
    ◆ Used when epithelium has features suggestive of dysplasia, but the changes are insufficient to be unequivocally diagnostic

- ◆ Often occurs in regenerating or inflamed mucosa
- ◆ Also used to describe mucosa with cytologic atypia that differs from that usually seen in dysplasia (e.g., sessile serrated polyp-like change, microvesicular mucinous metaplasia)
- — Low-grade dysplasia
  - ◆ Characterized by changes similar to those present in an adenomatous polyp, including hyperchromatic, enlarged nuclei with preserved polarity
  - ◆ Mucinous differentiation is decreased
  - ◆ Dystrophic goblet cells (cytoplasmic vacuole is not in communication with the lumen)
  - ◆ Atypia may focally reach the surface
- — High-grade dysplasia
  - ◆ Prominent nuclear pleomorphism with hyperchromatic, often rounded nuclei that are stratified throughout the cell
  - ◆ Atypia extends to the surface
  - ◆ Cytologic features resemble those of carcinoma but are confined by a basement membrane

Special Stains and Immunohistochemistry

- Noncontributory

Other Techniques for Diagnosis

- Immunostains for p53, β-catenin, and bcl-2 have been investigated
- Molecular techniques (e.g., loss of heterozygosity) are also described

Differential Diagnosis

- ▌ Inflammatory atypia
  - Characterized by nuclei with prominent nucleoli, but without overt pleomorphism typically associated with dysplasia
  - Nuclei tend to have round to oval, smooth external contours, have some uniformity, and mature toward the luminal surface
  - Cryptitis and crypt abscesses are often present
- ▌ Low-grade versus high-grade dysplasia
  - Distinction made by the degree of cytologic changes present
  - Typically high-grade lesions have marked nuclear pleomorphism, loss of nuclear polarity, and nuclear stratification that extends to the luminal surface and is readily discernible at low magnification; mitotic figures are often plentiful and may be atypical
  - High-grade dysplastic glands have extensive budding, and the surface may have a villiform pattern
  - Many surgeons perform total proctocolectomy with ileal pouch–anal anastomosis for low-grade or high-grade dysplasia
- ▌ DALM versus sporadic adenoma
  - Pathologic distinction between these two lesions is not possible

- Characteristics favoring DALM include
  - — Patients younger than 40 years with history of ulcerative colitis of long duration (>10 years)
  - — Large lesion (>1 cm) in an area of proven endoscopic or histologic colitis with dysplasia in the adjacent flat mucosa
  - — Positive for p53 (not sensitive or specific enough for clinical use)
  - — Negative for bcl-2 (not sensitive or specific enough for clinical use)
  - — Chromosome 3p loss of heterozygosity (not generally available)
- Characteristics favoring a sporadic adenoma include
  - — Patients older than 40 years with colitis symptoms of shorter duration
  - — Small size (<1 cm)
  - — Pedunculated polyp outside proven areas of endoscopic colitis without dysplasia in adjacent mucosa
  - — Negative for p53 (not sensitive or specific enough for clinical use)
  - — Positive for bcl-2 positivity (not sensitive or specific enough for clinical use)
  - — No loss of heterozygosity for chromosome 3p (not generally available)
  - — Because sporadic adenomas and DALM cannot be separated pathologically, it is better to frame the issue as one of proper patient management. If the adenoma-like lesion occurs in an area uninvolved endoscopically by colitis, it should be considered a sporadic adenoma and treated by polypectomy alone. If the lesion occurs in an area involved endoscopically by colitis, it is best thought of as a dysplasia-associated lesion or mass. That said, there is increasing evidence that many such polypoid dysplasia lesions can be adequately treated by endoscopic polypectomy alone in IBD patients, provided careful patient selection criteria are applied, including the following: the patient is older than 40 years, the lesion is discretely defined endoscopically, excision of the lesion appears complete to the endoscopist, no other flat dysplasia is identified in the colon (one can use conservative management in patients with multiple adenoma-like dysplasia lesions), and the colon is relatively easy to survey (i.e., compliant patient, no inflammatory polyposis). Nevertheless, these patients should receive careful short-term endoscopic surveillance, and colectomy may be appropriate for patients not fulfilling these criteria

Selected References

Odze RD, Farraye FA, Hecht JL, Hornick, JL: Long-term follow-up after polypectomy for adenoma-like dysplastic lesions in ulcerative colitis. Clin Gastroenterol Hepatol 2:534-541, 2004.

Petras RE: The significance of adenomas in ulcerative colitis: Deciding when a colectomy should be performed. Inflamm Bowel Dis 5:306-308, 1999.

Rubin PH, Friedman S, Harpaz N, et al: Colonoscopic polypectomy in chronic colitis: Conservative management after endoscopic resection of dysplastic polyps. Gastroenterology 117:1295-1300, 1999.

Sigel JE, Petras RE, Lashner BA, et al: Intestinal adenocarcinoma in Crohn's disease: A report of 30 cases with a focus on coexisting dysplasia. Am J Surg Pathol 23:651-655, 1999.

Petras R, Mir-Madjlessi S, Farmer R: Crohn's disease and intestinal carcinoma: A report of 11 cases with emphasis on epithelial dysplasia. Gastroenterology 93:1307-1314, 1987.

Blackstone MO, Riddell RH, Rogers BHG, Levin B: Dysplasia-associated lesion or mass (DALM) detected by colonoscopy in long-standing ulcerative colitis: An indication for colectomy. Gastroenterology 80:366-374, 1981.

Other Forms of Colitis

Clinical Features

▌ Infectious colitis (acute self-limited colitis)
- Acute onset and short duration
- Constitutional symptoms, including fever
- History of travel or family members with febrile illness
- Bloody or watery diarrhea

▌ *Clostridium difficile*–associated pseudomembranous colitis
- Recent history of antibiotic administration
- Symptoms include diarrhea and abdominal pain
- Diagnosis is based on identification of *C. difficile* toxin in stool

Figure 6-69. **Resection specimen of acute ischemic colitis** showing patchy areas of ulcer and hemorrhage mimicking Crohn disease.

Figure 6-70. **Rigid proctoscopic view of solitary rectal ulcer syndrome.** The irregularly shaped ulcer is surrounded by heaped-up, firm mucosa.

- Endoscopy reports may describe typical pseudomembranes
- NAP-1 strain seen recently causes more serious illness and can be transmitted to otherwise healthy individuals

▌ Radiation colitis
- Usually associated with doses greater than 45,000 cGy

Figure 6-68. *Clostridium difficile*–**associated pseudomembranous colitis** showing patchy, creamy plaques with intervening erythematous colonic mucosa.

Figure 6-71. The focal active colitis pattern of injury in toxin-proved _Clostridium difficile_ infection. Note the neutrophils loose within the lamina propria unassociated with increased chronic inflammatory cells.

Figure 6-72. _Clostridium difficile_–**associated pseudomembranous colitis** showing the exploding crypt lesion. The nuclei and karyorrhectic debris are oriented in a curious linear fashion within the inflammatory pseudomembrane.

Figure 6-73. Radiation-induced colonic epithelial atypia showing cellular gigantism, a relatively low nuclear-to-cytoplasmic ratio, and cytoplasmic eosinophilia with vacuolization.

Figure 6-74. Acute ischemic colitis showing coagulative necrosis, mild acute inflammation, and karyorrhectic debris involving the surface with relative preservation of the deep crypt.

- May be potentiated by presence of diabetes, cardiovascular disease, concurrent chemotherapy
- Acute and chronic forms occur
- Symptoms include diarrhea and abdominal pain; bowel obstruction may occur in the chronic form

▍ Ischemic colitis
- Tends to occur in elderly patients with history of cardiovascular or atherosclerotic diseases
- Generally has an acute onset
- Patients may have abdominal pain, nausea, vomiting, diarrhea, or lower gastrointestinal bleeding
- Etiologies include vascular occlusive disease, mechanical obstruction, nonocclusive mesenteric ischemia, drugs that can cause ischemic-type damage (e.g., NSAIDs, oral contraceptives), and infections that can cause ischemic-type change (e.g., enterohemorrhagic _Escherichia coli_, _Clostridium difficile_)

▍ Lymphocytic and collagenous colitis
- Many cases have unknown pathogenesis; some are related to drugs (e.g., ticlopidine) or infection (e.g., Brainerd diarrhea)

Figure 6-75. Lymphocytic colitis shows an increase in chronic inflammatory cells within the lamina propria and intraepithelial lymphocytosis.

Figure 6-76. Collagenous colitis with increased subepithelial collagen plate, subepithelial vacuoles, and surface epithelial sloughing.

Figure 6-77. Solitary rectal ulcer syndrome. There is architectural distortion accompanied by fibromuscular obliteration of the lamina propria with capillary ectasia.

Figure 6-78. Defunctionalized rectum showing marked intramucosal lymphoid hyperplasia associated with surface epithelial atrophy.

Figure 6-79. Lymphocytic colitis with subepithelial giant cells.

- Patient typically presents with watery diarrhea
- Often patients are older than 50 years
- Collagenous colitis is 10 times more common in women
- It may be associated with immunologic diseases, osteoarthritis, or celiac disease
- Endoscopy is characteristically normal (thus diagnosis rests solely on microscopic findings; along with lymphocytic colitis, it is often referred to clinically as *microscopic colitis*)

- Mucosal prolapse syndromes
  - Syndromes include solitary rectal ulcer syndrome, localized colitis cystica profunda, prolapsing mucosal folds in diverticular disease cap polyposis, and inflammatory cloacogenic polyp
  - Many patients show abnormal function of anal and pelvic floor musculature
  - Usually middle-aged patients are affected and have constipation, history of difficult defecation, and passage of mucus or blood per rectum

Gross and Endoscopic Pathology

- Infectious colitis (acute self-limited colitis)
  - Ranges from mild mucosal edema and erythema to nonspecific ulcerative lesions resembling IBD
- *Clostridium difficile*–associated pseudomembranous colitis (antibiotic-associated colitis)
  - Typically segmental involvement with pseudomembranes
  - Superficial erosion
  - Patchy erythema
- Radiation colitis
  - Endoscopic findings include dusky mucosa, edema, and loss of superficial vascularity
- Ischemic colitis
  - Depends on severity of ischemia and ranges from mild increase in vascularity and pale, edematous mucosa to dark zones of mucosal hemorrhage to areas of frank green-gray necrosis; ulcers
- Microscopic colitis (lymphocytic and collagenous colitis)
  - By definition the endoscopic changes are minimal or absent; patchy erythema
- Mucosal prolapse syndromes
  - Mucosal erythema, ulcer, or polypoid lesion (isolated or multiple, cap polyposis)

Histopathology

- Infectious colitis (acute self-limited colitis)
  - Typically shows the focal active colitis pattern of inflammation
  - Lamina propria hemorrhage and congestion
  - Detachment and necrosis of surface epithelium
  - Withering of superficial aspects of crypts
  - Little glandular distortion or architectural atypia
  - Cryptitis and crypt abscesses
  - Neutrophils loose in the lamina propria without increased plasma cells
- *Clostridium difficile*–associated pseudomembranous colitis
  - Classically eruptive acute inflammatory exudate is seen on surface of intact inflamed mucosa
  - Superficial erosions may be present
  - May show infectious colitis pattern
- Radiation colitis
  - Acute changes include edema, vascular dilation, acute cryptitis, and superficial ulceration; usually patchy

- Atypical epithelial cells without an infiltrative pattern, with cellular gigantism, abundant eosinophilic cytoplasm with vacuoles, and possibly emperipolesis
  - Chronic changes are similar to chronic ischemia and include stromal fibrosis containing atypical fibroblasts and thickened subepithelial collagen, glandular atrophy and distortion, and vascular changes (fibrosis, intimal thickening, and enlarged endothelial cells with vesicular nuclei); architectural distortion can mimic chronic primary inflammatory bowel disease
- Ischemic colitis
  - Mild ischemia is characterized by superficial hemorrhage, patchy mucosal necrosis, dilated vessels, and regenerating crypts producing "decapitated" glands
  - Severe ischemic changes include crypt dropout, acute inflammation, acute cryptitis, and coagulative necrosis
  - In late lesions, the mucosa ulcerates and is replaced by granulation tissue and eventually fibrous tissue (scarring)
- Microscopic colitis (lymphocytic and collagenous colitis)
  - Lymphocytic colitis
    - Characterized by an absolute increase in the chronic inflammatory component in the lamina propria and increased intraepithelial lymphocytes (>15 per 100 enterocytes; normal is only 5 to 6 per 100)
  - Collagenous colitis
    - Combination of a thickened subepithelial collagen layer (≥15 μm) and increased mixed inflammatory infiltrate of the lamina propria, which tends to be displaced downward by the collagen
    - Intraepithelial lymphocytes are often present, and in some areas, the epithelium may be denuded, leaving fragments composed of only "naked" lamina propria
- Mucosal prolapse syndromes
  - Characteristic histology found in polypoid areas or mucosa adjacent to ulcers includes
    - Fibromuscular proliferation and lamina propria
    - Mucosal architectural change
    - Mucosal capillary ectasia
    - May have erosion with inflammatory pseudomembrane
    - Misplaced glands in muscularis mucosae or submucosa (so-called localized colitis cystica profunda)

Special Stains and Immunohistochemistry

- Trichrome stain highlights thickened subepithelial collagen band in collagenous colitis; usually not necessary
- Tenascin immunostaining is described in collagenous colitis; not used clinically

Other Techniques for Diagnosis

- Noncontributory

Differential Diagnosis

- Inflammatory bowel disease
  - Clinically patients have repeated bouts of abdominal pain, diarrhea that is often bloody, and fever over months (usually > 6 months)
  - Characterized by lymphoplasmacytic infiltrates that reach the crypt bases and by alterations in the glands (branching crypts, mucin depletion, and pyloric and Paneth cell metaplasia)
  - Granulomas are sometimes present in Crohn disease
- Diversion colitis and proctitis
  - Occurs in a segment of colon or rectum excluded from the fecal stream; most often a Hartmann pouch constructed at the time of resection of a proximal segment of colon
  - Some patients have mucus discharge or diarrhea
  - Histologic features include prominent lymphoid aggregates and follicles and a dense lymphoid infiltrate in lamina propria
  - Scattered neutrophilic infiltrate with foci of cryptitis and rare crypt abscesses may be seen
  - Crypt architecture is usually relatively normal early; diversion of some duration causes glandular atrophy
  - Diversion of proctitis changes can be superimposed on changes of ulcerative colitis or Crohn disease in patients originally resected for primary inflammatory bowel disease
  - Cured by resumption of fecal stream; can be treated with short-chain fatty acid enemas
- Mucinous adenocarcinoma
  - The misplaced glands and dissecting mucus in the muscularis mucosae and submucosa seen with localized colitis cystica profunda can closely mimic invasive mucinous adenocarcinoma
  - Features that favor mucosal prolapse syndromes include
    - Rounded, pushing external contour to misplaced glands and mucus
    - No epithelium in mucus pools or single discontinuous layer of epithelium at periphery
    - No dysplasia in misplaced epithelium
    - Lack of tumor desmoplasia
    - Presence of hemorrhage and hemosiderin deposits in nearby connective tissues
- Aberrant histologic features in microscopic colitis
  - Architectural change, subepithelial giant cells, cryptitis, Paneth cell metaplasia, ulcers, or inflammatory pseudomembranes are sometimes seen in cases otherwise typical for lymphocytic colitis or collagenous colitis
  - Histology (aberrant or otherwise) generally does not correlate with symptoms, results of treatment, or clinical outcome, with the following exceptions

- Cryptitis sometimes correlates with antibiotic use
- Paneth cell metaplasia correlates with severity of diarrhea in collagenous colitis
- Ulcers can be seen with concomitant NSAID use; ulcers may also indicate "fractured" colon in patients with collagenous colitis
- Inflammatory pseudomembranes may indicate comorbid *Clostridium difficile* infection but usually do not

Pearls

- Many conditions may mimic IBD; clinical impression is helpful when evaluating colonic biopsies
- Colonic biopsies with predominant acute inflammation in the absence of glandular changes generally indicate self-limited colitis rather than IBD
- Atypical stromal fibroblasts and associated glandular atrophy with mucosal capillary ectasia are clues to indicate radiation colitis
- Subepithelial collagen is abnormal when it is more than 15 µm thick and is diagnostic of collagenous colitis
- When cytoplasm is visible under the enterocyte nucleus, the section is tangential; do not mistake this for thickened subepithelial collagen (a common trap for the unwary)
- Be wary when diagnosing invasive, well-differentiated mucinous adenocarcinoma in the rectum; localized colitis cystica profunda must always be considered and ruled out

Selected References

Petras RE: Non-neoplastic intestinal disease. In Mills SE (ed): Sternberg's Diagnostic Surgical Pathology. 4th ed. Philadelphia, Lippincott Williams & Wilkins, 2004, pp 1475-1485.

Shaz BH, Reddy SI, Ayata G, et al: Sequential clinical and histopathological changes in collagenous and lymphocytic colitis over time. Mod Pathol 17:395-401, 2004.

Sherman A, Ackert JJ, Rajapaksa R, et al: Fractured colon: An endoscopically distinctive lesion associated with colonic perforation following colonoscopy in patients with collagenous colitis. J Clin Gastroenterol 38:341-345, 2004.

Yuan S, Reyes V, Bronner MP: Pseudomembranous collagenous colitis. Am J Surg Pathol 27:1375-1379, 2003.

Ayata G, Ithamukkala S, Sapp H, et al: Prevalence and significance of inflammatory bowel disease-like morphologic features in collagenous and lymphocytic colitis. Am J Surg Pathol 26:1414-1423, 2002.

Libbrecht L, Croes R, Ectors N, et al: Microscopic colitis with giant cells. Histopathology 40:335-338, 2002.

Wang N, Dumot JA, Achkar E, et al: Colonic epithelial lymphocytosis without a thickened subepithelial collagen table: A clinicopathologic study of forty cases supporting a heterogenous entity. Am J Surg Pathol 23:1068-1074, 1999.

Dignan CR, Greenson JK: Can ischemic colitis be differentiated from C. difficile colitis in biopsy specimens? Am J Surg Pathol 22:773-774, 1998.

Bryant DA, Mintz ED, Puhr ND, et al: Colonic epithelial lymphocytosis associated with an epidemic of chronic diarrhea. Am J Surg Pathol 20:1102-1109, 1996.

Kelly JK: Polypoid prolapsing mucosal folds in diverticular disease. Am J Surg Pathol 15:871-878, 1991.

Griffin P, Olmstead L, Petras R: Escherichia coli O157:H7-associated colitis: A clinical and histologic study of 11 cases. Gastroenterology 99:142-149, 1990.

Levine DS: "Solitary" rectal ulcer syndrome: Are "solitary" rectal ulcer syndrome and "localized" colitis cystica profunda analogous syndromes caused by rectal prolapse? Gastroenterology 92:243-253, 1987.

Norstrant TT, Kumar NB, Appelman HD: Histopathology differentiates acute self-limited colitis from ulcerative colitis. Gastroenterology 92:318-328, 1987.

Amebiasis

Clinical Features

- Worldwide distribution
- Uncommon in the United States, although occurs with increased frequencies in AIDS patients and homosexual men
- Most often due to *Entamoeba histolytica*
  — Invasive motile trophozoite
  — Characteristic cyst form (resists gastric acid, chlorination, and room-temperature storage)
- Symptoms vary widely and include
  — Dysentery with diarrhea and rectal bleeding, mimicking IBD

Figure 6-80. Amebiasis. The trophozoites of *Entamoeba histolytica* are larger than histiocytes and show an eccentrically placed circular nucleus. Some of the trophozoites have ingested red blood cells.

- Liver abscesses
- Colonic granulomatous masses that can mimic carcinoma
- Complications include colonic perforation and fistulas or liver abscesses

Gross and Endoscopic Pathology

- Early lesions form small oval ulcers with hyperemic overhanging edges and yellow exudate on base
- Patchy areas of erythema, erosions, and ulceration are especially common in the cecum, appendix, and rectosigmoid (mimics Crohn disease)

Histopathology

- Resected specimens contain ulcers that undermine the adjacent, intact mucosa, producing the characteristic flask shape
- Crypt abscesses and goblet cell depletion
- Biopsy specimens contain only nonspecific inflammation; the focal active colitis pattern of injury can be seen; erosions and ulcers may occur with associated fibrinous exudate, which contains diagnostic organisms (trophozoites)
  — Typical organisms are large (up to 40 μm) oval structures that have a small nucleus with large karyosome and abundant pink, vacuolated cytoplasm
  — Cytoplasm often contains ingested erythrocytes (*Entamoeba histolytica*)

Special Stains and Immunohistochemistry

- Iron hematoxylin in combination with PAS highlights ingested erythrocytes

Other Techniques for Diagnosis

- Serologic tests are available

Differential Diagnosis

▎ Inflammatory bowel disease
- Ulcerative colitis characteristically shows more diffuse colonic involvement with mucosal architectural distortion and lamina propria basal plasmacytosis
- Crohn disease (like amebiasis) may be patchy but is distinguished by fissuring ulcers rather than flask-shaped undermining ulcers. Ulcers of Crohn disease tend to have the long axis parallel to the long axis of the bowel. Amebic ulcers tend to have the long axis perpendicular to the long axis of the bowel
- IBD typically lacks fibrinous exudate containing diagnostic organisms
- Biopsy specimens in Crohn disease show focal active colitis pattern of injury, usually with some architectural distortion and increased basal lamina propria plasma cells

Pearls

- Always scan the biopsy section for trophozoites when discrete ulcers and fibrinous exudates are present
- Trophozoites must be distinguished from histiocytes, which are smaller, but have a larger nucleus and stain less intensely with PAS

Selected References

Calderaro A, Villanacci V, Bommezzadri S, et al: Colonic amoebiasis and spirochetosis: Morphological, ultrastructural and microbiological evaluation. J Gastroenterol Hepatol 22:64-67, 2007.

Allason-Jones E, Mindel A, Sargeunt P, Williams P: Entamoeba histolytica as a commensal intestinal parasite in homosexual men. N Engl J Med 315:353-356, 1986.

Merritt RJ, Coughlin E, Thomas DW, et al: Spectrum of amebiasis in children. Am J Dis Child 136:785-789, 1982.

Connor DH, Neafle RC, Meyers WM: Amebiasis. In Binford CH, Connor DH (eds): Pathology of Tropical and Extraordinary Diseases, vol 1. Washington, DC, Armed Forces Institute of Pathology, 1976.

Other Intestinal Parasitic Infestations

Clinical Features

▌ *Strongyloides stercoralis*
- Diarrhea, malabsorption; autoinfection can be fatal in immunocompromised patients
- Diagnosis usually made by identifying larvae in stool
- Infective form found in soil and can penetrate intact skin

▌ *Aonchotheca (Capillaria) philippinensis*
- Protein-losing enteropathy; found in Asia, Middle East, and Africa

Figure 6-81. Gross photograph of *Diphyllobothrium* species. This worm was removed endoscopically.

Figure 6-82. Strongyloidiasis with autoinfection. The crypt shows an infiltrating infective filiform larva of *Strongyloides stercoralis*. The lamina propria shows prominent infiltration with eosinophilic leukocytes.

Figure 6-83. *Trichuris trichiura*. Note the characteristic egg morphology in this adult worm removed during endoscopy.

- Diagnosis usually made by identifying eggs, larvae, or worms in stool

▌ *Trichuris trichiura* (whipworm)
- Often asymptomatic but has been associated with abdominal pain and diarrhea; may cause rectal prolapse

▌ *Enterobius vermicularis* (pinworm)
- Nocturnal perianal itching caused by gravid females migrating to perianal skin to deposit eggs

Figure 6-84. *Enterobius vermicularis.* This appendectomy specimen showing acute suppurative appendicitis contains an intraluminal worm with the characteristic lateral alae. Intraluminal bacteria suggestive of *Actinomyces* species are also present.

▌ *Diphyllobothrium latum* (fish tapeworm)
  ● From raw or undercooked fish
  ● Usually asymptomatic but may cause intestinal obstruction, vitamin B_{12} deficiency, and pernicious anemia
▌ *Ankylostoma duodenale* or *Necator americanus* (hookworm)
  ● May have itching at skin site of entry; wheezing and bronchitis when larvae migrates through lungs
  ● Signs and symptoms of anemia (e.g., pallor, tachycardia)
▌ Schistosomiasis
  ● Can cause colitis or bowel obstruction

Gross and Endoscopic Pathology

▌ *Strongyloides stercoralis*
  ● Worms bury themselves in duodenum and jejunum
▌ *Aonchotheca (Capillaria) philippinensis*
  ● Worms infest jejunum and upper ileum
▌ *Trichuris trichiura*
  ● Adults are about 4 cm in length and reside in cecum and ascending colon
▌ *Enterobius vermicularis*
  ● Adults live in cecum; gravid females migrate to anus at night to deposit eggs
  ● Commonly found in the appendix resection specimen
▌ *Diphyllobothrium latum*
  ● Adults can be up to 10 m in length
  ● Found in small intestine
▌ *Ankylostoma duodenale* or *Necator americanus*
  ● About 10 mm; live in small intestine
▌ Schistosomiasis
  ● Focal ulcers, stricture, inflammatory polyps

Histopathology

▌ *Strongyloides stercoralis*
  ● May see eosinophilic granulomatous reaction
  ● May see adult female or eggs in small bowel biopsy specimen
  ● In cases of autoinfection, can see filariform larvae in bowel wall
▌ *Aonchotheca (Capillaria) philippinensis*
  ● Only rarely described in biopsy specimens
  ● Morphologic resemblance to those of trichuriasis
▌ *Trichuris trichiura*
  ● Often extracted at endoscopy; "whip" morphology can be seen on H&E-stained section
  ● Ova have polar plugs
▌ *Enterobius vermicularis*
  ● Can be seen and extracted at endoscopy
  ● Lateral alae visible on cross section of worm; eggs with characteristic morphology
▌ *Diphyllobothrium latum*
  ● Whole mount demonstrates typical morphology; operculate eggs have aopercular knob
▌ *Ankylostoma duodenale* or *Necator americanus*
  ● May cause eosinophilic enteritis; diagnosis made usually by identification in stool
▌ Schistosomiasis
  ● Marked inflammatory reaction to eggs

Special Stains and Immunohistochemistry

  ● Noncontributory

Other Techniques for Diagnosis

  ● Noncontributory

Selected References

Meyers WM, Neafie RC, Marty AM, Wear DJ (eds): Pathology of Infectious Diseases, vol 1. Helminthiases. Washington, DC, Armed Forces Institute of Pathology, American Registry of Pathology, 2000.
Gutierrez Y, Bhatia P, Garbadawala ST, et al: Strongyloides stercoralis eosinophilic granulomatous enterocolitis. Am J Surg Pathol 20:603-612, 1996.
Gutierrez Y: Diagnostic pathology of parasitic infections with clinical correlations. Philadelphia, Lea & Febiger, 1990.
Milder JE, Walzer PD, Kilgore G, et al: Clinical features of *Strongyloides stercoralis* infection in an endemic area of the United States. Gastroenterology 80:1481-1488, 1981.

Lymphangiectasia

Clinical Features

  ● Primary or secondary forms exist
    — Primary form is typically seen in children and is caused by a congenital obstruction of the lymphatics
    — Secondary form is associated with many conditions, including retroperitoneal fibrosis,

Figure 6-85. Artifact mimicking lymphangiectasia. The surface epithelium has pulled away from the basement membrane, creating an artifactual space mimicking dilated lymphatics.

pericarditis, pancreatitis, gastrointestinal malignancy, and sarcoidosis
- Symptoms include protein-losing enteropathy, obstruction
- Treatment generally is focused on the underlying condition

Gross and Endoscopic Pathology

- Often form small mucosal elevations that expand the mucosal folds
- Small cysts that may exude milky, chylous fluid
- Small lesions are generally incidental findings

Histopathology

- Primary and secondary forms have same histologic features
- Small multiloculated cysts lined by flat endothelium surrounded by a variable amount of ill-defined supportive stroma
- No red blood cells in the open channels

Special Stains and Immunohistochemistry

- Factor VIII or CD34: lining cells are negative

Other Techniques for Diagnosis

- Noncontributory

Differential Diagnosis

- Must be distinguished from fixation-induced separation of basement membrane from surface epithelium, which can produce an artifactual space; occasional dilated mucosal lacteals are of no clinical significance
- ▌ Pneumatosis intestinalis
  - Multiple air-filled cysts, most of which are devoid of an endothelial lining
  - Surrounding tissue has wide variability in inflammatory reaction (related to underlying condition); often contains leukocytes, eosinophils, plasma cells, macrophages, and foreign-body giant cells
- ▌ Hemangioma
  - Generally forms a discrete mass
  - Can be distinguished from lymphangiectasia by the presence of red cells in the open channels
- ▌ Lymphangioma
  - Discrete mass lesion composed of microscopic cysts lined by flat endothelium
  - Loose, myxoid connective tissue stroma surrounds cysts

Pearls

- Primary lymphangiectasis is a rare condition, and protein loss is the predominating clinical presentation

Selected References

Kuroda Y, Katoh H, Ohsato K: Cystic lymphangioma of the colon. Report of a case and review of the literature. Dis Colon Rectum 27:679-682, 1984.

Vardy PA, Lebenthal E, Shwachman H: Intestinal lymphangiectasia: A reappraisal. Pediatrics 55:842-851, 1975.

Waldmann TA: Protein-losing enteropathy. Gastroenterology 50:422-443, 1966.

Pneumatosis Intestinalis

Clinical Features

- Gas-filled cysts in the intestines that are related to either underlying pulmonary disease (chronic form) or infection by gas-forming intestinal organisms (acute form)
- Chronic form more common in adults; acute form more common in infants
- May be found anywhere in the intestines
- Symptoms are usually related to underlying disease
  - Infants: usually coexists with necrotizing enterocolitis, producing severe gastrointestinal complications
  - Adults: diarrhea, flatulence, and excess stool mucus
- Complications include obstruction, volvulus, hemorrhage, and rarely pneumoperitoneum

Figure 6-86. Pneumatosis cystoides intestinalis involving sigmoid colon. The surface mucosa shows scattered ischemic changes. The cut section reveals the distended mural gas cysts.

- Classic radiographic sign is rings of gas in the small or large bowel wall

Gross and Endoscopic Pathology

- Generally a diffuse process but may be localized
- Forms cysts in the mucosa, submucosa, or serosa of small or large intestine
- Cysts are usually near mesenteric border
- Cysts range from 1 mm to several centimeters, often appearing like serosal bubbles
- Submucosal cysts may be imperceptible from the surface but generally cause intestinal crepitance
- Cut surface reveals numerous tiny cysts resulting in a honeycomb appearance

Histopathology

- Multiple air-filled cysts, most of which are devoid of an endothelial lining
- Surrounding tissue has wide variability in inflammatory reaction (related to underlying condition); often contains leukocytes, eosinophils, plasma cells, macrophages, and foreign-body giant cells
- Mucosa is usually normal

Special Stains and Immunohistochemistry

- Gram stain rarely detects bacteria around cysts in acute form

Other Techniques for Diagnosis

- Noncontributory

Differential Diagnosis

▌ Lymphangiectasia
- Microscopic cysts in the small or large intestine with endothelial lining

- Lacks discrete inflammatory component (especially eosinophils and foreign-body giant cells) surrounding cysts

Pearls

- Cysts are thought to form secondary to traumatic rupture of gas into bowel (such as induced by coughing) or to proliferation of gas-forming organisms (such as *Clostridium perfringens*, *Enterobacter aerogenes*, and *Escherichia coli*)

Selected References

Heng Y, Schuffler MD, Haggit RC, Rohrmann CA: Pneumatosis intestinalis: A review. Am J Gastroenterol 90:1747-1758, 1995.

Galandiuk S, Fazio VW: Pneumatosis cystoides intestinalis. Dis Colon Rectum 29:358, 1986.

Galandiuk S, Fazio VW, Petras R: Pneumatosis cystoides intestinalis in Crohn's disease: A report of two cases. Dis Colon Rectum 28:951-956, 1985.

Melanosis Coli

Clinical Features

- Associated with chronic laxative ingestion (anthraquinones, cascara, sagrada, aloes, senna, frangula, rhubarb) that induces apoptosis
- Patients generally have a history of constipation

Figure 6-87. Severe melanosis coli (resection specimen).

Gross and Endoscopic Pathology

- Dark brown to black mucosal pigmentation
- Primarily involves the right colon
- Severe cases may involve entire colon, appendix, and terminal ileum

Histopathology

- Lipofuscin deposits in lamina propria histiocytes
- Pigments are granular, refractile, and golden-brown and form clusters between intact glands
- Draining lymph nodes may contain similar pigments
- Occasionally nonspecific inflammation or microgranulomas (containing pigment) present; the latter can cause confusion with Crohn disease

Special Stains and Immunohistochemistry

- Melanosis coli pigment is positive with PAS, AFB, and Fontana-Masson stains
- Perl reaction negative
- Prussian blue (iron) stain negative

Other Techniques for Diagnosis

- Noncontributory

Differential Diagnosis

▮ Brown bowel syndrome (ceroidosis)
- Lipofuscin deposits are in the smooth muscle cells of the muscularis mucosae, muscularis propria, and vascular walls rather than in lamina propria histiocytes
- Patients often have vitamin E deficiency (often seen in celiac sprue or cystic fibrosis) and are typically symptomatic (abdominal pain and diarrhea)

Pearls

- Presence of the coarse, brown pigments in the lamina propria that are Prussian blue (iron) stain negative and Fontana-Masson stain positive indicates melanosis coli
- Hemosiderin deposits in the lamina propria are positive for Prussian blue (iron) stain
- Brown granular deposits (lipofuscin) in the smooth muscle cells indicate brown bowel syndrome

Selected References

Walker NI, Bennett RE, Axelsen RA: Melanosis coli: A consequence of anthraquinone-induced apoptosis of colonic epithelial cells. Am J Pathol 131:465-476, 1988.

Gallager RL: Intestinal ceroid deposition—"brown bowel syndrome." A light and electron microscopic study. Virchows Arch A Pathol Anat Histol 389:143-151, 1980.

Smith B: Pathologic changes in the colon produced by anthraquinone purgatives. Dis Colon Rectum 16:455-458, 1973.

Gastrointestinal Polyps

Clinical Features

- Typically occur in the colon
- Most common are hyperplastic polyps, inflammatory polyps, and adenomas

Figure 6-88. Endoscopic view of hyperplastic polyp. Hyperplastic polyps are typically small (<5 mm) and are about the same color as the surrounding colonic mucosa.

Figure 6-89. Endoscopic view of pedunculated tubulovillous adenoma.

Figure 6-92. Traditionally defined serrated adenoma. These polyps are typically pedunculated and left sided and demonstrate epithelial dysplasia. The serration imparts a resemblance to hyperplastic polyp. Serrated adenoma typically shows gastric foveolar change and eosinophilic cytoplasmic changes.

Figure 6-90. Hyperplastic polyp. Histologic section shows elongate crypts lined by evenly distributed goblet cells and absorptive cells. The crypts and surface epithelium have a serrated appearance. The surface basement membrane shows focal hyalinization. Mitotic figures are seen in the crypt base.

Figure 6-93. Sessile serrated polyp showing branded crypts, deep crypt dilation, horizontal orientation of crypts, and an irregular distribution of goblet cells.

Figure 6-91. Colonic adenoma with high-grade dysplasia demonstrating full-thickness stratification and a focal cribriform pattern.

▮ Hyperplastic polyp
- More common in men
- Most common colonic polyp
- In the colon, hyperplastic polyps are 3 to 10 times more common than adenomas
- Almost always asymptomatic

▮ Inflammatory polyp (pseudopolyps)
- Occur in setting of chronic, ulcerating colitis, such as ulcerative colitis, Crohn disease, trauma and prolapse, and infectious colitis; may also occur adjacent to mucosal injury (e.g., surgical anastomosis)

▮ Adenomas
- Thought to precede development of many carcinomas
- When multiple (>10), *may* indicate a genetic syndrome (e.g., FAP, attenuated FAP, and MYH-associated polyposis syndrome)
- Generally exhibit slow growth with 10-year doubling time
- Prevalence is thought to be around 35% in Western civilizations
- Prevalence increases dramatically after 40 years of age (peak, 60 to 70 years)

Figure 6-94. Sessile serrated polyp with inverted histology. The regenerative zone of the sessile serrated polyp is enveloped by smooth muscle fibers of the muscularis mucosae; some parts of the polyp have herniated into the submucosa.

- Presence of one adenoma is associated with a 40% to 55% risk for additional adenomas
- Risk for presence of villous architecture and for higher-grade dysplasia increases with multiple adenomas
- Risk for new adenomas is 20% to 60% within 3 to 10 years after initial polypectomy
- Symptoms include
  — Bleeding; however, adenomas smaller than 1 cm are usually asymptomatic, except those in the rectosigmoid area, which may bleed
  — Larger and villous lesions may produce mucinous diarrhea or constipation
  — Ominous signs are obstruction and abdominal pain
- Detection of small sigmoid or rectal adenomas is indication for full colonoscopy

Gross and Endoscopic Pathology

▌ Hyperplastic polyp
- Typically smaller than 0.5 cm but rarely larger than 1 cm (larger polyps must be distinguished from sessile serrated polyps; see "Differential Diagnosis")
- Often on crest of mucosal folds
- Often multiple

▌ Inflammatory polyp
- Small, sessile nodules with smooth surfaces; some with variable shapes
- Often multiple

▌ Adenomas
- Most are exophytic, mucosal protrusions

- Three endoscopic types: pedunculated, sessile, flat and depressed
- Gross architecture is related to histologic type
  — Tubular adenomas are usually small, round, and pedunculated
  — Tubulovillous adenomas are larger
  — Villous adenomas are more likely sessile, flat, or on a short, broad pedicle
- Larger adenomas are more likely to be hemorrhagic
- Flat adenomas are difficult to detect endoscopically and are small, plaquelike mucosal discolorations
- Estimated 1% of adenomas smaller than 1 cm contain cancer, compared with 45% of adenomas larger than 2 cm

Histopathology

▌ Hyperplastic polyp
- Characterized by serrated, convoluted (sawtooth pattern) luminal border (due to an increased number of mature colonocytes per unit area)
- Slight expansion of the mitotically active basal cell zone, limited to the lower half of the crypt (so-called bottom-up atypia)
- No dysplasia
- Mixture of absorptive cells and goblet cells

▌ Inflammatory polyp
- Mixture of inflamed stromal tissue and hyperplastic epithelium in variable proportions
- Sometimes exhibits an ulcerated surface and exuberant granulation tissue reaction containing mixed inflammation
- Dilated epithelial cysts in various stages of degeneration and regeneration—at times simulating adenomatous change
- Inflammatory polyp with bizarre stromal cells
  — Designation used for occasional inflammatory polyps that contain large, bizarre spindle or polygonal stromal cells; usually a surface phenomenon

▌ Adenomas
- Three types: tubular, tubulovillous, villous
- Small, pedunculated adenomas are usually tubular or tubulovillous
- Larger, sessile adenomas usually have a villous component
- Many exceptions exist; thus, large, pedunculated tubular adenomas and small, sessile villous adenomas are found
- All adenomas, by definition, are composed of dysplastic epithelium, characterized by cells with enlarged, hyperchromatic, stratified nuclei and decreased mucin; increased mitotic figures extending to the upper areas of the crypt
- Most adenomas demonstrate some evidence of maturation into mucin-secreting cells called *oligomucous cells*; these cells have variable amounts of mucus, and thus some goblet cells are usually present

- Degree of dysplasia is determined by evidence of maturation
  — Low-grade dysplasia: slightly stratified spindle or oval nuclei with apical cytoplasm (roughly half of the total cell height) and evidence of goblet cell formation
  — High-grade dysplasia: full-thickness, stratified, round nuclei and little cytoplasm (most nuclei reach the gland lumen) with greater nuclear pleomorphism and little goblet cell differentiation
  — The term *high-grade dysplasia* is sometimes expanded to include more complex cribriform pattern (adenocarcinoma in situ) or cases with infiltration of carcinoma cells into the lamina propria or muscularis mucosae alone (so-called intramucosal adenocarcinoma) that lack submucosal invasion
  — With increasing degrees of dysplasia, dystrophic goblet cells occur; these occur in epithelium with stratified nuclei resulting in goblet cells above the basal layer, simulating signet rings
- Dysplastic epithelium appears first on the superficial surface and eventually replaces the deeper epithelium (so-called top-down atypia)
- Adenomatous epithelium in the submucosa simulating invasive carcinoma (so-called pseudoinvasion) occurs in 2% to 10% of pedunculated polyps, particularly those in the sigmoid colon with long (>1 cm) stalks; thought to arise following torsion resulting in hemorrhage, inflammation, fibrosis, or increased pressure causing herniation of the adenomatous epithelium through defects in the muscularis mucosae
- Pseudoinvasion is recognized by
  — Presence of lamina propria around adenomatous glands or by identifying direct connection to mucosa
  — Hemosiderin deposits and fibrosis rather than desmoplasia
  — Lack of malignant cytology
  — Rounded contours to malpositioned glands without infiltration
- Tubular adenoma
  — Most common (more than 70%)
  — Composed of tubular glands (similar to normal colonic glands), but lined by dysplastic epithelium
  — Tubular architecture constitutes more than 80% of adenoma
- Villous adenoma
  — Composed of slender, finger-like, epithelial fronds and deep crypts extending outward from the muscularis mucosae
  — Fronds contain vascular cores and are lined by adenomatous epithelium
  — Villous architecture composes more than 80% of adenoma

- Tubulovillous adenoma
  — Mixture of both tubular and villous architecture
  — Villous architecture composes roughly 20% to 80% of the adenoma
- Mixed hyperplastic and adenomatous polyp
  — Relatively rare
  — Discrete areas of both hyperplastic and adenomatous histology with a sharp demarcation between the two
  — Most examples likely represent dysplasia in a sessile serrated polyp
- Traditionally defined serrated adenoma
  — True adenoma (with epithelial dysplasia) characterized by serration
  — Lining cells are less mature than in hyperplastic polyps often showing eosinophilic cytoplasm or gastric foveolar metaplasia, and show superficial mitotic figures, nuclear polarity, high nuclear-to-cytoplasmic ratio, and nuclear pleomorphism; however, the cells have abundant mucin
  — May be admixed with areas of hyperplastic polyp, sessile serrated polyp, and classic adenomatous polyp
  — Usually left sided and pedunculated

Special Stains and Immunohistochemistry

▌ Hyperplastic polyp
- Trichrome stain or collagen IV immunostain demonstrates a thickened subepithelial collagen zone
- Carcinoembryonic antigen (CEA) is overexpressed in hyperplastic polyps

▌ Inflammatory polyp
- Stromal cells (including bizarre stromal cells) are CEA, cytokeratin, and mucin negative; positive for vimentin and muscle-specific actin (MSA)

Other Techniques for Diagnosis

- Noncontributory

Differential Diagnosis

▌ Sessile serrated polyp
- Also known by a number of synonyms, including *giant* or *large hyperplastic polyp*, *polyp with epithelial serrated proliferation*, and *sessile serrated adenoma*
- Typically right-sided, large (>1 cm), sessile, and often poorly circumscribed
- May mimic enlarged mucosal fold
- Polyps containing four or more of the following characteristics should be classified as sessile serrated polyp and differentiated from hyperplastic polyp
  — Basal crypt dilation
  — Crypt branching
  — Horizontal orientation of crypts
  — Inverted histology (glands malpositioned into muscularis mucosae or submucosa)
  — Prominent serration
  — Epithelial-to-stromal ratio exceeding 50%

— No surface basement membrane thickening
— Persistent nuclear enlargement, atypia, and nucleoli in the upper third of crypt
— Mitosis figures in upper third of crypt
— Abnormal patchy distribution of dystrophic goblet cells
- May be specific precursor lesion of sporadic microsatellite instability–high (MSI-H) colorectal carcinoma
- Polyp type seen in hyperplastic (serrated) polyposis syndrome
- Data suggest that patients with this type of polyp, if it is incompletely excised or associated with similar unsampled polyps, may benefit from a shorter surveillance interval (e.g., 1 to 2 years) because the transition to carcinoma may occur faster in the serrated polyp pathway than in the adenoma carcinoma sequence
- Hamartomatous polyps
- Regenerative change
  - Can be seen with mucosal trauma and prolapse or in inflammatory polyps
  - Regenerative epithelium usually shows increased nuclear size, cytoplasmic basophilia, and increased mitoses restricted to the basal half of the crypt with more mature goblet cells and absorptive cells at the surface

Pearls

- Inflammatory polyp
  - To avoid misdiagnosis of neoplasia, carefully evaluate stromal cells (particularly in small biopsies and when the epithelium is atrophic or regenerative), looking for fibromuscular hyperplasia and ectatic capillaries, which are often seen in inflammatory polyps
- Adenomas
  - Biologically, adenomatous growth is thought to progress sequentially, through a continuum: low-grade dysplasia, high-grade dysplasia, carcinoma in situ, intramucosal carcinoma, and invasive carcinoma
  - Clinically the important distinctions are size, villous component, and presence of high-grade dysplasia or carcinoma
    - Carcinoma cells that infiltrate into the muscularis mucosae or lamina propria alone (intramucosal adenocarcinoma) have virtually no risk for metastasis; many advocate classifying these lesions as high-grade dysplasia
    - Degree of dysplasia correlates with cancer risk; high-grade dysplasia carries a risk for progression several times higher than that of low-grade dysplasia
    - Only when the carcinoma cells infiltrate through the muscularis mucosae into the submucosa or beyond are they considered invasive (and clinically significant)

— Invasion of submucosa is recognized by an infiltrative pattern to the neoplastic glands accompanied by tumor desmoplasia
— Desmoplasia accompanies invasion of at least the submucosa, but it cannot be used to identify the actual depth of invasion in a biopsy specimen
- Pathology report should include
  - Highest degree of dysplasia present in the biopsy specimen and presence of villous component
  - Degree of differentiation and distance from the margin, if invasive carcinoma is present, as well as the presence or absence of vascular and lymphatic invasion

Selected References

Goldstein NS: Small colonic microsatellite unstable adenocarcinomas and high-grade epithelial dysplasias in sessile serrated adenoma polypectomy specimens: A study of eight cases. Am J Clin Pathol 125:132-145, 2006.

Sheridan TB, Fenton H, Lewin MR, et al: Sessile serrated adenomas with low- and high-grade dysplasia and early carcinomas: An immunohistochemical study of serrated lesions "caught in the act." Am J Clin Pathol 126:564-571, 2006.

Winawer SJ, Zauber AG, Fletcher RH, et al: Guidelines for colonoscopy surveillance after polypectomy: A consensus update by the US Multi-Society Task Force on Colorectal Cancer and the American Cancer Society. Gastroenterology 130:1872-1885, 2006.

Snover DC, Jass JR, Fenoglio-Preiser C, Batts KP: Serrated polyps of the large intestine: A morphologic and molecular review of an evolving concept. Am J Clin Pathol 124:380-391, 2005.

Jass JR: Hyperplastic polyps and colorectal cancer: is there a link? Clin Gastroenterol Hepatol 2:1-8, 2004.

Goldstein NS, Bhanot P, Odish E, Hunter S: Hyperplastic-like colon polyps that preceded microsatellite-unstable adenocarcinomas. Am J Clin Pathol 119:778-796, 2003.

Riddell RH, Petras RE, Williams GT, Sobin LH: Tumors of the intestines. Atlas of Tumor Pathology Third Series, Fascicle #32. Washington, DC, Armed Forces Institute of Pathology, 2003.

Hawkins NJ, Ward RL: Sporadic colorectal cancers with microsatellite instability and their possible origin in hyperplastic polyps and serrated adenomas. J Natl Cancer Inst 93:1307-1313, 2001.

Volk EE, Goldblum JR, Petras RE, et al: Management and outcome of patients with invasive carcinoma arising in colorectal polyps. Gastroenterology 109:1801-1807, 1995.

Sporadic Adenomas and Adenocarcinoma of the Large Intestine

Classification

- Many different molecular pathways to colorectal carcinoma described
  - About 85% are derived through the chromosomal instability pathway
    - Cancers are often DNA aneuploid by flow cytometry

Figure 6-95. Microsatellite instability high colorectal carcinoma. These cancers are typically right sided and large.

Figure 6-97. Medullary adenocarcinoma. This histologic pattern of colonic carcinoma is characterized by syncytial groups of highly anaplastic epithelial cells without lumen formation. A brisk peritumoral lymphocytic response is present.

Figure 6-96. Gross resection specimen of ulcerated carcinoma of sigmoid colon.

Figure 6-98. Endometriosis involving the sigmoid colon. Note the endometrial glands and stroma within the submucosa.

- ◆ Demonstrate abnormalities of chromosomes 5, 17, and 18
- ◆ FAP-related colorectal carcinomas arise by this pathway
- — About 15% arise in the mutator phenotype pathway

- ◆ Cancers are DNA diploid
- ◆ Cancers demonstrate epiphenomenon referred to as *microsatellite instability*
- ◆ Colorectal carcinoma complicating Lynch syndrome arises by this pathway

- Lynch syndrome
  - Individuals with germline mutations of DNA mismatch repair genes (e.g., *hMLH1, hMSH2, hPMS2, hMSH6, hPMS1*)
  - About 15-fold increased risk for colorectal carcinoma compared with the general population
    - Cancers occur on average in patients 20 years younger than colorectal carcinoma of the general population
  - Increased risk for other carcinomas, including endometrium, ovary, stomach, urinary tract, biliary tract, central nervous system, and small bowel
  - Can be suspected clinically based on Amsterdam criteria
    - Three or more relatives with Lynch syndrome–related tumors
    - Colorectal carcinoma in two generations
    - One or more Lynch syndrome–related tumors occurring in a patient younger than 50 years
    - Kindred fulfilling Amsterdam criteria but without mutation of a known mismatch repair gene are referred to as having *familial colorectal cancer syndrome type X*

Clinical Features

- Incidence is about 153,000 new cases and 52,000 deaths/year, accounting for 10% of cancer deaths in the United States in 2007
- Peak incidence between 60 to 79 years of age; fewer than 20% occur in patients younger than 50 years of age
- High incidence in populations with diet rich in animal fat and sedentary lifestyle
- Increased risk with chronic inflammatory bowel disease
- Symptoms include
  - Anemia: when present in an elderly male, colon cancer is suspected until proved otherwise
  - Location dependent
    - Right-sided tumors: enlarge without direct symptoms, but bleed easily, thus causing indirect symptoms, including anemia and fatigue
    - Left-sided tumors (where colon caliber is smaller): produce melena, constipation, and diarrhea (change in bowel habits)

Gross and Endoscopic Pathology

- ▌Adenocarcinoma
  - Patulous right colon tends to produce larger exophytic tumors, generally without causing obstruction
  - Tumors in the smaller-caliber distal colon evolve into annular "napkin ring" tumors
  - Can be fungating, ulcerated, or necrotic masses

- Lynch syndrome and sporadic MSI-H colorectal carcinoma tend to be right sided (75%), can be multiple and tend to be large and bulky

Histopathology

- ▌Adenocarcinoma
  - Histology can be similar regardless of location
  - Infiltration of glands of variable differentiation lined by anaplastic epithelial cells
  - Lining cells are fully stratified and have large hyperchromatic nuclei and prominent nucleoli
  - Prominent mitotic activity often with atypical forms
  - Invasion promotes a characteristic robust desmoplastic tissue reaction, imparting the hard gross consistency
    - Grade I
      - Composed predominantly of well-formed glands in a desmoplastic stroma
    - Grade II
      - Less well-formed glands with focal cribriform architecture
    - Grade III
      - Tumor grows in solid sheets with no distinct gland formation
- ▌Mucinous adenocarcinoma
  - Accounts for about 10% of colorectal malignancies
  - Production of excess mucin with associated malignant epithelial glands and free-floating, malignant cells
  - Generally agreed that 75% to 80% of the tumor must be mucinous to be linked to a worse prognosis
  - Worse prognosis, presumably due to the greater penetration imparted by the mucin
- ▌Lynch syndrome and sporadic MSI-H colorectal cancer
  - Can have a prominent lymphoid component, including peritumoral lymphocytes (so-called Crohn-like reaction) and increased intratumoral lymphocytes
  - Tend to be poorly differentiated (e.g., undifferentiated or medullary carcinoma)
  - Mucinous and signet ring cell histology over-represented
- ▌Uncommon types of colorectal cancer include neuroendocrine carcinoma (including small cell carcinoma), adenosquamous carcinoma, squamous carcinoma, pleomorphic giant cell carcinoma, and carcinosarcoma

Special Stains and Immunohistochemistry

- Immunohistochemistry for mismatch repair gene proteins hMLH1, hMSH2, hPMS2, and hMSH6 is commercially available

Other Techniques for Diagnosis

- PCR tests for microsatellite instability or immunohistochemistry for mismatch repair gene

protein should be performed on cancers fulfilling modified Bethesda criteria, which include
  — Patient younger than 50 years
  — Synchronous or metachronous Lynch syndrome–related tumors regardless of age
  — Colorectal carcinoma with MSI-H histology in a patient younger than 60 years
  — Colorectal carcinoma in a patient with a first-degree relative with a Lynch syndrome–related tumor (<50 years of age) or first degree relative with a colorectal adenoma (<40 years of age)
  — Colorectal carcinoma in a patient with two or more relatives with a Lynch syndrome–related tumor regardless of age
- Microsatellite instability testing or immunohistochemistry for mismatch repair gene proteins probably should be done on all colorectal carcinomas because
  — There is a survival advantage for MSI-H colorectal carcinoma stage for stage compared with MSI-low and MSI stable cancer
  — MSI-H predicts for metachronous carcinomas
  — MSI-H predicts poor response to fluorouracil-based chemotherapy regimens; MSI-H may be associated with a better response to irinotecan-based chemotherapy regimen
  — MSI-H testing aids in the detection of Lynch syndrome because more than 40% of probands patients are older than 50 years, and almost 25% of Lynch syndrome patients do not fulfill Amsterdam or Bethesda guidelines
- Gene sequencing for mismatch repair genes may be indicated in some patients with MSI-H by PCR and some with abnormal immunohistochemistry

Differential Diagnosis

▌ Endometriosis
- Often involves the colon and rectum (15% to 20% of endometriosis cases); occasionally involves the small intestine
- Typically an incidental finding; generally asymptomatic but occasionally may cause a polyp or bowel obstruction and can mimic carcinoma
- Endometriomas are usually ill-defined masses smaller than 4 or 5 cm; typically involve the serosa and subserosa but may extend through to the mucosa and bulge into the lumen
- Characterized histologically by the presence of endometrial glands and stroma
- Biopsy of the mucosa is often negative unless the mucosa is eroded

▌ Metastatic carcinoma
- No surface component
- Bulk of tumor cells in submucosa
- Immunohistochemistry for CK7 and CK20 can sometimes help differentiate a primary colorectal adenocarcinoma from a metastasis

Pearls

- Prognosis: although symptomatic at a smaller size, left-sided neoplasms are more often high stage at diagnosis and thus have poorer prognosis (5-year survival rates are 100%, 80%, 60%, and 10% for stages I, II, III, and IV, respectively)

Selected References

Jass JR: Classification of colorectal cancer based on correlation of clinical, morphological and molecular features. Histopathology 50:113-130, 2007.

Lindor NM, Petersen GM, Hadley DW, et al: Recommendations for the care of individuals with an inherited predisposition to Lynch syndrome: A systematic review. JAMA 296:1507-1517, 2006.

Hampel H, Frankel WL, Martin E, et al: Screening for the Lynch syndrome (hereditary nonpolyposis colorectal cancer). N Engl J Med 352:1851-1860, 2005.

Carethers JM, Smith EJ, Behling CA, et al: Use of 5-fluorouracil and survival in patients with microsatellite-unstable colorectal cancer. Gastroenterology 126:394-401, 2004.

Umar A, Boland CR, Terdiman JP, et al: Revised Bethesda Guidelines for hereditary nonpolyposis colorectal cancer (Lynch syndrome) and microsatellite instability. J Natl Cancer Inst 96:261-268, 2004.

Riddell RH, Petras RE, Williams GT, Sobin LH: Tumors of the intestines. Atlas of Tumor Pathology Third Series, Fascicle #32, Washington, DC, Armed Forces Institute of Pathology, 2003.

American Gastroenterological Association: Medical position statement: Hereditary colorectal cancer and genetic testing. Gastroenterology 121:195-197, 2001.

Polyposis Syndromes

Clinical Features

- Includes syndromes associated with the development of both neoplastic and hamartomatous (non-neoplastic) polyps

Figure 6-99. Colonic resection specimen from a patient with familial adenomatous polyposis. This close-up view shows numerous adenomas.

Figure 6-100. Colonic resection specimen from a patient with juvenile polyposis syndrome. Some of the polyps have typical juvenile polyp morphology (pedunculated with a smooth red surface). Some show unusual forms with finger-like multilobulated shapes.

Figure 6-101. Endoscopic photograph of the colon in Cronkhite-Canada syndrome showing diffuse edematous expansion of the colonic mucosa and focal polyp formation with an adherent exudate.

Figure 6-102. One-gland adenoma in familial adenomatous polyposis.

Figure 6-103. Peutz-Jeghers polyp of the colon illustrating the arborizing hamartomatous overgrowth of the muscularis mucosae.

Figure 6-104. Juvenile polyp of the colon demonstrating edematous and inflammatory expansion of the lamina propria associated with mucosal microcyst formation.

Figure 6-105. Cronkhite-Canada syndrome. The polyp (*center right*) is a localized accentuation of a diffuse mucosal abnormality characterized by edema, chronic inflammation, and microcyst formation.

Figure 6-106. Mucosal ganglioneuroma composed of spindle cells and scattered ganglion cells.

Figure 6-107. Colonic resection specimen from a patient with hyperplastic (serrated) polyposis syndrome. Many polyps have the typical morphology of hyperplastic polyps. Some polyps are large (>1 cm). Some show unusual morphology, such as plaques or abnormal thickening of mucosal folds.

— FAP and variants
— Peutz-Jeghers syndrome
— Juvenile polyposis
— Phosphatase and tensin homologue (PTEN) polyposis syndrome (e.g., Ruvalcaba-Myhre-Smith syndrome, Cowden disease)
— Cronkhite-Canada syndrome

▌ FAP
• Autosomal dominant transmission with nearly complete penetrance
• Affects about 1 in 7000 to 1 in 30,000 live births
• Adenomas may occur before 1 year of age but usually begin around puberty

Figure 6-108. Benign fibroblastic polyp (perineurioma) of the colon. The spindle cell proliferation within the lamina propria is associated with hyperplastic polyp-like mucosal changes.

• Without colonic resection, development of invasive carcinoma of colon or rectum and death from colorectal carcinoma are inevitable
• FAP-associated gene has been identified on chromosome 5 (5q21), called *APC* (adenomatous polyposis coli) gene
  — Specific mutations within the gene generally correlate with severity of the disease and associated conditions
  — Mutations near the 3′ and 5′ end of the gene and within exon 9 cause a mild form of the disease called *attenuated FAP*
• Associated conditions
  — Congenital hypertrophy of the retinal pigment epithelium
  — Upper gastrointestinal polyps in stomach and small bowel; small bowel adenomas, particularly the periampullary area, can progress to carcinoma (which is the cause of death in more than 20% of patients after colectomy)
  — Mandibular osteomas and other dental and skin lesions and cysts
  — Abdominal desmoid tumors
  — Carcinoma at extraintestinal sites (e.g., papillary thyroid carcinoma and hepatoblastoma)
• Presenting symptoms in patients not in surveillance include bleeding and anemia; symptomatic patients are much more likely to harbor colorectal carcinoma
• No gender preference; all races are affected equally
• Gardner syndrome

— Variant of FAP characterized by osteomas, fibromatosis, and epidermal cysts

— High frequency of thyroid and duodenal cancer

- Turcot syndrome
  — Rare variant of FAP coexisting with medulloblastoma
  — Some Turcot syndrome patients have germline mutations of the mismatch repair genes (Lynch syndrome) coexisting with glial neoplasms, usually glioblastoma multiforme
- Muir-Torre syndrome
  — Rare autosomal dominant disorder associated with mutations of mismatch repair genes
  — Generally fewer than 100 adenomas, which are frequently in the proximal colon
  — Associated with basal cell carcinoma, sebaceous carcinoma, and squamous cell carcinoma
- MYH-associated polyposis syndrome
  — Mutation of *mutY* homologue (MYH), a base excision repair gene
  — Autosomal recessive inheritance
  — Afflicted patients acquire somatic mutation of *APC* gene at a high rate
  — Can mimic FAP and attenuated FAP

▌ Peutz-Jeghers syndrome
- Genetic disorder characterized by gastrointestinal hamartomas and skin and mucosal hyperpigmentation; diagnostic criteria include a histologically confirmed Peutz-Jeghers polyp and two of the following
  — Family history of Peutz-Jeghers syndrome
  — Hyperpigmented lesions of skin and mucous membrane
  — Small intestinal polyposis
- Autosomal dominant with variable penetrance
- Far less common than FAP
- Gastrointestinal polyps and pigmented skin and mucosal lesions present in infancy
- Associated with extraintestinal malignancies, especially involving the pancreas, gonads, and breast; associated with ovarian sex cord tumor with annular tubules and testicular Sertoli cell tumors

▌ Juvenile polyps and juvenile polyposis syndrome
- Isolated juvenile polyps
  — Usually children
  — May have up to five small (<2 cm) polyps in colon and rectum
  — Prone to autoamputation
- Juvenile polyposis syndrome
  — Defined as six or more juvenile polyps in the colon and rectum, patient with juvenile polyps throughout the gastrointestinal tract, any juvenile polyp in a patient with a positive family history of juvenile polyposis syndrome
  — Familial and nonfamilial forms exist
  — Nonfamilial form is associated with other congenital abnormalities in 20% of cases

— Several varieties of familial juvenile polyposis exist with different inheritance patterns, usually autosomal dominant, and involve different areas of the gastrointestinal tract

— Juvenile polyps occur in about 3 in 100,000 patients younger than 10 years

— Patients with juvenile polyposis become symptomatic early in childhood with bleeding (80% of cases) or symptoms of obstruction; polyp may prolapse into anal canal

▌ PTEN-associated polyposis syndrome
- Cowden disease
  — Rare autosomal dominant disease characterized by hamartomas and neoplasms, mainly of face, thyroid, and gastrointestinal tract
  — Equal sex distribution
  — Most lesions are benign
  — Lesions occur between 20 and 40 years of age
  — Breast carcinoma occurs in up to half of affected patients
- Ruvalcaba-Myhre-Smith syndrome (Bannayan-Riley-Ruvalcaba syndrome)
  — Presents in childhood with macrocephaly, mental deficiency, unusual craniofacial appearance, pigmented macules on the penis, and gastrointestinal polyps

▌ Cronkhite-Canada syndrome
- Unknown etiology
- Rare adult, nonfamilial (nonhereditary), gastrointestinal polyposis syndrome
- Onset typically occurs in late adulthood
- Associated with alopecia, skin hyperpigmentation, and nail dystrophy; hair loss can be total and usually occurs rapidly
- Symptoms include diarrhea, abdominal pain, and protein and weight loss
- Mortality rate is 60%, due to cachexia

Gross and Endoscopic Pathology

▌ FAP
- In fully developed cases, the colon is carpeted with adenomas
- Sizes range from not grossly visible to larger than 1 cm
- Average number of polyps is generally more than 1000; exceptions include attenuated FAP and MYH-associated polyposis syndrome that usually demonstrate less than 100 polyps

▌ Peutz-Jeghers syndrome
- Pigmented lesions resemble freckles; on lips, buccal mucosa, and perianal skin
- Polyps occur throughout the gastrointestinal tract, with small bowel (96% of cases) and colon (30% of cases) most commonly affected
- Usually less than 50 polyps
- Polyps range in size from several millimeters to greater than 5 cm

■ Juvenile polyposis syndrome
- Six to several hundred polyps most commonly seen in the colon or stomach
- Size ranges from smaller than 1 mm to about 5 cm
- Nearly 90% are within 20 cm of the anus
- Most are pedunculated; unusual shapes
- Surface ulceration is common (accounts for bleeding episodes)
- Lobulated, globoid, gray-red, mushroom-like masses

■ PTEN-associated polyposis syndrome
- Cowden disease
  — Numerous facial abnormalities occur, including beaked nose, arched palate, and retinal gliomas
  — About 70% of patients have gastrointestinal polyps, which may be anywhere from esophagus to rectum
  — Polyps can resemble hyperplastic or trauma- and prolapse-related polyps grossly and endoscopically
  — Facial trichilemmomas, together with gastrointestinal polyps, is considered diagnostic
- Ruvalcaba-Myhre-Smith syndrome
  — Pigmented macules on penis
  — Gastrointestinal polyps similar to Cowden disease

■ Cronkhite-Canada syndrome
- Polyps develop anywhere from esophagus to rectum
- Most polyps are found in the stomach and colon
- Presentation varies from tiny mucosal granularity, which can mimic primary inflammatory bowel disease, to edematous mucosal folds to pedunculated polyps
- Polyps often have gelatinous appearance to cut section because of cyst formation

Histopathology

■ FAP
- Polyps have histologic features identical to those of sporadic adenomas (tubular, tubulovillous, and villous adenomas)
- Earliest lesion consists only of dysplastic epithelium lining one (so-called one-gland adenoma) or several crypts
- Small intestinal polyps are also adenomas composed of dysplastic epithelium; gastric polyps may be adenomas (rare in Western countries) or fundic gland polyps

■ Peutz-Jeghers syndrome
- Represents hamartomatous overgrowth of the muscularis mucosae
- Characterized by an exophytic proliferation composed of epithelium and lamina propria lining intervening treelike or arborizing fascicles of smooth muscle
- Smooth muscle fibers branch out and thin peripherally
- Foci of dysplasia rarely seen
- Mild lamina propria edema with mild mixed inflammatory infiltrate can be present

■ Juvenile polyposis syndrome
- Represents hamartomatous overgrowth of the lamina propria
- Composed of resident benign glands, often focally dilated into cysts, which may be empty or contain mucus; cysts are lined by hyperplastic or atrophic epithelium
- Intervening stroma is inflamed, edematous, and generally devoid of smooth muscle
- Surface is often lined by attenuated glandular epithelium and is often ulcerated or focally replaced by granulation tissue
- Ganglioneuromatous proliferation (ganglion cells and hypertrophic nerves) can occur; there are histologic overlaps with PTEN polyposis syndrome
- Can have atypical histology with epithelial overgrowth; dysplasia reported in up to 20% of patients and some polyps may even contain malignancy

■ PTEN-associated polyposis syndromes (Cowden disease and Ruvalcaba-Myhre-Smith syndrome)
- Gastrointestinal polyps may be of the juvenile polyp type; some resemble solitary rectal ulcer syndrome
- Ganglioneuromas can be seen

■ Cronkhite-Canada syndrome
- Histologic features virtually identical to those of juvenile polyps
- Polyps often have cysts lined by atrophic epithelium
- Rarely, adenomatous change and carcinoma can develop
- Intervening mucosa is abnormal, showing edematous expansion of lamina propria; eosinophils can be prominent

Special Stains and Immunohistochemistry
- Noncontributory

Modern Techniques for Diagnosis

■ FAP and Gardner syndrome
- Truncated protein assay is largely replaced by gene sequencing to determine precise location of the mutation within the *APC* gene (5q 21-22)

■ Peutz-Jeghers syndrome
- About 70% linked to mutation in *STK-11* (*LKB1*; 19q13.3)

■ Juvenile polyposis
- Some kindred link to mutations of *MADH-4* (*SMAD-4*; 18q21.1) and *BMPR1A* (10q22.3)

■ PTEN-associated polyposis syndrome
- Cowden disease linked to mutations of *PTEN* gene (10q22-23)
- Ruvalcaba-Myhre-Smith syndrome linked to mutation of *PTEN* gene (10q23.3)

Differential Diagnosis

■ Sporadic juvenile and Peutz Jeghers polyps
  ● Histologically identical to their nonsyndromatic counterparts
  ● Diagnosis of the polyposis syndromes requires knowledge of the clinical and family history, the presence of polyps elsewhere in the gastrointestinal tract, and associated conditions
■ Intestinal ganglioneuromatosis
  ● Most ganglioneuromas seen in practice are isolated
  ● Can be seen in juvenile polyposis syndrome, PTEN polyposis syndromes, tuberous sclerosis, neurofibromatosis, and MEN-IIB
■ Hyperplastic (serrated) polyposis syndrome
  ● Defined as five or more hyperplastic polyps proximal to the sigmoid colon, of which two are larger than 1 cm; or any number of hyperplastic polyps proximal to the sigmoid colon in an individual with a first-degree relative with known hyperplastic polyposis syndrome or a patient with more than 30 hyperplastic polyps with any size and location in the colon and rectum
  ● About half of patients reported with hyperplastic polyposis syndrome have had complicating colorectal carcinoma
  ● Polyp types vary
  ● Typical hyperplastic polyps can be seen; polyps typical of sessile serrated polyp are common, and sessile serrated polyps admixed with areas of dysplasia (serrated adenoma) may occur
  ● Familial forms may represent an inherited predisposition to DNA hypermethylation
■ Traditionally defined serrated adenoma
  ● Usually isolated and pedunculated, involving left colon
  ● Serration may mimic hyperplastic polyp or sessile serrated polyp
  ● Characterized by gastric metaplasia, eosinophilic cytoplasmic change, and epithelial dysplasia
■ Benign fibroblastic polyp and colorectal perineurioma
  ● Solitary or multiple; may be found throughout the gastrointestinal tract
  ● Proliferation of small, tightly packed spindle cells within the lamina propria, often oriented parallel to the muscularis mucosae
  ● Frequently coexists with hyperplastic polyp-like epithelial changes
  ● Negative for S-100 protein and other neural markers
  ● Positive for epithelial membrane antigen

Pearls

■ FAP
  ● Patients with more than 10 cumulative adenomas should be studied for FAP and related syndromes

■ Juvenile polyposis syndrome
  ● Biopsies in patients with known history of juvenile polyposis should be carefully screened for dysplasia
  ● Juvenile polyps are usually isolated and sporadic and not part of a polyposis syndrome; they are the most common pediatric gastrointestinal polyp and are prone to autoamputation

Selected References

Jass JR: Gastrointestinal polyposes: Clinical, pathological and molecular features. Gastroenterol Clin N Am 26:927-946, 2007.

Galiatsatos P, Foulkes WD: Familial adenomatous polyposis. Am J Gastroenterol 101:385-398, 2006.

Giardiello FM, Trimbath JD: Peutz-Jeghers syndrome and management recommendations. Clin Gastroenterol Hepatol 4:408-415, 2006.

Lefevre JH, Rodriguez CM, Mourra N, et al: Implication of MYH in colorectal polyposis. Ann Surg 244:874-879; discussion, 879-880, 2006.

Zamecnik M, Chlumska A: Perineurioma vs. fibroblastic polyp of the colon. Am J Surg Pathol 30:1337-1339, 2006.

Burt R, Neklason DW: Genetic testing for inherited colon cancer. Gastroenterology 125:1696-1716, 2005.

Schreibman IR, Baker M, Amos C, McGarrity TJ: The hamartomatous polyposis syndromes: A clinical and molecular review. Am J Gastroenterol 100:476-490, 2005.

Hyman NH, Anderson P, Blasyk H: Hyperplastic polyposis and the risk of colorectal cancer. Dis Colon Rectum 47:2101-2104, 2004.

Lipton L, Tomlinson I: The multiple colorectal adenoma phenotype and MYH, a base excision repair gene. Clin Gastroenterol Hepatol 8:633-638, 2004.

Riddell RH, Petras RE, Williams GT, Sobin LH: Tumors of the intestines. Atlas of Tumor Pathology, Third Series, Fascicle #32. Washington, DC, Armed Forces Institute of Pathology, 2003.

Aaltonen LA, Jass JR, Howe JR: Juvenile polyposis. In Hamilton SR, Aaltonen LA (eds): World Health Organization Classification of Tumours of the Digestive System. Lyon, IARC Press, 2000, pp 130-133.

Burt R, Jass JR: Hyperplastic polyposis. In Hamilton SR, Aaltonen LA (ed): World Health Organization Classification of Tumours: Pathology and Genetics: Tumours of the Digestive System. Lyon, IARC Press, 2000, pp 135-136.

Lynch HT, Smyrk T, McGinn T, et al: Attenuated familial adenomatous polyposis (AFAP): A phenotypically and genotypically distinctive variant of FAP. Cancer 76:2427-2433, 1995.

Sarre R, Frost A, Jagelman D, et al: Gastric and duodenal polyps in familial adenomatous polyposis: A prospective study of the nature and prevalence of upper gastrointestinal polyps. Gut 28:306-314, 1987.

Gastrointestinal Mesenchymal Neoplasms

Clinical Features

● Historically, spindle cell neoplasms of the gastrointestinal tract were thought to arise from

Figure 6-109. Endoscopic view of a gastric gastrointestinal stromal tumor illustrating a spherical mass with intact mucosa.

Figure 6-110. Cross section of a resected small intestinal gastrointestinal stromal tumor showing areas of hemorrhagic degeneration.

Figure 6-111. Epithelioid gastrointestinal stromal tumors are composed of round cells with peripheral clear cytoplasm.

Figure 6-112. Desmoid tumor of the small bowel showing a proliferation of uniform spindle cells without atypia infiltrating the mesenteric adipose tissue.

Figure 6-113. Benign leiomyoma of colonic muscularis mucosae showing haphazard intertwining fascicles of plump smooth muscle cells.

smooth muscle and were thus termed *leiomyoma*, *leiomyosarcoma*, or *leiomyoblastoma*

- Subsequently, ultrastructural and immunohistochemical studies demonstrated that cells composing these tumors were either undifferentiated or only rarely showed evidence of smooth muscle or neural differentiation, or both
- Currently most of these stromal tumors are thought to arise from or are differentiated toward interstitial

Figure 6-114. Benign schwannoma involving the stomach showing the prominent cuffing of lymphocytes (Crohn-like reaction).

Figure 6-115. Granular cell tumor of the stomach showing round and elongated spindle cells with variably shaped small nuclei and prominent eosinophilic cytoplasmic granules.

cell of Cajal; a cell that may control motility (intercalating between autonomic nerves and muscle cells), possibly explaining the prior studies showing neural and muscle differentiation

- Currently, stromal tumors of the gastrointestinal tract are generally split into two groups
  - Recognizable diagnostic entities identical to soft tissue tumors found elsewhere in the body (e.g., schwannoma, leiomyoma)

Figure 6-116. Glomus tumor of the stomach is composed of small cells surrounding angulated dilated blood vessels. The glomus tumor cells are round and uniform, with basophilia, cytoplasm, and a centrally placed nucleus. Cellular borders are typically sharply defined.

Figure 6-117. Clear cell sarcoma with multinucleated giant cells involving the small intestine. This mimicker of gastrointestinal stromal tumor is composed of highly cellular malignant spindle cells with scattered osteoclast-like giant cells.

  - Spindle cell neoplasms, most of which overexpress CD117 (c-Kit) and are referred to as *gastrointestinal stromal tumors (GISTs)*
- GIST
  - Account for 0.1% to 1% of all gastrointestinal tumors
  - Histologic features overlap with other mesenchymal tumors
  - Most common in the stomach and small intestine
    - Most patients are older (50 to 70 years of age)
    - About 50% of these tumors ulcerate and bleed
    - The tumor may occur in young women (<20 years) alone or may be associated with Carney triad, which includes

Figure 6-118. Endoscopic photograph of duodenum with follicular lymphoma. Notice the variably sized mucosal polyps (lymphomatous polyposis).

Figure 6-120. Follicular lymphoma showing prominent *bcl-2* immunostaining.

Figure 6-119. Follicular lymphoma involving duodenum showing small cleaved cells in a follicular arrangement.

Figure 6-121. Colonic resection specimen demonstrating lymphomatous polyposis. The polyps themselves are spherical and attached to the mucosal folds by a small pedicle. Larger polyps show central ulceration.

- ◆ Epithelioid GIST
- ◆ Pulmonary chondroma
- ◆ Extra-adrenal paraganglioma

Gross and Endoscopic Pathology

▮ GIST

- Both benign and malignant tumors are spherical, well-circumscribed, submucosal or mural tumors that extend into the gastrointestinal lumen; mucosa over lesion may ulcerate
- Cut surface is smooth, pink-white, and firm; may have a lobulated or whorled appearance

- Focal areas of hemorrhage, necrosis, or small cyst formation may be seen
- Malignant tumors may have fleshy, tan-pink parenchyma with soft, necrotic areas
  — Some tumors may be large with an infiltrative, destructive growth pattern

Histopathology

▌ GIST

- Histologically composed of spindle cells of varying cellularity, hyperchromasia, and nuclear pleomorphism
- May be composed of epithelioid cells (epithelioid GIST)
- Pathologic factors do not necessarily correlate with clinical behavior
- Consensus approach to prognostic groups is recommended
  - Tumors smaller than 2 cm containing less than 5 mitoses/50 hpf are considered at very low risk for aggressive behavior
  - Low-risk tumors measure 2 to 5 cm in greatest cross-dimension and contain less than 5 mitoses/50 hpf
  - Intermediate-risk tumors include tumors smaller than 5 cm that have 6 to 10 mitoses/50 hpf and tumors measuring 5 to 10 cm but have less than 5 mitoses/50 hpf
  - Tumors larger than 5 cm with more than 5 mitoses/10 hpf, any tumor larger than 10 cm, and any tumor with more than 10 mitoses/50 hpf fall into a high-risk group for aggressive behavior
- These consensus risk groups have prognostic significance
  - Risk for an adverse outcome varies with site
    - ◆ The proportion of aggressive behavior in gastric tumors ranges from 0% in the very–low-risk group, 1.8% in the low-risk group, 7.3% in the intermediate-risk group, and 45.9% in the high-risk group
    - ◆ For small bowel tumors, aggressive behavior had been observed in 0% in the very–low-risk group, 4.3% in the low-risk group, 24.6% in the intermediate-risk group, and 77.2% in the high-risk group
    - ◆ Colorectal GISTs are rare, with most patients falling into a high-risk group and with 75% having acted in an aggressive fashion; aggressive behavior has only rarely been observed in colorectal GISTs demonstrating very–low-, low-, or intermediate-risk group characteristics
  - Adjuvant chemotherapy with imatinib may be indicated for high-risk GIST

Special Stains and Immunohistochemistry

▌ GIST

- Since introduction of imatinib as effective treatment for metastatic GIST, tumors should be shown to overexpress CD117 (c-Kit) by immunohistochemistry, preferentially as part of an immunohistochemical panel including CD34, desmin, actin, and S-100 protein (or other melanoma markers)

- Scattered cells can be positive for SMA and vimentin
- Spindle cells are positive for CD34 in more than 80% of cases
- Small percentage of GISTs are positive for S-100 protein

Other Techniques for Diagnosis

- Activating mutations in *KIT* genes are detected in exons 11, 9, 13, and 17; these may have prognostic significance. About 85% of patients with exon 11 mutation have at least a partial response to imatinib; whereas only half of patients with exon 9 mutations respond. Patients with exon 13 or 17 mutations rarely respond to imatinib

Differential Diagnosis

▌ CD117-negative GIST

- About 4% of tumors with typical GIST morphology fail to overexpress c-Kit, CD117, or C34 by immunohistochemistry
  - These tumors often show GIST-associated chromosomal abnormalities (monosomy of chromosome 14 or 14q deletion)
  - About 72% show *PDGFRA* mutation
  - About 12% have *KIT* gene mutation
  - Epithelioid GISTs are over-represented, as are omental and peritoneal GISTs
  - Some patients respond to imatinib

▌ Spindle cell carcinoma

- Characterized by areas of epithelial differentiation and by cytokeratin immunoreactivity

▌ Malignant fibrous histiocytoma (MFH)

- May resemble high-grade GIST
- MFH is characterized by presence of storiform architecture and large amounts of collagen (highlighted with trichrome stain)

▌ Fibromatosis

- Characterized by an orderly proliferation of bland, wavy spindle cells, often extending into the mucosa, bowel wall, or mesenteric fat with an infiltrative border
- Lacks fascicular arrangement of typical smooth muscle tumors
- No cellular atypia
- Can have keloid-like areas
- Usually lacks mitosis figures
- May give false-positive CD117 immunostaining; this varies by immunostaining technique

▌ True smooth muscle tumor

- Rare, most often encountered in esophagus or muscularis mucosae of colon and rectum
- Leiomyomas are typically well circumscribed with pushing borders; composed of interlacing fascicles of plump spindle cells with cigar-shaped nuclei and minimal mitotic activity
- Leiomyosarcomas are rare but most often described in the stomach, small bowel, or colon

— Hypercellular tumors with haphazard arrangement of spindle, oval, or rounded cells; bizarre giant cells may be intermixed
— Infiltrative growth and high mitosis rate
— Necrosis common
— Must prove smooth muscle origin (e.g., SMA immunohistochemistry) and must rule out GIST with immunohistochemistry for CD117 and CD34

▮ Inflammatory myofibroblastic tumor
  ● Usually contains admixture of spindle cells and inflammatory cells with plasma cells
  ● Negative for immunoreactive CD117 and CD34; scattered cells positive for SMA and desmin
▮ Schwannoma
  ● Typical Antoni A and Antoni B areas with hyalinized blood vessels
  ● Often demonstrates a prominent cuffing by lymphoid aggregates
  ● Stains positive for S-100 protein; CD117 and CD34 immunostains variable
▮ Solitary fibrous tumor
  ● Highly cellular spindle cell tumor associated with deposits of collagen
  ● CD34 immunostain positive; negative for CD117
▮ Granular cell tumor
  ● Composed of spindle and epithelioid cells with granular basophilic cytoplasm
  ● Strong S-100–positive immunostaining; negative for CD117
▮ Glomus tumor
  ● Tumor cells are small and sharply defined, showing solid arrangements around dilated blood vessels
  ● Robust SMA immunostaining; negative for CD117 and CD34
▮ Osteoclast-rich tumor resembling clear cell sarcoma
  ● Can mimic GIST
  ● CD117 negative; positive for S-100 protein and stain variably for cytokeratin and melanoma markers (e.g., HMB-45, melan-A)

Selected References

Hassan I, You YN, Dozois EJ, et al: Clinical, pathologic, and immunohistochemical characteristics of gastrointestinal stromal tumors of the colon and rectum: Implications for surgical management and adjuvant therapies. Dis Colon Rectum 49:609-615, 2006.

Miettinen M, Fetsch JF: Evaluation of biological potential of smooth muscle tumours. Histopathology 48:97-105, 2006.

Miettinen M, Makhlouf H, Sobin LH, Lasota J: Gastrointestinal stromal tumors of the jejunum and ileum: A clinicopathologic, immunohistochemical, and molecular genetic study of 906 cases before imatinib with long-term follow-up. Am J Surg Pathol 30:477-489, 2006.

Rubin BP: Gastrointestinal stromal tumours: An update. Histopathology 48:83-96, 2006.

Diment J, Tamborini E, Casali P, et al: Carney triad: Case report and molecular analysis of gastric tumor. Human Pathol 36:112-116, 2005.

Miettinen M, Sobin LH, Lasota J: Gastrointestinal stromal tumors of the stomach: A clinicopathologic, immunohistochemical, and molecular genetic study of 1765 cases with long-term follow-up. Am J Surg Pathol 29:52-68, 2005.

Medeiros F, Corless CL, Duensing A, et al: KIT-negative gastrointestinal stromal tumors: Proof of concept and therapeutic implications. Am J Surg Pathol 28:889-894, 2004.

Rodriguez JA, Guarda LA, Rosai J: Mesenteric fibromatosis with involvement of the gastrointestinal tract: A GIST simulator: a study of 25 cases. Am J Clin Pathol 121:93-98, 2004.

Miettinen M, Kopczynski J, Makhlouf HR, et al: Gastrointestinal stromal tumors, intramural leiomyomas, and leiomyosarcomas in the duodenum: A clinicopathologic, immunohistochemical, and molecular genetic study of 167 cases. Am J Surg Pathol 27:625-641, 2003.

Riddell RH, Petras RE, Williams GT, Sobin LH: Tumors of the intestines. Atlas of Tumor Pathology Third Series, Fascicle #32. Washington, DC, Armed Forces Institute of Pathology, 2003.

Zambrano E, Reyes-Mugica M, Franchi A, Rosai J: An osteoclast-rich tumor of gastrointestinal tract with features resembling clear cell sarcoma of soft parts: reports of 6 cases of a GIST simulator. Int J Surg Pathol 11:75-81, 2003.

Miettinen M, Sarlomo-Rikala M, Sobin LH, Lasota J: Gastrointestinal stromal tumors and leiomyosarcomas in the colon: A clinicopathologic, immunohistochemical and molecular genetic study of 44 cases. Am J Surg Pathol 24:1339-1352, 2000.

Intestinal Lymphoma

Clinical Features

● Gastrointestinal tract is most common extranodal site of lymphoma (stomach is most common gastrointestinal site, followed by small intestine and then colon)

Figure 6-122. Mantle cell lymphoma involving the small intestine showing monotonous cells with a distinctive rim of cytoplasm. A small nucleolus is present in many of the cells.

Figure 6-123. Mantle cell lymphoma. Cyclin D1 immunostain.

Figure 6-124. Pleomorphic enteropathy-associated T-cell lymphoma showing atypical lymphocytes of various sizes and shapes.

- Most are B-cell lymphomas
- By definition, distant nodes, peripheral blood, bone marrow, and other extranodal sites are uninvolved initially in primary intestinal lymphoma
- Patients present with abdominal pain, weight loss, intestinal obstruction, acute abdomen
■ Follicular lymphoma
  - Rarely primary in the gastrointestinal tract
  - Usually causes obstruction
  - Can present as a polyp or lymphomatous polyposis
  - Composed of small cleaved (centrocyte-like) cells; can have admixed larger cells
  - Translocation at t(14;18) causes overexpression of *bcl-2*
■ Mantle cell lymphoma
  - Usually presents with widespread lymphadenopathy and frequent bone marrow involvement

- Gastrointestinal tract involved in 10% to 20% of patients; clinically occult involvement in up to 80% of patients
- Can present with a mass, diffuse mucosal thickening, or lymphomatous polyposis
- Composed of atypical small cleaved lymphocytes surrounding germinal centers and effacing them
- Express CD20; coexpress CD5
- Translocation at t(11;14) causes overexpression of cyclin D1, which is considered definitional
■ Extranodal marginal B-cell lymphoma of MALT type (also see gastric lymphoma, earlier)
  - Can present as lymphomatous polyposis
  - Immunoproliferative small intestinal disease (IPSID, Mediterranean lymphoma) considered a variant
    — Can be associated with α heavy-chain disease
■ Enteropathy-associated T-cell lymphoma
  - Most (if not all) cases associated with active or latent celiac sprue or refractory celiac sprue; typically affects patients in fifth to sixth decades
  - Causes small intestinal ulcers and strictures
  - Poor prognosis
  - Two histologic types
    — Pleomorphic lymphoma (80% of cases); cells are CD3 positive, TIA-1 negative, CD56 negative, CD4 negative, CD5 negative, CD8 positive in 20% of cases
    — Monomorphic small to medium cells; cells are 90% CD56 positive, 80% CD8 positive

Other Techniques for Diagnosis

- Flow cytometry, gene rearrangement studies, and cytogenetics are crucial for the classification of lymphomas
- Extranodal marginal zone B-cell lymphoma of MALT type
  — Flow cytometry: CD19 and CD20 positive; CD5, CD10, and CD23 negative
  — Fluorescent in situ hybridization (FISH) for t(11;18), t(14;18), trisomy 3, and 18q21 rearrangements
- Mantle cell lymphoma
  — Flow cytometry: CD5, bcl-2, and cyclin D1 positive; CD10 and CD23 negative
  — FISH for t(11;14)

Differential Diagnosis

- The main differential diagnosis is between benign reactive conditions and different variants of lymphoma
- Benign lymphoid hyperplasia in the gastrointestinal tract
  — Grossly or endoscopically present with multiple tan-white mucosal nodules 0.1 to 0.5 cm
  — May be anywhere in bowel but most common in ileum (Peyer patches), duodenum, and rectum (so-called rectal tonsil)

— Composed of variably sized lymphoid nodules with germinal centers; germinal centers have reactive changes, including tingible body macrophages, mitoses, nuclear debris, and phagocytosis

— Mixed inflammatory background consisting of small lymphocytes, plasma cells, and histiocytes

— Remember that children often have marked lymphoid hyperplasia of the terminal ileum

— No immunoglobulin light-chain restriction; no B-cell gene rearrangements

Pearls

- Procure tissue for flow cytometric analysis or gene rearrangement studies in all suspected cases of lymphoma
- Lymphoepithelial lesions are suggestive of MALT lymphoma
- Ulcerated lesions in the jejunum (especially with a history of celiac sprue) are suggestive of enteropathy-associated T-cell lymphoma

Selected References

Banks PM: Gastrointestinal lymphoproliferative disorders. Histopathology 50:42-54, 2007.

Cellier C, Cerf-Bensussan N: Treatment of clonal refractory celiac disease or cryptic intraepithelial lymphoma: A long road from bench to beside. Clin Gastroenterol Hepatol 4:1320-1321, 2006.

Kodama T, Ohshima K, Nomura K, et al: Lymphomatous polyposis of the gastrointestinal tract, including mantle cell lymphoma, follicular lymphoma and mucosa-associated lymphoid tissue lymphoma. Histopathology 47:467-478, 2005.

Riddell RH, Petras RE, Williams GT, Sobin LH: Tumors of the intestines. Atlas of Tumor Pathology Third Series, Fascicle #32. Washington, DC, Armed Forces Institute of Pathology, 2003.

Anal Canal

Anal Neoplasia

- Proper classification requires careful clinical assessment
  - Lesions below the dentate line should be classified according to World Health Organization typing of skin tumors and should be treated accordingly

Clinical Features

▌ Condyloma acuminatum
- More common in men, particularly homosexual men
- Other risk factors include
  - Cervical and vulvar condyloma
  - HIV infection
  - Pregnancy
  - Diabetes mellitus

Figure 6-125. Endoscopic view of "rectal tonsil" demonstrating a large intraluminal polyp involving the rectum.

Figure 6-126. Lymphoid hyperplasia of the rectum shows follicular hyperplasia and scattered islands of pale-staining histiocytes.

Figure 6-127. Condyloma acuminatum involving the anal canal and perianal skin (clinical photograph).

Figure 6-128. Resection specimen of anal squamous carcinoma. The focally ulcerated lesion undermines the rectal mucosa.

Figure 6-130. Basaloid carcinoma of the anal canal showing insular-type infiltration, peripheral palisading of neoplastic cells, and retraction artifact.

Figure 6-129. Squamous carcinoma in situ, Bowen type, showing full-thickness squamous epithelial atypia.

Figure 6-131. High-grade neuroendocrine carcinoma of the low rectum and anal canal, large cell type (chromogranin immunostain).

▌ Intraepithelial squamous neoplasia
  ● Can occur in anal canal and perianal skin
  ● Includes anal canal intraepithelial neoplasia (AIN), bowenoid dysplasia, and squamous carcinoma in situ, Bowen type (Bowen disease [BD])
  ● AIN and BD are associated with HPV infection
  ● Bowenoid dysplasia can occur as a multifocal macular lesion in young patients; often referred to as *bowenoid papulosis*
  ● AIN is usually a single lesion and is more common in older women

  ● BD, a form of squamous cell carcinoma in situ, typically affects elderly patients in whom it presents with itching and burning
▌ Anal carcinoma
  ● Arise from anal canal
  ● About 80% to 90% are squamous cell carcinomas or variant squamous cell carcinomas
  ● Anal canal carcinomas arise above the dentate line
  ● Symptoms include rectal bleeding and pain
  ● Anal canal carcinomas occur at all ages (predominantly 40 to 60 years) and are more common in young men and older women
  ● Risk factors for anal canal carcinoma include
    — Condyloma acuminatum
    — Anal intraepithelial neoplasia and BD

Figure 6-132. Paget disease of perianal skin. The epidermis contains individual and groupings of large pale vacuolated cells with some gland formation.

— Crohn disease
— Immunodeficient state

Gross and Endoscopic Pathology

▌ Condyloma acuminatum
  ● Varies from single, small exophytic growths to cauliflower-like masses covering large areas
▌ Intraepithelial squamous neoplasia
  ● AIN: flat, generally single lesion in older patients
  ● BD: slightly raised, scaly, reddish plaque
▌ Anal carcinoma
  ● Arises near dentate line
  ● May present as submucosal nodule or be diffusely infiltrative
  ● May infiltrate prostate gland, vagina, or bladder

Histopathology

▌ Condyloma acuminatum
  ● Acanthotic, papillomatous lesions with hyperkeratosis, koilocytotic atypia, and variable dysplasia; can be flat
  ● Discrete transition from adjacent normal squamous epithelium
  ● Variable chronic inflammation
  ● HPV-16 and HPV-18 are associated with high-grade dysplasia

▌ Intraepithelial squamous neoplasia
  ● AIN
    — Thickened epithelium with variable degree of undifferentiated basal cell proliferation (analogous to cervical intraepithelial neoplasia) showing epithelial dysplasia
    — Variable chronic inflammatory response
  ● Bowenoid dysplasia and bowenoid papulosis
    — Sharply demarcated area of acanthosis and hyperkeratosis with frequent parakeratosis and some degree of superficial maturation
    — Koilocytotic atypia is usually present
  ● BD
    — Plaquelike, full-thickness atypical and dyskeratotic squamous cells
    — Marked nuclear pleomorphism, giant cells, and koilocytotic atypia are often present
    — Unlike bowenoid papulosis, BD more commonly involves adjacent sweat ducts and is less well demarcated
▌ Anal carcinoma
  ● Most are variants of squamous carcinomas
  ● About 50% of anal canal tumors are nonkeratinizing and are poorly differentiated
  ● Tumors arising in the anal transitional zone have also been termed *basaloid, cloacogenic,* and *transitional carcinoma*
  ● Squamous variants contain syncytial cells in nests and cords, often with central keratinization; a basaloid, transitional, and keratinizing squamous cell carcinoma pattern often coexists; sarcomatoid carcinoma and evidence of neuroendocrine or rhabdomyoblastic differentiation may be seen
  ● Basaloid pattern
    — Characterized by peripheral palisading in tumor islands, although typically less than in basal cell carcinoma of skin
  ● Other patterns of anal carcinoma include mucoepidermoid, adenoid cystic, colorectal-type adenocarcinoma, and undifferentiated carcinoma with neuroendocrine features, large cell and small cell type

Special Stains and Immunohistochemistry

  ● A high proliferation rate with Ki-67 immunostain and overexpression of p16 correlate with high-grade AIN
  ● Immunoreactive p53 is often overexpressed in high-grade AIN and invasive squamous carcinoma
  ● High-grade squamous carcinoma, especially the basaloid variant, can mimic high-grade neuroendocrine carcinoma and lymphoma; immunostaining for LCA, cytokeratin, and neuroendocrine markers (e.g., chromogranin and synaptophysin) can be helpful

Other Techniques for Diagnosis

- Identification and typing of HPV in condyloma, dysplasia, and anal cancer by in situ hybridization or PCR can be done but is not used clinically

Differential Diagnosis

▍ Verrucous carcinoma
- Differentiated from invasive well-differentiated carcinoma by its bulbous growth that pushes into the underlying stroma, compared with the infiltrative growth pattern of conventional squamous carcinoma
- Distinction from condyloma acuminatum is arbitrary; however, both require complete surgical excision
- Size greater than 2 cm and presence of fistulas and complex sinuses argue strongly for verrucous carcinoma over conventional squamous carcinoma

▍ Paget disease
- Characterized by an intraepithelial proliferation of large, pale cells similar to those seen in melanoma; can mimic BD
- Paget cells contain mucin and are PAS, mucicarmine, and Alcian blue stain positive; immunohistochemistry for CEA is often positive
- Can represent classic apocrine-type Paget disease but can also be seen in association with primary rectosigmoid adenocarcinoma, primary anal canal adenocarcinoma; although clinical assessment is paramount, immunostaining for CK7, CK20, and gross cystic disease protein can help differentiate these entities pathologically

▍ Adenocarcinoma involving the anal canal
- Adenocarcinoma involving the anal canal can represent downward extension of rectal adenocarcinoma, can arise primarily in the anal canal or perianal duct and glands, or can complicate a chronic perianal fistula
  — Primary adenocarcinoma of the anal canal shows no surface component and can have nonintestinal morphology
- Adenocarcinoma in chronic anorectal fistula usually occurs in men with a long history of perianal disease; almost all cases reported have been mucinous adenocarcinoma

▍ Malignant melanoma
- Rare tumors; make up 1% of all primary melanomas and less than 1% of all anal tumors
- May contain large intraepithelial pale cells mimicking those of Paget and Bowen disease
- Adjacent squamous mucosa may demonstrate in situ melanoma with pagetoid melanocytes
- Positive immunostain for S-100 protein and HMB-45 and melan-A aid in diagnosis
- Tumor cells negative for mucin, cytokeratin, and CEA

Pearls

- If confronted with a tumor in the anal canal that is difficult to classify on routine H&E-stained sections, always remember the possibility of malignant melanoma
  — The anal canal is the third most common site for melanoma; frequently mimics a hemorrhoid clinically
  — Histologic appearance of anal melanoma can mimic solitary rectal ulcer syndrome, sarcoma, lymphoma, basaloid carcinoma, and high-grade neuroendocrine carcinoma
  — Immunostains for S-100 protein, HMB-45, and melan-A should be considered

Selected References

Balachandra B, Marcus V, Jass JR: Poorly differentiated tumours of the anal canal: A diagnostic strategy for the surgical pathologist. Histopathology 50:163-174, 2007.

Shepherd NA: Anal intraepithelial neoplasia and other neoplastic precursor lesions of the anal canal and perianal region. Gastroenterol Clin N Am 36:969-988, 2007.

Bernick PE, Klimstra DS, Shia J, et al: Neuroendocrine carcinomas of the colon and rectum. Dis Colon Rectum 47:163-169, 2004.

Colquhoun P, Nogueras JJ, Dipasquale B, et al: Interobserver and intraobserver bias exists in the interpretation of anal dysplasia. Dis Colon Rectum 45:453-458, 2002.

Riddell R, Petras RE, Williams G, Sobin L: Tumors of the small intestine, colon, and anus. Atlas of Tumor Pathology Third Series, Fascicle #32. Washington, DC, Armed Forces Institute of Pathology, 2003, pp 251-278.

Vermiform Appendix

Developmental Abnormalities

- The appendix can be congenitally absent or hypoplastic

Figure 6-133. Mucocele of the vermiform appendix. The opened normal appendiceal lumen (*right*) is adjacent to a well-defined mucin-containing cyst.

- Duplications can occur, usually in association with cecal duplication
- Diverticula are seen, but most are acquired from obstructive lesions of the appendix

Appendicitis

Clinical Features

- May occur at any age; peak age in teenage years and young adulthood
- About 10% of people in the United States are affected during their life
- Elderly patients have higher mortality and complication rates
- Presentation includes periumbilical pain that radiates to the right lower abdominal quadrant, rebound tenderness, fever, and leukocytosis
- About 15% of appendices that are resected for a preoperative diagnosis of acute appendicitis are normal

Gross Pathology

- Typically the serosa is dull, hyperemic, and coated by fibrinous exudate and adhesion, and it may contain a discrete focus of perforation
- Cut surface may be frankly necrotic; lumen often contains blood-tinged pus
- When perforation is present, the mesoappendix is often congested and tense
- Appendiceal lumen may contain a fecalith

Histopathology

- Variable histologic features depend on the duration of inflammation
- Early lesions contain mild acute inflammation at the crypt bases with small mucosal erosions
- Advanced lesions contain submucosal and mural abscesses and extensive mucosal ulceration
- Gangrenous lesions show complete mural necrosis with acute periappendicitis

Special Stains and Immunohistochemistry

- Noncontributory

Other Techniques for Diagnosis

- Noncontributory

Differential Diagnosis

▌ Mucocele
- Term should be used only as a gross description
- Characterized by cystic dilation of the appendix by mucus and is almost always associated with neoplastic process (mucinous cystadenoma or cystadenocarcinoma)
- Existence of non-neoplastic cysts called *retention cysts* is debated; these are characterized by cystic

appendices (<1 cm) that are lined by atrophic or normal (nondysplastic) epithelium
▌ Adenocarcinoma
- Mucinous adenocarcinoma is characterized by mucin-filled, neoplastic cysts lined by malignant, papillary mucinous epithelium with invasion
- Nonmucinous adenocarcinoma is identical to colorectal adenocarcinoma

Pearls

- Acute appendicitis is due to a combination of infection and luminal obstruction with ischemic damage, which in turn has many causes, including luminal fecalith (most common), lymphoid hyperplasia (often related to viral infection), foreign bodies, parasites (particularly *Enterobius vermicularis*), and fungi

Selected References

Blair NP, Bugis SP, Turner LJ, MacLoed MM: Review of the pathologic diagnoses of 2,216 appendectomy specimens. Am J Surg 165:618-620, 1993.

Butler C: Surgical pathology of acute appendicitis. Hum Pathol 12:870-878, 1981.

Appendiceal Neoplasms

Clinical Features

▌ Mucocele
- Gross term only
- Cystic dilation of the appendix by mucus caused by either a neoplastic or rarely an apparent non-neoplastic process; cysts larger than 1 cm should be considered neoplastic until proved otherwise
- Most are secondary to mucinous cystadenoma or cystadenocarcinoma; pseudomyxoma peritonei may

Figure 6-134. Mucinous cystadenoma of the appendix showing a villous adenoma similar to that seen in the colon.

Figure 6-135. Invasive well-differentiated adenocarcinoma arising in association with a mucinous cystadenoma of the appendix (mucinous cystadenocarcinoma). There is an infiltrating pattern to the neoplastic glands, which are surrounded by a tumor desmoplasia.

Figure 6-136. Myxoglobulosis of the vermiform appendix. The resected dilated appendix contained these intraluminal pearl-like globules along with a mucinous cystadenoma.

occur if neoplastic process dissects through the wall of the appendix
- Non-neoplastic cysts, called *retention mucoceles*, are controversial, measure less than 1 cm, and are generally caused by sterile obstruction of the appendiceal lumen
▌ Mucinous cystadenoma
- Occurs in adults (mean age, 53 years; peak, seventh decade)
- Most present as mucoceles in asymptomatic patients
- About 20% to 25% are associated with separate primary colonic adenocarcinoma

- Often causes symptoms of appendicitis, palpable mass, or pseudomyxoma peritonei
▌ Adenocarcinoma
- Uncommon in the appendix
- Typically found in adults 50 to 60 years old
- Often presents with symptoms of acute appendicitis; may cause pseudomyxoma peritonei
- Rarely recognized preoperatively

Gross and Endoscopic Pathology

▌ Mucocele
- Cystic dilation of the appendix caused by accumulation of mucus
- Generally larger than 1 cm
▌ Mucinous cystadenoma
- Often sausage-like appendix
- Mucin-filled diverticula may be present
▌ Adenocarcinoma
- Usually forms a mass at base of the appendix
- Fungating mass with abundant mucus and necrosis
- May obliterate appendix, making exact site of origin difficult to determine

Histopathology

▌ Mucinous cystadenoma
- Lined by columnar cells showing epithelial dysplasia, most often low grade
- Abundant mucus fills and dilates the appendiceal lumen
- Can extend into diverticula with rupture
- Hyalinization of appendiceal wall and dystrophic calcification commonly seen
- Can be associated with pseudomyxoma peritonei
▌ Adenocarcinoma
- Mucinous cystadenocarcinoma
  — Neoplastic glands infiltrate appendiceal wall with tumor desmoplasia
  — Coexists with precursor mucinous cystadenoma
  — Can be associated with pseudomyxoma peritonei
- Nonmucinous adenocarcinoma
  — Identical to colorectal adenocarcinomas
▌ Pseudomyxoma peritonei
- Peritoneal accumulation of gelatinous ascites caused by benign or malignant neoplasms of the vermiform appendix
- Often composed of virtually acellular pools of mucus
- Prognosis varies depending on extent of pseudomyxoma (localized better than diffuse), status of primary tumor (benign better than malignant), cellularity within the mucus of the pseudomyxoma (no or few epithelial cells better than cellular mucus), and degree of dysplasia (low-grade dysplasia better than high-grade dysplasia and adenocarcinoma)
  — Even with diffuse intraperitoneal disease, patients with a benign primary tumor, low cellularity within the mucus, and low-grade dysplasia have a 70% 10-year survival rate

- — Patients usually die of sepsis and bowel obstruction and not cancer
- — In woman, pseudomyxoma peritonei can occur with concomitant ovarian mucinous tumors; the vermiform appendix is the primary site in all cases

Special Stains and Immunohistochemistry

- PAS, mucicarmine, and Alcian blue stains are all positive in mucinous tumors (generally unnecessary)

Other Techniques for Diagnosis

- Cases of pseudomyxoma peritonei with coexisting ovarian mucinous tumor have been studied with CK7, CK20, and *K-ras*; results usually support appendiceal origin of the tumors

Differential Diagnosis

▌ Ruptured acute appendicitis
- Characterized by acute inflammation, mural necrosis, and acute periappendicitis without dissecting mucus, neoplastic epithelium, or desmoplastic tissue reaction

▌ Myxoglobulosis
- May present with mucocele
- Term is applied to intraluminal pearl-like globules that are often calcified
- Histologically, eosinophilic laminations with calcification are seen
- Can coexist with appendiceal mucinous neoplasia

Pearls

- Because many appendiceal neoplasms present with acute appendicitis, all appendectomy specimens should be carefully examined grossly to detect subtle mural lesions or tumors; routine histologic examination of appendiceal margin of excision is highly recommended

Selected References

Young RH: Pseudomyxoma peritonei and selected other aspects of the spread of appendiceal neoplasms. Semin Diagn Pathol 21:134-150, 2004.

Riddell RH, Petras RE, Williams GT, Sobin LH: Tumors of the intestines. Atlas of Tumor Pathology, Third Series, Fascicle #32. Washington, DC, Armed Forces Institute of Pathology, 2003.

Szych C, Staebler A, Connolly DC, et al: Molecular genetic evidence supporting the clonality and appendiceal origin of pseudomyxoma peritonei in women. Am J Pathol 154:1849-1855, 1999.

Ronnett BM, Kurman RJ, Shmookler BM, et al: The morphologic spectrum of ovarian metastases of appendiceal adenocarcinomas: A clinicopathologic and immunohistochemical analysis of tumors often misinterpreted as primary ovarian tumors or metastatic tumors from other gastrointestinal sites. Am J Surg Pathol 21:1144-1155, 1997.

Ronnett BM, Kurman RJ, Zahn CM, et al: Pseudomyxoma peritonei in women: A clinicopathologic analysis of 30 cases with emphasis on site of origin, prognosis, and relationship to ovarian mucinous tumors of low malignant potential. Hum Pathol 26:509-524, 1995.

Ronnett BM, Zahn CM, Kurman RF, et al: Disseminated peritoneal adenomucinosis and peritoneal mucinous carcinomatosis: A clinicopathologic analysis of 109 cases with emphasis on distinguishing pathologic features, site of origin, prognosis, and relationship to "pseudomyxoma peritonei." Am J Surg Pathol 19:1390-1408, 1995.

Nitecki SS, Wolff BG, Schlinkert R, et al: The natural history of surgically treated primary adenocarcinoma of the appendix. Ann Surg 219:51-57, 1994.

Young RH, Gilks CB, Sculy RE: Mucinous tumors of the appendix associated with mucinous tumors of the ovary and pseudomyxoma peritonei: A clinicopathologic analysis of 22 cases supporting an origin in the appendix. Am J Surg Pathol 15:415-429, 1991.

Gonzalez JE, Hann SE, Trujillo YP: Myxoglobulosis of the appendix. Am J Surg Pathol 12:962-966, 1988.

Carcinoids and Other Nonepithelial Tumors of the Vermiform Appendix

Clinical Features

▌ Carcinoid tumors
- Many are asymptomatic
- Can present with signs and symptoms of acute appendicitis

Gross and Endoscopic Pathology

- Present as a nodule or thickening of appendiceal wall

Histopathology

- Three variants described
- — Insular: typical midgut pattern of carcinoid tumor, well-demarcated variably sized islands composed of cells with uniform polygonal shape, little nuclear pleomorphism or mitotic activity with eosinophilic granular cytoplasm

Figure 6-137. Carcinoid tumor of the appendix, midgut pattern with insular groupings of carcinoid tumor cells showing cytoplasmic granules, round nuclei, and a coarsely granular chromatin pattern.

Figure 6-138. Tubular carcinoid of the appendix composed of ribbons and small tubular structures.

Figure 6-139. Appendiceal goblet cell carcinoid (microglandular goblet cell adenocarcinoma). Note the insular growth pattern of neoplastic cells showing prominent signet ring cell differentiation resembling mature goblet cells.

— Tubular: dominant glandlike pattern sometimes with columns or ribbons and acinar arrangement of small neoplastic endocrine cells that lack pleomorphism, have little or no mitotic activity
— Goblet cell carcinoid
  ◆ A misnomer; *crypt cell carcinoma* or *microglandular goblet cell adenocarcinoma* is the preferred name because these terms better reflect the true nature of the tumor
  ◆ Small, well-defined clusters and strands and microglandular collections of mucus-secreting epithelial cells that resemble goblet cells infiltrate the appendiceal wall
  ◆ Positive with pan-cytokeratin immunostains; usually negative for neuroendocrine markers

such as chromogranin or synaptophysin, or can show scattered rare neuroendocrine cells
  ◆ Solid areas of growth, a complex infiltrative pattern, nuclear atypia with increased numbers of mitoses figures, and dissecting mucus usually signal dedifferentiation into a higher grade of adenocarcinoma

Special Stains and Immunohistochemistry

- Mucin stains can be done with goblet cell carcinoid but are usually not necessary
- Chromogranin and synaptophysin immunohistochemistry is helpful, especially in the differential diagnosis of tubular carcinoid versus carcinoma

Other Techniques for Diagnosis

- Noncontributory

Differential Diagnosis

- Fibrous obliteration of the lumen and appendiceal neuroma
  — These spindle cell proliferations can contain scattered neuroendocrine cells that represent hyperplasia
  — A definite insular or tubular growth pattern, extension of the cells into the muscularis propria or beyond, or the presence of a gross nodule indicates carcinoid tumor
- Tubular carcinoma versus well-differentiated adenocarcinoma
  — Immunohistochemistry for chromogranin and synaptophysin helpful
- Signet ring cell carcinoma versus goblet cell carcinoid
  — Signet ring cell carcinoma is more infiltrative, with increased pleomorphism and larger nuclei
- Neurofibroma, granular cell tumor, paraganglioma, ganglioneuroma, gastrointestinal stromal tumor, sarcoma, and lymphoma have been described primarily within the vermiform appendix but are extremely rare

Pearls

- Composite tumor with areas that look like conventional adenocarcinoma will act like conventional adenocarcinoma
- Discovery of carcinoid and variant tumors is usually a surprise in an appendectomy specimen removed either incidentally or for acute appendicitis; therefore, routine examination of the appendiceal margin or resection is recommended
- Indications for right hemicolectomy for appendiceal carcinoid tumor include size greater than 2 cm, invasion beyond muscularis propria, venous invasion, incomplete excision (e.g., positive margin of resection), and coexisting adenocarcinoma

Selected References

Modlin IM, Kidd M, Latich I, et al: Current status of gastrointestinal carcinoids. Gastroenterology 128:1717-1751, 2005.

Young RH: Pseudomyxoma peritonei and selected other aspects of the spread of appendiceal neoplasms. Semin Diag Pathol 21:134-150, 2004.

Riddell RH, Petras RE, Williams GT, Sobin LH: Tumors of the intestines. In Atlas of Tumor Pathology, Third Series, Fascicle 32. Washington, DC, Armed Forces Institute of Pathology, 2003.

Burke AP, Sobin LH, Federspiel BH, et al: Goblet cell carcinoids and related tumors of the vermiform appendix. Am J Clin Pathol 94:27-35, 1990.

Burke AP, Sobin LH, Federspiel BH, et al: Appendiceal carcinoids: Correlation of histology and immunohistochemistry. Mod Pathol 2:630-637, 1989.

Secondary Malignancies in the Gastrointestinal Tract

Gastrointestinal Metastatic Disease

Clinical Features

▮ Esophagus
  ● Primary tumors of the lungs, pharynx, thyroid, and stomach may invade the esophagus directly
  ● Breast, kidney, testicular, prostate, and pancreatic neoplasms can metastasize to the esophagus
  ● Breast cancer may produce strictures due to extensive lymphatic infiltration
  ● Melanoma metastasizes to the gastrointestinal tract in 43% of cases

▮ Stomach
  ● Stomach is a more common site of metastases than small or large bowel

Figure 6-140. Resection specimen of large cell lymphoma involving the small intestine showing a stricturing and ulcerating mass lesion with a homogeneous, fleshy cut surface.

  ● Most common gastric metastases are melanomas and carcinomas of the lung and breast
  ● Gastric metastases often have a targetoid endoscopic appearance due to extensive central necrosis (features particularly notable on radiologic examination)

▮ Small intestine
  ● Because primary small bowel tumors are so uncommon, metastases (carcinomas and sarcomas) are the most common tumors of the small bowel
  ● Larger tumors are often polypoid, causing obstruction, intussusception, or perforation
  ● Tumors near the ampulla may represent secondary involvement of the intestine by pancreaticobiliary adenocarcinoma; primary ampullary malignancies usually arise in a preexisting adenoma and have a better prognosis than pancreatitis biliary carcinoma
  ● Malignant melanoma is the most common small bowel metastasis and often produces obstruction
  ● About 5% of testicular tumors metastasize to the gastrointestinal tract
  ● Sarcomas only rarely metastasize to the small bowel
  ● Bronchogenic squamous carcinoma has a propensity to metastasize to the proximal jejunum

▮ Large intestine
  ● Most common spread of metastases to the colon is by peritoneal seeding, particularly at the pouch of Douglas (anterior wall of rectum)
  ● Prostatic carcinoma may directly invade the rectum, producing gastrointestinal rather than urinary symptoms
  ● Anal melanomas may extend into the rectum
  ● Most common colonic metastases in males are from noncolonic gastrointestinal tumors and lung carcinomas
  ● Most common colonic metastases in females are from ovarian, breast, and lung carcinomas
  ● Colonic metastases are often asymptomatic, but with large tumors, obstruction and bleeding may occur

▮ Appendix
  ● Patients with mucinous tumors of the ovary may have a concurrent mucinous neoplasm in the appendix; all represent appendiceal primary tumors
  ● Other metastatic tumors reported include breast, stomach, cervix, and lung

Gross and Endoscopic Pathology

▮ Esophagus
  ● Nonspecific

▮ Stomach
  ● Often have multiple tumors that commonly show extensive central necrosis

▮ Small intestine
  ● Intramural masses form submucosal nodules and eventually produce bulging polypoid masses
  ● Tumors may be circumferential
  ● Black tumors in the small intestine suggest melanoma; however, melanoma is often amelanotic

- Fleshy cut sections are typical for lymphoma
- Ovarian metastases are most likely to present with carcinomatosis
- Ampullary tumors should be examined carefully to detect any residual adenoma (making the lesion more likely a primary small bowel neoplasm, rather than pancreatic)
▌ Large intestine
  - Metastasis is suggested by a mural-centered mass not involving the overlying mucosa

Histopathology

▌ Esophagus
  - Metastatic carcinoma including breast carcinoma preferentially involves the submucosal lymphatics and leaves overlying mucosa intact
▌ Stomach
  - Breast carcinoma may be diffusely infiltrative and difficult to distinguish from a primary poorly differentiated adenocarcinoma, diffuse type of Lauren
▌ Small intestine
  - Ampullary tumors that are primary may have residual adenoma
  - Pancreatic primary tumors with secondary involvement of the duodenum grow as an infiltrating, well-differentiated glandular proliferation or as highly anaplastic carcinoma with marked desmoplasia if high grade; often have non-neoplastic duodenal mucosa on the surface
▌ Large intestine
  - Primary colonic tumors may be distinguished from metastatic adenocarcinoma (such as lung) by the presence of extensive necrosis containing nuclear fragments (so-called dirty necrosis) along with lack of a surface component and predominant mural location

Special Stains and Immunohistochemistry

- In all cases, immunohistochemical markers unique to a specific site outside the gastrointestinal tract are helpful to diagnose a metastasis (e.g., TTF-1 for lung primary)

- Estrogen receptor (ER) and progesterone receptor (PR) testing should be performed on a metastatic breast carcinoma, but these immunostains are not specific for breast cancer
- CEA and CA-125 immunostains may be used to determine whether a gastrointestinal tumor is primary (CEA positive) or ovarian (CA-125 positive)
- S-100 protein and HMB-45 are typically positive in metastatic malignant melanoma
- Primary colonic carcinoma
  — More likely to be positive for CEA and cytokeratin 20 and negative for cytokeratin 7
- Pulmonary adenocarcinoma
  — Tends to be positive for cytokeratin 7 and TTF-1 and negative for cytokeratin 20

Other Techniques for Diagnosis

- Noncontributory

Differential Diagnosis

- Clinical history is important
- Regardless of the site, tumors in the gastrointestinal tract that are not mucosal based or that predominantly involve the bowel wall and serosa should be considered potentially metastatic

Pearls

- Any small intestinal malignancy outside the ampullary region is more likely to be a metastatic tumor than a primary tumor

Selected References

Berezauski K, Stastny J, Kornstein M, et al: Cytokeratin 7 and 20 and carcinoembryonic antigen in ovarian and colonic carcinoma. Mod Pathol 9:426, 1995.

Adair C, Ro JY, Sahin AA, et al: Malignant melanomas metastatic to gastrointestinal tract: A clinico-pathologic study. Int J Surg Pathol 2:3, 1994.

Telerman A, Gerard B, van den Hevle B, et al: Gastrointestinal metastases from extra-abdominal tumors. Endoscopy 17:99-101, 1985.

Matthew M. Yeh and Paul E. Swanson

7 Hepatobiliary System

Viral Hepatitis

Clinical Features

▌ Hepatitis A virus (HAV)
  ● Single-stranded RNA (ssRNA) virus (picornavirus)
  ● Transmission route: fecal-oral
  ● Incubation: 2 to 6 weeks
  ● Self-limited
  ● Not associated with chronic carrier state, chronic hepatitis, or hepatocellular carcinoma (HCC)

▌ Hepatitis B virus (HBV)
  ● Partially circular double-stranded DNA virus (hepadnavirus)
  ● Transmission route: perinatal, sexual, and parenteral
  ● Incubation: 6 to 8 weeks
  ● Chronic infection (10%): persistent serum hepatitis B surface antigen (HBsAg) more than 6 months after diagnosis
  ● Associated with chronic hepatitis, fulminant hepatitis, cirrhosis, and HCC
  ● Anti-HBsAg confers long-term immunity

411

▌ Hepatitis C virus (HCV)
- ssRNA virus (flavivirus like)
- Transmission route: parenteral
- Incubation: 6 to 12 weeks
- Highest rate of chronic hepatitis (60% to 80%) and persistent infection
- Associated with cirrhosis and HCC
- Anti-HCV does not confer immunity
- Serum transaminases: fluctuating

▌ Hepatitis D (delta agent) virus
- Defective RNA virus requiring HBsAg (envelope protein) for infectivity
- Transmission route: parenteral
- Associated with cirrhosis and HCC

▌ Hepatitis E virus
- ssRNA virus
- Water-borne infection

- Incubation: 6 weeks
- Virion shed in stools
- Usually self-limited
- High mortality rate among pregnant women

▌ Hepatitis G virus
- Nonpathogenic

Gross Pathology
- Noncontributory

Histopathology
▌ Acute viral hepatitis
- Injury is predominantly hepatocellular in the acini (zone 3)
- General features
  — Predominantly lymphocytic infiltrate, usually conspicuous in zone 3
  — Swollen hepatocytes with rarefied and granular cytoplasm
  — Apoptotic hepatocytes showing pyknotic nuclear remnants, shrunken and dense cytoplasm
  — Liver cell dropout with replacement by small groups of lymphocytes and macrophages
- Specific features
  — HAV: perivenular cholestasis; hepatitis with periportal inflammation (interface hepatitis) and dense portal infiltrate, including abundant plasma cells; or extensive microvesicular steatosis
  — HBV: ground-glass hepatocytes (indicating abundant HBsAg in the hepatocytes—evidence of viral infection)

▌ Chronic viral hepatitis
- Persistent liver injury with positive viral serology and abnormally high serum aminotransferase of >6 months' duration
- Injury is accentuated in the portal and periportal regions
- General features
  — Portal inflammatory infiltrate predominantly composed of lymphocytes with or without interface hepatitis of varying severity
  — Spotty or confluent necrosis with or without bridging necrosis
  — Portal fibrous expansion, periportal fibrosis, bridging fibrosis to cirrhosis (stages 1 to 4)
- Specific features
  — HBV: ground-glass hepatocytes
  — HCV: lymphoid aggregates or follicles with or without germinal centers, focal macrovesicular steatosis, damaged interlobular bile ducts

Special Stains and Immunohistochemistry
- Immunohistochemistry for hepatitis B core antigen (HBcAg), HBsAg, and hepatitis B early antigen (HBeAg)

Figure 7-1. A, Ground-glass hepatocytes in hepatitis B. B, Chronic hepatitis C. Classic lymphoid aggregates with focal mild interface hepatitis.

Other Techniques for Diagnosis

- Electron microscopy: HBsAg in hepatocyte cytoplasm (22-nm spheres and rods)

Differential Diagnosis

- Serologic markers of viral infection are virtually essential to establish or exclude the diagnosis
- ▌ Alcoholic hepatitis
  - Clinical history is important
  - Fatty change is typical but not always present
  - Many ballooned hepatocytes and Mallory hyaline are usually seen
  - Megamitochondria are a common finding
  - Lobular inflammatory foci (usually rich in neutrophils)
  - Perivenular and pericellular fibrosis (chicken-wire pattern)
- ▌ Nonalcoholic steatohepatitis (NASH)
  - Significant steatosis is present, predominantly macrovesicular
  - Zone 3 injury pattern with lobular inflammatory foci
  - Ballooned hepatocytes and Mallory hyaline are typical findings
  - Megamitochondria are a common finding
  - Perivenular and pericellular fibrosis (chicken-wire pattern)
- ▌ Autoimmune hepatitis
  - Serologic markers important (positive antinuclear antibody [ANA], anti–smooth muscle antibody [ASMA], and liver-kidney microsomal antibody [LKM])
  - Coexistent autoimmune diseases are common
  - Prominent plasma cells in the portal and periportal region or deep within the parenchyma
  - Marked interface hepatitis and parenchymal activity
  - Bridging necrosis is common and may form hepatitis rosettes
- ▌ Epstein-Barr virus (EBV) hepatitis
  - Seen more often after transplantation
  - Marked sinusoidal lymphoplasmacytic inflammatory infiltrate characteristically in single-file arrangement
  - Marked hepatocellular regeneration
- ▌ Primary biliary cirrhosis (PBC)
  - Bile ductular reaction
  - Florid duct lesion with granuloma
  - Damage and loss of interlobular bile duct
  - Positive antimitochondrial antibody (AMA)
  - Cholestatic picture
- ▌ Primary sclerosing cirrhosis
  - Bile ductular reaction
  - Periductal fibrosis and loss of interlobular bile duct
  - Association with ulcerative colitis is common
  - Characteristic beading on endoscopic retrograde cholangiopancreatography (ERCP)
- ▌ Drug hepatitis
  - Clinical history is important (time course of drug use)
  - Negative serologic markers of viral infection

Pearls

- Serologic markers of viral infection as well as the pattern of hepatic enzyme elevations are most important in distinguishing the many causes of hepatitis

Selected References

Batts KP, Ludwig J: Chronic hepatitis: An update on terminology and reporting. Am J Surg Pathol 19:1409-1417, 1995.

Goodman ZD, Ishak KG: Histopathology of hepatitis C infection. Semin Liver Dis 15:70-81, 1995.

Ishak KG: Chronic hepatitis: Morphology and nomenclature. Mod Pathol 7:690-713, 1994.

Gerber MA, Thung SN: The diagnostic value of immunohistochemical demonstration of hepatitis viral antigens in the liver. Hum Pathol 18:771-774, 1987.

Sciot R, Van Damme B, Desmet VJ: Cholestatic features in hepatitis A. J Hepatol 3:172-181, 1986.

Nonviral Infections

Clinical Features

- High mortality rate
- Patients often have fever and right upper quadrant tenderness
- Surgical drainage is often required
- Bacterial abscesses are caused by portal spread of extrahepatic infection with *Staphylococcus aureus*, *Salmonella typhi*, and syphilis
- Parasitic abscesses are caused by *Entamoeba histolytica*, *Echinococcus* species, malaria, *Leishmania* species, *Ascaris lumbricoides*, and liver flukes (e.g., *Clonorchis sinensis*, *Fasciola hepatica*, and *Opisthorchis viverrini*)

Gross Pathology

- Bacteremic spread through arterial or portal system: multiple, soft, grossly necrotic lesions
- Bacteremic spread by direct extension or trauma: solitary, large, soft, grossly necrotic lesions
- ▌ Syphilis
  - Single or multiple soft well-circumscribed lesions (gummas) that eventually scar, resulting in hepar lobatum, which grossly resembles cirrhosis
- ▌ Entamebiasis
  - Well-circumscribed lesion containing thick, dark material
- ▌ Echinococcal (hydatid) cyst
  - Space-occupying cystic lesion with internal daughter cysts
- ▌ Ascariasis
  - Numerous foul-smelling cavities

Figure 7-2. A, Bacterial abscess. Low-power view shows liver parenchyma with marked necrosis. **B, Amebic abscess.** Liver tissue showing necrotic debris with trophozoites at the center of the microphotograph.

▮ Malaria and leishmaniasis
  ● Hepatomegaly (secondary Kupffer cell hyperplasia)

Histopathology

▮ Bacterial
  ● Marked neutrophilic infiltrate with hepatocyte destruction
▮ Syphilis
  ● Congenital: neonatal hepatitis
  ● Tertiary: gummas (granulomatous abscesses), which heal as dense scars
▮ Entamebiasis
  ● Necrotic debris with trophozoites at the periphery
▮ Echinococcal infection
  ● Outer laminated non-nuclear layer, inner nucleated germinal layer with attached capsules containing numerous scolices that are released into the cyst cavity and give rise to daughter cysts
  ● Secondary cholangitis results from obstruction of intrahepatic bile ducts

▮ Ascariasis
  ● Necrotic debris with granulomatous and eosinophilic response to degenerated parasites
▮ Liver flukes
  ● Biliary epithelial hyperplasia, cholangitis, and periductal fibrosis
▮ Malaria
  ● Kupffer cell hyperplasia and phagocytosis of ruptured erythrocytes
▮ Leishmaniasis
  ● Kupffer cell hyperplasia and phagocytosis of organisms (Donovan bodies)

Special Stains and Immunohistochemistry

  ● Gram stain: helps highlight bacteria
  ● Warthin-Starry or Dieterle stain: syphilis
  ● Giemsa stain to identify amastigotes: leishmaniasis
  ● Direct examination for *Echinococcus* species scolices and liver flukes

Other Techniques for Diagnosis

  ● Culture may help identify organism

Differential Diagnosis

  ● See earlier for specific infection characteristics

Pearls

  ● Amebic abscesses are more likely to spread into the thoracic cavity
  ● Echinococcal cysts should be removed intact

Selected References

Koneman EW, Allen SD, Woods GL, et al (eds): Color Atlas and Textbook of Diagnostic Microbiology, 6th ed. Philadelphia, Lippincott Williams & Wilkins, 2005, pp 1244-1326.
Bissada AA, Bateman J: Pyogenic liver abscesses: A 7-year experience in a large community hospital. Hepatogastroenterology 38:17-20, 1991.

Drug-Induced Liver Disease

Clinical Features

  ● Clinical history important (e.g., ingesting an agent known to cause liver disease)
  ● An appropriate time interval between exposure and onset of disease
  ● Resolution of the lesion after withdrawal
  ● Can be acute or chronic

Histopathology

  ● Different agents may result in different liver injury patterns; for example
    — Zone 3 hepatocellular necrosis: acetaminophen
    — Mimicking acute viral hepatitis: antituberculous drugs, anesthetics, herbal medicine, nonsteroidal anti-inflammatory drugs

— Cholestasis with duct damage and duct loss: amoxicillin and clavulanic acid (Augmentin)

— Vanishing bile duct: chlorpromazine, amoxicillin and flucloxacillin, haloperidol

— Microvesicular steatosis: valproic acid, tetracycline, nucleoside analogues, salicylate (Reye syndrome)

— Hypertrophic hepatic stellate cells and perivenular and pericellular fibrosis: hypervitaminosis A

— Veno-occlusive disease: pyrrolizidine alkaloids or chemotherapeutic agents associated with bone marrow transplantation

— Steatohepatitis-like: amiodarone, tamoxifen

- Drug toxicity should always enter the differential diagnosis when abundant eosinophils or epithelioid granulomas are present

Special Stains and Immunohistochemistry

- Noncontributory

Other Techniques for Diagnosis

- Noncontributory

Differential Diagnosis

▌ Viral hepatitis
  - Positive serologic markers or viral nucleic acids
  - Immunohistochemistry may help to detect viral antigens (e.g., HBV, cytomegalovirus [CMV], herpes simplex virus [HSV], EBV)
▌ Autoimmune hepatitis
  - Positive ANA, ASMA, and anti-LKM
  - Prominent plasma cells
  - Responds to corticosteroid
▌ Biliary obstruction
  - Image studies may help
▌ PBC
  - Positive AMA
  - Florid duct lesion

Pearls

- Careful correlation of past and present history is essential, including use of herbal remedies and over-the-counter medications
- Rule out other liver diseases

Selected References

Geller SA, Petrovic LM: Effects of drugs and toxins on the liver. In Geller SA, Petrovic LM (eds): Biopsy Interpretation of the Liver. Philadelphia, Lippincott Williams & Wilkins, 2004, pp 111-124.

Zimmerman HJ, Ishak KG: Hepatic injury due to drugs and toxins. In MacSween RNM, Burt AD, Portmann BC, et al (eds): Pathology of the Liver, 4th ed. Edinburgh, Churchill Livingstone, 2002, pp 621-709.

Scheuer PJ, Lefkowitch JH: Drugs and toxins. In Scheuer PJ, Lefkowitch JH (eds): Liver Biopsy Interpretation. London, WB Saunders, 2000, pp 134-150.

Zimmerman HJ. Hepatotoxicity: The Adverse Effects of Drugs and Other Chemicals on the Liver, 2nd ed. Philadelphia, Lippincott Williams & Wilkins, 1999.

Alcoholic Liver Disease and Alcoholic Steatohepatitis

Clinical Features

- Nonspecific symptoms including malaise, anorexia, weight loss, and tender hepatomegaly with mild elevation of serum bilirubin and alkaline phosphatase
- About 20% to 25% of heavy drinkers develop alcoholic steatohepatitis

Gross Pathology

- Early: large, soft, greasy, yellow liver
- Late: shrunken, mottled, red-brown liver with bile staining
- End-stage: cirrhosis

Histopathology

- Steatosis
- Zone 3 injury pattern
- Ballooning degeneration
- Lobular inflammatory infiltrates, especially rich in neutrophils
- Mallory hyaline and megamitochondria
- Perivenular and pericellular fibrosis
- Bile ductular reaction

Special Stains and Immunohistochemistry

- Noncontributory

Other Techniques for Diagnosis

- Noncontributory

Differential Diagnosis

- Clinical history is essential
▌ Chronic viral hepatitis
  - Positive serologic markers of viral infection
  - Hepatocellular injury and initiation of fibrosis are more marked in the periportal areas, as opposed to steatohepatitis (perivenular and pericellular fibrosis and hepatocellular injury predominantly in zone 3 region)
  - Mallory hyaline more common in steatohepatitis
▌ Fatty liver of pregnancy
  - Typically occurs in third trimester of pregnancy
  - Steatosis is microvesicular
▌ Nonalcoholic steatohepatitis
  - Steatosis is essential
  - Glycogenated nuclei more common
  - Mallory hyaline and bile ductular reaction less common

Figure 7-3. Steatohepatitis. A, Macrovesicular fat with ballooned hepatocyte and lobular inflammatory infiltrate. **B,** Mallory hyaline is present in the ballooned hepatocytes with associated inflammatory foci. **C,** Pericellular and perisinusoidal fibrosis (chicken-wire pattern).

- Sclerosing hyaline necrosis or veno-occlusive lesion not common

Pearls

- Major pathologic effects of alcohol are caused by interference with lipid metabolism, mitochondrial damage, and cytoskeletal injury
- Genetically determined susceptibility is thought to account for the fact that only 20% to 25% of heavy drinkers develop alcoholic steatohepatitis, whereas individuals with minimal to no alcohol intake may develop histologically identical nonalcoholic steatohepatitis

Selected References

Geller SA, Petrovic LM: Alcoholic liver disease. In Geller SA, Petrovic LM (eds): Biopsy Interpretation of the Liver. Philadelphia, Lippincott Williams & Wilkins, 2004, pp 134-149.

Brunt EM: Alcoholic and nonalcoholic steatohepatitis. Clin Liver Dis 6:399-420, 2002.

Scheuer PJ, Lefkowitch JH: Fatty liver and lesions in the alcoholic. In Scheuer PJ, Lefkowitch JH (eds): Liver Biopsy Interpretation. London, WB Saunders, 2000, pp 111-133.

Nonalcoholic Fatty Liver Disease and Nonalcoholic Steatohepatitis

Clinical Features

- A manifestation of the metabolic (insulin resistance) syndrome
- Risk factors: central obesity, hyperglycemia, type II diabetes, arterial hypertension, and hypertriglyceridemia
- NASH is the progressive lesion of nonalcoholic fatty liver disease (NAFLD)
- Histologically, NASH is almost identical to alcoholic steatohepatitis but occurs in individuals who do not have significant alcohol history

Gross Pathology

- Early: large, soft, greasy, yellow liver
- Late: shrunken, mottled, red-brown liver with bile staining
- End-stage: cirrhosis

Histopathology

▌ Nonspecific steatosis in NAFLD
  - Predominantly macrovesicular fatty change
  - Typically starts in a zone 3 centrilobular pattern
▌ NASH
  - Begins as a zone 3 injury pattern consisting predominantly of macrovesicular steatosis, ballooned hepatocytes, and lobular inflammation

- Pigmented macrophages and acidophile bodies can be seen
- Cytoplasmic Mallory hyaline (fibrillary eosinophilic material composed of intermediate cytokeratin filaments associated with ubiquitin, a protein from cytoskeletal injury)
- Zone 3 perivenular and pericellular fibrosis (chicken-wire pattern), which progresses to central-portal bridging
- Cirrhosis (end-stage disease)

Special Stains and Immunohistochemistry

- Immunohistochemical stains for ubiquitin and p62 have been developed to identify Mallory hyaline

Other Techniques for Diagnosis

- Noncontributory

Differential Diagnosis

- Clinical history is essential
▌Chronic viral hepatitis
- Positive serologic markers of viral infection
- Inflammation is more accentuated in the portal and periportal areas
- Fibrosis initiates in portal regions
- Mallory hyaline is more common in steatohepatitis
▌Fatty liver of pregnancy
- Typically occurs in third trimester of pregnancy
- Steatosis is microvesicular
▌Biliary obstruction (especially PBC)
- Mallory hyaline may be present and would most likely be seen in periportal as opposed to pericentral areas
▌Wilson disease
- Mallory hyaline may be present and would most likely be seen in periportal as opposed to pericentral areas
- Marked copper overload
▌Indian childhood cirrhosis
- Occurs almost exclusively in India
- Mallory hyalines are often present
- Steatosis conspicuously absent
- Marked copper overload

Pearls

- Presence of Mallory hyaline associated with lobular inflammatory infiltrates and steatosis (predominantly macrovesicular) in a zone 3 injury pattern suggests alcoholic or nonalcoholic steatohepatitis
- Mallory hyaline may be present in other pathologic processes, including chronic cholestatic disease, Wilson disease, Indian childhood cirrhosis, and even HCCs (about 10%)

Selected References

Brunt EM: Nonalcoholic steatohepatitis: Pathologic features and differential diagnosis. Semin Diagn Pathol 22:330-338, 2005.

Kleiner DE, Brunt EM, Van Natta M, et al: Design and validation of a histological scoring system for nonalcoholic fatty liver disease. Hepatology 41:1313-1321, 2005.

Brunt EM: Nonalcoholic steatohepatitis: Definition and pathology. Semin Liver Dis 21:3-16, 2001.

Acute Fatty Liver of Pregnancy

Clinical Features

- Onset typically occurs during third trimester of pregnancy
- Bleeding, nausea and vomiting, jaundice, and occasionally coma
- Usually resolves after delivery

Gross Pathology

- Greasy, small, pale-yellow liver

Histopathology

- Microvesicular steatosis
- Canalicular and intrahepatocytic cholestasis may occur
- Portal tract inflammation may be prominent

Special Stains and Immunohistochemistry

- Oil red O (on frozen-section slide) demonstrates microvesicular fat droplets

Other Techniques for Diagnosis

- Noncontributory

Figure 7-4. Acute fatty liver of pregnancy. Marked microvesicular transformation of hepatocytes.

Differential Diagnosis

- Clinical history is essential
- ❚ Drug toxicity
  - May show similar histologic features (e.g., tetracycline, valproic acid, nucleoside analogues), which are all associated with microvesicular fatty change
  - Clinical history is required for definitive distinction
- ❚ Reye syndrome
  - Also shows microvesicular steatosis
  - History of aspirin use
  - Associated with encephalopathy
- ❚ HCV
  - Typically shows macrovesicular steatosis
  - Shows lobular hepatitis and portal lymphoid aggregates
- ❚ Alcoholic steatohepatitis
  - Mallory hyaline is typically prominent and often associated with a neutrophilic infiltrate

Pearls

- Onset during pregnancy, usually third trimester
- Pathogenesis: defective intramitochondrial fatty acid oxidation

Selected References

Riely CA: Acute fatty liver of pregnancy. Semin Liver Dis 7:47-54, 1987.

Rolfes DB, Ishak KG: Liver disease in pregnancy. Histopathology 10:555-570, 1986.

Kaplan MM: Acute fatty liver of pregnancy. N Engl J Med 313:367-370, 1985.

Rolfes DB, Ishak KG: Acute fatty liver of pregnancy: A clinicopathologic study of 35 cases. Hepatology 5:1149-1158, 1985.

Figure 7-5. Hemochromatosis. A, Hepatocytes containing a large amount of iron. **B,** Prussian blue stain is strongly positive, highlighting the massive iron deposits.

Hemochromatosis

Clinical Features

- Abnormal accumulation of iron in liver, pancreas, myocardium, and other organs
- Hereditary: homozygous recessive
- Acquired: multiple transfusions, Bantu hemosiderosis (alcoholic beverages brewed in iron drums in sub-Saharan Africa)
- Most often presents in men older than 40 years
- Liver is the most severely affected organ
- Classic triad: cirrhosis, skin pigmentation, and diabetes mellitus (not as common now owing to early diagnosis and treatment)
- Patients may also have abdominal pain, cardiac dysfunction, and atypical arthritis
- Laboratory studies show increased serum iron and ferritin
- Increased risk for developing HCC

Gross Pathology

- Enlarged liver with dark-brown pigmentation
- Ultimately micronodular cirrhosis with persistent dark-brown pigmentation

Histopathology

- Early: hemosiderin granules in cytoplasm of periportal hepatocytes
- Middle
  - Progressive involvement of lobule and eventually bile duct epithelium and Kupffer cells, resulting in hepatocyte necrosis, portal inflammation, and portal and bridging fibrosis
  - Lobular inflammation typically absent
- Late: fibrous septa develop over years with progression to micronodular cirrhosis with intense hemosiderin pigmentation

Special Stains and Immunohistochemistry

- Prussian blue stain for iron highlights increased iron deposition

Other Techniques for Diagnosis

- Hepatic iron index (HII): currently the definitive test; biochemical quantitation of hepatic iron in fresh tissue or paraffin block calculated as micromoles iron per gram dry weight divided by patient's age
  — Homozygotes: HII greater than 2 (may be greater than 40)
  — Heterozygotes: less than 2
  — Normal individuals: less than 1
- Human leukocyte antigen (HLA) gene analysis: hemochromatosis gene is HLA-H located on the short arm of chromosome 6
  — Most common mutation is cysteine to tyrosine at amino acid 282

Differential Diagnosis

▍Hemosiderosis
- Patients typically have a cause for secondary iron overload (e.g., multiple transfusions, porphyria cutanea tarda, or chronic dietary iron overload as in Bantu siderosis)

Pearls

- Iron is directly hepatotoxic; no inflammatory mediators released
- Women are less commonly affected and present later as a result of physiologic blood loss during menstruation and pregnancy
- Treatment is reduction of iron overload by phlebotomy

Selected References

Brunt EM: Pathology of hepatic iron overload. Semin Liver Dis 25:392-401, 2005.

Deugnier YM, Turlin B, Powell LW, et al: Differentiation between heterozygotes and homozygotes in genetic hemochromatosis by means of a histologic hepatic iron index: A study of 192 cases. Hepatology 17:30-34, 1993.

Deugnier YM, Loreal O, Turlin B, et al: Liver pathology in genetic hemochromatosis: A review of 135 cases and their bioclinical correlations. Gastroenterology 104:228-234, 1992.

Bacon BR, Britton RS: The pathology of hepatic iron overload: a free radical-mediated process. Hepatology 11:127-137, 1990.

Wilson Disease

Clinical Features

- Abnormal accumulation of copper in liver, brain, eyes, and other organs
- Variable age of onset
- Autosomal recessive
- Laboratory findings include decreased serum ceruloplasmin, increased hepatic copper, increased urinary excretion of copper
- Serum copper levels not helpful
- Most commonly presents with acute or chronic liver disease
- Neuropsychiatric symptoms also frequent at presentation secondary to involvement of basal ganglia
- Kayser-Fleischer rings are diagnostic (green-brown deposits of copper in Descemet membrane in limbus of cornea)

Gross Pathology

- Liver eventually becomes cirrhotic

Histopathology

- Excessive copper granule in hepatocytes can only be seen with special stain
- Mild to moderate fatty change
- Focal hepatocyte necrosis
- Glycogen vacuoles in hepatocyte nuclei
- Mallory hyaline in periportal hepatocytes
- Acute and chronic hepatitis
- Cirrhosis following chronic hepatitis
- Rarely, massive liver necrosis

Special Stains and Immunohistochemistry

- Rhodanine stain for copper positive
- Orcein stain for copper-associated protein positive

Figure 7-6. Wilson disease. High-power view shows liver cells containing cytoplasmic copper pigment.

Other Techniques for Diagnosis

- Biochemical quantitation of hepatic copper in fresh tissue or paraffin block (more than $250 \mu g$ copper/1 g dry liver)

Differential Diagnosis

▌ Viral hepatitis
- Serologic markers are positive
- No accumulation of copper

▌ Chronic obstructive cholestasis
- Lesser degree of copper accumulation

Pearls

- Normally free copper is absorbed in the stomach and duodenum, weakly bound to albumin, transferred to hepatocytes, and incorporated into α_2-globulin to form ceruloplasmin, which is re-secreted into plasma; senescent ceruloplasmin is taken up by hepatocytes, degraded by lysosomes, and excreted into bile
- Wilson disease gene is *ATP7B* on chromosome 13 and encodes a transmembrane copper-transporting adenosine triphosphatase (ATPase) located on canalicular membrane of hepatocytes
- Treatment is copper chelation with D-penicillamine

Selected References

Ludwig J, Moyer TP, Rakela J: The liver biopsy diagnosis of Wilson's disease: Methods in pathology. Am J Clin Pathol 102:443-446, 1994.

Stremmel W, Meyerrose KW, Niederau C, et al: Wilson disease: Clinical presentation, treatment and survival. Ann Intern Med 115:720-726, 1991.

Sternlieb I: Perspectives on Wilson's disease. Hepatology 12:1234-1239, 1990.

Stromeyer FW, Ishak KG: Histology of the liver in Wilson's disease: A study of 34 cases. Am J Clin Pathol 73:12-24, 1980.

α_1-Antitrypsin Deficiency

Clinical Features

- Variable age of onset
- Autosomal recessive disease caused by mutations of the polymorphic Pi (protease inhibitor) gene on chromosome 14
- Absent or decreased Pi activity results in unchecked activity of neutrophilic elastase leading to pulmonary emphysema (destruction of elastic fibers supporting alveolar spaces)
- The mutant polypeptide is abnormally folded, blocking its movements from the endoplasmic reticulum to Golgi and accumulating in the endoplasmic reticulum of hepatocytes

Figure 7-7. α_1-Antitrypsin deficiency. Hepatocytes containing intracytoplasmic eosinophilic globules (periodic acid–Schiff stain with diastase).

- In some patients, there is liver disease without pulmonary emphysema owing to functional mutant forms that inhibit neutrophil elastase but that are not appropriately degraded in hepatocytes
- Clinical hepatic presentations range from
  - Neonatal hepatitis with cholestatic jaundice
  - Young adults with recurrent attacks of hepatitis that either resolve or lead to chronic hepatitis and cirrhosis
  - Middle-aged to older adults with cirrhosis after a clinically silent course
- Increased risk for HCC, especially in homozygous patients
- Successful liver transplantation is curative

Gross Pathology

- Noncontributory

Histopathology

- Round to oval, variably sized eosinophilic globules most concentrated in periportal hepatocytes
- Otherwise variable histologic features
  - Neonatal hepatitis with or without cholestasis
  - Chronic hepatitic picture
  - Cirrhosis

Special Stains and Immunohistochemistry

- Eosinophilic globules are positive for PAS and resistant to diastase digestion

Other Techniques for Diagnosis

- Identification of mutant protein by electrophoresis
- About 75 variants identified and named alphabetically according to migration on isoelectric gel

- Normal genotype is PiMM
- PiZZ is most clinically significant genotype (results from amino acid substitution of Glu to Lys) and shows the highest association with carcinoma
- Patients with PiMZ genotype have 50% normal α_1-antitrypsin and 50% mutant form
- Other mutant alleles include S (reduced levels of α_1-antitrypsin but no clinical disease) and null (no detectable protein)

Differential Diagnosis

▌ Other types of chronic hepatitis and cirrhosis include viral, drug, and autoimmune hepatitis, but they do not demonstrate the PAS-positive and diastase-resistant globules that are characteristic of α_1-antitrypsin deficiency

Pearls

- α_1-Antitrypsin deficiency is one of the few liver diseases that can still be diagnosed in an end-stage liver explant because of the PAS-positive and diastase-resistant globules that remain in the hepatocyte cytoplasm
- This is a multifactorial disease in which there are heterogeneous genetic mutations, resulting in highly variable clinical presentations even among members of individual families

Selected References

Cohen C, Derose PB: Liver cell dysplasia in alpha 1-antitrypsin deficiency. Mod Pathol 7:31-36, 1994.

Deutsch J, Becker H, Aubock L: Histopathological features of liver disease in alpha-1-antitrypsin deficiency. Acta Paediatr 393(Suppl):8-12, 1994.

Propst T, Propst A, Dietze O, et al: Alpha-1-antitrypsin deficiency and liver disease. Dig Dis 12:139-149, 1994.

Lomas DA, Evans DL, Finch JT, et al: The mechanism of Z alpha 1-antitrypsin accumulation in the liver. Nature 57:605-607, 1992.

Autoimmune Hepatitis

Clinical Features

- Young and middle-aged women (female-to-male ratio of 7:3)
- Often associated with extrahepatic autoimmune disorders such as rheumatoid arthritis, thyroiditis, Sjögren syndrome
- Hyperglobulinemia
- Characterized by serum autoantibodies, classically ANA, ASMA, soluble liver antigen (SLA), and anti-LKM1
- Negative viral serologic markers
- Responsive to immunosuppressive therapy

Figure 7-8. Autoimmune hepatitis. Prominent portal and periportal infiltrate of plasma cells.

Gross Pathology

- Noncontributory

Histopathology

- Significant portal and periportal inflammatory infiltrate with lymphocytes and plasma cells (prominent plasma cells are the hallmark)
- Marked lobular inflammatory infiltrate with prominent plasma cells deep in the parenchyma
- Prominent interface hepatitis
- Bridging necrosis is common
- Severe hepatocellular injury with hepatitic rosette formation and syncytial giant hepatocytes

Special Stains and Immunohistochemistry

- Noncontributory

Other Techniques for Diagnosis

- Noncontributory

Differential Diagnosis

- Clinical correlation is important in the differential diagnosis of this disease
▌ Chronic viral hepatitis
  - Positive serologic markers
  - Plasma cells less prominent
  - Milder lobular hepatitis and interface hepatitis (especially in HCV)
  - No association with autoimmune diseases

Pearls

- Most frequent in young women and associated with hyperglobulinemia and various serologic markers of autoimmune disease

- Rosette formation, although not specific, is highly suggestive of autoimmune hepatitis
- This is one of the few forms of chronic hepatitis that responds well to immunosuppressive therapy

Selected References

Washington MK: Autoimmune liver disease: Overlap and outliers. Mod Pathol 20:S15-S30, 2007.

Czaja AJ: Autoimmune hepatitis: Evolving concepts and treatment strategies. Dig Dis Sci 40:435-456, 1995.

Johnson PJ, McFarlane IG: Meeting report. International Autoimmune Hepatitis Group. Hepatology 18:998-1005, 1993.

Bach N, Thung SN, Schaffner F: The histologic changes of chronic hepatitis C and autoimmune hepatitis: A comparative study. Hepatology 15:572-577, 1992.

Primary Biliary Cirrhosis

Clinical Features

- Most commonly occurs in middle-aged women
- Serum AMAs in more than 90% of cases
- Insidious onset, with pruritus being the most common presenting symptom and jaundice developing later
- Elevated serum alkaline phosphatase, with hyperbilirubinemia developing later
- Chronic and progressive, with cirrhosis developing only after many years

Figure 7-9. Primary biliary cirrhosis. A portal tract shows granulomatous inflammation, chronic inflammatory infiltrate, and paucity of bile ducts.

Gross Pathology

- Early: unremarkable
- Late: finely granular capsule; bile-stained parenchyma
- Ultimately liver becomes cirrhotic (biliary type cirrhosis)

Histopathology

- Variability in stages of lesions (i.e., coexistence of different stages in single specimen)
- *Stage I (florid duct lesion)*: focal destruction of small and medium-sized bile ducts by granulomatous inflammation; bile duct epithelium irregular and hyperplastic; dense portal tract infiltrate of lymphocytes, macrophages, plasma cells, and eosinophils
- *Stage II (ductular reaction)*: scarring; disappearance of small bile ducts; scarring of medium-sized bile ducts; proliferation of bile ductules in portal tracts; inflammation and interface hepatitis of adjacent periportal hepatic parenchyma
- *Stage III (scarring)*: small and medium-sized ducts scarce; little inflammation in fibrous septa or parenchyma; lymphoid aggregates with or without PAS-positive material representing residual basement membrane material in areas where ducts had been
- *Stage IV (cirrhosis)*: cirrhosis, often with a jigsaw pattern

Special Stains and Immunohistochemistry

- Noncontributory

Other Techniques for Diagnosis

- Noncontributory

Differential Diagnosis

- Primary sclerosing cholangitis (PSC)
  - Characterized by periductal fibrosis and typical ERCP findings
  - Lacks the florid duct lesion seen in PBC
  - Occurs in young men as opposed to middle-aged women
  - Negative AMA
  - Often associated with ulcerative colitis
- Autoimmune hepatitis–PBC overlap syndrome
  - AMA and ANA positive with histologic features of both PBC and autoimmune hepatitis (more than the usual degree of lobular hepatitis, interface hepatitis, and plasma cell infiltrate)
- Autoimmune cholangitis
  - Histologically identical to PBC
  - Patients are AMA negative and ANA positive
- Graft-versus-host disease and liver transplant rejection
  - Clinical history important
  - Both can cause bile duct injury, lymphocytic cholangitis, and vanishing bile duct syndrome, which can resemble PBC

Pearls

- AMAs are against E2 subunit of pyruvate dehydrogenase complex on interlobular bile ducts in PBC
- Generally believed to be an autoimmune disease
- Liver transplantation is definitive treatment

Selected References

Berk PD: Primary biliary cirrhosis, Parts I and II. Semin Liver Dis 17:1-250, 1997.

Lacerda MA, Ludwig J, Dickson ER, et al: Antimitochondrial antibody-negative primary biliary cirrhosis. Am J Gastroenterol 90:247-249, 1995.

Mahl TC, Shockcor W, Boyer JL: Primary biliary cirrhosis: Survival of a large cohort of symptomatic and asymptomatic patients followed for 24 years. J Hepatol 20:707-713, 1994.

Sherlock S: Primary biliary cirrhosis: Clarifying the issues. Am J Med 96(Suppl):27S-33S, 1994.

Primary Sclerosing Cholangitis

Clinical Features

- More common in males in the third to fifth decades
- Characteristic beaded appearance of intrahepatic biliary tree by contrast radiography (ERCP) due to irregular strictures and secondary dilations of affected bile ducts
- About 70% of cases are associated with ulcerative colitis (conversely, only 4% of patients with ulcerative colitis have PSC)
- Elevated alkaline phosphatase and bilirubin
- Increased risk of cholangiocarcinoma (terminal event in about 10% of patients with PSC)

Gross Pathology

- Early: unremarkable
- Late: bile-stained, biliary-type cirrhosis

Histopathology

- Characterized by fibroinflammatory stricture of the bile ducts anywhere from the ampulla of Vater to the interlobular bile ducts
- *Stage I (portal)*: concentric periductal fibrosis and lymphocytic inflammation in portal tracts
- *Stage II (periportal)*: fibrosis extends into periportal parenchyma, interface hepatitis, and bile ductular reaction
- *Stage III (septal)*: obliteration of bile ducts and bridging fibrosis
- *Stage IV (cirrhotic)*: biliary-type cirrhosis (jigsaw pattern)
- Features of chronic cholestasis, especially pseudoxanthomatous changes, are commonly seen

Special Stains and Immunohistochemistry

- Noncontributory

Figure 7-10. Primary sclerosing cholangitis. A, Histologic section of a portal field showing concentric periductal fibrosis. **B,** Histologic section of a portal field showing chronic inflammation and obliteration of the bile duct.

Other Techniques for Diagnosis

- Noncontributory

Differential Diagnosis

- Well-differentiated cholangiocarcinoma
  - Heterogeneity of cells within individual glands
  - Perineural invasion often seen
  - Radiologic information is helpful
- PBC
  - Occurs more commonly in middle-aged women
  - Typically positive for AMA
  - Florid duct lesions followed by absence of bile duct as opposed to the fibroinflammatory obliteration of ducts seen in PSC
- Extrahepatic or large duct intrahepatic biliary obstruction
  - Can give rise to a secondary sclerosing cholangitis similar to PSC

- Features suggestive of secondary cholangitis include marked ductular reaction and severe cholestasis with inspissated bile, which is often green and laminated
- Often see marked pseudoxanthomatous change and rapid onset (months) of biliary cirrhosis

Pearls

- Associated with chronic inflammatory bowel disease, particularly ulcerative colitis
- Increased risk for cholangiocarcinoma
- Characterized by fibroinflammatory obliteration of small and medium-sized bile ducts
- Liver transplantation is curative; however, disease may recur in transplanted liver

Selected References

Angulo P, Lindor KD: Primary sclerosing cholangitis. Hepatology 30:325-332, 1999.

Harnois DM, Lindor KD: Primary sclerosing cholangitis: Evolving concepts in diagnosis and treatment. Dig Dis 15:23-41, 1997.

Lee YM, Kaplan MM: Primary sclerosing cholangitis. N Eng J Med 332:924-933, 1995.

Ueno Y, LaRusso NF: Primary sclerosing cholangitis. J Gastroenterol 29:531-543, 1994.

Liver Transplantation Pathology

Clinical Features

- Indications for liver transplantation include end-stage chronic liver disease, acute liver failure, and hepatic neoplasm
- The main complications of liver transplantation include surgical complications involving vascular or biliary structures, allograft rejection, recurrent diseases, acquired diseases, and complications of immunosuppressive therapy (opportunistic infections, post-transplantation lymphoproliferative diseases, and drug toxicities)

Gross Pathology

- Hyperacute and humoral allograft rejection: massive hemorrhagic necrosis
- Graft ischemia in early post-transplantation period: irregular geographic areas of infarction with a surrounding hemorrhagic border
- Ischemic bile duct necrosis: necrotic and bile-stained portal regions with surrounding centrilobular cholestasis

Histopathology

- Acute (cellular) rejection in allograft
  - Portal inflammation, bile duct damage, and endotheliitis are the characteristic histologic triad

Figure 7-11. A, Acute cellular rejection. Portal inflammation, endotheliitis, and lymphocytic cholangitis. **B, Chronic rejection.** Loss of interlobular bile ducts in the portal tract.

  - Portal inflammatory infiltrate includes large lymphocytes, activated blast cells, plasmacytoid cells, macrophages, neutrophils, and eosinophils
  - The previous cell types are also involved in mediating bile duct damage and endotheliitis

Special Stains and Immunohistochemistry

- Noncontributory

Other Techniques for Diagnosis

- Noncontributory

Differential Diagnosis

▌ Recurrent HCV
- Typical portal infiltrate in recurrent chronic HCV rarely seen within first month after transplantation
- Endotheliitis usually milder
- Lymphocytic cholangitis usually milder and more localized

▌ Post-transplantation lymphoproliferative disease
  - Immunohistochemistry demonstrates clonal population of the lymphoid infiltrate and EBV-associated proteins
  - In situ hybridization demonstrates EBV nucleic acids
▌ Chronic (ductopenic) rejection in allograft
  - Loss of interlobular bile ducts
  - Obliterative arteriopathy with intimal aggregates of lipid-laden foamy macrophages in large and medium-sized arteries
  - Centrilobular necrosis is a common finding

Special Stains and Immunohistochemistry

  - CK7 for staining bile ductal epithelium
  - PAS with diastase to stain basement membrane of the bile duct

Other Techniques for Diagnosis

  - Noncontributory

Differential Diagnosis

▌ Recurrent PSC
  - Periductal fibrosis present
  - Typical ERCP finding
  - Portal and periportal fibrosis
▌ Recurrent PBC
  - Florid duct lesion
  - Portal inflammation
  - Portal and periportal fibrosis

Pearls

  - A definitive diagnosis of ductopenic rejection is established with a formal count of at least 20 portal tracts showing loss of interlobular bile ducts from more than 50% of portal tracts (serial biopsies may be required to warrant adequate sampling and confident diagnosis)
  - A diagnosis of rejection needs to be distinguished from other complications such as ischemia, biliary obstruction, infection, drug injury, and recurrent diseases

Selected References

Hubscher SG, Portmann BC: Transplantation pathology. In Burt AD, Portmann BC, Ferrell LD (eds): MacSween's Pathology of the Liver, 5th ed. London, Churchill Livingstone, 2007, pp 815-880.

Batts KP: Acute and chronic hepatic allograft rejection: Pathology and classification. Liver Transpl Surg 5:S21-29, 1999.

Jones KD, Ferrell LD: Interpretation of biopsy findings in the transplant liver. Semin Diagn Pathol 15:306-317, 1998.

Demetris AJ, Batts KP, Dhillon AP, et al: Banff schema for grading liver allograft rejection: An international consensus document. Hepatology 25:658-663, 1997.

Cirrhosis

Clinical Features

  - Etiology: virtually all chronic liver diseases, including viral hepatitis, autoimmune hepatitis, alcoholic liver disease, nonalcoholic fatty liver disease, chronic biliary diseases, hemochromatosis, Wilson disease, α_1-antitrypsin deficiency, drugs, metabolic disorders, and cryptogenic disorders
  - May be clinically silent
  - Anorexia, weight loss, and weakness; ultimately debilitating
  - Death due to progressive hepatic failure, complications of portal hypertension, or HCC

Gross Pathology

  - Early: enlarged with or without greasy surface
  - Late: shrunken with diffuse nodularity

Histopathology

  - Diffuse nodules of regenerating hepatocytes surrounded by fibrous bands
  - Arteries, bile ductules, and inflammatory infiltrate within fibrous septa
  - Irregular ("jigsaw" pattern) nodules in biliary-type cirrhosis

Special Stains and Immunohistochemistry

  - Trichrome: useful for determining the extent and pattern of fibrosis
  - Reticulin: useful for identifying thickened hepatic plates within regenerative nodules (two or three cell layers thick)

Other Techniques for Diagnosis

  - Noncontributory

Figure 7-12. Cirrhosis. Nodular appearance of liver architecture surrounded by fibrous septa (trichrome stain).

Differential Diagnosis

- Distinguishing cirrhosis from other entities is important but may be sometimes challenging in a biopsy specimen because some histologic features may overlap
- High-grade dysplastic nodules
  - Plates more than two cells thick or areas of pseudoglandular formation may be seen
  - Cytologic atypia with high nuclear-to-cytoplasmic ratio, hyperchromatic nuclei, irregular nuclear contour, and rare mitoses
- HCC
  - Nuclear atypia with increased nuclear-to-cytoplasmic ratio, hyperchromatic nuclei, and frequent mitotic activity
  - Absence of portal tracts in the nodules
  - Thick trabeculae or pseudoglandular formation and increased unpaired arteries may be seen
- Congenital hepatic fibrosis
  - Large bands of collagen dividing liver into geographic areas
  - Preservation of spatial relationships between vessels; therefore, not truly nodular
  - Morphologically similar to biliary type cirrhosis
  - Usually without inflammation or hepatocellular regeneration
- Nodular regenerative hyperplasia
  - Generalized or multiple hyperplastic parenchymal nodules without significant fibrosis
  - Associated with myeloproliferative disorders, rheumatic diseases, chronic venous congestion, and drugs such as corticosteroids and chemotherapeutic agents
- Focal nodular hyperplasia
  - Focal, distinct hypervascular lesion on image study
  - Central scar
  - Thickened arteries within fibrous septa
- Subcapsular fibrosis
  - Fibrosis does not extend down into the liver parenchyma

Pearls

- World Health Organization definition: cirrhosis is a diffuse process characterized by fibrosis and the conversion of normal liver architecture into structurally abnormal nodules
- Cirrhosis is the end stage of myriad different liver diseases, and the etiology is not always apparent in the explanted liver of end-stage disease

Selected References

Geller SA, Petrovic LM: Cirrhosis, hepatic fibrosis, and noncirrhotic portal hypertension. In Geller SA, Petrovic LM (eds): Biopsy Interpretation of the Liver. Philadelphia, Lippincott Williams & Wilkins, 2004, pp 228-238.

Scheuer PJ, Lefkowitch JH: Cirrhosis. In Scheuer PJ, Lefkowitch JH (eds): Liver Biopsy Interpretation. London, WB Saunders, 2000, pp 173-190.

Focal Nodular Hyperplasia

Clinical Features

- Most common in women in third to fifth decades
- Can occur in both genders and any age group, including childhood
- Female-to-male ratio: adults, 2:1; children, 4:1
- Usually found incidentally at surgery or during image studies for unrelated symptoms
- Distinctively hypervascular by arteriography
- Liver function tests usually normal
- Oral contraceptive use not an apparent etiologic factor
- Multiple focal nodular hyperplasia can be associated with hemangiomas, meningiomas, astrocytomas, and arterial dysplasia in other organs

Gross Pathology

- Well circumscribed but not encapsulated
- Lighter color than adjacent liver
- Often subcapsular
- Any size, but usually less than 5 cm in diameter
- Characteristic central stellate scar

Histopathology

- Nodules of hepatocytes with large central stellate scar
- Hepatocytes adjacent to the fibrous septa may show chronic cholestatic changes

Figure 7-13. Focal nodular hyperplasia. Nodules of hepatocytes with large central stellate scar. Fibrous septa contain thickened vessels, numerous bile ductules, and a varying degree of inflammatory cell infiltration.

- All components of normal liver lobule present (i.e., central veins and portal triads)
- Fibrous septa contain thickened vessels, numerous bile ductules, and varying degree of inflammatory cell infiltration
- Pseudoxanthomatous change (chronic cholestasis) adjacent to the fibrous septa

Special Stains and Immunohistochemistry

- Rhodanine stain to demonstrate accumulation of copper or Victoria blue stain to demonstrate copper-binding protein

Other Techniques for Diagnosis

- Noncontributory

Differential Diagnosis

❚ Hepatocellular adenoma
- No fibrous septa and bile ductules
- Cells arranged in sheets or thick plates without portal tracts
- No central scar
- Frequently see areas of infarction or hemorrhage
- Most occur in women; associated with oral contraceptive use
❚ Nodular regenerative hyperplasia
- Diffuse process involving the entire liver
- No fibrous septa or central scar
- Clinically associated with a wide variety of extrahepatic disorders
❚ Well-differentiated HCC
- Cells arranged in sheets or plates without portal tracts
❚ Cirrhosis
- Generalized regenerative nodules surrounded by fibrous bands
- Arising in the background of underlying liver disease

Pearls

- Most characteristic features include central stellate scar, broad septa containing proliferating bile ducts, and the presence of all components of normal liver lobule

Selected References

Makhlouf HR, Abdul-Al HM, Goodman ZD: Diagnosis of focal nodular hyperplasia of the liver by needle biopsy. Hum Pathol 36:1210-1216, 2005.

Nguyen BN, Flejou JF, Terris B, et al: Focal nodular hyperplasia of the liver: A comprehensive pathologic study of 305 lesions and recognitions of new histologic forms. Am J Surg Pathol 23:1441-1454, 1999.

Ishak KG, Goodman ZD, Stocker JT: Benign hepatocellular tumors. In Atlas of Tumor Pathology, 3rd series, fascicle 31. Washington, DC, Armed Forces Institute of Pathology, 2001, pp 9-48.

Hepatic Adenoma

Clinical Features

- Characteristically affects women of child-bearing age
- Related to oral contraceptive use; decreasing incidence related to use of low-dose contraception
- Liver function tests usually within reference range
- Large tumors at risk for rupture or hemorrhage, may present as abdominal emergency
- Symptoms include epigastric and acute abdominal pain, the latter associated with rupture
- Hypovascular by arteriography

Gross Pathology

- Any size; may measure up to 30 cm in diameter
- Usually solitary, well-defined, partially encapsulated, bulging mass
- Often subcapsular
- Multiple lesions uncommon; >10 adenomas indicates adenomatosis
- Different color from surrounding liver (yellow to tan or brown)
- Areas of necrosis or hemorrhage common

Histopathology

- Thick plates of tightly packed, well-differentiated, glycogen-rich hepatocytes with abundant eosinophilic cytoplasm
- No portal triads or central veins
- Fibrous septa do not contain bile ducts
- Intracellular and canalicular bile may be seen
- Lipid often conspicuous
- Kupffer cells and stellate cells often seen
- Mitoses rare

Special Stains and Immunohistochemistry

- *Hep*atocyte antigen in *par*affin (HepPar-1) positive
- Low-molecular-weight keratin positive; pattern resembles normal liver (accentuation of subplasmalemmal cytoplasm)

Figure 7-14. Hepatic adenoma. Proliferation of uniform liver cells characteristically lacking portal tracts.

- Occasional cases with "capillarization" of sinusoids (CD34 positivity similar to HCC)

Other Techniques for Diagnosis

- Noncontributory

Differential Diagnosis

▌ Focal nodular hyperplasia
- Central stellate scar
- Portal triads and central veins present
- Bile ducts in fibrous septa; bile ductular reaction pattern often prominent

▌ Nodular regenerative hyperplasia
- Diffuse process
- Clinically associated with a wide variety of extrahepatic disorders

▌ Well-differentiated HCC
- Liver cell plates are more than three cells thick
- Tumor cells show significant nuclear pleomorphism with increased nuclear-to-cytoplasmic ratio
- Increased mitotic activity
- Absence of Kupffer cells

Pearls

- Focal process with absence of normal portal elements
- Composed of normal-appearing hepatocytes
- Difficult to separate from low-grade HCC in a needle biopsy
- Never occurs in cirrhosis (by convention); similar lesions in cirrhosis classified as low-grade dysplasia (macroregenerative nodule)

Selected References

DeCarlis L, Pirotta V, Rondinara GF, et al: Hepatic adenoma and focal nodular hyperplasia: Diagnosis and criteria for treatment. Liver Transpl Surg 3:160-165, 1997.

Resnick MB, Kozakewich HP, Perez-Atayde AR: Hepatic adenoma in the pediatric age group: Clinicopathological observations and assessment of cell proliferative activity. Am J Surg Pathol 19:1181-1190, 1995.

Goodman ZD, Mikel W, Lubbers PR, et al: Kupffer cells in hepatocellular adenomas. Am J Surg Pathol 11:191-196, 1987.

Hepatocellular Carcinoma

Clinical Features

- Common carcinoma worldwide (eighth overall in women; fifth in men); strongly correlated with relative incidence of hepatitis B
- Most common primary hepatic malignancy in adults
- Most patients in Western countries are older than 50 years
- Fibrolamellar variant typically occurs in patients younger than 30 years
- Male-to-female ratio about 4:1

Figure 7-15. Hepatocellular carcinoma. A, Well-differentiated type. Neoplastic liver cells with large nuclei, prominent nucleoli, and fine granular cytoplasm arranged in a trabecular pattern. **B, Poorly differentiated type.** Note greater variation in cord size and nuclear size. **C, Fibrolamellar type.** Prominent fibrosis arranged in lamellar fashion around the neoplastic hepatocytes.

- Patients often present with abdominal pain, ascites, or hepatomegaly; early disease typically asymptomatic
- Elevated serum α-fetoprotein (AFP) in 60% to 80% of cases
- Serum AFP more than 100 times normal is diagnostic if malignant germ cell neoplasm is excluded

- Numerous associated factors, including cirrhosis, HBV (especially *Hbx* gene product) and HCV, fatty liver disease, obesity, diabetes, hemochromatosis, progestational agents, anabolic steroids, thorium dioxide (Thorotrast), aflatoxins, ataxia-telangiectasia, α_1-antitrypsin deficiency, tyrosinemia, schistosomiasis
- DNA ploidy abnormalities (especially 8p loss of heterozygosity [LOH]), microsatellite instability, altered β-catenin expression, dysplasia, increases in transforming growth factor-α (TGF-α) and AFP expression, and increased proliferative activity often precede malignant transformation

Gross Pathology

- Soft, yellow-green or reddish nodules
- Highly variable in size
- Solitary, multinodular, and diffuse types
- Increasing numbers of small carcinomas (lesions <3 cm) detected as a result of advances in diagnostic imaging techniques or examination of liver explants
- Advanced cases often associated with portal vein invasion or metastasis at diagnosis

Histopathology

- Three classic patterns: trabecular, acinar, and solid
  — Trabecular
    ◆ Cords greater than three cells thick lined by flat endothelial cells and lacking Kupffer cells
  — Acinar
    ◆ Results from central degeneration of otherwise solid trabeculae eventually replaced by pseudoglandular spaces containing colloid-like material or bile
    ◆ May also represent dilated canaliculi
  — Solid
    ◆ Results from compression artifact or scarring; least common of three patterns
- Bile production by tumor cells is pathognomonic
- Neoplastic cells are variable in size, although typically large and polygonal, with central vesicular nuclei and prominent nucleoli
- Cytoplasm is finely granular and often markedly basophilic
- Cytoplasmic and nuclear inclusions of different types are common; intranuclear inclusions are typically eosinophilic
- Highly pleomorphic cells with bizarre nuclei may occupy large areas
- Clear cells may predominate
- Carcinoma cell cords and clusters are surrounded by a network of sinusoidal vessels
- Bile canaliculi are present (grade dependent)
- Grading is based on degree of resemblance to normal liver

- Adjacent liver is typically cirrhotic
- Fibrolamellar variant (distinctive histology)
  — Shows a prominent lamellar fibrous stroma
  — Composed of oncocytic-appearing malignant hepatocytes
  — Occurs in a noncirrhotic liver
- Mixed HCC and cholangiocarcinoma is uncommon; requires elements of trabecular pattern HCC and distinct fields of unequivocal glandular differentiation (see also "Special Stains and Immunohistochemistry")

Special Stains and Immunohistochemistry

- AFP highly specific but insensitive (<25% of cases positive)
- HepPar-1 (a urea cycle mitochondrial enzyme) highly sensitive for normal and neoplastic hepatocytes; specific in the proper histologic context, although metaplastic and neoplastic intestinal cells may also be positive
- Selected anti–thyroid transcription factor-1 (anti–TTF-1) antibodies label cytoplasm (not nucleus) of normal and neoplastic hepatocytes due to common epitope in TTF-1 on a novel mitochondrial peptide
- Glypican-3 may distinguish between non-neoplastic and neoplastic hepatocytes
- Low-molecular-weight keratins (keratins 8 and 18) positive, often with accentuation of subplasmalemmal cytoplasm
- Keratin 7 occasionally positive
- Keratins 17 and 19 generally negative or only faintly positive
- Epithelial membrane antigen (EMA) typically negative, except in mixed HCC and cholangiocarcinoma; similar result with mucicarmine stains
- Polyclonal carcinoembryonic antigen (CEA) labels a non-CEA bile moiety; accentuates canaliculi. Similar result with antibodies to CD10, multidrug-resistant p-glycoprotein, and occasionally villin
- Sinusoids often CD34 positive (so-called capillarization of sinusoids)
- Monoclonal CEA typically negative

Other Techniques for Diagnosis

- Electron microscopy: demonstration of bile canaliculi is pathognomonic of hepatocellular differentiation, but not HCC
  — Bile canaliculi show stubby microvilli and cell junctions of tight and intermediate types
  — Tumor cells resemble normal adult hepatocytes; typically numerous mitochondria, abundant electron-dense glycogen particles, and intracytoplasmic bile products
- Flow cytometry: aneuploidy correlates with higher grade but is also seen in dysplasia and is therefore not diagnostic of malignancy

Differential Diagnosis

- In general, HCC resembles normal liver in its platelike growth and cytology
- ▮ Macroregenerative nodule in cirrhosis
  - Presence of bile duct epithelial cells and chronic inflammation
  - Absence of trabecular pattern
  - Absence of significant cytologic atypia
- ▮ High-grade dysplasia in cirrhosis
  - Disordered lobular architecture, but generally three or fewer cells in cords
  - Focally prominent nuclear atypia
  - Retention of portal elements
  - Ki-67 proliferative index intermediate between cirrhosis and carcinoma
  - TGF-α expression intermediate between cirrhosis and carcinoma
- ▮ Cholangiocarcinoma
  - Absence of bile production
  - Glandular differentiation; positive for CEA and mucicarmine
  - Positive for EMA; negative for HepPar-1 and glypican-3
  - Keratin 19 typically present; keratins 8 and 18 (CAM 5.2) positive
  - Villin in brush-border pattern
  - Focal or variable CDX2 immunoreactivity
- ▮ Focal nodular hyperplasia
  - Liver cell plates less than three cells thick
  - Cells have a normal nuclear-to-cytoplasmic ratio
  - Absence of mitotic activity
  - Central stellate scar
  - Retention of portal elements; bile ductular reaction
- ▮ Hepatic adenoma
  - Liver cell plates less than three cells thick
  - Slightly increased nuclear-to-cytoplasmic ratio, but no bizarre nuclei
  - Absent or rare typical mitotic figures
  - Kupffer cells present
- ▮ Hepatoblastoma
  - Typically seen in young children
  - Small polygonal or round cells; may resemble fetal liver
  - Macrotrabecular pattern uncommon; closest resemblance to HCC
  - Strong AFP immunoreactivity
- ▮ Metastatic endocrine carcinoma
  - Cords and ribbons mimic low-grade HCC
  - Low-grade lesions have uniform round to oval nuclei
  - Mitotic activity variable
  - Granular cytoplasm typically positive for synaptophysin or CD56; may be chromogranin positive or positive for organ-specific endocrine peptides
- ▮ Metastatic nonendocrine neoplasms
  - Sharply demarcated from adjacent liver; often with hyperemic rim

- Uninvolved liver is typically normal (noncirrhotic)
- Selected immunoprofile compatible with specific lineage (remember melanoma); metastatic carcinoma often resembles primary cholangiocarcinoma

Pearls

- Extremely helpful features: platelike growth of tumor cells separated by vascular sinusoids and bile production
- Reactivity for HepPar-1 characteristic
- Stage is most important prognostic determinant
- Fibrolamellar variant is associated with a better prognosis
- Glypican-3 may be a useful marker for identifying low-grade HCC in needle biopsies

Selected References

Yeh MM, Larson AM, Campbell JS, et al: The expression of transforming growth factor-alpha in cirrhosis, dysplastic nodules, and hepatocellular carcinoma: An immunohistochemical study of 70 cases. Am J Surg Pathol 31:681-689, 2007.

Pang Y, von Turkovich M, Wu H, et al: The binding of thyroid transcription factor 1 and hepatocyte paraffin 1 to mitochondrial proteins in hepatocytes: A molecular and immunoelectron microscopic study. Am J Clin Pathol 125:722-726, 2006.

Brechot C: Pathogenesis of hepatitis B-virus-related hepatocellular carcinoma: Old and new paradigms. Gastroenterology 127(Suppl 1):556-561, 2004.

Maeda T, Adachi E, Kajiyama K, et al: Combined hepatocellular and cholangiocarcinoma: Proposed criteria according to cytokeratin expression and analysis of clinicopathologic features. Hum Pathol 26:956-964, 1995.

Hepatoblastoma

Clinical Features

- Most common liver neoplasm in children
- Occurs almost exclusively in infants
- About one third are associated with a variety of congenital anomalies, syndromes, or other childhood tumors: Beckwith-Wiedemann syndrome and familial adenomatous polyposis
- Serum AFP is often elevated
- Patients may present with virilization; result of ectopic sex hormone production
- Uncommon presentation: sexual precocity in boys with elevated serum and urine human chorionic gonadotropin (HCG)

Gross Pathology

- Solitary, unencapsulated, often large mass measuring up to 25 cm in diameter

Figure 7-16. Hepatoblastoma. Tumor is composed of spindle cells with an embryonal appearance. Notice entrapped hepatocytes in the center of the photomicrograph.

- Variegated cut surface with areas of necrosis, cystic changes, and hemorrhage
- Normal surrounding liver

Histopathology

- Two types: epithelial (75%) and mixed epithelial and mesenchymal (25%)
▌ Epithelial type
- Components are *fetal* and *embryonal*, both invariably present in varying proportions and often intermingled
    — Fetal component
        ◆ Fetal-type cells are polygonal and large with round to oval nuclei and with single nucleoli and clear or granular cytoplasm
        ◆ Cells are organized into irregular plates with bile canaliculi and sinusoids
        ◆ Commonly associated with extramedullary hematopoiesis
    — Embryonal component
        ◆ Embryonal-type cells are smaller and elongated with hyperchromatic nuclei and scant cytoplasm
        ◆ Predominantly solid pattern with rosette-like clusters, cords, ribbons, and rarely tubules
- Variants of epithelial: anaplastic small cell and macrotrabecular
    — Anaplastic small cells arranged in sheets; histologically similar to neuroblastoma
    — Macrotrabecular component resembles HCC
- Intestinal-type glandular elements and areas of squamous metaplasia (often highly keratinized) uncommon
- Multinucleated giant cells may be associated with hormone production
▌ Mixed epithelial and mesenchymal type
- Fetal and embryonal epithelium component admixed with mesenchymal elements

- Mesenchymal component is usually osteoid, cartilage, or undifferentiated spindled cells
- Osteoid areas are typically keratin positive (metaplastic, not true mesenchyme)
- Other elements, such as striated muscle, and neural tissue, are rarely seen

Special Stains and Immunohistochemistry

- Keratin low molecular weight (keratins 8 and 18) and pan-keratin typically positive
- EMA typically positive
- HepPar-1 positive
- CEA positive
- AFP positive in fetal and embryonal cells
- Neuron-specific enolase (NSE), S-100 protein, and chromogranin often positive
- Bcl-2 variably positive

Other Techniques for Diagnosis

- Electron microscopy: immature hepatocytes in epithelial areas
- Flow cytometry: fetal type shows diploid DNA content; embryonal and anaplastic small cell are aneuploid in 50% of cases
- Cytogenetics
    — Complex karyotypes with gains of chromosomes 2 and X
    — 11p15 LOH in Beckwith-Wiedemann syndrome
    — Trisomy 2q and 20
- *Wnt* signaling pathway abnormalities (β-catenin and adenomatous polyposis coli [APC] mutations)
- Rarely *TP53* mutations

Differential Diagnosis

▌ Metastatic primitive tumor of infancy (nephroblastoma and neuroblastoma)
- Clinical history (i.e., evidence of primary) is essential
- Immunohistochemical stains may be of value in proper histologic context
    — WT-1 in nephroblastoma; keratin variable
    — Endocrine markers in the absence of keratin in neuroblastoma
▌ HCC of childhood
- Generally resembles normal adult liver with platelike growth of tumor cells separated by CD34-positive vascular sinusoids
- Bile production by tumor cells

Pearls

- Hepatoblastoma is thought to arise from a multipotential blastema
- Poor prognostic indicators include age less than 1 year, large size, involvement of vital structures, predominance of anaplastic small cells or macrotrabeculae, and aneuploidy

Selected References

Schnater JM, Kohler SE, Lamers WH, et al: Where do we stand with hepatoblastoma? A review. Cancer 98:668-678, 2003.

Douglass EC: Hepatic malignancies in childhood and adolescence (hepatoblastoma, hepatocellular carcinoma, and embryonal sarcoma). Cancer Treat Res 92:201-212, 1997.

Raney B: Hepatoblastoma in children: A review. J Pediatr Hematol Oncol 19:418-422, 1997.

Abenoza P, Manivel JC, Wick MR, et al: Hepatoblastoma: An immunohistochemical and ultrastructural study. Hum Pathol 18:1025-1035, 1987.

Bile Duct Hamartoma (von Meyenburg Complex)

Clinical Features

- Usually incidental finding at surgery or autopsy
- Part of a spectrum of ductal plate malformations of the liver
- Often associated with polycystic liver or kidney disease

Gross Features

- Multiple white nodules up to several millimeters in diameter scattered throughout the liver
- Grossly mimics metastatic tumor

Histopathology

- Focal, well-demarcated lesions composed of a variable number of ductal structures embedded in a hyalinized stroma
- Ductal structures are variably dilated and may have bile in the ductal lumens

Figure 7-17. Bile duct hamartoma. Variable number of ductal structures embedded in a hyalinized stroma. The ductal structures are variably dilated and may have microcystic dilation with bile in the ductal lumens. The ductal lumens are lined by a flattened or cuboidal epithelium.

- Ductal lumens are lined by a flattened or cuboidal epithelium
- No cytologic atypia

Special Stains and Immunohistochemistry

- Noncontributory

Other Techniques for Diagnosis

- Noncontributory

Differential Diagnosis

- **▌ Peribiliary gland hamartoma (bile duct adenoma)**
  - Usually single
  - Composed of small tubular structures with no dilatation or bile
- **▌ Mesenchymal hamartoma**
  - Usually solitary
  - Prominent myxoid stroma
  - Contains hepatocyte islands
  - Bile rarely present within the ducts
- **▌ Metastatic neoplasm**
  - Histologically and cytologically malignant
  - Clinical history important

Pearls

- A result of bile ductal plate malformation
- Often associated with polycystic liver or kidney disease
- Usually incidental finding

Selected References

Goodman ZD, Terracciano LM: Tumours and tumour-like lesions of the liver. In Burt AD, Portmann BC, Ferrel LD (eds): MacSween's Pathology of the Liver, 5th ed. London, Churchill Livingstone, 2007, pp 761-814.

Ishak KG, Goodman ZD, Stocker JT: Benign cholangiocellular tumors. In Atlas of Tumor Pathology, 3rd series, fascicle 31. Washington, DC, Armed Forces Institute of Pathology, 2001, pp 49-70.

Peribiliary Gland Hamartoma (Bile Duct Adenoma)

Clinical Features

- Usually asymptomatic and found incidentally at intra-abdominal surgery or autopsy
- Benign behavior

Gross Pathology

- Solitary, round or ovoid, well-demarcated but unencapsulated tumors, usually less than 1 cm in size
- Gray, white, yellow to tan in color, and firm in consistency

Histopathology

- Small tubules and acini with slight branching and tortuosity

Figure 7-18. Peribiliary gland hamartoma (bile duct adenoma). Proliferation of packed uniform tubular structure.

- Minimal luminal dilation and no cystic changes
- Tubules lined by single layer of cuboidal to columnar cells
- No bile in lumens
- May contain intracytoplasmic mucin
- No communication between tubular structures and interlobular bile ducts
- Fibrous stroma, which may be cellular or hyalinized
- Normally spaced portal tracts often present

Special Stains and Immunohistochemistry

- Noncontributory

Other Techniques for Diagnosis

- Noncontributory

Differential Diagnosis

▌ Bile duct hamartoma
- Typically multiple
▌ Mesenchymal hamartoma
- Primarily found in infants
- Often cystic
- Myxoid stroma
- Contains cords of hepatocytes
▌ Well-differentiated carcinoma (metastatic or cholangiocarcinoma)
- Variably pleomorphic cells within single gland
- Increased nuclear-to-cytoplasmic ratio

Pearls

- Hamartoma of peribiliary glands (small accessory glands of the major bile ducts)
- Not associated with dysplasia or malignancy

Selected References

Goodman ZD, Terracciano LM: Tumours and tumour-like lesions of the liver. In Burt AD, Portman BC, Ferrell LD (eds): MacSween's Pathology of the Liver, 5th ed. London, Churchill Livingstone, 2007, pp 761-814.

Bhathal PS, Hughes NR, Goodman ZD: The so-called bile duct adenoma is a peribiliary gland hamartoma. Am J Surg Pathol 20:858-864, 1996.

Allaire GS, Rabin L, Ishak KG, et al: Bile duct adenoma: a study of 152 cases. Am J Surg Pathol 12:708-715, 1988.

Biliary Cystadenoma and Cystadenocarcinoma

Clinical Features

- Relatively rare neoplasm
- Almost exclusively a neoplasm of women
- Predominantly arises within the liver but may arise in the extrahepatic biliary tree, including the gallbladder

Gross Pathology

- Solitary and multilocular cystic neoplasm containing mucinous or clear fluid
- Multiple lobules of varying size
- Inner lining smooth, glistening, trabecular, or with papillary excrescences

Histopathology

▌ Cystadenoma
- Lined by single layer of tall columnar cells that focally may become cuboidal, flattened, or even papillary
- Almost always mucinous
- Intestinal metaplasia with goblet cells can be present
- Densely cellular ovarian-like stroma is a feature that hepatobiliary cystadenoma shares with mucinous cystic neoplasm in the pancreas
- Ovarian-like stroma is exclusively present in women
- Varying degrees of dysplasia in the cystic epithelium may be seen, and it can develop into invasive cystadenocarcinoma
▌ Cystadenocarcinoma
- Most arise from preexisting cystadenoma
- Often show ovarian-type stroma in women
- Cytologic atypia, mitosis, and invasion of underlying stroma

Special Stains and Immunohistochemistry

- Keratin (7 and 19) and CEA: epithelial lining is positive
- Mucicarmine and Alcian blue: may demonstrate cytoplasmic mucin in epithelial cells
- Vimentin, smooth muscle actin (SMA), inhibin, estrogen receptor, and progesterone receptor: stromal component is positive

Other Techniques for Diagnosis

- Noncontributory

Differential Diagnosis

▌ Developmental cysts
- Unilocular
- No nuclear atypia
▌ Biliary papillomatosis
- No ovarian-type stroma

Figure 7-19. A, Biliary cystadenoma. The cyst is lined by a layer of tall columnar epithelium that focally may become cuboidal or flattened. **B, Biliary cystadenoma.** High-power photomicrograph showing the columnar epithelium resembling biliary epithelium with cytoplasmic mucin and an underlying ovarian-like stroma. **C, Cystadenocarcinoma.** Notice the stratification of the epithelium, and stromal invasion. (Courtesy of Dr. Zachary Goodman, Armed Forces Institute of Pathology, Washington, DC.)

- Also affects men
- Communicating with bile ducts

Pearls

- May arise from ectopic ovarian tissue or from embryonic foregut rests

Selected References

Weihing RR, Shintaku IP, Geller SA, Petrovic LM: Hepatobiliary and pancreatic mucinous cystadenocarcinomas with mesenchymal stroma: Analysis of estrogen receptors/progesterone receptors and expression of tumor-associated antigens. Mod Pathol 10:372-379, 1997.

Devaney K, Goodman ZD, Ishak KG: Hepatobiliary cystadenoma and cystadenocarcinoma: A light microscopic and immunohistochemical study of 70 patients. Am J Surg Pathol 18:1078-1091, 1994.

Wheeler DA, Edmondson HA: Cystadenoma with mesenchymal stroma (CMS) in the liver and bile ducts: A clinicopathologic study of 17 cases, 4 with malignant change. Cancer 56:1434-1445, 1985.

Biliary Papillomatosis (Intraductal Papillary Neoplasia of Liver)

Clinical Features

- Uncommon papillary neoplasm of the biliary tree
- May be solitary or may spread extensively along the biliary tree within or outside of the liver, including the gallbladder
- A biliary counterpart of intraductal papillary mucinous tumor (IPMT) in the pancreas
- Symptoms of biliary obstruction
- Curative resection difficult with frequent recurrence

Gross Pathology

- Dilated bile ducts with polypoid excrescences
- May contain inspissated mucus
- Histopathology
  - The involved bile ducts are dilated, containing papillary growth of columnar epithelial cells overlying fibrovascular stalks
  - Lining epithelial cells may mimic biliary epithelium or show gastric or intestinal metaplasia
  - Mucin production may be present
  - Lining epithelial cells may show varying degrees of dysplasia and may progress to invasive carcinoma

Special Stains and Immunohistochemistry

- Noncontributory

Other Techniques for Diagnosis

- Noncontributory

Differential Diagnosis

- Biliary cystadenoma
  - Ovarian-type stroma

Figure 7-20. Biliary papillomatosis. A, The bile duct is dilated and filled with papillary outgrowth of epithelium. **B,** Higher power shows the lining epithelial cells with mucin production.

- Almost exclusively occurs in women
- No communication with bile duct

Pearls

- Clinicopathologic features are similar to those of IPMT of the pancreas
- Geographic predilection; most large series reported in East Asia, where hepatolithiasis and clonorchiasis infestation are common

Selected References

Goodman ZD, Terracciano LM: Tumours and tumour-like lesions of the liver. In Burt AD, Portmann BC, Ferrell LD (eds): MacSween's Pathology of the Liver, 5th ed. London, Churchill Livingstone, 2007, pp 761-814.

Zen Y, Fujii T, Itatsu K, et al: Biliary papillary tumors share pathological features with intraductal papillary mucinous neoplasm of the pancreas. Hepatology 44:1333-1343, 2006.

Shibahara H, Tamada S, Goto M, et al: Pathologic features of mucin-producing bile duct tumors: Two histopathologic categories as counterparts of pancreatic intraductal papillary-mucinous neoplasms. Am J Surg Pathol 28:327-338, 2004.

Nakanuma Y, Sasaki M, Ishikawa A, et al: Biliary papillary neoplasm of the liver. Histol Histopathol 17:851-861, 2002.

Cholangiocarcinoma: Intrahepatic, Extrahepatic, and Hilar (Klatskin Tumor)

This tumor arises from (or differentiates as) bile duct epithelium and is classified as either intrahepatic or extrahepatic. Hilar (Klatskin) tumors are generally considered extrahepatic. The main differences are in clinical presentation and gross appearance.

Clinical Features

- Average age at presentation is 60 years
- Equal frequency in men and women
- More common in Southeast Asian countries
- Often preceded by biliary hyperplasia or dysplasia
- Risk factors include ulcerative colitis, sclerosing cholangitis, thorium dioxide (Thorotrast) exposure, *Clonorchis sinensis* infestation, intrahepatic bile duct lithiasis, and a variety of congenital anomalies of intrahepatic and extrahepatic bile ducts
- Most cases not associated with cirrhosis or hepatitis
- Normal serum AFP, elevated serum CEA
- Intrahepatic tumors present with abdominal pain and weight loss
- Hilar tumors often present as small lesions because their location results in early biliary obstruction
- Extrahepatic tumors also present with jaundice and ascites but tend to be larger than hilar lesions at presentation
- Frequently metastasizes to regional and peripancreatic lymph nodes
- Generally poor prognosis

Figure 7-21. Cholangiocarcinoma. A characteristic feature of this lesion is the infiltrating nature of the glands surrounded by a marked desmoplastic stromal reaction.

Gross Pathology

- Intrahepatic
  - Gray-white, tough, scirrhous mass with finger-like extensions along major bile ducts and lymphatics
  - Can be large
  - Often multifocal
- Extrahepatic
  - Nodular or flat sclerotic lesions with deep penetration into the bile duct wall; less commonly polypoid superficial lesions
- Klatskin tumor (hilar)
  - Begins at hepatic duct junction and spreads along segments of biliary tree
  - Large green liver with collapse of gallbladder and extrahepatic ducts is characteristic

Histopathology

- Usually well-differentiated mucin-secreting adenocarcinomas with abundant fibrous stroma
- Typically do not show necrosis
- Heterogeneity of cells within same gland
- Increased nuclear-to-cytoplasmic ratio
- Prominent nucleoli
- Concentric layering of cellular stroma around neoplastic glands
- Spreads between hepatic plates (sinusoidal growth) and along ducts and nerves
- Stromal and perineural invasion; vascular invasion less common than in HCC
- Metaplastic and dysplastic changes may be seen in adjacent biliary epithelium
- Sarcomatoid differentiation rare
- Occasionally admixed with trabeculae of neoplastic hepatocytes (mixed cholangiocarcinoma and HCC)

Special Stains and Immunohistochemistry

- Mucicarmine and PAS with diastase (PAS-D) positive
- EMA, keratins 7 and 19 positive
- Villin positive with brush-border accentuation; CD10 similar pattern
- CDX2 variable or weak reactivity
- CEA positive (will be positive with polyclonal anti-CEA but lacks the canalicular staining of HCC)
- Epidermal growth factor receptor protein (EGFR) positive (but so, too, HCC)
- C-erbB-2 positive, especially in PSC-related lesions

Other Techniques for Diagnosis

- Electron microscopy: nonspecific glandular characteristics
- Molecular studies
  - Expression of *C-myc, C-ras, c-erbB-2* oncogenes related to tumor differentiation (not diagnostically useful)
  - High incidence of *C-ras* oncogene mutation

  - Decreased β-catenin expression
  - Elevated *cox-2* expression

Differential Diagnosis

❚ HCC
- Positive for low-molecular-weight keratin (with subplasmalemmal accentuation)
- Positive for HepPar-1, glypican-3
- Canalicular staining with polyclonal anti-CEA and CD10
- Sinusoidal endothelium CD34 positive
- Negative with monoclonal anti-CEA
- Absence of mucin
- Often resembles normal liver with thicker plates and cytologic pleomorphism; bile production

❚ Metastatic adenocarcinoma
- More common in liver than cholangiocarcinoma
- Clinical history important
- Virtually all colonic metastases show intraluminal necrosis

❚ Epithelioid hemangioendothelioma
- Intracytoplasmic vacuoles; occasionally contain red blood cells
- Less often keratin positive
- Vascular markers positive

Pearls

- Perineural invasion is a helpful diagnostic feature, particularly on frozen section
- Clusters of small acini (periluminal sacculi of Beale) normally present in the extrahepatic duct wall should not be mistaken for invasive carcinoma

Selected References

Shaib YH, Davila JA, McGlynn K, El-Serag HB: Rising incidence of intrahepatic cholangiocarcinoma in the United States: A true increase? J Hepatol 40:472-477, 2004.

Thuluvath PJ, Rai R, Venbrux AC, et al: Cholangiocarcinoma: A review. Gastroenterologist 5:306-315, 1997.

Tada M, Omata M, Ohto M: High incidence of ras gene mutation in intrahepatic cholangiocarcinoma. Cancer 69:1115-1118, 1992.

Voravud N, Foster CS, Gilbertson JA, et al: Oncogene expression in cholangiocarcinoma and in normal hepatic development. Hum Pathol 20:1163-1168, 1989.

Qualman ST, Haupt HM, Bauer TW, et al: Adenocarcinoma of the hepatic duct junction: A reappraisal of the histologic criteria of malignancy. Cancer 53:1545-1551, 1984.

Gallbladder Carcinoma

Clinical Features

- Marked female predominance
- Age peak in seventh decade; uncommon in patients younger than 50 years
- Higher incidence in Latin American countries
- Increased risk with cholelithiasis

Figure 7-22. Adenocarcinoma of gallbladder. A, High-power view shows the transition between normal mucosa and malignant epithelium. **B,** Both in situ carcinoma and infiltrating carcinoma are evident in this photomicrograph.

- Other risk factors include porcelain gallbladder (end-stage calcifying cholecystitis), cholecystenteric fistula, anomalous pancreaticobiliary duct anastomosis, ulcerative colitis, adenomatous polyposis coli, and Gardner syndrome (APC mutations)
- Can present with right upper quadrant pain and anorexia
- More commonly found incidentally after cholecystectomy for cholelithiasis
- Increased serum alkaline phosphatase levels

Gross Pathology

- Two growth patterns
  - Diffuse growth (two thirds of cases)
  - Polypoid or papillary mass (one third of cases)
- Diffuse pattern can be mistaken for cholecystitis
- Carcinomatous gallbladders often contain calculi and exhibit marked mural fibrosis

Histopathology

- Commonly associated with hyperplasia, gastric or intestinal metaplasia, dysplasia, or carcinoma in situ of adjacent mucosa

- Carcinoma in situ can extend into cystic duct and Aschoff-Rokitansky sinuses and *should not be mistaken for invasion*
- Most commonly invasive cancers are tubular adenocarcinomas that resemble cholangiocarcinoma
- Well-formed glands with wide lumens lined by one or more layers of highly atypical columnar or cuboidal cells surrounded by concentrically arranged cellular stroma
- Mucin production
- Characteristically better differentiated architecturally than cytologically
- Characteristically grows along nerves
- Regional lymph node metastases common
- Foci of intestinal differentiation common
- Choriocarcinoma-like elements rarely reported
- Other types: high-grade endocrine (small cell), adenosquamous, squamous (exceptionally rare), low-grade endocrine, and sarcomatoid

Special Stains and Immunohistochemistry

- Keratins 7 and 19 strongly positive; more likely than typical intrahepatic and extrahepatic cholangiocarcinoma to coexpress keratin 20
- CEA strongly positive
- Villin positive with brush-border accentuation
- CDX2 weak or variable
- AFP occasionally positive

Other Techniques for Diagnosis

- Electron microscopy: adenocarcinoma cells show pleomorphic microvilli, mucin vacuoles, and abundant lysosomes (nonspecific features)
- Overexpression of *TP53* in most cases; more common in high-grade tumors; more common in gallbladder tumors than in extrahepatic cholangiocarcinomas

Differential Diagnosis

▌Cholangiocarcinoma
  - Similar immunohistochemical staining pattern (although less often keratin 20 positive)
  - Gross specimen and clinical information necessary to differentiate
▌HCC
  - CEA negative except for bile canaliculi when using polyclonal antibodies, owing to cross-reactivity with non-CEA bile-associated glycoprotein
  - Subplasmalemmal accentuation with low-molecular-weight keratin antibodies
  - Absence of mucin
▌Metastatic tumors
  - Rare in gallbladder
  - Most reported cases are melanoma, breast carcinoma, or renal cell carcinoma

Pearls

- Most important prognostic indicator is stage; low-stage lesions are effectively limited to those detected incidentally at cholecystectomy
- Thought to arise from a sequence of intestinal metaplasia, dysplasia, and in situ carcinoma

Selected References

Lee RG, Emond J: Prognostic factors and management of carcinomas of the gallbladder and extrahepatic bile ducts. Surg Oncol Clin N Am 6:639-659, 1997.

Abi-Rached B, Neugut AI: Diagnostic and management issues in gallbladder carcinoma. Oncology 9:19-24, 1995.

Kamel D, Paakko P, Nuorva K, et al: P53 and c-erbB-2 protein expression in adenocarcinomas and epithelial dysplasias of the gallbladder. J Pathol 70:67-72, 1993.

Yamaguchi K, Enjoji M: Carcinoma of the gallbladder. Cancer 62:1425-1432, 1988.

Hepatic Metastases

Clinical Features

- Metastatic disease overall more common than primary hepatic malignancy
- Liver is a common site for metastases from many primary sites, particularly the colon, breast, pancreas, lung, kidney, and stomach
- Sarcomas and malignant melanomas also metastasize to the liver
- Primary tumors of gallbladder, extrahepatic bile ducts, pancreas, and stomach frequently involve the liver by direct extension
- Resection with possibility of cure may be indicated for single or multiple liver metastases from the colon
- Liver metastasis from the breast is considered evidence of systemic disease and is not an indication for resection
- Metastases are relatively rare in cirrhotic livers

Gross Pathology

- Hepatic metastases are usually discrete and well demarcated (grossly and histologically) from adjacent liver parenchyma; often with a hyperemic rim
- May be single or multiple, occasionally with infiltrative growth; may mimic either intrahepatic cholangiocarcinoma or HCC
- Diffusely infiltrative patterns may resemble primary liver tumors
- Occasionally metastases from the breast, prostate, or stomach can spread through the liver as small punctate lesions simulating cirrhosis
- Colonic metastases are usually multiple large nodules with marked central umbilication on the surface of the liver

Histopathology

- Depends on the primary malignancy
- Colon: prominent central necrosis in metastatic glandular lumens; mucin production can be abundant and may undergo calcification
- Squamous cell carcinoma: polygonal cells with abundant eosinophilic cytoplasm; may keratinize. If basaloid cells predominate, think upper aerodigestive or anal origin
- Lung and breast: often medium-sized nodules without extensive necrosis or hemorrhage and with early central umbilication; may be histologically indistinguishable if poorly differentiated
- Gallbladder: cluster around gallbladder bed and diminish in size with infiltration of hepatic parenchyma
- Malignant melanoma: large epithelioid or spindled cells with prominent nucleoli with or without pigment
- Prostate: epithelial cells with prominent nucleoli; acinar differentiation may not be conspicuous in some cases

Special Stains and Immunohistochemistry

- Immunohistochemical stains are relevant in both the clinical and histologic context. In selected cases, an immunohistochemical profile may confirm or augment the histologic and clinical impression. Useful examples include (but are not limited to)
  — Keratin 20 without keratin 7; villin (brush border); uniform CDX2: *lower intestinal tract*
  — Keratin 7 with variable or absent keratin 20; villin (brush border), keratin 17 or 19, weak or variable CDX2: *upper gastrointestinal tract and pancreaticobiliary* (additional markers, including mesothelin and MUC 1, 2, 4, 5AC, and 6 may also be of value)
  — Keratin 7 without keratin 20; TTF-1 and surfactant A positive; CDX2 and villin negative: *pulmonary*
  — Keratin 7 and 20; CEA; high-molecular-weight keratin (including keratin 5/6; p63; absent CDX2: *urothelial*
  — Keratin 7 and 20 negative; CD10, EMA, PAX2 positive: *conventional type renal*
  — Keratin 7 and 20 negative; high-molecular-weight and p63 negative; prostate-specific antigen or prostatic acid phosphatase positive: *prostatic*
  — Thyroglobulin, TTF-1 positive; surfactant negative: *thyroidal*
  — Gross cystic disease fluid protein-15, mammaglobin, S-100 protein positive; estrogen and progesterone receptor positive: *mammary*
  — Keratin 7, p53, CA-125, WT-1, estrogen receptor protein positive; CEA negative: *mullerian (serous*

more likely WT-1 positive; mucinous are CA-125 negative with an overall profile similar to intestinal carcinoma)
— S-100 protein, GCDFP-15, androgen receptor protein positive; estrogen receptor protein negative: *salivary ductal* (other salivary gland lesions often coexpress S-100 protein and myoepithelial markers p63, SMA, and calponin)
— S-100 protein, HM-B45, melan-A, tyrosinase, microphthalmia transcription factor (MiTF) positive; keratin negative: *melanocytic*
— Synaptophysin, chromogranin A, NSE, CD56, CD57 positive; keratin variable; TTF-1 variable: *endocrine* (selected endocrine neoplasms have unique profiles, including calcitonin and TTF-1 in medullary thyroid and insulin, glucagon, somatostatin, and others in pancreatic)
- Likelihood that immunohistochemistry will be helpful is inversely related to grade of metastatic lesion

Other Techniques for Diagnosis

- Not likely to contribute

Pearls

- Metastasis more common than primary hepatic malignancy
- Clinical history is most important, although some histologic patterns and selected immunohistochemical profiles may provide useful diagnostic information
- Number of metastases is important in the context of some cancers, especially colorectal adenocarcinoma, because some patients might be eligible for resection
- Gland formation with extensive central necrosis is characteristic of colonic metastases

Selected References

Kakar S, Gown AM, Goodman ZD, Ferrell LD: Best practices in diagnostic immunohistochemistry: Hepatocellular carcinoma versus metastatic neoplasm. Arch Pathol Lab Med 131:1648-1654, 2007.
Sardi A, Akbarov A, Conaway G: Management of primary and metastatic tumors to the liver. Oncology 10:911-925, 1996.

Peliosis Hepatis

Clinical Features

- Associated with use of anabolic steroids, oral contraceptives, thiopurines, and danazol
- Resolves after discontinuation of causative drugs
- Associated with hepatic infection by *Bartonella henselae* (causative organism of bacillary angiomatosis) in HIV-infected patients

Gross Pathology

- Liver parenchyma with focal blood lakes

Histopathology

- Large, intraparenchymal, blood-filled spaces and cysts surrounded by hepatocytes
- Blood-filled spaces without lining cells
- Disruption of sinusoids
- In *Bartonella*-associated cases: myxoid perisinusoidal stroma with clumps of granular material

Special Stains and Immunohistochemistry

- Reticulin stain demonstrates disruption of sinusoidal reticulin fibers
- Warthin-Starry stain positive in granular *Bartonella*-associated deposits

Other Techniques for Diagnosis

- Noncontributory

Differential Diagnosis

▌ Sinusoidal dilation
- Lacks cystic and cavernous change
- Sinusoidal reticulin intact
▌ Hemangioma
- Dilated vascular spaces lined by flattened endothelial cells
- Endothelial cells are CD31, CD34, factor VIII–related antigen (von Willebrand factor) and *Ulex europaeus I* positive

Pearls

- Most commonly related to use of androgenic anabolic steroids
- Associated with *Bartonella henselae,* especially in HIV-positive patients

Selected References

Koehler JE, Sanchez MA, Garrido CS: Molecular epidemiology of Bartonella infections in patients with bacillary angiomatosis-peliosis. N Engl J Med 337:1876-1883, 1997.
Cavalcanti R: Impact and evolution of peliosis hepatis in renal transplant recipients. Transplantation 58:315-316, 1994.
Se KL: Liver pathology associated with the use of anabolic-androgenic steroids. Liver 12:73-79, 1992.
Perkocha LA: Clinical and pathological features of bacillary peliosis hepatis in association with human immunodeficiency virus infection. N Engl J Med 323:1581-1586, 1990.

Hemangioma

Clinical Features

- Most common hepatic neoplasm (in as many as 20% of autopsy cases)
- Typically asymptomatic
- Lesions larger than 4 cm may present with abdominal distention, mass, or pain
- Usually diagnosed in adulthood

Figure 7-23. Liver hemangioma. Low-power photomicrograph of a liver section shows classic hemangioma composed of dilated vascular spaces.

Gross Pathology

- Usually solitary; most less than 4 cm
- Well-circumscribed, spongy, red-brown lesion
- Typically subcapsular

Histopathology

- Vascular spaces lined by single layer of bland endothelial cells
  — Capillary: consists of small, thin-walled, anastomosing capillary-like vessels
  — Cavernous: consists of large irregular, dilated vascular spaces
- Intralesional thrombosis is common; Masson-like lesions may suggest a diagnosis of angiosarcoma
- Connective tissue stroma often shows areas of sclerosis and calcification

Special Stains and Immunohistochemistry

- Vascular markers (CD31, CD34, podoplanin, *Ulex europaeus I*, factor VIII–related antigen, and von Willebrand factor) positive
- Keratin negative

Other Techniques for Diagnosis

- Noncontributory

Differential Diagnosis

- ▌Peliosis hepatis
  - Consists of blood lakes without endothelial lining
- ▌Angiosarcoma
  - Multiple spongy hemorrhagic nodules with ill-defined borders
  - Lining cells are large and show significant cytologic atypia
  - Often has a high mitotic rate; occasional atypical mitotic figures
- ▌Juvenile hemangioendothelioma
  - Capillary-like vascular proliferation with plump endothelial cells

- Occasional mitotic figures
- Central fibrous scar
- Focal necrosis
- ▌Epithelioid hemangioendothelioma
  - Multiple hepatic nodules with ill-defined borders
  - Poorly defined vascular channels lined by atypical epithelioid cells

Pearls

- Usually incidental
- Most are cavernous type
- Large or symptomatic lesions should be surgically excised

Selected References

Iqbal N, Saleem A: Hepatic hemangioma: A review. Tex Med 93:48-50, 1997.

Semelka RC, Sofka CM: Hepatic hemangiomas. Mag Reson Imaging Clin N Am 5:241-253, 1997.

Stanley P, Geer GD, Miller JH, et al: Infantile hepatic hemangiomas: Clinical features, radiologic investigations, and treatment of 20 patients. Cancer 64:936-949, 1989.

Infantile Hemangioendothelioma

Clinical Features

- Rare
- About 90% diagnosed in first year of life, male predominance
- Presents as abdominal mass or hepatomegaly
- Most symptomatic patients die from
  — Arteriovenous shunt with risk for high-output congestive heart failure
  — Rupture
- Multicentricity precludes surgery; vascular ligation or embolization common means of treatment
- May involute or regress

Gross Pathology

- May be solitary or multicentric
- Marked variation in size (microscopic to greater than 15 cm)
- Central scar

Histopathology

- Capillary-like small vascular proliferation in periphery of lesion
- Lining endothelial cells plump, focally epithelioid
- Occasional mitotic figures identified
- Hypovascular stroma in center of lesion
- Central necrosis and calcification

Special Stains and Immunohistochemistry

- Vascular markers positive
- Keratin negative

Other Techniques for Diagnosis

- Noncontributory

Differential Diagnosis

❚ Capillary hemangioma
- Bland endothelial cells
- Lacks central scar

❚ So-called infantile angiosarcoma
- May be a variant of infantile hemangioendothelioma
- Endothelial cells more pleomorphic or kaposiform; may show intravascular budding
- Aggressive local infiltration, metastasis

❚ Angiosarcoma
- Increased nuclear atypia and mitotic activity
- Focal sinusoidal involvement

Selected Reference

Dehner LP, Ishak KG: Vascular tumours of the liver in infants and children: A study of 30 cases and review of the literature. Arch Pathol 92:101-111, 1971.

Epithelioid Hemangioendothelioma

Clinical Features

- Middle-aged patients, female predominance
- Slow growing
- Calcifications commonly seen by imaging studies
- Surgical excision often precluded by multifocal nature of lesion; liver transplantation effective means of treatment
- About 40% rate of recurrence
- About 30% may also involve spleen, lymph nodes, lung, or bone (metastasis versus metachronous primary disease)

Figure 7-24. Epithelioid hemangioendothelioma. Proliferation of vascular channels lined by atypical epithelioid cells. Notice the sclerotic background.

Gross Pathology

- Hepatic nodules with ill-defined borders; 70% of cases multifocal
- Central scarlike areas with myxoid or calcified stroma

Histopathology

- Poorly defined vascular channels lined by atypical epithelioid tumor cells
- Central scars contain dendritic tumor cells with vacuolated cytoplasm and only slight nuclear atypia
- Sparing of portal tracts
- Infiltrative borders
- Myxoid or sclerotic background

Special Stains and Immunohistochemistry

- Vascular markers (CD31, CD34, factor VIII-related antigen, *Ulex europaeus I*) positive
- Keratin (low molecular weight) occasionally positive
- Villin negative

Other Techniques for Diagnosis

- Electron microscopy: Weibel-Palade bodies

Differential Diagnosis

❚ Angiosarcoma
- Sinusoidal involvement
- Increased nuclear atypia and mitotic activity

❚ Cholangiocarcinoma
- No blood-filled spaces
- True gland formation
- Keratin 7 and 19 and CEA positive
- Villin positive with brush-border pattern
- Vascular markers negative

❚ Metastatic carcinoma
- Keratin positive
- Vascular markers negative

❚ Malignant melanoma
- Nests and individual cells with prominent macronucleoli
- Melanin pigment occasionally seen
- S-100 protein, HMB-45, melan-A, tyrosinase, MiTF positive

Pearls

- Prognosis is more favorable than for angiosarcoma
- May involve several different organs at diagnosis (30% of cases)

Selected References

Fujii T, Zen Y, Sato Y, et al: Podoplanin is a useful marker for epithelioid hemangioendothelioma of the liver. Mod Pathol 21:125-130, 2008.

Kelleher MB, Iwatsuki S, Sheahan DG: Epithelioid hemangioendothelioma of liver: Clinicopathological correlation of 10 cases treated by orthotopic liver transplantation. Am J Surg Pathol 13:999-1008, 1989.

Ishak KG, Sesterhenn IA, Goodman MZD, et al: Epithelioid hemangioendothelioma of the liver: A clinicopathologic and follow-up study of 32 cases. Hum Pathol 15:839-852, 1984.

Angiosarcoma

Clinical Features

- Most common in men during the sixth and seventh decades
- Abdominal pain or hepatomegaly in most cases
- Associated with exposure to thorium dioxide (Thorotrast, a radiographic contrast material), vinyl chloride (plastics), arsenic, and anabolic steroids
- Latency period of many years
- Poor prognosis; metastasis at diagnosis not uncommon

Gross Pathology

- Multiple, spongy hemorrhagic nodules with ill-defined borders

Histopathology

- Variable patterns
- Growth of markedly atypical endothelial cells along existing sinusoids (often seen with other patterns)
- Predominantly cavernous with pseudopapillary projections of pleomorphic spindled to epithelioid mesenchymal cells and admixed hemorrhage
- Occasional solid tumor cell nests without appreciable vascular spaces
- Individual malignant cells may be seen in adjacent hepatic parenchyma

Special Stains and Immunohistochemistry

- Vascular markers (CD31, CD34, podoplanin, factor VIII–related antigen, podoplanin, and *Ulex europaeus I*) positive
- Keratin typically negative, but variable reactivity in some cases
- Villin negative

Other Techniques for Diagnosis

- Electron microscopy: Weibel-Palade bodies
- Molecular studies: *K-ras-2* oncogene point mutations in vinyl chloride–associated cases

Differential Diagnosis

- ▌ HCC
  - Neoplastic cells positive for keratin and HepPar-1
  - Negative for vascular markers (beware prominent CD34-positive sinusoidal endothelium)
- ▌ Cholangiocarcinoma
  - Neoplastic cells positive for keratin, villin (brush-border pattern), and CEA
  - Negative for vascular markers
- ▌ Epithelioid hemangioendothelioma
  - Less prominent vascular differentiation
  - Does not involve hepatic sinusoids
  - Typically shows less cytologic atypia and a low mitotic rate
  - Intracytoplasmic vacuoles may be present
- ▌ Metastatic carcinoma
  - Neoplastic cells positive for keratins
  - Negative for vascular markers

Pearls

- Increased risk associated with Thorotrast, vinyl chloride, and arsenic exposure
- Sinusoidal growth pattern characteristic
- Well-differentiated lesions may mimic benign vascular lesions; poorly differentiated lesions may be difficult to distinguish histologically from epithelial neoplasms
- Poor prognosis

Selected References

Lee FI, Smith PM, Bennett B, et al: Occupationally related angiosarcoma of the liver in the United Kingdom 1972-1994. Gut 39:312-318, 1996.

Ohsawa M, Kanno H, Aozasa K, et al: Use of immuno-histochemical procedures in diagnosing angiosarcoma: Evaluation of 98 cases. Cancer 75:2867-2874, 1995.

Selby DM, Stocker JT, Ishak KG: Angiosarcoma of the liver in childhood: A clinicopathologic and follow-up study of 10 cases. Pediatr Pathol 12:485-498, 1992.

Tamburro CH: Relationship of vinyl monomers and liver cancers: Angiosarcoma and hepatocellular carcinoma. Semin Liver Dis 4:158-169, 1984.

Figure 7-25. Angiosarcoma. Dilated vascular channels lined by pleomorphic, neoplastic, and endothelial cells.

Mesenchymal Hamartoma

Clinical Features

- Rare benign lesion
- Presents during first 2 years of life

Figure 7-26. Mesenchymal hamartoma. Proliferation of loose connective tissue, dilated vessels, and scattered branching bile ducts.

- Rare in adolescents and young adults
- Male-to-female ratio, 2:1
- Presents with abdominal swelling and palpable abdominal mass
- Related to polycystic disease, congenital hepatic fibrosis, and bile duct hamartoma
- Etiology uncertain (developmental anomaly versus ischemia versus neoplasm)

Gross Pathology

- Solitary spherical nodule
- Large (>1 kg) soft fluctuant mass with a smooth surface
- Multiple cystic spaces filled with thin or viscous fluid
- Solid areas are variable: white and fibrous, yellow and myxoid, or brown and liver-like

Histopathology

- Low-power appearance resembles fibroadenoma
- Loose, edematous, myxoid connective tissue with dilated lymphatics, vessels, and fluid-filled spaces
- Scattered disorganized and elongated branching bile ducts
- Scattered hepatocellular nodules
- Extramedullary hematopoiesis is common

Special Stains and Immunohistochemistry

- Noncontributory

Other Techniques for Diagnosis

- Electron microscopy: connective tissue component (myo)fibroblastic; admixed normal liver elements
- Flow cytometry: occasionally aneuploid

Differential Diagnosis

- Bile duct adenoma
  - Tubular structures with small or no lumens
  - Lacks distinctive mesenchymal septa

- No liver cell islands
- May secrete mucin
- Bile duct hamartoma
  - Characteristically multiple
  - Composed of complex bile ducts in a fibrous stroma background
- Embryonal (undifferentiated) sarcoma
  - Found in prepubertal children
  - Entirely mesenchymal tumor with few entrapped bile ducts
  - Phenotypically diverse malignant cells
  - Extensive necrosis

Pearls

- Mesenchymal hamartoma is a localized abnormality of ductal plates that is typically congenital
- Thought to arise in connective tissue of portal triads

Selected References

Craig JR: Mesenchymal tumors of the liver: Diagnostic problems for the surgical pathologist. Pathology 3:141-160, 1994.

DeMaioribus CA, Lally KP, Sim K, et al: Mesenchymal hamartoma of the liver. Arch Surg 125:598-600, 1990.

Stocker JT, Ishak KG: Mesenchymal hamartoma of the liver. Pediatr Pathol 1:245-267, 1983.

Embryonal (Undifferentiated) Sarcoma

Clinical Features

- Childhood neoplasm most common between ages 5 and 10 years; rare in adults
- No gender predilection
- No serum AFP elevation
- Presents with abdominal distention and weight loss
- Poor prognosis despite aggressive therapy

Gross Pathology

- Single, large, soft globular mass (10 to 30 cm)
- Variegated, solid, and cystic cut surface; pretreatment imaging studies often characteristic
- Fibrous pseudocapsule
- May show hemorrhage and necrosis

Histopathology

- Extensive necrosis; islands of viable neoplasm generally in periphery
- Loosely arranged pleomorphic spindled or stellate cells
- Scattered histiocytoid, fibrohistiocytoid, and myofibroblastic cells
- Fibroblast-like or smooth muscle–like fascicles or bundles of cells
- Minority population of cells resembling rhabdomyoblasts
- Scattered bizarre multinucleated giant cells
- Compact areas of more uniform round cells may be seen

Figure 7-27. Embryonal (undifferentiated) sarcoma. Loosely arranged proliferation of spindle to oval cells with eosinophilic cytoplasm. Atypical mitosis is evident in the center portion of the photomicrograph.

- Variably sized eosinophilic globules in neoplastic cell cytoplasm and extracellular matrix
- Abundant acid mucopolysaccharide matrix
- Cystic, fluid-filled spaces secondary to degeneration are common
- Intermingled dilated benign bile ducts (entrapped), usually in periphery
- Extramedullary hematopoiesis in about 50% of cases

Special Stains and Immunohistochemistry

- PAS-D and α_1-antitrypsin: eosinophilic globules are positive
- Vimentin diffusely positive
- Keratin (pan-keratins and low-molecular-weight keratin) may be focally positive

Other Techniques for Diagnosis

- Electron microscopy: neoplastic cells show mesenchymal differentiation, including spindle-shaped cells with minimal cytoplasmic organelles and no desmosomal junctions
- Complex karyotype

Differential Diagnosis

▌ Pleomorphic sarcoma (so-called malignant fibrous histiocytoma)
  - Typically occurs in elderly patients
  - Positive for SMA (variable) and for histiocyte and lysosomal markers (CD68 and others)

▌ Primary and metastatic hepatic sarcomas and other spindle cell neoplasms
  - Rarely encountered
  - Monodirectional differentiation in an appropriate histologic context; examples include (but are not limited to)
    — SMA and desmin: *leiomyosarcoma*
    — Muscle-specific actin, desmin, and caldesmon: *rhabdomyosarcoma* (spindled embryonal, solid alveolar, and pleomorphic variants)
    — SMA, HMB-45, and melan-A: *angiomyolipoma*
    — CD117 and CD34: *gastrointestinal stromal tumor*
    — S-100 protein, HMB-45, melan-A, tyrosinase, and MiTF: *melanoma*

▌ Anaplastic small cell hepatoblastoma
  - Found in younger children
  - Elevated serum AFP
  - Monomorphic neoplastic cells

▌ HCC with sarcomatoid differentiation
  - Elevated serum AFP
  - Areas of typical HCC usually present (*beware limited sampling in biopsies*)
  - Sarcomatoid areas more densely cellular than embryonal sarcoma
  - Positive for keratin and HepPar-1

▌ Mesenchymal hamartoma
  - Composed of benign elements
  - Close association between mesenchymal and ductal components

Pearls

- Radiographic appearance of untreated lesion characteristic
- Must be considered in older prepubertal children with hepatic masses
- Purely mesenchymal neoplasm with phenotypic diversity
- Characteristic PAS-positive eosinophilic globules

Selected References

Stocker JT: An approach to handling pediatric liver tumors. Am J Clin Pathol 109(4 Suppl 1):S67-72, 1998.

Craig JR: Mesenchymal tumors of the liver: Diagnostic problems for the surgical pathologist. Pathology 3:141-160, 1994.

Aoyama C, Hachitanda Y, Sato JK, et al: Undifferentiated (embryonal) sarcoma of the liver: A tumor of uncertain histogenesis showing divergent differentiation. Am J Surg Pathol 15:615-624, 1991.

Ralph H. Hruban and Mehmet Guler

8

Pancreas

Non-neoplastic Conditions

Chronic Pancreatitis

Clinical Features

- Defined by irreversible loss of pancreatic parenchyma and function caused by inflammation
- Patients present with recurrent attacks of abdominal and back pain and evidence of loss of pancreatic function, including exocrine insufficiency (malabsorption and steatorrhea) and diabetes mellitus
- Alcohol abuse is the leading cause of chronic pancreatitis in Western countries; other common causes include obstruction of the ducts by calculi, and hereditary pancreatitis; cystic fibrosis is the leading

cause of chronic pancreatitis in the pediatric population
- Chronic pancreatitis has a poor long-term prognosis with a 20-year mortality rate of 50%
- Chronic pancreatitis can clinically, radiologically, and pathologically mimic pancreatic cancer
- Pancreatic cancer can cause chronic pancreatitis, and long-standing chronic pancreatitis, particularly hereditary pancreatitis, can increase the risk for developing pancreatic cancer
- Autoimmune (lymphoplasmacytic sclerosing) pancreatitis is associated with elevated serum immunoglobulin G4 (IgG4) levels and other autoimmune diseases such as chronic sclerosing sialadenitis (Küttner tumor), primary sclerosing

Figure 8-1. Chronic pancreatitis. Low-power view shows fibrosis and acinar dropout; however, the lobular architecture is maintained (*left*). Note the aggregation of islets (*right*).

Figure 8-2. Autoimmune pancreatitis. A, Characteristic mixed duct-centric inflammation. **B,** Venulitis with partial involvement of the vein.

cholangitis, inflammatory bowel disease, retroperitoneal fibrosis (Ormond disease), and Riedel thyroiditis

Gross Pathology

- Diffuse atrophy of the gland with firm white fibrosis
- Early chronic pancreatitis may produce a localized ill-defined masslike lesion that may mimic pancreatic cancer
- When caused by alcohol abuse, there may be associated pseudocysts and intraductal calculi
- Autoimmune pancreatitis often affects the head of the pancreas

Histopathology

- Defined by inflammation with destruction of pancreatic parenchyma and replacement by fibrous connective tissue and fat
- Lobular architecture of the parenchyma is retained
- Remaining ductal epithelium can be atrophic or reactive
- Residual islets of Langerhans may aggregate, producing enlarged islets that can mimic a neoplasm
- Autoimmune (lymphoplasmacytic sclerosing) pancreatitis is characterized by a duct-centric mixed plasma cell–rich inflammatory infiltrate, interstitial fibrosis, and venulitis

Special Stains and Immunohistochemistry

- Noncontributory

Modern Techniques for Diagnosis

- Genetic testing for inherited mutations in the *PRSS1* gene available for familial pancreatitis

Differential Diagnosis

▮ Infiltrating ductal adenocarcinoma
- Haphazard arrangement of glands with loss of lobular architecture at low power
- Glands immediately adjacent to muscular vessels
- Perineural invasion
- Vascular invasion
- Variation in the area of nuclei in a single gland by more than 4 to 1 (*4-to-1 rule*)
- Incomplete lumens
- Luminal necrosis

▮ Well-differentiated pancreatic endocrine neoplasm
- Larger size and tendency to produce a single hormone (monoclonal)

Pearls

- Chronic pancreatitis can clinically and pathologically mimic pancreatic cancer, yet the two entities are treated vastly differently
- Growth pattern and location are the two most helpful features in distinguishing reactive from neoplastic glands
- Autoimmune pancreatitis is important to recognize because it may respond to treatment with steroids
- Avoid overdiagnosing the aggregated islets of Langerhans in chronic pancreatitis as a neuroendocrine neoplasm

Selected References

Hruban RH, Pitman MB, Klimstra DS: Tumors of the pancreas. In Atlas of Tumor Pathology, 4th Series, Fascicle 6. Washington, DC, American Registry of Pathology and Armed Forces Institute of Pathology, 2007.

Zhang L, Notohara K, Levy MJ, et al: IgG4-positive plasma cell infiltration in the diagnosis of autoimmune pancreatitis. Mod Pathol 20:23-28, 2007.

Klöppel G, Maillet B: Pathology of acute and chronic pancreatitis. Pancreas 8:659-670, 1993.

Pancreatic Pseudocyst

Clinical Features

- Accounts for 75% of cystic lesions of the pancreas
- Pathologic release of pancreatic enzymes causes the localized digestion of intrapancreatic and extrapancreatic tissues
- A complication of acute pancreatitis, often in the setting of chronic alcoholic pancreatitis
- May spontaneously resolve, may become infected, or may perforate adjacent organs

Gross Pathology

- Cysts are usually solitary
- Often involves peripancreatic tissues such as the lesser omental sac, the retroperitoneum between the stomach and transverse colon, and the space between the stomach and the liver
- Cysts are filled with hemorrhagic necrotic debris rich in pancreatic enzymes
- Associated with peripancreatic hemorrhagic fat necrosis
- Cysts range in size from 2 to 30 cm

Histopathology

- Cysts contain necrotic and hemorrhagic debris with hemosiderin-laden macrophages
- Cysts lack a true epithelial lining
- Cysts are lined by granulation and fibrous connective tissue

Special Stains and Immunohistochemistry

- Noncontributory

Other Techniques for Diagnosis

- Noncontributory

Differential Diagnosis

▮ Cystic neoplasms of the pancreas
- Cystic neoplasms have a true epithelial lining and typically contain mucinous or serous fluid
- Solid pseudopapillary neoplasms can contain hemorrhagic and necrotic debris, but they will have poorly cohesive epithelial cells surrounding delicate branching blood vessels

Pearls

- Suspect a mimicker of a pseudocyst if the patient does not have a clinical history of acute or chronic pancreatitis, and when the pancreatic parenchyma is normal
- Extensive sampling may be necessary to demonstrate an epithelial lining in a cystic neoplasm
- Cyst fluid amylase levels should be high in pseudocysts

Selected References

Hruban RH, Pitman MB, Klimstra DS: Tumors of the pancreas. In Atlas of Tumor Pathology, 4th Series, Fascicle 6. Washington, DC, American Registry of Pathology and Armed Forces Institute of Pathology, 2007.

Klöppel G: Pseudocysts and other non-neoplastic cysts of the pancreas. Semin Diagn Pathol 17:7-15, 2000.

Sanfey H, Aguilar M, Jones RS: Pseudocysts of the pancreas, a review of 97 cases. Am Surg 60:661-668, 1994.

Lymphoepithelial Cyst

Clinical Features

- Often an incidental finding
- Rare, with only about 50 cases reported
- Predominantly seen in men, with a 4:1 male-to-female ratio
- Mean age about 55 years

Gross Pathology

- Unilocular or multilocular
- Mean size about 5 cm
- Well-demarcated, filled with keratinaceous (cheesy) debris
- Cysts with thin walls

Histopathology

- Cysts lined by mature keratinizing squamous epithelium
- Subepithelial layer of lymphoid tissue often with germinal center formation
- *No* skin adnexal structures and *no* components with other directions of differentiation

Special Stains and Immunohistochemistry

- Noncontributory

Other Techniques for Diagnosis

- Noncontributory

Differential Diagnosis

▪ Mature cystic teratoma (dermoid cyst)
  - In addition to the squamous epithelium, these have skin adnexal structures and often mature mesenchymal elements such as cartilage

▪ Epidermoid cyst in heterotopic spleen
  - Distinctive cystic lesion can also be lined by mature squamous epithelium

Pearls

- The keratinous debris can resemble the necrotic contents of a pseudocyst
- Unlike their counterparts in the head and neck, no relationship to immunosuppression and Epstein-Barr virus (EBV) infection has been found
- Although their pathogenesis is unknown, one proposal is squamous metaplasia of an obstructed, inflamed, and dilated duct

Selected References

Hruban RH, Pitman MB, Klimstra DS: Tumors of the pancreas. In Atlas of Tumor Pathology, 4th Series, Fascicle 6. Washington, DC, American Registry of Pathology and Armed Forces Institute of Pathology, 2007.

Adsay NV, Hasteh F, Cheng JD, et al: Lymphoepithelial cysts of the pancreas: A report of 12 cases and a review of the literature. Mod Pathol 15:492-501, 2002.

Neoplasms of the Exocrine Pancreas

Serous Cystic Neoplasms

Clinical Features

- Slightly more common in women than in men, with a female-to-male ratio of 7:3
- Mean age about 65 years
- Can be associated with the von Hippel-Lindau (VHL) disease
- Present nonspecifically as large abdominal masses

Figure 8-3. Lymphoepithelial cyst. The cyst is lined by mature squamous epithelium with an underlying lymphoid infiltrate.

Figure 8-4. Serous cystadenoma. The relatively small cysts are lined by a single layer of glycogen-rich cuboidal epithelial cells with round uniform nuclei.

- Most are benign, with only a few case reports of aggressive behavior

Gross Pathology

- Can be composed of innumerable small cysts (microcystic) or a few larger cysts (macrocystic)
- Can be solid (solid serous adenoma)
- Can be combined with a well-differentiated pancreatic endocrine neoplasm (especially in patients with VHL disease)
- Well demarcated, often with a central stellate scar
- Cysts are thin walled and contain watery, straw-colored fluid

Histopathology

- Cysts are lined by a flat cuboidal epithelium with optically clear cytoplasm and round uniform nuclei
- Mitoses and nuclear pleomorphism are not seen
- Septa are composed of relatively acellular fibrous connective tissue
- Solid variant is composed of sheets and nests of cells cytologically identical to the more common cystic variety

Special Stains and Immunohistochemistry

- Cells contain abundant glycogen and therefore stain with periodic acid–Schiff (PAS) stain, and this staining is sensitive to diastase digestion
- Epithelial cells label with antibodies to cytokeratin (AE1/AE3 and CAM5.2), and one third label with epithelial membrane antigen
- Immunolabeling for carcinoembryonic antigen (CEA) is negative

Other Techniques for Diagnosis

- Electron microscopy demonstrates abundant intracellular glycogen
- Some, especially those that arise in association with VHL disease, harbor mutations in the *VHL* gene

Differential Diagnosis

▌ Mucinous cystic neoplasm
  - Cysts have a thick wall and contain gooey tenacious mucin
  - Cysts are lined by tall columnar cells containing large quantities of mucin
  - Cysts have distinctive ovarian-type stroma
▌ Intraductal papillary mucinous neoplasm
  - Cysts contain tenacious mucin
  - Cysts are lined by tall columnar cells containing mucin
  - Cysts communicate with larger pancreatic ducts
▌ Metastatic renal cell carcinoma
  - Nuclear atypia and prominent nucleoli
  - Immunolabel for vimentin, renal cell carcinoma marker (RCCma), and CD10

▌ Lymphangioma
  - Flat cells lining spaces
  - Associated lymphoid aggregates in cyst walls
  - Express CD31 and factor VIII–related antigen

Pearls

- The relationship of the cysts to the pancreatic ducts, the thickness of the cyst walls, and the cyst contents can be used to support the diagnosis
- Radiologic feature of a central stellate scar can be characteristic
- Serous cystadenocarcinomas are extremely rare and can be distinguished from benign serous neoplasms only by their aggressive behavior (spread to other organs)

Selected References

Hruban RH, Pitman MB, Klimstra DS: Tumors of the pancreas. In Atlas of Tumor Pathology, 4th Series, Fascicle 6. Washington, DC, American Registry of Pathology and Armed Forces Institute of Pathology, 2007.

Galanis C, Zamani A, Cameron JL, et al: Resected serous cystic neoplasms of the pancreas: A review of 158 patients with recommendations for treatment. J Gastrointest Surg 11:820-826, 2007.

Compton CC: Serous cystic tumors of the pancreas. Semin Diagn Pathol 17:43-55, 2000.

Mucinous Cystic Neoplasms

Clinical Features

- Much more common in women than in men with a female-to-male ratio of 20:1
- Mean age about 45 years
- Present nonspecifically as a large abdominal mass
- One third are associated with an invasive adenocarcinoma

Figure 8-5. Mucinous cystic neoplasm with low-grade dysplasia. The cyst is lined by tall columnar cells with abundant intracellular mucin. Note the characteristic ovarian-type stroma.

Figure 8-6. Mucinous cystic neoplasm with high-grade dysplasia. The mucin-producing epithelium is now architecturally complex, and there is significant nuclear pleomorphism.

- Presence or absence of an associated invasive carcinoma drives prognosis

Gross Pathology

- Most occur in the body or tail of the pancreas
- Usually solitary and multilocular
- Composed of large, 1- to 3-cm, thick-walled cysts containing tenacious mucin
- Cysts do not communicate with the larger pancreatic ducts
- Lining of the cysts can be smooth, or prominent papillary structures can project into the lumens

Histopathology

- Cysts are lined by tall columnar epithelium with varying degrees of cytologic and architectural atypia
- Noninvasive tumors are classified into low-grade dysplasia, moderate dysplasia, and high-grade dysplasia
- Dysplasia and even invasive cancer can be focal
- The stroma is cellular and is histologically similar to ovarian stroma
- One third have an associated invasive ductal adenocarcinoma

Special Stains and Immunohistochemistry

- PAS, PAS with diastase treatment, and mucicarmine positive
- Epithelium labels with antibodies to cytokeratin and CEA
- Stroma labels with antibodies to inhibin, and to progesterone and estrogen receptors

Other Techniques for Diagnosis

- May harbor *K-ras2* and *TP53* gene mutations
- Most noninvasive mucinous cystic neoplasms have intact dpc4 expression, whereas half of the invasive

cancers associated with mucinous cystic neoplasms show loss of dpc4 expression

Differential Diagnosis

- Intraductal papillary mucinous neoplasm
  - Located in the head more frequently than in the body or tail of the gland
  - Cysts connect to the larger pancreatic ducts
  - Have a paucicellular stroma, not the ovarian-type stroma
- Serous cystic neoplasm
  - Cysts contain thin, watery, straw-colored fluid
  - Cysts are usually smaller (microcystic) and have a thinner wall
  - The tumor has a central stellate scar
  - Cysts are lined by cuboidal glycogen-rich cells
- Pseudocyst
  - Cysts contain hemorrhagic and necrotic material
  - Cysts lack an epithelial lining

Pearls

- The epithelium can be partially denuded; in these cases, the diagnosis is suggested by the presence of ovarian-type stroma
- Because an invasive carcinoma can arise focally in these neoplasms, they should be entirely resected and thoroughly, if not completely, sampled for histologic examination

Selected References

Hruban RH, Pitman MB, Klimstra DS: Tumors of the pancreas. In Atlas of Tumor Pathology, 4th Series, Fascicle 6. Washington, DC, American Registry of Pathology and Armed Forces Institute of Pathology, 2007.

Goh BK, Tan YM, Chung YF, et al: A review of mucinous cystic neoplasms of the pancreas defined by ovarian-type stroma: Clinicopathological features of 344 patients. World J Surg 30:2236-2245, 2006.

Wilentz RE, Albores-Saavedra J, Hruban RH: Mucinous cystic neoplasms of the pancreas. Semin Diagn Pathol 17:31-42, 2000.

Zamboni G, Scarpa A, Bogina G, et al: Mucinous cystic tumors of the pancreas: Clinicopathological features, prognosis, and relationship to other mucinous cystic tumors. Am J Surg Pathol 23:410-422, 1999.

Intraductal Papillary Mucinous Neoplasms

Clinical Features

- Slightly more common in men than in women, with a male-to-female ratio of 1.5:1
- Mean age about 65 years
- Arise in the head of the gland more commonly than in the body or tail
- Imaging may reveal a dilated main pancreatic duct

Figure 8-7. Intraductal papillary mucinous neoplasm. Low-power view shows a distended pancreatic duct filled with complex papillary structures lined by mucin-producing columnar cells.

- May present with symptoms of chronic pancreatitis or symptoms of intermittent pancreatic duct obstruction
- One third have an associated invasive adenocarcinoma
- Presence or absence of an invasive component drives prognosis
- May be multifocal

Gross Pathology

- Most arise in the head of the gland
- Can be multifocal
- Cysts communicate with the larger pancreatic ducts
- Main duct–type involves the main pancreatic duct; branch duct–type involves a side branch of the main duct
- Lining of the cysts can be relatively flat or may have large papillae

Histopathology

- Cysts are lined by tall columnar epithelium with abundant intracellular and extracellular mucin
- Neoplastic epithelium involves preexisting ducts
- Noninvasive neoplasms are classified into low-grade dysplasia, moderate dysplasia, and high-grade dysplasia
- Stroma is paucicellular
- One third are associated with an invasive adenocarcinoma
- The invasive carcinoma can be a tubular (ductal) adenocarcinoma or a colloid (mucinous noncystic) adenocarcinoma; the designation "colloid" should be reserved for invasive adenocarcinomas, with at least 80% colloid differentiation

Special Stains and Immunohistochemistry

- PAS, PAS with diastase treatment, and mucicarmine positive
- Epithelium labels with antibodies to cytokeratin and CEA
- Intestinal type expresses the mucin MUC2; pancreatobiliary type expresses the mucin MUC1

Other Techniques for Diagnosis

- The prevalence of mutations in the *K-ras2* and *TP53* genes increases with increasing degrees of dysplasia
- Dpc4 expression is usually intact, especially in those that are noninvasive and have intestinal differentiation

Differential Diagnosis

▌ Mucinous cystic neoplasm
  - Arises in women more often than in men
  - Arises in the body and tail more often than in the head
  - Cysts do not communicate with the larger pancreatic ducts
  - Characteristic ovarian-type stroma
▌ Pancreatic intraepithelial neoplasia (PanIN)
  - Smaller (<0.5 cm)
  - Short, stubby papillae relative to the long, finger-like papillae of intraductal papillary mucinous neoplasms
  - Express the mucin MUC1

Pearls

- Can be multifocal
- Bivalving a resected specimen along a probe placed in the main pancreatic duct can help determine the relationship of the cysts to the duct system
- These neoplasms should be sampled extensively because the presence or absence of invasion is the most important prognosticator
- Colloid and mucinous differentiation in the invasive component portends a better prognosis

Selected References

Hruban RH, Pitman MB, Klimstra DS: Tumors of the pancreas. In Atlas of Tumor Pathology, 4th Series, Fascicle 6. Washington, DC, American Registry of Pathology and Armed Forces Institute of Pathology, 2007.

Sohn TA, Yeo CJ, Cameron JL, et al: Intraductal papillary mucinous neoplasms of the pancreas: An updated experience. Ann Surg 239:788-797, 2004.

Chari ST, Yadav D, Smyrk TC, et al: Study of recurrence after surgical resection of intraductal papillary mucinous neoplasm of the pancreas. Gastroenterology 123:1500-1507, 2002.

Adsay NV, Merati K, Andea A, et al: The dichotomy in the preinvasive neoplasia to invasive carcinoma sequence in the pancreas: Differential expression of MUC1 and MUC2 supports the existence of two separate pathways of carcinogenesis. Mod Pathol 15:1087-1095, 2002.

Pancreatic Intraepithelial Neoplasia

Clinical Features

- Too small to be detected reliably using available imaging techniques
- Believed to be a precursor to invasive ductal adenocarcinoma of the pancreas
- More common in the head of the gland than in the tail
- More common in elderly patients
- More common in pancreata with an invasive carcinoma than in pancreata without a neoplasm

Gross Pathology

- Almost always too small to be appreciated grossly

Histopathology

- Epithelial proliferations within the smaller pancreatic ducts
- May be flat or papillary
- Papillae are short and stubby
- Classified into PanIN-1, PanIN-2, and PanIN-3 based on the degree of architectural and cytologic dysplasia
- Lobular units downstream of PanINs often show lobulocentric atrophy and scarring, presumably due to obstructive effects of exuberant duct epithelium

Special Stains and Immunohistochemistry

- Express the mucin MUC1

Other Techniques for Diagnosis

- Progressive Accumulation of genetic alterations with activating *K-ras2* gene mutations observed in low-grade PanINs (PanIN-1 lesions), inactivation of *p16/CDKN2A* in intermediate lesions (PanIN-2), and *TP53* and *SMAD4* loss in high-grade lesions (PanIN-3)

Differential Diagnosis

- Intraductal papillary mucinous neoplasm
  - Grossly visible lesions
  - Long, finger-like papillae
  - Abundant intracellular and extracellular mucin production
  - Some express the mucin MUC2
- Invasive ductal adenocarcinoma
  - Loss of lobular architecture at low power
  - Glands immediately adjacent to muscular vessels
  - Perineural invasion
  - Vascular invasion
  - Variation in the area of nuclei in a single gland by more than 4 to 1
  - Incomplete lumens
  - Luminal necrosis

Pearls

- Avoid overstating the clinical significance of PanIN lesions. PanINs, particularly low-grade PanINs, are common in the population, particularly the elderly population. Thus, presence of a PanIN lesion at a margin in a resection for an invasive carcinoma is of unknown significance and in most cases should not prompt further surgery
- Avoid misdiagnosing the lobulocentric atrophy (see "Chronic Pancreatitis") surrounding PanIN lesions as invasive carcinoma with desmoplasia. The overall lobular pattern should always be intact

Selected References

Hruban RH, Takaori K, Klimstra DS, et al: An illustrated consensus on the classification of pancreatic intraepithelial neoplasia and intraductal papillary mucinous neoplasms. Am J Surg Pathol 28:977-987, 2004.

Hruban RH, Adsay NV, Albores-Saavedra J, et al: Pancreatic intraepithelial neoplasia: A new nomenclature and classification system for pancreatic duct lesions. Am J Surg Pathol 25:579-586, 2001.

Invasive Ductal Adenocarcinoma and Its Variants

Clinical Features

- Most patients are between 60 and 80 years old
- Strikes men slightly more than women
- Patients are usually not diagnosed until after the cancer has spread
- Most common symptoms include epigastric pain radiating to the back, weight loss, and painless jaundice
- The 5-year survival rate is less than 5%

Figure 8-8. Pancreatic intraepithelial neoplasia. This papillary proliferation of epithelial cells projects into the lumen of a small duct. The papillae are shorter than those of intraductal papillary mucinous neoplasms.

Figure 8-9. Well-differentiated infiltrating adenocarcinoma. Medium-power view shows a haphazard arrangement of the glands and the associated desmoplastic stroma.

Figure 8-11. Colloid carcinoma. Neoplastic glands float in large pools of extracellular mucin.

Figure 8-10. Well-differentiated infiltrating adenocarcinoma. This gland is immediately adjacent to a muscular vessel, a clue to the diagnosis of invasive carcinoma.

Figure 8-12. Undifferentiated carcinoma with osteoclast-like giant cells. High-power view shows a neoplasm composed of large osteoclast-like giant cells with uniform nuclei and the adjacent pleomorphic neoplastic cells.

Gross Pathology

- Most arise in the head of the pancreas (65%)
- Firm, poorly defined sclerotic mass
- Can undergo cystic degeneration
- Often obstruct the pancreatic and bile ducts, resulting in upstream dilation of these ducts

Histopathology

▌ Ductal adenocarcinoma
  - Atypical gland-forming epithelial cells infiltrating into the stroma
  - Loss of lobular architecture at low power
  - Glands immediately adjacent to muscular vessels
  - Perineural invasion

- Vascular invasion
- Variation in the area of nuclei in a single gland by more than 4 to 1
- Incomplete lumens
- Luminal necrosis

▌ Adenosquamous carcinoma
  - Invasive carcinoma with both glandular and squamous differentiation
  - At least 30% of the neoplasm should have squamous differentiation

▌ Colloid carcinoma
  - Prominent extracellular mucin production with neoplastic cells floating in pools of extracellular mucin

- By definition, at least 80% of the neoplasm has colloid differentiation
- Almost always arises in association with an intraductal papillary mucinous neoplasm
■ Hepatoid carcinoma
  - Large pink cells with prominent liver differentiation, including the formation of trabeculae and sometimes even bile production
  - May express HepPar-1
  - Need to exclude a liver primary
■ Medullary carcinoma
  - Poorly differentiated carcinoma with syncytial growth pattern, pushing borders, and an associated lymphocytic infiltrate
  - Shows microsatellite instability
■ Signet ring cell carcinoma
  - Infiltrating, round, noncohesive cells with prominent intracytoplasmic mucin vacuole
  - Need to exclude gastric and breast primaries before making the diagnosis in the pancreas
■ Undifferentiated carcinoma
  - Epithelial neoplasm with no definite direction of differentiation
  - Cells may be large and bizarre in shape (anaplastic), they may be spindle shaped (sarcomatoid), or they may have a combination of glandular and spindle cell elements (carcinosarcoma)
■ Undifferentiated carcinoma with osteoclast-like giant cells
  - Neoplastic atypical mononuclear epithelial cells admixed with large non-neoplastic osteoclast-like giant cells

Special Stains and Immunohistochemistry

- Mucicarmine and PAS (with and without diastase) stains highlight intracellular and extracellular mucin
- Immunolabeling for cytokeratin (7 and 19) is positive, as is labeling for CEA, CA-19.9, and MUC1
- Loss of dpc4 expression observed in 55%

Other Techniques for Diagnosis

- Infiltrating ductal adenocarcinomas often harbor mutations in the *K-ras2*, *TP53*, *p16/CDKN2A*, and *SMAD4/DPC4* genes
- Medullary carcinomas frequently are microsatellite unstable

Differential Diagnosis

■ Chronic pancreatitis
  - Lobular arrangement maintained
  - No perineural or vascular invasion
  - No glands next to muscular vessels
  - No luminal necrosis
  - Complete lumens
  - Only mild nuclear pleomorphism (<4:1)
  - Intact dpc4 expression, negative for CEA

■ Acinar cell carcinoma
  - Cellular neoplasm with less desmoplastic stroma
  - Acinar formations with basally placed nuclei and granular apical cytoplasm
  - Single prominent nucleoli
  - Expresses trypsin and chymotrypsin
  - Negative for cytokeratin 7
■ Pancreatoblastoma
  - Squamoid nests
  - Cellular neoplasm with less desmoplastic stroma
  - Acinar formations with basally placed nuclei and granular apical cytoplasm
  - Single prominent nucleoli
  - Expresses trypsin and chymotrypsin
■ Solid pseudopapillary neoplasm
  - Occurs predominantly in young women
  - Does not form true lumens
  - Eosinophilic globules
  - Positive for CD10
  - Nuclear labeling for β-catenin
■ Well-differentiated pancreatic endocrine neoplasm
  - Cellular neoplasm with less desmoplastic stroma
  - Cells nest or form trabeculae
  - Uniform nuclei with salt-and-pepper chromatin
  - Positive for synaptophysin and chromogranin
  - Negative for cytokeratin 7
■ Metastases to the pancreas
  - Clinical history of another primary
  - Morphology unusual for a pancreatic primary including clear cells (renal primary) and signet ring cells (gastric or breast primary)
  - Melanin pigment (melanoma)
  - Absence of an intraductal papillary mucinous neoplasm or PanIN lesions

Pearls

- Despite their hugely different prognoses, adenocarcinoma of the pancreas can be difficult to distinguish from reactive glands of chronic pancreatitis; location of the glands is the single most helpful feature
- Rule out metastases to the pancreas before diagnosing a primary signet ring cell carcinoma of the pancreas
- Pancreatic carcinoma has a poor prognosis, primarily because it is clinically detected so late; early detection strategies would be expected to be helpful in management and treatment

Selected References

Hruban RH, Pitman MB, Klimstra DS: Tumors of the pancreas. In Atlas of Tumor Pathology, 4th Series, Fascicle 6. Washington, DC, American Registry of Pathology and Armed Forces Institute of Pathology, 2007.

Adsay NV, Bandyopadhyay S, Basturk O, et al: Chronic pancreatitis or pancreatic ductal adenocarcinoma? Semin Diagn Pathol 21:268-276, 2004.

Sharma S, Green KB: The pancreatic duct and its arteriovenous relationship: An underutilized aid in the diagnosis and distinction of pancreatic adenocarcinoma from pancreatic intraepithelial neoplasia: A study of 126 pancreatectomy specimens. Am J Surg Pathol 28:613-620, 2004.

Klöppel G, Hruban RH, Longnecker DS, et al: Ductal adenocarcinoma of the pancreas. In Hamilton SR, Aaltonen LA (eds): World Health Organization Classification of Tumours. Pathology and Genetics: Tumours of the Digestive System. Lyon, IARC Press, 2000, pp 221-230.

Acinar Cell Carcinoma

Clinical Features

- Mostly in adults with a mean age of about 60 years
- Occurs in males more than females, with a male-to-female ratio of 3.5:1
- Presenting signs and symptoms include weight loss, abdominal pain, nausea, and vomiting
- About 15% present with metastatic fat necrosis, arthralgias, and peripheral eosinophilia caused by the release of lipase from the neoplasm

Gross Pathology

- Large, well-circumscribed masses in head or tail of the pancreas (mean, 10 cm)

Histopathology

- Most architecturally form acinar structures with basally oriented nuclei and granular apical cytoplasm
- Some form solid sheets of cells without well-formed acini
- Nuclei are relatively uniform and contain single prominent nucleoli

Special Stains and Immunohistochemistry

- Immunolabel for trypsin, chymotrypsin, and lipase
- May have focal endocrine differentiation (if >25%, classify as mixed acinar-endocrine)

Figure 8-13. Acinar cell carcinoma. Although this particular example does not form well-defined acini, the single prominent nucleolus provides a clue to the diagnosis.

- Immunolabel for cytokeratin (AE1/AE3 and CAM5.2)

Other Techniques for Diagnosis

- In contrast to ductal Adenocarcinomas, acinar cell carcinomas rarely have *K-ras2* gene mutations

Differential Diagnosis

- ▌ Pancreatoblastoma
  - Presence of squamoid nests distinguishes pancreatoblastoma from acinar cell carcinomas
- ▌ Well-differentiated pancreatic endocrine neoplasm
  - Salt-and-pepper nuclei
  - Usually does not have a single prominent nucleoli
  - Diffusely expresses chromogranin and synaptophysin
- ▌ Solid pseudopapillary neoplasm
  - Occurs predominantly in young women
  - Does not form true lumens
  - Eosinophilic globules
  - Positive for CD10
  - Nuclear labeling for β-catenin
- ▌ Ductal adenocarcinoma
  - Less cellular neoplasm with prominent desmoplastic stroma
  - Gland formation with mucin production
  - Nuclear pleomorphism
  - Express cytokeratin 7; negative for trypsin, chymotrypsin, and lipase

Pearls

- Neoplastic cells with single prominent nucleoli should suggest the diagnosis of an acinar carcinoma
- Some grow as sheets of cells and do not form well-defined acini
- Mixed endocrine-acinar carcinomas should be considered aggressive neoplasms similar to the pure acinar variety

Selected References

Hruban RH, Pitman MB, Klimstra DS: Tumors of the pancreas. In Atlas of Tumor Pathology, 4th Series, Fascicle 6. Washington, DC, American Registry of Pathology and Armed Forces Institute of Pathology, 2007.

Ordonez NG: Pancreatic acinar cell carcinoma. Adv Anat Pathol 8:144-159, 2001.

Klimstra DS, Heffess CS, Oertel JE, Rosai J: Acinar cell carcinoma of the pancreas: A clinicopathologic study of 28 cases. Am J Surg Pathol 16:815-837, 1992.

Pancreatoblastoma

Clinical Features

- Most occur in children
- Associated with Beckwith-Wiedemann syndrome and familial adenomatous polyposis (FAP)
- Presents clinically as large abdominal mass
- Some patients have elevated α-fetoprotein levels

Figure 8-14. Pancreatoblastoma. Cells with acinar differentiation admixed with squamoid nests.

Selected References

Hruban RH, Pitman MB, Klimstra DS: Tumors of the pancreas. In Atlas of Tumor Pathology, 4th Series, Fascicle 6. Washington, DC, American Registry of Pathology and Armed Forces Institute of Pathology, 2007.

Abraham SC, Wu TT, Klimstra DS, et al: Distinctive molecular genetic alterations in sporadic and familial adenomatous polyposis-associated pancreatoblastomas: Frequent alterations in the APC/beta-catenin pathway and chromosome 11p. Am J Pathol 159:1619-1627, 2001.

Klimstra DS, Wenig BM, Adair CF, Heffess CS: Pancreatoblastoma: A clinicopathologic study and review of the literature. Am J Surg Pathol 19:1371-1389, 1995.

Neoplasms of the Endocrine Pancreas

Well-Differentiated Pancreatic Endocrine Neoplasms

Clinical Features

- Functional well-differentiated pancreatic endocrine neoplasms (PENs) are associated with a clinical syndrome caused by the release of endocrine hormones by the neoplasm
- Functional PENs include insulinomas (hypoglycemia), glucagonomas (necrotizing migratory erythema, stomatitis, and diabetes), gastrinomas (duodenal ulceration), and vasoactive intestinal polypeptide-secreting tumors, or *VIPomas* (watery diarrhea, hypokalemia, and achlorhydria)
- Nonfunctional PENs may synthesize endocrine hormones but do not produce a clinical syndrome
- Associated with multiple endocrine neoplasia type I (MEN I)
- Microadenomas are smaller than 0.5 cm
- Size, mitotic rate, large vessel invasion, and spread to lymph nodes and other organs are all prognosticators

Gross Pathology

- Arise in the head, body, and tail
- Are well demarcated
- Are usually solid and soft, but some are cystic

Histopathology

- Nested or trabecular pattern of growth
- Uniform, salt-and-pepper nuclei
- Amyloid deposition can be seen, especially in insulin-producing neoplasms
- Psammoma bodies are typically associated with somatostatin-producing neoplasms

Special Stains and Immunohistochemistry

- Grimelius and Fontana-Masson stains positive
- Immunolabel with antibodies to chromogranin, synaptophysin, and CD56
- May immunolabel for specific hormones (e.g., insulin, glucagon)

Gross Pathology

- Large, well-circumscribed masses in head or tail of the pancreas (mean, 10 cm)

Histopathology

- By definition, at least two components must be present: neoplastic cells with acinar differentiation, and squamoid nests
- May also have cells with endocrine and ductal differentiation
- Stromal and primitive components may also be seen

Special Stains and Immunohistochemistry

- Acinar component positive for trypsin, chymotrypsin, and lipase
- Endocrine component, if present, expresses chromogranin and synaptophysin
- Squamoid nests often not immunoreactive

Other Techniques for Diagnosis

- Most have loss of heterozygosity of a highly imprinted region of chromosome 11p near the *WT-2* locus

Differential Diagnosis

▍ Acinar cell carcinoma
- Usually in older patients
- Does not have squamoid nests
- Otherwise remarkably similar

▍ Well-differentiated pancreatic endocrine neoplasm
- Salt-and-pepper nuclei
- Usually does not have single prominent nucleoli
- Diffusely expresses chromogranin and synaptophysin

Pearls

- Should be thought of in children
- Squamoid nests are key to the diagnosis

Figure 8-15. Well-differentiated pancreatic endocrine neoplasm. Low-power view shows nests of uniform cells with salt-and-pepper chromatin.

- Immunolabel for cytokeratin (AE1/AE3 and CAM5.2), usually cytokeratin 7 negative

Other Techniques for Diagnosis

- MEN I syndrome is caused by inherited (germline) mutations in the *MEN1* gene on chromosome 11q13

Differential Diagnosis

▌ Solid pseudopapillary neoplasm
- Found predominantly in young women
- Eosinophilic globules
- Poorly cohesive cells
- Cholesterol clefts
- Positive for CD10
- Nuclear labeling for β-catenin

▌ Ductal adenocarcinoma
- Less cellular neoplasm with prominent desmoplastic stroma
- Gland formation with mucin production
- Nuclear pleomorphism
- Expresses cytokeratin 7; negative for chromogranin, synaptophysin, and CD56

▌ Acinar cell carcinoma
- Acinar formations with basally placed nuclei and granular apical cytoplasm
- Single prominent nucleoli
- Expresses trypsin and chymotrypsin
- Acinar cell carcinoma can have a significant component with endocrine differentiation (mixed acinar-endocrine neoplasms), but the presence of histologic features of acinar cell carcinoma (acinar formation and large cells with prominent nucleoli) should distinguish these more aggressive neoplasms from the more indolent endocrine neoplasms

▌ Pancreatoblastoma
- Squamoid nests
- Acinar formations with basally placed nuclei and granular apical cytoplasm

- Single prominent nucleoli
- Positive for trypsin and chymotrypsin

▌ Islet aggregation in chronic pancreatitis
- Background of chronic pancreatitis
- Small focal lesions
- Polyclonal endocrine hormone production

Pearls

- Large neoplasms tend to be nonfunctioning because patients with functional neoplasms usually come to clinical attention early in their disease
- These are not staged
- Behavior is difficult to predict, and all pancreatic endocrine neoplasms larger than 0.5 cm should be considered potentially malignant
- Size, mitotic rate, large vessel invasion, lymph node metastases, invasion into another organ, and distant metastases are all prognosticators
- Although functioning gastrinomas causing Zollinger-Ellison syndrome do arise in the pancreas, they are most often duodenal. When a hormone is expressed, insulin is the most common among neuroendocrine neoplasms arising in the pancreas
- Multiple synchronous or metachronous neoplasms may be observed in patients with MEN-I

Selected References

Hruban RH, Pitman MB, Klimstra DS: Tumors of the pancreas. In Atlas of Tumor Pathology, 4th Series, Fascicle 6. Washington, DC, American Registry of Pathology and Armed Forces Institute of Pathology, 2007.

Klimstra DS, Perren A, Oberg K, et al: Pancreatic endocrine tumours: Non-functioning tumours and microadenomas. In DeLellis RA, Lloyd RV, Heitz PU, Eng C (eds): Pathology and Genetics of Tumours: Endocrine Organs. Lyon, IARC Press, 2004, pp 201-204.

Undifferentiated Endocrine Neoplasms (Small Cell Carcinoma)

Clinical Features

- Rare neoplasm, occurring primarily in adults
- Occurs more often in males than females
- May be associated with a paraneoplastic syndrome such as Cushing syndrome
- Need to rule out a lung primary metastatic to the pancreas
- Extremely aggressive

Gross Pathology

- Solid, white, poorly defined, often with necrosis

Histopathology

- Small, round blue cell neoplasm
- Nuclear molding

- Minimal cytoplasm, inconspicuous nucleoli
- Extremely high mitotic rate (>50 mitosis/10 high-power fields)

Special Stains and Immunohistochemistry

- Express cytokeratin, synaptophysin, and chromogranin
- High labeling index with Ki-67

Other Techniques for Diagnosis

- Noncontributory

Differential Diagnosis

▪ Pulmonary small cell carcinoma metastatic to the pancreas
  - Clinical history, imaging of the lungs
▪ Well-differentiated pancreatic endocrine neoplasm
  - Lower proliferative rate (<2 mitoses/10 high-power fields)
  - Uniform and more intense expression of synaptophysin and chromogranin
▪ Lymphoma
  - Uniform, more dispersed sheets of round blue cells
  - Lacks expression of neuroendocrine markers
  - Expresses lymphoid markers (e.g., CD45)
▪ Primitive neuroectodermal tumors (PNETs) and other round blue cell tumors of infancy and childhood
  - Occur more commonly in pediatric patients
  - Specific immunohistochemical and cytogenetic findings
    — PNETs express CD99 and harbor the t(11;22)(q24;q12) translocation
    — Intra-abdominal desmoplastic round cell tumors express desmin and harbor the t(11;22)(p13;q12) translocation
    — Rhabdomyosarcomas express MyoD

Pearls

- Small cell cancer of the lung must be excluded before establishing a pancreatic primary

Selected Reference

Manabe T, Miyashita T, Ohshio G, et al: Small carcinoma of the pancreas: Clinical and pathologic evaluation of 17 patients. Cancer 62:135-141, 1988.

Neoplasms of Uncertain Direction of Differentiation

Solid Pseudopapillary Neoplasms

Clinical Features

- Most occur in young women in their 20s and 30s, with a female-to-male ratio of 10:1 and a mean age of 30 years
- Present with nonspecific symptoms related to a large abdominal mass
- Rarely rupture and produce hemoperitoneum
- Slow-growing, low-grade malignancy

Gross Pathology

- May arise in the head, body, or tail of the gland
- Solitary, relatively large (mean size, 10 cm), well-demarcated masses
- Soft-white to yellow, with areas of hemorrhage and cystic degeneration

Histopathology

- Uniform poorly cohesive cells
- Nuclear grooves
- Delicate branching blood vessels

Figure 8-16. Solid pseudopapillary neoplasm. A, Low-power view shows uniform, poorly cohesive cells surrounding delicate blood vessels. **B,** Hyaline globules are a feature of these tumors.

- Hyaline globules
- Foam cells
- Cholesterol clefts

Special Stains and Immunohistochemistry

- Label with antibodies to CD10
- Nuclear labeling with antibodies to β-catenin
- Hyaline globules label with antibodies to α₁-antitrypsin

Other Techniques for Diagnosis

- β-Catenin gene mutations result in the nuclear accumulation of the β-catenin protein

Differential Diagnosis

- Well-differentiated pancreatic endocrine neoplasm
  - Cells nest or form trabeculae
  - Salt-and-pepper chromatin
  - Expresses synaptophysin and chromogranin
  - Membranous labeling with β-catenin
- Ductal adenocarcinoma
  - Less cellular neoplasm with prominent desmoplastic stroma
  - Gland formation with mucin production
  - Nuclear pleomorphism
  - Expresses cytokeratin 7, negative for CD10
  - Membranous labeling with β-catenin
- Acinar cell carcinoma
  - Acinar formations with basally placed nuclei and granular apical cytoplasm
  - Single prominent nucleoli
  - Label with antibodies to trypsin and chymotrypsin
- Pancreatoblastoma
  - Squamoid nests
  - Acinar formations with basally placed nuclei and granular apical cytoplasm
  - Single prominent nucleoli
  - Positive for trypsin and chymotrypsin

Pearls

- Should be at the top of the differential for a pancreatic neoplasm in a woman in her 20s or 30s
- Touch preparations can highlight the delicate vasculature and poorly cohesive cells
- Hyaline globules are a clue to the diagnosis
- Although vascular invasion is seen and should be documented as portending a possible poorer prognosis, metastasis to liver and peritoneum is rare

Selected References

Hruban RH, Pitman MB, Klimstra DS: Tumors of the pancreas. In Atlas of Tumor Pathology, 4th Series, Fascicle 6. Washington, DC, American Registry of Pathology and Armed Forces Institute of Pathology, 2007.

Abraham SC, Klimstra DS, Wilentz RE, et al: Solid-pseudopapillary tumors of the pancreas are genetically distinct from pancreatic ductal adenocarcinomas and almost always harbor beta-catenin mutations. Am J Pathol 160:1361-1369, 2002.

Klimstra DS, Wenig BM, Heffess CS: Solid-pseudopapillary tumor of the pancreas: A typically cystic carcinoma of low malignant potential. Semin Diagn Pathol 17:66-80, 2000.

Metastases to the Pancreas

Clinical Features

- History of a cancer in another organ

Gross Pathology

- Can be multiple

Histopathology

- Clear cell neoplasm in metastatic renal cell carcinoma
- Signet ring cell neoplasm in metastatic gastric carcinoma and lobular carcinoma of the breast
- Melanin in metastatic melanoma

Special Stains and Immunohistochemistry

- CD10 and RCCma positive in metastatic renal cell carcinoma
- Gross cystic disease fluid protein (GCDFP), estrogen and progesterone receptor positive in metastatic mammary carcinoma
- S-100 protein, HMB-45, and melan-A positive in metastatic melanoma

Other Techniques for Diagnosis

- Noncontributory

Differential Diagnosis

- Ductal adenocarcinoma
  - Prominent desmoplastic stroma
  - Adjacent PanIN or intraductal papillary mucinous neoplasm
  - Expresses cytokeratin 7
  - About 55% have loss of dpc4

Pearls

- Know the patient's history
- Radiology is crucial to the correct diagnosis
- Differentiation of pancreatic, biliary, and upper gastrointestinal tract neoplasms is difficult at best if one relies only on immunohistochemistry

Selected Reference

Adsay NV, Andea A, Basturk O, et al: Secondary tumors of the pancreas: An analysis of a surgical and autopsy database and review of the literature. Virchows Arch 444:527-535, 2004.

Sylvia L. Asa and Sandra E. Fischer

9

Adrenal Gland

Adrenal Cortical Insufficiency (Addison Disease)

Clinical Features

▋ Primary adrenal cortical insufficiency
  ● Etiology
    — Autoimmune etiology in 75% to 90% of cases, with circulating autoantibodies to endocrine antigens (21-OH, P-450scc, and 17-OH)
    — Other causes include infectious diseases including tuberculosis, hemorrhage (sepsis), metastatic tumors, amyloidosis, adrenoleukodystrophy, and drugs
  ● Signs and symptoms: weakness, fatigue, salt craving, hypotension, anorexia and weight loss, hyperpigmentation (due to elevated adrenocorticotropic hormone [ACTH] and other pro-opiomelanocortin fragments)
  ● Biochemistry: decreased production of cortisol and aldosterone, elevated levels of ACTH and renin; hyponatremia and hyperkalemia may be seen as a result of decreased aldosterone
  ● Therapy: corticosteroid and mineralocorticoid replacement; fatal if not treated

▋ Secondary adrenal cortical insufficiency
  ● Etiology: inadequate stimulation of the adrenal cortex as a result of low corticotropin-releasing hormone (CRH) or ACTH
    — May be seen after prolonged suppression of the hypothalamic-pituitary-adrenal axis by exogenous glucocorticoids or associated with destructive lesions of the hypothalamus or the pituitary gland
  ● Signs and symptoms: weakness, fatigue, anorexia, weight loss, hypopigmentation
  ● Biochemistry: aldosterone levels are typically normal, and hyperpigmentation does not occur

Gross Pathology

● Idiopathic form characterized by pale, irregular, shrunken adrenal gland, often weighing less than 2 to 3 g, with marked thinning of the cortical zone; severe atrophy may impair gross recognition of the adrenal glands
● Secondary forms often associated with adrenal enlargement and infiltration by inflammation or tumor

Figure 9-1. A, Addison disease due to tuberculosis infection. Tissue destruction due to tuberculosis infection results in adrenal enlargement, but the gland is replaced by necrotic yellow material. No normal tissue is identified. The surrounding fat is unremarkable. **B, Addison disease due to tuberculosis infection.** Caseating granuloma with giant cell reaction present in the adrenal cortex. **C, Addison disease due to autoimmune inflammation.** The adrenal is atrophic; the cortex is almost completely lost, and there is focal inflammation surrounding the residual medulla. **D, Addison disease due to autoimmune inflammation.** Inflammatory cells replace the cortex, and fibrosis is evident between the few residual cortical cells.

Histopathology

- Idiopathic form exhibits marked atrophy of the adrenal cortex, with intact medulla surrounded by fibrous tissue containing few small islands of atrophic cortical cells; lymphoid infiltrate is often present
- Infiltrative forms due to inflammation or malignancy

Special Stains and Immunohistochemistry

- Special stains for microorganisms: may identify organisms in cases of infectious etiology

Other Techniques for Diagnosis

- Noncontributory

Differential Diagnosis

- One must distinguish between primary and secondary adrenal insufficiency

- If primary, one must attempt to determine etiology
    - Inflammatory; rule out infectious
    - Metastatic tumor
    - Amyloidosis (rare)

Pearls

- First described by Addison in 1855
- Must have destruction of more than 90% of adrenal gland before symptoms develop
- Immune form associated with autoimmune polyglandular syndromes (APS) type 1 and type 2 (Schmidt syndrome); APS type 1 is caused by mutations in the *AIRE-1* gene

Selected References

Shulman DI, Palmert MR, Kemp SF: Adrenal insufficiency: Still a cause of morbidity and death in childhood. Pediatrics 119:e484-494, 2007.

Fujieda K, Tajima T: Molecular basis of adrenal insufficiency. Pediatr Res 57:62R-69R, 2005.

Ten S, New M, Maclaren N: Clinical review 130: Addison's disease 2001. J Clin Endocrinol Metab 86:2909-2922, 2001.

Peterson P, Uibo R, Krohn KJE: Adrenal autoimmunity: Results and developments. Trends Endocrinol Metab 11:285-290, 2000.

Congenital Adrenal Hyperplasia (Adrenogenital Syndrome)

Clinical Features

- Etiology
  - Autosomal recessive disorder of cortisol biosynthesis resulting in impaired glucocorticoid feedback inhibition at the hypothalamic and pituitary levels, increased serum levels of CRH and ACTH, and adrenal hyperplasia
  - Results from a defect in one of the five enzymatic steps involved in steroid synthesis; 90% to 95% of cases are caused by deficiency of 21-hydroxylase, resulting in marked elevation of 17-hydroxyprogesterone, the main substrate for the enzyme
  - Unusual causes: 20,22-desmolase deficiency, 17α-hydroxylase deficiency, 3β-hydroxysteroid dehydrogenase deficiency, or 11β-hydroxylase deficiency
  - Congenital lipoid adrenal hyperplasia
    - The most severe form of congenital adrenal hyperplasia (CAH), in which the synthesis of all gonadal and adrenal cortical steroids is markedly impaired
    - Lipoid CAH may be caused by the defect in either the steroidogenic acute regulatory (StAR) protein or the P-450scc

- Epidemiology
  - Classic form occurs in 1 of 5000 to 15,000 live births
  - Nonclassic form occurs in 0.3% of the white population
- Signs and symptoms
  - Most common cause of ambiguous genitalia in newborn females; clinical presentation correlates with severity of 21-OH deficiency
  - Classic form
    - Can present as salt-wasting form or simple virilizing type
    - Newborn females typically show virilization at birth as a result of increased circulating androgens (clitoral hypertrophy and pseudohermaphroditism)
    - Postpubertal females have oligomenorrhea, hirsutism, and acne
    - Newborn males usually present with salt-losing crisis within days to weeks after delivery due to decreased synthesis of aldosterone (hypovolemia, hyperreninemia, and hyperkalemia can be life threatening)
    - Males later show enlargement of external genitalia and precocious puberty
  - Nonclassic form
    - Affected individuals are normal at birth and do not have cortisol and aldosterone deficiency
    - Develop signs of androgen excess (virilization) in late childhood or puberty
    - Presentation in heterozygotes: asymptomatic
- Therapy
  - Pharmacologic treatment involves glucocorticoid and mineralocorticoid replacement and the use of androgen and estrogen antagonists

  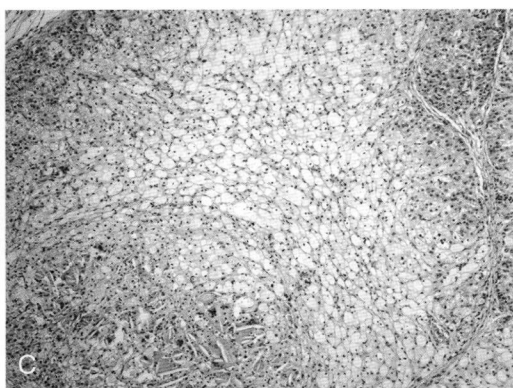

Figure 9-2. A, Congenital adrenal hyperplasia due to 21-hydroxylase deficiency. The adrenal glands are diffusely enlarged with lipid-depleted cortex. **B, Congenital adrenal hyperplasia due to 21-hydroxylase deficiency.** Microscopic examination of the diffusely enlarged gland shows a prominent cortex with poor zonation, and predominantly compact cells. **C, Lipoid congenital adrenal hyperplasia.** The adrenal cortex is thickened by large clear adrenal cortical cells containing increased amount of lipid with focal cholesterol clefts and multinucleated giant histiocytes. (**A,** Photo courtesy of Dr. Glenn P. Taylor, Hospital for Sick Children, Toronto.)

— Bilateral adrenalectomy performed in selected cases

— Gene therapy studies underway

Gross Pathology

- Bilateral adrenal gland enlargement with diffuse thickening of the cortex
- Adrenal glands may weigh up to 10 to 15 times normal weight
- Adrenals show a convoluted surface owing to numerous redundant folds

Histopathology

- Thickened adrenal cortex involving zona glomerulosa, zona fasciculata, and especially zona reticularis; poorly defined zonation
- Most cortical cells have lipid-depleted (compact) cytoplasm owing to sustained ACTH stimulation
- In lipoid CAH, the gland enlargement results from the accumulation of cholesterol esters in adrenal cortical cells; further damage with cell rupture and foreign-body granulomatous reaction to cholesterol clefts can be seen focally

Special Stains and Immunohistochemistry

- Noncontributory

Other Techniques for Diagnosis

- Genetic testing for 21-hydroxylase deficiency, or rarely 20,22-desmolase deficiency, 17α-hydroxylase deficiency, 3β-hydroxysteroid dehydrogenase deficiency, or 11β-hydroxylase deficiency

Differential Diagnosis

▌Adrenal cortical adenoma
- Is a discrete adrenal cortical nodule rather than diffuse hypertrophy, and usually unilateral

Pearls

- Defective adrenomedullary organogenesis owing to lack of glucocorticoids results in epinephrine deficiency and hypoglycemia
- Several reported cases of cortical adenomas and cortical carcinomas developing in children with congenital adrenal hyperplasia; may be related to persistent ACTH stimulation
- Adrenal cortical tumors may be seen developing in the testis of patients with congenital cortical hyperplasia; believed to arise from ectopic adrenal cortical rests

Selected References

Ogilvie CM, Crouch NS, Rumsby G, et al: Congenital adrenal hyperplasia in adults: A review of medical, surgical and psychological issues. Clin Endocrinol 64:2-11, 2006.

Merke DP, Bornstein SR: Congenital adrenal hyperplasia. Lancet 365:2125-2136, 2005.

Speiser PW, White PC: Congenital adrenal hyperplasia. N Engl J Med 349:776-788, 2003.

Merke DP, Bornstein SR, Avila NA, Chrousos GP: Future directions in the study and management of congenital adrenal hyperplasia due to 21-hydroxylase deficiency. Ann Intern Med 136:320-334, 2002.

White PC: Congenital adrenal hyperplasias. Best Pract Res Clin Endocrinol Metab 15:17-41, 2001.

Adrenal Cortical Hyperplasia

Clinical Features

- Two forms: primary (ACTH independent) and secondary (ACTH dependent)
- Etiology: depends on primary versus secondary
  - Primary adrenal cortical hyperplasia: due to germline mutations
    - ◆ Activating mutations of the ACTH receptor; illegitimate expression of membrane receptors (GIP receptor, β-adrenergic receptor, and LH receptor), and activating mutations of *GNAS* 1 in McCune-Albright syndrome result in ACTH-independent macronodular hyperplasia (AIMAH)
    - ◆ Inactivating germline mutations of the *PRKAR1A* and *PDE11A* genes are found in Carney complex and isolated primary pigmented nodular adrenal cortical disease (PPNAD)
    - ◆ Bilateral adrenal hyperplasia also seen in multiple endocrine neoplasia type I (MEN I) syndrome and familial adenomatous polyposis
  - Secondary (ACTH-dependent) hyperplasia: due to ACTH excess from primary pituitary disease (corticotroph adenoma or hyperplasia) or ectopic ACTH production by tumors at other sites
- Signs and symptoms
  - Primary disorders may present with a variety of endocrine syndromes including Cushing syndrome, Conn syndrome, or virilization
  - Secondary disorder presents with severe Cushing syndrome, usually typical when pituitary dependent, and atypical (prominent wasting and pigmentation) when due to ectopic production by other malignancies
- Biochemistry
  - Variable, depending on clinical manifestations (Cushing, Conn, and virilization syndromes); ACTH levels usually low (suppressed) except in secondary forms
- Therapy
  - Treatment of primary source of ACTH excess in secondary cases
  - Medical therapy to reduce glucocorticoid hypersecretion with ketoconazole, other drugs

Figure 9-3. A, Macronodular adrenal cortical hyperplasia. Gross photograph showing multiple adrenal cortical nodules. **B, Diffuse adrenal cortical hyperplasia.** Gross photograph showing a normal adrenal gland (*top*) and a diffusely enlarged gland with a lipid-depleted cortex in a patient with ectopic adrenocorticotropic hormone syndrome (*bottom*). **C, Macronodular adrenal cortical hyperplasia.** Classic nodular adrenal cortical hyperplasia with multiple poorly defined cortical nodules composed of clear and compact cells. **D, Zona glomerulosa hyperplasia.** The adrenal gland is lined by a continuous layer of zona glomerulosa that is normally discontinuous. The cells are small and are on average five nests in thickness (*inset*).

— Laparoscopic adrenalectomy for removal of adrenals followed by replacement therapies

Gross Pathology

- Non-neoplastic (polyclonal) condition consisting of nodular or diffuse hyperplasia of the adrenal cortex
- Degree of enlargement dependent on cause
  - Severe when due to ectopic ACTH or in ACTH-independent macronodular hyperplasia (AIMAH)
  - Mild to moderate with pituitary-dependent ACTH excess or PPNAD
  - Grossly undetectable when due to zona glomerulosa hyperplasia with Conn syndrome
- Almost always bilateral except for rare pigmented nodules showing prominent brown-black discoloration, which are more commonly unilateral
- Nodular form may show micronodules (<1 cm) or macronodules (>1 cm)
- Combination of nodular and diffuse types may be seen

Histopathology

- Adrenal cortex with diffuse hyperplasia or multinodular architecture
- Vague alveolar or trabecular pattern
- Cells are uniform in size with small, round nuclei
- Cells have vacuolated (clear) or eosinophilic (compact) granular cytoplasm
- Areas of lipomatous metaplasia may be seen
- Zona glomerulosa hyperplasia limited to periphery of gland, characterized by continuous layer of nests of cells with scant cytoplasm averaging five nests in thickness

- Mixture of large clear cells and small compact cells in AIMAH; pigmented nodules show enlarged, globular cortical cells with variable amounts of granular dark-brown pigment
- Cortical atrophy and disorganization of the normal zonation between nodules in PPNAD, as opposed to AIMAH, which shows characteristic interlobular hyperplasia

Special Stains and Immunohistochemistry

- PPNAD nodules stain positive for synaptophysin and 17α-hydroxylase cytochrome P-450; 3β-hydroxysteroid dehydrogenase staining is dominant in AIMAH nodules

Other Techniques for Diagnosis

- Noncontributory

Differential Diagnosis

▌ Adrenal cortical adenoma
- Presence of solitary, unilateral lesions with evidence of autonomous growth favors adenoma
- Presence of small nodules adjacent to a larger nodule favors adrenal hyperplasia
- Definitive distinction between nodular hyperplasia and adrenal cortical adenoma can often be difficult or even impossible

Pearls

- Hyperplasia of the adrenal cortex (micronodular and diffuse) has been reported in cases of familial hyperaldosteronism type I (glucocorticoid-remediable aldosteronism), an autosomal dominant disorder caused by a hybrid gene formed by crossover between the ACTH-responsive regulatory portion of 11β-hydroxylase (*CYP11B1*) gene and the coding region of the aldosterone synthase (*CYP11B2*) gene. As a result, there is ACTH-responsive ectopic secretion of aldosterone in the zona fasciculata

Selected References

Cazabat L, Ragazzon B, Groussin L, Bertherat J: PRKAR1A mutations in primary pigmented nodular adrenocortical disease. Pituitary 9:211-219, 2006.

Makras P, Toloumis G, Papadogias D, et al: The diagnosis and differential diagnosis of endogenous Cushing's syndrome. Hormones 5:231-250, 2006.

Christopoulos S, Bourdeau I, Lacroix A: Clinical and subclinical ACTH-independent macronodular adrenal hyperplasia and aberrant hormone receptors. Horm Res 64:119-131, 2005.

Libe R, Bertherat J: Molecular genetics of adrenocortical tumors, from familial to sporadic diseases. Eur J Endocrinol 153:477-487, 2005.

Mulatero P, Dluhy RG, Giacchetti G, et al: Diagnosis of primary aldosteronism: From screening to subtype differentiation. Trends Endocrinol Metab 16:114-119, 2005.

Adrenal Cortical Adenoma

Clinical Features

- Etiology
  - Most are sporadic with no known genetic basis
  - Association with familial disease (MEN I, familial hyperaldosteronism, and congenital adrenal hyperplasia) can occur
  - Comparative genomic hybridization studies have demonstrated genetic alterations in 30% to 60% of adrenal adenomas; losses on chromosomes 2, 11q, and 17p, and gains on chromosomes 4 and 5 are the most common
  - *TP53* and *K-ras* mutations and loss of heterozygosity (LOH) of 11p15 and ACTH receptor are rare events in adenomas
- Signs and symptoms
  - Most adrenal cortical adenomas are asymptomatic (nonfunctional) and found incidentally
  - Patients may present with Cushing syndrome or hyperaldosteronism (Conn syndrome); virilization is rarely associated with adenomas, and feminization in males is almost exclusively a sign of malignancy (see "Adrenal Cortical Carcinoma")
  - Adenomas associated with Cushing syndrome and primary hyperaldosteronism are usually small and solitary; can rarely be multiple and bilateral
- Biochemistry
  - Variable, depending on clinical manifestations (Cushing, Conn, and virilization syndromes); ACTH levels usually low (suppressed), except in Conn syndrome
- Therapy
  - Laparoscopic tumor removal is the preferred treatment

Gross Pathology

- Adenomas associated with Cushing syndrome or hyperaldosteronism are usually solitary and unilateral and weigh less than 50 g
- Well-defined tumors appear encapsulated
- Adenomas associated with Conn syndrome have a characteristic bright-yellow or golden-yellow color
- Adenomas associated with Cushing syndrome may be bright yellow or tan
- All adenomas may show focal hemorrhage or necrosis (typically in larger lesions)
- Rarely, adenomas are diffusely pigmented black (pigmented adenoma)
- Oncocytic adrenal cortical adenomas have a dark-tan to mahogany-brown cut surface

Histopathology

- Circumscribed tumor with pushing borders, lacks true capsule

Figure 9-4. A, Adrenal cortical adenoma associated with Conn syndrome. Gross photograph shows that the tumor is well delineated and bright golden-yellow. The adjacent adrenal is unremarkable. **B, Adrenal cortical adenoma associated with Cushing syndrome.** Gross photograph shows that the nodule is well delineated and yellow with focal hemorrhage, and the adjacent gland shows marked atrophy. **C, Adrenal cortical adenoma with pigmentation ("black adenoma").** Gross photograph shows that the nodule is well delineated and dark black owing to pigment deposition. **D, Adrenal cortical adenoma associated with Conn syndrome.** On microscopy, there is a large, well-delineated but unencapsulated clear cell adenoma, and the adjacent gland has zona glomerulosa hyperplasia (see Fig. 9-3D).

Continued

- Typically has trabecular or alveolar (nesting) architecture
- Tumor cells are large and have round, regular nuclei with small, dotlike nucleoli; focal pleomorphism and large prominent nucleoli may be seen
- Absent or rare mitotic activity; never atypical mitoses
- Cytoplasm is abundant and "clear" or "compact"
  — In adenomas associated with Conn syndrome, cytoplasm is clear, lipid rich, and vacuolated; spironolactone bodies (small eosinophilic laminated intracytoplasmic inclusions) may develop in cells of the zona glomerulosa, typically if patient is treated with spironolactone; these are best seen with the Luxol fast blue (LFB) stain
  — In adenomas associated with Cushing syndrome, cytoplasm may be clear or eosinophilic

(compact), and in most tumors, both types may be seen
- Pigmented adenomas have cells with eosinophilic cytoplasm containing prominent granular yellow-brown pigment (lipofuscin)
- Oncocytic adenomas have cells with abundant granular eosinophilic cytoplasm; focal marked nuclear pleomorphism and nuclear pseudoinclusions may be seen
- Histologic appearance of the tumor cannot reliably predict accompanying clinical presentation; examination of the adjacent nontumorous gland is more helpful
  — Atrophy of the normal cortex indicates Cushing syndrome with suppression of ACTH
  — In patients with Conn syndrome, there may occasionally be hyperplasia of the zona glomerulosa (paradoxical hyperplasia)

Figure 9-4. cont'd. E, Adrenal cortical adenoma associated with Conn syndrome. On microscopy, the tumor cells have abundant clear cytoplasm. **F, Adrenal cortical adenoma associated with Cushing syndrome.** On microscopy, there is a large, well-delineated but unencapsulated adenoma, and the adjacent gland exhibits marked atrophy with complete loss of the zona reticularis, indicating lack of adrenocorticotropic hormone stimulation. **G, Adrenal cortical adenoma associated with Cushing syndrome.** On microscopy, the adenoma has mixed clear and compact cell morphology with small round nuclei and abundant cytoplasm that varies from chromophobic to eosinophilic. **H, Adrenal cortical adenoma, pigmented type.** High-power view showing proliferation of a monomorphic population of adrenal cortical cells with large amounts of eosinophilic cytoplasm containing yellow-brown pigment.

Special Stains and Immunohistochemistry

- LFB for spironolactone bodies
- Immunohistochemistry for enzymes involved in steroidogenesis can distinguish function, but this is not used diagnostically
- MIB1 or Ki-67 labeling index usually below 2.5

Other Techniques for Diagnosis

- Electron microscopy
  - Cells contain abundant lipid and prominent smooth endoplasmic reticulum; mitochondria are also numerous
  - Mitochondrial morphology correlates with function: aldosterone-producing cells (zona glomerulosa differentiation) have flat, platelike, "lamellar" cristae, whereas glucocorticoid and sex steroid-producing cells (zona reticularis and fasciculata) have round or spherulated cristae

  - Pigmented adenomas contain many electron-dense granules consistent with lipofuscin
  - Spironolactone bodies are composed of concentric whorls of membranes

Differential Diagnosis

- Adrenal cortical carcinoma
  - Usually large mass with gross evidence of hemorrhage and necrosis
  - Infiltrative borders typically invading into surrounding tissue
  - Tumor cells show marked pleomorphism and frequent mitotic activity

Pearls

- Histologic appearance of adrenal cortical adenoma cannot be used to predict associated endocrine

Figure 9-4. cont'd. I, Adrenal cortical adenoma associated with Conn syndrome. The Luxol fast blue stain highlights spironolactone bodies. **J, Adrenal cortical adenoma associated with Conn syndrome.** Electron microscopy shows that the tumor cells have abundant smooth endoplasmic reticulum; the mitochondria have flat platelike cristae, consistent with zona glomerulosa differentiation and mineralocorticoid production; and there are lamellated spironolactone bodies. **K, Adrenal cortical adenoma associated with Cushing syndrome.** Electron microscopy shows that the tumor cells have abundant smooth endoplasmic reticulum, and the mitochondria have tubulovesicular cristae, consistent with differentiation as steroid-producing cells. **L, Adrenal cortical adenoma, pigmented type.** Electron microscopy shows that the tumor cells have abundant smooth endoplasmic reticulum and numerous mitochondria, and there are large electron-dense granules consistent with complex lysosomes containing lipofuscin.

abnormality or syndrome, although the adjacent adrenal cortex may show atrophy (Cushing syndrome), or hyperplasia of the zona glomerulosa (Conn syndrome)
- Treatment is typically resection of the adrenal gland containing the adenoma

Selected References

Young WF Jr: The incidentally discovered adrenal mass. N Engl J Med 356:601-610, 2007.

Libe R, Bertherat J: Molecular genetics of adrenocortical tumors, from familial to sporadic diseases. Eur J Endocrinol 153:477-487, 2005.

Mulatero P, Dluhy RG, Giacchetti G, et al: Diagnosis of primary aldosteronism: From screening to subtype differentiation. Trends Endocrinol Metab 16:114-119, 2005.

Ribeiro RC, Figueiredo B: Childhood adrenocortical tumours. Eur J Cancer 40:1117-1126, 2004.

Koch CA, Pacak K, Chrousos GP: Genetics of endocrine disease: The molecular pathogenesis of hereditary and sporadic adrenocortical and adrenomedullary tumors. J Clin Endocrinol Metab 87:5367-5384, 2002.

Adrenal Cortical Carcinoma

Clinical Features

- Etiology
  — Sporadic adrenal cortical carcinoma is most common; however, it also occurs in hereditary syndromes: Li-Fraumeni, Beckwith-Wiedemann, MEN I, Carney complex, and hereditary isolated glucocorticoid deficiency syndrome
  — Sporadic carcinomas can harbor similar molecular defects, including germline and somatic mutations of *TP53*, and 17p13 LOH; rare *Menin* mutations, but frequent 11q13 LOH; 17q22-24 LOH (*PRKAR1A*); 11p15 LOH and *IGF-II* overexpression; 18p11 LOH (*MC2-R*)
- Epidemiology
  — Rare tumor; occurs in about 1 per 1 million population
  — Typically presents in fourth and fifth decades of life; less common in pediatric population
  — Equal incidence in males and females
- Signs and symptoms
  — Usually presents as incidental finding or associated with abdominal or flank pain; may present with a palpable abdominal mass or with evidence of distant metastasis
  — About 79% of carcinomas secrete hormones, and most functional tumors secrete cortisol with marked virilization owing to co-secretion of 17-ketosteroids and dehydroepiandrosterone (DHEA)
  — Less often, virilization in women and feminization in men can result from secretion of free testosterone and androstenedione, respectively
  — Mineralocorticoid excess is rare; however, combined secretion of cortisol and mineralo-corticoid can occur
- Therapy
  — Tumor removal is the preferred treatment

Gross Pathology

- Usually large tumors weighing between 100 and 1000 g; may measure more than 20 cm (average, 14 to 15 cm)
- Irregular, variegated, tan-yellow mass with infiltrative borders
- Extension into adjacent soft tissue or surrounding organs is common
- Cut surface often shows extensive hemorrhage and necrosis

Histopathology

- Characteristic pattern is that of broad trabeculae with anastomosing architecture
- Other common patterns include solid or alveolar architecture
- Infiltrative growth pattern
- Tumor cells may resemble normal adrenal cortical cells; however, there is marked nuclear atypia, atypical and frequent mitoses (more than 5/50 high-power fields), vascular and extra-adrenal invasion, and necrosis
- Although uncommon, intracytoplasmic eosinophilic hyaline globules may be seen and are better visualized with periodic acid–Schiff (PAS) staining
- Broad fibrous bands are a characteristic feature
- Diagnostic features of malignancy include size (weight, >100 g), vascular invasion, and metastasis

Special Stains and Immunohistochemistry

- Vimentin, inhibin-α, steroidogenic factor-1 (SF-1), and melan-A positive
- Cytokeratin may be negative or weakly positive
- Synaptophysin may be positive
- Chromogranin: negative
- Ki-67 labeling index may be helpful to separate adenomas from carcinomas and has prognostic relevance
- Cyclin E: positive staining correlates with advanced stage

Other Techniques for Diagnosis

- Electron microscopy: prominent rough and smooth endoplasmic reticulum; mitochondria with spherulated cristae; intracellular lipid droplets may be seen. These features are useful to characterize metastatic lesions as derived from adrenal cortex
- Cytogenetic studies: 17p13 LOH, 11p15 uniparental disomy (UPD), and *IGF-II* overexpression are consistent findings

Differential Diagnosis

▌ Metastasis
- Separating adrenal cortical carcinoma from metastatic carcinomas from kidney and liver usually can be done using markers normally expressed in the adrenal cortex, including D11, SF-1, inhibin-α, and melan-A

▌ Adrenal cortical adenoma
- Is usually much smaller and lacks prominent hemorrhage or necrosis, pleomorphism, atypical mitotic figures, and vascular invasion

▌ Pheochromocytoma
- Typically has solid nesting architecture (Zellballen) with indiscreet cell borders, abundant intracytoplasmic hyaline globules, strong

Figure 9-5. Adrenal cortical carcinoma. A, Gross photograph showing a large yellow tumor with areas of hemorrhage, necrosis, and cystic degeneration. **B** to **D,** On microscopy, the tumor is composed of a solid proliferation of neoplastic cells with moderately eosinophilic cytoplasm. There are areas of fibrosis (**B**), necrosis (**C**), and cytologic atypia (**D**). **E,** Electron microscopy characterizes the malignancy with prominent mitosis (*top right*) as derived from steroid-secreting cells by the prominence of smooth endoplasmic reticulum and the numerous large mitochondria with spherulated cristae.

synaptophysin and chromogranin positivity, and S-100 protein highlighting sustentacular cells surrounding Zellballen

Pearls

- Adrenal cortical carcinoma has a high mortality rate, with death typically occurring within 2 to 3 years
- Large size, vascular invasion, and high mitotic rate are features of a more aggressive tumor
- Typical sites of metastasis include liver, lung, and lymph nodes

Selected References

Libe R, Fratticci A, Bertherat J: Adrenocortical cancer: Pathophysiology and clinical management. Endocr Relat Cancer 14:13-28, 2007.

Allolio B, Fassnacht M: Clinical review: Adrenocortical carcinoma: clinical update. J Clin Endocrinol Metab 91:2027-2037, 2006.

Pan CC, Chen PC, Tsay SH, Ho DM: Differential immunoprofiles of hepatocellular carcinoma, renal cell carcinoma, and adrenocortical carcinoma. Appl Immunohistochem Mol Morphol 13:347-352, 2005.

Saeger W, Fassnacht M, Chita R, et al: High diagnostic accuracy of adrenal core biopsy: Results of the German and Austrian adrenal network multicenter trial in 220 consecutive patients. Hum Pathol 34:180-186, 2003.

Terzolo M, Boccuzi A, Bovio S, et al: Immunohistochemical assessment of Ki-67 in the differential diagnosis of adrenocortical tumors. Urology 57:176-182, 2001.

Adrenal Medullary Hyperplasia

Clinical Features

- Etiology: usually associated with MEN IIA and MEN IIB syndromes
  - MEN IIA (Sipple syndrome) autosomal dominant syndrome includes medullary carcinoma of thyroid, pheochromocytoma, and parathyroid hyperplasia
  - MEN IIB autosomal dominant syndrome includes medullary carcinoma of thyroid; pheochromocytoma; neuromas of the lip, mucous membranes, and gastrointestinal tract; and parathyroid hyperplasia
  - Occasionally associated with cystic fibrosis or Beckwith-Wiedemann syndrome
  - Not seen in other familial pheochromocytoma syndromes (von Hippel-Lindau disease, neurofibromatosis)
- Signs and symptoms
  - May resemble pheochromocytoma with paroxysmal hypertension, diaphoresis, and tachycardia
- Biochemistry
  - Elevated urinary catecholamine and metanephrine levels
- Therapy
  - Surgical resection of one or both adrenal glands is often indicated in both familial and sporadic forms

Gross Pathology

- Usually bilateral, with increased adrenal gland weight
- May be diffuse or have nodular architecture
- Nodules must be less than 1 cm to be considered hyperplasia (nodules greater than 1 cm are considered pheochromocytoma)
- Nodules are typically distinct and have a gray-tan cut surface

Histopathology

- Diffuse expansion of the medulla into the tail of the gland, with or without nodule formation, and with an increased medulla-to-cortex ratio
- Enlarged cells with or without pleomorphism and increased mitotic activity may be seen

Figure 9-6. Adrenal medullary hyperplasia. A, Low-power view showing the adrenal gland with a diffusely hyperplastic medulla that extends all the way to the end of the wing. There is a suggestion of nodularity to the medulla. **B,** Low-power view showing the adrenal gland with nodules of hyperplastic medulla.

- Hyaline globules are commonly seen in patients with MEN II
- No reliable morphologic criteria distinguish hyperplasia from pheochromocytoma apart from size, which is the best indicator for distinguishing these two entities

Special Stains and Immunohistochemistry

- Noncontributory

Other Techniques for Diagnosis

- Flow cytometry: tumor cells are usually diploid
- Germline mutation of the *ret* proto-oncogene can be detected by cytogenetic studies in MEN II patients

Differential Diagnosis

- Distinction between nodular adrenal medullary hyperplasia and pheochromocytoma is currently based on the size of the lesion

Pearls

- Armed Forces Institute of Pathology (AFIP) has designated adrenal medulla nodules less than 1 cm as medullary hyperplasia and nodules greater than 1 cm as pheochromocytoma
- Medullary hyperplasia is believed to be the initial pathologic change in the adrenal gland, leading subsequently to the development of pheochromocytoma

Selected References

Carney JA: Familial multiple endocrine neoplasia: The first 100 years. Am J Surg Pathol 29:254-274, 2005.

Qupty G, Ishay A, Peretz H, et al: Pheochromocytoma due to unilateral adrenal medullary hyperplasia. Clin Endocrinol (Oxford) 47:613-617, 1997.

Montgomery TB, Mandelstam P, Tachman ML, et al: Multiple endocrine neoplasia type IIb: A description of several patients and review of the literature. J Clin Hypertens 3:31-49, 1987.

DeLellis RA, Wolfe HJ, Gagel RF, et al: Adrenal medullary hyperplasia: A morphometric analysis in patients with familial medullary thyroid carcinoma. Am J Pathol 83:177-196, 1976.

Carney JA, Sizemore GW, Sheps SG: Adrenal medullary disease in multiple endocrine neoplasia, type 2: Pheochromocytoma and its precursors. Am J Pathol 66:279-290, 1976.

Pheochromocytoma

Clinical Features

- Etiology
  - Although classic teaching indicated that only 10% of pheochromocytomas were hereditary, recent studies show that almost half of pheochromocytomas are hereditary; a small percentage of these are bilateral or multifocal, involving extra-adrenal paragangliomas
  - Germline mutations in *VHL* (3p26-25), resulting in von Hippel-Lindau disease; *RET* (10q11.2), resulting in MEN II; *NF1* (17q11.2), resulting in neurofibromatosis type 1 syndrome; or the succinate dehydrogenase genes *SDHD* (11q23) and *SDHB* (1p36.1-35), resulting in familial paraganglioma syndrome
- Epidemiology
  - Sporadic tumors are usually diagnosed in patients aged 40 to 50 years, whereas hereditary forms are most often detected before age 40 years
- Signs and symptoms
  - Clinical presentation is paroxysmal and results from the direct actions of secreted catecholamines, including hypertension, tachycardia, pallor, headache, and anxiety; up to 25% of pheochromocytomas are asymptomatic
  - Anesthesia and tumor manipulation most often elicit a catecholamine crisis, but several drugs and food can also induce paroxysms
- Biochemistry
  - Diagnosis is made or confirmed based on measurements of urinary and plasma catecholamines, urinary metanephrines, and urinary vanillylmandelic acid (VMA)
- Imaging techniques
  - Computed tomography or magnetic resonance imaging and localization with functional ligands such as ^{123}I-MIBG
- Therapy
  - Laparoscopic tumor removal is the preferred treatment, after preoperative blocking of the effects of secreted catecholamines

Gross Pathology

- Variable size and weight (from few grams to >2000 g)
- Round to oval, sharply circumscribed mass that is often encapsulated
- Cut surface shows a soft, variegated appearance with a dusky red-brown color
- Marked hemorrhage and necrosis may be seen; occasionally central cystic degeneration is seen
- Compression of the adjacent adrenal gland is common; tumor may cause marked attenuation of the adrenal gland around the tumor

Histopathology

- Tumor cells are arranged in well-defined nests, Zellballen appearance
- Distinct nests of tumor cells surrounded by thin strands of fibrovascular stroma that may (rarely) contain amyloid
- Rim of sustentacular cells may be seen at periphery of cell nests
- Tumor cells have varying size and shape with round nuclei, prominent nucleoli, and granular amphophilic to basophilic cytoplasm
- Nuclei often show inclusion-like structures due to intranuclear cytoplasmic invaginations

Figure 9-7. Pheochromocytoma. A, The intra-adrenal tumor has a characteristic dusky appearance due to the marked vascular congestion of this lesion. **B,** The adrenal cortex (*right*) is compressed by a tumor composed of nests of neoplastic cells surrounded by delicate strands of fibrovascular stroma. **C,** High-power view showing solid nests, or Zellballen, of polygonal neoplastic cells with poorly defined cell borders and abundant basophilic granular cytoplasm. **D,** Immunohistochemical stains such as synaptophysin and chromogranin confirm the diagnosis of a neuroendocrine lesion, but positivity for tyrosine hydroxylase characterizes this as a pheochromocytoma or paraganglioma. **E,** Immunohisto-chemical localization of S-100 protein decorates sustentacular cells that surround the nests of tumor cells. **F,** Electron microscopy identifies abundant electron-dense membrane-bound secretory granules of variable size and shape.

- Marked pleomorphism with bizarre tumor giant cells and numerous mitotic figures may be seen; *these features are not diagnostic of malignant behavior*
- Occasional tumors of patients with von Hippel-Lindau disease have marked stromal edema and lipid degeneration
- Tumors of patients with MEN II may be associated with adrenal medullary hyperplasia and may be multiple or bilateral
- Composite pheochromocytoma is a pheochromocytoma with areas resembling neuroblastoma, ganglioneuroblastoma (GNB), or typical ganglioneuroma

Special Stains and Immunohistochemistry

- Chromogranin positive
- Synaptophysin positive
- Tyrosine hydroxylase positive
- S-100 protein: immunoreactivity of sustentacular cells surrounding Zellballen; stain often decreases in malignant tumors
- Neurofilament and serotonin may show positivity
- HMB-45 may show focal or faint positivity
- Ki-67 may be helpful to assess proliferative activity

Other Techniques for Diagnosis

- Electron microscopy: cells contain numerous neurosecretory granules
- Cytogenetic studies: allelic losses on chromosomes 1p, 3p, 3q, 17p, and 22q are common in hereditary and nonhereditary pheochromocytomas

Differential Diagnosis

▌Adrenal cortical adenoma
- Typically, adenomas appear golden-yellow on gross examination; pheochromocytomas with lipid degeneration can have a similar gross appearance, but stains for chromogranin and synaptophysin are diagnostic

▌Neuroblastoma
- Typically found in children younger than 4 years; composed of small round blue cells often with pseudorosette formation

Pearls

- Malignant behavior cannot be determined based on morphologic findings; only presence of distant metastases proves malignancy
- Metastatic spread through lymphatic or hematogenous pathways most commonly involves lymph nodes, bones (particularly ribs and spine), lung, and liver
- Benign, surgically treated tumors have a 5-year survival rate of more than 95%; the 5-year survival rate of patients with malignant pheochromocytoma is about 44%

- Pheochromocytoma is rare in children and is most often extra-adrenal, multifocal, and associated with hereditary syndromes
- Tyrosine hydroxylase immunoreactivity in pheochromocytomas is helpful to rule out neuroendocrine carcinomas

Selected References

Benn DE, Robinson BG: Genetic basis of phaeochromocytoma and paraganglioma. Best Pract Res Clin Endocrinol Metab 20:435-450, 2006.

Lenders JWM, Eisenhofer G, Mannelli M, Pacak K: Phaeochromocytoma. Lancet 366:665-675, 2005.

Elder EE, Elder G, Larsson C: Pheochromocytoma and functional paraganglioma syndrome: No longer the 10% tumor. J Surg Oncol 89:193-201, 2005.

Gimm O: Pheochromocytoma-associated syndromes: Genes, proteins and functions of RET, VHL and SDHx. Fam Cancer 4:17-23, 2005.

Salmenkivi K, Heikkila P, Haglund C, Arola J: Malignancy in pheochromocytomas. APMIS 112:551-559, 2004.

Ganglioneuroma

Clinical Features

- Etiology
  — Ganglioneuromas can present as de novo tumors or may arise from neuroblastomas and GNBs that underwent spontaneous maturation or after treatment with chemotherapy
- Epidemiology
  — Rare benign tumors found in older individuals; the median age at diagnosis ranges from 5.5 to 10 years; with a slight female predominance (1.5:1)
  — The most common locations are the posterior mediastinum (41%), retroperitoneum (37%), adrenal gland (21%), and neck (8%)
  — Most common tumor of sympathetic nervous system in adults
- Signs and symptoms
  — Most often manifests as an asymptomatic mass
  — May present with symptoms of catecholamine excess, rarely with diarrhea
- Biochemistry
  — Elevated VMA and homovanillic acid (HVA) levels
  — Increased secretion of vasoactive intestinal peptide (VIP) or serotonin may cause diarrhea
- Therapy
  — Tumor removal is the preferred treatment

Gross Pathology

- Large, well circumscribed, although a true capsule is uncommon
- Measure from 1 cm to more than 15 cm; average about 8 cm
- Firm consistency with homogeneous, solid, tan-yellow to gray-white cut surface
- Occasionally multifocal

Figure 9-8. A, Ganglioneuroma. High-power view showing characteristic proliferation of spindle cells with wavy nuclei. Several classic ganglion cells are present in the center of the field. **B, Composite pheochromocytoma and ganglioneuroma.** The lesion consists of two components: a typical pheochromocytoma (*left*) and spindle cell ganglioneuroma (*right*).

Histopathology

- Composed entirely of ganglion cells and stromal elements represented by Schwann cells and mature fibrous tissue
- Ganglion cells have compact eosinophilic cytoplasm with distinct cell borders and a single eccentric nucleus with a prominent nucleolus; may contain granular golden-brown pigment (neuromelanin)
- Variable numbers of ganglion cells may be present; few may be seen, making distinction from neurofibroma difficult
- Mitotic activity and necrosis are absent
- Mast cells may be present, although tumor does not contain neuroblasts or intermediate cells

Special Stains and Immunohistochemistry

- S-100 protein positive
- Synaptophysin: ganglion cells positive

Other Techniques for Diagnosis

- Electron microscopy: ganglion cells have an eccentric nucleus with a prominent nucleolus; cytoplasm shows peripheral rough endoplasmic reticulum, and neurosecretory granules

Differential Diagnosis

▌ Neurofibroma
- Lacks ganglion cell differentiation

Pearls

- Ganglioneuroma is believed to be the fully differentiated counterpart of peripheral neuroblastic tumors

- Considered a benign tumor; however, malignant transformation to malignant peripheral nerve sheath tumor (MPNST) has been reported
- Thorough sampling needed to rule out less well-differentiated areas; all friable or hemorrhagic areas must be submitted for microscopic examination

Selected References

Mounasamy V, Thacker MM, Humble S, et al: Ganglioneuromas of the sacrum: A report of two cases with radiologic-pathologic correlation. Skel Radiol 35:117-121, 2006.

Mora J, Gerald WL: Origin of neuroblastic tumors: clues for future therapeutics. Exp Rev Mol Diagn 4:293-302, 2004.

Lonergan GJ, Schwab CM, Suarez ES, Carlson CL: Neuroblastoma, ganglioneuroblastoma, and ganglioneuroma: Radiologic-pathologic correlation. Radiographics 22:91-134, 2002.

Joshi VV: Peripheral neuroblastic tumors: Pathologic classification based on recommendations of International Neuroblastoma Pathology Committee (modification of Shimada classification). Pediatr Dev Pathol 3:184-199, 2000.

Marchevsky AM: Mediastinal tumors of peripheral nervous system origin. Semin Diagn Pathol 16:65-78, 1999.

Ganglioneuroblastoma

Clinical Features

- Epidemiology
  - Most often seen in patients 2 to 4 years old, and exceedingly rare after the age of 10 years; occur with equal frequency in boys and girls
- Signs and symptoms
  - Patients often present with an abdominal mass or with abdominal tenderness

— Most common tumor site is the abdomen, followed by the mediastinum, neck, and lower extremity
- Therapy
  — Prognosis and response to therapy is significantly more favorable than those of neuroblastoma

Gross Pathology

- Well-circumscribed mass with a variegated cut surface
- Tumor appearance varies depending on the amount of mature to immature elements, ranging from predominantly solid to cystic
- Firm tan-white areas (better differentiated component) and hemorrhagic areas (poorly differentiated component) may be seen
- Granular calcifications are often present

Histopathology

- Shows histologic features similar to those of neuroblastoma, except that ganglion cell differentiation is present
- Variable amounts of neuroblastoma and ganglioneuroma are seen in the same tumor; typically the ganglioneuromatous component is in excess of 50% of the tumor
- Subtypes (International Neuroblastoma Pathology Committee)
  — *GNB: nodular classic* (abrupt transition between the neuroblastomatous nodule and the surrounding ganglioneuromatous component)
  — *GNB: nodular atypical* (no nodules are seen on gross or microscopic examination; ganglioneuromatous component is present as a thin rim; metastasis shows neuroblastomatous features)
  — *GNB: intermixed* (tumor is composed predominantly of gangliomatous component with well-delineated microscopic foci of neuroblastomatous component)
- These categories have prognostic significance: nodular has an unfavorable prognosis; intermixed has favorable prognosis

Special Stains and Immunohistochemistry

- Neuron-specific enolase (NSE) positive
- Neurofilament positive
- Chromogranin positive
- Synaptophysin positive
- S-100 protein positive in spindle cell population

Other Techniques for Diagnosis

- Electron microscopy: cells with abundant filiform cell processes; cytoplasm showing distinct neurosecretory granules and neurotubules

Differential Diagnosis

- Neuroblastoma
  - Has single population of small to medium-sized blue cells with no ganglion cells or evidence of differentiation
- Ganglioneuroma
  - Has a spindle cell population in a loose, myxoid background with distinct ganglion cells and no component of neuroblastoma

Pearls

- GNBs are transitional tumors of sympathetic cell origin that contain elements of both neuroblastoma and ganglioneuroma
- It has been suggested that nodular GNB evolves as a result of clonal proliferation of more aggressive malignant tumor cells in a neuroblastomatous component of what originally was a GNB of intermixed type maturing ganglioneuroma
- Nodules of nodular GNB may be identified by imaging studies and present with higher levels of urinary excretion of catecholamines compared with intermixed GNB and ganglioneuroma

Selected References

Guo YK, Yang ZG, Li Y, et al: Uncommon adrenal masses: CT and MRI features with histopathologic correlation. Eur J Radiol 62:359-370, 2007.
Rha SE, Byun JY, Jung SE, et al: Neurogenic tumors in the abdomen: Tumor types and imaging characteristics. Radiographics 23:29-43, 2003.
Shimada H, Umehara S, Monobe Y, et al: International neuroblastoma pathology classification for prognostic evaluation of patients with peripheral neuroblastic tumors. Cancer 92:2451-2461, 2001.
Joshi VV: Peripheral neuroblastic tumors: Pathologic classification based on recommendations of International Neuroblastoma Pathology Committee (modification of Shimada classification). Pediatr Dev Pathol 3:184-199, 2000.

Neuroblastoma

Clinical Features

- Etiology
  — Malignant tumor of sympaticoadrenal lineage of the neural crest that can develop anywhere in the sympathetic nervous system
  — Genomic amplification of *MYCN* is common and consistently associated with poor outcome
  — Other biologic variables include deletions of 1p (25% to 35%), allelic loss of 11q (35% to 45%), and gain of 17q
- Epidemiology
  — Incidence of about 8 per 1×10^6 population; most common extracranial solid tumor of childhood

Figure 9-9. Neuroblastoma. A, The adrenal gland is replaced by a circumscribed, round to oval mass with a variegated, lobular appearance, invading into the kidney. **B,** Low-power view showing a monomorphic proliferation of small blue cells and adjacent residual adrenal cortex. **C,** High-power view showing a monomorphic proliferation of small blue cells with fine granular chromatin and indistinct cytoplasmic borders. Notice the fibrillary background. (**A,** Photo courtesy of Dr. Glenn P. Taylor, Hospital for Sick Children, Toronto.)

— Accounts for more than 7% of malignancies in patients younger than 15 years; more than 85% occur in children younger than 4 years

— Can occur in a variety of locations, with adrenal gland being most common site (50% to 80%)

— Other common sites include posterior mediastinum (about 15%)

- Signs and symptoms

— About 40% of patients present with localized disease ranging from an incidental adrenal mass discovered on prenatal ultrasound to large and invasive tumors

— Classic signs of disseminated neuroblastoma include periorbital ecchymoses (raccoon eyes), proptosis, or both, due to metastasis to the bony orbit

— Paraneoplastic syndromes include (1) intractable diarrhea and failure to thrive secondary to secretion of VIP and (2) opsoclonus-myoclonus syndrome (2% to 4%)

- Biochemistry

— May produce catecholamines with increased levels of urinary VMA

- Therapy

— Surgery, chemotherapy, radiotherapy, and biotherapy, as well as observation alone in selected cases, are used according to risk group based on the presence or absence of unfavorable biologic features

Gross Pathology

- Typically circumscribed, round to oval mass, often with a variegated, lobular cut surface; usually tan to gray-white

- May be variable in size ranging from less than 1 cm to greater than 10 cm

- Usually solitary and unicentric, but bilateral cases have been reported

- Typically solid but occasionally shows cystic degeneration

- Often shows marked hemorrhage, necrosis, or calcification

- Invasion into adjacent organs and soft tissue may be seen

Histopathology

- Cellular, small round blue cell tumor with vague lobular architecture

- Nodular aggregates of tumor cells separated by delicate fibrovascular septa

- Prominent Homer-Wright pseudorosettes (round spaces surrounded by palisading peripheral nuclei and filled with a faintly eosinophilic fibrillary matrix) may be seen

- Fibrillar matrix representing neuritic cell processes; resembles neuropil of the central nervous system

- Cells are medium sized and round to oval with high nuclear-to-cytoplasmic ratio and scant cytoplasm; hyperchromatic nuclei have stippled chromatin and inconspicuous nucleoli

- Hemorrhage and microcalcifications are common findings

- Variable mitotic activity

- Microscopic grading criteria (International Neuroblastoma Pathology Committee [INPC]): the criteria divide tumors into subtypes

— *Neuroblastoma, undifferentiated:* small, medium, or large round neuroblasts showing lack of differentiation or neuropil by routine light microscopy

— *Neuroblastoma, undifferentiated, pleomorphic subtype:* neuroblasts are large, with pleomorphic

nuclei, prominent nucleoli, and moderate to abundant cytoplasm (some cells may have rhabdoid features); no neuropil
— *Neuroblastoma, poorly differentiated:* less than 5% neuroblasts show synchronous differentiation toward ganglion cells
— *Neuroblastoma, differentiating:* more than 5% neuroblasts show synchronous differentiation toward ganglion cells
- Mitosis karyorrhexis index (MKI) is based on percentage seen in 10 high-power fields (total of 5000 cells): less than 2% (low), 2% to 4% (intermediate), and more than 4% (high)
- Assessment of the MKI is crucial because it is used to determine prognostic categories (unfavorable versus favorable histology) in combination with the tumor differentiation and age of the patient (Table 9-1)

Special Stains and Immunohistochemistry

- NSE positive
- Neurofilament positive
- S-100 protein: spindle cell population positive
- Chromogranin positive
- Synaptophysin positive
- Cytokeratin positive
- Negative for desmin, myoglobin, vimentin, leukocyte common antigen (LCA), and CD99

Other Techniques for Diagnosis

- Electron microscopy: characteristically shows cytoplasmic filaments, dense-core neurosecretory granules, and microtubules

- Cytogenetic studies: *MYCN* and 1p deletion by fluorescent in situ hybridization technique and DNA index by flow cytometry

Differential Diagnosis

▌ GNB
- Has evidence of differentiation in the form of ganglion cells, which may appear normal or abnormal

▌ Rhabdomyosarcoma
- A rare tumor, usually arising in or around kidney, composed of large tumor cells with eccentric nuclei and prominent nucleoli; large eosinophilic cytoplasmic inclusions are often seen
- Immunohistochemical stains: positive for cytokeratin, negative for NSE, chromogranin, and synaptophysin

▌ Malignant lymphoma
- Composed of diffuse sheets of atypical lymphoid cells without fibrovascular septa; lacks rosette formation and has no fibrillary matrix
- CD45 (LCA) positive; negative for NSE, chromogranin, and synaptophysin

▌ Ewing sarcoma
- Typically found in long bones and occasionally in soft tissue
- Tumor cells frequently show intracytoplasmic glycogen (PAS positive) and are positive for CD99, negative for chromogranin and synaptophysin
- This tumor has a characteristic t(11;22) translocation

▌ Nephroblastoma (Wilms tumor)
- Shows triphasic pattern consisting of blastema, stromal, and epithelial components
- Is negative for synaptophysin, chromogranin, and NSE

Pearls

- DNA index is a prognostic marker for patients younger than 2 years with disseminated disease: near-diploid DNA content is associated with genomic instability and worse outcome, whereas hyperdiploidy (often near-triploidy) appears to be favorable
- May exhibit familial incidence (1% to 2%); may be associated with Hirschsprung disease, congenital central hypoventilation, pheochromocytoma, and neurofibromatosis type 1
- *4S disease* refers to stage 4S (S, special) that occurs in 5% of patients showing small localized primary tumors with metastasis in liver, skin, or bone marrow that almost always spontaneously regress (massive hepatomegaly can cause respiratory compromise in infants younger than 2 months) (Table 9-2)

Table 9-1. Prognosis for Neuroblastoma

Age (yr)	Differentiation	Mitosis Karyorrhexis Index	Prognostic Category
<1.5	Undifferentiated	Any	Unfavorable histology
<1.5	Poorly differentiated or differentiating	Low or intermediate	Favorable histology
<1.5	Any	High	Unfavorable histology
1.5 to 5	Undifferentiated or poorly differentiated	Any	Unfavorable histology
1.5 to 5	Differentiating	Low	Favorable histology
1.5 to 5	Differentiating	Intermediate or high	Unfavorable histology
>5	Any	Any	Unfavorable histology

Table 9-2. Neuroblastoma Risk Groups for Pediatric Oncology Group and Children's Group Clinical Protocols

INS Stage	Age (yr)	*MYCN* Status	INPC Classification	DNA Ploidy	Risk Group
1	0-21	Any	Any	Any	Low
2A, 2B	<1	Any	Any	Any	Low
	>1-21	Not amplified	Any	—	Low
	>1-21	Amplified	FH	—	Low
	>1-21	Amplified	UH	—	High
3	<1	Not amplified	Any	Any	Intermediate
	<1	Amplified	Any	Any	High
	>1-21	Not amplified	FH	—	Intermediate
	>1-21	Not amplified	UH	—	High
	>1-21	Amplified	Any	—	High
4	<1	Not amplified	Any	Any	Intermediate
	<1	Amplified	Any	Any	High
	>1-21	Any	Any	—	High
4S	<1	Not amplified	FH	>1	Low
	<1	Not amplified	Any	1	Intermediate
	<1	Not amplified	UH	Any	Intermediate
	<1	Amplified	Any	Any	High

FH, favorable histology; INPC, International Neuroblastoma Pathology Committee; INS, International Staging System; UH, unfavorable histology.

Selected References

Maris JM, Hogarty MD, Bagatell R, Cohn SL: Neuroblastoma. Lancet 369:2106-2120, 2007.

Shimada H, Umehara S, Monobe Y, et al: International neuroblastoma pathology classification for prognostic evaluation of patients with peripheral neuroblastic tumors. Cancer 92:2451-2461, 2001.

Goto S, Umehara S, Gerbing RB, et al: Histopathology (International Neuroblastoma Pathology Classification) and MYCN status in patients with peripheral neuroblastic tumors. Cancer 92:2699-2708, 2001.

Joshi VV: Peripheral neuroblastic tumors: Pathologic classification based on recommendations of International Neuroblastoma Pathology Committee (modification of Shimada classification). Pediatr Dev Pathol 3:184-199, 2000.

Thorner PS, Squire JA: Molecular genetics in the diagnosis and prognosis of solid pediatric tumors. Pediatr Dev Pathol 1:337-365, 1998.

Figure 9-10. Malignant melanoma. High-power view showing large pleomorphic cells with abundant eosinophilic cytoplasm, large nuclei, and prominent nucleoli.

Primary Malignant Melanoma

Clinical Features

- First observation in 1946; rare tumor with rigid diagnostic criteria
  - Only one adrenal gland involved
  - No medical history of melanoma or pigmented lesion
  - No evidence of endocrine disorders
  - Unequivocal histologic features of melanoma

- Epidemiology
  - Highly aggressive tumor that affects middle-aged adults; usually locally advanced with renal adhesions by the time of diagnosis
- Signs and symptoms
  - Presents as flank tenderness or palpable tumor; radiologic features are not specific

- Therapy
  - Surgical treatment (usually nephroadrenalectomy) is poorly effective, with a mortality rate near 100% in 2 years

Gross Pathology

- Unilateral brown to black tumor of variable size (8 to 17 cm)
- Cut surface often shows areas of hemorrhage and necrosis
- Gross appearance resembles pheochromocytoma

Histopathology

- Typical microscopic findings of malignant melanoma
  - Large polygonal or spindle cells with marked nuclear polymorphism
  - Prominent nucleoli
  - Presence of abundant melanin pigment

Special Stains and Immunohistochemistry

- S-100 protein positive
- HMB-45 positive
- Microphthalmia transcription factor positive
- Cytokeratin negative

Other Techniques for Diagnosis

- Electron microscopy: true melanin pigment seen in melanosomes or premelanosomes

Differential Diagnosis

▎ Pigmented adrenal cortical adenoma
  - Usually associated with Cushing syndrome or primary hyperaldosteronism (Conn syndrome)
  - Composed of cells with eosinophilic cytoplasm with a variable amount of golden-brown pigment (lipofuscin)
  - S-100 protein and HMB-45 negative, but melan-A positive
▎ Metastatic melanoma
  - More common; it is often bilateral but otherwise similar to primary melanoma: a primary lesion can only be diagnosed if there is no current or history of malignant melanocytic lesion of skin
▎ Pigmented pheochromocytoma
  - Exhibits immunoreactivity for neuroendocrine markers (chromogranin-A, synaptophysin), and on electron microscopy, cells contain numerous neurosecretory granules
  - Also positive for HMB-45, and sustentacular cells show reactivity for S-100 protein

Pearls

- The histogenesis of primary adrenal melanoma is not fully elucidated. The pluripotent neural crest cells appear to link malignant melanoma and the adrenal medulla because they serve as precursors

of melanocytes, neurons, glial cells of the peripheral nervous system, and adrenal chromaffin cells
- Both the argentaffin reaction and its disappearance after oxidative treatment are features shared by other nonmelanotic brown pigments, such as lipofuscin and neuromelanin

Selected References

Bastide C, Arroua F, Carcenac A, et al: Primary malignant melanoma of the adrenal gland. Int J Urol 13:608-610, 2006.

Granero LE, Al-Lawati T, Bobin JY: Primary melanoma of the adrenal gland, a continuous dilemma: Report of a case. Surg Today 34:554-556, 2004.

Bellezza G, Giasanti M, Cavaliere A, Sidoni A: Pigmented "black" pheochromocytoma of the adrenal gland: A case report and review of the literature. Arch Pathol Lab Med 128:e125-128, 2004.

Amerigo J, Roig J, Pulido F, et al: Primary malignant melanoma of the adrenal gland. Surgery 126:107-111, 1999.

Myelolipoma

Clinical Features

- Etiology
  - A proliferation of hematopoietic elements
- Epidemiology
  - Usually found in older individuals (fifth to seventh decades); incidence in autopsy series between 0.08% and 2%
  - Adrenal gland is the most common site
- Signs and symptoms
  - More than 50% of cases are asymptomatic and found incidentally; large tumors may present with flank or abdominal tenderness, constipation, vomiting, or as a palpable mass
  - Rarely may be associated with Cushing syndrome or Conn syndrome, usually associated with adrenal cortical adenoma

Gross Pathology

- Variable size and weight; range in size from few centimeters to greater than 30 cm
- Soft, fleshy, well-circumscribed tumor with pushing border
- Variable color with tan-yellow and red-brown areas
- Large lesion may show areas of hemorrhage or necrosis; rarely, small cyst formation may be seen

Histopathology

- Composed of normal-appearing hematopoietic elements with all three cell lines typically represented (resembles normal bone marrow)
- Variable amount of mature adipose tissue is seen
- Compression of normal appearing adrenal cortex is seen at periphery

Figure 9-11. Myelolipoma. A, This large lesion has tan and red areas admixed with pale-yellow adipose tissue. The compressed adrenal is bright yellow (*top*). **B,** Classic features include the presence of bone marrow elements and adipose tissue.

Special Stains and Immunohistochemistry
- Noncontributory

Other Techniques for Diagnosis
- Noncontributory

Differential Diagnosis
▌ Lipoma
  - Is rarely found in adrenal gland and is composed solely of mature adipose tissue; lacks bone marrow elements

Pearls
- May be found in extra-adrenal sites, including liver, retroperitoneum, and stomach
- Occasionally associated with hypertension, similar to pheochromocytoma
- Etiology is controversial. The embolization of hematopoietic stem cells and ectopic myeloid hyperplasia has been implicated in the etiology. In addition, transformation of the zona reticularis into bone marrow tissue has been observed in mature rats after treatment with testosterone

Selected References
Guo YK, Yang ZG, Li Y, et al: Uncommon adrenal masses: CT and MRI features with histopathological correlation. Eur J Radiol 62:359-370, 2007.

Elsayes KM, Mukundam G, Narra VR, et al: Adrenal masses: MR imaging features with pathologic correlation. Radiographics 24(Suppl 1):S73-86, 2004.

Lam KY, Lo CY: Adrenal lipomatous tumours: A 30 year clinicopathological experience at a single institution. J Clin Pathol 54:707-712, 2001.

Yildiz L, Akpolat I, Erzurumlu K, et al: Giant adrenal myelolipoma: Case report and review of the literature. Pathol Int 50:502-504, 2000.

Adrenal Cysts and Pseudocysts

Clinical Features
- Etiology
  — A heterogeneous group of lesions: true cysts versus pseudocysts
- Epidemiology
  — Rare (incidence between 0.06% and 0.18% in autopsy series, and about 5% of incidentally discovered adrenal lesions by computed tomography and magnetic resonance imaging)
  — Found at any age, with increased incidence in fourth to sixth decades; occur more frequently in women than men
  — Usually unilateral with no tendency to occur in either side
- Signs and symptoms
  — Mostly asymptomatic; in the case of large size can present with gastrointestinal symptoms, lumbar or back pain, and palpable abdominal mass
  — Acute symptoms can occur due to rupture, cyst hemorrhage, or infection
  — May clinically and radiographically mimic retroperitoneal or adrenal neoplasms
- Therapy
  — Treatment depends on the underlying pathology, size of the cyst, associated symptoms, and occurrence of complications (small asymptomatic

Figure 9-12. Pseudocyst of the adrenal gland. A, The adrenal cortex is intact, and there is a large cyst containing yellow necrotic material. **B,** Section showing adrenal cortex with an underlying hemorrhagic and cystic lesion containing necrotic material. Notice the lack of epithelial lining.

cysts with benign angiographic features can be managed by percutaneous aspiration and watch and follow)

Gross Pathology

- Typically of small size; can reach sizes of up to 30 cm
- Usually uniloculated; rarely multiloculated
- Cyst wall is composed of fibrotic tissue; areas of calcification may be seen
- Contains serous or serosanguineous fluid
- Cyst may contain clotted blood or degenerated thrombus (hemorrhagic cysts)
- Pushing border with compression of the adjacent adrenal gland parenchyma

Histopathology

- Four main groups: endothelial cysts (45%); pseudocysts (39%); epithelial cysts (9%); and parasitic cysts (7%)
  — Endothelial and epithelial cysts have true walls lined with endothelium and epithelium, respectively (true cysts)
  — Endothelial cysts include lymphangiomatous, angiomatous, and hamartomatous subtypes
  — Epithelial cysts are divided into cystic adenomas, glandular or retention cysts, and cystic transformation of embryonal remnants
  — Pseudocysts arise after an episode of a prior adrenal hemorrhage and subsequent clot formation and are characterized by a fibrotic wall without a well-defined endothelial or epithelial lining
  — Parasitic cysts are usually echinococcal in origin (hydatid cyst)

- ◆ Mature adipose tissue or foci of myelolipomatous metaplasia are occasionally seen
- ◆ Rim of compressed adrenal gland may be seen at the periphery

Special Stains and Immunohistochemistry

- Factor VIII: highlights endothelial cell lining
- Elastic: may find elastic fibers within the fibrotic cyst wall

Other Techniques for Diagnosis

- Noncontributory

Differential Diagnosis

▌Myelolipoma
- Typically forms a solid mass with a tan-yellow to red-brown cut surface and is composed entirely of mature adipose tissue and hematopoietic elements; cysts may rarely be seen but are typically small
▌Adrenal cysts
- May show focal myelolipomatous differentiation but also have a fibrotic wall that is filled with proteinaceous debris, blood, or thrombus material

Pearls

- Hemorrhagic cysts may be associated with Beckwith-Wiedemann syndrome
- Cyst wall showing factor VIII and elastic positivity supports vascular and lymphatic nature of this lesion
- Pseudocysts tend to have mural, rimlike calcification more commonly than endothelial cysts, which tend to contain septal calcification

Selected References

Guo YK, Yang ZG, Li Y, et al: Uncommon adrenal masses: CT and MRI features with histopathological correlation. Eur J Radiol 62:359-370, 2007.

Carvounis E, Marinis A, Arkadopoulos N, et al: Vascular adrenal cysts. Arch Pathol Lab Med 130:1722-1724, 2006.

Sanal HT, Kocaoglu M, Yildirim D, et al: Imaging features of benign adrenal cysts. Eur J Radiol 60:465-469, 2006.

Elsayes KM, Mukundam G, Narra VR, et al: Adrenal masses: MR imaging features with pathologic correlation. Radiographics 24(Suppl 1):S73-86, 2004.

Tanuma Y, Kimura M, Sakai S: Adrenal cyst: A review of the Japanese literature and report of a case. Int J Urol 8:500-503, 2001.

Metastatic Tumors

Clinical Features

- Epidemiology
  - Most common tumors of the adrenal gland
  - Bilateral adrenal gland involvement is found in about 50% of cases
  - Lung is most common primary tumor site, followed by stomach, esophagus, liver, bile ducts, pancreas, large intestine, kidney, and breast
- Signs and symptoms
  - About 90% are asymptomatic, affect elderly patients, and are diagnosed as part of multiorgan metastases

Figure 9-13. A, Metastatic adenocarcinoma. Gross photo showing complete replacement of the adrenal gland by a metastatic adenocarcinoma. **B, Metastatic hepatocellular carcinoma.** The adrenal cortex is compressed (*left*), and the tumor resembles an adrenal cortical adenoma; however, the presence of bile pigment is characteristic of hepatocellular carcinoma. **C, Metastatic renal cell carcinoma.** The adrenal cortex and medulla (*left*) are infiltrated by a clear cell tumor that forms tubules. **D, Metastatic renal cell carcinoma.** The adrenal cortex (*left*) stains for inhibin A, but the tumor (*right*) is negative for this marker.

— Patients may present with Addison disease (adrenal insufficiency) or peritoneal hemorrhage

Gross Pathology

- Often multifocal nodular disease
- Solitary lesions may mimic primary adrenal cortical carcinoma
- Typically involves adrenal cortex and often shows extension into adjacent adipose tissue
- Tumors may occasionally show extension into vena cava
- Brown or black discoloration should raise suspicion of a metastatic melanoma

Histopathology

- Depends on primary site of malignancy
- Adenocarcinomas and squamous cell carcinomas are the most common subtypes
- Lung and breast metastases typically show poorly differentiated carcinoma; squamous or glandular differentiation may be seen in metastatic lung carcinoma
- Metastatic melanoma composed of large, polygonal cells with pleomorphic nuclei and prominent nucleoli; melanin pigment may be seen

Special Stains and Immunohistochemistry

- See "Differential Diagnosis"

Other Techniques for Diagnosis

- Noncontributory

Differential Diagnosis

- The use of markers normally expressed in the adrenal cortex, including D11, SF-1, inhibin-α, and melan-A, can be helpful in distinguishing primary from metastatic carcinomas
- Clinical history is important

▌ Metastatic malignant melanoma
  - Distinction from primary malignant melanoma can be challenging (see "Primary Malignant Melanoma")
▌ Metastatic hepatocellular carcinoma
  - Can be difficult to distinguish from adrenal cortical cell carcinoma. Hepatocellular carcinoma is positive for HepPar-1, canalicular polyclonal carcinoembryonic antigen (pCEA), and canalicular CD10 by immunohistochemistry
▌ Metastatic renal cell carcinoma (clear cell)
  - Must be distinguished from adrenal cortical cell carcinoma
  - Often there is adrenal gland involvement by direct extension of a renal cell carcinoma; renal cell carcinoma is immunoreactive for RCC, CD10, vimentin, and cytokeratin

Pearls

- Fine-needle aspiration is useful in diagnosing adrenal gland metastases

Selected References

Pan CC, Chen PC, Tsay SH, Ho DM: Differential immunoprofiles of hepatocellular carcinoma, renal cell carcinoma, and adrenocortical carcinoma. Appl Immunohistochem Mol Morphol 13:347-352, 2005.

Saeger W, Fassnacht M, Chita R, et al: High diagnostic accuracy of adrenal core biopsy: Results of the German and Austrian Adrenal Network Multicenter Trial in 220 consecutive patients. Hum Pathol 34:180-186, 2003.

Lam KY, Lo CY: Metastatic tumours of the adrenal glands: A 30-year experience in a teaching hospital. Clin Endocrinol 56:95-101, 2002.

Page DL, DeLellis RA, Hough AJ: Tumors of the adrenal. In Atlas of Tumor Pathology, 2nd Series, Fascicle 23. Washington, DC, Armed Forces Institute of Pathology, 1995.

Cristina Magi-Galluzzi and Ming Zhou

10

Ureter, Urinary Bladder, and Kidney

Ureter

Ureteritis Cystica et Glandularis

Clinical Features

- One of the most common non-neoplastic urothelial proliferations
- Believed to be a reactive urothelial proliferation that develops after an inflammatory stimulus
- Typically asymptomatic and found incidentally

Gross Pathology

- Nodular cobblestone appearance due to numerous small, superficial, fluid-filled cysts

Histopathology

▌ Ureteritis cystica
- Von Brunn nests (small nests of normal urothelial cells within lamina propria) with central lumens (cystic dilation) lined by urothelial cells
▌ Ureteritis glandularis
- Von Brunn nests with central lumens lined by columnar cells

Special Stains and Immunohistochemistry

- Noncontributory

Other Techniques for Diagnosis

- Noncontributory

Differential Diagnosis

▌ Urothelial hyperplasia
- Increase in number of layers of urothelial cells
- Does not show nesting of urothelial cells
▌ Von Brunn nests
- Lack central cystic dilation

Pearls

- Believed by some to be a normal feature of the urothelial mucosa
- Most believe that an inflammatory stimulus is needed
- Must be considered in the differential diagnosis of ureteral and renal pelvic filling defects

Selected References

Hochberg DA, Motta J, Brodherson MS: Cystitis glandularis. Urology 51:112-113, 1998.
Duffin TK, Regan JB, Hernandez-Graulau JM: Ureteritis cystica with 17-year followup. J Urol 151:142-143, 1994.
Petersen UE, Kvist E, Friis M, Krogh J: Ureteritis cystica. Scand J Urol Nephrol 25:1-4, 1991.

Urothelial Carcinoma (Transitional Cell Carcinoma)

Clinical Features

- Relatively rare in the ureter; constitutes 2% to 5% of urothelial neoplasms

Figure 10-1. A, Low-grade papillary urothelial carcinoma of the ureter. The neoplasm shows a nodular and inverted growth pattern. Cells show minimal anaplasia; the nuclei are uniformly enlarged with mild differences in shape, contour, and chromatin distribution. **B, High-grade urothelial carcinoma of the ureter.** Ulceration and denudation of the urothelium are often seen in high-grade tumors of the ureter. Cells are large and irregular with moderate to marked nuclear pleomorphism. Infiltration of the underlying subepithelial connective tissue is common.

- Similar etiologic and pathogenic agents as in bladder urothelial carcinoma: tobacco smoking is the most common risk factor; higher association with analgesic abuse
- Clinical features are comparable to lesions arising in the urinary bladder and include hematuria and flank pain

- More commonly results in urinary obstruction
- Can occur in any portion of the ureter; distal third is most common

Gross Pathology

- Low-grade tumors typically have a papillary architecture with delicate papillary fronds over the ureteral surface
- Higher-grade tumors often lack papillary architecture and show nodular, polypoid, or sessile pattern
- Ureteral wall is typically thickened and may show significant narrowing
- Ulceration and hemorrhage are often seen in high-grade tumors

Histopathology

▌ Low-grade papillary urothelial carcinoma (World Health Organization and International Society of Urological Pathology [WHO/ISUP] 2003 system)
- Exophytic growth pattern characterized by slender papillary fronds with obvious fibrovascular cores, frequent branching, and minimal fusion
- The papillae are lined by urothelium that shows an orderly appearance with easily recognizable variations in architectural and cytologic features
- Cells usually show minimal anaplasia; the nuclei are uniformly enlarged, with mild differences in shape, contour, and chromatin distribution
- Mitoses are infrequent

▌ High-grade papillary urothelial carcinoma (WHO/ISUP 2003 system)
- May lack a distinct papillary architecture, although papillary remnants may persist
- The papillae are frequently fused and branching
- The pattern of disorder is predominant, with easily recognizable variations in architectural and cytologic features
- Cells are large and irregular with a spectrum of nuclear pleomorphism ranging from moderate to marked; nucleoli may be prominent
- Bizarre or multinucleated tumor cells may be seen
- High mitotic activity; numerous atypical forms are often seen
- Usually infiltrates the underlying subepithelial connective tissue or muscularis propria and grows in solid cords or nests
- Reactive desmoplastic stroma surrounds infiltrating nests of tumor cells
- Squamous differentiation is seen in more than 20% of cases

Special Stains and Immunohistochemistry

- Cytokeratin (high molecular weight and CK7) and p63 positive
- Carcinoembryonic antigen (CEA) positive (especially in high-grade tumors)

Other Techniques for Diagnosis

- Cytogenetic studies: similar findings as in urothelial carcinoma of the bladder

Differential Diagnosis

▌ Inverted papilloma
- Minimal cytologic atypia and low mitotic activity
- Lacks invasion into the muscularis propria

▌ Fibroepithelial polyp
- Typically solitary with a short, thin stalk
- Consists of a polyp of loose fibroconnective and fibrovascular tissue covered by normal-appearing urothelium

Pearls

- Urine cytology is helpful in evaluating ureteral lesions
- Prognosis is related to tumor stage (depth of invasion), grade (histologic and cytologic features), and multifocality (presence of synchronous tumor in the renal pelvis)

Selected References

Lehmann J, Suttmann H, Kovac I, et al: Transitional cell carcinoma of the ureter: Prognostic factors influencing progression and survival. Eur Urol 51:1281-1288, 2007.

Korkes F, Silveira TS, Castro MG, et al: Carcinoma of the renal pelvis and ureter. Int Braz J Urol 32:648-653, 2006.

Urinary Bladder

Cystitis

Infectious Cystitis

- Infectious cystitis can be caused by various microorganisms, including bacteria, fungi, viruses, and parasites
- Diagnosis relies primarily on urinalysis, urine culture, and empirical anti-microbial therapy

Bacterial Cystitis

Clinical Features

- Most common cause of cystitis
- Much more common in sexually active women between ages 20 and 40 years owing to a short urethra
- Associated with bacteria such as *Escherichia coli* and *Klebsiella*, *Streptococcus*, *Staphylococcus*, *Proteus*, and *Pseudomonas* species
- Urine culture is often able to isolate organism
- Predisposing conditions include structural abnormalities of the genitourinary tract (including bladder exstrophy, urethral malformation), calculi, urine stasis, and systemic diseases, such as diabetes, chronic renal disease, and immunosuppression
- Patients present with urinary frequency, urgency, and dysuria; hematuria may be seen

Gross Pathology

- Bladder mucosa is edematous with areas of erythema; hemorrhagic mucosa may be seen
- Fibrinous exudate with mucosal ulceration often develops

Histopathology

- Ulcerated bladder mucosa covered by fibrinous exudate consisting of abundant neutrophils
- Neutrophils typically extend into lamina propria
- Abscess may form
- Urothelium may be hyperplastic or metaplastic and can show reactive atypia
- Late findings include granulation tissue and bladder wall fibrosis

Special Stains and Immunohistochemistry

- Noncontributory

Other Techniques for Diagnosis

- Noncontributory

Differential Diagnosis

▌ Low-grade papillary urothelial carcinoma
- Typically shows papillary architecture with increased cytologic atypia
- Acute and chronic inflammation may be seen; however, the neutrophilic infiltrate is typically much greater in bacterial cystitis

▌ Noninfectious cystitis
- Features of polypoid cystitis, follicular cystitis, giant cell cystitis, or hemorrhagic cystitis
- No acute inflammatory cell infiltrate
- Urine culture is negative

▌ Interstitial cystitis
- Shows chronic inflammatory infiltrate with numerous mast cells
- Urine culture is negative

Pearls

- Bacteria almost always gain access into the bladder through ascending route
- Negative urine culture does not rule out diagnosis of bacterial cystitis

Selected References

Sussman M, Gally DL: The biology of cystitis: Host and bacterial factors. Annu Rev Med 50:149-158, 1999.

Roberts JA: Pathophysiology of bacterial cystitis. Adv Exp Med Biol 462:325-338, 1999.

Malakoplakia

Clinical Features

- Most commonly found in the bladder; may be seen in the ureter, renal pelvis, testis, gynecologic tract, gastrointestinal tract, and lung
- Typically found in women; peak incidence in fifth decade
- Rarely seen in children
- Most patients present with typical symptoms of urinary tract infection
- Often culture *Escherichia coli* or other bacteria from the urine

Gross Pathology

- Multiple soft, yellow-white, nodular plaques measuring less than 2 cm
- Involves mucosal surface

Histopathology

- Accumulation of histocytes filled with abundant eosinophilic granular cytoplasm (von Hansemann histiocytes) in the superficial lamina propria, typically underlying an intact urothelial layer
- Michaelis-Gutmann bodies (small round basophilic intracytoplasmic or extracytoplasmic laminated structures with a bull's-eye appearance) are found within histiocytes as well as within the interstitium
- Michaelis-Gutmann bodies are formed by precipitation of calcium or iron on bacteria or bacterial fragments
- Extensive fibrosis and marked acute and chronic inflammation may be seen

Special Stains and Immunohistochemistry

- Von Kossa calcium and Perl Prussian blue: Michaelis-Gutmann bodies positive

Figure 10-2. Malakoplakia. The lamina propria contains numerous histocytes with a large amount of eosinophilic granular cytoplasm and intracytoplasmic inclusions (Michaelis-Gutmann bodies).

- Periodic acid-Schiff (PAS) stain: von Hansemann and Michaelis-Gutmann bodies positive

Other Techniques for Diagnosis

- Electron microscopy: Michaelis-Gutmann bodies consist of a dense core surrounded by a homogeneous zone composed of myelin figures; measure 5 to 10 μm in diameter

Differential Diagnosis

▌ Xanthogranulomatous cystitis
- Lacks Michaelis-Gutmann bodies
▌ Langerhans cell histiocytosis
- Histiocytes positive for CD1a and S-100

Pearls

- Terminology derived from the Greek words *plakos* (plaque) and *malakos* (soft)
- Believed to result from impairment of the ability of mononuclear cells to kill phagocytosed bacteria
- Must identify Michaelis-Gutmann bodies to make diagnosis

Selected References

Pusl T, Weiss M, Hartmann B, et al: Malacoplakia in a renal transplant recipient. Eur J Intern Med 17:133-135, 2006.

Tam VK, Kung WH, Li R, Chan KW: Renal parenchymal malacoplakia: A rare cause of ARF with a review of recent literature. Am J Kidney Dis 41:E13-17, 2003.

Dobyan DC, Truong LD, Eknoyan G: Renal malakoplakia reappraised. Am J Kidney Dis 22:243-252, 1993.

Noninfectious Cystitis (Polypoid Cystitis, Follicular Cystitis, Giant Cell Cystitis)

Clinical Features

- Patients may present with urinary frequency, urgency, or dysuria
- Polypoid cystitis is often seen in patients with indwelling bladder catheters
- Follicular cystitis is frequently seen in patients with bladder carcinoma and urinary tract infection
- *Giant cell cystitis* is not a clinical entity; rather, it is a term used to describe the presence of atypical stromal cells in the lamina propria of the bladder
- Noninfectious cystitis is occasionally seen after radiation treatment

Gross Pathology

▌ Polypoid cystitis
- Small polypoid mucosal lesions (may mimic bladder carcinoma)
▌ Follicular cystitis
- Mucosa showing erythematous gray-white nodules
▌ Giant cell cystitis
- Usually subtle finding; erythematous bladder mucosa may be seen

Figure 10-3. Giant cell cystitis. The lamina propria shows atypical large stromal cells with bipolar or multipolar tapering eosinophilic processes and multiple, enlarged hyperchromatic nuclei.

Histopathology

▊ Polypoid cystitis
  ● Broad fronds covered by benign-appearing transitional cells
  ● Lamina propria is edematous, with chronic inflammation and congested blood vessels
▊ Follicular cystitis
  ● Lamina propria contains scattered lymphoid follicles, usually with germinal centers
▊ Giant cell cystitis
  ● Atypical large stromal cells with bipolar or multipolar tapering eosinophilic processes and enlarged hyperchromatic nuclei (degenerative atypia); cells often contain multiple nuclei
  ● Mitoses are absent or rare

Special Stains and Immunohistochemistry

  ● Noncontributory

Other Techniques for Diagnosis

  ● Noncontributory

Differential Diagnosis

▊ Bacterial cystitis
  ● Inflammatory component consists of acute inflammatory cells
  ● Bladder culture may yield positive results
▊ Low-grade papillary urothelial carcinoma
  ● May be confused with polypoid cystitis
  ● Typically shows branching delicate papillae rather than broad fronds
  ● Papillae are covered by atypical urothelial cells, which is much more pronounced than is seen in polypoid cystitis
▊ Malignant lymphoma
  ● Must be distinguished from follicular cystitis

  ● Lymphomatous infiltrate typically shows a diffuse rather than follicular architecture
▊ Sarcoma
  ● Must be distinguished from giant cell cystitis
  ● Sarcomatous stromal cells have higher degree of nuclear atypia; mitoses are commonly found

Pearls

  ● Removal of the irritant (catheter, toxin) typically results in resolution of cystitis
  ● Often these conditions are asymptomatic and found incidentally

Selected References

Hansson S, Hanson E, Hjalmas K, et al: Follicular cystitis in girls with untreated asymptomatic or covert bacteriuria. J Urol 143:330-332, 1990.

Young RH: Papillary and polypoid cystitis: A report of eight cases. Am J Surg Pathol 12:542-546, 1988.

Ekelund P, Anderstrom C, Johansson SL, Larsson P: The reversibility of catheter-associated polypoid cystitis. J Urol 130:456-459, 1983.

Treatment-Related Cystitis

Clinical Features

  ● Bacillus Calmette-Guérin (BCG) cystitis is associated with intravesical instillation of BCG used in the treatment of urothelial carcinoma in situ (CIS) and high-grade papillary urothelial carcinoma
  ● Radiation cystitis may be acute or chronic and can occur whenever the bladder is included in the treatment field
  ● Hemorrhagic cystitis is associated with radiation and chemotherapy; also seen with various chemical toxins (cyclophosphamide, busulfan) and viral infection (adenovirus in children), or may be idiopathic

Gross Pathology

▊ Granulomatous cystitis secondary to BCG therapy (BCG cystitis)
  ● Partially or entirely denuded bladder mucosa
▊ Radiation cystitis
  ● Hyperemic and edematous bladder mucosa with thickened mucosal folds
▊ Hemorrhagic cystitis
  ● Hemorrhagic and edematous bladder mucosa

Histopathology

▊ BCG cystitis
  ● Superficial lamina propria shows discrete noncaseating granulomas containing epithelioid histiocytes and multinucleated giant cells
  ● Granulomas are associated with intense lymphocytic infiltrate

Figure 10-4. Radiation cystitis. A, The lamina propria shows edema, hyperemia, and thickened mucosal folds. The urothelium shows superficial ulceration and atypical cytologic features. The stroma contains extravasated erythrocytes, inflammation, and occasional bizarre multinucleated giant cells. **B,** Late changes include superficial ulceration and dilated blood vessels with fibrinous exudate.

- Urothelium may show nonspecific reactive atypia or may be denuded
- Radiation cystitis
  - Lamina propria shows edema, hyperemia, and dilated blood vessels with fibrin
  - Urothelium may show desquamation, superficial ulceration, and atypical cytologic features mimicking CIS
  - Bizarre giant cells and multinucleated cells are often present
  - Stroma contains extravasated erythrocytes, inflammation, and hemosiderin deposition
  - Late changes include collagenization of the lamina propria, myointimal proliferation or hyalinization of the arteriole's media, and often ulceration with fibrinous exudate

- Hemorrhagic cystitis
  - Lamina propria shows hemorrhage and congested blood vessels
  - Urothelium shows regenerative changes including nuclear pleomorphism
  - Healing may result in hyperplastic urothelium with papillae formation
  - Repeated bouts may result in a fibrotic, contracted bladder

Special Stains and Immunohistochemistry

- Acid-fast stain rarely reveals the presence of microorganisms in BCG cystitis

Other Techniques for Diagnosis

- Noncontributory

Differential Diagnosis

- Bacterial cystitis
  - Inflammatory component consists of acute inflammatory cells
  - Bladder culture may yield positive results
- Urothelial CIS
  - Cytologic atypia and architectural distortion are more pronounced and mitoses are frequently found

Pearls

- Acute symptoms of radiation cystitis may appear 4 to 6 weeks after initiation of treatment; late symptoms appear as late as 10 years later
- Pathologist must be aware that these changes may be seen with a remote radiation or chemotherapy history
- Accurate clinical history is key to avoiding misdiagnosis

Selected References

Shelley MD, Wilt TJ, Court J, et al: Intravesical bacillus Calmette-Guerin is superior to mitomycin C in reducing tumour recurrence in high-risk superficial bladder cancer: A meta-analysis of randomized trials. BJU Int 93:485-490, 2004.

Chan TY, Epstein JI: Radiation or chemotherapy cystitis with "pseudocarcinomatous" features. Am J Surg Pathol 28:909-913, 2004.

Hoffman JA, Shah AJ, Ross LA, Kapoor N: Adenoviral infections and a prospective trial of cidofovir in pediatric hematopoietic stem cell transplantation. Biol Blood Marrow Transplant 7:388-394, 2001.

Interstitial (Hunner) Cystitis

Clinical Features

- Classically occurs in middle-aged and elderly women
- Interstitial cystitis is manifested by sensory hypersensitivity; patients present with urinary frequency, urgency, nocturia, suprapubic pressure, and pelvic and bladder pain

- Hematuria may be seen
- Urine is sterile and thus bladder culture is negative

Gross Pathology

- Cystoscopy shows small areas of hemorrhage and small linear ulcerations in the mucosa (Hunner ulcer)
- Scarring of bladder mucosa is often noted
- Long-standing cases may result in a fibrotic, contracted bladder with markedly diminished capacity
- Usually affects dome and posterolateral bladder walls

Histopathology

- Nonulcerative or early disease
  — Multiple microhemorrhages are present within the lamina propria (glomerulations)
- Classic phase (Hunner ulcer)
  — Single or multiple patches of reddened ulcerated or denuded bladder mucosa with fibrinous exudate often seen admixed with chronic inflammatory cells, including lymphocytes, plasma cells, and mast cells
  — Characteristic feature is increase in mast cells within the mucosa, lamina propria, and muscularis propria
  — Hemorrhage, edema, congestion, and fibrosis are also seen
  — Occasionally there is no ulceration of the mucosa; only chronic inflammation, edema, hemorrhage, and granulation tissue are seen

Special Stains and Immunohistochemistry

- Noncontributory

Other Techniques for Diagnosis

- Noncontributory

Differential Diagnosis

▌ Flat urothelial CIS
- Denuding CIS exhibits ulceration, vascular congestion, and inflammation resembling interstitial cystitis
- Multiple tissue sections should be examined to search for atypical cells

▌ Bacterial cystitis
- Inflammatory component consists of acute inflammatory cells
- No increase in mast cells
- Bladder culture may yield positive results

▌ Noninfectious cystitis
- Features of polypoid cystitis, follicular cystitis, giant cell cystitis, or hemorrhagic cystitis
- No increase in mast cells

Pearls

- The histologic features are nonspecific and must be correlated with clinical impression

- Exclude CIS before rendering a diagnosis of interstitial cystitis

Selected References

Sant GR, Kempuraj D, Marchand JE, Theoharides TC: The mast cell in interstitial cystitis: Role in pathophysiology and pathogenesis. Urology 69(4 Suppl):34-40, 2007.

Mayer R: Interstitial cystitis pathogenesis and treatment. Curr Opin Infect Dis 20:77-82, 2007.

Chai TC, Keay S: New theories in interstitial cystitis. Nat Clin Pract Urol 1:85-89, 2004.

Moldwin RM, Sant GR: Interstitial cystitis: A pathophysiology and treatment update. Clin Obstet Gynecol 45:259-272, 2002.

Cystitis Cystica et Glandularis

Clinical Features

- Common non-neoplastic lesion of the bladder
- Believed to be induced by chronic inflammatory stimulus
- Found most commonly in adults; occasionally seen in children
- Cystoscopically may occasionally mimic carcinoma

Gross Pathology

▌ Cystitis cystica
- Small submucosal cysts filled with clear yellow fluid

▌ Cystitis glandularis
- May not always be grossly visible
- Occasionally see irregular nodular mucosa

Figure 10-5. Cystitis cystica et glandularis. The lamina propria shows cystically dilated glands lined by urothelial cells (*right*). In some cases, the epithelial lining undergoes glandular metaplasia with intestinal-type goblet cells (*left*). This variant is called *cystitis glandularis with intestinal metaplasia.*

Histopathology

- Cystitis cystica
  - Von Brunn nests within the lamina propria showing central cystic dilation with spaces lined by transitional or low cuboidal epithelium
  - Cysts are often filled with pale eosinophilic fluid
- Cystitis glandularis
  - Epithelial lining of von Brunn nests undergoes glandular metaplasia
  - Glands are lined by cuboidal to columnar cells without anaplasia
  - Cells may contain mucin; occasionally, goblet cells are present
  - If the epithelium acquires intestinal-type goblet cells, this variant is called *cystitis glandularis with intestinal metaplasia* (colonic metaplasia)

Special Stains and Immunohistochemistry

- Reactive urothelium shows CK20 immunoreactivity in only the umbrella cell layer
- Predominantly negative p53 nuclear staining; occasional weak positivity is shown in the basal and parabasal intermediate cells
- CD44 can be overexpressed in the entire reactive urothelium or can be focally positive in intermediate cells

Other Techniques for Diagnosis

- Noncontributory

Differential Diagnosis

- Urothelial carcinoma, nested variant
  - Florid von Brunn nests can be differentiated from nested variant of urothelial carcinoma by its lobular or linear array of the nests, flat noninfiltrative base, and lack of cytologic atypia
- Adenocarcinoma
  - Rare bladder neoplasm
  - Atypical glands lined by stratified pleomorphic cells with infiltration into the muscular layer
  - Signet ring cells may be seen

Pearls

- Florid von Brunn nests, cystitis cystica, and cystitis glandularis are closely related reactive changes that may be seen in any portion of the urothelial tract
- Cystitis cystica et glandularis has no direct association with bladder cancer; coincidental coexistence may be seen
- Cystitis glandularis may be confused with adenocarcinoma, especially if extravasated mucin is present
- Believed to be associated with chronically irritated bladders; may resolve if source of inflammation is removed

Selected References

Tamas EF, Epstein JI: Detection of residual tumor cells in bladder biopsy specimens: Pitfalls in the interpretation of cytokeratin stains. Am J Surg Pathol 31:390-397, 2007.

Volmar KE, Chan TY, De Marzo AM, Epstein JI: Florid von Brunn nests mimicking urothelial carcinoma: A morphologic and immunohistochemical comparison to the nested variant of urothelial carcinoma. Am J Surg Pathol 27:1243-1252, 2003.

McKenney JK, Desai S, Cohen C, Amin MB: Discriminatory immunohistochemical staining of urothelial carcinoma in situ and non-neoplastic urothelium: An analysis of cytokeratin 20, p53, and CD44 antigens. Am J Surg Pathol 25:1074-1078, 2001.

Young RH, Bostwick DG: Florid cystitis glandularis of intestinal type with mucin extravasation: A mimic of adenocarcinoma. Am J Surg Pathol 20:1462-1468, 1996.

Nephrogenic Adenoma

Clinical Features

- Most cases involve the bladder; occasionally found in the urethra, ureter, or renal pelvis
- Found in young adults with a male predominance (2:1)
- About half of the cases are found after genitourinary surgery, including renal transplantation
- Also associated with calculi, trauma, and cystitis
- Often asymptomatic, although patients frequently present with hematuria or dysuria

Gross Pathology

- Usually found over the posterior bladder wall
- May present as a papillary or polypoid exophytic mass or velvety lesion
- Sessile forms make up about 25% to 30% of cases
- Papillary structures usually measure less than 1 cm; may rarely measure greater than 5 cm

Histopathology

- Classic histologic pattern is that of small tubules resembling renal tubules
- May also see papillary architecture
- Tubules are lined by hobnail cells resembling endothelial-lined vascular spaces
- Tubules are often surrounded by a layer of hyalinized basement membrane
- Cells with oxyphilic or clear cytoplasm, or signet ring–like cells, may also be seen
- Mitotic activity is rare
- Pale eosinophilic secretions are often found within the tubules
- A variable degree of acute and chronic inflammation and stromal edema are common in the background

Special Stains and Immunohistochemistry

- Cytokeratin 7 (CK7) and PAX2 positive in the tubular lining cells

Figure 10-6. Nephrogenic adenoma. A, Proliferation of small tubules lined by cuboidal epithelium. No mitotic activity or nuclear pleomorphism is noted. Tubules are often surrounded by a layer of hyalinized basement membrane. Pale eosinophilic secretions are often found within the tubules. **B,** Papillary fronds lined by cuboidal eosinophilic cells with occasional hobnail features.

- Focal and weak prostate-specific antigen (PSA) and prostatic acid phosphatase (PAP) expression is detected in a subset of cases
- Most cases positive for α-methylacyl coenzyme A racemase (AMACR) and negative for high-molecular-weight cytokeratin (34BE12)

Other Techniques for Diagnosis
- Noncontributory

Differential Diagnosis
▪ Prostatic and clear cell adenocarcinoma
- Not typically associated with other clinical conditions
- Tubules with prominent nucleoli sometimes situated within muscle bundles
- Usually much larger
- Shows greater cytologic atypia and high mitotic rate

▪ Low-grade papillary urothelial carcinoma
  - Papillae are covered by neoplastic urothelial cells rather than benign-appearing cuboidal cells
  - Nested variant of urothelial carcinoma exhibits greater atypia and increased mitoses at the deep invasive fronts
▪ Capillary hemangioma
  - Negative for CK7 and positive for endothelial markers, such as CD31

Pearls
  - Benign metaplastic process rather than a neoplastic condition

Selected References

Tong GX, Melamed J, Mansukhani M, et al: PAX2: A reliable marker for nephrogenic adenoma. Mod Pathol 19:356-363, 2006.
Gupta A, Wang HL, Policarpio-Nicolas ML, et al: Expression of alpha-methylacyl-coenzyme A racemase in nephrogenic adenoma. Am J Surg Pathol 28:1224-1229, 2004.
Mazal PR, Schaufler R, Altenhuber-Muller R, et al: Derivation of nephrogenic adenomas from renal tubular cells in kidney-transplant recipients. N Engl J Med 347:653-659, 2002.

Flat Urothelial Lesions

Urothelial Hyperplasia

Clinical Features
- Rare benign urothelial lesion; it may be seen in the flat mucosa adjacent to low-grade papillary urothelial lesion

Gross Pathology
- Noncontributory

Histopathology
- Thickened urothelial mucosa without cytologic atypia
- Marked thickening, rather than a specific number of cell layers, is needed for the diagnosis of flat hyperplasia

Special Stains and Immunohistochemistry
- Noncontributory

Modern Techniques for Diagnosis
- Frequent deletions of chromosome 9 detected by fluorescence in situ hybridization (FISH) have been previously reported in urothelial hyperplasias found in patients with papillary bladder cancer

Differential Diagnosis
▪ Urothelial dysplasia
  - Variable, often appreciable, loss of cell polarity with nuclear crowding and cytologic atypia that is not severe enough to merit a diagnosis of CIS

▌ Urothelial CIS
  - Pleomorphism, prominent nucleoli throughout the urothelium; and upper-level mitoses

Pearls

- Regarded in the 2003 WHO/ISUP classification as a lesion without malignant potential
- Molecular analysis has shown that urothelial hyperplasia in bladder cancer patients may be chronically related to papillary tumors
- In the absence of an associated papillary urothelial neoplasm, no treatment or follow-up is required

Selected References

van Oers JM, Adam C, Denzinger S, et al: Chromosome 9 deletions are more frequent than FGFR3 mutations in flat urothelial hyperplasias of the bladder. Int J Cancer 119:1212-1215, 2006.

Epstein JI: Urothelial hyperplasia. In Eble JN, Sauter G, Epstein JI, Sesterhann IA (eds): World Health Organization Classification of Tumours: Pathology and Genetics: Tumors of the Urinary System and Male Genital Organs. Lyon, IARC Press, 2004, p 111.

Hartmann A, Moser K, Kriegmair M, et al: Frequent genetic alterations in simple urothelial hyperplasias of the bladder in patients with papillary urothelial carcinoma. Am J Pathol 154:721-727, 1999.

Urothelial Dysplasia

Clinical Features

- De novo dysplasia affects predominantly middle-aged men presenting occasionally with irritative bladder symptoms with or without hematuria

Figure 10-7. Urothelial dysplasia. The urothelium shows nuclear crowding and cytologic atypia. The cells have mildly altered chromatin distribution, slightly enlarged nuclei, inconspicuous nucleoli, and rare mitoses.

Gross Pathology

- Lesion may be inapparent or associated with erythema, erosion, or rarely ulceration

Histopathology

- Variable, often appreciable, loss of cell polarity with nuclear crowding and cytologic atypia that is not severe enough to merit a diagnosis of CIS
- Cells may have mildly altered chromatin distribution, slightly enlarged nuclei, inconspicuous nucleoli, and rare mitoses
- Thickness of the urothelium is usually normal but may also be increased or decreased
- Lamina propria may contain increased inflammatory cells or neovascularity
- May involve von Brunn nests

Special Stains and Immunohistochemistry

- Aberrant CK20 expression
- Overexpression of p53 and Ki-67

Other Techniques for Diagnosis

- Alteration of chromosome 9 and *p53* allelic losses have been demonstrated

Differential Diagnosis

▌ Urothelial CIS
  - Typically shows pleomorphism and prominent nucleoli throughout the urothelium
  - Increased mitotic activity with upper-level mitosis
▌ Reactive inflammatory atypia
  - Presence of acute and chronic inflammation

Pearls

- Dysplasia in patients with noninvasive papillary neoplasms indicates urothelial instability and a marker for progression or recurrence
- De novo dysplasia progresses to urothelial neoplasia in 5% to 19% of patients

Selected References

Amin MB, McKenney JK: An approach to the diagnosis of flat intraepithelial lesions of the urinary bladder using the World Health Organization/International Society of Urological Pathology consensus classification system. Adv Anat Pathol 9:222-232, 2002.

Hartmann A, Schlake G, Zaak D, et al: Occurrence of chromosome 9 and p53 alterations in multifocal dysplasia and CIS of human urinary bladder. Cancer Res 62:809-818, 2002.

Urothelial Carcinoma In Situ

Clinical Features

- Patients are usually in their fifth or sixth decade
- Asymptomatic or symptomatic with dysuria, frequency, urgency, or even hematuria

Figure 10-8. Urothelial carcinoma in situ. The entire thickness of the urinary bladder epithelium is replaced by neoplastic cells. There is complete loss of polarity, marked crowding, and pleomorphism. Nuclei are hyperchromatic and have a coarse or condensed chromatin distribution.

- CIS is commonly multifocal and may be diffuse
- De novo (primary) CIS accounts for less than 1% to 3% of urothelial neoplasms but is seen with 45% to 65% of invasive urothelial carcinomas

Gross Pathology

- Bladder mucosa may be unremarkable or erythematous and edematous

Histopathology

- Urothelial CIS is a nonpapillary (i.e., flat) lesion in which the surface epithelium contains cells that are cytologically malignant
- The term *carcinoma in situ* is synonymous with *high-grade intraurothelial neoplasia*
- *Nuclear anaplasia* is identical to *high-grade papillary urothelial carcinoma*
- Urothelium may be denuded, diminished in thickness, of normal thickness, or even hyperplastic
- There may be complete loss of polarity, marked crowding, and pleomorphism
- Nuclei are frequently hyperchromatic and have a coarse or condensed chromatin distribution

Special Stains and Immunohistochemistry

- CK20: diffuse strong cytoplasmic staining
- p53: Nuclear staining may be diffuse throughout the full thickness
- CD44: expression limited to residual basal cell layer or negative

Other Techniques for Diagnosis

- Chromosome 9 deletions and *p53* allelic losses have been demonstrated frequently

Differential Diagnosis

▎ Urothelial dysplasia
  - Cytologic atypia is not severe enough to merit a diagnosis of CIS
  - Lacks pleomorphism (comparable to high-grade papillary carcinoma), discohesion, or mitoses in the upper urothelium
▎ Reactive atypia
  - Lacks nuclear pleomorphism
  - Presence of acute and chronic inflammation

Pearls

- De novo CIS is less likely than secondary CIS to progress to invasive disease
- BCG immunotherapy remains the most effective treatment and prophylaxis for CIS, reducing short-term tumor recurrence by about 20%, long-term recurrence by about 7%, disease progression, and mortality

Selected References

Yin H, He Q, Li T, Leong AS: Cytokeratin 20 and Ki-67 to distinguish carcinoma in situ from flat non-neoplastic urothelium. Appl Immunohistochem Mol Morphol 14:260-265, 2006.

Amling CL: Diagnosis and management of superficial bladder cancer. Curr Probl Cancer 25:219-278, 2001.

McKenney JK, Desai S, Cohen C, Amin MB: Discriminatory immunohistochemical staining of urothelial carcinoma in situ and non-neoplastic urothelium: an analysis of cytokeratin 20, p53, and CD44 antigens. Am J Surg Pathol 25:1074-1078, 2001.

Papillary Urothelial Lesions

Papillary Urothelial Hyperplasia

Clinical Features

- Typically discovered on routine follow-up cystoscopy for papillary urothelial neoplasms

Gross Features

- Benign focally elevated lesion identified at cystoscopy, described as papillary, raised, sessile, or bleblike

Histopathology

- Undulating urothelium arranged into mucosal narrow papillary folds of varying heights
- The urothelium within papillary hyperplasia and the adjacent flat mucosa are often thicker than normal
- Cytologic findings are similar to those characteristic of normal urothelium

Special Stains and Immunohistochemistry

- Noncontributory

Other Techniques for Diagnosis

- Noncontributory

Differential Diagnosis

▌ Urothelial papilloma
- Well-developed, branching fibrovascular cores of a papillary neoplasm are evident

Pearls

- Patients should be followed because papillary hyperplasia likely represents the precursor lesion to low-grade papillary urothelial neoplasms

Selected References

Swierczynski SL, Epstein JI: Prognostic significance of atypical papillary urothelial hyperplasia. Hum Pathol 33:512-517, 2002.

Taylor DC, Bhagavan BS, Larsen MP, et al: Papillary urothelial hyperplasia: A precursor to papillary neoplasms. Am J Surg Pathol 20:1481-1488, 1996.

Urothelial Papilloma

Clinical Features

- Benign papillary urothelial tumor lined by normal-appearing urothelium
- Slightly more common in men
- Tends to occur in younger patients and is seen in children
- Usually presents with gross hematuria

Gross Features

- Urothelial papillomas typically have a simple papillary architecture

Figure 10-9. Urothelial papilloma. Papillary fronds are lined by normal-appearing urothelium. Superficial umbrella cells are often prominent, with abundant eosinophilic cytoplasm and vacuolization.

Histopathology

- Papillary fronds are lined by normal-appearing urothelium, lacking atypia
- Usually have a simple, minimally branching arrangement, slender fibrovascular stalks, with a predominantly exophytic pattern
- Superficial umbrella cells are often prominent, with abundant eosinophilic cytoplasm and vacuolization
- Mitoses are rare or absent

Special Stains and Immunohistochemistry

- Cytokeratin 20: confined to the umbrella cells, similarly to normal urothelium

Other Techniques for Diagnosis

- Noncontributory

Differential Diagnosis

▌ Papillary neoplasm of low malignant potential (PUNLMP)
- Thickened urothelium
- Mitoses may be present but are confined to the basal layers

Pearls

- Rarely recur; can progress to higher-grade disease
- Complete transurethral resection is treatment of choice

Selected References

Magi-Galluzzi C, Epstein JI: Urothelial papilloma of the bladder: A review of 34 de novo cases. Am J Surg Pathol 28:1615-1620, 2004.

McKenney JK, Amin MB, Young RH: Urothelial (transitional cell) papilloma of the urinary bladder: A clinicopathologic study of 26 cases. Mod Pathol 16:623-629, 2003.

Inverted Papilloma

Clinical Features

- Rare benign urothelial tumor of unknown etiology
- More common in males and occurs at all ages; median age is 55 years
- Typically involves the bladder at the trigone, bladder neck, or prostatic urethra
- Frequently presents with hematuria

Gross Pathology

- Typically solitary flat or slightly raised polypoid mass with smooth contours
- Usually minimal exophytic component
- Most are less than 3 cm in diameter

Histopathology

- Anastomosing cords or islands of urothelium showing minimal cytologic atypia; rare mitotic activity

Figure 10-10. Inverted papilloma. A, The tumor originates from the surface urothelium and extends down into the underlying lamina propria. It forms anastomosing cords or islands of urothelium. **B,** The urothelial cells show minimal cytologic atypia.

- Tumor originates from the surface urothelium and extends down into the underlying lamina propria but not into the muscular bladder wall
- Small cystic spaces and true glandular differentiation with a layer of mucin-secreting cells may be seen
- Minimal stromal component that lacks inflammation

Special Stains and Immunohistochemistry
- Noncontributory

Other Techniques for Diagnosis
- Noncontributory

Differential Diagnosis
▪ Urothelial carcinoma
  - Typically shows an exophytic papillary architecture
  - Increased cytologic atypia and increased mitotic activity
  - Invasive growth pattern is often noted

▪ Florid proliferation of von Brunn nests
  - Round nests without the anastomosing pattern

Pearls
- Relationship between inverted papilloma and low-grade papillary urothelial carcinoma is not fully understood
- Inverted papilloma is best treated by transurethral resection; occasional recurrences have been reported
- Occasionally, coexistence with papillary urothelial carcinoma has been described, although it is unresolved whether there is an increased risk for this relationship

Selected References

Sung MT, MacLennan GT, Lopez-Beltran A, et al: Natural history of urothelial inverted papilloma. Cancer 107:2622-2627, 2006.

Ho H, Chen YD, Tan PH, et al: Inverted papilloma of urinary bladder: Is long-term cystoscopic surveillance needed? A single center's experience. Urology 68:333-336, 2006.

Broussard JN, Tan PH, Epstein JI: Atypia in inverted urothelial papillomas: Pathology and prognostic significance. Hum Pathol 35:1499-1504, 2004.

Papillary Urothelial Neoplasm of Low Malignant Potential

Clinical Features
- Papillary urothelial neoplasm lined by urothelium with minimal atypia
- Slightly more common in men
- Mean age at diagnosis is 64.6 years (range, 29 to 94 years)
- Usually presents with gross or microscopic hematuria

Figure 10-11. Papillary urothelial neoplasm of low malignant potential. A discrete and slender papillary frond lined by a thickened multilayered urothelium with minimal to absent cytologic atypia.

Gross Features

- Small to 2-cm papillary tumor

Histopathology

- Discrete and slender papillary fronds lined by a thickened multilayered urothelium with minimal to absent cytologic atypia
- Cell density appears to be increased compared with normal
- Polarity is preserved
- Mitoses are rare and have a basal location

Special Stains and Immunohistochemistry

- Cytokeratin 20: confined to the umbrella cells

Other Techniques for Diagnosis

- Noncontributory

Differential Diagnosis

- ▌ Noninvasive low-grade papillary urothelial carcinoma
  - Scattered cells with enlarged hyperchromatic nuclei
  - More than rare mitotic figures
- ▌ Urothelial papilloma
  - Lining urothelium is of normal thickness

Pearls

- Recurrence is at a lower frequency than with papillary carcinoma
- Transurethral resection is the treatment of choice

Selected References

Jones TD, Cheng L: Papillary urothelial neoplasm of low malignant potential: Evolving terminology and concepts. J Urol 175:1995-2003, 2006.

Fine SW, Humprey PA, Dehner LP, et al: Urothelial neoplasms in patients 20 years or younger: A clinicopathological analysis using the world health organization 2004 bladder consensus classification. J Urol 174:1976-1980, 2005.

Campbell PA, Conrad RJ, Campbell CM, et al: Papillary urothelial neoplasm of low malignant potential: Reliability of diagnosis and outcome. BJU Int 93:1228-1231, 2004.

Noninvasive Low-Grade Papillary Urothelial Carcinoma

Clinical Features

- Papillary neoplasm lined by urothelium with easily recognizable variation in architectural and cytologic features
- Slightly more common in men
- Mean age at diagnosis is 69.2 (range, 28 to 90 years)
- Usually presents with gross or microscopic hematuria

Gross Features

- In most cases, the papillary tumor is single

Figure 10-12. Noninvasive low-grade papillary urothelial carcinoma. A slender papillary frond lined by an orderly urothelium with easily recognizable variations in architectural and cytologic features. The nuclei are uniformly enlarged, with mild differences in shape, contour, and chromatin distribution.

Histopathology

- Slender papillary fronds showing frequent branching and minimal fusion
- Orderly appearance with easily recognizable variations in architectural and cytologic features
- Nuclei are uniformly enlarged with mild differences in shape, contour, and chromatin distribution
- Mitoses are infrequent and may occur at any level

Special Stains and Immunohistochemistry

- Expression of p53 and Ki-67 is intermediate between PUNLMP and high-grade urothelial carcinoma

Other Techniques for Diagnosis

- Allelic loss of multiple chromosome loci has been reported

Differential Diagnosis

- ▌ Papillary urothelial neoplasm of low malignant potential
  - Monotonous bland-appearing cells, lacking scattered cells with enlarged hyperchromatic nuclei
  - Rare mitotic figure
- ▌ High-grade papillary urothelial carcinoma
  - High degree of cytologic atypia with architectural distortion

Pearls

- Recurrence is common and occurs in about 48% to 71% of patients
- Progression to invasion and cancer deaths occurs in less than 5% of cases
- Transurethral resection is treatment of choice; multifocal or recurrent disease is sometimes treated with intravesical immunotherapy

Selected References

Vardar E, Gunlusoy B, Minareci S, et al: Evaluation of p53 nuclear accumulation in low- and high-grade (WHO/ISUP classification) transitional papillary carcinomas of the bladder for tumor recurrence and progression. Urol Int 77:27-33, 2006.

Wu XR: Urothelial tumorigenesis: A tale of divergent pathways. Nat Rev Cancer 5:713-725, 2005.

Noninvasive High-Grade Papillary Urothelial Carcinoma

Clinical Features

- Papillary neoplasm characterized by a disorderly appearance of urothelium resulting from marked architectural and cytologic abnormalities, recognizable at low magnification
- Usually presents with gross or microscopic hematuria

Gross Features

- Appearance varies from papillary to nodular and solid sessile lesion

Histopathology

- Papillae are frequently fused and branching, although some may be delicate; extensive denudation may be present
- Cytologically, there is a spectrum of pleomorphism ranging from moderate to marked
- There is marked variation in nuclear polarity, size, shape, and chromatin pattern; nucleoli may be prominent
- Mitotic figures, including atypical forms, are frequently seen at all levels of the urothelium

Special Stains and Immunohistochemistry

- Detection of p53 and Ki-67 is more frequent than in low-grade urothelial carcinoma

Other Techniques for Diagnosis

- Deletion of chromosome 9p appears to be an early event in the development of papillary urothelial carcinoma

Differential Diagnosis

▌ Low-grade papillary urothelial carcinoma
  - Mild degree of cytologic atypia with lack of architectural distortion

Pearls

- Invasion both within the papillary cores and at the base of the lesions should be ruled out

Selected References

Owens CL, Epstein JI: Significance of denuded urothelium in papillary urothelial lesions. Am J Surg Pathol 31:298-303, 2007.

MacLennan GT, Kirkali Z, Cheng L: Histologic grading of noninvasive papillary urothelial neoplasms. Eur Urol 51:889-897, 2007.

Yin H, Leong AS: Histologic grading of noninvasive papillary urothelial tumors: Validation of the 1998 WHO/ISUP system by immunophenotyping and follow-up. Am J Clin Pathol 121:679-687, 2004.

Invasive Urothelial Carcinoma

Clinical Features

- Typically found in elderly individuals with a mean age greater than 65 years

Figure 10-13. Noninvasive high-grade papillary urothelial carcinoma. Papillae are frequently fused and branching. Cytologically, there is moderate to marked pleomorphism with marked variation in nuclear polarity, size, shape, and chromatin pattern.

Figure 10-14. High-grade urothelial carcinoma invading lamina propria. Foci of invasion are characterized by urothelial nests within the lamina propria.

- More frequently seen in men (3:1)
- Associated with tobacco smoking, toxic chemicals (including nitrosamines), drugs (phenacetin, cyclophosphamide), and infections (*Schistosoma haematobium*)
- Most common presenting symptom is painless hematuria
- Patients may have flank pain and obstructive symptoms

Gross Features

- Tumors usually involve the lateral or posterior bladder walls; occasionally involve the bladder dome
- Low-grade tumors typically have a papillary architecture appearing as multiple finger-like fronds over the bladder mucosa (see "Noninvasive Low-Grade Papillary Urothelial Carcinoma")
- Higher-grade tumors often lack papillary architecture and show nodular, polypoid, or sessile pattern (see "Noninvasive High-Grade Papillary Urothelial Carcinoma"); focal remnants of papillary architecture may persist
- Bladder wall is typically thickened, firm, and gray-white
- Ulceration and hemorrhage is often seen in the high-grade tumors

Histopathology

▮ Urothelial carcinoma invading lamina propria (pT1)
- Foci of invasion are characterized by urothelial nests, clusters, or single cells within the papillary cores or lamina propria
- Grow in solid cords or nests; nuclear palisading is often seen at periphery of nests
- Reactive desmoplastic stroma surrounds infiltrating nests of tumor cells
- Foci of invasive tumor may be associated with retraction artifact, mimicking vascular invasion

▮ Urothelial carcinoma invading muscularis propria (pT2)
- Usually nonpapillary tumors infiltrate the underlying muscularis propria
- Muscularis propria invasion is diagnosed when carcinoma infiltrates between thick distinct fascicles of muscle bundles
- Muscle invasion may or may not elicit a desmoplastic stromal response
- Even in cases of noninvasive disease, the pathologist should note whether muscularis propria is present in the biopsy specimen

▮ Urothelial carcinoma invading adipose tissue and surrounding organs (pT3 and pT4)
- Adipose tissue is often present between detrusor muscle bundles; thus, the presence of tumor in fat in a biopsy does not necessarily equate with involvement of perivesical fat

▮ Urothelial carcinoma: histologic variants
- Infiltrating urothelial carcinoma with squamous differentiation
  — Most common pattern of the divergent differentiation in urothelial carcinoma
  — Occurs in 21% of urothelial carcinomas of the bladder and 44% of tumors of the renal pelvis
  — Clinical significance of squamous differentiation remains uncertain
- Infiltrating urothelial carcinoma with glandular differentiation
  — Tubular or enteric glands with mucin secretions may be present in about 6% of urothelial carcinoma of the bladder
- Infiltrating urothelial carcinoma, nested variant
  — Aggressive neoplasm, with 70% of the patients dead 4 to 40 months after diagnosis, despite therapy
  — This variant has a deceptively benign appearance that closely resembles von Brunn nests infiltrating the lamina propria
- Infiltrating urothelial carcinoma, micropapillary variant
  — Resembles papillary serous carcinoma of the ovary
  — Surface of the tumors shows slender, delicate papillary and villiform processes, often with a central vascular core
  — Invasive portion is characterized by minute nests of cells or fine papillae contained within tissue retraction spaces, simulating lymphatic spaces
  — Tumors are invariably muscle invasive, high grade
- Infiltrating urothelial carcinoma, lymphoepithelioma like
  — Proportion of lymphoepithelioma-like carcinoma should be reported
  — Behavior is uncertain because only few cases have been reported
  — Pure form of lymphoepithelioma-like carcinoma is responsive to chemotherapy

Grading of Urothelial Carcinoma

- See "Noninvasive Low-Grade Papillary Urothelial Carcinoma" and "Noninvasive High-Grade Papillary Urothelial Carcinoma"

Special Stains and Immunohistochemistry

- Cytokeratin (high molecular weight, CK7, CK20) positive
- Positive for p63 and Leu-M1 (CD15)
- CEA positive (especially in high-grade tumors)

Other Techniques for Diagnosis

- Cytogenetic studies: deletion of chromosome 9p is associated with superficial disease; abnormalities involving chromosome 17p are associated with disease progression

Differential Diagnosis

- Polypoid cystitis
  - Must be distinguished from low-grade papillary transitional cell carcinoma
  - Usually shows wider papillary structures and stromal edema
  - Urothelium may show reactive atypia but usually less dysplasia than in transitional cell carcinoma
- Von Brunn nests
  - Must be distinguished from the nested variant of urothelial carcinoma
  - Presence of muscle invasion, smaller and irregularly invading crowded nests
  - Tendency for increasing atypia in the deeper portion of the lesion
- Nephrogenic adenoma
  - Must be distinguished from the glandular component of urothelial carcinoma with glandular differentiation
  - Classic histologic pattern is that of small tubules resembling renal tubules
  - Papillary architecture can be confused with urothelial carcinoma
  - Papillae and tubules are lined by benign cuboidal cells
- Inverted papilloma
  - Minimal cytologic atypia and low mitotic activity
  - Lacks invasion into the muscularis propria
- Squamous cell carcinoma
  - Pure squamous lesions lacking a urothelial component
  - If a urothelial component is seen, the lesion should be classified as urothelial carcinoma with squamous differentiation
- Lymphoma
  - Must be distinguished from the lymphoepithelioma-like variant of urothelial carcinoma
  - Islands of high-grade epithelial cells are not seen
  - Cytokeratin is diffusely negative
  - Leukocyte common antigen (LCA) is diffusely positive
- Prostatic adenocarcinoma
  - Must be distinguished from poorly differentiated bladder cancer
  - Specimen is often obtained from the trigone or bladder neck
  - Negative for p63 and thrombomodulin
  - PSA, prostate-specific acid phosphatase (PSAP), and p501s (protein) positive

Pearls

- Urine cytology is a valuable tool for management of patients with bladder cancer (best used to monitor therapeutic response)
- Superficial urothelial tumors include tumors confined to the lamina propria (stage T1); invasive cancer includes lesions that have invaded the superficial muscularis propria (detrusor muscle) (stage T2a) or deep muscularis propria (stage T2b), perivesical tissue (stage T3), and contiguous organs or tissues (stage T4)
- Low-grade urothelial carcinoma when completely excised virtually never metastasizes
- Pathologist must comment on whether the biopsy material contains muscularis propria (detrusor muscle) and also whether there is muscularis propria invasion
- Superficial tumors have traditionally been treated with transurethral resection, and muscle invasive tumors have required radical cystectomy

Selected References

Magi-Galluzzi C, Zhou M, Epstein JI: Neoplasms of the urinary bladder. In Genitourinary Pathology: A Volume in Foundations in Diagnostic Pathology Series. Philadelphia, Churchill Livingstone, 2007, pp 176-189.

Tamas EF, Nielsen ME, Schoenberg MP, Epstein JI: Lymphoepithelioma-like carcinoma of the urinary tract: A clinicopathological study of 30 pure and mixed cases. Mod Pathol 20:828-834, 2007.

Lopez-Beltran A, Cheng L: Histologic variants of urothelial carcinoma: Differential diagnosis and clinical implications. Hum Pathol 37:1371-1388, 2006.

Lopez-Beltran A, Sauter G, Gasser T, et al: Infiltrating urothelial carcinoma. In Eble JN, Sauter G, Epstein JI, Sesterhenn IA (eds): World Health Organization Classification of Tumours: Pathology and Genetics: Tumours of the Urinary System and Male Genital Organs. Lyon, IARC Press, 2004, pp 93-109.

Samaratunga H, Khoo K: Micropapillary variant of urothelial carcinoma of the urinary bladder: A clinicopathological and immunohistochemical study. Histopathology 45:55-64, 2004.

Other Neoplastic Conditions

Villous Adenoma

Clinical Features

- Rare glandular neoplasm of the urinary bladder that histologically mimics its enteric counterpart
- Occurs in elderly patients (mean age, 65 years)
- Most common locations are the urachus, dome, and trigone
- Patients often present with hematuria and irritative symptoms, occasionally with mucosuria
- Often coexists with in situ or invasive adenocarcinoma

Gross Features

- Papillary tumor indistinguishable from papillary urothelial carcinoma

Histopathology

- Blunt finger-like papillary architecture with central fibrovascular core, lined by pseudostratified columnar epithelium

Figure 10-15. Villous adenoma. A, A neoplasm with blunt finger-like papillary architecture with a central fibrovascular core, lined by pseudostratified columnar epithelium. **B,** Epithelial cells display nuclear stratification, crowding, hyperchromasia, and occasional prominent nucleoli.

● Epithelial cells display nuclear stratification, crowding, hyperchromasia, and occasional prominent nucleoli

Special Stains and Immunohistochemistry

● CK20, CK7, and CEA positive
● Epithelial membrane antigen (EMA) and acid mucin stains frequently positive

Other Techniques for Diagnosis

● Noncontributory

Differential Diagnosis

▌ Well-differentiated adenocarcinoma of the colon or bladder
  ● Degree of cytologic atypia similar to analogous colonic lesions
  ● Invasion into lamina propria

Pearls

● Presence of villous adenoma histology in a limited biopsy does not entirely exclude the possibility of adenocarcinoma, and complete excision is essential

Selected References

Seibel JL, Prasad S, Weiss RE, et al: Villous adenoma of the urinary tract: A lesion frequently associated with malignancy. Hum Pathol 33:236-241, 2002.
Chan TY, Epstein JI: In situ adenocarcinoma of the bladder. Am J Surg Pathol 25:892-899, 2001.

Adenocarcinoma

Clinical Features

● Rare bladder neoplasm constituting less than 2% of all bladder tumors
● Divided into two groups
  — Nonurachal adenocarcinoma
    ◆ Accounts for two thirds of adenocarcinoma of the bladder
    ◆ Found in adults with a mean age of 60 years
    ◆ Most common presenting symptom is gross hematuria, followed by dysuria
    ◆ Up to 40% of patients have metastatic disease at time of diagnosis
    ◆ Occasionally associated with *Schistosoma haematobium* (less common association than with squamous cell carcinoma)
    ◆ About 15% of tumors arise in patients with nonfunctioning bladder, and 85% are associated with exstrophy
  — Urachal adenocarcinoma
    ◆ Primary carcinoma derived from the urachal remnants
    ◆ Occurs in the fifth and sixth decades; mean patient age is 50 years
    ◆ Mucosuria occurs in about 25% of cases

Gross Features

▌ Nonurachal adenocarcinoma
  ● Typically an exophytic, papillary, ulcerating mass arising from the bladder mucosa
  ● Usually involves the trigone or posterior bladder wall
  ● Often shows infiltrative margins
  ● May be sessile and cause a diffuse thickening of the bladder wall (resembles linitis plastica of the stomach); overlying bladder mucosa may be intact, leading to negative biopsies (signet ring cell variant)
▌ Urachal adenocarcinoma
  ● Most form discrete masses over the dome of the bladder
  ● May involve urachal remnants, forming a large mass in the anterior abdominal wall

- Overlying bladder mucosa may be intact or ulcerated
- Cut surface of the mass often shows abundant mucin

Histopathology

▮ Urachal and nonurachal adenocarcinomas
  - Mucinous carcinoma with pools of mucin containing single and groups of neoplastic cells (often resembles colonic adenocarcinoma)
  - Neoplastic glands with an infiltrative growth pattern
  - Glands are lined by large pleomorphic cells with vesicular chromatin and prominent nucleoli; nuclear stratification is also common
  - Signet ring cells may be seen
  - CIS or intestinal metaplasia may be seen in nonurachal adenocarcinoma
▮ Urachal adenocarcinomas
  - Criteria to classify a tumor as urachal adenocarcinoma
    - ◆ Location in the dome or anterior wall of the bladder
    - ◆ Sharp demarcation between tumor and normal surface epithelium
    - ◆ Lack of in situ adenocarcinoma
    - ◆ Typically, adjacent mucosa lacks prominent cystitis glandularis
    - ◆ Bulk of tumor is in the bladder wall rather than luminal
    - ◆ Exclusion of primary adenocarcinoma located elsewhere that has spread secondarily to the bladder

Special Stains and Immunohistochemistry

- CK20 and CEA positive
- CK7 variably positive
- Leu-M1 (CD15) positive
- Villin positive in the enteric type
- CDX2 and nuclear staining for β-catenin negative

Other Techniques for Diagnosis

- Noncontributory

Differential Diagnosis

▮ Cystitis cystica et glandularis
  - Small submucosal cysts with benign cytologic features
  - Typically small lesions without deep infiltration
▮ Nephrogenic adenoma
  - About 50% of cases found after genitourinary surgery
  - Composed of small uniform tubules resembling proximal tubules in the kidney
  - Usually much smaller than adenocarcinoma
▮ Endometriosis
  - Composed of endometrial glands and stroma
  - Hemosiderin-laden macrophages often seen
▮ Metastatic adenocarcinoma
  - Presence of primary adenocarcinoma at distant site must be ruled out

Pearls

- Intestinal metaplasia is precursor lesion in most nonurachal adenocarcinomas
- Treatment of urachal adenocarcinoma includes en bloc resection of the bladder, including the entire urachal tract and umbilicus
- Treatment of nonurachal adenocarcinoma includes cystectomy or cystoprostatectomy with pelvic lymph node dissection
- Overall prognosis is poor for both types

Selected References

Wright JL, Porter MP, Li CI, et al: Differences in survival among patients with urachal and nonurachal adenocarcinomas of the bladder. Cancer 107:721-728, 2006.

Siefker-Radtke A: Urachal carcinoma: Surgical and chemotherapeutic options. Expert Rev Anticancer Ther 6:1715-1721, 2006.

Raspollini MR, Nesi G, Baroni G, et al: Immunohistochemistry in the differential diagnosis between primary and secondary intestinal adenocarcinoma of the urinary bladder. Appl Immunohistochem Mol Morphol 13:358-362, 2005.

Siefker-Radtke AO, Gee J, Shen Y, et al: Multimodality management of urachal carcinoma: The M. D. Anderson Cancer Center experience. J Urol 169:1295-1298, 2003.

Squamous Cell Carcinoma

Clinical Features

- Can involve the urinary bladder, renal pelvis, or occasionally the ureter
- Prevalence varies significantly depending on region of the world; it accounts for less than 5% of bladder carcinomas in areas where infection with *Schistosoma haematobium* is not endemic and 75% in areas where infection is endemic
- Typically affects adults, with a slight male predominance
- Patients typically have a long duration of symptoms of cystitis and often have gross hematuria
- Bladder calculi and indwelling bladder catheters increase risk; tobacco is an important risk factor

Gross Pathology

- Typically large solid tumors, often filling the bladder lumen and infiltrating the bladder wall
- Extensive necrosis is common

Histopathology

- Well-differentiated form consists of well-defined islands of squamous cells with prominent intercellular bridges and minimal pleomorphism; keratin formation is typically abundant
- Poorly differentiated form consists of sheets of neoplastic cells with marked cytologic atypia and focal squamous differentiation

- Squamous metaplasia often seen in adjacent epithelium
- Keratinizing squamous metaplasia or leukoplakia is often seen

Special Stains and Immunohistochemistry
- Noncontributory

Other Techniques for Diagnosis
- Noncontributory

Differential Diagnosis
▍ Urothelial carcinoma with squamous differentiation
  - If urothelial component is present, the tumor should not be classified as a squamous cell carcinoma
  - Urothelial CIS may be present, which is not seen in a pure squamous cell carcinoma
▍ Metastatic squamous cell carcinoma
  - Presence of squamous cell carcinoma from local (cervix) or distant site must be ruled out
▍ Squamous papilloma
  - Lack of cytologic atypia and invasion
▍ Condyloma
  - Presence of koilocytic cells

Pearls
- Constitute about 5% of all malignant bladder tumors
- Overall 5-year survival is 56%: 67% for patients with organ-confined tumor, and 19% for non–organ-confined tumor
- Treatment consists of radial cystectomy or cystoprostatectomy
- Overall poor prognosis
- Commonly develop local recurrence rather than distant metastases
- Metastases when present often involve bone

Selected References

Kassouf W, Spiess PE, Siefker-Radtke A, et al: Outcome and patterns of recurrence of nonbilharzial pure squamous cell carcinoma of the bladder: A contemporary review of the University of Texas M. D. Anderson Cancer Center experience. Cancer 110:764-769, 2007.

El-Sebaie M, Zaghloul MS, Howard G, Mokhtar A: Squamous cell carcinoma of the bilharzial and non-bilharzial urinary bladder: A review of etiological features, natural history, and management. Int J Clin Oncol 1091:20-25, 2005.

Small Cell Carcinoma

Clinical Features
- Constitutes less than 1% of primary bladder tumors
- Typically found in elderly men, with a 4:1 male-to-female ratio
- Most common presenting complaint is gross hematuria
- Patients often have extensive local involvement or distant metastases at time of presentation

Gross Pathology
- Variable size, ranging from 2 cm up to greater than 10 cm
- May have solid or papillary architecture
- Hemorrhage, necrosis, and mucosal ulceration are common

Histopathology
- Resembles small cell carcinoma of other sites
- Uniform population of small to medium-sized cells with nuclear molding, scant cytoplasm, and nuclei with finely stippled chromatin and inconspicuous nucleoli
- Nuclei are hyperchromatic and show prominent folding
- Chromatin is dispersed and nucleoli are inconspicuous
- Mitotic activity is prominent
- Diagnosis can be made on morphologic grounds alone, even if neuroendocrine differentiation cannot be demonstrated immunohistochemically
- Rarely see well-differentiated variant, which has features of carcinoid, including an organoid pattern

Special Stains and Immunohistochemistry
- Neuron-specific enolase (NSE), synaptophysin, and CD56 positive
- Chromogranin positive in one third of cases
- Cytokeratin typically positive, occasionally nonreactive
- LCA negative

Other Techniques for Diagnosis
- Electron microscopy: tumor cells contain numerous dense core neurosecretory granules

Differential Diagnosis
▍ Metastatic small cell carcinoma
  - Clinical correlation is needed to exclude presence of primary small cell carcinoma at distant site
  - Identification of urothelial component, including urothelial CIS, supports a bladder primary
▍ Malignant lymphoma
  - Consists of atypical lymphoid population
  - Positive staining for LCA
  - Negative staining for cytokeratin, synaptophysin, and chromogranin

Pearls
- Aggressive behavior with poor prognosis
- Overall 5-year survival rate for patients with local disease has been reported as low as 8%

• Treatment includes radical cystectomy or cystoprostatectomy in addition to multiagent chemotherapy

Selected References

Wang X, MacLennan GT, Lopez-Beltran A, Cheng L: Small cell carcinoma of the urinary bladder: Histogenesis, genetics, diagnosis, biomarkers, treatment, and prognosis. Appl Immunohistochem Mol Morphol 15:8-18, 2007.

Choong NW, Quevedo JF, Kaur JS: Small cell carcinoma of the urinary bladder: The Mayo Clinic experience. Cancer 103:1172-1178, 2005.

Cheng L, Pan CX, Yang XJ, et al: Small cell carcinoma of the urinary bladder: A clinicopathologic analysis of 64 patients. Cancer 101:957-962, 2004.

Inflammatory Myofibroblastic Tumor and Inflammatory Pseudotumor

Clinical Features

• Typically found in patients in second through fifth decades
• Slightly more common in women
• Usually presents with gross hematuria

Gross Pathology

• Typically pedunculated, nodular mass ranging in size from 2 to 5 cm and extending into the bladder lumen
• May occasionally be sessile and extend into the underlying tissue

Histopathology

• Characterized by myofibroblastic cells resembling tissue culture fibroblasts arranged in fascicles or more haphazardly

• Background usually contains a sparse inflammatory component consisting of lymphocytes and plasma cells; eosinophils may also be numerous
• Prominent network of thin-walled blood vessels in an edematous or myxoid stroma with little to moderate collagen deposition is common
• Spindle cells may show focal pleomorphism
• Mitotic figures may be present and even frequent, but they are not atypical
• Infiltration into the muscularis propria may occur

Special Stains and Immunohistochemistry

• ALK protein positive in two thirds of cases
• Cytokeratin: variable staining pattern
• Vimentin positive
• Smooth muscle actin (SMA) often positive
• Desmin typically negative

Other Techniques for Diagnosis

• Translocation involving chromosome 2p23, site of the *ALK* gene

Differential Diagnosis

▎ Carcinosarcoma
  • Malignant epithelial and malignant mesenchymal components
  • Numerous mitotic figures
  • Lacks inflammatory background
  • Lacks network of thin-walled blood vessels
▎ Leiomyosarcoma
  • Overall rare; however, it is the most common bladder sarcoma in older adults
  • Usually shows infiltrative margins
  • Typically shows cytologic atypia and increased mitotic activity with atypical mitotic figures
  • More commonly shows immunohistochemical evidence of smooth muscle differentiation

Pearls

• Benign spindle cell neoplasm; cured by conservative surgery
• Most common misdiagnosis is that of a sarcoma or sarcomatoid carcinoma

Figure 10-16. Inflammatory myofibroblastic tumor. The neoplasm is composed of a proliferation of spindle cells with a mixed inflammatory background.

Selected References

Lott S, Lopez-Beltran A, MacLennan GT, et al: Soft tissue tumors of the urinary bladder. Part I: Myofibroblastic proliferations, benign neoplasms, and tumors of uncertain malignant potential. Hum Pathol 38:807-823, 2007.

Sukov WR, Cheville JC, Carlson AW, et al: Utility of ALK-1 protein expression and ALK rearrangements in distinguishing inflammatory myofibroblastic tumor from malignant spindle cell lesions of the urinary bladder. Mod Pathol 20:592-603, 2007.

Montgomery EA, Shuster DD, Burkart AL, et al: Inflammatory myofibroblastic tumors of the urinary tract: A clinicopathologic study of 46 cases, including a malignant example inflammatory fibrosarcoma and a subset associated with high-grade urothelial carcinoma. Am J Surg Pathol 30:1502-1512, 2006.

Tsuzuki T, Magi-Galluzzi C, Epstein JI: ALK-1 expression in inflammatory myofibroblastic tumor of the urinary bladder. Am J Surg Pathol 28:1609-1614, 2004.

Rhabdomyosarcoma

Clinical Features

- Relatively common malignant neoplasm in children younger than 15 years
- Most common bladder tumor of childhood
- Typically found before the age of 5 years
- Slightly more common in boys (male-to-female ratio of 3:2)
- Most tumors are of embryonal subtype and exophytic (polypoid), with or without a botryoid component
- Rare in adults, usually of the pleomorphic type
- Typically presents with hematuria or bladder outlet obstruction

Gross Pathology

- Embryonal rhabdomyosarcoma can be divided into two basic forms with prognostic impact
  — Polypoid, mostly intraluminal, associated with favorable prognosis (grapelike clusters, botryoid subtype)
  — Deeply invasive tumors with a worse prognosis
- Typically occurs at the bladder trigone

Histopathology

- Tumor cells are small and round with scant cytoplasm and hyperchromatic nuclei
- Typically, a loose myxoid background is seen
- Large cells with abundant eosinophilic cytoplasm and cross-striations (strap cells) may be seen

Special Stains and Immunohistochemistry

- Myogenin (myf4) and MyoD1 positive
- Desmin and pan-actin (HHF35) positive, but not specific
- Myosin and myoglobin can be negative
- Cytokeratin negative

Other Techniques for Diagnosis

- Electron microscopy: thin actin and thick myosin filaments forming hexagonal pattern

Differential Diagnosis

▌ Sarcomatoid carcinoma (carcinosarcoma)
- Consists of malignant epithelial and malignant spindle cell components
- Islands of cells with epithelial differentiation are seen
- Cytokeratin positivity in the epithelial component

▌ Inflammatory myofibroblastic tumor (IMT)
- Background usually contains a sparse inflammatory component
- Prominent network of thin-walled blood vessels in an edematous or myxoid stroma
- Mitotic figures may be present and even frequent, but they are not atypical
- ALK-1 protein expression

Pearls

- Treatment includes surgery, radiation therapy, and chemotherapy; combination therapy has greatly improved survival in children
- Constitute greater than 75% of bladder tumors in children
- Most common mesenchymal tumor of the urinary bladder

Selected References

Sukov WR, Cheville JC, Carlson AW, et al: Utility of ALK-1 protein expression and ALK rearrangements in distinguishing inflammatory myofibroblastic tumor from malignant spindle cell lesions of the urinary bladder. Mod Pathol 20:592-603, 2007.

Ferrer FA, Isakoff M, Koyle MA: Bladder/prostate rhabdomyosarcoma: Past, present and future. J Urol 176:1283-1291, 2006.

Carcinosarcoma (Sarcomatoid Carcinoma with and without Heterologous Elements)

Clinical Features

- Rare tumors of the urinary bladder
- Primarily affects elderly adults (seventh and eighth decades)
- Usually presents with hematuria or bladder outlet obstruction
- May rarely involve the ureter, renal pelvis, and bladder diverticulum
- Previous history of carcinoma treated by radiation or exposure to cyclophosphamide therapy is common

Gross Pathology

- Typically a large polypoid mass measuring up to 10 to 12 cm in diameter with infiltrative margins

Histopathology

- Biphasic malignant neoplasm exhibiting morphologic or immunohistochemical evidence of epithelial and mesenchymal differentiation; presence or absence of heterologous elements should be mentioned in the diagnosis
- Malignant epithelial component is composed of a urothelial, glandular, or small cell component showing a variable degree of differentiation

- Mesenchymal component usually consists of a pleomorphic, undifferentiated high-grade spindle cell neoplasm
- Most common heterologous element is osteosarcoma followed by chondrosarcoma, rhabdomyosarcoma, leiomyosarcoma, liposarcoma

Special Stains and Immunohistochemistry

- Cytokeratin (low molecular weight): epithelioid component is positive; some positivity in mesenchymal component may be seen
- EMA may be positive but less frequently than cytokeratin
- Vimentin: mesenchymal component is positive
- SMA may be positive in areas of smooth or striated muscle differentiation

Other Techniques for Diagnosis

- Noncontributory

Differential Diagnosis

▋ Urothelial carcinoma
  - Malignant urothelial cells without malignant spindle cell component
  - Vimentin negativity
▋ Inflammatory myofibroblastic tumor and postoperative spindle cell nodule
  - Seen in association with recent therapeutic intervention; thus, clinical history is important
  - Most involve the genital tract of women or periprostatic tissue of men
  - Reactive, highly cellular spindle cell proliferation
  - Often show myxoid background with scattered small blood vessels and sparse neutrophilic infiltrate
  - May have high mitotic rate; no abnormal mitoses
▋ Malignant spindle cell tumors, including leiomyo-sarcoma
  - Primary sarcoma of the bladder is rare in adults
  - Lacks epithelial component
  - Negative for cytokeratin and EMA

Pearls

- Cytokeratin staining in both the epithelial and mesenchymal components supports a single cell line precursor theory
- Epithelial component may be a minority of the tumor; thus, extensive sectioning is required to identify an in situ or invasive epithelial component
- Aggressive tumor with poor prognosis
- Treatment consists of radical cystectomy or cystoprostatectomy; patients may also receive chemotherapy

Selected References

Gronau S, Menz CK, Melzner I, et al: Immunohistomorphologic and molecular cytogenetic analysis of a carcinosarcoma of the urinary bladder. Virchows Arch 440:436-440, 2002.

Lopez-Beltran A, Pacelli A, Rothenberg HJ, et al: Carcinosarcoma and sarcomatoid carcinoma of the bladder: Clinicopathological study of 41 cases. J Urol 159:1497-1503, 1998.

Metastatic Tumors and Secondary Extension

Clinical Features

- Metastases to the bladder or ureter are rare
- Most metastatic lesions are secondary to direct extension from tumors of the prostate, lower intestinal tract, and female genital tract
- Common primary tumors that metastasize to the bladder include breast, colon, and kidney carcinomas and malignant melanoma

Gross Pathology

- Often multiple tumors, typically located in the submucosa
- Focal ulceration of the urothelium overlying the mass may be seen

Histopathology

- Typically located within the bladder wall in a submucosal location
- Presence of a poorly differentiated tumor sparing the urothelial mucosa should raise suspicion of a possible metastasis
- Glandular differentiation is typically seen in metastatic colonic carcinoma; gland formation may also be seen in metastatic prostate carcinoma

Special Stains and Immunohistochemistry

- PSA, PSAP, p501s positive in metastatic prostate carcinoma
- S-100, melan-A, and HMB-45 positive in metastatic melanoma
- Villin and CDX2 positive in metastatic colonic carcinoma

Other Techniques for Diagnosis

- Noncontributory

Differential Diagnosis

- Clinical history is important, especially the presence of a prostate carcinoma in men or a gynecologic tumor in women

Pearls

- Bladder metastases are most frequently a late event and are almost always associated with disseminated disease

Selected References

Suh N, Yang XJ, Tretiakova MS, et al: Value of CDX2, villin, and alpha-methylacyl coenzyme A racemase immunostain in the distinction between primary adenocarcinoma of the bladder and secondary colorectal adenocarcinoma. Mod Pathol 18:1217-1222, 2005.

Helpap B, Ayala AG, Grignon DJ, et al: Metastatic tumors and secondary extension in urinary bladder. In Eble JN, Sauter G, Epstein JI, Sesterhenn IA (eds): World Health Organization Classification of Tumours: Pathology and Genetics: Tumours of the Urinary System and Male Genital Organs. Lyon, France, IARC Press, 2004, pp 148-149.

Bates AW, Baithun SI: Secondary neoplasms of the bladder are histological mimics of nontransitional cell primary tumors: Clinicopathological and histological features of 282 cases. Histopathology 36:32-40, 2000.

Kidney

Renal Dysplasia

Clinical Features

- Refers to the presence of a metanephric structure with aberrant nephronic differentiation
- Two main theories have been considered in its pathogenesis
  — A primary failure of ureteric bud activity
  — Disruption produced by fetal urinary flow impairment
- Most often sporadic, but it may be syndromic and develop as part of a multiple malformation syndrome or chromosomal anomaly, some of which are hereditary
- Almost always accompanied by other urinary tract abnormalities
- Dysplastic kidneys are usually nonfunctional
- Large cystic dysplastic kidneys typically present as a palpable mass in a newborn; diagnosis confirmed by ultrasound
- Small dysplastic kidneys may remain asymptomatic for many years
- Bilateral disease results in oligohydramnios (Potter syndrome) and neonatal death from pulmonary hypoplasia

Gross Pathology

- Unilateral or bilateral involvement may be seen
- Distorted renal parenchyma with numerous variably sized cysts
- Dysplastic kidneys usually enlarged; may occasionally be small

Histopathology

- Characteristic features include markedly disorganized kidney parenchyma with islands of cartilage and dysplastic ducts lined with columnar epithelium and surrounded by collars of spindle cells
- Cystic spaces lined by flattened epithelium
- Rudimentary glomeruli may be seen

Special Stains and Immunohistochemistry

- Noncontributory

Figure 10-17. Renal dysplasia. A, Markedly disorganized kidney parenchyma with dysplastic ducts lined with columnar epithelium and surrounded by collars of spindle cells. **B,** Island of cartilage and cystic spaces lined by flattened epithelium. Few glomeruli are seen.

Other Techniques for Diagnosis

- If multiple malformations are detected in a pediatric autopsy, it is important to obtain tissue for karyotype analysis

Differential Diagnosis

- Infantile polycystic kidney disease (autosomal recessive)
  - Often results in stillbirth or early neonatal death
  - Cysts are in the cortex and medulla and do not congregate at the papillary tips
  - Cartilaginous metaplasia and other dysplastic elements are never seen
- Medullary cystic disease (autosomal dominant)
  - Patients present with renal failure in first or second decade
  - Cysts are located at the corticomedullary junction
- Medullary sponge kidney
  - Typically found in children or adolescents; not found at birth

- Ectasia of the papillary collecting ducts of one or more renal pyramids
- Renal function normal
- Rare progression to end-stage renal disease

Pearls

- Usually associated with congenital genitourinary abnormalities, including ureteral atresia
- Many investigators believe that renal dysplasia is associated with in utero urinary tract obstruction
- Unilateral disease is typically treated by nephrectomy
- Bilateral renal dysplasia ultimately results in renal failure

Selected References

Bisceglia M, Galliani CA, Senger C, et al: Renal cystic disease: A review. Adv Anat Pathol 13:26-56, 2006.

Woolf AS, Price KL, Scambler PJ, Winyard PJ: Evolving concepts in human renal dysplasia. J Am Soc Nephrol 15:998-1007, 2004.

Bonsib SM, Koontz P: Renal maldevelopment: A pediatric renal biopsy study. Mod Pathol 10:1233-1238, 1997.

Infantile (Autosomal Recessive) Polycystic Kidney Disease

Clinical Features

- Found in 1 in 10,000 to 50,000 live births
- Usually results in stillbirth or early neonatal death

Figure 10-18. Infantile polycystic kidney. Characteristic dilated collecting ducts located perpendicular to the renal cortex.

- Abdominal distention due to massively enlarged kidneys
- Lungs may be poorly developed and hypoplastic owing to compression of the thoracic organs; fatal in 75% of cases
- Associated with congenital hepatic fibrosis in patients who survive infancy

Gross Pathology

- Always bilateral disease
- Massively enlarged kidneys with smooth external surface
- Renal parenchyma shows numerous small cysts involving the cortex and medulla
- Cysts are radially arranged and are oriented perpendicular to the renal capsule
- Calyceal system is normal

Histopathology

- Dilated collecting ducts lined by uniform cuboidal cells
- Normal-appearing nephrons seen between cysts

Special Stains and Immunohistochemistry

- Noncontributory

Modern Techniques for Diagnosis

- Cytogenetic studies: single gene (*PKHD1*) mutation on chromosome 6p21-23: encodes for polyductin or fibrocystin

Differential Diagnosis

- ▌ Dysplastic kidney
  - Markedly disorganized kidney parenchyma with islands of cartilage and dysplastic ducts lined with columnar epithelium and surrounded by collars of spindle cells
- ▌ Medullary cystic disease
  - Presents with renal failure in first or second decade
  - Kidneys are typically small
  - Cysts are located primarily at the corticomedullary junction
- ▌ Medullary sponge kidney
  - Typically found in children or adolescents; not found at birth
  - Multiple small cysts involving pyramids and renal papillae
  - Rare progression to end-stage kidney disease

Pearls

- Autosomal recessive disease
- Poor prognosis; often causes death in utero or shortly after birth
- Most cases are associated with multiple epithelium-lined cysts in the liver

Selected References

Garcia-Gonzalez MA, Menezes LF, Piontek KB, et al: Genetic interaction studies link autosomal dominant and recessive polycystic kidney disease in a common pathway. Hum Mol Genet 16:1940-1950, 2007.

Rossetti S, Harris PC: Genotype-phenotype correlations in autosomal dominant and autosomal recessive polycystic kidney disease. J Am Soc Nephrol 18:1374-1380, 2007.

Yoder BK: Role of primary cilia in the pathogenesis of polycystic kidney disease. J Am Soc Nephrol 18:1381-1388, 2007.

Zerres K, Rudnik-Schoneborn S, Deget F, et al: Autosomal recessive polycystic kidney disease in 115 children: Clinical presentation, course and influence of gender. Acta Paediatr 85:437-445, 1996.

Medullary Sponge Kidney

Clinical Features

- Congenital renal malformation
- Rare condition found sporadically in about 1 in 5000 live births
- Unknown etiology
- Children and adolescents are typically asymptomatic
- Usually detected in adults being evaluated for nephrolithiasis
- Patients usually have normal renal function; rare progression to chronic renal failure

Gross Pathology

- Kidneys are typically of normal size
- Characterized by ectasia along the intrapyramidal or intrapapillary portion of the medullary collecting duct
- Cysts, typically measuring less than 0.5 cm, communicate with the collecting ducts

Histopathology

- Cysts lined by transitional, columnar, or occasionally squamous epithelium

Figure 10-19. Medullary sponge kidney. Multiple small cysts lined by columnar epithelium. The interstitium contains fibrous tissue and chronic inflammatory cells.

- Small foci of interstitial fibrosis and chronic inflammation may be seen, but significant cortical scarring is absent

Special Stains and Immunohistochemistry

- Noncontributory

Other Techniques for Diagnosis

- Noncontributory

Differential Diagnosis

- **▌** Medullary cystic disease
  - Typically presents with renal failure in first or second decade
  - Cysts located at corticomedullary junction
- **▌** Dysplastic kidney
  - Presents with renal failure early in life (bilateral disease)
  - Islands of cartilage and dysplastic ducts lined with columnar epithelium and surrounded by collars of spindle cells are characteristic
- **▌** Infantile polycystic kidney disease
  - Usually results in stillbirth or early neonatal death
  - Cysts are radially arranged and located in the cortex and medulla rather than at the tips of the papillae

Pearls

- Rare progression to end-stage renal disease; may develop urolithiasis or pyelonephritis
- Cysts originate from the collecting ducts
- Associated with hemihypertrophy in about 10% of cases

Selected References

Lee S, Jang YB, Kang KP, et al: Medullary sponge kidney. Kidney Int 70:979, 2006.

Indridason OS, Thomas L, Berkoben M: Medullary sponge kidney associated with congenital hemihypertrophy. J Am Soc Nephrol 7:1123-1130, 1996.

Medullary Cystic Kidney Disease and Familial Juvenile Nephronophthisis

Clinical Features

- Four variants exist
  — Sporadic (20%): nonfamilial
  — Familial juvenile nephronophthisis: autosomal recessive
  — Renal-retinal dysplasia (15%): autosomal recessive
  — Adult-onset medullary cystic disease (15%): autosomal dominant
- Accounts for 10% to 20% of renal failure in childhood
- Patients typically present with renal failure in the first or second decade

- Patients have polyuria and polydipsia as a result of salt wasting; develop uremia and growth retardation
- Most patients develop end-stage renal disease within 5 years of diagnosis

Gross Pathology

- Bilateral disease
- Kidneys are usually small and often have a contracted, granular surface
- Cysts are typically numerous and involve the corticomedullary junction
- Cysts are small, with a diameter of less than 2 cm

Histopathology

- Cysts are lined by flattened or squamous epithelium
- Atrophic tubules, hyalinized glomeruli, significant interstitial fibrosis, and chronic inflammation are characteristically seen in the cortex

Special Stains and Immunohistochemistry

- Noncontributory

Other Techniques for Diagnosis

- Cytogenetic studies: two predisposing genes have been localized: *MCKD1* on chromosome 1q21, and *MCKD2* on chromosome 16p12

Differential Diagnosis

▌ Medullary sponge kidney
- Typically presents later in life
- Patients have normal renal function
- Cysts involve the medullary pyramids and renal papillae and communicate with the collecting ducts

▌ Dysplastic kidney
- Patients present with renal failure early in life (bilateral disease)
- Dysplastic ducts and metaplastic cartilage are characteristic

▌ Infantile polycystic kidney disease
- Usually results in stillbirth or early neonatal death
- Cysts located in cortex and medulla, not at papillary tips

Pearls

- Cysts are characteristically seen at the corticomedullary junction
- Renal failure is result of cortical tubulointerstitial disease rather than the cyst formation
- Dialysis or renal transplantation is only current treatment
- Does not recur after renal transplantation

Selected References

Hildebrandt F, Omram H: New insights: Nephronophthisis-medullary cystic kidney disease. Pediatr Nephrol 16:168-176, 2001.

Aridon P, DeFusco M, Ballabio A, Casari G: Identification of a new locus for medullary cystic disease, on chromosome 16p12. Am J Hum Genet 64:1655-1660, 1990.

Adult (Autosomal Dominant) Polycystic Kidney Disease

Clinical Features

- Found in 1 in 400 to 1000 live births
- One of the leading causes of end-stage renal disease in adults; found in 5% to 10% of all patients on dialysis
- Family history in about 70% to 75% of affected persons

Figure 10-20. Adult polycystic kidney. A, Grossly the kidneys are markedly enlarged and show numerous cysts in the cortex and medulla. **B,** Multiple cysts lined by flat cuboidal epithelium, some of which contain proteinaceous material.

- Typically presents in fourth to fifth decade after sufficient renal parenchyma destruction has occurred and renal failure has developed
- Usually presents with hematuria (secondary to stones, tumor, or infection) and proteinuria
- Chronic flank pain is common
- Patients often develop urinary tract infections
- Extrarenal manifestations include
  — Intracranial berry aneurysms, hypertension, colonic diverticula, extrarenal cysts (pancreatic, hepatic), and cardiac valve abnormalities including mitral valve prolapse

Gross Pathology

- Early in disease, kidneys are of normal size with few cysts in cortex and medulla
- Progression of disease leads to marked bilateral kidney enlargement with an increase in the size and number of cysts (may weigh up to 4 kg each)
- Kidneys have an irregular contour due to numerous peripheral cysts
- Cysts range in size from a few millimeters up to several centimeters; typically contain hemorrhagic or clear yellow fluid

Histopathology

- Cysts are lined by single layer of flat to cuboidal epithelium
- Small papillary projections may be seen
- Cysts contain proteinaceous material; calcified deposits often seen
- Intervening kidney tissue typically shows interstitial fibrosis, lymphocytic infiltrate, tubular atrophy, and glomerular and vascular sclerosis
- Frequently associated with renal epithelial tumors (renal cell carcinoma [RCC])

Special Stains and Immunohistochemistry

- Noncontributory

Other Techniques for Diagnosis

- Cytogenetic studies
  — Abnormality associated with chromosome 16 (16q13.3) in 85% of patients (involves *PKD1* gene, which encodes a protein named polycystin 1)
  — Mutation involving chromosome 4 (4q21-23) in about 15% of cases (*PKD2* gene, which encodes a protein named polycystin 2)

Differential Diagnosis

▌ Acquired cystic disease
- Patients typically have chronic renal failure and are on dialysis before cysts develop
- Cysts are typically located in the cortex

- Lacks family history, which is typically present in polycystic kidney disease
- No associated extrarenal manifestations

Pearls

- Autosomal dominant disorder with high penetrance
- Almost 100% penetrance if patient lives to 80 years of age
- End-stage kidney disease is found in about 50% of patients by age 60 years
- Renal transplantation is curative when patient develops end-stage kidney disease

Selected References

Torres VE, Harris PC, Pirson Y: Autosomal dominant polycystic kidney disease. Lancet 369:1287-1301, 2007.
Yoder BK: Molecular pathogenesis of autosomal dominant polycystic kidney disease. Expert Rev Mol Med 8:1-22, 2006.
Calvet JP, Grantham JJ: The genetics and physiology of polycystic kidney disease. Semin Nephrol 21:107-123, 2001.

Acquired Cystic Disease

Clinical Features

- Common finding in patients receiving hemodialysis or peritoneal dialysis
- Presence of cysts increases as time on dialysis increases
- Occasionally seen in patients with chronic renal insufficiency who are not on dialysis
- Pathogenesis of cyst formation remains largely unknown
- Often remains asymptomatic; may present with gross or microscopic hematuria

Figure 10-21. Acquired cystic disease. There is a wide variation in the size of cysts (from 1 mm up to several centimeters). Cysts are typically cortical, and there must be more than five to distinguish from incidental simple cysts.

- Cyst formation is associated with increased risk for RCC

Gross Pathology

- Wide variation in size of cysts, from 1 mm up to several centimeters
- Cysts are usually numerous; must be more than five to distinguish from incidental simple cysts
- Cysts are typically cortical
- Cysts usually contain clear serous fluid; may contain hemorrhagic fluid
- Presence of solid areas suggests possible development of RCC

Histopathology

- Cysts are lined by single epithelial cell layer
- Epithelial lining may become hyperplastic and may occasionally develop into an adenoma or carcinoma
- If development of a tumor with clear cell change is seen, the diagnosis of clear cell carcinoma should be made
- Papillary projections may be seen in adenoma or carcinoma; correct characterization depends on size and cytologic features
- Malignant tumors may develop in cystic areas or in adjacent kidney parenchyma
- Adjacent kidney parenchyma shows changes of end-stage kidney disease, including interstitial fibrosis, hyalinized glomeruli, and tubular atrophy

Special Stains and Immunohistochemistry

- Noncontributory

Other Techniques for Diagnosis

- Noncontributory

Differential Diagnosis

▌Adult polycystic kidney disease
- Kidneys are markedly enlarged and show numerous cysts in the cortex and medulla
- Family history is often present
- Found in third through fifth decades in patients without history of dialysis

Pearls

- Typically associated with hemodialysis or peritoneal dialysis
- Increased time on dialysis increases likelihood of cyst development
- Increased risk for subsequent development of RCC
- Patients are typically asymptomatic and do not require specific treatment
- Computed tomography is recommended to periodically evaluate cysts and look for development of suspicious masses

Selected References

Koljima Y, Takahara S, Miyake O, et al: Renal cell carcinoma in dialysis patients: A single center experience. Int J Urol 13:1045-1048, 2006.

Savaj S, Liakopoulos V, Ghareeb S, et al: Renal cell carcinoma in peritoneal dialysis patients. Int Urol Nephrol 35:263-265, 2003.

Xanthogranulomatous Pyelonephritis

Clinical Features

- Subacute to chronic inflammatory lesion typically forming single or multiple mass lesions often mimicking a renal neoplasm
- Usually unilateral
- *Proteus* species and *Escherichia coli* are the most common infective agents
- Most common presenting complaints are flank pain, fever, and flank mass
- Nephrolithiasis is found in up to 70% of patients

Gross Pathology

- Kidney has dilated, thickened pelvis containing a staghorn calculus
- Yellow nodular tumor masses replace renal pyramids
- Suppurative inflammation and edema begin within pelvic mucosa and sinus fat, resulting in pelvicaliceal ulceration and fat necrosis
- Nodules may become confluent and eventually involve renal capsule, perinephric fat, and retroperitoneal tissue
- Diffuse form is most common; segmental form is polar and more common in children

Figure 10-22. Xanthogranulomatous pyelonephritis. Collection of lipid-laden macrophages in a background of acute and chronic inflammatory cells.

Histopathology

- Xanthogranulomatous nodules have a zonal pattern
  - Central nidus of necrotic debris and neutrophils (microabscesses) with admixture of inflammatory cells, including lymphocytes and plasma cells
  - Surrounding sheets of lipid-laden macrophages with abundant clear cytoplasm (may resemble clear cell RCC)
  - Multinucleated giant cells and spindled fibroblasts surrounding macrophages (may resemble sarcomatoid carcinoma)

Special Stains and Immunohistochemistry

- CD68: macrophages positive
- Cytokeratin negative
- Vimentin positive in reactive fibrous tissue

Other Techniques for Diagnosis

- Noncontributory

Differential Diagnosis

- ❙ Clear cell RCC
  - Sheets of clear cells often with vague alveolar architecture
  - Lacks inflammatory component
  - Vimentin, cytokeratin, and CA9 (carbonic anhydrase IX) positive
  - CD68 negative
- ❙ Sarcomatoid carcinoma
  - Polypoid mass often filling the bladder lumen
  - Islands of cells with epithelial differentiation
  - Cytokeratin positive and CD68 negative
- ❙ Malakoplakia
  - Typically found in the urinary bladder
  - Michaelis-Guttman bodies are characteristic

Pearls

- May clinically, radiologically, and pathologically mimic RCC

Selected References

Hendrickson RJ, Lutfiyya WL, Karrer FM, et al: Xanthogranulomatous pyelonephritis. J Pediatr Surg 41:e15-17, 2006.

Zorzos I, Moutzouris V, Korakianitis G, Katsou G: Analysis of 39 cases of xanthogranulomatous pyelonephritis with emphasis on CT findings. Scand J Urol Nephrol 37:342-347, 2003.

Hoeffel JC, Chastagner P, Boman F, et al: Misleading leads: Focal xanthogranulomatous pyelonephritis in childhood. Med Pediatr Oncol 30:122-124, 1998.

Angiomyolipoma

Clinical Features

- Most cases are sporadic; 20% of cases are associated with tuberous sclerosis

Figure 10-23. Angiomyolipoma. Classic angiomyolipoma of the kidney showing mature adipose tissue, smooth muscle, and blood vessels.

- Most patients with tuberous sclerosis develop angiomyolipoma
- Tumors associated with tuberous sclerosis are usually asymptomatic; tumors are found earlier because these patients are evaluated for kidney tumors
- Sporadic cases are larger, and patients present with hematuria or flank or abdominal pain; rarely, retroperitoneal hemorrhage may occur

Gross Pathology

- Sporadic cases are typically single and unilateral
- Cases associated with tuberous sclerosis are typically multiple and bilateral
- Tumors are well circumscribed but unencapsulated
- Variegated appearance consisting of vascular and adipose tissue and gray-white solid areas corresponding to the smooth muscle component
- Necrosis is rarely seen, but hemorrhage is common

Histopathology

- Triphasic tumor consisting of smooth muscle, mature adipose tissue, and thick-walled hyalinized blood vessels in varying proportion
- One component may predominate
- Atypical features may occasionally be seen, including nuclear pleomorphism and mitosis
- Smooth muscle areas may show epithelioid differentiation with cells having abundant eosinophilic cytoplasm and large nuclei with prominent nucleoli

Special Stains and Immunohistochemistry

- Melanocytic markers positive
- Smooth muscle markers positive in smooth muscle component
- Epithelial markers negative

Other Techniques for Diagnosis

- Noncontributory

Differential Diagnosis

▋ Malignant spindle cell tumors, including leiomyosarcoma
- Lack triphasic appearance
- Poorly circumscribed tumors with infiltrative borders
- Unequivocal high-grade, malignant cytologic features
- Negative for melanocytic markers

Pearls

- Tumor in the renal vein or in regional lymph nodes occasionally seen, but this is not a sign of malignant transformation
- Need to sample these tumors extensively to rule out presence of coexisting RCC
- Must recognize that fatty tissue is part of lesion and not interpret as invasion into perirenal adipose tissue

Selected References

Roma AA, Magi-Galluzzi C, Zhou M: Differential expression of melanocytic markers in myoid, lipomatous, and vascular components of renal angiomyolipomas. Arch Pathol Lab Med 131:122-125, 2007.

Rakowski SK, Winterkorn EB, Paul E, et al: Renal manifestations of tuberous sclerosis complex: Incidence, prognosis, and predictive factors. Kidney Int 70:1777-1782, 2006.

L'Hostis H, Deminiere C, Ferriere JM, Coindre JM: Renal angiomyolipoma: A clinicopathologic, immunohistochemical, and follow-up study of 46 cases. Am J Surg Pathol 23:1011-1020, 1999.

Papillary Adenoma

Clinical Features

- Usually an incidental finding
- Often seen in patients receiving long-term hemodialysis and associated with acquired cystic disease; also more common in kidneys scarred from chronic pyelonephritis
- Occasionally associated with von Hippel-Lindau disease

Gross Pathology

- Cortical tumors smaller than 5 mm
- Soft, well-circumscribed mass with yellow to gray cut surface
- Pushing borders occasionally compressing the adjacent kidney parenchyma

Histopathology

- Tubular, papillary, or tubulopapillary architecture; tubular pattern is most common
- Lacks distinct capsule but does not have an infiltrative border

Figure 10-24. Papillary adenoma. Small tumor (<5 mm) with papillary architecture. It lacks a distinct capsule but does not have an infiltrative border.

- Typically consist of densely packed tubules lined by small regular cuboidal cells with round to oval nuclei; low-grade nuclei similar to Fuhrman nuclear grades 1 and 2
- Nuclei show coarse chromatin and inconspicuous nucleoli
- Mitotic activity is rare
- Cells have high nuclear-to-cytoplasmic ratio with scant cytoplasm
- Psammomatous calcifications and foamy histiocytes may be present
- 2004 WHO classification of renal tumors regards any tumor as papillary adenoma when cortical tumor is composed of closely packed tubules with or without papillary architecture and no more than 5 mm in greatest dimension
- Cells are small, regular, and cuboidal with round to oval low-grade nuclei and rare or no mitotic activity
- No areas of clear cell differentiation

Special Stains and Immunohistochemistry

- Noncontributory

Other Techniques for Diagnosis

- Cytogenetic studies: may be associated with trisomy 7 or 17, loss of Y chromosome in male patients

Differential Diagnosis

▋ Low-grade papillary renal cell carcinoma (PRCC)
- May be histologically indistinguishable from papillary adenoma; thus, the size (5 mm) becomes the sole criterion that separates the two. However, one needs to be aware that the size may not be perfectly correlated with the biologic behavior
▋ Metanephric adenoma
- Usually larger
- Consists of tightly packed small acini
- Cells are small and have scant cytoplasm

- A panel of immunohistochemical stains (CK7, WT-1, and AMACR) can aid the differential diagnosis, with metanephric adenoma positive for WT-1 and negative for CK7 and AMACR, whereas papillary adenoma is positive for CK7 and AMACR but negative for WT-1

Pearls

- Definitive criteria to distinguish papillary adenoma from RCC are arbitrarily defined
- 2004 WHO criteria define cytologically benign tumor smaller than 5 mm and of low nuclear grade as adenoma, and tumor larger than 5 mm or of high nuclear grade as carcinoma

Selected References

Wang KL, Weinrach DM, Luan C, et al: Renal papillary adenoma: A putative precursor of papillary renal cell carcinoma. Hum Pathol 38:239-246, 2007.

Eble JN, Moch H: Papillary adenoma of the kidney. In Eble JN, Sauter G, Epstein JI, Sesterhann IA (eds): World Health Organization Classification of Tumours: Pathology and Genetics: Tumors of the Urinary System and Male Genital Organs. Lyon, IARC Press, 2004, p 41.

Ligato S, Ro JY, Tamboli P, et al: Benign tumors and tumor-like lesions of the adult kidney. Adv Anat Pathol 6:1-11, 1999.

Grignon DJ, Eble JN: Papillary and metanephric adenomas of the kidney. Semin Diagn Pathol 15:41-53, 1998.

Metanephric Adenoma

Clinical Features

- Rare benign kidney tumor
- Female predominance with a female-to-male ratio of 2:1
- Found in childhood through adulthood, most commonly in the fifth decade
- About 50% of cases symptomatic with hematuria and abdominal pain
- About 10% to 15% of cases with polycythemia

Figure 10-25. Metanephric adenoma. Proliferation of tubulopapillary structures within an acellular stroma background. Note the sharp border with the kidney.

Gross Pathology

- Unilateral, solitary, well-circumscribed but unencapsulated tumor
- Variable size ranging from less than 1 cm up to 15 cm (mean, 5 cm)
- Cut surface shows soft, fleshy, tan-yellow tissue
- Hemorrhage and necrosis may be seen

Histopathology

- Pushing border with no capsule or infiltration into surrounding kidney parenchyma
- Ordered array of small, tightly packed acini separated by acellular stroma
- Papillary architecture may be seen
- Focal solid areas consisting of small round cells (blastema-like areas) infrequently seen
- Tumor cells are small and uniform with round to oval nuclei and scant cytoplasm
- Nuclei show delicate chromatin and inconspicuous nucleoli
- Rare to absent mitotic activity
- Microcalcifications may be seen

Special Stains and Immunohistochemistry

- Cytokeratin: AE1/3 positive in 50%, but CK7 usually negative
- CD56 negative
- AMACR positive in 10%
- WT-1 positive

Other Techniques for Diagnosis

- Electron microscopy: cells have basal lamina and microvilli
- Flow cytometry: tumor cells almost always diploid

Differential Diagnosis

▌ Differentiated nephroblastoma (epithelial-predominant Wilms tumor)
- Has a tumor capsule and may show a distinct triphasic pattern with blastema, stromal, and epithelial components after careful sampling
- Elongated or columnar nuclei with frequent mitotic activity
- Positive for CD56 and CD57

▌ PRCC, solid variant
- Often have a tumor capsule
- Tumor cells have more abundant cytoplasm
- Foamy histiocytes and hemosiderin deposition common
- CK7 and AMACR positive, but WT-1 negative

Pearls

- Benign renal epithelial neoplasm probably representing the benign end of the metanephric tumors that also include Wilms tumor
- No reports of local recurrence or distant metastases

- May represent complete maturation of Wilms tumor; alternatively, metanephric adenoma may develop into Wilms tumor, as in neuroblastoma-ganglioneuroblastoma-ganglioneuroma sequence

Selected References

Argani P: Metanephric neoplasms: The hyperdifferentiated, benign end of the Wilms tumor spectrum? Clin Lab Med 25:379-392, 2005.

Brunelli M, Eble JN, Zhang S, et al: Metanephric adenoma lacks the gains of chromosomes 7 and 17 and loss of Y that are typical of papillary renal cell carcinoma and papillary adenoma. Mod Pathol 16:1060-1063, 2003.

Muir TE, Cheville JC, Lager DJ: Metanephric adenoma, nephrogenic rests, and Wilms' tumor: A histologic and immunophenotypic comparison. Am J Surg Pathol 25:1290-1296, 2001.

Renal Oncocytoma

Clinical Features

- Accounts for about 5% to 10% of kidney tumors in adults
- Most are asymptomatic, although flank pain may be a presenting complaint; hematuria may be seen
- Computed tomography or magnetic resonance imaging may identify central scar (spoke-wheel appearance)

Gross Pathology

- Well-circumscribed, homogeneous cortical tumor
- Mahogany-brown cut surface
- Often shows a central, irregular fibrous scar (about 40% of cases)
- Focal hemorrhage may be seen
- No grossly evident necrosis
- No renal vein invasion
- Bilateral or multicentric in 2% to 3% of cases

Histopathology

- Three histologic variants
  - Classic (most common)
  - Organoid pattern with well-defined nests of tumor cells
    - ◆ Edematous, myxoid, or hyalinized stroma
    - ◆ Confluent nests of tumor cells can be seen at the periphery of the lesion; nests of tumor cells should be outlined by interlacing framework of thin fibrous septa
  - Tubulocystic
    - ◆ Variably sized tubular and cystic structures
    - ◆ Spaces often contain eosinophilic secretion
- Mixed pattern
  - Composed of both organoid and tubular architecture
  - Tumor cells have finely granular eosinophilic cytoplasm

Figure 10-26. Oncocytoma. A, The tumor is composed of well-defined nests of tumor cells with abundant eosinophilic granular cytoplasm in an edematous stroma. **B,** High-power view shows the classic cytoplasmic and nuclear features of renal oncocytoma.

  - Round nuclei with smooth, regular contour and evenly distributed chromatin
  - Presence of nucleoli is variable; may be absent or prominent
  - Absence of mitotic figures
  - Focally pleomorphic cells with hyperchromatic smudged nuclei may be seen
- Other unusual features
  - Focal extension into perirenal fat, which has no adverse effect on the prognosis
  - Focal cytoplasmic clearing, especially in a scarred area
- Histologic features that should never be seen include
  - Gross extension into perirenal adipose tissue or gross vascular invasion
  - Papillary architecture
  - Sarcomatous or spindle cell areas
  - Atypical mitotic figures
  - Positive for colloidal iron stain

Special Stains and Immunohistochemistry

- CK7 stains single cells or clusters of cells
- Vimentin and Hale colloidal iron stain negative

Other Techniques for Diagnosis

- Electron microscopy: cells have abundant, evenly distributed mitochondria and a paucity of other organelles
- Flow cytometry: usually diploid
- Cytogenetic studies
  — Most oncocytomas are composed of a mixed population of cells with normal and abnormal karyotypes
  — Some cases display loss of chromosomes 1 and 14
  — Occasionally, t(5;11) is observed

Differential Diagnosis

▌ Clear cell RCC with eosinophilic cytoplasm
  - Eosinophilic cytoplasm can be seen in high-grade clear cell RCC, but presence of clear cells or papillary structures precludes the diagnosis of oncocytoma
  - Nuclear grade is usually high and mitosis is readily identifiable
  - CK7 negative but vimentin positive
▌ Chromophobe RCC, eosinophilic variant
  - Sheetlike compact growth pattern
  - "Raisinoid" nuclei and perinuclear halos
  - CK7 diffusely positive; Hale colloidal iron positive

Pearls

- Believed to arise from the intercalated cells of collecting ducts
- Oncocytomas are benign tumors; previous reports of malignant oncocytomas are almost certain RCC misdiagnosed as oncocytomas
- Most common histologic features include well-defined nests of eosinophilic tumor cells separated by fine, delicate fibrous bands and a central fibrous scar
- Hybrid oncocytic tumors with features of both oncocytoma and chromophobe RCC can be seen in patients with Birt-Hogg-Dube syndrome

Selected References

Wu SL, Kothari P, Wheeler TM, et al: Cytokeratins 7 and 20 immunoreactivity in chromophobe renal cell carcinomas and renal oncocytomas. Mod Pathol 15:712-717, 2002.

Tickoo SK, Amin MB: Discriminant nuclear features of renal oncocytoma and chromophobe renal cell carcinoma: Analysis of their potential utility in the differential diagnosis. Am J Clin Pathol 110:782-787, 1998.

Amin MB, Crotty TB, Tickoo SK, Farrow GM: Renal oncocytoma: A reappraisal of morphologic features with clinicopathologic findings in 80 cases. Am J Surg Pathol 21:1-12, 1997.

Renal Cell Carcinoma, Clear Cell Type

Clinical Features

- The most common variant of renal epithelial tumors, accounting for 2% of all malignancies and about 70% of RCCs
- Occur primarily in adults (sixth to seventh decades)
- Male predominance (2:1)
- Hematuria is single most common presenting sign
- Less than 10% present with classic triad of flank mass, pain, and hematuria

Gross Pathology

- Solitary renal cortical mass
- Bilaterality and multifocality more common in familial syndrome
- Well-circumscribed, lobulated with golden-yellow cut surface
- Cystic change, hemorrhage, necrosis, and calcification often present

Histopathology

- Alveolar nests and sheets of clear cells interspersed by delicate vascular network
- Other patterns are also seen, including trabecular, microcystic, and occasionally pseudopapillary or tubular
- Sarcomatoid differentiation is often in the form of spindle cells

Special Stains and Immunohistochemistry

- Cam 5.2, AE1/3, EMA, vimentin, CD10, CA9, and RCC antigen positive
- Keratin 34BE12 negative
- S-100 or CEA only rarely positive

Figure 10-27. Renal cell carcinoma, clear cell type. Nests and sheets of clear cells interspersed by a delicate vascular network.

Other Techniques for Diagnosis

- Electron microscopy
  - Abundant cytoplasmic lipid and glycogen
  - Tubular differentiation: microlumens, microvilli, and brush border
- Molecular genetics
  - Chromosome 3p deletion in most sporadic clear cell RCCs
  - Mutation of the *VHL* gene in 34% to 56%, and promoter methylation in 20% of sporadic cases

Differential Diagnosis

▌ Chromophobe RCC
- Nonencapsulated mass with a homogeneous, light-brown cut surface
- Translucent and reticulated, not clear, cytoplasm
- Hale colloidal iron positive
- CK7 diffusely positive

▌ PRCC
- Histiocytes and intracellular hemosiderin usually present
- CK7, AMACR positive
- CA9 negative
- Trisomy 7 and 17, loss of Y chromosome in male patients

▌ Adrenocortical carcinoma
- Flocculated, not "water clear," cytoplasm
- EMA and cytokeratin negative
- Inhibin and calretinin positive

▌ Epithelioid angiomyolipoma
- May have other components, such as fat or dysmorphic vessels
- Multinucleated epithelioid cells are characteristic
- Negative for epithelial markers, but positive for melanocytic markers, such as HMB-45, melan-A, tyrosinase, MiTF

Pearls

- Most common histologic subtype of RCC
- Clear cytoplasm due to rich cytoplasmic glycogen and lipid contents
- Chromosome 3p alteration is the most common genetic change
- *VHL* gene and genes in hypoxia-inducible pathway play critical role in the pathogenesis

Selected References

Zhou M, Roma A, Magi-Galluzzi C: The usefulness of immunohistochemical markers in the differential diagnosis of renal neoplasms. Clin Lab Med 25:247-257, 2005.

Jones TD, Eble JN, Cheng L: Application of molecular diagnostic techniques to renal epithelial neoplasms. Clin Lab Med 25:279-303, 2005.

Cheville JC, Lohse CM, Zincke H, et al: Comparisons of outcome and prognostic features among histologic subtypes of renal cell carcinoma. Am J Surg Pathol 27:612-624, 2003.

Amin MB, Amin MB, Tamboli P, et al: Prognostic impact of histologic subtyping of adult renal epithelial neoplasms: An experience of 405 cases. Am J Surg Pathol 26:281-291, 2002.

Avery AK, Beckstead J, Renshaw AA, Corless CL: Use of antibodies to RCC and CD10 in the differential diagnosis of renal neoplasms. Am J Surg Pathol 24:203-210, 2000.

Renal Cell Carcinoma, Papillary Type

Clinical Features

- Comprises about 10% to 15% of all RCCs; mostly sporadic, less than 5% associated with hereditary PRCC syndrome that involves the *c-met* gene on chromosome 7q31
- Signs and symptoms similar to clear cell RCC
- More likely to be bilateral or multiple than other RCCs
- Significantly better outcome than that of the clear cell type

Gross Pathology

- Solitary, well-circumscribed cortical mass
- Fibrous pseudocapsule
- Necrosis and hemorrhage common
- More likely to be bilateral or multifocal than other RCCs

Histopathology

- Papillae and tubulopapillary structures with true fibrovascular cores
- Solid pattern due to tightly compact growth of papillae
- Foamy histiocytes expanding papillary core characteristic
- Psammoma bodies common

Figure 10-28. Renal cell carcinoma, papillary type. Papillae and tubulopapillary structures with true fibrovascular cores. Foamy histiocytes expanding papillary core are characteristic.

- Subdivided into two types based on morphology
  — Type 1: papillae lined with single layer of cells, usually low-grade nuclear features, and scant cytoplasm
  — Type 2: pseudostratified nuclei of higher nuclear grade and abundant eosinophilic cytoplasm
- Sarcomatoid differentiation in 5% cases

Special Stains and Immunohistochemistry

- Pan-cytokeratin and low-molecular-weight cytokeratin positive
- CK7 positive in 80% of type I cases and 20% type II cases
- EMA and vimentin positive in 50% of cases
- CD10 and RCC antigen positive in most cases

Other Techniques for Diagnosis

- Cytogenetics: trisomy or tetrasomy 7 and 17 and loss of Y chromosome are the most common cytogenetic changes

Differential Diagnosis

▌ Papillary adenoma
- By WHO criteria, smaller than 5 mm and low nuclear grade (Fuhrman nuclear grade 1 or 2)
▌ Metanephric adenoma
- Sharp circumscription from the kidney parenchyma without capsule
- Tightly packed tumor cells form small acini, tubulopapillary structures
- Tumor cells with scant cytoplasm, uniform nuclei without mitosis or nucleoli
- CK7 negative, but WT-1 positive
▌ Differentiated nephroblastoma (epithelial-predominant Wilms tumor)
- Has a tumor capsule and may show a distinct triphasic pattern with blastemal, stromal, and epithelial components after careful sampling
- Elongated or columnar nuclei with frequent mitotic activity
- CD56 and CD57 positive
▌ RCC associated with Xp11.2/TFE3 translocation
- Often affects children and young adults
- Papillary structures lined by tumor cells with abundant clear to granular cytoplasm
- Psammomatous calcification and hyalinized fibrovascular cores present
- Most epithelial markers, including cytokeratins and EMA, negative
- Positive TFE3 stain confirmatory
▌ Collecting duct carcinoma
- Involving central region of the kidney
- Irregular, small glands and ducts in a loose collagenous chronically inflamed desmoplastic stroma
- Cells lining glands are high grade with pleomorphic nuclei; typically have hobnail appearance
- Associated tubular epithelial dysplasia

Pearls

- Second most common RCC subtypes
- Significantly better prognosis than clear cell RCC
- Trisomy 7 and 17 and loss of Y chromosome are characteristic, but lacks *VHL* mutation

Selected References

Eble JN, McCredie MR, Bethwaite PB, et al: Morphologic typing of papillary renal cell carcinoma: Comparison of growth kinetics and patient survival in 66 cases. Hum Pathol 32:590-595, 2001.

Amin MB, Corless CL, Renshaw AA, et al: Papillary (chromophil) renal cell carcinoma: Histomorphologic characteristics and evaluation of conventional pathologic prognostic parameters in 62 cases. Am J Surg Pathol 21:621-635, 1997.

Delahunt B, Eble JN: Papillary renal cell carcinoma: A clinicopathologic and immunohistochemical study of 105 tumors. Mod Pathol 10:537-544, 1997.

Renal Cell Carcinoma, Chromophobe Type

Clinical Features

- About 5% of RCCs
- Presents similarly to clear cell RCC
- Most are sporadic; familial cases associated with Birt-Hogg-Dube syndrome
- Significantly better prognosis than clear cell RCC

Gross Pathology

- Solitary, spherical, well-circumscribed, pseudoencapsulated mass
- Homogeneous, tan or light-brown cut surface

Figure 10-29. Renal cell carcinoma, chromophobe type. Proliferation of compact cells with finely reticulated pale cytoplasm and prominent cell membrane. Koilocytic nuclear atypia, with a wrinkled nuclear membrane and perinuclear halo, and binucleation are common.

Histopathology

- Two histologic variants
  - Classic: cells with finely reticulated pale cytoplasm with prominent cell membrane
  - Eosinophilic: smaller cells with intense eosinophilic cytoplasm and prominent cell membrane
- Koilocytic nuclear atypia with wrinkled nuclear membrane and perinuclear halo
- Binucleation common
- Thick hyalinized blood vessels

Special Stains and Immunohistochemistry

- CK7 and EMA diffusely positive
- RCC antigen variably positive
- CD10 and S-100A1 negative
- Hale colloidal iron stain positive

Other Techniques for Diagnosis

- Electron microscopy
  - Abundant cytoplasmic microvesicles
  - Eosinophilic variant: abundant mitochondria, few microvesicles
- Molecular genetics
  - Extensive chromosomal loss, most frequently involving chromosomes 1, 2, 6, 10, 13, 17, and 21

Differential Diagnosis

❙ Clear cell RCC
- No koilocytic nuclear atypia or prominent cell membrane
- Hale colloidal iron stain negative
- CK7 negative

❙ Oncocytoma
- Uniform nuclei without koilocytic nuclear atypia or prominent cell membranes
- Hale colloidal iron stain highlights lumina, not the entire tumor cells
- CK7 stains single cells or small clusters of cells
- S-100A1 positive

Pearls

- Third most common RCC subtype
- Significantly better prognosis than clear cell RCC; most patients are cured by nephrectomy
- Extensive chromosomal loss, distinct from clear cell and PRCC

Selected References

Li G, Barthelemy A, Feng G, et al: S100A1: A powerful marker to differentiate chromophobe renal cell carcinoma from renal oncocytoma. Histopathology 50:642-647, 2007.

Abrahams NA, MacLennan GT, Khoury JD, et al: Chromophobe renal cell carcinoma: A comparative study of histological, immunohistochemical and ultrastructural features using high throughput tissue microarray. Histopathology 45:593-602, 2004.

Tickoo SK, Amin MB, Zarbo RJ: Colloidal iron staining in renal epithelial neoplasms, including chromophobe renal cell carcinoma: Emphasis on technique and patterns of staining. Am J Surg Pathol 22:419-424, 1998.

Thoenes W, Störkel S, Rumpelt HJ, et al: Chromophobe cell renal carcinoma and its variants: A report on 32 cases. J Pathol 155:277-287, 1988.

Multilocular Cystic Renal Cell Carcinoma

Clinical Features

- Rare variant (5%) of clear cell RCC
- Excellent prognosis; surgical resection is curative

Gross Pathology

- Well-circumscribed, entirely cystic mass of small and large cysts with serous or hemorrhagic content

Figure 10-30. Multilocular cystic renal cell carcinoma. A, A cystic mass of small and large cysts with serous or hemorrhagic content. No solid expansile nodules of tumor cells are noted. **B,** Small collections of clear epithelial cells within fibrous septa.

- Occasionally calcified
- No solid expansile nodules of tumor cells

Histopathology

- Cysts lined by single layer of cells
- Small collections of clear epithelial cells within fibrous septa

Special Stains and Immunohistochemistry

- Identical to clear cell RCC

Other Techniques for Diagnosis

- Identical to clear cell RCC

Differential Diagnosis

▎ Cystic nephroma
- Striking female predominance
- No clear cells within fibrous septa
- Hyalinized or cellular stroma resembling ovarian stroma

▎ RCC with extensive cystic change
- Presence of solid, expansile tumor nodules of any size excludes diagnosis of multilocular cystic RCC

Pearls

- A variant of clear cell RCC with excellent prognosis after surgical resection
- Strict diagnostic criteria should be applied to ensure the prognostic significance associated with the diagnosis: no solid expansile tumor nodule of any size is allowed

Selected References

Suzigan S, Lopez-Beltran A, Montironi R, et al: Multilocular cystic renal cell carcinoma: A report of 45 cases of a kidney tumor of low malignant potential. Am J Clin Pathol 125:217-222, 2006.

Eble JN, Bonsib SM: Extensively cystic renal neoplasms: cystic nephroma, cystic partially differentiated nephroblastoma, multilocular cystic renal cell carcinoma, and cystic hamartoma of renal pelvis. Semin Diagn Pathol 15:2-20, 1998.

Collecting Duct Carcinoma (Carcinoma of the Collecting Ducts of Bellini)

Clinical Features

- Rare, comprising about 0.1% of RCCs
- Flank mass, pain, and hematuria
- One third have metastasis at presentation

Gross Pathology

- Medullary location
- Light-gray, white cut surface with invasive borders
- Necrosis, hemorrhage, and cystic changes may be present

Figure 10-31. Collecting duct carcinoma. Tubular and tubulopapillary structures with tapered ends in an inflamed desmoplastic stroma.

Histopathology

- Highly infiltrative border
- Tubular and tubulopapillary structure with tapered ends
- Inflamed desmoplastic stroma
- High-grade nuclear features, brisk mitosis
- Intraluminal and intracytoplasmic mucin may be present
- Tubular epithelial dysplasia in adjacent kidney parenchyma

Special Stains and Immunohistochemistry

- Low- and high-molecular-weight keratin, CK7, CEA, peanut agglutinin (PNA), and *Ulex europaeus* agglutinin (UEA) positive
- CD10 negative

Other Techniques for Diagnosis

- Electron microscopy: well-formed cell junctions, short apical microvilli, and prominent basal lamina
- Molecular genetics: not well characterized

Differential Diagnosis

▎ PRCC
- Typically located in the cortex
- Well circumscribed with a tumor capsule
- Histiocytes and hemosiderin deposition in papillary cores
- Lack inflamed desmoplastic stroma
- High-molecular-weight cytokeratin and *Ulex* species negative

▎ Urothelial carcinoma with glandular features
- Histology and immunoprofile similar to collecting duct carcinoma
- Urothelial carcinoma in renal calyces or pelvis favors the diagnosis of urothelial carcinoma

▎ Renal medullary carcinoma
- Affects exclusively patients with sickle trait or disease
- Sickle cells may be found within the tumor vessels

▌ Metastatic carcinoma
  ● History of primary carcinoma
  ● Often multifocal with concentration at the corticomedullary junction
  ● Extensive involvement of perinephric fat and intravascular permeation

Pearls

● Rare, highly aggressive renal tumor
● Diagnosis is difficult and often is one of exclusion
● Consider this entity in the presence of a high grade tumor with features reminiscent of PRCC, urothelial carcinoma, and clear cell RCC

Selected References

Tokuda N, Naito S, Matsuzaki O, et al: Collecting duct (Bellini duct) renal cell carcinoma: A nationwide survey in Japan. J Urol 176:40-43, 2006.

Peyromaure M, Thiounn N, Scotté F, et al: Collecting duct carcinoma of the kidney: A clinicopathological study of 9 cases. J Urol 170:1138-1140, 2003.

Chao D, Zisman A, Pantuck AJ, et al: Collecting duct renal cell carcinoma: Clinical study of a rare tumor. J Urol 167:71-74, 2002.

Renal Medullary Carcinoma

Clinical Features

● Typically presents with gross hematuria; may present with abdominal or flank pain
● Almost always associated with sickle cell trait or sickle cell disease in a patient younger than 40 years

Gross Pathology

● Ill-defined, poorly circumscribed mass predominantly located in the renal medulla, but often involving most of the renal parenchyma
● Typically extends into the calyces and pelvis and often invades into the perirenal adipose tissue
● Firm to rubbery lobulated tumor with tan-gray cut surface
● Typically shows extensive hemorrhage and necrosis

Histopathology

● Characteristically shows a reticular growth pattern; reminiscent of testicular yolk sac tumor on low-power examination
● Often shows areas with a more compact adenoid cystic appearance
● Solid sheets of poorly differentiated tumor cells are also commonly present
● Tumor cells have clear or vesicular nuclei with prominent nucleoli
● Desmoplastic stroma in the form of mucoid, myxoid, or edematous areas are typical findings
● Stroma typically shows variable degrees of inflammatory cells

Figure 10-32. Renal medullary carcinoma. A, Proliferation of compact neoplastic ductlike structures resembling adenoid cystic carcinoma. **B,** High-power view shows neoplastic cells with a large amount of eosinophilic cytoplasm, pleomorphic nuclei with vesicular chromatin pattern, and prominent nucleoli. Sickled red cells are seen.

● Most tumors show areas of hemorrhage and necrosis
● Lymphatic and vascular invasion is usually present
● Sickled red cells typically seen

Special Stains and Immunohistochemistry

● Cytokeratin typically positive
● High-molecular-weight cytokeratin negative

Other Techniques for Diagnosis

● Noncontributory

Differential Diagnosis

▌ Collecting duct carcinoma
  ● Clinical history critical: patients have no sickle cell trait or disease
  ● Irregular, small glands and ducts in an inflamed desmoplastic stroma
  ● Cells lining glands are high grade with pleomorphic nuclei; typically have hobnail appearance

Pearls

- Previously referred to as *collecting duct carcinoma*, but now recognized as a unique entity
- Lymph node metastases are common at time of presentation; involvement of liver and lung is also common
- Radical nephrectomy is treatment of choice; however, it is an aggressive tumor, and most patients die within 1 year after diagnosis

Selected References

Swartz MA, Karth J, Schneider DT, et al: Renal medullary carcinoma: Clinical, pathologic, immunohistochemical, and genetic analysis with pathogenetic implications. Urology 60:1083-1089, 2002.

Figenshau RS, Easier JW, Ritter JH, et al: Renal medullary carcinoma. J Urol 159:711-713, 1998.

Avery RA, Harris JE, Davis CJ Jr, et al: Renal medullary carcinoma: Clinical and therapeutic aspects of a newly described tumor. Cancer 78:128-132, 1996.

Mucinous Tubular and Spindle Cell Carcinoma

Clinical Features

- Wide range of age (17 to 82 years; mean, 53 years)
- Female predominance
- Most tumors are asymptomatic and detected incidentally
- Prognosis favorable; best regarded as a low-grade carcinoma

Gross Pathology

- Well-circumscribed, homogeneous, tan-white to pinkish cut surfaces

Figure 10-33. Mucinous tubular and spindle cell carcinoma. Elongated and compressed tubules are present in a background of extracellular mucinous material.

Histopathology

- Comprising variable amounts of three components: elongated and compressed tubules, spindle-shaped epithelial cells, and a background extracellular mucinous material
- Nuclei are bland, spherical, or oval with inconspicuous nucleoli
- Necrosis, foamy histiocytes, and chronic inflammation may be present

Special Stains and Immunohistochemistry

- Cytokeratins CAM5.2, AE1/3, CK7, and CK19 positive
- AMACR positive
- Markers of proximal tubules, including CD10 and villin, negative

Other Techniques for Diagnosis

- Molecular genetics: cytogenetic changes distinct from PRCC and clear cell RCC

Differential Diagnosis

- Collecting duct carcinoma
  - Irregular, small glands and ducts in an inflamed desmoplastic stroma
  - Cells lining glands are high grade with pleomorphic nuclei; typically have hobnail appearance
- PRCC, solid variant
  - Compressed tubulopapillary structures forming solid or glomeruloid pattern
  - Lacks spindle cell and mucinous components
  - CK7, AMACR, and CD10 positive
- Sarcomatoid RCC
  - Nondescript spindle cells, often with high nuclear grade
  - Characteristic areas of preexisting RCC often seen after extensive sampling

Pearls

- Recently described low-grade carcinoma classically comprising mucinous stroma, compressed tubules, and bland spindle cells
- Immunohistochemically similar but genetically distinct from PRCC

Selected References

Shen SS, Ro JY, Tamboli P, et al: Mucinous tubular and spindle cell carcinoma of kidney is probably a variant of papillary renal cell carcinoma with spindle cell features. Ann Diagn Pathol 11:13-21, 2007.

Fine SW, Argani P, DeMarzo AM, et al: Expanding the histologic spectrum of mucinous tubular and spindle cell carcinoma of the kidney. Am J Surg Pathol 30:1554-1560, 2006.

Cossu-Rocca P, Eble JN, Delahunt B, et al: Renal mucinous tubular and spindle carcinoma lacks the gains of chromosomes 7 and 17 and losses of chromosome Y that are prevalent in papillary renal cell carcinoma. Mod Pathol 19:488-493, 2006.

Brandal P, Lie AK, Bassarova A, et al: Genomic aberrations in mucinous tubular and spindle cell renal cell carcinomas. Mod Pathol 19:186-194, 2006.

Ferlicot S, Allory Y, Comperat E, et al: Mucinous tubular and spindle cell carcinoma: A report of 15 cases and a review of the literature. Virchows Arch 447:978-983, 2005.

Renal Cell Carcinoma Associated with Xp11.2/TFE3 Translocation

Clinical Features

- Predominantly affects children and young adults
- Defined by several different translocations involving chromosome Xp11.2, all resulting in gene fusions involving the *TFE3* gene
- The alveolar soft part locus (ASPL)-TFE3 carcinomas and those in adults characteristically present at advanced stage

Gross Pathology

- Similar to clear cell RCC
- Solitary cortical mass with tan-yellow cut surface, foci of hemorrhage and necrosis

Histopathology

- Papillary structures lined with clear cells are the most distinctive feature
- Nested pattern made up of cells with abundant acidophilic cytoplasm is common
- Histology may vary with different chromosomal translocations
  — ASPL-TFE3: less compact, nested pattern; cells with voluminous clear to eosinophilic cytoplasm,

Figure 10-34. Renal cell carcinoma associated with Xp11.2/TFE3 translocation. The distinctive feature is the presence of papillary structures lined with cells with voluminous clear to eosinophilic cytoplasm, discrete cell borders, vesicular chromatin, and prominent nucleoli.

discrete cell borders, vesicular chromatin, and prominent nucleoli; psammoma bodies and hyaline nodules frequent
  — PRCC-TFE3: compact, nested pattern; less abundant cytoplasm, fewer psammoma bodies and hyaline nodules

Special Stains and Immunohistochemistry

- TFE3 confirmatory
- EMA focally positive or negative
- CAM5.2 and vimentin commonly positive
- CD10 and RCC antigen consistently positive

Other Techniques for Diagnosis

- Cytogenetics: chromosomal translocation involving the *TFE3* gene on Xp11.2 and several partner genes, including *PRCC* on 1q21, *ASPL* on 17q25, *PSF* on 1p34, and *NonP* on X chromosome

Differential Diagnosis

▌ Clear cell RCC
- Exceedingly rare in patients younger than 25 years
- Nests of clear cells separated by delicate fibrovascular septa; papillary structures with clear cells rarely seen
- Epithelial markers positive, but TFE3 negative

▌ PRCC
- RCC in children and young adults often has unusual morphology, including papillary architecture
- No alveolar or nested architecture, or clear cells
- TFE3 negative

Pearls

- Although RCC is rare in children and young adults, translocation-associated RCC accounts for 24% to 40% of RCC in this age group
- Most characteristic histologic feature is papillary structures lined with clear cells
- TFE3 immunostain is confirmatory

Selected References

Argani P, Olgac S, Tickoo SK, et al: Xp11 translocation renal cell carcinoma in adults: Expanded clinical, pathologic, and genetic spectrum. Am J Surg Pathol 31:1149-1160, 2007.

Meyer PN, Clark JI, Flanigan RC, Picken MM: Xp11.2 translocation renal cell carcinoma with very aggressive course in five adults. Am J Clin Pathol 128:70-79, 2007.

Argani P, Ladanyi M: Translocation carcinomas of the kidney. Clin Lab Med 25:363-378, 2005.

Bruder E, Passera O, Harms D, et al: Morphologic and molecular characterization of renal cell carcinoma in children and young adults. Am J Surg Pathol 28:1117-1132, 2004.

Argani P, Lal P, Hutchinson B, Lui MY, et al: Aberrant nuclear immunoreactivity for TFE3 in neoplasms with TFE3 gene fusions: A sensitive and specific immunohistochemical assay. Am J Surg Pathol 27:750-761, 2003.

Argani P, Antonescu CR, Illei PB, et al: Primary renal neoplasms with the ASPL-TFE3 gene fusion of alveolar soft part sarcoma:

a distinctive tumor entity previously included among renal cell carcinomas of children and adolescents. Am J Pathol 159:179-192, 2001.

Renal Cell Carcinoma Associated with Neuroblastoma

Clinical Features

- Rare: less than two dozen cases reported in the literature
- Occurs in long-term survivors of childhood neuroblastoma
- Diagnosis of neuroblastoma at 2 years of age; median age at diagnosis of RCC, 13.5 years

Gross Pathology

- Either kidney or both kidneys can be affected

Histopathology

- Morphologically heterogeneous, with some tumors showing solid and papillary architecture, cells with abundant eosinophilic cytoplasm
- Many tumors have typical clear cell appearance

Special Stains and Immunohistochemistry

- EMA, vimentin, CK8, CK18, and CK20 usually positive
- CK7, CK14, and CK19 negative

Other Techniques for Diagnosis

- Genetically different from other RCC types

Differential Diagnosis

- ▌ RCC with eosinophilic cytoplasm
  - Many RCCs, including clear cell and papillary types, may have abundant eosinophilic cytoplasm, especially in high-grade tumors
  - History of neuroblastoma is key to the diagnosis of postneuroblastoma RCC

Pearls

- Recently described RCC that affects survivors of childhood neuroblastoma
- Genetically different from other RCC types

Selected References

Dhall D, Al-Ahmadie HA, Dhall G, et al: Pediatric renal cell carcinoma with oncocytoid features occurring in a child after chemotherapy for cardiac leiomyosarcoma. Urology 70:178.e13-178.e15, 2007.

Koyle MA, Hatch DA, Furness PD III, et al: Long-term urological complications in survivors younger than 15 months of advanced stage abdominal neuroblastoma. J Urol 166:1455-1458, 2001.

Medeiros LJ, Palmedo G, Krigman HR, et al: Oncocytoid renal cell carcinoma after neuroblastoma: A report of four cases of a distinct clinicopathologic entity. Am J Surg Pathol 23:772-780, 1999.

Renal Cell Carcinoma, Sarcomatoid Type

Clinical Features

- Sarcomatoid differentiation can occur in all histologic subtypes of RCC and currently is not considered a distinctive subtype
- Sarcomatoid differentiation is considered a poor prognostic sign

Gross Pathology

- Tumor is large with bulging, lobulated, soft and gray-white, fleshy cut surface
- Sarcomatoid component may appear firm and fibrous without hemorrhage and necrosis

Histopathology

- Sarcomatoid component is composed of nondescript malignant spindle cells
- Many resemble malignant fibrous histiocytoma
- Patterns reminiscent of leiomyosarcoma, fibrosarcoma, angiosarcoma, or rhabdomyosarcoma rarely seen
- Carcinomatous component may be separate or admixed with the sarcomatous component

Special Stains and Immunohistochemistry

- Immunohistochemistry: heterogenous staining patterns with variable cytokeratin and EMA staining in the spindle cells
- RCC markers, including CD10 and RCC antigen, usually negative in sarcomatous areas

Other Techniques for Diagnosis

- Noncontributory

Differential Diagnosis

- ▌ RCC with scar and granulation tissue
  - RCC, especially clear cell type, may have granulation tissue and scar within the tumor
  - Fibroblastic reaction may be mistaken for sarcomatous differentiation
  - Fibroblasts do not exhibit cytologic atypia
- ▌ Mucinous tubular and spindle cell carcinoma
  - Elongated compressed tubules and spindle cells in a mucinous, myxoid background
  - Spindle cells have bland cytology and lack atypia
- ▌ Primary renal sarcoma
  - Rare
  - Diagnosis can be established only after extensive sampling and immunohistochemical stains to rule out sarcomatoid RCC with a minor epithelial component

Pearls

- Sarcomatous differentiation can occur in all types of RCC

- Indicative of poor prognosis, regardless of the histologic subtypes of underlying RCC, or the extent of sarcomatous component
- Graded as Fuhrman nuclear grade 4

Selected References

Kwak C, Park YH, Jeong CW, et al: Sarcomatoid differentiation as a prognostic factor for immunotherapy in metastatic renal cell carcinoma. J Surg Oncol 95:317-323, 2007.

Cheville JC, Lohse CM, Zincke H, et al: Sarcomatoid renal cell carcinoma: An examination of underlying histologic subtype and an analysis of associations with patient outcome. Am J Surg Pathol 28:435-441, 2004.

de Peralta-Venturina M, Moch H, Amin M, et al: Sarcomatoid differentiation in renal cell carcinoma: A study of 101 cases. Am J Surg Pathol 25:275-284, 2001.

Renal Cell Carcinoma, Unclassified Type

Clinical Features

- RCC that does not fit into any subtype of 2004 WHO classification
- Heterogeneous group of tumors with divergent clinical, morphologic, immunohistochemical, ultrastructural, or genetic characteristics

Gross Pathology

- Variable

Histopathology

- Histologic features that would fit into more than one category, including tumors with features of both oncocytoma and chromophobe RCC, clear cell RCC with papillary architecture, and PRCC with clear cells
- High-grade carcinoma
- Sarcomatoid RCC with no recognizable or classifiable epithelial elements

Special Stains and Immunohistochemistry

- Noncontributory

Other Techniques for Diagnosis

- Noncontributory

Differential Diagnosis

▌ Renal cell carcinoma with predominantly sarcomatoid differentiation
- Renal cell carcinoma with the epithelial component overrun by the sarcomatoid elements
- Extensive sampling of the tumor may reveal the coexisting epithelial component

▌ Metastatic carcinoma to the kidney
- Patient often has a previous history of malignancy
- Metastatic tumor nodules are often multiple and concentrated along the corticomedullary junction
- Immunohistochemistry, especially lineage-specific markers (thyroid transcription factor-1 [TTF-1] for lung and thyroid, thyroglobulin for thyroid, and CDX2 for gastrointestinal tract), may aid the differential diagnosis

Pearls

- "Wastebasket" for those cases of RCC that do not fit into any entities defined in the 2004 WHO classification
- Poorly differentiated and sarcomatoid carcinomas have aggressive behavior

Selected References

Amin MB, Amin MB, Tamboli P, et al: Prognostic impact of histologic subtyping of adult renal epithelial neoplasms: An experience of 405 cases. Am J Surg Pathol 26:281-291, 2002.

Zisman A, Chao DH, Pantuck AJ, et al: Unclassified renal cell carcinoma: Clinical features and prognostic impact of a new histological subtype. J Urol 168:950-955, 2002.

Cystic Nephroma (Multilocular Cyst)

Clinical Features

- Middle-aged adults
- Marked female predominance
- Usually asymptomatic

Gross Pathology

- Solitary, encapsulated, and well circumscribed
- Thin-walled, multiloculated cyst
- Cystic spaces do not communicate with renal pelvis
- Focal hemorrhage is often seen

Histopathology

- Cysts are lined by single layer of flattened or cuboidal or low columnar cells with clear or eosinophilic cytoplasm

Figure 10-35. Cystic nephroma. Multiple cystic structures lined by a single layer of flattened or cuboidal cells.

- Stromal component is hyalinized or cellular, which resembles ovarian stroma
- Renal nephron elements within stromal component should not be seen

Special Stains and Immunohistochemistry

- Cellular stroma positive for estrogen receptor (ER) and progesterone receptor (PR)

Other Techniques for Diagnosis

- Noncontributory

Differential Diagnosis

▮ Cystic RCC
- Shows focal areas of clear cells characteristic of clear cell RCC

▮ Cystic renal dysplasia
- History of urinary obstruction or ureteral duplication
- Primitive renal tubules and fetal cartilage

▮ Benign (non-neoplastic) renal cysts
- Abnormal renal architecture
- Remnant nephrons in the septa

Pearls

- Pediatric cystic nephroma and cystic partially differentiated nephroblastoma are benign neoplasms currently considered to be a part of the spectrum of nephroblastoma

Selected References

Turbiner J, Amin MB, Humphrey PA, et al: Cystic nephroma and mixed epithelial and stromal tumor of kidney: A detailed clinicopathologic analysis of 34 cases and proposal for renal epithelial and stromal tumor (REST) as a unifying term. Am J Surg Pathol 31:489-500, 2007.

Eble JN, Bonsib SM: Extensively cystic renal neoplasms: Cystic nephroma, cystic partially differentiated nephroblastoma, multilocular cystic renal cell carcinoma and cystic hamartoma of renal pelvis. Semin Diagn Pathol 15:2-20, 1998.

Mixed Epithelial and Stromal Tumor of the Kidney

Clinical Features

- Rare benign tumor with striking female predominance
- Flank mass and pain, hematuria, or symptoms of urinary tract infection
- Estrogen imbalance is suspected etiologically

Gross Pathology

- Frequent central location in the kidney
- Well-circumscribed mass, frequently herniating into the renal pelvis
- Mixed solid and cystic cut surface

Figure 10-36. Mixed epithelial and stromal tumor of the kidney.
A, Biphasic neoplasm with epithelial and stromal elements.
B, Epithelial elements consist of cysts of variable sizes and tubules lined with flat, cuboidal, or low columnar cells. **C,** Stromal component is variably cellular, from hypocellular collagen-rich, to hypercellular ovarian stroma–like, to smooth muscle bundles.

Histopathology

- Biphasic: epithelial and stromal elements
  — Epithelial elements: cysts of variable sizes and tubules lined with flat, cuboidal, or low columnar cells; focal clear cells may be present
  — Stromal elements: variably cellular, from hypocellular collagen-rich to hypercellular, ovarian stroma–like, to smooth muscle bundles; fat may be present

Special Stains and Immunohistochemistry

- CK and vimentin positive in epithelial elements
- Vimentin, actin, desmin, ER, and PR positive in stromal elements

Other Techniques for Diagnosis

- Noncontributory

Differential Diagnosis

- ▌ Cystic nephroma
  - Mixed epithelial and stromal tumor and cystic nephroma are currently considered to fall in the morphologic spectrum of the same entity (renal epithelial and stroma tumor)
  - Cystic nephroma is morphologically much simpler, without complex tubular and glandular structure or epithelial and stromal interaction
- ▌ Cystic RCC
  - Shows focal areas of clear cells identical to those of clear cell RCC

Pearls

- Predominantly female patients with history of estrogen imbalance
- Currently considered as renal epithelial and stromal tumor along with cystic nephroma

Selected References

Turbiner J, Amin MB, Humphrey PA, et al: Cystic nephroma and mixed epithelial and stromal tumor of kidney: A detailed clinicopathologic analysis of 34 cases and proposal for renal epithelial and stromal tumor (REST) as a unifying term. Am J Surg Pathol 31:489-500, 2007.

Adsay NV, Eble JN, Srigley JR, et al: Mixed epithelial and stromal tumor of the kidney. Am J Surg Pathol 24:958-970, 2000.

Renomedullary Interstitial Cell Tumor and Medullary Fibroma

Clinical Features

- Almost always asymptomatic lesions found incidentally in kidneys removed for other reasons or found at autopsy
- Found in up to 40% of autopsies

Figure 10-37. Renomedullary interstitial cell tumor and medullary fibroma. Well-circumscribed nodule composed of haphazardly arranged, benign-appearing spindle cells.

Gross Pathology

- Well-circumscribed, firm, gray-white nodules in the kidney medulla
- Usually less than 0.5 cm in diameter
- Several nodules occasionally seen in the same kidney

Histopathology

- Well-circumscribed nodule composed of haphazardly arranged, benign-appearing spindle cells
- Typically paucicellular tumor with a loose collagenous or myxoid stroma
- Entrapped medullary tubules can be found at the periphery
- No mitotic activity or features of malignancy should be present

Special Stains and Immunohistochemistry

- Noncontributory

Other Techniques for Diagnosis

- Noncontributory

Differential Diagnosis

- ▌ Leiomyoma
  - Rare renal tumor
  - Found in the cortex or capsule; not in renal medulla
  - Shows cytologic features similar to those of smooth muscle tumors at other sites

Pearls

- Cell of origin is the renomedullary interstitial cell, which plays a role in blood pressure control
- Lesions are almost always asymptomatic

Selected References

Tamboli P, Ro JY, Amin MB, et al: Benign tumors and tumor-like lesions of the adult kidney. Part II: Benign mesenchymal and mixed neoplasms, and tumor-like lesions. Adv Anat Pathol 1:47-66, 2000.

Dall'Era M, Das S: Benign medullary fibroma of the kidney. J Urol 164:2018, 2000.

Juxtaglomerular Cell Tumor and Renin-Secreting Tumor

Clinical Features

- Benign kidney tumor with differentiation toward the modified smooth muscle cells of the juxtaglomerular apparatus adjacent to the afferent arteriole at the hilus of the glomerulus
- Most commonly presents in patients younger than 30 years
- Slight female predominance
- All patients have hypertension, which is corrected in most cases by removal of the tumor
- Elevated renin level is characteristic; increased aldosterone levels with hypokalemia may occur

Gross Pathology

- Unilateral and solitary, well-circumscribed neoplasm in the cortex
- Cut surface shows a solid gray-white mass occasionally with small cystic spaces

Histopathology

- Classically has a diffuse architecture; trabecular or glomeruloid pattern may be seen
- Polygonal to spindle-shaped cells with oval bland nuclei
- Cells have moderate to abundant granular pink cytoplasm
- Loose myxoid stroma with scattered lymphocytic infiltrate
- Typically shows prominent vasculature with hemangiopericytoma-like pattern
- Mitotic activity is rare

Special Stains and Immunohistochemistry

- SMA, muscle-specific actin, and CD31 positive
- Renin positive
- Cytokeratin, desmin, S-100, HMB-45 negative

Other Techniques for Diagnosis

- Electron microscopy: rhomboid, renin-specific crystalline structures

Differential Diagnosis

▌ Clear cell RCC
- Lacks hypertension as a presenting symptom
- Typically found in older patients
- Composed of sheets of clear cells with distinct cell borders

Pearls

- Small tumors can be localized by serum renin level in the renal vein
- Tumor is best treated surgically, typically with nephrectomy
- Blood pressure returns to normal levels after surgical resection
- No reports of local recurrence or metastases regardless of type of surgical resection

Selected References

Martin SA, Mynderse LA, Lager DJ, Cheville JC: Juxtaglomerular cell tumor: A clinicopathologic study of four cases and review of the literature. Am J Clin Pathol 116:854-863, 2001.

Hasegawa A: Juxtaglomerular cells tumor of the kidney: A case report with electron microscopic and flow cytometric investigation. Ultrastruct Pathol 21:201-208, 1997.

Nephroblastoma (Wilms Tumor)

Clinical Features

- Common solid tumor of childhood; 90% found before age 6 years; peak, ages 2 to 5 years
- Rarely found in adults or neonates
- About 10% associated with dysmorphic syndromes
  - WAGR syndrome (Wilms tumor, aniridia, genital anomalies, and mental retardation; deletion of chromosome 11p13 involving *WT-1* gene): 30% of patients develop Wilms tumor
  - Denys-Drash syndrome (point mutation in *WT-1* gene): 90% risk for Wilms tumor
  - Beckwith-Wiedemann syndrome (hemihypertrophy, macroglossia, omphalocele, visceromegaly, *WT-2* locus on 11p15)
  - Familial nephroblastoma (17q12-21 and 19q13.3-13.4)
- Patients usually present with an abdominal mass or abdominal tenderness; may present with hematuria, hypertension, or rarely peritoneal symptoms if spontaneous rupture has occurred
- Treatment includes surgical resection, chemotherapy, and radiation
- Prognosis depends on tumor stage, histologic features, and patient age at time of diagnosis

Gross Pathology

- Typically single, well-circumscribed mass with lobulated appearance
- Variegated, bulging, pale-gray to tan-pink cut surface typically with extensive hemorrhage and necrosis; cyst formation may be seen
- Must carefully examine for evidence of spread into renal pelvis, renal vein, ureter, or perirenal adipose tissue
- Perirenal lymph node involvement may be found

Figure 10-38. Nephroblastoma (Wilms tumor). A, Wilms tumor showing a classic triphasic pattern consisting of blastemal, stromal, and epithelial elements. **B,** Wilms tumor showing a classic epithelial component.

Histopathology

- Classically shows triphasic pattern consisting of blastemal, stromal, and epithelial components
- Biphasic or even monophasic tumors occasionally found
- Blastemal component is arranged in diffuse sheets or thin cords or as nodular aggregates; peripheral palisading of nuclei may be seen
- Blastema consists of small, round cells with hyperchromatic nuclei showing coarse chromatin and scant cytoplasm
- Frequent mitotic activity is common
- Diffuse pattern shows poorly cohesive cells with infiltrative growth pattern
- Stroma is typically myxoid or fibromyxoid; differentiation toward skeletal muscle or less commonly cartilage, bone, fat, or neural tissue may be seen

- Epithelial component is in the form of poorly formed tubules to well-developed tubular or papillary structures
- Foci of squamous metaplasia or mucinous epithelium are not uncommon
- Nuclear anaplasia
  - Presence of polyploidy multipolar mitotic figures, or nuclear enlargement with hyperchromasia (nuclei are more than 3 times the size of adjacent non-neoplastic nuclei)
  - Associated with responsiveness to therapy, rather than tumor aggressiveness

Special Stains and Immunohistochemistry

- Vimentin highlights blastemal component
- WT-1: very low level or no expression in stromal area; diffuse expression in blastemal and early epithelial differentiation; patchy and variable expression in differentiated epithelium

Other Techniques for Diagnosis

- Electron microscopy
  - Can help distinguish between the tumors in the small round blue cell category (lymphoma, neuroblastoma) when only limited tissue is available
  - Shows cellular features resembling those of the developing metanephrons
  - Blastemal cells have numerous organelles with many desmosomes, intermediate filaments, mitochondria, and cilia
- Cytogenetic studies
  - One third of sporadic Wilms tumors harbor *WT-1* deletion, and 10% harbor point mutation

Differential Diagnosis

▌ Neuroblastoma
- Most commonly found in the adrenal gland
- Homer-Wright pseudorosettes often seen
- Positive for chromogranin, synaptophysin, and NSE; negative for WT-1
▌ Synovial sarcoma
- Most cases are monophasic with short intersecting fascicles
- Cystic structures lined with hobnail cells
- WT-1 negative
- t(X;18) translocation with SYT/SSX fusion transcripts
▌ Primitive neuroectodermal tumor
- Grossly poorly circumscribed
- Primitive round cells with variable rosette formation
- CD99 positive and WT-1 negative
▌ Rhabdoid tumor
- Often presents with metastatic disease
- Tumor cells have large nucleoli and cytoplasmic inclusions
- Lacks triphasic pattern; no blastemal component

▌Mesoblastic nephroma
  - Typically found within first 3 months of life
  - Composed of interlacing fascicles of bland spindle cells infiltrating among normal-appearing kidney structures

Pearls

- Embryonal neoplasm derived from nephrogenic blastemal cells
- Hereditary cases are more commonly bilateral
- All tumors must be generously sampled to determine presence and extent of tumor anaplasia
- Anaplastic nephroblastoma is virtually never encountered in infants
- Common sites of metastasis include regional lymph nodes, lung, and liver
- Younger age at time of diagnosis is associated with better prognosis
- Overall good prognosis; cure rate is about 90% after surgery, chemotherapy, and radiation

Selected References

Parham DM, Roloson GJ, Feely M, et al: Primary malignant neuroepithelial tumors of the kidney: A clinicopathologic analysis of 146 adult and pediatric cases from the National Wilms' Tumor Study Group Pathology Center. Am J Surg Pathol 25:133-146, 2001.

Beckwith JB: Nephrogenic rests and the pathogenesis of Wilms' tumor: Developmental and clinical considerations. Am J Med Genet 79:268-273, 1998.

Beckwith JB: New developments in the pathology of Wilms' tumor. Cancer Invest 15:153-162, 1997.

Charles AK, Mall S, Watson J, Berry PJ: Expression of the Wilms' tumour gene WT1 in the developing human and in pediatric renal tumours: An immunohistochemical study. Mol Pathol 50:138-144, 1997.

Nephrogenic Rests and Nephroblastomatosis

Clinical Features

- Nephrogenic rests are present in 25% to 40% of nephrectomy specimens with nephroblastoma
- *Nephroblastomatosis* refers to multifocal or diffuse nephrogenic rests
- Finding of nephrogenic rests increases the likelihood of subsequent development of nephroblastoma in the opposite kidney

Gross Pathology

- Hyperplastic nephrogenic rests form irregular subcortical or intraparenchymal yellow-tan lesions
- Nephroblastomatosis may cause diffuse cortical enlargement

Histopathology

- Nephrogenic rests are divided into perilobar and intralobar types
- Perilobar nephrogenic rests are composed of blastemal or tubular patterns and little stroma at the periphery of the renal lobe
- Intralobar nephrogenic rests are ill-defined, stroma-rich lesions placed randomly within the renal lobe

Special Stains and Immunohistochemistry

- Noncontributory

Other Techniques for Diagnosis

- Noncontributory

Differential Diagnosis

▌Nephroblastoma
  - Presence of a fibrous tumor capsule
  - Expansile and rounded contour

Pearls

- Finding of nephrogenic rests increases the likelihood of subsequent development of nephroblastoma in the opposite kidney
- The non-neoplastic kidney has to be sampled carefully

Selected References

Hennigar RA, O'Shea PA, Grattan-Smith JD: Clinicopathologic features of nephrogenic rests and nephroblastomatosis. Adv Anat Pathol 8:276-289, 2001.

Beckwith JB: Nephrogenic rests and the pathogenesis of Wilms' tumor: Developmental and clinical considerations. Am J Med Genet 79:268-273, 1998.

Cystic Partially Differentiated Nephroblastoma

Clinical Features

- Occurs with greater frequency in boys than in girls
- Almost all patients are younger than 24 months
- Palpable abdominal mass is the most common presentation

Gross Pathology

- Large, well-circumscribed mass with a fibrous pseudocapsule
- Cystic with variably sized cysts separated by thin septa
- No expansile solid component

Histopathology

- Cysts are lined with flattened, cuboidal, or hobnail epithelium or lack lining, undifferentiated and differentiated mesenchyme, blastema, and nephroblastomatous epithelial elements within the septa
- Termed *pediatric cystic nephroma* when no nephroblastomatous elements are present

Special Stains and Immunohistochemistry

- Noncontributory

Other Techniques for Diagnosis

- Noncontributory

Differential Diagnosis

▌ Cystic nephroblastoma
- Presence of solid, expansile tumor nodule

Pearls

- Pediatric cystic nephroma is considered different from the adult cystic nephroma

Selected References

Eble JN, Bonsib SM: Extensively cystic renal neoplasms: Cystic nephroma, cystic partially differentiated nephroblastoma, multilocular cystic renal cell carcinoma, and cystic hamartoma of renal pelvis. Semin Diagn Pathol 15:2-20, 1998.

Joshi VV, Beckwith JB: Multilocular cyst of the kidney (cystic nephroma) and cystic, partially differentiated nephroblastoma: Terminology and criteria for diagnosis. Cancer 64:466-479, 1989.

Mesoblastic Nephroma

Clinical Features

- Most common congenital renal neoplasm; diagnosis typically made within first 3 months of life
- Uncommon in children older than 1 year old; rarely found in adults
- Almost all infants present with an abdominal mass
- May occasionally recur; rare reports of metastases

Gross Pathology

- Centered in the renal sinus
- Classic mesoblastic nephroma: small with firm, whorled cut surface resembling leiomyoma
- Cellular mesoblastic nephroma: large, frequently soft and cystic with foci of hemorrhage and necrosis

Figure 10-39. Mesoblastic nephroma. Proliferation of spindle cells infiltrating around renal structures.

Histopathology

- Classic variant resembling benign fibromatosis; composed of interlacing fascicles of bland fibroblastic cells with infrequent mitoses; locally invasive, extending into adjacent renal fat
- Cellular variant, identical to infantile fibrosarcoma; composed of sheets or ill-defined fascicles of densely packed plump cells with high mitotic activity; less invasive with pushing margins
- Mixed pattern recognized when features of both are present in a single tumor

Special Stains and Immunohistochemistry

- Vimentin positive
- SMA positive

Other Techniques for Diagnosis

- Electron microscopy: prominent network of endoplasmic reticulum
- Cytogenetics: cellular variant has trisomy 11 or t(12;15)(p13;q25)

Differential Diagnosis

▌ Nephroblastoma (Wilms tumor)
- Blastemal component not present in mesoblastic nephroma
- Usually found in children older than 1 year of age
- Often bilateral

▌ Clear cell sarcoma
- Typically found in older patients
- Classic histologic pattern consists of cords of uniform spindle-shaped cells with round to oval nuclei and a moderate amount of clear to pale cytoplasm in a collagenous background
- Often metastasizes to bone or other sites

▌ Rhabdoid tumor
- Often presents with metastatic disease
- Angiolymphatic invasion is often readily identified
- Tumor cells show nuclear pleomorphism and have large nucleoli and eosinophilic cytoplasmic inclusions

Pearls

- Treatment is surgical resection; complete resection renders excellent prognosis
- Tumor may recur; metastases are uncommon
- Risk for recurrence and metastasis includes cellular histology, stage III and higher disease, and involvement of intrarenal or sinus vessels

Selected References

Dal Cin P, Lipcsei G, Hermand G, et al: Congenital mesoblastic nephroma and trisomy 11. Cancer Genet Cytogenet 103:68-70, 1998.

Rubin BP, Chen CJ, Morgan TW, et al: Congenital mesoblastic nephroma t(12;15) is associated with ETV6-NTRK3 gene fusion: Cytogenetic and molecular relationship to congenital (infantile) fibrosarcoma. Am J Pathol 153:1451-1458, 1998.

Truong LD, Williams R, Ngo T, et al: Adult mesoblastic nephroma: Expansion of the morphologic spectrum and review of literature. Am J Surg Pathol 22:827-839, 1998.

Mascarello JT, Cajulis TR, Krous HF, Carpenter PM: Presence or absence of trisomy 11 is correlated with histologic subtype in congenital mesoblastic nephroma. Cancer Genet Cytogenet 77:50-54, 1994.

Pettinato G, Manivel JC, Wick MR, Dehner LP: Classical and cellular (atypical) congenital mesoblastic nephroma: A clinicopathologic, ultrastructural, immunohistochemical, and flow cytometric study. Hum Pathol 20:682-690, 1989.

Clear Cell Sarcoma

Clinical Features

- Rare renal tumor; about 5% of all pediatric kidney tumors
- Typically presents between ages 6 months and 5 years
- Presents with an abdominal mass; metastasis often present at time of presentation
- Common sites of metastasis include bone, brain, lung, liver, soft tissue, and lymph nodes

Gross Pathology

- Solitary tumor with variable size and weight; typically large
- Appears well circumscribed, with compression of adjacent kidney parenchyma
- Uniform tan-white to gray appearance
- Often shows cystic areas
- Focal necrosis and hemorrhage may be seen but are rarely prominent

Histopathology

- Classic pattern: cords of cells with pale cytoplasm and pale, vesicular nuclei separated by delicate, regularly spaced fibrovascular arcades

Figure 10-40. Clear cell sarcoma. Proliferation of cells with pale cytoplasm and pale, vesicular nuclei separated by a delicate, regularly spaced fibrovascular arcade.

- Subtly infiltrating kidney-tumor interface with entrapment and separation of nephrons and tubules at the periphery
- Histologic variants: myxoid, sclerosing, cellular, epithelioid, spindle cell, and palisading patterns

Special Stains and Immunohistochemistry

- Vimentin positive
- Cytokeratin negative

Other Techniques for Diagnosis

- Electron microscopy: primitive cells with abundant cytoplasmic processes and few poorly formed cell junctions; prominent collagen

Differential Diagnosis

▌ Nephroblastoma (Wilms tumor)
  - Shows heterologous cell types
  - Blastemal component is not present in clear cell sarcoma
▌ Mesoblastic nephroma
  - Typically discovered at birth; almost always before 1 year of age
  - Composed of bland spindle cells without significant clear cell differentiation
  - Stroma often shows dilated staghorn vessels
  - Rarely metastasizes
▌ Rhabdoid tumor
  - Highly cellular tumor composed of large cells with prominent nucleoli and large eosinophilic cytoplasmic inclusions
  - Cytokeratin positive

Pearls

- This highly aggressive tumor has a poor prognosis
- Metastases to bone and other extrapulmonary sites are common
- Treatment includes surgical resection and chemotherapy

Selected References

Schuster AE, Schneider DT, Fritsch MK, et al: Genetic and genetic expression analyses of clear cell sarcoma of the kidney. Lab Invest 83:1293-1299, 2003.

Argani P, Perlman EJ, Breslow NE, et al: Clear cell sarcoma of the kidney: A review of 351 cases from the National Wilms Tumor Study Group Pathology Center. Am J Surg Pathol 24:4-18, 2000.

Sotelo-Avila C, Gonzalez-Crussi F, Sadowinski S, et al: Clear cell sarcoma of the kidney: A clinicopathologic study of 21 patients with long-term follow-up evaluation. Hum Pathol 16:1219-1230, 1985.

Rhabdoid Tumor

Clinical Features

- About 2% of all pediatric renal neoplasms
- Male-to-female ratio of 1.5:1

- Mean age of 13 months; usually younger than 24 months
- Hematuria, hypercalcemia; 15% associated with posterior fossa primitive neuroectodermal tumor (PNET)
- Highly lethal; 75% of patients die within 1 year of diagnosis
- Widespread hematogenous and lymphatic metastases
- No effective therapy

Gross Pathology

- Moderately circumscribed, nonencapsulated mass
- Necrosis and hemorrhage common

Histopathology

- Sheets of uniform cells with
  — Large vesicular nuclei
  — Prominent nuclei and cytoplasmic inclusions

Special Stains and Immunohistochemistry

- Epithelial markers positive, with a characteristic pattern of focal but intense staining in a background of nonreactive cells

Other Techniques for Diagnosis

- Electron microscopy: cytoplasmic inclusions consist of aggregates of intermediate filaments
- Cytogenetic studies: inactivation of *hSNF5/INI1* gene on chromosome 22 constitutes a molecular hallmark of rhabdoid tumor of the kidney

Differential Diagnosis

▌ Nephroblastoma (Wilms tumor)
- Common solid tumor of childhood (typically in children ages 2 to 5 years)
- Typically shows a distinct triphasic pattern with blastemal, stromal, and epithelial components
▌ Mesoblastic nephroma
- Composed of interlacing fascicles of bland spindle cells
- Cells lack intracytoplasmic inclusions

Pearls

- Most common malignant tumor of childhood
- Cell of origin remains unknown
- Tumor cells resemble immature skeletal muscle but show no ultrastructural or immunohistochemical features of muscle differentiation
- Aggressive tumors; more than 50% of patients die within 1 year of diagnosis

Selected References

Savla J, Chen TT, Schneider NR, et al: Mutations of the hSNF5/INI1 gene in renal rhabdoid tumors with second primary brain tumors. J Natl Cancer Inst 92:648-650, 2000.

Schofield DE, Beckwith JB, Sklar J: Loss of heterozygosity at chromosome regions 22q11-12 and 11p15.5 in renal rhabdoid tumors. Genes Chromosomes Cancer 15:10-17, 1996.

Weeks DA, Beckwith JB, Mierau GW, Luckey DW: Rhabdoid tumor of kidney: A report of 111 cases from the National Wilms' Tumor Study Pathology Center. Am J Surg Pathol 13:439-458, 1989.

Metastatic Tumors

Clinical Features

- Kidney is a common site for metastases from other malignant tumors
- Most common primary sites include lung, skin (malignant melanoma), gastrointestinal tract, ovary, testes, and contralateral kidney

Gross Pathology

- Metastatic tumors in the kidney are typically multiple and often bilateral
- May involve the cortex or medulla

Histopathology

- Depends on primary site
- Typically shows poorly differentiated carcinoma; glandular or squamous differentiation may be seen in metastatic carcinomas from the lung or gastro-intestinal tract
- Malignant melanoma shows large, pleomorphic, polygonal cells with prominent nucleoli; melanin pigment may be seen

Special Stains and Immunohistochemistry

- S-100 protein and HMB-45 positive in metastatic melanoma

Other Techniques for Diagnosis

- Noncontributory

Differential Diagnosis

- Rarely have diagnostic difficulty with metastatic tumors involving the kidney because primary tumor is typically well-documented before development of kidney metastases

Pearls

- Primary tumor is usually known before development of renal metastases
- Prognosis is poor

Selected References

Murphy WM, Beckwith JB, Farrow GM: Tumors of the kidney, bladder and related urinary structures. In Atlas of Tumor Pathology, 3rd Series, Fascicle 11. Washington, DC, Armed Forces Institute of Pathology, 1994, pp 313-317.

Bracken RB, Chica G, Johnson DE, Luna M: Secondary renal neoplasms: an autopsy study. South Med J 72:806-807, 1979.

Michael R. Pins

11

Male Genitourinary System

Prostate Gland

Acute and Chronic Prostatitis

Clinical Features

- Clinical classification of acute and chronic prostatitis
  — Acute bacterial prostatitis
    ◆ Prostate is swollen and tender on palpation
    ◆ Often refractory to antibiotic therapy because the prostate is a "safe haven" for bacteria
    ◆ Patients may present with recurrent urinary tract infections
    ◆ Cultured organisms are the same as those seen in urinary tract infections (i.e., *Escherichia coli*, other gram-negative rods, and *Enterococcus* and *Staphylococcus* species)
  — Chronic bacterial prostatitis
    ◆ Same as acute prostatitis, but symptoms are of longer duration
  — Chronic abacterial prostatitis
    ◆ Most common form of clinical prostatitis
    ◆ Presents similar to acute and chronic bacterial prostatitis
    ◆ By definition, no organisms are cultured (idiopathic); however, infection by *Chlamydia*, *Ureaplasma*, or *Mycoplasma* species has been suggested
  — Granulomatous prostatitis
    ◆ Nonspecific (idiopathic) granulomatous type
      ◇ Patients are between 20 and 70 years of age (mean age, 60 years)
      ◇ Patients present with obstructive symptoms, dysuria, fever, and chills; may have a history of urinary tract infection
      ◇ Prostate on palpitation can be firm and indurated (may clinically mimic carcinoma)
      ◇ After bacillus Calmette-Guérin (BCG) therapy: history of intracystic BCG therapy for transitional cell carcinoma (TCC) may be remote
    ◆ Post-transurethral or postbiopsy granulomatous type: history of procedure up to 5 years ago
    ◆ Infectious granulomatous type: history of infection by any one of the following
      ◇ Bacteria (tuberculosis, syphilis, or brucella)
      ◇ Fungi (cryptococcosis, blastomycosis, or coccidioidomycosis)
      ◇ Viruses (herpes)
      ◇ Parasites (schistosomiasis, echinococcosis)
  — Malakoplakia
    ◆ Primarily affects men older than 50 years
    ◆ Symptoms include fever, frequency, dysuria, and hematuria
    ◆ Urine culture is often positive for *Escherichia coli*

Gross Pathology

- Acute and chronic bacterial and chronic abacterial prostatitis
  — Prostatic enlargement; may be soft and swollen
- Granulomatous prostatitis
  — Enlarged with firm, nodular parenchyma
  — Areas of infarction and necrosis with infectious granulomas often seen

Histopathology

- Acute and chronic bacterial prostatitis
  — Prominent neutrophilic infiltrate with abscess formation
  — Neutrophils and necrotic debris may fill prostatic ducts and acini

Figure 11-1. A, Chronic, focally acute prostatitis. Note the presence of reactive atypicality of the acinar epithelium in the form of conspicuous nucleoli. **B, Iatrogenic granulomatous prostatitis.** Noncaseating epithelioid granulomas and associated lymphocytic infiltrate in a patient receiving bacillus Calmette-Guérin therapy for urothelial cancer. **C, Iatrogenic granulomatous prostatitis.** Low-power view of palisading histiocytes after transurethral resection. Note the atrophic-appearing prostatic gland (*top left*).

— Reactive glandular epithelium showing mild cytologic atypia; nuclei with prominent nucleoli may be seen
— Glands may appear atrophic and have a pseudocribriform architecture owing to little glands budding off within lumen
— Stroma is edematous and hyperemic
- Chronic abacterial prostatitis
  — Presence of neutrophils and lymphocytes in prostatic ducts and epithelium
  — Reactive glandular epithelium showing mild cytologic atypia; nuclei with prominent nucleoli may be seen
  — May be associated with glandular atrophy
- Granulomatous prostatitis
  — Nonspecific (idiopathic) granulomatous type
    ◆ Admixture of histiocytes, plasma cells, eosinophils, neutrophils, lymphocytes, and giant cells
    ◆ Cells arranged in sheets around ruptured ducts and acini
  — Post-BCG therapy
    ◆ Mostly histiocytes and giant cells associated with ducts or acini
  — Post-transurethral or postbiopsy granulomatous type
    ◆ Central zone of fibrinoid necrosis surrounded by palisading histiocytes and some multi-nucleated giant cells
    ◆ Minimal chronic inflammatory infiltrate
    ◆ Eosinophilic infiltrate typically present after recent prostate surgery (1 month after resection)
  — Infectious granulomatous type
    ◆ Granulomatous inflammation, with or without necrosis
    ◆ Eosinophils often present with parasitic infection
  — Malakoplakia
    ◆ Hansemann cells: histiocytes with clear or eosinophilic cytoplasm arranged in sheets with surrounding mixed chronic inflammatory infiltrate
    ◆ Michaelis-Gutmann bodies: round, target-shaped structures found intracellularly and extracellularly

Special Stains and Immunohistochemistry

- Granulomatous prostatitis
  — Nonspecific granulomatous type
    ◆ Stains positively for histiocytic markers, negative for epithelial markers
  — Infectious granulomatous type
    ◆ May identify causative organism with special stains (Gomori methenamine silver [GMS], periodic acid–Schiff [PAS], acid-fast bacillus [AFB] stains)

— Malakoplakia
  ◆ Von Kossa calcium, iron, and PAS highlight Michaelis-Gutmann bodies

Other Techniques for Diagnosis

- Noncontributory

Differential Diagnosis

▎ Non-Hodgkin lymphoma
- Rare in the prostate gland
- Proliferation of neoplastic lymphoid cells that typically infiltrate the prostatic stroma in diffuse sheets while sparing the ducts and acini
- Infiltration into surrounding periprostatic tissues is common
- Monoclonal lymphoid population seen with flow cytometry and immunohistochemistry
- Most common tumor subtype is diffuse large cell lymphoma, B-cell type

▎ Poorly differentiated adenocarcinoma (Gleason grades 8 to 10)
- Infiltrating tumor composed of a diffuse and focally glandular proliferation
- Malignant cells have pleomorphic nuclei and prominent nucleoli
- Neoplastic glands lack basal cell layer (negative high-molecular-weight cytokeratin [HMWCK] staining)
- Inflammatory cell infiltrate is unusual in adenocarcinoma

▎ Sarcoidosis
- Patients typically have evidence of systemic disease; rare to have isolated prostate involvement
- Characterized by noncaseating granulomas composed of epithelioid histiocytes and giant cells
- Special stains for organisms are negative

Pearls

- Preferable to diagnose inflamed prostate specimens as having acute or chronic inflammation than as acute or chronic prostatitis (i.e., the latter are clinical diagnoses)
- Biopsy is not required because most prostatitis cases are effectively treated with antibiotics
- Patients with chronic prostatitis often have frequent recurrences, and histology correlates poorly with clinical findings (e.g., stromal and periglandular mononuclear cell infiltrates are normal in older men)
- All forms of prostatic disease may cause mild elevation of prostate-specific antigen (PSA)

Selected References

Nickel JC: Prostatitis: Myths and realities. Urology 51:362-366, 1998.

Roberts RO, Lieber MM, Bostwick DG, Jacobsen SJ: A review of clinical and pathological prostatitis syndromes. Urology 49:809-821, 1997.

van Iersel MP, Witjes WP, de la Rosette JJ, Oosterhof GO: Prostatic-specific antigen density: Correlation with histological diagnosis of prostate cancer, benign prostatic hyperplasia and prostatitis. Br J Urol 76:47-132, 1995.

Infarction

Clinical Features

- Patients may be asymptomatic or present with urinary retention and hematuria
- Typically occurs in a background of nodular hyperplasia

Gross Pathology

- In general, the greater the degree of nodular hyperplasia, the greater the likelihood of infarction
- Central pale-yellow zone surrounded by hyperemic tissue

Histopathology

- Acute infarction
  — Central coagulative necrosis with surrounding hemorrhage
  — Adjacent glands show reactive and metaplastic changes; typically squamous metaplasia
  — Reactive glandular epithelium is characterized by cells with enlarged nuclei, prominent nucleoli, and mitotic figures
- Remote infarction
  — Central fibrous scar with hemosiderin admixed with small glands often showing squamous metaplasia

Special Stains and Immunohistochemistry

- Noncontributory

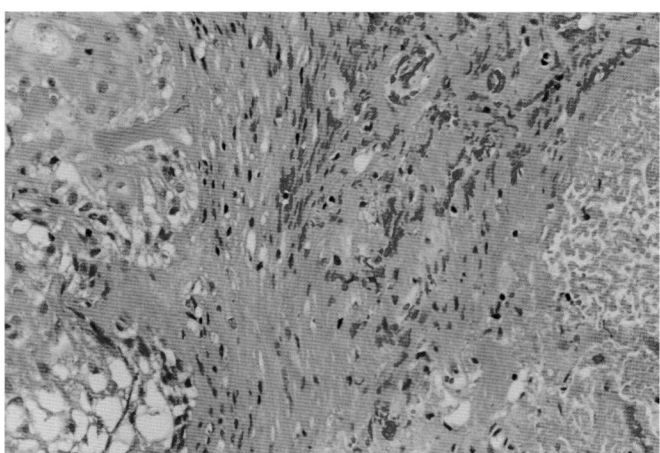

Figure 11-2. Prostatic infarct. Coagulative necrosis with hemorrhage (*right*) and early squamous metaplasia of prostatic glandular epithelium (*left*).

Other Techniques for Diagnosis

- Noncontributory

Differential Diagnosis

- ▌ Squamous cell carcinoma
  - Rare in the prostate gland
  - Infiltrative architecture composed of irregular nests or cords of malignant cells with squamous differentiation; areas of keratinization often seen
  - Typically have prominent desmoplastic changes in the surrounding stroma
- ▌ Prostatic adenocarcinoma, low grade
  - Low-power magnification reveals uniform proliferation of small glands with irregular contours and irregular stromal spacing
  - Neoplastic glands are lined by a single layer of epithelium (basal cell layer is absent)
  - Higher-power magnification demonstrates cuboidal or columnar cells with abundant cytoplasm, enlarged nuclei, and prominent nucleoli
  - Perineural infiltration is often present

Pearls

- Commonly seen at autopsy in men with marked hypotension who had had a urethral catheter in place

Selected References

Anjum I, Ahmed M, Assopardi A, Mufti GR: Prostatic infarction/ infection in acute urinary retention secondary to benign prostatic hyperplasia. J Urol 160:792-793, 1998.

Megyeri J, Varga J: Prostatic infarction. Int Urol Nephrol 7:315-319, 1975.

Hyperplasia

Clinical Features

- Common in males after 60 years of age
- Patients may have symptoms of urinary obstruction (inability to initiate or terminate urinary flow) or may be asymptomatic

Gross Pathology

- ▌ Benign (nodular) prostatic hyperplasia
  - Multilobulated surface
  - Variably sized nodules typically located around the prostatic urethra
  - Peripheral zone appears compressed and atrophic
  - Small foci of infarction may be seen
- ▌ Basal cell and clear cell cribriform hyperplasia
  - Often incidental finding associated with benign (nodular) hyperplasia
- ▌ Atypical adenomatous hyperplasia
  - Nonspecific gross features

Histopathology

- ▌ Benign (nodular) prostatic hyperplasia
  - Well-circumscribed, nonencapsulated nodules

Figure 11-3. A, Benign (nodular) prostatic hyperplasia. Low-power view of a gland-rich hyperplastic nodule. Other nodules (not shown) may be stroma rich. **B, Basal cell hyperplasia (BCH).** Subluminal cell proliferation of basal cells characterized by elongated nuclei, longitudinal nuclear grooves, conspicuous nucleoli, and amphophilic cytoplasm. BCH showing enlarged nucleoli (atypical basal cell hyperplasia) should not be confused with high-grade prostatic intraepithelial neoplasia.

- Composed of hyperplastic epithelial and stromal components
  - — Epithelial component
    - ◆ Large, irregularly shaped glands
    - ◆ Glands with a double cell layer and some with pseudostratification of secretory cells
    - ◆ Columnar cells with pale-staining granular cytoplasm
    - ◆ Papillae with fibrovascular cores
    - ◆ Chronic inflammatory infiltrate that surrounds glands
  - — Stromal component
    - ◆ Composed of fibroblasts and smooth muscle cells
- ▌ Basal cell proliferations
  - Basal cell hyperplasia (BCH)
    - — Typically an incidental finding

— Forms well-defined, small solid nests of basal cells or glandular structures; may have an infiltrative architecture

— Hyperplastic glands with proliferation of uniform basaloid cells that may occlude the glandular lumens

— Glands showing peripheral nuclear palisading

— Hypercellular, fibroblastic stroma

— Often seen together with typical benign (nodular) prostatic hyperplasia

- BCH with nucleolomegaly (atypical BCH)
  — Architecture is similar to that of BCH
  — Differentiating feature is basaloid cells with prominent nucleoli

■ Clear cell cribriform hyperplasia
- Almost always associated with benign (nodular) hyperplasia
- Characterized by distended acini arranged in a cribriform pattern
- Cells are cuboidal to columnar and have small hyperchromatic nuclei, indistinct nucleoli, and clear cytoplasm
- Basal cell layer is intact

■ Sclerosing adenosis
- Lobular or focally infiltrative glandular proliferation
- Glands may be round or compressed and have an angulated, slitlike appearance
- Glands have a double cell layer (may be difficult to appreciate) and a thickened basement membrane
- Cells contain medium-to-large nuclei with fine chromatin and typically indistinct nucleoli
- Stromal component contains plump spindle cells arranged randomly or in fascicles

■ Atypical adenomatous hyperplasia
- Architecturally similar to Gleason grade 1 or 2 adenocarcinoma
- Circumscribed proliferation of variably sized acini that may show focal infiltration at the periphery
- Tightly packed small glands intermixed with larger glands
- Basal cell layer may be discontinuous and indistinct but is usually focally present in at least some glands
- Glandular cells typically have pale to clear cytoplasm, small nuclei, and inconspicuous nucleoli; prominent nucleoli may occasionally be seen; however, macronucleoli (>3 μm) should not be present
- Corpora amylacea is often present (much less common in adenocarcinoma)

Special Stains and Immunohistochemistry

- HMWCK: highlights basal cell layer in benign (nodular) prostatic hyperplasia, BCH, clear cell cribriform hyperplasia, and sclerosing adenosis
- Muscle-specific actin (MSA) and S-100 protein positive for some basal and spindle cells in sclerosing adenosis (indicates myoepithelial differentiation)

Other Techniques for Diagnosis

- Noncontributory

Differential Diagnosis

■ Prostatic intraepithelial neoplasia (PIN)
- Glands are large and branched with intraluminal papillary projections
- Nuclei are elongated, pseudostratified, and perpendicular to the basement membrane

■ Prostatic adenocarcinoma, low grade
- Low-power microscopy reveals uniform proliferation of small glands with irregular contours and irregular stromal spacing
- Neoplastic glands are lined by a single layer of epithelium (basal cell layer is absent)
- Higher-power microscopy demonstrates cuboidal or columnar cells with abundant cytoplasm, enlarged nuclei, and prominent nucleoli
- Perineural infiltration is often present

■ Clear cell cribriform hyperplasia versus cribriform adenocarcinoma
- Cells in clear cell cribriform hyperplasia have distinct clear cytoplasm, small nuclei with indistinct nucleoli, and a prominent basal cell layer

Pearls

- Treatment for symptomatic hyperplasia is typically transurethral prostatectomy (TURP); occasionally treated with suprapubic prostatectomy
- May be treated with various drugs, including
  — Finasteride (androgen-converting enzyme inhibitor)
  — α_1-Adrenergic blockers
- Neoplastic nature of atypical adenomatous hyperplasia and its relationship to low-grade adenocarcinoma is an area of active investigation
- A diagnosis of carcinoma should not be made based on identification of a few malignant-appearing cells in a background clearly demonstrating atypical adenomatous hyperplasia

Selected References

Bostwick DG, Meiers I. Diagnosis of prostate carcinoma after therapy: Review 2007. Arch Pathol Lab Med 131:360-371, 2007.

Amin MB, Tamboli P, Verma M, Surgley JR: Postatrophic hyperplasia of the prostate gland: A detailed analysis of its morphology in needle biopsy specimens. Am J Surg Pathol 23:925-931, 1999.

Bostwick DG, Svigley J, Grignon D, et al: Atypical adenomatous hyperplasia of the prostate: Morphological criteria for its distinction from well-differentiated carcinoma. Hum Pathol 24:819-832, 1993.

Devaraj LT, Bostwick DG: Atypical basal cell hyperplasia of the prostate: Immunoprofile and proposed classification of basal cell proliferation. Am J Surg Pathol 17:645-659, 1993.

McNeal J: Pathology of benign prostatic hyperplasia: Insight into etiology. Urol Clin North Am 17:477-486, 1990.

Epithelial Metaplasia

Clinical Features

- Urothelial and transitional cell metaplasia
  - Describes a condition in which transitional epithelium is within the prostatic ducts and acini
  - Often seen in infants and neonates
  - Generally no clinical symptoms
- Squamous metaplasia
  - May be associated with infarction, estrogen therapy, androgen ablation, or radiation therapy
  - Common in neonates
  - Generally no clinical symptoms

Gross Pathology

- Nonspecific

Histopathology

- Urothelial and transitional cell metaplasia
  - Localized to peripheral prostatic ducts and acini
  - Urothelium admixed with alternating areas of cuboidal and columnar epithelium
  - Cells are spindle to ovoid to polygonal and have ovoid nuclei overlapping in a streaming manner; nuclei are uniform and have prominent nuclear grooves
  - May completely fill gland lumen forming a solid nest
  - Differs from normal urothelium by lack of umbrella cells and presence of eosinophilic secretory lining cells
- Squamous metaplasia
  - Squamous differentiation (polygonal cells with eosinophilic cytoplasm) with variable keratin formation and intercellular bridging
  - May be associated with infarcts and nodular prostatic hyperplasia; if associated with prostatic infarction, mild nuclear atypia may be seen
- Mucinous metaplasia
  - Haphazardly scattered or small groups of tall, mucin-filled goblet cells
  - Cells have small, dark, basally oriented nuclei and abundant mucin-filled cytoplasm
  - Can be found in association with normal and hyperplastic prostate glands, as well as in areas of urothelial metaplasia, BCH, or atrophy

Special Stains and Immunohistochemistry

- HMWCK positive in urothelial and transitional cells and squamous metaplasia
- Alcian blue and mucicarmine positive for intracytoplasmic acid mucin in mucinous metaplasia
- PAS positive for neutral mucin in mucinous metaplasia (diastase resistant)

Other Techniques for Diagnosis

- Noncontributory

Differential Diagnosis

- Transitional cell carcinoma
  - Carcinoma in situ (intraductal TCC) is typically present adjacent to the invasive component
  - Infiltrative component consists of single or small groups of cells showing hyperchromatic, pleomorphic nuclei with chromatin clumping, multiple nucleoli, and angulated nuclear borders
  - Mitotic figures and tumor necrosis are common
  - Desmoplasia is typically associated with the invasive stromal component
- Squamous and adenosquamous cell carcinoma
  - Rare in prostate gland
  - Infiltrative growth pattern composed of malignant cells with squamous features (keratin formation and intercellular bridging)
  - Must exclude secondary involvement from extraprostatic sites (e.g., urinary bladder)
  - Adenosquamous carcinoma composed of typical squamous cell carcinoma admixed with adenocarcinoma (patients usually have a history of radiation or hormonal therapy)
- Mucinous adenocarcinoma
  - At least 25% of tumor consists of extracellular mucin lakes
  - Neoplastic cells and glands float within lakes of extracellular mucin
  - Cribriform pattern is most common, with mucin within the gland lumina and dissecting between the stroma
  - Neoplastic cells have variable degree of cytologic atypia

Pearls

- None of the metaplastic cell types are associated with subsequent development of prostatic adenocarcinoma

Selected References

Yang XJ, Lecksell K, Short K, et al: Does long-term finasteride therapy affect the histologic features of benign prostatic tissue and prostate cancer on needle biopsy? PLEES Study Group. Proscar Long-Term Efficiency and Safety Study. Urology 53:696-700, 1999.

Sheaff MT, Baithum SI: Effects of radiation on the normal prostate gland. Histopathology 30:341-348, 1997.

Prostatic Intraepithelial Neoplasia

Clinical Features

- High-grade PIN is considered a premalignant condition based on morphologic, epidemiologic, and genetic features
- In autopsy series, high-grade PIN precedes carcinoma by 10 years and is common in the fourth decade of life
- Currently, high-grade PIN is associated with adenocarcinoma on rebiopsy in 25% of patients;

Figure 11-4. Prostatic intraepithelial neoplasia, high grade, flat type. Back-to-back glands lined by a single layer of epithelial cells with prominent nucleoli. Note the presence of attenuated basal cells (*inset*; high-molecular-weight cytokeratin immunohistochemical stain).

significantly less than the 50% association reported in patients biopsied in the late 1980s (see "Pearls")
- Presence of high-grade PIN mandates rebiopsy; however, it is unclear that chasing PIN has any benefit (i.e., it simply results in the detection of clinically insignificant prostate cancers)
- Clinical significance of low-grade PIN unclear; should not be diagnosed

Gross Pathology
- Nonspecific

Histopathology
- Low-grade PIN
  — Morphologic features not rigorously defined and subjective; should not be diagnosed
- High-grade PIN
  — Four patterns include tufted, cribriform, micropapillary, or flat
  — Cells have enlarged nuclei with prominent nucleoli
  — Basal cells are present but may be attenuated

Special Stains and Immunohistochemistry
- HMWCK and p63: basal cell layer is immunopositive but may be thin and attenuated
- α-Methylacyl coenzyme A racemase (AMACR): high-grade PIN may be positive but more apical and granular and less intense than carcinoma

Other Techniques for Diagnosis
- Morphometric studies: high-grade PIN and adenocarcinoma have similar cytologic features (i.e., nuclear area, nuclear perimeter size, nuclear shape, amount and distribution of chromatin, and nucleolar changes)

Differential Diagnosis
▌ Prostatic adenocarcinoma, low grade
  - Low-power magnification reveals a uniform compact proliferation of small glands with irregular contours and irregular stromal spacing
  - Neoplastic glands are lined by a single layer of epithelium (basal cell layer is absent)
  - Higher magnification demonstrates cuboidal or columnar cells with abundant cytoplasm, enlarged nuclei, and prominent nucleoli
  - Perineural infiltration is often present
  - Negative staining for HMWCK (no basal cell layer)

Pearls
- The decreasing association between high-grade PIN and carcinoma is due to
  — Increased number of cores performed per biopsy procedure with better targeting of peripheral zone
  — Changing patient population (younger, PSA screened) with lower prevalence or lower volume of adenocarcinoma; bayesian reasoning dictates that the positive predictive value of any test result (high-grade PIN on biopsy) is a function of the prevalence of disease (carcinoma) in the population being tested
- Diagnosis of high-grade PIN should be made conservatively (cells must show both nucleomegaly and nucleolomegaly)

Selected References
Iczkowski KA: Current Prostate Biopsy Interpretation. Criteria for cancer, atypical small acinar proliferation, high-grade prostatic intraepithelial neoplasia, and use of immunostains. Arch Pathol Lab Med 130:835-843, 2006.

Bostwick DG, Qian J: High-grade prostatic intraepithelial neoplasia. Mod Pathol 17:360-379, 2004.

Haggman MJ, Macosta JA, Wojno KJ, Oesterling JE: The relationship between prostatic intraepithelial neoplasm and prostate cancer: Critical issues. J Urol 158:12-22, 1997.

Bostwick DG, Pacelli A, Lopez-Beltran A: Molecular biology of prostatic intraepithelial neoplasia. Prostate 29:117-124, 1996.

Adenocarcinoma: Acinar (Conventional) and Distinct Subtypes (Colloid [Mucinous], Signet Ring Cell, Ductal Type, Foamy Gland, Carcinosarcoma [Sarcomatoid], Atrophic Type, Pseudohyperplastic)

Clinical Features
- Most common cause of cancer in men; second most common cause of cancer death after lung cancer
- One in five American men will be diagnosed with prostate cancer
- Occurs predominantly in men older than 50 years

Figure 11-5. A, Prostatic adenocarcinoma on needle core. Gleason score 3 + 2: pattern 3 based on variability in the size of the acini and pattern 2 based on good circumscription. **B, Findings pathognomonic for prostatic adenocarcinoma.** Circumferential perineural invasion (*top left*), extraprostatic invasion (*top right*), glomeruloid bodies (*bottom left*), and mucinous fibroplasia and collagenolysis (*bottom right*).

Continued

- More prevalent in black men and rare in Asians
- Familial predisposition exists
- Because of the typical location of prostatic carcinoma (posterior aspects of the peripheral zone), urinary symptoms occur late; asymptomatic tumors are often detected by digital rectal examination or after routine examination that detects elevated PSA
- Advanced disease may cause obstructive symptoms (difficulty initiating or terminating urination, frequency, or dysuria)

- Metastases to bone may cause osteoblastic or osteolytic lesions; however, in men, the demonstration of osteoblastic bone metastases is virtually diagnostic of metastatic prostate carcinoma
- Back pain is a common finding in patients with metastatic disease
- Screening methods
  — Digital rectal examination: cancer focus may be nonpalpable or indurated

Figure 11-5. cont'd. C, Variants of prostatic adenocarcinoma. Ductal type showing tall columnar cells with marked nucleomegaly and nucleolomegaly (*top left*), neuroendocrine carcinoma in a patient with a history of treated acinar-type adenocarcinoma (*top right*), signet ring cell type with individual cells diffusely infiltrating (*bottom left*), and mucinous type with intraluminal and interstitial mucin (*bottom right*).

— PSA levels greater than 4 ng/mL (some advocate 2 ng/mL) prompt biopsy
— Random bilateral biopsies now standard of care in select patients with nonpalpable disease
— Transrectal ultrasound with biopsy
- Elevated PSA is not sensitive or specific for prostatic cancer; other benign conditions, including inflammatory processes or nodular hyperplasia, may cause slight PSA elevation
- PSA levels do not distinguish between significant and insignificant cancers; identification of such biomarkers (e.g., EPCA-2) is an active area of research (see Flaig et al, 2007)
- Elevated PSA in patients after treatment for prostatic carcinoma is a useful indicator of recurrent or progressive disease
▌ Ductal-type adenocarcinoma
- Cystoscopy often shows a polypoid lesion with extension into prostatic urethra
- Patients may present with urinary obstruction symptoms earlier than patients with typical prostatic adenocarcinoma
▌ Carcinosarcoma (sarcomatoid)
- Associated with a previous or current high-grade prostatic adenocarcinoma
- May have a history of radiation therapy for prior adenocarcinoma of prostate
- Serum PSA may be normal or only slightly elevated

- Carcinosarcoma and sarcomatoid carcinoma are often used interchangeably; however, by convention
— *Carcinosarcoma* should be reserved for tumors that have distinct carcinomatous and sarcomatous elements by histology and immunohistochemistry
— *Sarcomatoid carcinoma* should be used for tumors that show a transition between the two elements

Gross Pathology

▌ Acinar (conventional) adenocarcinoma
- Often multifocal
- Preference for the posterior aspects of the peripheral zone (about 75% of tumors); this location renders tumor more likely to be palpable on digital rectal examination
- Small tumors typically show no gross abnormalities
- Neoplastic tissue is firm, gritty, and less spongy than the surrounding non-neoplastic prostate parenchyma; may show focal yellow discoloration
▌ Colloid (mucinous) adenocarcinoma
- Cut surface may be glistening or mucinous
▌ Ductal-type adenocarcinoma
- May have papillary or polypoid mass extending into urethra

Histopathology

▌ Acinar (conventional) adenocarcinoma
- Constitutes more than 95% of prostate cancer

- Low-power magnification
  - Haphazard proliferation of crowded, but uniform, small acini with irregular contours; typically has an infiltrative pattern
  - Occasionally the neoplastic glands are larger and have a papillary or cribriform architecture
  - High-grade tumors tend to grow in cords, nests, or sheets
  - See Gleason grading system (Table 11-1)

Table 11-1. Gleason Grading System

Characteristics

- Based on a low-power view of architectural growth patterns of the tumor
- Patterns are grouped into five grades based on a continuum of growth (1 through 5, with 1 being the most well differentiated)
- **Gleason score is the sum of the two most prevalent patterns**
- If only one pattern is present, it is multiplied by 2 to get the Gleason score
- Secondary pattern must occupy at least 5% of the tumor
- Grading aids in assessing malignant potential (invasiveness and metastases) and therapeutic decisions
- Final scores of 8 to 10 represent poorly differentiated, highly aggressive adenocarcinomas
- Final scores of 2 to 4 indicate a low malignant potential and are often of transition zone origin
- Good correlation between the prognosis and the degree of differentiation (i.e., Gleason grade)

Determination of Gleason Grade

- *Gleason grade 1:* Circumscribed nodule of uniform, closely packed neoplastic glands
- *Gleason grade 2:* Focally infiltrative glandular proliferation composed of more loosely arranged neoplastic glands
- *Gleason grade 3:* Infiltrative glandular proliferation composed of variably sized neoplastic glands that may form a cribriform pattern
- *Gleason grade 4:* Proliferation of fused and irregular glands with infiltrative growth pattern
- *Gleason grade 5:* Infiltrating tumor composed of individual or solid masses of neoplastic cells; often shows comedo necrosis (lacks glandular differentiation)

2005 International Society of Urological Pathology Consensus Conference on Gleason Grading of Prostatic Carcinoma Suggested Changes

- *Caveat:* Application of these changes may result in upgrading in as many as one fourth of needle core biopsies, yet these changes have few supporting clinical data.
- High-grade tumor of any amount is included in the final score
- Ill-defined glands with poorly formed lumens are Gleason grade 4
- Gleason grade 3 (cribriform pattern) is assigned only to glands of the same size or smaller-than-normal glands
- Lower-grade secondary patterns are ignored if they make up less than 5% of the tumor volume
- Foamy gland, colloid (mucinous), and small cell carcinoma variants and glomeruloid and mucinous fibroplasia (collagenous micronodule) patterns are not graded. Ductal-type and pseudohyperplastic adenocarcinoma variants should be grade 4 and 3, respectively

- High-power magnification
  - Acini are lined by a single layer of epithelial cells; basal cell layer is absent
  - Epithelial cells are cuboidal or columnar and have abundant amphophilic cytoplasm and enlarged, variably pleomorphic nuclei with one or more prominent macronucleoli
  - Mitotic figures are a helpful feature of malignancy but are uncommon, especially in low-grade tumors
  - Features pathognomonic for carcinoma include glomeruloid structures, mucinous fibroplasias (collagenous micronodules), circumferential perineural invasion, and extraprostatic extension
  - Blue-tinged mucinous material, amorphous eosinophilic material, and crystalloid within lumina of neoplastic glands (less common in benign glands) may be seen
  - Corpora amylacea is rare (much more common in benign conditions)
- Colloid (mucinous) adenocarcinoma
  - Uncommon variant
  - At least 25% of tumor consists of extracellular mucin lakes
  - Neoplastic cells and glands float within lakes of extracellular mucin
  - Cribriform pattern is most common, with mucin within the gland lumina and dissecting between stromal muscle fibers
  - Neoplastic cells have variable degrees of cytologic atypia
  - Typically associated with an acinar-type adenocarcinoma
  - Considered Gleason grade 4 and is associated with aggressive biologic behavior
- Signet ring cell adenocarcinoma
  - At least 25% of tumor consists of cells with a cytoplasmic vacuole that displaces the nucleus to the side
  - Cells diffusely infiltrate the stroma and invade perineural and vascular spaces as well as the prostatic capsule
  - Other patterns of prostatic adenocarcinoma in the same tumor are typically seen
- Ductal-type adenocarcinoma
  - Located in the larger periurethral prostatic ducts and usually found in association with acinar-type adenocarcinoma
  - Papillary and cribriform architecture composed of pseudostratified columnar cells; comedo necrosis may be seen
  - Neoplastic cells have atypical large nuclei with coarse chromatin and large nucleoli
  - Mitotic figures are common
  - Considered Gleason grade 4 (or 5 if comedo necrosis is present); some consider this a subset of acinar adenocarcinoma, Gleason grade 4

- Foamy gland adenocarcinoma
  - Histologically characterized by cells with abundant foamy cytoplasm and bland nuclei
  - May be underdiagnosed on needle core because of lack of nucleomegaly and nucleolomegaly
  - Usually associated with higher-Gleason-score acinar-type adenocarcinoma; therefore, prognostic significance per se unclear
- Pseudohyperplastic adenocarcinoma
  - Two patterns on low-power microscopy
    - Crowded glands lined by pseudostratified epithelium (truly pseudohyperplastic)
    - Large acini
  - High-power microscopy shows nucleomegaly and nucleolomegaly
  - May be underdiagnosed on needle core biopsy because the pseudostratified epithelium looks like hyperplasia or high-grade PIN on low-power microscopy and the large acinar pattern deviates from the more typical small acinar pattern
- Carcinosarcoma (sarcomatoid)
  - Biphasic tumor: admixture of carcinoma and sarcoma components
  - Sarcoma component consists of spindle cells with pleomorphic nuclei and high mitotic rate
  - Common sarcoma patterns
    - Malignant fibrous histiocytoma-like
    - High-grade sarcoma-like, not otherwise specified
    - Fibrosarcoma-like
    - Leiomyosarcoma-like
  - Elements resembling osteosarcoma, rhabdomyosarcoma, or chondrosarcoma may be present
  - Carcinoma component is usually high grade
- Atrophic-type adenocarcinoma
  - Glandular proliferation with an infiltrative growth pattern
  - Neoplastic cells have large nuclei with prominent nucleoli
  - Glands lack a basal cell layer
  - Generally associated with an adjacent acinar adenocarcinoma
- Treated adenocarcinoma
  - Androgen deprivation therapy
    - Smaller acini or single cells with loss of nucleolomegaly and cytoplasmic clearing (special stains may be required); residual carcinoma showing treatment effect should not be Gleason graded
    - Adjacent benign tissue shows stromal hyperplasia and gland involution with BCH and squamous metaplasia
  - Radiation therapy
    - Smaller acini or single cells with cytoplasmic vacuolization (special stains may be required); residual carcinoma showing treatment effect should not be Gleason graded
    - Adjacent benign tissue shows glandular atrophy, nucleomegaly, nucleolomegaly, and BCH

Special Stains and Immunohistochemistry

- AMACR
  - Sensitive and specific marker for conventional (acinar) prostate cancer; positive in 82% to 100% of cases
  - Less sensitive in low-grade and hormone-treated conventional prostate cancer and prostate cancer variants, such as foamy gland, pseudohyperplastic, atrophic-type, and ductal-type prostate cancers
  - Positive but less intense, noncircumferential or only focal in high-grade PIN, atypical adenomatous hyperplasia, atrophy, nephrogenic adenoma, and benign glands adjacent to cancer
  - AMACR is less useful in evaluating metastases because many tumors in other organs are immunopositive
- HMWCK and p63
  - Stains basal cell cytoplasm (HMWCK) and nuclei (p63); therefore, negative in adenocarcinoma because basal cells are absent
- PSA and prostatic acid phosphatase (PAP) positive for tumor cells of mucinous, signet ring cell, and ductal-type variants of adenocarcinoma; also positive in epithelial component of carcinosarcoma
- Carcinoembryonic antigen (CEA) positive in some ductal-type variants of carcinoma
- Vimentin: spindle cell component of carcinosarcoma positive
- Desmin, smooth muscle actin (SMA), and S-100 protein: variable positivity in spindle cell component of carcinosarcoma

Other Techniques for Diagnosis

- Genetic studies: familial studies have demonstrated an 8q24 genetic variant that may be associated with prostate cancer risk. TMPRSS2-ERG fusion has been identified as an early molecular event in the development of prostate cancer
- Flow cytometry: diploid tumors have a more favorable outcome than tumors that are aneuploid

Differential Diagnosis

- Sclerosing adenosis
  - Lobular or focally infiltrative glandular proliferation composed of glands with a double cell layer (may be difficult to appreciate) and a thickened basement membrane
  - Cells contain medium-sized to large nuclei with fine chromatin and indistinct nucleoli
  - Stromal component contains plump spindle cells arranged randomly or in fascicles
  - Cellular spindle cell component is positive for actin and S-100 protein (indicates myoepithelial differentiation)
- Atypical adenomatous hyperplasia (adenosis)
  - Architecturally similar to Gleason grade 1 or 2 adenocarcinoma

- Circumscribed proliferation of variably sized acini that may show focal infiltration at the periphery
- Tightly packed small glands intermixed with larger glands
- Basal cell layer may be discontinuous and indistinct but is usually focally present in at least some glands (positive staining for HMWCK)
- Glandular cells typically have pale to clear cytoplasm, small nuclei, and inconspicuous nucleoli; distinct nucleoli may occasionally be seen; however, macronucleoli (>3 μm) should not be present
- Corpora amylacea is often present (much less common in adenocarcinoma)
- Often seen adjacent to unequivocal adenocarcinoma

▐ PIN
- Usually large acini (invasive carcinoma usually small to medium-sized acini)
- Glands are large and branched and have intraluminal papillary projections
- Nuclei are elongated and pseudostratified and have large nuclei with prominent nucleoli
- Positive HMWCK staining of basal layer distinguishes this from carcinoma
- Often seen adjacent to unequivocal adenocarcinoma

▐ Glandular atrophy versus atrophic-type adenocarcinoma
- Atrophic glands may have a focally infiltrative architecture and thus may mimic atrophic-type adenocarcinoma
- Atrophic glands have open lumens and are lined by cells with an increased nuclear-to-cytoplasmic ratio and inconspicuous nucleoli
- Atrophic-type adenocarcinoma is associated with an adjacent acinar adenocarcinoma

▐ Clear cell cribriform hyperplasia versus cribriform adenocarcinoma
- Cells in clear cell cribriform hyperplasia have distinct clear cytoplasm, small nuclei with indistinct nucleoli, and a prominent basal cell layer

▐ Transitional cell carcinoma
- Typically, TCC involves the urethra or prostatic ducts in patients with a history of carcinoma in situ of the urinary bladder who have been treated conservatively
- Carcinoma in situ (intraductal TCC) is typically present adjacent to the invasive component
- Lacks glandular differentiation
- Mitotic figures and tumor necrosis are common
- Stains negative for PSA and PAP

Pearls

- Prostatic carcinoma is typically multifocal, and gross examination usually underestimates the extent of disease
- Tumors of the transitional zone are less aggressive than tumors of the peripheral zone
- Metastases typically involve the pelvic or para-aortic lymph nodes and axial skeleton (most commonly lumbar vertebrae)

- Only in recent years has a survival advantage been demonstrated with the onset of widespread PSA screening; however, this same advantage has also been observed in Europe, where PSA screening is less common
- AMACR staining quality may be affected by technologist expertise, run-to-run variability, and the use of monoclonal (P504S) versus polyclonal antibodies, with the latter showing more background staining
- Total androgen blockade therapy is commonly used as an adjunct to postradiation therapy for treatment of adenocarcinoma metastases
  — Luteinizing hormone–releasing hormone agonists (e.g., leuprolide)
  — Direct antiandrogens (e.g., flutamide)
- Endocrine therapy is used to deprive tumor cells of testosterone and is typically used in patients with widespread metastatic disease (orchiectomy or estrogen administration decreases or eliminates testicular production of testosterone)
- Cryotherapy and radiation implants are being used more frequently as alternatives to radical prostatectomy
- In general, the presence of lymph node metastases precludes radical prostatectomy
- Submission of tissue for evaluation should allow for the following (Table 11-2)

Table 11-2. Pathologic Staging Based on 2005 TNM System

Stage	Description
T1	**Microscopic disease (clinically nonpalpable and asymptomatic)**
T1a	Tumor in up to 5% of examined tissue
T1b	Tumor in more than 5% of examined tissue
T1c	Tumor identified in needle biopsy
T2	**Palpable tumor**
T2a	Tumor in less than half of one lobe
T2b	Tumor in more than half of one lobe
T2c	Tumor in both lobes
T3	**Extracapsular extension (still clinically localized)**
T3a	Unilateral or bilateral
T3b	Seminal vesicle invasion
T4	**Tumor invades adjacent structures (other than seminal vesicles), such as bladder neck, rectum, external sphincter, levator muscle, or pelvic wall**
N1	**Regional lymph nodes**
M1	**Distant metastases**
M1a	Nonregional lymph nodes
M1b	Bone involvement
M1c	Other sites

— Orientation and location of tumor
— Status of the prostate pseudocapsule (not involved, penetration without perforation, and extraprostatic extension)
— Extent and location of extraprostatic extension and seminal vesicle invasion, if applicable
— Postoperative measure of specimen volume for correlation with imaging studies
— Evaluation of tumor grade
● Ten-year survival rate for all stages of adenocarcinoma is about 50%
— Localized tumor: 10-year survival rate is 95%
— Adenocarcinoma with metastases to regional lymph nodes: 40% survival at 10 years
— Adenocarcinoma with metastases to distant organs: 10% survival at 10 years

Selected References

Berney DM, Fisher G, Kattan MW, et al: Pitfalls in the diagnosis of prostate cancer: Retrospective review of 1791 cases with clinical outcome. Histopathology 51:452-457, 2007.

Braeckman J, Michielsen D: Prognostic factors in prostate cancer. Rec Results Cancer Res 175:25-32, 2007.

Flaig TW, Nordeen SK, Lucia S, et al: Conference report and review: Current status of biomarkers potentially associated with prostate cancer outcomes. J Urol 177:1229-1237, 2007.

Gudmundsson J, Sulem P, Manolescu A, et al: Genome-wide association study identifies a second prostate cancer susceptibility variant at 8q24. Nat Genet 39:631-637, 2007.

Leman E, Cannon G, Trock B, et al: EPCA-2: A highly specific serum marker for prostate cancer. Urology 69:714-720, 2007.

Lapointe J, Kim YH, Miller MA, et al: A variant of TMPRSS2 isoform and ERG fusion gene product in prostate cancer with implications for molecular diagnosis. Mod Pathol 20:463-473, 2007.

Bostwick DG, Meiers I: Atypical small acinar proliferation in the prostate: Clinical significance in 2006. Arch Pathol Lab Med 130:952-957, 2006.

Guimaraes MS, Billis A, Quintal MM, et al: The impact of the 2005 International Society of Urological Pathology (ISUP) consensus conference on standard Gleason grading of prostatic carcinoma (abstract). Lab Invest 86:639, 2006.

Iczkowski KA: Current prostate biopsy interpretation: Criteria for cancer, atypical small acinar proliferation, high-grade prostatic intraepithelial neoplasia, and use of immunostains. Arch Pathol Lab Med 130:835-843, 2006.

Srigley JR and Members of the Cancer Committee, College of American Pathologists: Updated protocol for the examination of specimens from patients with carcinomas of the prostate gland. Arch Pathol Lab Med 130:936-946, 2006.

Epstein JI, Allsbrook WC, Amin MB, Egevad LL, and the ISUP Grading Committee: The 2005 International Society of Urological Pathology (ISUP) consensus conference on Gleason grading of prostatic carcinoma. Am J Surg Pathol 29:1228-1242, 2005.

Adley BP, Yang XJ: Application of alpha-methylacyl coenzyme A racemase immunohistochemistry in the diagnosis of prostate cancer: A review. Anal Quant Cytol Histol 27:1-12, 2005.

Amin M, Boccon-Gibod L, Egevad LL, et al: Prognostic and predictive factors and reporting of prostate carcinoma in prostate needle biopsy specimens. Scand J Urol Nephrol 39:20-33, 2005.

Basal Cell Carcinoma

Clinical Features

● Basal cell tumors consist of a spectrum of disease ranging from BCH to atypical BCH to basal cell adenoma to basal cell carcinoma (some authors refer to basal cell tumors with a cribriform architecture as *adenoid basal cell tumor* or *adenoid cystic carcinoma*)
● Serum PSA and PAP levels are typically not elevated
● Benign and malignant basal cell lesions are relatively uncommon (reported in less than 6% to 9% of cases); benign basal cell proliferations make up most of them

Gross Pathology

● Nonspecific

Histopathology

▮ Basal cell carcinoma
● Infiltrative clusters of basaloid cells
● Often have prominent desmoplastic stromal response
● Must demonstrate one or more of the following features: necrosis, perineural invasion, or infiltration outside prostatic capsule
▮ Cribriform basal cell tumors (adenoid basal cell tumor)
● Histologic features similar to those of adenoid cystic carcinoma of the salivary glands
● Cells form poorly circumscribed, infiltrative nodules surrounded by a loose or myxoid stroma
● Nests show peripheral nuclear palisading around adenoid cystlike spaces that contain mucinous, eosinophilic, or hyaline material
● Focal squamous differentiation with keratin production may be seen
● Basaloid cells are uniform and have round hyperchromatic nuclei
● Perineural invasion is rare
● Low malignant potential; no reports of metastasis (believed by some authors to be part of BCH and adenoma)

Special Stains and Immunohistochemistry

● PSA and PAP typically positive
● HMWK: focal weak positivity in basaloid cells

Other Techniques for Diagnosis

● Noncontributory

Differential Diagnosis

▮ Sclerosing adenosis
● Lobular or focally infiltrative proliferation composed of glands with a double cell layer (may be difficult to appreciate) and a thickened basement membrane

- Cells contain medium-sized to large nuclei with fine chromatin and indistinct nucleoli
- Cellular spindle cell stroma with evidence of myoepithelial differentiation demonstrated by positive staining for S-100 protein and MSA
▌ Atypical adenomatous hyperplasia
  - Circumscribed proliferation of variably sized acini that may show focal infiltration at the periphery
  - Tightly packed small glands intermixed with larger glands
  - Some glands may show a basal cell layer (positive for HMWCK)
  - Glandular cells typically have pale to clear cytoplasm, small nuclei, and inconspicuous nucleoli; prominent nucleoli may occasionally be seen; however, macronucleoli (>3 μm) should not be present
▌ Adenocarcinoma, cribriform type
  - Typical cytologic features of malignancy, including cuboidal or columnar cells with abundant amphophilic cytoplasm, enlarged nuclei, and one or more prominent macronucleoli
  - Absence of basal cell layer (negative for HMWCK)

Pearls

- Typically treated with transurethral resection; controversy still exists regarding treatment for basal cell carcinoma
- Basal cell lesions in the prostate form a spectrum of disease behavior that is typically benign
- Malignant behavior in adenoid basal cell tumor has not been demonstrated

Selected References

Ali TZ, Epstein JI: Basal cell carcinoma of the prostate: A clinicopathologic study of 29 cases. Am J Surg Pathol 31:697-705, 2007.

Tan PH, Billis A: Basal cell carcinoma. In Eble JN, Sauter G, Epstein JI, Sesterhenn IA (eds): World Health Organization Classification of Tumours: Pathology and Genetics: Tumours of the Urinary System and Male Genital Organs. Lyon, IARC Press, 2004, p 206.

Devaraj LT, Bostwick DG: Atypical basal cell hyperplasia of the prostate: Immunoprofile and proposed classification of basal cell proliferation. Am J Surg Pathol 17:645-659, 1999.

Neuroendocrine (Small Cell) Carcinoma

Clinical Features

- Rarely occurs de novo; patients usually have a history of treated prostate cancer
- Most show no evidence of hormonal secretion; however, paraneoplastic syndromes can occur
  — Cushing syndrome (most common)
  — Malignant hypercalcemia
  — Syndrome of inappropriate antidiuretic hormone (SIADH)
  — Eaton-Lambert syndrome
- May have minor elevations of serum PSA
- Metastasizes through hematogenous (liver, brain) rather than lymphatic channels

Gross Pathology

- Nonspecific

Histopathology

- Histologic features similar to those of small cell carcinoma of the lung
- Necrosis is commonly seen in small cell carcinoma
- Typical acinar pattern of adenocarcinoma is present in more than 50% of cases; the neuroendocrine component should not be assigned a Gleason score

Special Stains and Immunohistochemistry

- Neuron-specific enolase (NSE), chromogranin, and cytokeratin typically positive
- PSA and PAP: often negative or only focally positive
- AMACR: 50% positive
- Secretory products may be present within neoplastic cells
  — Adrenocorticotropic hormone (ACTH), serotonin, calcitonin, human chorionic gonadotropin (HCG), thyroid-stimulating hormone (TSH), and bombesin

Other Techniques for Diagnosis

- Electron microscopy: neuroendocrine cells contain round, regular membrane-bound neurosecretory granules, measuring 100 to 400 nm

Differential Diagnosis

▌ Metastatic small cell carcinoma from bladder or lung
  - Clinical history is important
  - Lacks associated acinar adenocarcinoma that is usually seen in primary neuroendocrine carcinoma of the prostate gland
  - Thyroid transcription factor-1 (TTF-1) immunostain not useful
▌ Non-Hodgkin lymphoma
  - Primary prostatic lymphoma is rare
  - Neoplastic lymphoid population infiltrating around ducts and acini (typically spares prostatic glands)
  - Infiltration into surrounding periprostatic tissue is common
  - Positive for leukocyte common antigen (LCA)
  - Negative for cytokeratin, NSE, chromogranin, and other neuroendocrine markers

Pearls

- Many acinar-type prostatic adenocarcinomas show immunohistochemical evidence of neuroendocrine differentiation, the significance of which is unknown
- Neuroendocrine carcinoma of the prostate may respond to small cell carcinoma–directed chemotherapy but is clinically aggressive

- Neuroendocrine carcinoma is more aggressive when androgen receptors are expressed (10 months' survival time versus more than 30 months' survival time)

Selected References

Yao JL, Madeb R, Bourne P, et al: Small cell carcinoma of the prostate: An immunohistochemical study. Am J Surg Pathol 30:705-712, 2006.

di Sant'Agnese PA, Egevad L, Epstein JI, et al: Neuroendocrine tumors. In Eble JN, Sauter G, Epstein JI, Sesterhenn IA (eds): World Health Organization Classification of Tumours: Pathology and Genetics: Tumours of the Urinary System and Male Genital Organs. Lyon, IARC Press, 2004, pp 207-208.

Transitional Cell Carcinoma

Clinical Features

- Rare primary prostate gland tumor (represents 1% to 3% of primary prostatic gland malignancies)
- Common symptoms include hematuria or urinary obstruction
- PSA not elevated
- Three modes of prostatic involvement
  — Primary tumor of prostatic urethra, ducts, or acini
  — Secondary mucosal involvement from a prior or currently active bladder cancer
  — Direct invasion from bladder cancer infiltrating through the bladder wall

Gross Pathology

- Nodular proliferation in prostatic urethra
- Nonspecific nodular architecture with involvement of prostatic ducts and acini

Histopathology

- Carcinoma in situ (intraductal TCC) is typically present adjacent to the invasive component; may involve the urethra, the prostatic ducts and acini, and occasionally the ejaculatory ducts and seminal vesicles
- Infiltrative component consists of small groups or single cells with hyperchromatic, pleomorphic nuclei with chromatin clumping, multiple nucleoli, and angulated nuclear borders
- Mitotic figures and tumor necrosis are common
- Elicits a desmoplastic stromal reaction
- Pagetoid spread and squamous metaplasia may be seen

Special Stains and Immunohistochemistry

- HMWCK, CK7, and CK20 variably positive
- PSA and PAP negative

Other Techniques for Diagnosis

- Noncontributory

Differential Diagnosis

▌ Prostatic adenocarcinoma
  - Gleason grade 5 adenocarcinoma with comedo necrosis may be difficult to distinguish from TCC
  - Focal gland formation can typically be found after careful evaluation of multiple sections
  - Not associated with TCC in situ
  - Positive for PSA, PAP, or AMACR

Pearls

- Typically TCC involves the urethra or prostatic ducts in patients with a history of carcinoma in situ of the bladder who have been treated
- Prostatic urethra urothelial carcinoma involving the prostate can rarely be mucinous (urothelial mucinous adenocarcinoma of the prostate)
- Prostatic stromal involvement by TCC is by definition stage T4 disease and carries a poor prognosis
- Radical cystoprostatectomy is the typical treatment

Selected References

Osunkoya AO, Epstein JI: Primary mucin-producing urothelial-type adenocarcinoma of prostate: Report of 15 cases. Am J Surg Pathol 31:1323-1329, 2007.

Palou J, Baniel J, Klotz L, et al: Urothelial carcinoma of the prostate. Urology 69:50-61, 2007.

Grignon DJ: Urothelial carcinoma. In Eble JN, Sauter G, Epstein JI, Sesterhenn IA (eds): World Health Organization Classification of Tumours: Pathology and Genetics: Tumours of the Urinary System and Male Genital Organs. Lyon, IARC Press, 2004, pp 202-204.

Squamous Cell Carcinoma and Adenosquamous Carcinoma

Clinical Features

- Rare in the prostate gland
- Typically found in older age group (mean age of about 70 years)
- Two clinical scenarios
  — Primary, de novo squamous cell carcinoma
  — Associated with treated (radiation or hormone ablation) adenocarcinoma
- Serum PSA and PAP are usually normal
- Metastatic bone lesions osteolytic, in contrast to adenocarcinoma, which causes osteoblastic bone lesions
- Most commonly associated with squamous cell carcinoma of the urinary bladder
- May be associated with *Schistosoma haematobium* infection

Gross Pathology

- Nonspecific

Figure 11-6. Primary squamous cell carcinoma of the prostate. A, Cross sections showing nodular growth replacing the gland. Low-power (**B**) and high-power (**C**) photomicrographs showing infiltrative squamous cell carcinoma with keratinization.

Histopathology

- Similar histologic features to squamous cell carcinoma of other sites
- Malignant squamous cells arranged in cords and nests with an infiltrative architecture
- Two forms of carcinoma
  - — Pure squamous carcinoma
    - ◆ Rare
    - ◆ Infiltrative growth pattern composed of malignant cells with squamous features (keratin formation and intercellular bridging)
    - ◆ No gland formation
    - ◆ No patient history of radiation or hormonal therapy
    - ◆ Must exclude secondary involvement from extraprostatic sites (e.g., bladder)
  - — Adenosquamous carcinoma
    - ◆ Admixture of adenocarcinoma and squamous cell carcinoma
    - ◆ Typically associated with a history of radiation or hormonal therapy

Special Stains and Immunohistochemistry

- PSA and PAP are positive in glandular component of adenosquamous carcinoma; pure squamous cell carcinoma is typically negative

Other Techniques for Diagnosis

- Noncontributory

Differential Diagnosis

- ▌ Squamous metaplasia
  - Commonly associated with prostatic infarction
  - Lacks significant cytologic atypia and tumor necrosis
- ▌ Prostatic primary
  - Much more common to have a squamous cell carcinoma in the prostate gland as metastatic disease or direct extension from adjacent organs (i.e., urinary bladder) than as a prostatic primary

Pearls

- Behaves in an aggressive manner (mean survival of 14 months, regardless of therapy)
- Unresponsive to androgen-deprivation therapy

Selected References

Van der Kwast TH: Squamous neoplasms. In Eble JN, Sauter G, Epstein JI, Sesterhenn IA (eds): World Health Organization Classification of Tumours: Pathology and Genetics: Tumours of the Urinary System and Male Genital Organs. Lyon, IARC Press, 2004, pp 205-206.

Gattuso P, Carson HJ, Candel A, et al: Adenosquamous carcinoma of the prostate. Hum Pathol 26:123-126, 1995.

Moskovitz N, Munichor M, Bolkier M, et al: Squamous cell carcinoma of the prostate. Urol Int 51:181-183, 1993.

Phyllodes Tumor

Clinical Features

- Rare neoplasm
- Wide age range
- Patients present with symptoms associated with prostatic enlargement, which include urinary obstruction, hematuria, and dysuria

Gross Pathology

- Multinodular solid, gray-white mass
- Cut surface may be spongy or cystic
- Variable size; may be larger than 25 cm in diameter

Histopathology

- Biphasic tumor composed of epithelial and stromal components
  - Epithelial cells are cuboidal to columnar, arranged in a double-layer lining glands, cysts, or slitlike spaces
  - Stellate to spindle stromal cells arranged in a loose, myxoid background
- Glandular or cystic spaces compressed by cellular stroma into a leaflike configuration
- Likelihood of recurrence and malignant behavior is associated with a high stromal to epithelial ratio (stromal hypercellularity), cellular atypia, and high mitotic rate

Special Stains and Immunohistochemistry

- Vimentin: stromal component is typically positive
- PSA and PAP: epithelial cell may be positive
- SMA negative

Figure 11-7. Prostatic phyllodes tumor. Proliferation of specialized prostatic stroma bulging into prostatic glands and creating clefted spaces.

Other Techniques for Diagnosis

- Noncontributory

Differential Diagnosis

- Stromal hyperplasia
  - Benign prostatic hyperplasia nodule with stromal overgrowth may be large
  - Lacks epithelial component and leaflike configuration
- Giant multilocular prostatic cystadenoma
  - Solitary cystic tumor with a surrounding dense fibrous stroma
  - Numerous, variably sized cystic spaces lined by benign-appearing prostatic epithelium
  - Lacks leaflike configuration
- Postoperative spindle cell proliferation
  - Rare reactive spindle cell proliferation that may occur after transurethral prostate resection (previously resected prostate tissue must show no evidence of a mesenchymal or spindle cell tumor)
  - Benign cytologic features and variable mitotic rate (uniform cells with no nuclear pleomorphism and no atypical mitotic figures)
  - Lacks epithelial component
- Solitary fibrous tumor of the prostate
  - Low-power view has variable cellularity and lacks leaflike configuration
  - High-power view has spindled cells insinuating themselves into bands of collagen
- Leiomyoma or leiomyosarcoma
  - Monophasic hypercellular spindle cell neoplasm without epithelial component
  - Positive for SMA and desmin
- Sarcomatoid carcinoma
  - Malignant spindle cell proliferation admixed with a malignant epithelial component
  - Spindle cell component may predominate; cytokeratin positivity, the distinguishing feature, may be weak and focal

Pearls

- Most are cured by surgical resection and follow a benign clinical course; however, biologic behavior is difficult to predict based on histologic features
- Tumors with overtly malignant stromal component have given rise to distant metastases (most commonly lung and bone)
- Diagnosis on needle biopsy may be difficult

Selected References

Hansel DE, Herawi M, Montgomery E, Epstein JI: Spindle cell lesions of the prostate. Mod Pathol 20:148-158, 2007.

Herawi M, Epstein JI: Specialized stromal tumors of the prostate: A clinicopathologic study of 50 cases. Am J Surg Pathol 30:694-704, 2006.

Cheville J, Algaba F, Boccon-Gibod L, et al: Mesenchymal Tumors. In Eble JN, Sauter G, Epstein JI, Sesterhenn IA (eds):

World Health Organization Classification of Tumours: Pathology and Genetics: Tumours of the Urinary System and Male Genital Organs. Lyon, IARC Press, 2004, pp 209-211.

Pins MR, Campbell SC, Laskin WB, et al: Solitary fibrous tumor of the prostate: A report of two cases and review of the literature. Arch Pathol Lab Med 125:274-277, 2001.

Rhabdomyosarcoma

Clinical Features

- Most common sarcoma of the prostate
- Occurs primarily between birth and 6 years of age
- Most common in the head and neck, followed by the genitourinary tract
- About 20% of childhood cases occur in the genitourinary tract
- Rare cases reported in older men
- Presents with pelvic mass and urethral obstruction
- Pelvic mass may cause bladder displacement and rectal compression

Gross Pathology

- Large, gray-white mass typically measuring 5 to 10 cm
- Appears grossly circumscribed but is typically infiltrative microscopically

Histopathology

- Embryonal rhabdomyosarcoma
  - Most common subtype
  - Mixture of sheets of primitive, undifferentiated, round to spindle cells admixed with haphazardly arranged rhabdomyoblasts in a myxoid stroma
  - Primitive cells are small and round with dark nuclei and minimal cytoplasm
  - Variable numbers of strap cells, with or without cross-striations
  - Variable mitotic activity
- Alveolar, botryoid, and pleomorphic patterns
  - These patterns are rare
  - Botryoid pattern consists of polypoid fragments covered with urothelium that often extends into the urethra or bladder

Special Stains and Immunohistochemistry

- Vimentin, MSA, desmin, and myoglobin positive
- Stains negatively for cytokeratin, LCA, NSE, PSA, and PAP

Other Techniques for Diagnosis

- Electron microscopy: rhabdomyoblasts have cytoplasmic myofilaments and Z bands
- Flow cytometry: tumor cells are typically aneuploid

Differential Diagnosis

- Must rule out metastasis from other primitive childhood small round blue cell tumors

- Non-Hodgkin lymphoma
  - Typically found in older age groups
  - Neoplastic lymphoid cells infiltrating stroma in diffuse sheets or patches; ducts and acini are typically spared
  - Positive for LCA
  - Composed of a monoclonal lymphoid population

Pearls

- Presence of strap cells or rhabdomyoblasts is diagnostic
- Treatment typically consists of surgery, chemotherapy, and radiotherapy
- Three-year survival rate is 70% with combined-therapy regimen

Selected References

Hansel DE, Herawi M, Montgomery E, Epstein JI: Spindle cell lesions of the prostate. Mod Pathol 20:148-158, 2007.

Ferrer FA, Isakoff M, Koyle MA: Bladder / prostate rhabdomyosarcoma: Past, present and future. J Urol 176:1283-1291, 2006.

Lymphoma

Clinical Features

- Most common in older men (mean age, 60 years)
- Presents with urinary obstruction symptoms
- Primary lymphoma involves the prostate gland without extraglandular involvement (i.e., liver, spleen, lymph nodes, peripheral blood)
- Secondary involvement of the prostate gland by a systemic lymphoma is more common than primary prostate lymphoma
- Systemic symptoms (fever, chills, night sweats, and weight loss) are infrequent and typically seen only in patients with disseminated disease

Gross Pathology

- Diffuse enlargement of the prostate gland
- Tan, homogeneous, rubbery parenchyma

Histopathology

- Proliferation of neoplastic lymphoid cells that typically infiltrate the prostatic stroma in diffuse sheets while sparing the ducts and acini
- Infiltration into surrounding periprostatic tissues is common
- Most common subtype is diffuse large cell lymphoma, B-cell type; small cleaved cell lymphoma is also relatively common
- Hodgkin disease is rare

Special Stains and Immunohistochemistry

- LCA positive (non-Hodgkin lymphoma)
- Refer to Chapter 14 for specific immunohistochemistry profiles

Other Techniques for Diagnosis

- Flow cytometric immunophenotyping using fresh tissue is useful in documenting clonality and for subtyping lymphomas (refer to Chapter 14)

Differential Diagnosis

- Chronic prostatitis with follicular hyperplasia
  - Mixed inflammatory infiltrate with germinal center formation
  - Inflammation is typically within duct lumina and in the glandular epithelium
  - Nonclonal lymphocytic population
- Granulomatous prostatitis
  - Admixture of histiocytes, plasma cells, eosinophils, neutrophils, lymphocytes, and giant cells
  - Inflammatory cells cause destruction of the prostatic ducts and acini
- Neuroendocrine carcinoma
  - Characteristic prostatic adenocarcinoma associated with a neuroendocrine carcinoma, which may range from a low-grade neuroendocrine carcinoma (carcinoid) to a small cell undifferentiated carcinoma (oat cell carcinoma)
  - Areas of necrosis are typical in small cell carcinoma
  - Positive for cytokeratin, NSE, chromogranin, and other neuroendocrine markers
  - Negative for LCA
- Rhabdomyosarcoma
  - Typically found in younger age group
  - Mixture of sheets of primitive, undifferentiated, round to spindle cells admixed with haphazardly arranged rhabdomyoblasts in a myxoid stroma
  - Positive for MSA, desmin, and myoglobin
  - Negative for LCA

Pearls

- Surgery is used mainly for relief of urinary obstruction symptoms
- Poor prognosis; death typically results within 2 years of diagnosis

Selected References

Araki K, Kubota Y, Lijima Y, et al: Indolent behaviour of low-grade B-cell lymphoma of mucosa-associated lymphoid tissue involved in salivary glands, renal sinus and prostate. Scand J Urol Nephrol 32:234-236, 1998.

Bostwick DG, Mann RB: Malignant lymphomas involving the prostate: A study of 13 cases. Cancer 56:2932-2938, 1985.

Testis

Cryptorchidism

Clinical Features

- Usually unilateral (75%)
- Occurs in 3% to 4% of term infants and in up to 20% of premature infants

Figure 11-8. Cryptorchidism. Complete tubular sclerosis and mild Leydig cell hyperplasia.

- Undescended testicles typically descend by 3 months of age (<1% remain undescended at 1 year of age)
- Associated with an inguinal hernia in 10% to 20% of cases
- Most cryptorchid testes are found in the inguinal canal
- Right testicle is more commonly involved
- Patients with undescended and surgically descended cryptorchid testes have decreased fertility and increased risk for certain germ cell and non–germ cell tumors
- Normal descent of testes is under hormonal control

Gross Pathology

- Cryptorchid testes are smaller and softer than normal testes

Histopathology

- Histologic changes in cryptorchid testis occur by age 2 years
- Seminiferous tubules may be small or ring shaped and have areas of tubular sclerosis or atrophy
- Spermatogonia may be decreased in number and irregularly distributed or totally absent
- Sertoli cells are increased in number; Leydig cell hyperplasia may be prominent
- Interstitium is typically widened and edematous
- Normally descended testis contralateral to the cryptorchid testis often shows many of the same histologic features

Special Stains and Immunohistochemistry

- Noncontributory

Other Techniques for Diagnosis

- Noncontributory

Differential Diagnosis

- Causes of testicular maldescent include anatomic abnormalities of the gubernaculum, hormonal dysfunction, mechanical impairment, and gonadal dysgenesis

Pearls

- Testicles normally descend from their intra-abdominal location to the scrotum in two phases, both of which are under hormonal control; defects in the transabdominal phase are much less common than defects in the inguinal or scrotal phase
- Patients with cryptorchidism have a 5 to 10 times higher risk for testicular malignancy than the general population; orchiopexy does not reduce the risk for cancer but does make detection easier
- Most common consequence is infertility
- Early orchiopexy (surgical placement of the testis in the scrotum) may have positive effect on fertility; orchiopexy after 4 years of age does not increase fertility

Selected Reference

Virtanen HE, Bjerknes R, Cortes D, et al: Cryptorchidism: Classification, prevalence, and long-term consequences. Acta Paediatr 96:611-616, 2007.

Hydrocele

Clinical Features

- Most are idiopathic; may be associated with inguinal hernia, scrotal trauma, orchitis, or testicular tumors
- May be secondary to congenital lack of closure of the processus vaginalis, resulting in a communication with the peritoneal cavity
- Characterized by accumulation of serous fluid between the parietal and visceral tunica vaginalis
- Patients present with a testicular mass that transilluminates
- Occasionally patients present with acute testicular enlargement secondary to hemorrhage; lack of transillumination may necessitate orchiectomy

Gross Pathology

- Clear serous fluid-filled cavity compresses adjacent testis
- Hemorrhage or infection may cause fluid to become opaque
- Tunica may be thickened in long-standing lesions

Histopathology

- Fluid-filled cavity lined by flattened or cuboidal mesothelial cells
- Mesothelium may be hyperplastic or cytologically atypical

Special Stains and Immunohistochemistry

- Noncontributory

Other Techniques for Diagnosis

- Noncontributory

Differential Diagnosis

- ▌ Spermatocele
  - Usually located near rete testis or caput epididymis
  - Contains spermatozoa
- ▌ Mesothelial cyst
  - Usually located anterior or lateral to testis
  - May arise within the tunica vaginalis, tunica albuginea, epididymis, or rarely the spermatic cord
  - May be multiloculated

Selected Reference

Haynes JH: Inguinal and scrotal disorders. Surg Clin North Am 86:371-381, 2006.

Orchitis

Clinical Features

- ▌ Viral orchitis
  - Mumps is most common; coxsackievirus B is also relatively common
  - Although the mumps viral syndrome occurs primarily in adolescent children, mumps orchitis is seen in postpubertal individuals
  - Manifests with testicular pain
  - Usually appears shortly after or during the viral syndrome, which includes parotitis
  - Testicular involvement is seen in 15% to 30% of mumps infections
  - May be bilateral
  - Infrequent in childhood
- ▌ Bacterial orchitis
  - *Escherichia coli* is most common causative agent
  - May be acute or chronic

Figure 11-9. Idiopathic granulomatous orchitis. Intratubular, non-necrotizing granulomas.

- Usually associated with infection elsewhere in the genitourinary tract
▎ Granulomatous orchitis
  - Usually a chronic process
  - Associated with a variety of organisms; often associated with systemic or extratesticular infection
  - May be idiopathic

Gross Pathology

- Acute: testicle is swollen and edematous
- Chronic: testicle is firm and often has a thickened tunica

Histopathology

▎ Viral orchitis
  - Acute inflammation seen during acute infection
  - Long-term infection results in patchy interstitial fibrosis and atrophy of seminiferous tubules; often involves both testes
▎ Bacterial orchitis
  - Often associated with bacterial epididymitis
  - Prominent neutrophilic infiltrate with abscess formation
  - Chronic bacterial orchitis may show granulomatous inflammation; lacks intratubular giant cells
▎ Syphilitic orchitis
  - Characterized by edema and diffuse lymphoplasmacytic inflammation
  - Defining features include obliterative endarteritis with perivascular lymphocytes and plasma cells
  - Gumma formation may be seen

Special Stains and Immunohistochemistry

- Stains for microorganisms can be useful to identify bacteria and fungi

Other Techniques for Diagnosis

- Noncontributory

Differential Diagnosis

▎ Infectious granulomatous orchitis
  - Specific agents (e.g., mycobacteria, brucellosis, fungi) must be demonstrated by special stains, culture, or serology
▎ Noninfectious granulomatous orchitis
  - Sarcoidosis
    — Isolated (i.e., nonsystemic) testicular involvement is extremely rare
    — Characterized by noncaseating granulomas composed of epithelioid histiocytes and giant cells
  - Idiopathic granulomatous orchitis
    — No organisms are identified
▎ Seminoma
  - Diagnostic foci of classic seminoma at least focally present
  - Placental alkaline phosphatase (PLAP) immunopositivity seen in seminoma cells

- Can elicit a significant granulomatous inflammatory reaction
▎ Malakoplakia
  - Diagnostic Michaelis-Gutmann bodies readily demonstrated by iron or calcium stain
  - Often associated with chronic *Escherichia coli* infection

Pearls

- Healing infection typically shows prominent granulation tissue and fibrosis
- Tuberculosis may involve the testes; more common in underdeveloped countries or immunocompromised patients

Selected Reference

Yap RL, Jang TL, Gupta R, et al: Xanthogranulomatous orchitis. Urology 63:176-177, 2006.

Malakoplakia

Clinical Features

- Typically presents with testicular enlargement with or without tenderness
- Often associated with chronic bacterial infections, particularly *Escherichia coli*
- Rarely seen in children

Gross Pathology

- Testicular enlargement with focal areas of firm, tan-yellow tissue

Histopathology

- Normal testicular architecture is obscured by a mixed inflammatory infiltrate including abundant macrophages with abundant eosinophilic cytoplasm (von Hansemann histiocytes)
- Destruction of the seminiferous tubules
- Intracytoplasmic and extracellular laminated concretions represent Michaelis-Gutmann bodies

Special Stains and Immunohistochemistry

- Von Kossa calcium and Prussian blue stains highlight Michaelis-Gutmann bodies
- PAS stains eosinophilic, undigested, bacterial debris in macrophage cytoplasm

Other Techniques for Diagnosis

- Electron microscopy may demonstrate bacilli in core of Michaelis-Gutmann bodies

Differential Diagnosis

▎ Idiopathic granulomatous orchitis
  - Usually has significant giant cell component
  - Lacks Michaelis-Gutmann bodies
▎ Lymphoma
  - Clonal lymphocytic proliferation, usually large cell lymphoma, B-cell type

Figure 11-10. Testicular malakoplakia. A, Hemisected testis showing nodular, tan tissue replacing testicular parenchyma with marked peritesticular fibrosis. **B,** High-power photomicrograph showing a mixed inflammatory infiltrate composed mainly of macrophages with abundant eosinophilic cytoplasm. **C,** A von Kossa histochemical stain for calcium nicely highlights Michaelis-Gutmann bodies.

- Characteristic interstitial growth pattern with sparing of the seminiferous tubules
- Lacks Michaelis-Gutmann bodies
∎ Seminoma with granulomatous response
  - Diagnostic seminoma is at least focally present
  - PLAP-immunopositive seminoma cells
  - Lacks Michaelis-Gutmann bodies

Pearls

- Chronic inflammatory disorder
- Many organs may be involved; urinary bladder is most commonly affected

Selected References

Waisman J: Malakoplakia outside the urinary tract. Arch Pathol Lab Med 131:1512, 2007.

Kostakopoulos A, Giannakopoulos S, Demonakou M, Deliveliotos C: Malakoplakia of the testis. Int Urol Nephrol 29:461-463, 1997.

Ramani P, Krishnaswami H: Testicular malakoplakia. Scand J Urol Nephrol 27:557-558, 1993.

Torsion

Clinical Features

- Torsion of the spermatic cord is the most common cause of testicular infarction

Figure 11-11. Testicular torsion. Hemisected orchiectomy specimen showing a venous-type hemorrhagic infarct involving testis and epididymis (*top*).

- Trauma and lesions of the spermatic cord vessels may also cause infarction
- Compression of the spermatic cord veins with continued arterial inflow can lead to venous infarction
- Patients typically present with acute onset of testicular pain

Gross Pathology

- Early vascular compromise is manifested by testicular congestion and swelling
- Infarcted testes are enlarged and consist of soft, necrotic, hemorrhagic tissue

Histopathology

- Changes range from intense congestion to extravasation of blood into the testicular interstitium and epididymis
- Eventually the entire testis becomes necrotic and hemorrhagic

Special Stains and Immunohistochemistry

- Noncontributory

Other Techniques for Diagnosis

- Noncontributory

Differential Diagnosis

▌ Germ cell tumor with extensive necrosis and hemorrhage
- Foci of typical germ cell tumor is almost invariably present somewhere in the testis; identification may require several histologic sections

Pearls

- If surgical intervention is delayed for more than 8 hours the testis is usually not viable

Selected References

Rosenstein D, McAninch JW: Urologic emergencies. Med Clin North Am 688:495-518, 2004.

Hadziselimovic F, Snyder H, Duckett J, Howards S: Testicular histology in children with unilateral testicular torsion. J Urol 136:208-210, 1986.

Male Infertility

Clinical Features

- In general, infertility is defined as lack of conception after 1 year of unprotected coitus
- Male factors are responsible for 40% to 50% of infertile couples
- In general, male infertility is broken down into pretesticular (hormonal), testicular (75% of cases), and post-testicular (obstruction of outflow) causes

Gross Pathology

- Testicular atrophy

Histopathology

- Seminiferous tubules
  - Show similar changes regardless of underlying cause
  - Tubular hyalinization

Figure 11-12. Sertoli-only tubule. Loss of germinal epithelium and persistence of Sertoli cells characterized by elongated cytoplasmic processes and pyramidal nuclei with prominent nucleoli.

- Germinal epithelium
  - May show arrest at any stage (spermatogonia → primary spermatocytes → secondary spermatocytes → spermatids → spermatozoa)
  - May be completely attenuated with only Sertoli cells remaining (Sertoli-only syndrome)
- Interstitium
  - May show varying degrees of fibrosis
  - Leydig cell hypoplasia or hyperplasia may be present
- Blood vessels
  - Atherosclerosis is a common cause of low sperm count, particularly in older individuals

Special Stains and Immunohistochemistry

- PLAP may be necessary to identify intratubular germ cells

Other Techniques for Diagnosis

- Noncontributory

Differential Diagnosis

- Causes of male infertility are numerous and include inflammatory, reactive or reparative, iatrogenic, infectious, and vascular-related processes
- Pathologic findings, which are often nonspecific, must be viewed in the context of the clinical evaluation

Pearls

- Many genetic syndromes are associated with infertility, including Klinefelter syndrome, Down syndrome, and Prader-Willi syndrome; also, structural abnormalities of the Y chromosome are associated
- Endocrine dysfunction, including Cushing syndrome, diabetes mellitus, and hyperprolactinemia, may result in infertility

- Prostate cancer treated with chemotherapy, radiation, or surgery may render the patient infertile
- Treatment of infertility is variable and depends on the patient's underlying condition

Selected References

McLachlan RI, Raipert-De Meyts E, Hoei-Hansen CE, et al: Histologic evaluation of the human testis—approaches to optimising the clinical value of the assessment: Mini review. Hum Reprod 22:2-16, 2007.

Nistal M, Paniaqua R: Non-neoplastic diseases of the testis. In Bostwick DG, Eble JN (eds): Urologic Surgical Pathology. Philadelphia, Mosby–Year Book, 1997, pp 496-535.

Intratubular Germ Cell Neoplasia

Clinical Features

- Originally called *carcinoma in situ*
- May be found in testicular biopsies performed on patients at high risk for germ cell tumors (high-risk conditions include cryptorchidism, prior testicular germ cell tumor, family history, gonadal dysgenesis, and androgen insensitivity syndrome)
- Considered a precursor lesion to germ cell neoplasia
- Almost invariably seen in orchiectomy specimens removed for germ cell neoplasia

Gross Pathology

- Typically has an unremarkable gross appearance; features associated with cryptorchidism, such as atrophy or fibrosis, may be seen

Histopathology

- Neoplastic intratubular germ cells typically form a single layer along the seminiferous tubules and may involve the rete testis

Figure 11-13. Intratubular germ cell neoplasia, usual type. Large malignant cells with vacuolated cytoplasm scattered along the basement membrane of the seminiferous tubules. Note the absence of spermatogenesis. Placental alkaline phosphatase immunohistochemical stain highlights the malignant germ cells (*inset*).

- Malignant germ cells are pleomorphic and have abundant vacuolated cytoplasm, large nuclei with coarse chromatin, and two or more nucleoli
- Spermatogenesis is severely diminished or absent in the affected tubule

Special Stains and Immunohistochemistry

- PLAP positive
- PAS positive, diastase sensitive (tumor cell cytoplasm contains glycogen)

Other Techniques for Diagnosis

- Noncontributory

Differential Diagnosis

▌ Germinal epithelium with maturation arrest
- May show some PAS positivity but is almost invariably PLAP negative
- Cells lack significant nuclear pleomorphism

Pearls

- May be seen in all germ cell tumors except yolk sac tumor and teratoma; not seen in spermatocytic seminoma
- Careful histologic evaluation is necessary because intratubular germ cell neoplasia may have a patchy distribution
- Bouin fixative is better than formalin for detection of intratubular germ cell neoplasia

Selected References

Del Vecchio MT, Epistolato MC, Tripodi SA, et al: Intratubular germ cell neoplasia of unclassified type. Anal Quant Cytol Histol 28:157-170, 2006.

Reuter VE: Origins and molecular biology of testicular germ cell tumors. Mod Pathol 18(Suppl 2):S51-60, 2005.

Ulbright TM: Germ cell tumors of the gonads: A selective review emphasizing problems in differential diagnosis, newly appreciated, and controversial issues. Mod Pathol 18(Suppl 2):S61-79, 2005.

Seminoma

Clinical Features

- Most common pure testicular germ cell neoplasm
- Typically occurs between 30 and 40 years of age (10 years older than nonseminomatous germ cell tumors); rare before puberty
- Presents as a painless testicular mass; may cause dull aching sensation
- Elevated HCG in 7% to 25% of cases (due to presence of syncytiotrophoblastic cells); α-fetoprotein (AFP) levels are usually normal

Gross Pathology

- Multinodular with bulging, cream to tan, fleshy cut surface

Figure 11-14. Seminoma. Monotonous population of cells with clear to eosinophilic cytoplasm and prominent, centrally placed nucleoli associated with a mild lymphocytic infiltrate in the thin, fibrous septa.

- Tumor typically replaces entire testis
- Yellow foci of necrosis may be seen in large tumors
- Extension into paratesticular structures occurs in 10% of cases
- Foci of punctate hemorrhage may indicate admixed syncytiotrophoblastic elements

Histopathology

- Composed of diffuse sheets of tumor cells with intervening branching fibrous septa; cells may be loosely cohesive, giving an appearance of cystlike or tubular spaces
- Interstitial growth pattern with preservation of seminiferous tubules may be seen at the periphery of the tumor
- Tumor cells are round to polyhedral and have pale to clear cytoplasm with well-defined cell borders; uniform, round to oval nuclei with finely granular chromatin and one or two prominent nucleoli
- Infrequent mitotic activity
- Nearly all tumors contain a lymphocytic infiltrate composed predominantly of T cells; lymphoid infiltrate is most dense in the perivascular areas and in the fibrous septa
- Granulomas consisting of small clusters of epithelioid histiocytes and multinucleated giant cells are seen in about 50% of cases
- Pagetoid spread may be seen within seminiferous tubules or rete testis
- Many tumors show scarring with hyalinized deposits of collagen; ossification of the fibrous septa can occur
- Single cells or small groups of syncytiotrophoblasts may be seen in 10% to 20% of cases and are often associated with foci of hemorrhage
- Anaplastic seminoma
  — Higher cellularity with increased nuclear pleomorphism
  — Three or more mitoses per high-power field (hpf)
- Prominent giant cells

Special Stains and Immunohistochemistry

- PLAP positive
- Cytokeratin: immunopositivity may be seen with frozen tissue but is usually not seen in formalin-fixed, paraffin-embedded samples
- PAS: cytoplasmic positivity due to intracytoplasmic glycogen
- HCG: syncytiotrophoblastic cells are positive
- Epithelial membrane antigen (EMA) uniformly negative

Other Techniques for Diagnosis

- Cytogenetic studies: isochromosome 12p is almost always present
- DNA content is usually aneuploid in the range of triploid to hypotetraploid

Differential Diagnosis

▪ Embryonal carcinoma
  - Typically has a tubular or papillary architecture
  - Tumor cells have poorly defined borders and pleomorphic nuclei with prominent macronucleoli
  - Lacks regular fibrous septa and prominent lymphocytic infiltrate
  - Usually shows greater positivity for cytokeratin and weaker PLAP staining
▪ Yolk sac tumor
  - Variable tumor architecture, which commonly is microcystic or solid
  - Usually shows hyaline globules and extracellular basement membrane material
  - Lacks fibrous septa and dense lymphoid infiltrate
  - Positive for cytokeratin and AFP
▪ Lymphoma
  - Typically occurs in older population
  - More frequently bilateral
  - Interstitial growth pattern with lymphomatous infiltrate surrounding seminiferous tubules
  - Not associated with intratubular germ cell neoplasia
  - Negative for PLAP
▪ Sertoli cell tumor
  - Rare tumors accounting for less than 1% of testicular neoplasms
  - Typically has a tubular growth pattern
  - Cells have clear cytoplasm, which is due to the presence of lipid rather than glycogen
  - Not associated with intratubular germ cell neoplasia
▪ Choriocarcinoma
  - Unlike choriocarcinoma, the syncytiotrophoblastic cells of seminoma are not associated with cytotrophoblasts and are not arranged in nodular aggregates

Pearls

- Identical tumor in the ovary is called *dysgerminoma*
- Seminomas that have a greater lymphocytic infiltrate may be associated with a better prognosis
- Combined orchiectomy plus radiation leads to a 95% cure rate in low-stage patients

Selected References

Schmoll HJ, Souchon R, Krege S, et al: European consensus on diagnosis and treatment of germ cell cancer: A report of the European Germ Cell Cancer Consensus Group (EGCCCG). Ann Oncol 15:1377-1399, 2004.

Woodward PJ, Heidenreich A, Looijenga LHJ, et al: Germ cell tumors. In Eble JN, Sauter G, Epstein JI, Sesterhenn IA (eds): World Health Organization Classification of Tumours: Pathology and Genetics: Tumours of the Urinary System and Male Genital Organs. Lyon, IARC Press, 2004, pp 221-249.

Cheville JC: Classifications and pathology of testicular germ cell and sex cord-stromal tumors. Urol Clin North Am 26:595-609, 1999.

Spermatocytic Seminoma

Clinical Features

- Rare germ cell tumor that occurs only in the testis
- Typically affects patients aged 50 to 60 years
- Patients present with painless, often long-standing testicular enlargement
- Not associated with cryptorchidism or other forms of germ cell neoplasia
- Serum tumor markers are not elevated
- Excellent prognosis

Gross Pathology

- Typically multinodular
- May measure up to 15 cm; typically 2 to 5 cm
- Variable cut surface with areas of fleshy, white tissue, mucoid material, hemorrhage, and cystic degeneration

Histopathology

- Polymorphous population of cells arranged in sheets, cords, or small nests
  - Small cells: 6 to 8 μm, smudged chromatin, and scant cytoplasm
  - Intermediate cells: 15 to 20 μm, scant cytoplasm, and round nuclei with granular or filamentous chromatin
  - Giant cells: 50 to 100 μm, uninucleate or multinucleate, and may show filamentous chromatin
- Lacks a lymphoid infiltrate, granulomas are not seen and not associated with intratubular germ cell neoplasia

Figure 11-15. Spermatocytic seminoma. A, Hemisected orchiectomy specimen showing nodules with a glistening cut surface and cystic spaces separated by fibrous septa. **B,** Characteristic small, intermediate, and large cell types. Note the absence of lymphocytes in the fibrous septa.

Special Stains and Immunohistochemistry

- Cytokeratin: positivity may be seen in a perinuclear, dotlike pattern
- PAS negative (cells do not contain glycogen)
- PLAP may be focally positive
- Cells are negative for vimentin, SMA, desmin, AFP, HCG, CEA, and LCA

Other Techniques for Diagnosis

- Electron microscopy: tumor cells have intercellular bridges, macula adherens-type junctions, and filamentous chromosomes with lateral fibrils
- Characteristically lacks isochromosome 12p

Differential Diagnosis

▍ Classic seminoma
  - Affects younger patients
  - May be associated with other germ cell tumor types

- Composed of a single cell type and cells contain abundant cytoplasmic glycogen
- Fibrous septa with prominent lymphoid infiltrate
- Strong PLAP positivity

Pearls

- Not associated with intratubular germ cell neoplasia
- Orchiectomy alone is curative; essentially no metastatic potential

Selected References

Schmoll HJ, Souchon R, Krege S, et al: European consensus on diagnosis and treatment of germ cell cancer: A report of the European Germ Cell Cancer Consensus Group (EGCCCG). Ann Oncol 15:1377-1399, 2004.

Woodward PJ, Heidenreich A, Looijenga LHJ, et al: Germ cell tumors. In Eble JN, Sauter G, Epstein JI, Sesterhenn IA (eds): World Health Organization Classification of Tumours: Pathology and Genetics: Tumours of the Urinary System and Male Genital Organs. Lyon, IARC Press, 2004, pp 221-249.

Embryonal Carcinoma

Clinical Features

- Common component of mixed germ cell tumors (present in 85% of cases)
- Pure embryonal carcinoma is rare, accounting for less than 5% of testicular germ cell neoplasms
- Presents as a testicular mass; gynecomastia or clinically evident metastasis is seen in 40% of patients at presentation
- Serum AFP and HCG may be slightly elevated (related to yolk sac tumor and choriocarcinoma components in mixed tumors); pure embryonal carcinoma is negative

Figure 11-16. Embryonal carcinoma. Glandular and diffuse growth of cells with marked pleomorphism and associated hemorrhage.

Gross Pathology

- Poorly circumscribed, variegated, gray-white mass with areas of hemorrhage and necrosis
- Tumor typically does not replace entire testis

Histopathology

- Cohesive clusters of primitive, anaplastic epithelial cells are seen in three major patterns: solid, tubular-glandular, and papillary
- Tumor cells have abundant cytoplasm and large, vesicular, pleomorphic nuclei with prominent macronucleoli; cell borders are ill defined, and the nuclei appear crowded or overlapping
- Foci of coagulative necrosis are common
- Mitotic rate is high, and karyorrhectic fragments are frequently seen
- Teratocarcinoma
  — Used to describe a mixed germ cell tumor composed of embryonal carcinoma and teratoma

Special Stains and Immunohistochemistry

- Cytokeratin strongly positive
- PLAP: patchy positivity is seen in more than 85% of cases
- CD30 (Ki-1) typically positive
- EMA negative

Other Techniques for Diagnosis

- Cytogenetic studies
  — Isochromosome 12p is often found
  — Interstitial deletion 12(p13;q22) is found in nonseminomatous germ cell neoplasms
- DNA index ranges from 1.4 to 1.6 (significantly lower than in seminoma)

Differential Diagnosis

▮ Seminoma
- Typically arranged in solid sheets; lacks glands, tubules, or papillae
- Tumor cells have well-defined borders with more uniform, evenly spaced nuclei
- Weaker cytokeratin immunopositivity and stronger reactivity for PLAP

▮ Yolk sac tumor
- Variable tumor architecture, which commonly is microcystic or solid
- Usually shows hyaline globules and extracellular basement membrane material
- Lacks fibrous septa and dense lymphoid infiltrate
- Positive for cytokeratin and AFP
- Commonly seen together as part of a mixed germ cell tumor (distinction between the two components may be difficult)

▮ Choriocarcinoma
- Predominantly hemorrhagic background
- Strongly immunopositive for HCG

Pearls

- Embryonal carcinoma is a frequent component of mixed germ cell tumors and is rarely seen as a pure tumor
- Intratubular germ cell neoplasia is frequently seen in association with embryonal carcinoma
- Poor prognostic factors include older age, high elevations of serum tumor markers (lactate dehydrogenase), and higher tumor stage
- Overall, more aggressive than seminomas

Selected References

Schmoll HJ, Souchon R, Krege S, et al: European consensus on diagnosis and treatment of germ cell cancer: A report of the European Germ Cell Cancer Consensus Group (EGCCCG). Ann Oncol 15:1377-1399, 2004.

Woodward PJ, Heidenreich A, Looijenga LHJ, et al: Germ cell tumors. In Eble JN, Sauter G, Epstein JI, Sesterhenn IA (eds): World Health Organization Classification of Tumours: Pathology and Genetics: Tumours of the Urinary System and Male Genital Organs. Lyon, IARC Press, 2004, pp 221-249.

Yolk Sac Tumor

Clinical Features

- Most common testicular tumor in children younger than 3 years
- Pure yolk sac tumor occurs in children from birth to 9 years, with a median age of 18 months; rare in adults
- In adults, yolk sac tumor usually occurs as a component of mixed germ cell tumor
- Patients typically present with a painless testicular mass
- Almost all patients have an elevated AFP level

Gross Pathology

- Nonencapsulated, solid, gray-white to tan, homogeneous mass with a myxoid or gelatinous cut surface; cystic change may be seen
- In adults, because yolk sac tumor is usually only one component of a mixed germ cell tumor, the appearance is variable and may include areas of hemorrhage or necrosis

Histopathology

- Numerous patterns are recognized in yolk sac tumor and include mixed and transitional forms of the following
  - Microcystic (most common pattern)
    - Microcystic appearance results from the presence of intracellular vacuoles, which gives the tumor a lacelike or reticular pattern
    - Extracellular spaces surrounded by cords of tumor cells may be seen

Figure 11-17. Yolk sac tumor. A, Tubuloalveolar and diffuse architectural patterns shown here represent just two of many described for yolk sac tumor. Note the brightly eosinophilic, intracytoplasmic, hyaline globules. **B,** A Schiller-Duval body with characteristic fibrovascular core.

  - Vacuolated cells have compressed nuclei, which resemble lipoblasts
  - Surrounding stroma is often myxoid
  - Solid and myxomatous patterns are often combined with the microcystic subtype
  - Solid (common pattern)
    - Composed of sheets of uniform cells with pale to clear cytoplasm and well-defined borders
    - Prominent thin-walled blood vessels may be present
    - May have a focal microcystic pattern
    - No lymphoid component or fibrous septa
  - Myxomatous (common pattern)
    - Consists of cytokeratin-positive epithelioid to spindle cells in a myxoid stroma
    - Prominent vascular network

◆ Typically intermixed with the microcystic pattern
— Endodermal sinus
  ◆ Characteristic Schiller-Duval or glomeruloid bodies (formed by a central blood vessel and rim of fibrous tissue surrounded by malignant epithelium); seen in about half of cases
  ◆ May be a component in any of the other patterns
— Papillary
  ◆ Papillae are lined by cuboidal, low columnar, or hobnail cells and project into cystic spaces
  ◆ Papillae may have well-formed or inconspicuous fibrovascular cores
  ◆ Frequently intermixed with the endodermal sinus pattern
— Glandular and alveolar
  ◆ Focally present in up to 30% of cases
  ◆ Composed of round or tubular glands that may show a simple or complex pattern
  ◆ May show areas of polyvesicular vitelline, myxomatous, solid, or microcystic patterns
— Macrovesicular
  ◆ Coalescence of microcystic spaces forms large, round to irregular cystic spaces
  ◆ Frequently has an adjacent microcystic pattern
— Polyvesicular vitelline
  ◆ Round, irregular, or dumbbell-shaped vesicular structures lined by flat, bland epithelium
  ◆ Abundant myxoid and loose fibrous stroma
— Hepatoid
  ◆ Present in up to 20% of cases; often only small, scattered foci
  ◆ Composed of polygonal, eosinophilic cells with vesicular nuclei and prominent nucleoli, arranged in sheets or trabeculae (resembles hepatocellular carcinoma)
  ◆ Contains abundant AFP
  ◆ Hyaline globules are common
— Sarcomatoid (uncommon pattern)
  ◆ Composed of a cellular proliferation of cytokeratin-positive spindle cells
  ◆ Often intermixed with the microcystic pattern but may be associated with any of the other subtypes
  ◆ Tumor cells in all patterns may have intracellular, round, hyaline globules, ranging from 1 μm to more than 50 μm in diameter

Special Stains and Immunohistochemistry

- Cytokeratin: strong diffuse positivity
- PLAP: variable positivity in 40% to 85% of cases
- Vimentin: immunopositivity is seen in the spindle cells of the myxomatous and sarcomatoid patterns
- AFP: patchy, cytoplasmic immunopositivity in 50% to 100% of cases; intense staining is seen in areas with a hepatoid pattern

- α1-Antitrypsin: 50% of cases are positive
- Intracellular hyaline globules are PAS positive, diastase resistant, and usually negative for AFP

Other Techniques for Diagnosis

- Electron microscopy: epithelial cells with junctional complexes, occasional apical microvilli, flocculent material in dilated endoplasmic reticulum, and cytoplasmic glycogen; electron-dense, non–membrane-bound bodies correspond to the hyaline globules
- Adult cases are almost all aneuploid and may show isochromosome 12p
- Childhood cases lack the isochromosome 12p, and about 30% are diploid

Differential Diagnosis

▌ Seminoma
- Unlike in seminoma, the solid pattern of yolk sac tumor lacks the prominent lymphoid component and the fibrous septa
▌ Embryonal carcinoma
- May show transitional patterns that are similar to those of yolk sac tumor but is typically composed of more pleomorphic, atypical cells
- Commonly seen together as part of a mixed germ cell tumor (distinction between the two components may be difficult)
- Positive for CD30 (Ki-1); negative for AFP
▌ Juvenile granulosa cell tumor
- Typically found in infants younger than 5 months
- May show architectural pattern similar to that of yolk sac tumor
- Tumor cells lack intracellular hyaline globules
- No Schiller-Duval bodies
- Negative for AFP

Pearls

- Also called *endodermal sinus tumor*
- Pediatric yolk sac tumor is the most common testicular neoplasm in prepubertal children; constitutes about 80% of testicular tumors in children
- Not associated with cryptorchidism
- Five-year survival rate about 90%
- In adults, up to 45% of nonseminomatous germ cell tumors have yolk sac tumor elements

Selected References

Schmoll HJ, Souchon R, Krege S, et al: European consensus on diagnosis and treatment of germ cell cancer: A report of the European Germ Cell Cancer Consensus Group (EGCCCG). Ann Oncol 15:1377-1399, 2004.

Woodward PJ, Heidenreich A, Looijenga LHJ, et al: Germ cell tumors. In Eble JN, Sauter G, Epstein JI, Sesterhenn IA (eds): World Health Organization Classification of Tumours: Pathology and Genetics: Tumours of the Urinary System and Male Genital Organs. Lyon, IARC Press, 2004, pp 221-249.

Teratoma

Clinical Features

- Pure teratoma occurs in children with a mean age of 20 months; unusual in children older than 4 years
- Childhood tumors are frequently found by parent or during routine physical examination
- Teratomatous elements are found in 50% of mixed germ cell tumors in adults
- Pure mature teratomas in prepubertal children do not metastasize

Gross Pathology

- Typically 5 to 10 cm
- Variable appearance with solid areas and multiple cysts (<1 cm in diameter) containing watery to mucoid fluid
- Semitranslucent nodules of gray-white cartilage may be seen
- Immature areas are typically composed of fleshy or hemorrhagic tissue

Histopathology

- Consists of any combination of mature or immature ectodermal, endodermal, and mesodermal elements including cartilage, smooth and skeletal muscle, neuroglia, enteric-type glands, squamous epithelial islands, respiratory or transitional epithelium, fetal neuroepithelium, undifferentiated blastema, or embryonic tubules
- Somatic-type malignancies (carcinoma or sarcoma) may occur and show expansile or infiltrative overgrowth of the teratomatous elements

Special Stains and Immunohistochemistry

- Immunohistochemical reactivity is as expected for the various tissue types present
- AFP: positivity may be seen in enteric or respiratory glands or liver-like tissue
- CEA and α_1-antitrypsin: epithelial areas may show positivity

Other Techniques for Diagnosis

- Tumors usually have an aneuploid DNA content in the hypotriploid range
- Cytogenetic studies: isochromosome 12p may be seen

Differential Diagnosis

▐ Dermoid cyst
- Predominantly cystic tumor composed of epidermis and adnexal structures such as hair follicles and sebaceous glands; a controversial entity
- No immature elements

▐ Epidermoid cyst
- Benign cyst with a lining of keratinizing squamous epithelium without associated adnexal structures

▐ Mixed germ cell tumor
- Much more common in postpubertal patients
- Adequate sampling is needed to determine the presence of other germ cell tumor components

▐ Somatic-type malignancy (carcinoma or sarcoma)
- Somatic-type malignancy arising in a teratoma (i.e., immature elements in a teratoma can look like a carcinoma or a sarcoma)
- Must show infiltrative or expansile overgrowth of the teratoma
- Amount of overgrowth required has not been rigorously defined

Pearls

- Second most common testicular germ cell tumor in children
- Some cases have associated congenital anomalies, including spina bifida, retrocaval ureters, hemihypertrophy, and inguinal hernia
- Prepubertal patients with pure mature teratoma are cured by orchiectomy
- Postpubertal patients rarely, if ever, have pure mature teratoma (metastases may resemble the original tumor or be composed of other germ cell elements
- All teratomas in postpubertal males are potentially malignant

Selected References

Schmoll HJ, Souchon R, Krege S, et al: European consensus on diagnosis and treatment of germ cell cancer: A report of the European Germ Cell Cancer Consensus Group (EGCCCG). Ann Oncol 15:1377-1399, 2004.

Figure 11-18. Teratoma. Low-power view showing mixed epithelial and stromal elements. Immature elements should not be confused with a somatic malignancy such as a carcinoma or sarcoma.

Woodward PJ, Heidenreich A, Looijenga LHJ, et al: Germ cell tumors. In Eble JN, Sauter G, Epstein JI, Sesterhenn IA (eds): World Health Organization Classification of Tumours: Pathology and Genetics: Tumours of the Urinary System and Male Genital Organs. Lyon, IARC Press, 2004, pp 221-249.

Ulbright TM: Gonadal teratomas: A review and speculation. Adv Anat Pathol 11:10-23, 2004.

Choriocarcinoma

Clinical Features

- Typically a component of mixed germ cell tumors; pure choriocarcinoma is extremely rare
- Patients present between the second and third decades; not reported before puberty
- Patients often present with symptoms secondary to metastases to lung, brain, or gastrointestinal tract; testicular tumor may be occult
- Serum HCG is usually highly elevated

Figure 11-19. A, Choriocarcinoma. Bilaminar distribution of syncytiotrophoblasts and cytotrophoblasts with associated hemorrhage. **B, Mixed germ cell tumor.** Hemisected orchiectomy specimen showing characteristically heterogeneous cut surface with solid, hemorrhagic, and necrotic areas.

Gross Pathology

- Testis may appear normal externally
- Often forms a small tumor with focal hemorrhage and necrosis
- Tumor regression may leave only a fibrous scar

Histopathology

- Characterized by an intimate mixture of cytotrophoblasts and syncytiotrophoblasts
  — Cytotrophoblasts: mononucleated cells with pale to clear cytoplasm and well-defined cell borders
  — Syncytiotrophoblasts: large, multinucleated cells with smudged chromatin and vacuolated, eosinophilic cytoplasm
- Hemorrhage and necrosis are typically prominent
- Angioinvasion is commonly seen
- Typically seen as a component of a mixed germ cell tumor; pure tumors are rare
- Teratocarcinoma: used to describe a mixed germ cell tumor composed of embryonal carcinoma and teratoma

Special Stains and Immunohistochemistry

- HCG: immunopositivity is strongest in syncytiotrophoblasts and weak or absent in cytotrophoblasts
- Cytokeratin and EMA typically positive
- CEA and PLAP may be positive

Other Techniques for Diagnosis

- Electron microscopy: syncytiotrophoblasts have prominent rough endoplasmic reticulum and interdigitating microvilli on the cell surface; desmosomes are seen in both cytotrophoblasts and syncytiotrophoblasts

Differential Diagnosis

▎ Mixed germ cell tumor containing foci of choriocarcinoma
- Adequate sampling is needed to differentiate pure choriocarcinoma from the much more common mixed germ cell tumor containing foci of choriocarcinoma

▎ Seminoma
- Syncytiotrophoblasts occurring in a seminoma are scattered as single cells or small clusters without any associated cytotrophoblastic cells
- Degenerated cells in other germ cell tumors, particularly embryonal carcinoma, may resemble syncytiotrophoblasts but are HCG negative

Pearls

- Choriocarcinoma has almost always metastasized at the time of presentation
- Pure choriocarcinoma carries a worse prognosis than other germ cell tumors; mixed germ cell tumors with choriocarcinoma components have a worse

prognosis than those without choriocarcinoma elements
- Radiation therapy is ineffective, but choriocarcinoma is chemosensitive

Selected References

Schmoll HJ, Souchon R, Krege S, et al: European consensus on diagnosis and treatment of germ cell cancer: A report of the European Germ Cell Cancer Consensus Group (EGCCCG). Ann Oncol 15:1377-1399, 2004.

Woodward PJ, Heidenreich A, Looijenga LHJ, et al: Germ cell tumors. In Eble JN, Sauter G, Epstein JI, Sesterhenn IA (eds): World Health Organization Classification of Tumours: Pathology and Genetics: Tumours of the Urinary System and Male Genital Organs. Lyon, IARC Press, 2004, pp 221-249.

Leydig Cell Tumor

Clinical Features

- Classified as a sex cord–stromal tumor
- Makes up about 3% of all testicular tumors
- Two peaks of incidence: children between 5 and 10 years of age (not seen before 2 years of age) and adults between ages 20 and 60 years
- Children present with isosexual pseudoprecocious puberty, and 10% have gynecomastia
- Adults present with testicular swelling; 30% have gynecomastia
- Associated with cryptorchidism and testicular atrophy
- Malignant behavior is seen in 10% of cases; benign behavior in prepubertal patients

Gross Pathology

- Well-circumscribed, solid or lobulated intratesticular nodule 2 to 5 cm in diameter
- Variably yellow, brown, or tan cut surface
- Hemorrhage and necrosis are uncommon

Histopathology

- Tumor cells are typically arranged in solid sheets; less commonly, nests or pseudoglandular pattern
- Cells are polygonal and have round nuclei with prominent central nucleoli and abundant eosinophilic cytoplasm
- Intracytoplasmic lipofuscin pigment can be seen, particularly in postpubertal patients
- Rod-shaped intracytoplasmic crystals of Reinke are seen in about 40% of cases
- Accumulated lipid may produce cells with clear, finely vacuolated cytoplasm
- Mitotic activity is typically low; ≥3 mitoses/10 hpf has been correlated with malignant behavior

Special Stains and Immunohistochemistry

- Vimentin and androgenic hormones: variable positivity

Figure 11-20. Leydig cell tumor. A, Hemisected orchiectomy specimen showing small, well-circumscribed, brown parenchymal nodule. **B,** Sheets of bland cells with a large amount of eosinophilic cytoplasm, rounded nuclei, and prominent nucleoli.

Other Techniques for Diagnosis

- Electron microscopy: cells have features of steroid synthesis, including lipid droplets, prominent smooth endoplasmic reticulum, and mitochondria with tubular cristae; crystals of Reinke appear as sharp geometric shapes, such as hexagons or rhomboid structures
- DNA aneuploidy can be seen in clinically benign tumors but has been associated with malignant behavior

Differential Diagnosis

▌ Leydig cell hyperplasia
- May form nodules but has an interstitial pattern with preservation of the seminiferous tubules
- May be multifocal
- Lacks crystals of Reinke

▌ Large cell calcifying Sertoli cell tumor
- Often bilateral and multifocal
- Cells have abundant eosinophilic cytoplasm and are arranged in a myxoid or collagenous stroma that is frequently calcified or ossified
- Lacks crystals of Reinke

Seminoma
- Must be differentiated from Leydig cell tumor with clear cells
- Tumor cells are round to polyhedral and have pale to clear cytoplasm with well-defined cell borders; uniform, round to oval nuclei with finely granular chromatin and one or two prominent nucleoli
- Tumor cells have abundant intracytoplasmic glycogen
- Fibrous septa with lymphoid component surrounding tumor cells
- PLAP positive

Pearls

- Sex cord–stromal tumor composed of androgen-producing cells
- Tumor may elaborate androgens or estrogens
- Prepubescent children present with pseudoprecocious puberty and have a uniformly benign course
- Most tumors (90%) behave in a benign fashion; 10% are invasive and produce metastases
- Tumor size, mitotic index, cytologic atypia, necrosis, angiolymphatic invasion, and infiltration into paratesticular structures have all been associated with malignant behavior

Selected References

Al-Agha OM, Axiotis CA: An in-depth look at Leydig cell tumor of the testis. Arch Pathol Lab Med 131:311-317, 2007.

Sesterhenn IA, Jacobsen GK, Cheville J, et al: Sex cord gonadal stromal tumours. In Eble JN, Sauter G, Epstein JI, Sesterhenn IA (eds): World Health Organization Classification of Tumours: Pathology and Genetics: Tumours of the Urinary System and Male Genital Organs. Lyon, IARC Press, 2004, pp 250-258.

Young RH: Sex cord-stromal tumors of the ovary and testis: Their similarities and differences with consideration of selected problems. Mod Pathol Suppl 18(Suppl 2):S81-98, 2005.

Sertoli Cell Tumor

Clinical Features

- Rare sex cord–stromal tumor constituting about 1% of testicular neoplasms
- Can occur at any age but most common in middle age
- Patients typically present with a testicular mass; gynecomastia or impotence due to estrogen production may be presenting complaint
- Children may develop gynecomastia but usually do not have isosexual pseudoprecocious puberty
- About 10% are malignant; malignancy can occur in prepubescent children
- Sclerosing variant presents without hormonal symptoms and is uniformly benign
- Large cell calcifying variant occurs in patients younger than 20 years and is a component of Carney syndrome in 40% of cases

Figure 11-21. Sertoli cell tumor. A, Hemisected orchiectomy specimen showing a homogeneous, rubbery cut surface. **B,** Tubular arrangement of cells with vacuolated cytoplasm in a collagenous background.

- Intratubular large cell–hyalinizing Sertoli cell neoplasia may be associated with Peutz-Jeghers syndrome

Gross Pathology

- Solid, gray-white nodule typically smaller than 3 cm
- Large cell calcifying variant, usually tan-yellow with gritty calcifications; multifocal and bilateral in 40% of cases

Histopathology

- Tumor cells are typically arranged in a trabecular pattern and form cordlike structures resembling immature seminiferous tubules
- Tumor cells usually have clear or vacuolated cytoplasm owing to lipid accumulation and oval nuclei with moderate-sized nucleoli
- Sclerosing variant
  — Has dense collagenous stroma

- Large cell calcifying variant
  - Composed of cells with abundant eosinophilic cytoplasm in a myxoid or collagenous stroma that is frequently calcified or ossified

Special Stains and Immunohistochemistry

- Cytokeratin and vimentin positive
- Sclerosing variant usually positive for vimentin and negative for cytokeratin

Other Techniques for Diagnosis

- Electron microscopy: cells have features of steroid synthesis, including lipid droplets, prominent smooth endoplasmic reticulum, and mitochondria with tubular cristae; adjacent cells are connected by desmosomes; perinuclear arrays of filaments (Charcot-Böttcher filaments) are pathognomonic for Sertoli cell differentiation and are present in all variants

Differential Diagnosis

❚ Seminoma
- Typically arranged in solid sheets rather than tubules
- Tumor cells have abundant intracytoplasmic glycogen instead of lipid
- Fibrous septa with prominent lymphoid infiltrate
- Typically shows adjacent intratubular germ cell neoplasia
❚ Adenomatoid tumor versus sclerosing Sertoli cell tumor
- Adenomatoid tumor forms a paratesticular mass
- Adenomatoid tumor is strongly positive for cytokeratin
❚ Androgen insensitivity syndrome or testicular feminization
- Patients may develop a nodular lesion of closely packed tubules lined by Sertoli cells, but these nodules also contain intervening Leydig cells

Pearls

- Rare sex cord–stromal tumor
- Malignant behavior in up to 10% of cases
- Charcot-Böttcher filaments are pathognomonic for Sertoli cell differentiation
- Diagnosis of large cell calcifying Sertoli cell tumor should prompt an investigation for other components of Carney syndrome

Selected References

Giglio M, Medica M, De Rose AF, et al: Testicular Sertoli cell tumors and relative sub-types: Analysis of clinical and prognostic features. Urol Int 70:205-210, 2003.

Sesterhenn IA, Jacobsen GK, Cheville J, et al: Sex cord gonadal stromal tumours. In Eble JN, Sauter G, Epstein JI, Sesterhenn IA (eds): World Health Organization Classification of Tumours: Pathology and Genetics: Tumours of the Urinary System and Male Genital Organs. Lyon, IARC Press, 2004, pp 250-258.

Granulosa Cell Tumor

Clinical Features

- Rare sex cord–stromal tumor with adult and juvenile subtypes
- Adult type
  - Least common sex cord–stromal tumor
  - Occurs in patients 15 to 75 years old
  - Presents with a testicular mass and is frequently associated with gynecomastia
  - Benign behavior; essentially no metastatic potential
- Juvenile type
  - Most common non–germ cell tumor of neonates
  - Restricted to infants younger than 5 months
  - Presents with a testicular mass without hormonal symptoms
  - May be associated with gonadal dysgenesis or sex chromosome anomalies
  - Malignant behavior has not been reported

Gross Pathology

- Solitary gray, yellow to tan nodule with solid and cystic areas
- May be up to 10 cm in diameter

Histopathology

❚ Adult type
- Microfollicular or solid pattern
- Characterized by Call-Exner bodies (small follicles containing eosinophilic material and nuclear debris)
- Tumor cells have round to oval nuclei, often with characteristic nuclear grooves and scant, pale cytoplasm
- Mitotic figures are uncommon

Figure 11-22. Granulosa cell tumor, juvenile type. Follicle-like structure consisting of uniformly bland cells and partially lined by eosinophilic material.

▌ Juvenile type
- Follicular, solid, or mixed pattern
- Basophilic material within follicles is mucicarmine positive
- Solid areas may have a hyalinized, collagenous stroma
- Tumor cells are round to polyhedral and have hyperchromatic nuclei with identifiable nucleoli and abundant pale to eosinophilic cytoplasm
- Mitoses may be frequent

Special Stains and Immunohistochemistry

- Cytokeratin (predominantly 8 and 18) positive
- Vimentin positive
- Mucicarmine
  — Intrafollicular material in juvenile granulosa cell tumors is positive
  — Adult granulosa cell tumors are mucicarmine negative

Other Techniques for Diagnosis

- Noncontributory

Differential Diagnosis

▌ Carcinoid tumor
- May resemble adult granulosa cell tumors, but the tumor cells lack nuclear grooves and have characteristic granular chromatin
- Positive for neuroendocrine immunohistochemical markers

▌ Yolk sac tumor
- May have a cystic or solid pattern and thus resemble juvenile granulosa cell tumors
- Tumor cells typically have characteristic intracellular hyaline globules
- May show characteristic Schiller-Duval bodies
- Positive for AFP

Pearls

- Juvenile-type granulosa cell tumor in adults is rare
- Juvenile-type granulosa cell tumor is the most common non–germ cell tumor in infants
- Malignant behavior is not seen in the juvenile type of testicular granulosa cell tumor

Selected References

Hisano M, Souza FM, Malheiros, et al: Granulosa cell tumor of the adult testis: Report of a case and review of the literature. Clinics 61:77-80, 2006.

Young RH: Sex cord-stromal tumors of the ovary and testis: Their similarities and differences with consideration of selected problems. Mod Pathol 18(Suppl 2):S81-98, 2005.

Sesterhenn IA, Jacobsen GK, Cheville J, et al: Sex cord gonadal stromal tumours. In Eble JN, Sauter G, Epstein JI, Sesterhenn IA (eds): World Health Organization Classification of Tumours: Pathology and Genetics: Tumours of the Urinary System and Male Genital Organs. Lyon, IARC Press, 2004, pp 250-258.

Gonadoblastoma

Clinical Features

- Occurs in the abnormal, dysgenetic gonads of patients with an intersex syndrome or in undescended testes
- Phenotypically, male patients present in childhood or early adolescence
- Usually an incidental finding in gonads removed for other indications
- Bilateral involvement is seen in one third of cases
- Typically have a benign clinical course; however, in 10% to 50% of cases, there is an associated germ cell neoplasm

Figure 11-23. A, Gonadoblastic congeries. Germ cells in a patient with intratubular germ cell neoplasia (usual type) incidentally involving a Sertoli cell nodule or congeries. This should not be confused with gonadoblastoma. **B, Gonadoblastoma.** Mixed population of Sertoli cells and neoplastic germ cells associated with hyalinization and microcalcifications.

Gross Pathology

- Solid, gray to yellow-brown tumor, ranging in size from less than 1 mm up to several centimeters
- Cut surface may be soft, fleshy, or firm, or may appear chondroid
- May have scattered, gritty calcification or be almost totally calcified

Histopathology

- Germ cells and cells of sex cord–stromal differentiation arranged in well-defined nests with surrounding connective tissue stroma
- Cells surround amorphous eosinophilic material (hyaline)
- Germ cells resemble seminoma, immature testicular germ cells, or spermatogonia (large cells have vesicular nuclei with finely granular chromatin and prominent nucleoli); mitotically active
- Epithelial cells of sex cord–stromal origin resemble immature Sertoli or granulosa cells (small, uniform, round or elongated cells with scanty cytoplasm and pale nuclei); mitotically inactive
- May have foci of calcification or hyalinization
- An associated germ cell tumor may be seen

Special Stains and Immunohistochemistry

- PAS: seminoma-like cells are positive owing to abundant glycogen

Other Techniques for Diagnosis

- Electron microscopy: Sertoli-like sex cord cells may contain Charcot-Böttcher filaments

Differential Diagnosis

- Sertoli cell nodule with intratubular germ cell neoplasia
  - Usually a microscopic lesion in a non-dysgenetic gonad with foci of neoplastic germ cells variably distributed among the Sertoli cells

Pearls

- Although pure gonadoblastoma is a benign lesion, prognosis depends on the presence and behavior of any associated germ cell neoplasm
- Bilateral orchiectomy is recommended because of the high incidence of bilaterality of gonadoblastoma and risk for associated germ cell neoplasm

Selected Reference

Ulbright TM: Tumours containing both sex cord/gonadal stromal elements. Gonadoblastoma. In Eble JN, Sauter G, Epstein JI, Sesterhenn IA (eds): World Health Organization Classification of Tumours: Pathology and Genetics: Tumours of the Urinary System and Male Genital Organs. Lyon, IARC Press, 2004, pp 259-262.

Lymphoma

Clinical Features

- Primary testicular lymphoma is rare; subclinical testicular involvement in the late stages of disseminated disease is more common
- Lymphoma makes up about 5% of all testicular tumors
- Most common malignant testicular tumor in patients older than 50 years

Figure 11-24. Non-Hodgkin lymphoma, large cell type. A, Hemisected orchiectomy specimen with characteristic homogeneous tan-yellow cut surface in a 60+-year-old patient. **B,** Interstitial growth of malignant lymphoid cells surrounding and partially involving a hyalinized seminiferous tubule.

Gross Pathology

- Part or the entire testis is replaced by a single mass or multiple nodules
- Cut surface is cream to tan, soft, fleshy, and homogeneous
- Spread to the epididymis or spermatic cord is seen in up to 50% of cases

Histopathology

- Lymphoid infiltrate shows a characteristic interstitial growth pattern typically sparing the seminiferous tubules
- The most common histologic type is diffuse large cell lymphoma, B-cell type
- Follicular lymphoma and Hodgkin disease are rare in the testis

Special Stains and Immunohistochemistry

- B-cell lymphomas make up about 90% of testicular lymphomas
- Immunohistochemical markers are as expected for the various types of lymphoma

Other Techniques for Diagnosis

- As with other lymphomas, flow cytometry, molecular diagnostic techniques, and cytogenetics may be crucial (refer to Chapter 14)

Differential Diagnosis

▌ Seminoma
- Composed of glycogen-rich cells with well-defined borders and prominent lymphocytic infiltrate
- Positive for PLAP
▌ Chronic orchitis
- Contains a heterogeneous population of inflammatory cells consisting of lymphocytes, plasma cells, and neutrophils that typically involve the seminiferous tubules
- Long-term infection results in patchy interstitial fibrosis and atrophy of seminiferous tubules; often involves both testes

Pearls

- Lymphoma accounts for more than 50% of testicular tumors in men older than 60 years
- Primary lymphoma limited to the testis is rare

Selected References

Clemens JQ, Pins MR: Non-Hodgkin's lymphoma presenting as bilateral testicular and adrenal masses. J Urol 163:241-242, 2000.

Hyland J, Lasota J, Jasinki M, et al: Molecular pathological analysis of testicular diffuse large cell lymphomas. Hum Pathol 29:1231-1239, 1998.

Moller MB, d'Amore F, Christensen BE: Testicular lymphomas: A population-based study of incidence, clinicopathological correlation and prognosis. The Danish Lymphoma Study Group, LYFO. Eur J Cancer 30A:1760-1764, 1994.

Paratesticular Adnexa

Epididymitis

Clinical Features

- May be acute or chronic depending on inciting agent and duration of disease
- Acute cases present with unilateral painful swelling of the epididymis and scrotum
- Acute epididymitis may be caused by bacteria (enteric gram-negative rods, *Neisseria gonorrhoeae*, *Chlamydia trachomatis*), viruses (mumps, cytomegalovirus), or trauma
- Chronic epididymitis is associated with tuberculosis, leprosy, sarcoidosis, fungi, and sperm granulomas
- Usually occurs in conjunction with orchitis or after trauma
- Most cases are due to retrograde spread by urine reflux
- Rarely seen as a surgical specimen

Gross Pathology

- Acute infection: epididymis is thickened, congested, and edematous and has a variable fibrinopurulent exudate
- Chronic infection: epididymis is indurated and scarred; calcification or calculi may be seen

Histopathology

- Microscopic features vary depending on the causative agent
- Bacterial infection is associated with neutrophilic microabscesses, edema, and tubular destruction; xanthogranulomas may be seen
- Cases of *C. trachomatis* infection show minimally destructive periductal and intraepithelial inflammation
- Viral infection leads to vascular congestion, edema, and interstitial lymphocytic infiltrates
- Tuberculous epididymitis has prominent caseating granulomas
- Lepromatous epididymitis leprosy shows perivascular and perineural lymphocytic infiltrates with sheets of macrophages containing acid-fast organisms
- Typical noncaseating granulomas may be seen in sarcoidosis
- Fungi usually cause necrotizing granulomas and abscesses
- Traumatic epididymitis shows vascular congestion and patchy blood extravasation
- Sperm granulomas cause foreign-body–type reactions due to extravasated sperm

Special Stains and Immunohistochemistry

- Special stains for bacteria or fungi may be helpful
- Immunohistochemistry for *C. trachomatis* or viral agents may be performed

Other Techniques for Diagnosis

- Noncontributory

Differential Diagnosis

- Differential diagnosis depends on clinical features and identification of the specific inciting agent

Pearls

- Presentation and microscopic features depend on the inciting agent
- Urethral or epididymal aspirate smears and cultures are useful in identifying the causative agent
- Diagnosis is generally based on clinical symptoms and culture results
- Treatment is typically medical; rarely seen as a surgical specimen

Selected References

Gatti JM, Murphy PJ: Current management of the acute scrotum. Semin Pediatr Surg 16:58-63, 2007.

Wegner HE, Loy V, Dieckmann KP: Granulomatous orchitis: An analysis of clinical presentation, pathological anatomic features and possible etiologic factors. Eur Urol 26:56-60, 1994.

Mikuz G, Dajanov I: Inflammation of the testis, epididymis, peritesticular membranes and scrotum. Pathol Ann 17:101-128, 1982.

Lipoma

Clinical Features

- Accounts for up to 90% of spermatic cord tumors
- Usually occurs in adults but can be seen at all ages

Gross Pathology

- Well-circumscribed, lobulated mass of mature, yellow adipose tissue

Histopathology

- Composed of mature, variably sized adipocytes with no nuclear pleomorphism or mitotic activity; similar to that of lipoma at other sites
- Variants include angiolipoma and combinations of fibrous or myxoid types
- Hibernoma may rarely be seen

Special Stains and Immunohistochemistry

- Noncontributory

Other Techniques for Diagnosis

- Noncontributory

Differential Diagnosis

- Well-differentiated liposarcoma
  - Rare in this location
  - Greater nuclear pleomorphism and higher mitotic rate

- Distinction between true (i.e., neoplastic) lipoma and so-called lipoma of the cord associated with inguinal hernias (prolapsed portions of preperitoneal adipose tissue) is somewhat arbitrary

Pearls

- Most common paratesticular tumor

Selected Reference

Lioe TF, Biggart JD: Tumours of the spermatic cord and paratesticular tissue: A clinicopathological study. Br J Urol 71:600-606, 1993.

Adenomatoid Tumor

Clinical Features

- Most common neoplasm of the paratesticular tissues
- Seen at all ages; peak incidence between 20 and 40 years of age
- Typically located in lower pole of epididymis; may be found in tunica albuginea or spermatic cord
- Presents as a painless, unilateral, solitary, solid mass that does not transilluminate
- May extend into testis, but behavior is uniformly benign

Gross Pathology

- Usually smaller than 5 cm; solitary, gray-white, well-demarcated, firm nodule
- Cut surface is homogeneous and fibrous with a whorled appearance; occasional yellow areas may be seen

Histopathology

- Composed of two major components: epithelial-like cells and fibrous stroma

Figure 11-25. Adenomatoid tumor. Characteristic variably sized tubular structures with a pseudoinfiltrative growth pattern lined by bland, low cuboidal epithelial cells.

- Epithelial-like cells
  - Form networks of round, oval, or slitlike tubules, irregular cysts, or small cords
  - Cells lining the tubules may be flat, cuboidal, or low columnar and have round to oval nuclei and abundant dense cytoplasm
  - Cytoplasm may contain intracytoplasmic vacuoles, giving the appearance of signet ring cells
- Fibrous stroma
  - May be hyalinized or contain smooth muscle
  - Stroma often contains lymphoid aggregates or patchy lymphocytic infiltrate
  - Infiltrative border with extension into the testicular parenchyma may be present
  - Lymphoid aggregates may be seen within the tumor or at the periphery

Special Stains and Immunohistochemistry

- Cytokeratin: epithelial cells positive
- Alcian blue: may be positive (hyaluronidase sensitive)
- CEA, Leu-M1, and factor VIII negative

Other Techniques for Diagnosis

- Electron microscopy: numerous microvilli on the luminal surface of the epithelial-like cells with well-developed desmosomes on the lateral surfaces

Differential Diagnosis

▎ Metastatic carcinoma
  - Typically occurs in an older age group
  - Usually bilateral
  - Demonstrates frankly malignant cells that may show hyaluronidase-resistant positive mucin staining
▎ Adenocarcinoma of the rete testis
  - Rare tumor
  - Typically forms an ill-defined mass at the testicular hilum
  - May have a solid or tubulopapillary growth pattern
  - Composed of pleomorphic cells with large nuclei and prominent nucleoli
  - Poor prognosis
▎ Malignant mesothelioma
  - Highly cellular tumor composed of pleomorphic cells with high mitotic rate
  - Characteristic immunohistochemical profile

Pearls

- Firm, well-demarcated paratesticular mass with epithelial-like elements in a fibrous stroma
- Uniformly benign behavior

Selected References

Amin MB: Selected other problematic testicular and paratesticular lesions: Rete testis neoplasms and pseudotumors, mesothelial lesions, and secondary tumors. Mod Pathol 18(Suppl 2):S131-145, 2005.

Rubenstein RA, Dogra VS, Seftel AD, Resnick MI: Benign intrascrotal lesions. J Urol 171:1765-1772, 2004.

Papillary Cystadenoma of the Epididymis

Clinical Features

- Accounts for one third of primary epididymal tumors
- Age range is from 15 to 70 years, with a slight peak in the second and third decades of life
- May present as a small nodule in the head of the epididymis
- About 40% are bilateral
- May be seen in patients with von Hippel-Lindau disease

Gross Pathology

- Well-circumscribed, often encapsulated nodule, typically 1 to 5 cm in diameter
- Multicystic mass with a mottled gray-tan, yellow, and brown cut surface
- Fluid within the cysts may be clear, yellow, or hemorrhagic

Histopathology

- Composed of dilated ducts and cystic spaces with papillary projections
- Cystic spaces and papillae are lined by a single or double layer of cuboidal to tall columnar cells with clear or vacuolated cytoplasm
- Tumor cells are filled with glycogen and secretory droplets and have cilia at the luminal surface
- Stroma is densely fibrous with focal areas of hyalinization and patchy chronic inflammation
- Small foci of lipogranulomatous inflammation may be seen

Special Stains and Immunohistochemistry

- PAS: tumor cells are PAS positive, diastase sensitive because of their high glycogen content

Other Techniques for Diagnosis

- Noncontributory

Differential Diagnosis

▎ Papillary carcinoma
  - Tumors with extensive papillary projections may appear solid and must be differentiated from papillary carcinoma, which tends to be more cellular and shows a greater degree of pleomorphism

Pearls

- Almost two thirds of the cases of cystadenoma occur in patients with von Hippel-Lindau disease
- Clinical behavior is uniformly benign

Selected Reference

Kuhn MT, Maclennan GT: Benign neoplasms of the epididymis. J Urol 174:723, 2005.

Fibrous Pseudotumor

Clinical Features

- Second most common mass-forming lesion of the testicular adnexa (most common is adenomatoid tumor)
- Diffuse or localized proliferation involving the tunicae, epididymis, or spermatic cord
- Reported in patients ranging from 7 to 95 years of age; peak incidence in the third decade
- About 30% of patients report a history of trauma or epididymo-orchitis

Gross Pathology

- Firm, white cut surface
- In the localized form, there may be single or multiple nodules ranging from less than 0.5 cm up to almost 10 cm in diameter
- Diffuse form is characterized by a diffuse thickening of the involved tissues

Histopathology

- Characteristically shows a spindle cell proliferation with a whorled appearance and areas of hyalinized collagen
- Focal hypercellularity may be seen
- Stroma contains a variable inflammatory cell infiltrate consisting of lymphocytes, plasma cells, histiocytes, and scattered eosinophils
- Calcification and ossification may be present
- About half of the lesions may show features of fibroxanthoma, sclerosing lipogranuloma, or sclerosing hemangioma

Special Stains and Immunohistochemistry

- Cytokeratin, SMA, and S-100 protein negative

Other Techniques for Diagnosis

- Noncontributory

Differential Diagnosis

- Spindle cell mesothelioma
  - Consists of cells with eosinophilic cytoplasm in a background of cytokeratin-positive cells
  - Features of mesothelial cell origin seen on electron microscopy
- Idiopathic fibromatosis
  - Typically a more diffuse process with less inflammatory infiltrate
  - May be seen in association with fibromatosis of the retroperitoneum
- Sarcoma
  - Generally hypercellular neoplasm composed of malignant cells with pleomorphic nuclei

- High mitotic rate often with atypical forms
  - Less inflammatory cell infiltrate
- Leiomyoma and neurofibroma
  - Best differentiated with immunohistochemistry

Pearls

- Fibrous pseudotumor is a reactive, non-neoplastic fibrous proliferation that may clinically mimic a testicular neoplasm

Selected References

Polsky EG, Ray C, Dubilier LD: Diffuse fibrous pseudotumor of the tunica vaginalis testis, epididymis, and spermatic cord. J Urol 171:1625-1626, 2004.

Jones MA, Young RH, Scully RE: Benign fibromatous tumors of the testis and paratesticular region: A report of 9 cases with a proposed classification of fibromatous tumors and tumor-like lesions. Am J Surg Pathol 21:296-305, 1997.

Leiomyoma and Leiomyosarcoma

Clinical Features

- Leiomyoma
  - Relatively common tumor of the epididymis
  - Variable age range; rare in children
  - Associated with a hernia sac or hydrocele in up to 20% of cases
  - Bilateral in up to 40% of cases
- Leiomyosarcoma
  - More common in the spermatic cord than in the epididymis
  - Peak incidence in the sixth and seventh decades

Gross Pathology

- Leiomyoma
  - Well-defined, variably sized, round, firm, gray-white mass
  - Whorled, bulging, homogeneous cut surface
- Leiomyosarcoma
  - Similar to leiomyoma; more commonly has areas of necrosis and hemorrhage

Histopathology

- Leiomyoma
  - Spindle cell proliferation composed of interlacing bundles of uniform, spindled smooth muscle cells
  - Rare or absent mitotic activity
- Leiomyosarcoma
  - Cellular spindle cell proliferation that typically shows greater nuclear pleomorphism
  - High mitotic rate ($\geq$1 to 2 mitoses/hpf)
  - Hemorrhage and necrosis are common, especially in high-grade tumors
  - Definitive features to distinguish leiomyoma from low-grade leiomyosarcoma are lacking

Figure 11-26. Smooth muscle hyperplasia of testicular adnexa.
A, Hemisected orchiectomy specimen showing normal testicular parenchyma and an adjacent rubbery white mass involving the epididymis. **B,** Smooth muscle intimately associated with epididymal tissue with secondary dilation and squamous metaplasia.

Figure 11-27. Leiomyosarcoma. Radical orchiectomy specimen showing a rubbery, tan, lobulated mass in the midportion of the spermatic cord.

Special Stains and Immunohistochemistry

- Vimentin, SMA, and desmin positive

Other Techniques for Diagnosis

- Electron microscopy: cells have features of smooth muscle differentiation with bundles of thin filaments and pinocytotic vesicles

Differential Diagnosis

❚ Low-grade leiomyosarcoma versus leiomyoma
- See "Histopathology"
❚ Fibrous mesothelioma
- Negative for SMA

Pearls

- Mitotic rate appears to be the most reliable criterion to distinguish between leiomyoma and low-grade leiomyosarcoma; necrosis, high mitotic activity, hypercellularity, and marked nuclear pleomorphism suggest malignancy
- Treatment of both leiomyoma and leiomyosarcoma is typically orchiectomy; role of retroperitoneal dissection for leiomyosarcoma is controversial
- Leiomyosarcoma frequently recurs locally and often metastasizes; about one third of patients die from metastatic disease

Selected References

Berkmen F, Celebioglu AS: Adult genitourinary sarcomas: A report of seventeen cases and review of the literature. J Exp Clin Cancer Res 16:45-48, 1997.
Soosay GH, Parkinson MC, Paradinas J, Fisher C: Paratesticular sarcomas revisited: A review of cases in the British Testicular Tumour Panel and Registry. Br J Urol 77:143-146, 1996.
deLuise VP, Draper JW, Gray GF Jr: Smooth muscle tumors of the testicular adnexa. J Urol 5:685-688, 1976.

Liposarcoma

Clinical Features

- Most common paratesticular sarcoma in adults (overall, rare in this location)
- Typically found in adults between the ages of 40 and 90 years
- Presents as large, firm, slowly growing mass within the scrotum or inguinal canal

Gross Pathology

- Resembles lipoma; more often multinodular
- Cut surface is yellow and may be soft or firm
- Focal mucinous areas or necrosis may be seen

Histopathology

- Well-differentiated liposarcoma
  — Most common subtype
  — Composed of enlarged, mature adipocytes that typically have atypical, hyperchromatic nuclei

— Varying numbers of vacuolated lipoblasts
— Often have prominent areas of sclerosis
- Myxoid and pleomorphic liposarcomas may be seen but are less common in the paratesticular tissues

Special Stains and Immunohistochemistry

- Oil red O and Sudan black: lipoblasts contain intracellular lipid vacuoles that are positive with fat stains

Other Techniques for Diagnosis

- Cytogenetic studies: well-differentiated liposarcoma is associated with ring chromosome 12; myxoid liposarcoma is associated with t(12;16)

Differential Diagnosis

▌ Lipoma
- Much more common in this location
- Composed of benign-appearing, mature adipocytes with small, eccentric, compressed nuclei
- No lipoblasts

▌ Sclerosing lipogranuloma
- Generally occurs in younger patients
- May involve the penis, scrotum, spermatic cord, or perineum
- Granulomatous and mixed inflammatory infiltrate in a sclerotic background
- Scattered foreign-body giant cells

Pearls

- Most tumors are well differentiated; may recur after local excision
- Typically more indolent behavior compared to other sarcomas
- Poorly differentiated liposarcoma is rare in this location but may produce distant metastases
- Treatment is typically radical orchiectomy, usually without lymph node dissection; may rarely need to perform hemiscrotectomy to obtain negative margins

Selected References

Coleman J, Brennan MF, Alektiar K, Russo P: Adult spermatic cord sarcomas: Management and results. Ann Surg Oncol 10:669-675, 2003.

Montgomery E, Fisher C: Paratesticular liposarcoma: A clinicopathologic study. Am J Surg Pathol 27:40-47, 2003.

Berkmen F, Celebioglu AS: Adult genitourinary sarcomas: A report of seventeen cases and review of the literature. J Exp Clin Cancer Res 16:45-48, 1997.

Rhabdomyosarcoma

Clinical Features

- Most common malignant tumor of the spermatic cord; may be found in the epididymis or testicular tunicae
- About 60% of cases occur in the first two decades of life
- About 95% of patients present with a mass in the scrotum, with only rare involvement of the testicular parenchyma
- Frequent local recurrences and pelvic lymph node metastases are seen
- Prognosis for stage I or II disease is excellent after surgery and chemotherapy
- Most patients with stage III or IV die from the disease despite aggressive therapy

Gross Pathology

- Encapsulated, lobulated, smooth, gray-white, glistening mass that displaces the testicular parenchyma (typically does not invade testicular tissue)
- Tumor size ranges from 1 to 20 cm
- Focal hemorrhage and cystic degeneration may be seen

Histopathology

- Embryonal rhabdomyosarcoma
  — Most common subtype (makes up 90% of rhabdomyosarcomas in the paratesticular tissues)
  — Mixture of haphazardly arranged rhabdomyoblasts and undifferentiated primitive cells
  — Primitive cells are small and round with dark nuclei and minimal cytoplasm
  — Variable numbers of strap cells, with or without cross-striations, and bizarre "tadpole" cells
  — Spindle cell morphology appears to be more common in this location
  — Variable mitotic activity
- Alveolar, botryoid, and pleomorphic patterns are rare

Special Stains and Immunohistochemistry

- MSA, desmin, and myosin: rhabdomyoblasts are typically positive
- Cytokeratin negative

Other Techniques for Diagnosis

- Electron microscopy: rhabdomyoblasts have cytoplasmic myofilaments and Z bands

Differential Diagnosis

▌ Metastasis from other primitive childhood tumors (small round blue cell tumors)

Pearls

- Peak incidence occurs at about 10 years of age
- Common site of metastasis is retroperitoneal lymph nodes
- About 80% survival rate following radical orchiectomy, retroperitoneal lymph node dissection, adjuvant radiation therapy, and chemotherapy

Selected References

Berkmen F, Celebioglu AS: Adult genitourinary sarcomas: A report of seventeen cases and review of the literature. J Exp Clin Cancer Res 16:45-48, 1997.

Soosay GH, Parkinson MC, Paradinas J, Fisher C: Paratesticular sarcomas revisited: A review of cases in the British Testicular Tumour Panel and Registry. Br J Urol 77:143-146, 1996.

Malignant Mesothelioma of the Tunica Vaginalis

Clinical Features

- Rare tumor but second most common paratesticular malignancy
- Often associated with a hydrocele
- Bimodal age distribution with peaks in the third to fourth and sixth to eighth decades
- History of asbestos exposure may be present

Gross Pathology

- Solid or partially cystic tumor
- Multiple shaggy, friable nodules or diffuse thickening of the tunica vaginalis

Histopathology

- Similar histology to malignant mesothelioma of the lung
- Variable histologic features, including epithelial, spindle cell, or biphasic patterns
- Epithelial pattern is most common (70% to 80% of cases)
  - Complex structures have papillary projections, tubuloalveolar structures, and solid sheets of cells
  - Cells lining the papillary structures and tubuloalveolar spaces are usually rounded and cuboidal but may be flattened
  - Cells arranged in solid sheets often have an epithelioid appearance, with eosinophilic cytoplasm and large round central, vesicular nuclei with prominent nucleoli
  - Variable mitotic rate
  - Marked pleomorphism and bizarre cells are rare
  - Psammoma bodies may be seen in the papillary areas

Special Stains and Immunohistochemistry

- Cytokeratin 5 and 6, EMA, calretinin (nuclear more than cytoplasmic), GLUT1, telomerase, p53, vimentin positive
- CEA, Leu-M1 negative
- Alcian blue positive; PAS and mucicarmine negative

Other Techniques for Diagnosis

- Electron microscopy: tumor cells have long, slender microvilli; tonofilaments; desmosomes; and perinuclear mitochondria

Differential Diagnosis

- Benign reactive mesothelial proliferation
  - Commonly seen in hernia sacs
  - Usually small and solitary with simple papillary processes
  - Minimal cytologic atypia
- Florid atypical mesothelial hyperplasia
  - May show some features of malignancy: cytologic atypia, numerous mitoses, and tubulopapillary architecture
  - No true invasion of stroma other than superficial entrapment; cytokeratin stains may be helpful
  - Tends to be p53 and EMA immunonegative and desmin immunopositive
- Adenocarcinoma, metastatic or primary
  - Best differentiated with immunohistochemistry (CEA, Leu-M1, and mucin positivity) or electron microscopy (tumor cells have short microvilli)

Pearls

- Distinctive ultrastructural appearance with long, slender, straight microvilli
- Malignant mesothelioma of the tunica may represent an early manifestation of generalized mesothelioma of the peritoneum or pleura
- Superficial papillary tumors are almost always benign
- Typically behaves in an aggressive manner with frequent recurrence and metastases
- Radical inguinal orchiectomy is typical treatment with retroperitoneal lymph node dissection if clinically or radiographically positive nodes are found

Figure 11-28. Malignant mesothelioma of tunica. Neoplasm composed of complex tubuloalveolar structures lined by low cuboidal epithelium extending from the tunica (*bottom*).

Selected References

Winstanley AM, Landon G, Berney D, et al: The immunohistochemical profile of malignant mesotheliomas of the tunica vaginalis: A study of 20 cases. Am J Surg Pathol 30:1-6, 2006.

Amin MB: Selected other problematic testicular and paratesticular lesions: Rete testis neoplasms and pseudotumors, mesothelial lesions and secondary tumors. Mod Pathol 18:S131-145, 2005.

Churg A (Chairman), Colby TV (Secretary), Cagle P, Corson J, et al, for the US-Canadian Mesothelioma Reference Panel, including: The separation of benign and malignant mesothelial proliferations. Am J Surg Pathol 24:1183-1200, 2000.

Seminal Vesicle

Carcinoma of the Seminal Vesicle

Clinical Features

- Rare tumor occurring in patients older than 50 years
- Symptoms include urinary retention, dysuria, and hematuria
- Only a few cases diagnosed early enough for cure

Gross Pathology

- Infiltrative tumor that replaces the seminal vesicle and may extend into the prostate gland or contralateral seminal vesicle
- Obstruction of the urethra and one or both ureters is common
- Tumors may grow to 10 to 15 cm in diameter

Histopathology

- Most tumors are papillary adenocarcinomas; some may be undifferentiated or mucinous and elicit a desmoplastic stromal response
- Tumor cells are columnar or polygonal and have vesicular nuclei, clear cytoplasm, and variably prominent nucleoli
- In situ adenocarcinoma may be present in adjacent seminal vesicle epithelium

Special Stains and Immunohistochemistry

- Consistently CA-125 and CEA positive; PSA and PAP negative
- Usually CK7 and HMWCK positive; CK20 negative
- AMACR staining unknown

Other Techniques for Diagnosis

- Noncontributory

Differential Diagnosis

▌ Prostatic adenocarcinoma
- More commonly involves both seminal vesicles
- PSA and PAP positive; CA-125 negative

▌ Urinary bladder adenocarcinoma
- Best distinguished clinically depending on site of primary tumor
- CA-125 negative

▌ Transitional cell carcinoma
- Best distinguished clinically depending on site of primary tumor
- CK20 positive; CA-125 negative

Pearls

- Carcinoma of the seminal vesicle should only be diagnosed if it can be demonstrated that the tumor arises in the seminal vesicle (may invade the prostate gland or bladder from outside)
- Prostate, colon, and bladder must be ruled out as primary site of malignancy before diagnosis of primary seminal vesicle is made
- Overall, tumors involving both the prostate gland and the seminal vesicle are much more likely to be of prostatic origin
- May be impossible to determine site of primary tumor in infiltrative high-grade tumors that involve multiple organs
- Disease has aggressive clinical course with poor prognosis

Selected References

Egevad L, Ehrnstrom R, Hakansson U, Grabe M: Primary seminal vesicle carcinoma detected at transurethral resection of prostate. Urology 69:778.e11-778.e13, 2007.

Thiel R, Effert P: Primary adenocarcinoma of the seminal vesicles. J Urol 186:1891-1896, 2002.

Ormsby AH, Haskell R, Jones D, Goldblum JR: Primary seminal vesicle carcinoma: An immunohistochemical analysis of four cases. Mod Pathol 13:46-51, 2000.

Urethra

Urethral Polyps

Fibroepithelial Polyp

Clinical Features

- Rare lesion
- Occurs only in males
- Usually congenital
- Patients usually present between 3 and 9 years of age with hematuria, urinary retention, and infection

Gross Pathology

- Polypoid mass arising in the prostatic urethra adjacent to the verumontanum

Histopathology

- Polyp lined by urothelium with variable stromal inflammation

Figure 11-29. Urethral caruncle. Seen only in women but illustrated in this chapter for completeness. Inflamed urothelium and stroma associated with hemorrhage and vascular ectasia.

Figure 11-30. Nephrogenic adenoma arising in a urethral diverticulum. Variably sized glandular spaces lined by uniformly bland, low cuboidal epithelial cells in an edematous background.

- Surface ulceration may be seen
- Squamous metaplasia may be present

Caruncle

Clinical Features

- Found exclusively in women; usually in later life
- Patients present with a red, painful mass at the external urethral meatus and frequently have dysuria, urinary frequency, or obstruction

Gross Pathology

- Small (1 to 2 cm), pedunculated or sessile polypoid lesion in the distal urethra
- Fleshy, hemorrhagic appearance

Histopathology

- Polypoid mass lined by urothelial (transitional) or squamous epithelium that is often hyperplastic
- Lamina propria consists of loose fibroblastic connective tissue that is richly vascular and has extravasated red blood cells and mixed inflammation

Nephrogenic Adenoma

Clinical Features

- Arises in response to chronic irritation or trauma
- Most common in young adult males
- Usually incidental finding at endoscopy; may cause hematuria
- Benign condition with no increased risk for malignancy; coexistent adenocarcinoma occasionally seen

Gross Pathology

- Flattened erythematous plaque or discrete papillary lesion

Histopathology

- May show papillary or flat configuration
  - Flat lesions have a loose stroma with scattered mixed inflammatory cells and numerous small tubules lined by uniform cuboidal cells with hyperchromatic, round to oval nuclei
  - Papillae have similar lining cells with associated small stromal tubules and mixed inflammation
  - Pale eosinophilic secretions are often found within the tubules

Special Stains and Immunohistochemistry

- Tubular secretion may be PAS positive, diastase resistant, or mucicarmine positive
- Epithelial cells are negative for PSA and PAP

Other Techniques for Diagnosis

- Noncontributory

Differential Diagnosis

▌ Adenocarcinoma
- Usually much larger and more commonly causes clinical symptoms, including dysuria and hematuria
- Glandular structures are composed of pleomorphic cells with a high mitotic rate

Prostatic Urethral Polyp

Clinical Features

- Usually asymptomatic; may cause hematuria
- More commonly seen in adults but may present at earlier ages

Gross Pathology

- Small, discrete, velvet-like papillary growths

Histopathology

- Papillary fronds with thin fibrovascular cores
- Lined by prostatic acinar epithelium with abundant clear to eosinophilic cytoplasm
- Small basally oriented nuclei without conspicuous nucleoli

Special Stains and Immunohistochemistry

- PSA: epithelial cells are positive

Other Techniques for Diagnosis

- Noncontributory

Differential Diagnosis

- Cytologic features need to be carefully examined to distinguish prostatic urethral polyp from intraluminal extension of prostatic adenocarcinoma

Selected References

Demirican M, Ceran C, Karaman A, et al: Urethral polyps in children: A review of the literature and report of two cases. Int J Urol 13:841-843, 2006.

Chan JK, Chow TC, Tsui MS: Prostatic-type polyps of the lower urinary tract: Three histiogenic types? Histopathology 11:789-801, 1987.

Carcinoma of the Urethra

Clinical Features

- Rare tumor
- Most common in older women
- Usually located in the prostatic or membranous portion of the urethra
- Patients usually present with symptoms associated with urinary obstruction
- May have purulent or bloody discharge
- Tumors of the anterior urethra may be palpable

Gross Pathology

- On endoscopy, the tumor may have an exophytic growth pattern or an area of ulceration

Histopathology

- Usually squamous cell carcinomas; tumors with transitional cell differentiation may be seen
- Tumors of transitional cell type may be papillary or flat and may be of any histologic grade
- Squamous cell carcinomas are usually well to moderately differentiated with little keratinization; however, verrucous carcinomas may be seen in the distal urethra
- Spindle cell variants of both transitional cell and squamous cell carcinomas may occur

Special Stains and Immunohistochemistry

- Cytokeratin: positivity may aid in differentiating the spindle cell variant from sarcoma

Other Techniques for Diagnosis

- Noncontributory

Differential Diagnosis

- Secondary involvement of the urethra by TCC of the bladder is much more common than primary urethral carcinoma
- Intramucosal pagetoid spread of TCC may be seen in the urethra in association with TCC of the bladder but is rare in primary urethral carcinoma

Pearls

- Spread of a TCC of the bladder into the urethra is much more common than primary urethral carcinoma
- Overall these tumors are aggressive primarily, resulting in local destruction; they occasionally metastasize

Selected Reference

Mostofi FK, Davis CJ Jr, Sesterhenn IA: Carcinoma of the male and female urethra. Urol Clin North Am 19:347-358, 1992.

Adenocarcinoma of the Periurethral Glands

Clinical Features

- Rare tumor (only few reported cases)
- Appears to be more common in women
- May present with symptoms of urinary obstruction, hematuria, or dysuria
- Advanced tumors may present as a perineal mass with skin ulceration

Figure 11-31. Clear cell adenocarcinoma arising in a urethral diverticulum in a female. Hobnail cells with eosinophilic cytoplasm (eosinophilic variant of clear cell carcinoma).

Gross Pathology

- Tumors arising in Cowper glands involve the posterior urethra or perineum
- Tumors arising in the periurethral glands of Littre involve the anterior urethra

Histopathology

- Variety of growth patterns and cell types described
  — Tubular or papillary growth pattern with or without intracytoplasmic mucin
  — Cuboidal or columnar cells with eosinophilic to clear cytoplasm and large, hyperchromatic nuclei
  — Clear cell variant is composed of large clear cells with abundant cytoplasmic glycogen

Special Stains and Immunohistochemistry

- ▌Mucinous tumors
  - Positive for cytokeratin
  - Negative for PSA and PAP
- ▌Clear cell carcinoma
  - May show PAS positivity with diastase sensitivity

Other Techniques for Diagnosis

- Noncontributory

Differential Diagnosis

- ▌Prostatic or urothelial adenocarcinoma
  - Periurethral involvement by prostatic or urothelial adenocarcinoma can often be ruled out based on clinical history

Pearls

- These tumors are rare in men
- Urethral adenocarcinomas are more prevalent in women and may arise in a background of chronic irritation (i.e., diverticulum) and mucinous metaplasia or may arise from Skene glands or the periurethral glands of Littre

Selected References

Murphy DP, Pantuck AJ, Amenta PS, et al: Female urethral adenocarcinoma: Immunohistochemical evidence of more than one tissue of origin. J Urol 161:11881-11884, 1999.

Ullmann AS, Ross OA: Hyperplasia, atypia and carcinoma in-situ in prostatic periurethral glands. Am J Clin Pathol 47:497-504, 1967.

Penis

Penile Fibromatosis (Peyronie Disease)

Clinical Features

- Patients present with painful erection and bending or constriction of the erect penis
- Commonly affects middle-aged or older men; rare before the age of 40 years

Figure 11-32. Penile fibromatosis (Peyronie disease). Fascicles of mature fibroblasts with elongated, tapered nuclei.

- Associated with other superficial fibromatoses, including palmar or plantar sites (Dupuytren and Ledderhose disease, respectively) in 10% to 25% of patients
- Clinical course is variable; spontaneous resolution is seen in one third of patients

Gross Pathology

- Circumscribed, firm plaque or nodule on the dorsal surface of the penile shaft
- Inelasticity of the plaques causes penile curvature and pain with erection; may cause urethral constriction

Histopathology

- Proliferative (early) phase shows increased cellularity and less collagen compared with advanced lesions
- Tumor cells are bland with fibroblastic and myofibroblastic features; rarely have focal mitotic activity, associated inflammation, and giant cells
- Advanced lesions may show hyalinization with foci of bone or cartilage formation

Special Stains and Immunohistochemistry

- SMA: variable positivity (indicative of myofibroblastic differentiation)

Other Techniques for Diagnosis

- Cytogenetic studies: various nonrandom karyotypic abnormalities may be seen (commonly trisomy 3 or 8)

Differential Diagnosis

- Diagnosis is made based on characteristic clinical history and presentation

Pearls

- Histologic features are often less dramatic than clinical presentation

- May resolve spontaneously, remain stable for many years, or progress
- Treatment options include resection of the penile plaques, radiotherapy, or steroid injections
- May be related to scarring secondary to urethritis, coital trauma, or urethral instrumentation; often idiopathic

Selected References

Gonzalez-Cadavid NF, Rajfer J: Mechanisms of disease: New insights into the cellular and molecular pathology of Peyronie's disease. Nat Clin Pract Urol 2:291-297, 2005.

Greenfield JM, Levine LA: Peyronie's disease: Etiology, epidemiology and medical treatment. Urol Clin North Am 32:469-478, 2005.

Balanitis Xerotica Obliterans

Clinical Features

- Penile equivalent of vulvar lichen sclerosus
- Atrophy of the epidermis and dermal connective tissue of the genital skin
- Asymptomatic white patch on glans or prepuce; may involve the urethral meatus

Gross Pathology

- Clinically, affected skin is white and fibrotic

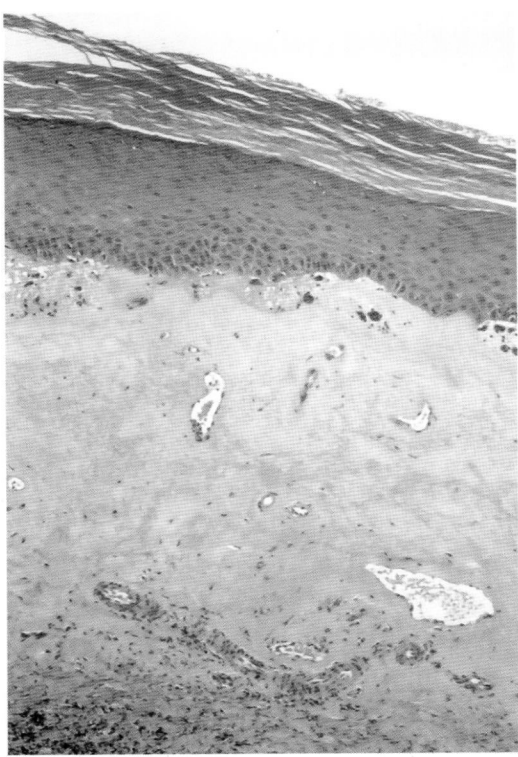

Figure 11-33. Balanitis xerotica obliterans. Characteristic subepithelial acellular collagenization with linear lymphocytic infiltrate. Epidermis may be normal or atrophic.

Histopathology

- Orthokeratotic hyperkeratosis, epidermal atrophy, upper dermal collagenization, and patchy lympho-plasmacytic infiltrate in the upper dermis

Special Stains and Immunohistochemistry

- Noncontributory

Other Techniques for Diagnosis

- Noncontributory

Differential Diagnosis

- Lichen simplex chronicus
  - Can show orthokeratotic hyperkeratosis, but unlike balanitis xerotica obliterans, it usually shows epidermal hyperplasia and no dermal collagenization
- Lichen planus
  - Prominent band of chronic inflammatory cells that can obscure the dermoepidermal junction
  - Balanitis xerotica obliterans has a less dense lymphocytic infiltrate
- Plasma cell (Zoon) balanitis (balanitis circumscripta plasmacellularis)
  - Clinically looks like squamous cell carcinoma in situ and occurs almost exclusively in uncircumcised men
  - Typically presents as a single bright-red patch on the glans or prepuce
  - Characterized by a distinct upper dermal band of plasma cells
  - Prominent dilated capillaries in the dermis
  - Lacks collagen deposition

Pearls

- Many of the same histopathologic features useful in the differential diagnosis of inflammatory lesions of the vulva are useful in the penis
- Variable treatment options include circumcision, laser ablation, steroid treatments, and antifungal agents
- May rarely progress to squamous cell carcinoma, particularly if persistent or not treated

Selected References

Pietrzak P, Hadway P, Corbishley CM, Watkin NA: Is the association between balanitis xerotica obliterans and penile carcinoma underestimated? Br J Urol Int 98:74-76, 2006.

Yesudian PD, Sugunendran H, Bates CM, O'Mahoney C: Lichen sclerosis. Int J STD AIDS 16:465-473, 2005.

Velazquez EF, Cubilla AL: Lichen sclerosis in 68 patients with squamous cell carcinoma of the penis: Frequent atypias and correlation with special carcinoma variants suggest a precancerous role. Am J Surg Pathol 27:1448-1453, 2003.

Condyloma Acuminatum (Genital Wart)

Clinical Features

- Most common tumor-like lesion of the penis
- Caused by human papillomavirus (HPV)
- Incidence of 5% among men aged 20 to 40 years

Gross Pathology

- Lesions are located on corona of glans, fossa navicularis, or penile meatus
- Involvement of penile shaft, scrotal skin, and perineum may be seen
- Lesions appear as pink to tan, flat, or papillary cauliflower-like nodules
- Can be large with pushing growth (giant condyloma of Buschke-Löwenstein)

Histopathology

- Exophytic growth with branching, papillary structures covered by hyperplastic squamous epithelium showing orderly maturation
- Koilocytes: cells with raisinoid, hyperchromatic, binucleated nuclei with perinuclear halos
- Hyperkeratosis and parakeratosis
- Minimal cytologic atypia with mitoses confined to the basal layer

Special Stains and Immunohistochemistry

- HPV can be demonstrated with immunohistochemistry
- HPV types 6 and 11 associated with nondysplastic genital warts

Other Techniques for Diagnosis

- In situ hybridization can demonstrate viral HPV DNA

Differential Diagnosis

- ▌ Verrucous carcinoma
  - Shows acanthosis, hyperkeratosis, parakeratosis, and sometimes koilocyte-like cells similar to condyloma
  - Typically has a broad invasive growth pattern at the deep margin
  - Not associated with HPV

Pearls

- Previous treatment with podophyllin or laser therapy may cause bizarre cytologic changes suggestive of malignancy
- Variable treatment consisting of podophyllin, laser therapy, radiation, or conservative surgical resection
- Patients with condyloma at increased risk for developing penile squamous cell carcinoma

Selected References

Nordenvall C, Chang ET, Adami HO, Ye W: Cancer risk among patients with condyloma acuminata. Int J Cancer 119:888-893, 2006.

Rubin MA, Kleter B, Zhou M, et al: Detection and typing of human papillomavirus DNA in penile carcinoma: Evidence for multiple independent pathways of penile carcinogenesis. Am J Pathol 159:1211-1218, 2001.

Penile Carcinoma In Situ: Erythroplasia of Queyrat

Clinical Features

- Usually occurs in men between the ages of 50 and 70 years
- Patients typically present with a plaque on the glans penis or prepuce
- Circumcision protects against the development of erythroplasia
- About 10% of cases progress to invasive squamous cell carcinoma

Figure 11-34. Condyloma acuminatum. Foreskin showing epidermal hyperplasia, hyperkeratosis, and parakeratosis with characteristic human papillomavirus cytopathic effect.

Figure 11-35. Erythroplasia of Queyrat or Bowen disease. Both show epithelium with full-thickness dysplasia.

Gross Pathology

- Shiny, elevated, red, velvety erythematous plaque on the glans or prepuce
- Solitary lesion in more than 50% of cases

Histopathology

- Squamous epithelium shows full-thickness dysplasia without invasion of the basement membrane
- Dysplastic cells demonstrate loss of polarity and lack normal maturation; cells have large, irregular hyperchromatic nuclei, multinucleation, and numerous typical and atypical mitotic figures
- Scattered dyskeratotic cells are seen throughout the epithelium
- Underlying lichenoid inflammation and vascular proliferation are common

Special Stains and Immunohistochemistry

- HPV demonstrable in up to 80% of lesions

Other Techniques for Diagnosis

- HPV DNA can be demonstrated with in situ hybridization techniques; HPV types 16 and 18 are most common

Differential Diagnosis

▌ Bowen disease
- Histologic features of erythroplasia of Queyrat and Bowen disease are almost identical; differentiation is based on clinical presentation and biologic behavior
▌ Bowenoid papulosis
- Affects younger men
- Often multifocal
- Typically shows slightly less dysplasia
- Does not progress to invasive squamous cell carcinoma

Pearls

- Unlike Bowen disease, erythroplasia is limited to the glans and prepuce and occurs in somewhat older patients
- About 10% incidence of progression to invasive squamous cell carcinoma

Penile Carcinoma In Situ: Bowen Disease

Clinical Features

- Usually occurs in men 40 to 60 years old
- Typically presents as a scaly plaque
- About 5% to 10% of cases progress to invasive squamous cell carcinoma
- Reported association with visceral (lung, gastrointestinal tract, and genitourinary tract) malignancies in up to 33% is debatable

Gross Pathology

- Crusted, sharply demarcated scaly plaque on the shaft of the penis

Histopathology

- Squamous epithelium has full-thickness dysplasia without invasion of basement membrane
- Dysplastic cells demonstrate loss of polarity and lack normal maturation; cells have large, irregular hyperchromatic nuclei, multinucleation, and numerous typical and atypical mitotic figures
- Scattered dyskeratotic cells are seen throughout the epithelium
- Underlying lichenoid inflammation and vascular proliferation are common
- Often has prominent hyperkeratosis and parakeratosis
- Commonly involves the pilosebaceous units

Special Stains and Immunohistochemistry

- HPV demonstrable in up to 80% of lesions

Other Techniques for Diagnosis

- HPV DNA can be demonstrated with in situ hybridization techniques; HPV types 16 and 18 are most common

Differential Diagnosis

▌ Erythroplasia of Queyrat
- Histologic features of erythroplasia of Queyrat and Bowen disease are almost identical; differentiation is based on clinical presentation and biologic behavior
▌ Bowenoid papulosis
- Affects younger men
- Often multifocal
- Typically shows slightly less dysplasia
- Does not progress to invasive squamous cell carcinoma

Pearls

- Unlike erythroplasia of Queyrat, Bowen disease arises on the skin of the penile shaft and occurs in somewhat younger patients
- About 5% to 10% incidence of progression to invasive squamous cell carcinoma
- Many authors use the term *Bowen disease* for carcinoma in situ of the skin and *erythroplasia of Queyrat* for carcinoma in situ of the glans penis

Selected Reference

Cubilla AL, Velazquez EF, Young RH: Epithelial lesions associated with invasive penile squamous cell carcinoma: A pathologic study of 288 cases. Int J Surg Pathol 12:351-364, 2004.

Bowenoid Papulosis

Clinical Features

- Usually seen in young adults (typically 20 to 40 years of age)
- Multiple papules or coalescent papules seen on the penile shaft or perineum
- Responds to topical therapy or local excision; may regress spontaneously
- Does not progress to invasive squamous cell carcinoma

Gross Pathology

- Multiple papules, 2 to 10 mm in diameter
- Papules may coalesce to form plaques resembling condyloma acuminatum

Histopathology

- Squamous epithelium showing variable degrees of acanthosis, papillomatosis, hyperkeratosis, and parakeratosis
- Scattered atypical keratinocytes and mitotic figures
- Shows more maturation than carcinoma in situ

Special Stains and Immunohistochemistry

- HPV: present in some cases (especially types 16 and 18)

Other Techniques for Diagnosis

- In situ hybridization techniques may demonstrate HPV DNA

Differential Diagnosis

▌ Bowen disease and erythroplasia of Queyrat
- Histologically, bowenoid papulosis is essentially identical to Bowen disease
- Unlike erythroplasia of Queyrat and Bowen disease, bowenoid papulosis affects younger men, is more often multifocal, shows somewhat less dysplasia, and does not progress to invasive squamous cell carcinoma

Pearls

- Does not progress to invasive squamous cell carcinoma
- Responds to local or topical therapy; may regress spontaneously

Selected References

Bhojwani A, Biyani CS, Nicol A, Powell CS: Bowenoid papulosis of the penis. Br J Urol 80:508, 1997.

Su CK, Shipley WU: Bowenoid papulosis: a benign lesion of the shaft of the penis misdiagnosed as squamous carcinoma. J Urol 157:1361-1362, 1997.

Squamous Cell Carcinoma

Clinical Features

- Accounts for less than 1% of malignancy in males, but accounts for up to 95% of penile malignancies
- Wide geographic variation; high rates in Uganda, Brazil, Jamaica, Mexico, and Haiti (areas where circumcision is not routinely practiced)
- Usually occurs in older men; rare before the age of 40 years
- Patients typically present with a slow-growing, exophytic or ulcerating penile mass; may have pain or difficulty voiding
- Risk factors include lack of circumcision, poor hygiene, phimosis, and HPV
- Extremely rare in men circumcised in infancy
- Retention of smegma or its derivatives may have an irritating effect
- Almost 50% of the patients have phimosis
- HPV type 11, 16, 18, or 30 can be demonstrated in about 50% of cases

Figure 11-36. A, Typical penile squamous cell carcinoma. Superficially invasive squamous cell carcinoma with keratinization. **B, Well-differentiated squamous cell carcinoma.** Tumor cells invade in a bulbous, pushing manner similar to that seen in a verrucous carcinoma; however, the degree of cytologic atypicality is too great for that diagnosis.

- Often clinically neglected and may metastasize to bilateral inguinal and iliac lymph nodes

Gross Pathology

- Exophytic or ulcerating mass arising on the glans or prepuce

Histopathology

- Well-differentiated invasive squamous cell carcinoma
  — Composed of atypical squamous cells that extend down from a thickened hyperkeratotic, papillomatous surface and infiltrate through the underlying basement membrane
  — Limited nuclear atypia and pleomorphism
  — Keratin pearls may be numerous
  — Intercellular bridges are prominent
- Higher-grade invasive squamous cell carcinoma
  — Composed of large cells with hyperchromatic nuclei and moderate to marked pleomorphism depending on grade
  — Ulcerated surface and invasive architecture with infiltration of the tumor through the basement membrane
  — Increased mitotic rate; atypical mitoses are common in poorly differentiated tumors
  — Poorly differentiated tumors typically have focal areas of necrosis
  — Fewer keratin pearls
- Two main growth patterns are seen: fungating-exophytic and ulcerating-infiltrative
- Exophytic tumors are usually well differentiated and have extensive keratinization
- Ulcerating tumors tend to be on the glans and are moderately or poorly differentiated
- Rare squamous cell carcinomas have a predominantly spindle cell pattern with marked nuclear pleomorphism and high mitotic rates with only focal areas of identifiable squamous differentiation

Special Stains and Immunohistochemistry

- Cytokeratin positive

Other Techniques for Diagnosis

- Electron microscopy: tumor cells have bundles of tonofilaments and desmosomes
- HPV DNA can be demonstrated by in situ hybridization
- Flow cytometric analysis of DNA ploidy and S-phase fractions may have prognostic significance

Differential Diagnosis

▌ Verrucous carcinoma
- Similar histologic characteristics as well-differentiated squamous cell carcinoma
- Typically has a broad pushing pattern of infiltration

- Low mitotic rate
- Much better prognosis with essentially no metastatic potential

▌ Penile sarcomas
- Various penile sarcomas enter into the differential diagnosis of poorly differentiated and spindle cell types of squamous cell carcinoma
- Sarcoma is typically cytokeratin negative

Pearls

- Squamous cell carcinoma accounts for most penile malignancies
- Wide variation in incidence based on geography and cultural practices
- Stage, specifically depth of invasion (epithelium, lamina propria, corpus spongiosum, corpus cavernosum), and lymph node status are prognostically important
- Almost 40% of patients have inguinal lymph node metastases at presentation; widespread metastases typically occur late in the course of disease

Selected References

Novarro G, Galfano A, De Marco V, et al: Prognostic factors in squamous cell carcinoma of the penis. Nat Clin Pract Urol 4:140-146, 2007.

Cubilla AL, Piris A, Pfanni R, et al: Anatomic levels. Important landmarks in penectomy specimens: A detailed anatomic and histologic study based on examination of 44 cases. Am J Surg Pathol 25:1091-1094, 2001.

Verrucous Carcinoma

Clinical Features

- Most commonly seen in middle-aged men
- Most arise in the coronal sulcus
- Behaves as a locally aggressive neoplasm; essentially no metastatic potential
- Not associated with HPV

Gross Pathology

- Large, fungating, warty tumor
- Surface of tumor is frequently ulcerated

Histopathology

- Endophytic and exophytic papillary growth consisting of acanthotic, hyperkeratotic, and parakeratotic squamous mucosa
- Minimal cytologic atypia and rare mitotic activity
- Deep margin of the tumor shows a pushing, broad area of infiltration
- True koilocytosis with large, wrinkled nuclei and perinuclear halos are not seen

Special Stains and Immunohistochemistry

- Consistent absence of HPV

Other Techniques for Diagnosis

- In situ hybridization fails to demonstrate HPV DNA

Differential Diagnosis

- Condyloma acuminatum and giant condyloma of Buschke-Löwenstein
  - True koilocytic atypia
  - Positive for HPV
- Invasive squamous cell carcinoma
  - Greater cytologic atypia, higher mitotic rate, and a more diffusely infiltrative growth pattern
- Hybrid tumors
  - Hybrid tumors with features of both well-differentiated squamous cell carcinoma and verrucous carcinoma may occur

Pearls

- True verrucous carcinomas with no metastatic potential are relatively rare
- May recur frequently and be locally destructive
- Tumors with features of both verrucous carcinoma and squamous cell carcinoma (so-called hybrid squamous-verrucous carcinoma) are relatively common

Selected Reference

Cubilla AL, Dillner J, Schellhammer PF, et al: Tumours of the penis: Verrucous carcinoma. In Eble JN, Sauter G, Epstein JI, Sesterhenn IA (eds): World Health Organization Classification of Tumours: Pathology and Genetics: Tumours of the Urinary System and Male Genital Organs. Lyon, IARC Press, 2004, p 286.

Penile Sarcoma

General Features

- Rare tumor composing less than 5% of penile malignancies
- As a group, penile sarcomas are the second most common penile malignancy
- Peak incidence is between 40 and 60 years of age; rhabdomyosarcoma may be seen in children
- Most present as nodules or masses on the penile shaft
- Most common histologic types include Kaposi sarcoma, epithelioid hemangioendothelioma, leiomyosarcoma, fibrosarcoma, and epithelioid sarcoma

Kaposi Sarcoma

Clinical Features

- About 20% of male patients with AIDS-related Kaposi sarcoma have penile lesions
- Tumors usually involve the glans or penile shaft
- Involvement of the glans or corpus spongiosum may cause urethral obstruction

Gross Pathology

- Red to purple patches, plaques, or nodules

Histopathology

- Patch stage
  - Dilated irregular vascular spaces, interspersed mononuclear cell infiltrate, extravasated red blood cells, and hemosiderin-laden macrophages
- Plaque stage
  - Vascular spaces become lined by plump spindle cells and there are variable perivascular spindle cell aggregates
- Nodular stage
  - Small and slitlike vascular spaces are scattered among sheets of plump spindle cells
  - Frequent mitotic activity, hemorrhage, and hemosiderin-laden macrophages

Pearls

- Usually associated with other systemic lesions seen in patients with HIV infection

Epithelioid Hemangioendothelioma

Clinical Features

- Rare vascular tumor that arises in the corpora cavernosum

Gross Pathology

- Red to purple, vaguely circumscribed, spongy nodule

Histopathology

- Anastomosing vascular spaces lined by plump to cuboidal cells with an epithelioid appearance
- Most are low grade, but some tumors may show marked pleomorphism, hemorrhage, and necrosis

Special Stains and Immunohistochemistry

- Immunohistochemical markers for vascular differentiation such as factor VIII, CD31, and CD34 may be useful

Other Techniques for Diagnosis

- Electron microscopy: Weibel-Palade bodies are characteristic of endothelial cell differentiation

Differential Diagnosis

- Poorly differentiated or metastatic carcinoma
  - Positive for cytokeratin and negative for vascular markers

Pearls

- Low-grade tumors usually follow an indolent course
- High-grade tumors have been reported to metastasize to lymph nodes, lung, liver, and bone

Leiomyosarcoma

Clinical Features

- Usually occurs in men between 40 and 70 years of age

Gross Pathology

- Well-circumscribed, superficial or deep-seated, tan-gray nodule
- Firm and whorled to myxoid cut surface

Histopathology

- Composed of interwoven fascicles of spindle cells
- Cigar-shaped nuclei with variable nuclear pleomorphism and hyperplasia
- At least 1 to 2 mitoses/hpf

Special Stains and Immunohistochemistry

- Tumor cells are positive for vimentin, desmin, and SMA

Other Techniques for Diagnosis

- Electron microscopy: cell cytoplasm contains bundles of thin filaments and pinocytotic vesicles with surrounding basal lamina

Pearls

- Superficial tumors arising from dermal smooth muscle respond well to local excision but may recur
- Deep tumors arising from the smooth muscle of the corpora tend to invade the urethra and metastasize early, leading to a poor prognosis despite radical surgery

Fibrosarcoma

Clinical Features

- Slowly growing, nontender mass on the dorsum of the shaft or glans

Gross Pathology

- Soft to firm mass with infiltrative borders and fleshy cut surface

Histopathology

- Spindle cell neoplasm with infiltrative borders
- Differentiation ranges from spindle cells growing in a well-ordered herringbone pattern to high-grade tumors with marked nuclear pleomorphism, frequent mitoses, and necrosis

Special Stains and Immunohistochemistry

- Vimentin positive
- Cytokeratin, desmin, and SMA negative

Other Techniques for Diagnosis

- Electron microscopy: bipolar spindle cells without intercellular junctions; organelles consist of rough endoplasmic reticulum and mitochondria

Differential Diagnosis

- ▌ Leiomyosarcoma
  - Positive for SMA
- ▌ Spindle cell variant of squamous cell carcinoma
  - At least focally cytokeratin positive
- ▌ Proliferative (early) phase of fibromatosis (Peyronie disease)
  - Only focal cytologic atypia

Epithelioid Sarcoma

Clinical Features

- Age range typically 20 to 40 years
- Patients present with a slow-growing, painless subcutaneous mass that may ulcerate the overlying skin
- May cause erectile pain or dysuria

Gross Pathology

- Gray to tan, firm nodules
- Central areas of necrosis and degeneration may be seen

Histopathology

- Cellular neoplasm with an infiltrative growth pattern and nodular architecture
- Tumor cells are arranged in nodules surrounded by hyalinized stroma and may have central necrosis and cystic degeneration
- Large, polygonal cells with abundant eosinophilic cytoplasm and vesicular nuclei with prominent nucleoli
- Frequent mitotic activity

Figure 11-37. Epithelioid sarcoma involving penile dermal tissue. Proliferation of polygonal cells with eosinophilic cytoplasm and associated with hyalinized bands of collagen and central necrosis.

Special Stains and Immunohistochemistry

- Vimentin positive
- Cytokeratin typically positive
- EMA: greater than 50% of cases are positive

Other Techniques for Diagnosis

- Noncontributory

Differential Diagnosis

▎ Ulcerating infiltrating squamous cell carcinoma
  - Positive for cytokeratin but negative for vimentin
▎ Ulcerating granulomatous reactions
  - Cells are positive for histiocytic markers
▎ Other spindle cell sarcomas
  - Negative for cytokeratin and EMA

Selected Reference

Katona TM, Lopez-Beltran A, MacLennan GT, et al: Soft tissue tumors of the penis: A review. Anal Quant Cytol Histol 28:193-206, 2006.

Scrotum

Idiopathic Scrotal Calcinosis

Clinical Features

- Idiopathic deposition of calcified nodules in the scrotal skin
- Calcification of dermal connective tissue may arise from eccrine duct cysts; however, residual cyst epithelium is often not apparent
- Typically found in young adults
- Multiple long-standing painless nodules up to 3 cm in diameter

Gross Pathology

- Hard, chalky, gray to white nodules
- Overlying skin is usually intact but may be ulcerated

Histopathology

- Dermal lesions consisting of granules and globules of calcific material
- Variable giant cell and granulomatous reaction

Special Stains and Immunohistochemistry

- Noncontributory

Other Techniques for Diagnosis

- Noncontributory

Differential Diagnosis

▎ Calcification of preexisting epidermal or pilar cyst
  - Presence of keratinaceous debris

Pearls

- Treatment may be unnecessary for asymptomatic lesions

Figure 11-38. A, Scrotal cyst. Dilated eccrine duct with intraluminal calcifications. **B, Scrotal calcinosis.** Calcified nodules embedded in a dense connective tissue matrix.

- Excision may be necessary for infected, recurrent, or extensive lesions

Selected References

Shah V, Shet T: Scrotal calcinosis results from calcification of cysts derived from hair follicles: A series of 20 cases. Am J Dermatopathol 29:172-175, 2007.
Yahya H, Rafindadi AH: Idiopathic scrotal calcinosis: A report of four cases and review of the literature. Int J Dermatol 44:206-209, 2005.

Paget Disease

Clinical Features

- Rare in this location
- Penile and scrotal Paget disease is usually associated with a primary visceral (bladder, prostate, urethra, or rectum) or perineal (skin adnexal) malignancy
- Typically occurs in the sixth and seventh decades of life
- Patients present with a scaly, eczematous lesion on the scrotum or penis

Figure 11-39. Penile Paget disease. Large atypical cells with clear cytoplasm showing intraepidermal spread.

Gross Pathology

- Scaly, indurated, eczematous plaque

Histopathology

- Low power shows single cells or clusters of atypical cells with radial and some degree of vertical intraepidermal spread
- Tumor cells have variable nuclear pleomorphism and vacuolated cytoplasm

Special Stains and Immunohistochemistry

- CEA positive
- S-100 protein negative
- PAS, mucicarmine, and Alcian blue stain positive (tumor cells contain intracytoplasmic neutral and acid mucopolysaccharides)

Other Techniques for Diagnosis

- Noncontributory

Differential Diagnosis

▌ Malignant melanoma
- Similar pattern of intraepidermal spread, but S-100 protein positive and CEA negative
- Lacks intracytoplasmic mucin
▌ Squamous cell carcinoma
- Can show a similar low-power pattern of spread
- Typically has greater degree of invasion with infiltration into underlying tissue

Pearls

- Visceral malignancy must be ruled out with any case of penile or scrotal Paget disease

Selected References

Yang WJ, Kim DS, Im YJ, et al: Extramammary Paget's disease of the penis and scrotum. Urol 65:972-975, 2005.

Van Randenborgh H, Paul R, Nahrig J, et al: Extramammary Paget's disease of penis and scrotum. J Urol 168:2540-2541, 2002.

Squamous Cell Carcinoma

Clinical Features

- First cancer linked to occupational exposure of 3'4'-benzpyrene
- Originally described in chimney sweeps; also seen in workers in other occupations with coal or petroleum exposure
- Typically occurs in sixth or seventh decade of life
- Ipsilateral inguinal lymphadenopathy is found at presentation in 50% of cases

Gross Pathology

- Early lesions are slow-growing, solitary papules or nodules
- Later lesions are ulcerated and have raised, rolled edges and a seropurulent discharge

Histopathology

- Well to moderately differentiated squamous cell carcinoma
- Keratinization is common
- Surrounding skin shows acanthosis, hyperkeratosis, and dysplasia

Special Stains and Immunohistochemistry

- Noncontributory

Other Techniques for Diagnosis

- Noncontributory

Differential Diagnosis

- Includes a wide variety of inflammatory and neoplastic skin lesions

Pearls

- Most common malignant tumor of the scrotum; much less frequent than penile squamous cell carcinoma
- First cancer linked to occupational exposure to a carcinogen
- Prognosis depends on stage; overall prognosis is poor (typically, 30% to 40% 5-year survival rate)

Selected References

Taniguchi S, Furukawa M, Kutsuna H, et al: Squamous cell carcinoma of the scrotum. Dermatol 193:253-254, 1996.

Andrews PE, Farrow GM, Oesterling JE: Squamous cell carcinoma of the scrotum: Long-term follow up of 14 patients. J Urol 146:1299-1304, 1991.

12

Female Reproductive System

12

Vulva

Inflammatory dermatologic diseases that affect hair-bearing skin elsewhere on the body may also occur on the vulva. The vulva is prone to skin infections because it is constantly exposed to secretions and moisture (see Chapter 2).

Lichen Sclerosus (Chronic Atrophic Vulvitis)

Clinical Features

- Most common in postmenopausal white women
- Tends to develop slowly but is insidious and progressive
- Treatment with topical testosterone, progesterone, or corticosteroids

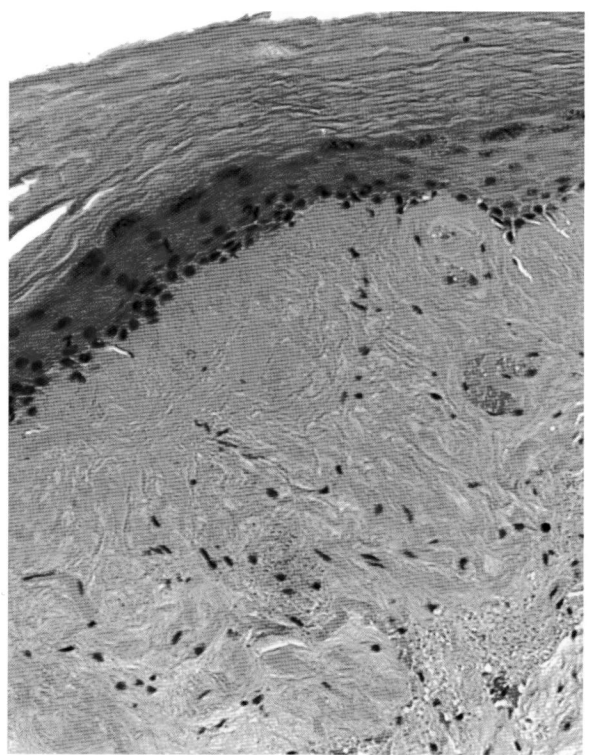

Figure 12-1. Lichen sclerosus. Loss of the rete pegs and collagenization of the dermis is evident.

Gross Pathology

- Flat, often symmetrical white plaques

Histopathology

- Thinned epidermis with blunting of rete ridges
- Hydropic degeneration of basal cells
- Dermal edema or collagenization
- Loss of melanocytes in affected areas
- Scattered bandlike lymphocytes underlying abnormal dermis

Special Stains and Immunohistochemistry

- MIB-1 index is elevated in the basal and parabasal cells

Other Techniques for Diagnosis

- Noncontributory

Differential Diagnosis

▌ Lichen planus
- Dense bandlike lymphoid infiltrate at dermoepidermal junction
- Other sites (mucosal and nonmucosal) often involved
- Colloid bodies (degenerated keratinocytes) may be present

Pearls

- Not recognized as a precancerous condition
- Confers a greater risk of subsequent carcinoma
- Associated with a greater than expected risk for subsequent carcinoma (1% to 4% of cases)

Selected References

Kadawo J: Vulval skin conditions. Nurs Stand 21:59, 2007.
Raspollini MR, Asirelli G, Moncini D, Taddei GL: A comparative analysis of lichen sclerosus of the vulva and lichen sclerosus that evolves to vulvar squamous cell carcinoma. Am J Obstet Gynecol 197:592-595, 2007.
Chiesa-Vottero A, Dvoretsky PM, Hart WR: Histopathologic study of thin vulvar squamous cell carcinomas and associated cutaneous lesions: A correlative study of 48 tumors in 44 patients with analysis of adjacent vulvar intraepithelial neoplasia types and lichen sclerosus. Am J Surg Pathol 30:310-318, 2006.
Jones RW, Sadler L, Grant S, et al: Clinically identifying women with vulvar lichen sclerosus at increased risk of squamous cell carcinoma: a case-control study. J Reprod Med 49:808-811, 2004.

Squamous Cell Hyperplasia and Lichen Simplex Chronicus

Clinical Features

- Adult women
- Commonly presents with focal vulvar pruritus
- Treated with topical corticosteroids and antipruritics

Gross Pathology

- Gray-white plaques, often edematous and excoriated

Histopathology

- Epithelial thickening, hyperkeratosis
- Normal maturation
- Squamous cell hyperplasia: no significant dermal changes
- Lichen simplex chronicus: collagenization of superficial dermis with underlying chronic inflammatory infiltrate

Special Stains and Immunohistochemistry

- Noncontributory

Other Techniques for Diagnosis

- Noncontributory

Differential Diagnosis

- Diagnosis of exclusion
- Chronic fungal infection
  - Periodic acid–Schiff (PAS) or silver stains will demonstrate organisms in the keratin layer
  - Intraepithelial inflammation

Pearls

- Vulvar squamous cell carcinomas are not generally associated with squamous cell hyperplasia and lichen simplex chronicus as precursor lesions

Selected References

Santos M, Montagut C, Mellado B, et al: Immunohistochemical staining for p16 and p53 in premalignant and malignant epithelial lesions of the vulva. Int J Gynecol Pathol 23:206-214, 2004.

Nascimento AF, Granter SR, Cviko A, et al: Vulvar acanthosis with altered differentiation: A precursor to verrucous carcinoma? Am J Surg Pathol 28:638-643, 2004.

Fox H, Wells M: Recent advances in the pathology of the vulva. Histopathology 42:209-216, 2003.

Vulvar Cysts

Clinical Features

- Generally asymptomatic
- Occur at any age
- Incidental finding on clinical examination

Gross Pathology

- Single or multiple thin-walled cysts several millimeters in diameter

Histopathology

- None of the cyst linings show epithelial atypia
- Epidermal inclusion cyst
  - As seen on the skin
  - Stratified squamous cornified epithelium
  - Prominent granular layer
  - Contains soft, yellow, keratinous debris
  - Epithelial lining may be flattened
- Bartholin duct cyst
  - Dilated segment of obstructed Bartholin gland duct
  - Noncornified squamous, transitional, or cuboidal lining
  - No keratinous debris in the lumen
- Mucinous cyst
  - Single layer of mucinous epithelial lining
  - Focal squamous metaplasia may be present

Figure 12-2. Squamous cell hyperplasia (ex-hyperplastic dystrophy). Hyperkeratosis, acanthosis, and mild chronic inflammation within the dermis.

Figure 12-3. Mucous cyst. Cystic space lined by simple mucus-secreting cells. Squamous metaplasia of the epithelium lining the cyst wall is evident.

■ Mesonephric-like cyst
  ● Single layer of cuboidal to columnar epithelial lining
  ● May be attenuated by pressure from cyst contents (clear fluid)
  ● Smooth muscle layer around basement membrane
■ Ciliated cyst
  ● Rare
  ● Ciliated and secretory columnar epithelial cell lining
  ● May show pseudostratification
  ● No muscle layer
  ● Absent cellularity of surrounding stroma
■ Mesothelial cyst
  ● Thin-walled cyst lined by a single layer of flattened mesothelial cells
■ Periurethral cyst
  ● Cyst lined by transitional cells

Special stains and Immunohistochemistry
  ● Noncontributory

Other Techniques for Diagnosis
  ● Noncontributory

Differential Diagnosis
■ Ciliated cyst versus endometriosis
  ● In endometriosis, the glands may be ciliated; however, endometrial-type stroma is necessary for diagnosis

Pearls
  ● None of the cysts listed above are associated with malignancy
  ● Surgical excision is curative

Selected References

Patil S, Sultan AH, Thakar R: Bartholin's cysts and abscesses. J Obstet Gynecol 27:241-245, 2007.
Hamada M, Kiryu H, Ohta T, Furue M: Ciliated cyst of the vulva. Eur J Dermatol 14:347-349, 2004.
Peters WA III: Bartholinitis after vulvovaginal surgery. Am J Obstet Gynecol 178:1143-1144, 1998.

Molluscum Contagiosum

Clinical Features
  ● Contagious DNA viral disease
  ● Spread by close contact
  ● Most lesions regress spontaneously

Gross Pathology
  ● Small, smooth papules, 3 to 6 mm
  ● Central umbilication
  ● Usually multiple and separate

Histopathology
  ● Brightly eosinophilic cytoplasmic inclusions with marked squamous hyperplasia
  ● In older lesions, the inclusions appear more basophilic

Figure 12-4. Molluscum contagiosum. Marked acanthosis with classic eosinophilic intracytoplasmic inclusions.

Special Stains and Immunohistochemistry
  ● Noncontributory

Other Techniques for Diagnosis
  ● None

Differential Diagnosis
  ● None

Pearls
  ● Most lesions regress spontaneously
  ● Central umbilication of papule is a helpful finding for clinical diagnosis
  ● Diagnosis may be made by cytology of scrapings from papule

Selected References

Trama JP, Adelson ME, Mordechai E: Identification and genotyping of molluscum contagiosum virus from genital swab samples by real-time PCR and Pyrosequencing. J Clin Virol 40:325-329, 2007.
Epstein WL: Molluscum contagiosum. Semin Dermatol 11:184-189, 1992.

Condyloma Acuminatum

Clinical Features
  ● Spread by sexual contact
  ● Human papilloma viruses (HPV) types 6 and 11 are the most common associated types

Figure 12-5. Condyloma acuminatum. A, Low-power view demonstrates a polypoid lesion associated with acanthosis and hyperkeratosis. **B,** High-power view shows classic koilocytotic cells with prominent perinuclear halos.

- Lesions turn white upon application of 3% to 5% acetic acid under colposcopic examination
- Usually asymptomatic

Gross Pathology

- Exophytic papular lesions
- Usually multiple and often confluent

Histopathology

- Koilocytes in superficial epithelial cells
  — Enlarged cells with perinuclear cytoplasmic clearing (halos)
  — Enlarged or pyknotic nuclei with irregular membranes (raisinoid)
  — Binucleate and multinucleate forms are common
- Epidermal hyperplasia
- Hyperkeratosis and parakeratosis
- Prominent granular cell layer
- Cytologic atypia is rarely present at the base of the lesion

Special Stains and Immunohistochemistry

- p16 INK4a assists in excluding aggressive HPV types (e.g., 16, 18, 31, 45)

Other Techniques for Diagnosis

- Polymerase chain reaction (PCR) or in situ hybridization (ISH): specific identification of HPV type, usually 6 or 11

Differential Diagnosis

▌ Vulvar intraepithelial neoplasia (VIN)
  - Usually flat lesions with or without koilocytic changes
  - Nuclear pleomorphism and hyperchromasia and abnormal mitoses
  - Cytologic atypia is present at the base of the lesion
▌ Squamous cell hyperplasia and lichen simplex chronicus
  - Lacks prominent granular layer
  - No koilocytes are present
  - Lacks HPV by PCR and DNA analysis
▌ Papilloma
  - Lacks hyperkeratosis
  - Lacks koilocytosis

Pearls

- HPV-6 is most commonly associated with condyloma acuminatum
- HPV-11 is not uncommon
- Most lesions regress spontaneously
- Progression to VIN and even to squamous cell carcinoma has been reported

Selected References

Srodon M, Stoler MH, Baber GB, Kurman RJ: The distribution of low and high-risk HPV types in vulvar and vaginal intraepithelial neoplasia (VIN and VAIN). Am J Surg Pathol 30:1513-1518, 2006.

Vinokurova S, Wentzensen N, Einenkel J, et al: Clonal history of papillomavirus-induced dysplasia in the female lower genital tract. J Natl Cancer Inst 97:1816-1821, 2005.

Vulvar Intraepithelial Neoplasia

Clinical Features

- Most common in premenopausal women
- Discolored, raised plaques, often white after application of (5%) acetic acid at colposcopic examination

Gross Pathology

- Flat or papular discolored lesions, often white but may be red, gray, brown, or black

Histopathology

▌ VIN 1 (low grade)
  - Nuclear pleomorphism and hyperchromasia involving the lower third of the epithelium
  - Increased mitotic activity in the lower third
  - *Flat condyloma* is a synonym of VIN 1

Figure 12-6. Vulvar intraepithelial neoplasia type 3. A, Vulvar skin with hyperkeratosis and finger-like projections showing severe nuclear atypia and lack of maturation. **B,** Full-thickness dysplasia of the epithelium with overlying parakeratosis. Notice the uniformity of the lesion.

▌ VIN 2 and 3 (high grade)
- Nuclear pleomorphism and hyperchromasia involving the lower two thirds (VIN 2) or full thickness (VIN 3) of the epithelium
- Binucleate and multinucleate cells are often present
- Atypical mitotic figures are readily identifiable
- Koilocytosis may be seen within or adjacent to the lesion

Special Stains and Immunohistochemistry
- p16 INK4a positive
- MIB-1 index high

Other Techniques for Diagnosis
- PCR, ISH: HPV-16 is commonly identified
- Ploidy: VIN lesions usually contain an aneuploid population of cells

Differential Diagnosis
▌ Paget disease
- Epidermis with scattered, highly atypical intraepithelial single cells resembling cells of adenocarcinoma
- Positive for mucin, *HER-2-neu*, and carcinoembryonic antigen (CEA)

Pearls
- VIN is usually multifocal, most often associated with HPV-16
- Bowenoid papulosis is essentially synonymous with VIN 3
- The term *erythroplasia of Queyrat* refers to VIN lesions in mucous membranes of the vulvar vestibule that are often red
- VIN, particularly low-grade lesions, may spontaneously regress, especially in young or pregnant women
- Local excision is the current recommended therapy

Selected References

Goffin F, Mayrand MH, Gauthier P, et al: High-risk human papillomavirus infection of the genital tract of women with a previous history or current high-grade vulvar intraepithelial neoplasia. J Med Virol 78:814-819, 2006.

Rodolakis A, Diakomanolis E, Vlachos G, et al: Vulvar intraepithelial neoplasia (VIN): Diagnostic and therapeutic challenges. Eur J Gynaecol Oncol 24:317-322, 2003.

Hart WR: Vulvar intraepithelial neoplasia: historical aspects and current status. Int J Gynecol Pathol 20:16-30, 2001.

Squamous Cell Carcinoma

Clinical Features
- Generally two patient populations
  — Young women with history of smoking and concomitant HPV-associated lesions
  — Postmenopausal women with well-differentiated squamous cell carcinoma and no evidence of HPV infection

Gross Pathology
- Superficially invasive: red papule, white plaque, or irregular ulcerated lesion
- Invasive: exophytic papillary mass or endophytic ulcer, usually solitary

Histopathology
- Full-thickness involvement of epithelium by pleomorphic cells with high nuclear-to-cytoplasmic ratio and mitotic activity

Figure 12-7. **Infiltrating squamous cell carcinoma. A,** Low-power view shows the characteristic pattern. Well-differentiated infiltrating squamous cell carcinoma featuring invasive sheets of tumor cells. **B,** High-power view shows infiltrating sheets of squamous cells with keratinization and prominent stromal reaction (desmoplasia).

- Atypical mitotic figures are often readily identifiable
- Microinvasive squamous cell carcinoma
  — Tumor depth less than 1 mm as measured from the basement membrane of the nearest dermal papilla to the point of deepest invasion by tumor
  — Less than 2 cm in diameter
- Invasive squamous cell carcinoma
  — Greater than 1 mm in depth of invasion
  — Variable degree of squamous differentiation, i.e., keratin pearl formation
    ◆ Gynecologic Oncology Group (GOG) grade 1: no undifferentiated cells; keratin pearls
    ◆ GOG grade 2: less than 50% undifferentiated cells
    ◆ GOG grade 3: greater than 50% undifferentiated cells
- Variants of squamous cell carcinoma
  — Squamous cell carcinoma with tumor giant cells
    ◆ Nonkeratinizing with pleomorphic multinucleate tumor giant cells

— Spindle cell squamous carcinoma
  ◆ Pleomorphic spindle cells that are keratin positive
— Acantholytic squamous cell carcinoma
  ◆ Pseudogland formation caused by acantholysis

Special Stains and Immunohistochemistry

- Cytokeratin positive
- p16 INK4a generally positive
- Mucin negative

Other Techniques for Diagnosis

- PCR, INH: HPV-16 detected in about 75% of tumors, especially in younger women with history of VIN
- Ploidy: most carcinomas are aneuploid

Differential Diagnosis

▌ Basaloid carcinoma
  - Endophytic invasion with densely hyalinized stroma
  - Nests and cords of cells with basaloid features surrounded by hyalinized stroma
  - Overlying squamous epithelium often shows VIN rather than carcinoma
  - Associated with synchronous or metachronous tumors of the vagina and cervix
▌ Verrucous carcinoma
  - Synonymous with giant condyloma of Buschke-Löwenstein
  - Exophytic growth resembling papilloma
  - No fibrovascular cores or cytologic atypia
  - Invasion is defined by large, cytologically bland, bulbous nests with pushing borders
▌ Warty (condylomatous) carcinoma
  - Squamous carcinoma with papillary exophytic growth
  - Fibrovascular fronds
  - Numerous koilocytes
  - Irregularly outlined nests of invasive tumor at base
▌ Basal cell carcinoma: as per basal cell carcinoma of skin
  - Adenoid pattern: in addition has tubular and glandlike differentiation
  - Basosquamous: includes foci of squamous cell carcinoma
▌ Amelanotic malignant melanoma
  - Negative for cytokeratin
  - Positive for S-100 protein, melan-A, and HMB-45 and pan-melanin markers
  - No keratinization or squamous pearl formation
▌ Epithelioid sarcoma
  - Absent intraepithelial component
  - Aggregates of atypical epithelioid cells resembling granulomas
  - Located deep in the mucosa near fascia
▌ Pseudoepitheliomatous hyperplasia
  - Bland cytology
  - Normally maturing squamous epithelium

- No stromal nests dissociated from basal layer
- Usually a reactive process
▌ Metastatic squamous cell carcinoma
  - Clinical history is important
  - Generally metastatic tumor will be present deep in the dermis
  - Most likely absent intraepidermal component

Pearls

- Important prognostic indicators are tumor thickness, depth of invasion, tumor diameter, and vascular and lymphatic space invasion
- The risk for inguinal node involvement increases significantly in tumors with a depth of invasion greater than 1 mm
- The invasive component is often better differentiated than the intraepithelial component
- Tumors with depth of invasion >1 to 2 mm have relatively low but unpredictable rates of inguinal node involvement
- Wide local excision appears to be the preferred treatment for superficially invasive carcinoma
- Tumors greater than 1 mm in depth could also be treated by partial or total vulvectomy with inguinal node dissection

Selected References

Hauspy J, Beiner M, Harley I, et al: Sentinel lymph node in vulvar cancer. Cancer 110:1015-1023, 2007.

Chiesa-Vottero A, Dvoretsky PM, Hart WR: Histopathologic study of thin vulvar squamous cell carcinomas and associated cutaneous lesions: A correlative study of 48 tumors in 44 patients with analysis of adjacent vulvar intraepithelial neoplasia types and lichen sclerosus. Am J Surg Pathol 30:310-318, 2006.

Malignant Melanoma

Clinical Features

- Most common in the labia and in older women
- High mortality rate even when localized
- Most often diagnosed when deeply invasive
- Local recurrences are frequent
- Overall 5-year survival between 40% and 50%

Gross Pathology

- Pigmented macule, papule, or plaque

Histopathology

- Similar to melanoma in other sites (see Chapter 2)

Special Stains and Immunohistochemistry

- S-100 protein, melan-A, and HMB-45 positive
- CEA negative

Other Techniques for Diagnosis

- Noncontributory

Differential Diagnosis

▌ Paget disease
  - More common in skin from the breast
  - Immunohistochemical profile (mucin and CEA positive; melan-A and HMB-45 negative) is the opposite of the profile for malignant melanoma
▌ VIN
  - Dysplastic cells fail to show prominent nucleoli
  - Commonly positive for p16 and negative for mucin, CEA, HMB-45, melan-A, and S-100 protein

Pearls

- Gross appearance of the lesion is characteristic
- Melanoma is a disease of older women

Selected References

Helm K, Findeis-Hosey J: Immunohistochemistry of pigmented actinic keratoses, actinic keratoses, melanomas in situ and solar lentigines with melan-A. J Cutan Pathol 35:931-934, 2008.

Ragnarsson-Olding BK, Kanter-Lewensohn LR, Lagerlof B, et al: Malignant melanoma of the vulva in a nationwide, 25-year study of 219 Swedish females: Clinical observations and histopathologic features. Cancer 86:1273-1284, 1999.

Bartholin Gland Carcinoma

Clinical Features

- Presents in older women
- Clinically may be mistaken for a cyst
- About 20% present with inguinal lymph node metastasis
- Treated by wide excision or vulvectomy with inguinal-femoral lymph node dissection

Gross Pathology

- Solid infiltrative tumor that occupies the anatomic site of the normal Bartholin gland

Histopathology

- Adenocarcinoma (>40%)
  — Generally nonspecific features of adenocarcinoma: malignant glands
  — Intracytoplasmic mucin
  — CEA-positive cells
- Squamous cell carcinoma (about 40%)
  — Usual appearance of squamous cell carcinoma (SCC)
- Adenoid cystic carcinoma (about 10%)
- Transitional cell carcinoma (about 5%)
- Adenosquamous carcinoma (about 5%)

Special Stains and Immunohistochemistry

- Cytokeratin positive
- CEA positive
- S-100 protein positive in adenoid cystic carcinoma

Figure 12-8. Bartholin gland adenocarcinoma. High-power view shows back-to-back neoplastic glands demonstrating nuclear stratification and hyperchromasia.

Other Techniques for Diagnosis
- None

Differential Diagnosis
▌ Metastatic adenocarcinoma versus primary Bartholin gland tumor
- Metastases are rare in this location
- May resemble organ of origin
- Clinical history is most important

▌ Skin adnexal adenocarcinoma versus Bartholin gland adenocarcinoma
- Usually well differentiated
- Morphologically the tumor resembles adnexal structure of origin

▌ Metastatic squamous cell carcinoma versus Bartholin gland squamous cell carcinoma
- Usually only weakly positive for CEA
- Clinical history is most important

Pearls
- Adenoid cystic type of Bartholin gland carcinoma generally has a better prognosis than other types
- Adenosquamous type generally has a worse prognosis than squamous cell carcinoma of vulva
- Adenocarcinoma has the highest rate of lymph node metastasis

Selected References
Woida FM, Ribeiro-Silva A: Adenoid cystic carcinoma of the Bartholin gland: An overview. Arch Pathol Lab Med 131:796-798, 2007.

Finnan MA, Barre G: Bartholin's gland carcinoma, malignant melanoma and other rare tumours of the vulva. Best Pract Res Clin Obstet Gynaecol 17:609-633, 2003.

Extramammary Paget Disease

Clinical Features
- Most common in postmenopausal white women
- Fluorescein is useful to visualize the lesion before excision
- Often presents with pruritus
- About 14% of cases are associated with primary breast carcinoma
- Most develop de novo in epidermis or adnexal structures
- Slowly progressive disease
- Not necessarily associated with underlying vulvar invasive cancer as in mammary Paget disease
- Therapy is wide local excision

Gross Pathology
- Pink to red eczematous patches with white foci due to hyperkeratosis

Histopathology
- Irregularly defined lesion often larger than clinical impression
- Abnormal cells in the epidermis concentrated in the basal layer but may also be present superficially and in skin appendages
- Intraepithelial tumor cells singly or in small groups
- Large cells with round nuclei often containing large nucleoli
- Pale cytoplasm or vacuolated signet ring cells
- Adenocarcinoma may be seen in underlying dermis in about 10% to 20% of cases

Special Stains and Immunohistochemistry
- PAS with diastase, mucin, and Alcian blue positive
- HER-2-neu positive
- Low-molecular-weight cytokeratin (LMWCK) and CEA positive

Figure 12-9. Paget disease. Paget cells with pale cytoplasm are present in the epidermis.

Other Techniques for Diagnosis

- Noncontributory

Differential Diagnosis

▍ VIN
- Usually associated with HPV infection
- More regular involvement of basal layer
- Smaller cells with less prominent nucleoli
- Negative for mucin, CEA, LMWCK, and HER-2-neu

▍ Superficial spreading malignant melanoma
- Positive for S-100 protein, melan-A, and HMB-45
- Negative for mucin, LMWCK, and HER-2-neu
- Cells may contain melanin pigment

Pearls

- Generally not associated with HPV
- Occasionally associated with underlying adenocarcinoma or primary breast carcinoma including Paget disease
- Mucin positivity is a helpful diagnostic feature
- Recurrences are frequent because lesions are often more extensive than can be appreciated clinically

Selected References

Petković S, Jeremić K, Vidakovic S, et al: Paget's disease of the vulva: A review of our experience. Eur J Gynaecol Oncol 27:611-612, 2006.

Kurman R, Norris H, Wilkinson E: Atlas of Tumor Pathology: Tumors of the Cervix, Vagina, and Vulva, 3rd Series, Fascicle 4. Washington DC, Armed Forces Institute of Pathology, 1992, pp 208-211.

Hidradenoma Papilliferum (Papillary Hidradenoma)

Clinical Features

- Occurs mainly in middle-aged women in the labia majora, labia minora, and perineum
- Adnexal origin (i.e., apocrine sweat glands)
- Vulva may contain tissue closely resembling breast (ectopic breast)
- Identical appearance to intraductal papillomas of the breast

Gross Pathology

- Round, firm, domed nodule that is 1 to 2 cm in diameter
- On occasion, slightly tender and ulcerated if neglected

Histopathology

- Complex papillary structures showing fine fibrovascular cores and a collagenous stroma
- Inner layer of columnar or cuboidal cells
- Basal layer of flattened myoepithelial cells underlies the epithelium

Figure 12-10. Papillary hidradenoma. Papillary structures with fibrovascular cores covered by two layers of cells: a basal layer of flattened myoepithelial cells and a luminal layer of tall columnar cells with decapitation secretions.

Special Stains and Immunohistochemistry

- S-100 protein positive in the myoepithelial cells
- PAS focally positive in the epithelial cells

Other Techniques for Diagnosis

- Noncontributory

Differential Diagnosis

▍ Adenocarcinoma
- Nuclear pleomorphism and mitotic figures
- Absence of myoepithelial layer

▍ Other skin and skin adnexal tumors
- The vulva and its adnexal structures may be affected by most skin tumors that occur in other sites (refer to Chapter 2 for detailed discussion)

Pearls

- The only cutaneous adnexal tumor that is seen in the vulva with any frequency

Selected References

Kazakov DV, Mikyskova I, Kutzner H, et al: Hidradenoma papilliferum with oxyphilic metaplasia: A clinicopathological study of 18 cases, including detection of human papillomavirus. Am J Dermatopathol 27:102-110, 2005.

Buhl A, Landow S, Lee YC, et al: Microcystic adnexal carcinoma of the vulva. Gynecol Oncol 82:571-574, 2001.

Granular Cell Myoblastoma (Granular Cell Tumor)

Clinical Features

- Peripheral nerve sheath tumor uncommon in the vulva

- Presents as a painless, slow-growing, subcutaneous mass
- Generally in the labia majora, clitoris, or mons pubis
- Local recurrences are common
- Malignant tumors are extremely rare

Gross Pathology

- Well-demarcated, firm mass

Histopathology

- Nonencapsulated; composed of irregular groups of polyhedral cells
- Cells display indistinct borders, numerous eosinophilic granules in the cytoplasm, and relatively small nuclei with hyperchromasia

Special Stains and Immunohistochemistry

- S-100 protein positive
- Myelin basic protein positive
- CEA positive

Other Techniques for Diagnosis

- Noncontributory

Differential Diagnosis

▍ Leiomyoma, neurofibroma, and dermatofibroma

Pearls

- Much more common in other locations (i.e., tongue)
- May enlarge rapidly during pregnancy
- Examination of the margins of resection is most important

Angiomyofibroblastoma

Clinical Features

- Benign tumor, rare
- May present as a Bartholin gland cyst or mass

Gross Pathology

- Well circumscribed
- Highly vascular

Histopathology

- Benign spindle cell stroma
- Numerous small vessels
- Perivascular hypercellularity
- Mast cells are usually present

Special Stains and Immunohistochemistry

- Vimentin and desmin positive
- Smooth muscle actin (SMA) negative
- S-100 protein negative

Other Techniques for Diagnosis

- Noncontributory

Differential Diagnosis

▍ Aggressive angiomyxoma
  - Less cellular
  - Numerous and muscular vessels in clusters
  - SMA positive

Pearls

- Treated by local excision

Selected Reference

Nasu K, Fujisawa K, Takai N, Miyakawa I: Angiomyofibroblastoma of the vulva. Int J Gynecol Cancer 12:228-231, 2002.

Aggressive Angiomyxoma

Clinical Features

- Usually arises in premenopausal women
- Locally aggressive subcutaneous tumor
- Wide local excision is the treatment of choice

Figure 12-11. Angiomyofibroblastoma. Spindle-shaped tumor cells with perivascular distribution. A prominent perivascular chronic inflammatory infiltrate is noted.

Figure 12-12. Aggressive angiomyxoma. Prominent myxoid stroma with small blood vessels is evident in this lesion.

Gross Pathology

- Soft gelatinous mass with ill-defined margins
- Clusters of vessels are visible on cut surface

Histopathology

- Myxoid stroma with benign spindled fibroblasts and myofibroblasts
- Numerous clustered medium-sized arterioles
- Entrapped fat, neural elements, or glandular elements may be present

Special Stains and Immunohistochemistry

- Factor VIII, CD34 positive in the vascular component of the tumor
- SMA: Spindle cells positive
- S-100 protein negative

Other Techniques for Diagnosis

- Noncontributory

Differential Diagnosis

- High-grade pleomorphic sarcoma (malignant fibrous histiocytoma)
  - Storiform pattern
  - Marked cytologic atypia with numerous mitotic figures
  - Diagnosis of exclusion
  - Vimentin and CD68 stains are positive and may be helpful
- Angiomyofibroblastoma
  - More cellular
  - Well-defined tumor margins
  - Lacks numerous clustered arterioles

Pearls

- Locally aggressive with significant rate of local recurrence

Selected References

Dierickx I, Deraedt K, Poppe W, Verguts J: Aggressive angiomyxoma of the vulva: A case report and review of literature. Arch Gynecol Obstet 277:483-487, 2008.

Abu JI, Bamford WM, Malin G, et al: Aggressive angiomyxoma of the perineum. Int J Gynecol Cancer 15:1097-1100, 2005.

Ribaldone R, Piantanida P, Surico D, et al: Aggressive angiomyxoma of the vulva. Gynecol Oncol 95:724-728, 2004.

Horiguchi H, Matsui-Horiguchi M, Fujiwara M, et al: Angiomyofibroblastoma of the vulva: Report of a case with immunohistochemical and molecular analysis. Int J Gynecol Pathol 22:277-284, 2003.

Leiomyosarcoma

Clinical Features

- Most common vulvar sarcoma but overall quite rare
- Occurs in women of any age
- Usually arises in labia majora
- Often presents with pain
- Treatment is wide excision
- Metastasis to lung and liver have been reported

Gross Pathology

- Well-defined firm mass with infiltrative edges
- Focal hemorrhage, necrosis, and cystic degeneration

Histopathology

- Interlacing bundles of smooth muscle cells with perinuclear clearing
- Coagulative necrosis
- Greater than 5 mitotic figures/10 high-power fields (hpf)
- Nuclear atypia

Special Stains and Immunohistochemistry

- Vimentin positive
- Cytokeratin: occasional positive cells
- Desmin and SMA positive
- S-100 protein negative

Other Techniques for Diagnosis

- Noncontributory

Differential Diagnosis

- Dermatofibrosarcoma protuberans
  - Storiform pattern
  - Rare cytologic atypia and mitotic figures
  - Negative for SMA
- High-grade pleomorphic sarcoma (malignant fibrous histiocytoma)
  - Marked cytologic atypia and many mitoses
  - Giant cells
  - Several patterns: interlacing fascicles, storiform
  - Vimentin and CD68 positivity are helpful, but not diagnostic
- Aggressive angiomyxoma
  - Multiple clusters of muscular arterioles
  - Generally lacks cytologic atypia and mitotic activity

Pearls

- Tumors >5 cm in diameter have a higher rate of recurrence
- Some tumors may have minimal cytologic atypia but infiltrative margins, coagulative necrosis, and mitotic count more than 5 mitotic figures/10 hpf

Selected References

Shankar S, Todd PM, Rytina E, Crawford RA: Leiomyosarcoma of the vulva. J Eur Acad Dermatol Venereol 20:116-117, 2006.

Nielsen GP, Rosenberg AE, Koerner FC, et al: Smooth-muscle tumors of the vulva: A clinicopathological study of 25 cases and review of the literature. Am J Surg Pathol 20:779-793, 1996.

Other Sarcomas

- The following mesenchymal tumors rarely arise in the vulvar subcutaneous tissue
  — Embryonal rhabdomyosarcoma, generally in children
  — Dermatofibrosarcoma protuberans
  — Malignant fibrous histiocytoma
  — Epithelioid sarcoma
  — Malignant rhabdoid tumor
  — Angiosarcoma
  — Hemangiopericytoma
  — Kaposi sarcoma
  — Alveolar soft part sarcoma
  — Malignant schwannoma (neural)
  — Liposarcoma
- In the vulva, these sarcomas are identical to their counterparts in soft tissue
- Refer to Chapters 2 and 17 for detailed discussion

Selected References

Ulutin HC, Zellars RC, Frassica D: Soft tissue sarcoma of the vulva: A clinical study. Int J Gynecol Cancer 13:528-531, 2003.

Kurman R, Norris H, Wilkinson E: Atlas of Tumor Pathology: Tumors of the Cervix, Vagina, and Vulva, 3rd Series, Fascicle 4. Washington DC, Armed Forces Institute of Pathology, 1992, pp 220-228.

Vagina

Both atresia and total absence of the vagina are extremely uncommon.

Fibroepithelial Polyp (Vaginal Polyp, Mesodermal Stromal Polyp)

Clinical Features

- Occurs in women of childbearing age
- Usually discovered incidentally during pelvic examination

Gross Pathology

- Soft polyp or papillary mass usually in the lower third of the vagina

Histopathology

- Squamous epithelium with underlying fibrovascular stroma
- Plump, cytologically atypical myofibroblasts may be present in the stroma
- Bizarre multinucleate giant cells may also be present
- Mitotic activity is generally low

Figure 12-13. Fibroepithelial polyp. Polypoid lesion composed of fibrous connective tissue covered by mature squamous epithelium.

Special Stains and Immunohistochemistry

- Vimentin positive
- Desmin negative

Other Techniques for Diagnosis

- Noncontributory

Differential Diagnosis

- Sarcoma botryoides
  - Patients are generally younger than 5 years
  - Population of small round blue undifferentiated cells
  - Cellular cambium layer
  - Rhabdomyoblasts
  - Invasion of overlying squamous epithelium

Pearls

- Clinically benign; important to recognize to avoid misdiagnosing as condyloma or sarcoma

Selected References

Eilber KS, Raz S: Benign cystic lesions of the vagina: A literature review. J Urol 170:717-722, 2003.

Kurman R, Norris H, Wilkinson E: Atlas of Tumor Pathology: Tumors of the Cervix, Vagina, and Vulva, 3rd Series, Fascicle 4. Washington DC, Armed Forces Institute of Pathology, 1992, pp 170-172.

Squamous Papilloma

Clinical Features

- Occurs at any age
- Usually asymptomatic

Gross Pathology

- Several millimeters or larger in diameter
- Clustered papillary lesions

Histopathology

- Single central fibrovascular core with papillary fronds
- Benign, normal squamous lining

Figure 12-14. Squamous papilloma. Papillary lesion lined by squamous epithelium.

Special Stains and Immunohistochemistry
- Noncontributory

Other Techniques for Diagnosis
- Noncontributory

Differential Diagnosis
▌ Condyloma acuminatum
- Arborizing architecture
- Koilocytosis
- HPV-6 or HPV-11
▌ Fibroepithelial polyp
- Thinner squamous lining
- Polypoid rather than papillary
- Prominent stroma with occasional large pleomorphic cells

Pearls
- Clinically benign; important to recognize to avoid misdiagnosing as condyloma or squamous cell carcinoma

Selected Reference

Kurman R, Norris H, Wilkinson E: Atlas of Tumor Pathology: Tumors of the Cervix, Vagina, and Vulva, 3rd Series, Fascicle 4. Washington DC, Armed Forces Institute of Pathology, 1992, p 141.

Vaginal Intraepithelial Neoplasia

Clinical Features
- Relatively rare compared with the incidence of cervical squamous intraepithelial lesions
- Usually occurs in postmenopausal women
- Frequently associated with squamous cell carcinomas of cervix or vulva

Figure 12-15. A, Vaginal intraepithelial neoplasia 2. Dysplastic cells occupy the lower two thirds of the epithelium. **B, Vaginal intraepithelial neoplasia 3.** The dysplastic cells are present throughout the full thickness of the epithelium. Notice the marked parakeratosis and lymphoplasmacytic response.

- HPV infection and cervical or vulvar intraepithelial neoplasia are risk factors
- Usually asymptomatic

Gross Pathology
- Roughened pink or white discolored epithelium
- Occasional gross abnormality

Histopathology
▌ Vaginal intraepithelial neoplasia (VAIN) 1 (low grade)
- Nuclear pleomorphism and hyperchromasia involving the lower third of the epithelium

- Increased mitotic activity in the lower third
- Flat condylomata acuminata are best classified as VAIN 1
▌ VAIN 2 and 3 (high grade)
  - Nuclear pleomorphism and hyperchromasia involving the lower two thirds (VAIN 2) or full thickness (VAIN 3) of the epithelium
  - Binucleate and multinucleate cells are often present
  - Atypical mitotic figures are readily identifiable
  - Koilocytosis may be seen within or adjacent to the lesion

Special Stains and Immunohistochemistry

- p16 INK4a

Other Techniques for Diagnosis

- HPV may be identified by PCR or ISH

Differential Diagnosis

▌ Atrophy
  - Thinned epithelium without squamous atypia or koilocytosis
  - No mitotic activity
▌ Immature squamous metaplasia
  - Nuclear pleomorphism is not dramatic
  - Minimal mitotic activity
▌ Radiation change
  - Preserved nuclear-to-cytoplasmic ratio
  - Vacuolated cytoplasm
  - Smudged chromatin
  - Multinucleation
  - Lack of mitotic activity
▌ Reactive atypia
  - Prominent nucleoli
  - Lack of nuclear membrane irregularities

Pearls

- Less than 10% progress to invasive carcinoma
- Laser ablation and topical 5-fluorouracil are alternative treatments

Selected References

Drodon M, Stoler MH, Baber GB, Kurman RJ: The distribution of low and high-risk HPV types in vulvar and vaginal intraepithelial neoplasia (VIN and VaIN). Am J Surg Pathol 30:1513-1518, 2006.

Jones RW, Rowan DM: Spontaneous regression of vulvar intraepithelial neoplasia 2-3. Obstet Gynecol 96:470-472, 2000.

Koutsky L: Epidemiology of genital human papillomavirus infection. Am J Med 102:3-8, 1997.

Squamous Cell Carcinoma

Clinical Features

- Most common malignant vaginal neoplasm, but rare
- One fiftieth the incidence of cervical squamous cell carcinoma

Figure 12-16. Infiltrating squamous cell carcinoma. Nests and clusters of neoplastic cells invade the stroma.

- Most common in postmenopausal women
- Treatment is radiation therapy

Gross Pathology

- Superficially invasive: red papule, white plaque, or irregular ulcerated lesion
- Invasive: exophytic papillary mass or endophytic ulcer, usually solitary

Histopathology

- Keratinizing with squamous pearl formation
- Superficially invasive tumor is defined as 3 mm or less depth of invasion without vascular space invasion
- Syncytial sheets of cells with variable amounts of eosinophilic cytoplasm
- Distinct cell borders
- Intercellular bridges may be seen
- Variants
  — Verrucous carcinoma
    ◆ Rare variant
    ◆ Bulbous solid masses composed of bland squamous cells that push into the stroma
    ◆ Generally koilocytes are not evident
    ◆ Lymph node metastasis is rare
  — Warty (condylomatous) carcinoma
    ◆ Squamous cell carcinoma with numerous koilocytes
    ◆ Exophytic growth

Special Stains and Immunohistochemistry

- Noncontributory

Other Techniques for Diagnosis

- Noncontributory

Differential Diagnosis

▌ Amelanotic malignant melanoma
  - Negative for cytokeratin
  - Positive for S-100 protein and HMB-45
  - Absent keratinization and squamous pearl formation
▌ Pseudoepitheliomatous hyperplasia
  - Bland cytology
  - Normally maturing squamous epithelium
  - Absent stromal nests dissociated from basal layer
  - Commonly a reactive process
▌ Metastatic squamous cell carcinoma
  - Clinical history is important
  - Generally metastatic tumor will be present deep in the submucosa
  - Absent overlying intraepithelial component

Pearls

  - Tumors with less than 3 mm depth of stromal invasion and also verrucous carcinomas have low rates of lymph node metastasis
  - Verrucous carcinomas should not be treated with radiation therapy because they are radioresistant and may transform to higher-grade squamous carcinoma

Selected References

Roma AA, Hart WR: Progression of simplex (differentiated) vulvar intraepithelial neoplasia to invasive squamous cell carcinoma: A prospective case study confirming its precursor role in the pathogenesis of vulvar cancer. Int J Gynecol Pathol 26:248-253, 2007.

Medeiros F, Nascimento AF, Crum CP: Early vulvar squamous neoplasia: Advances in classification, diagnosis, and differential diagnosis (review). Adv Anat Pathol 12:20-26, 2005.

Vaginal Adenosis

Clinical Features

  - Associated with diethylstilbestrol (DES) exposure, most frequently in utero
  - Occurs in about one third of women exposed to DES
  - Young women aged 30 to 50 most commonly are affected
  - Red granular spots that do not stain with iodine
  - Excessive mucous discharge is a common symptom
  - Glandular epithelium may be observed colposcopically
  - May occur without exposure

Gross Pathology

  - Red granular patches
  - Upper third of anterior wall is most common location

Histopathology

  - Mucous columnar epithelium resembling endocervical mucosa replaces squamous lining of vagina

Figure 12-17. Vaginal adenosis. Low-power view demonstrates glandular epithelium at the junction of the mucosa and submucosa or lamina propria in the vagina.

  - Mucinous glands are present in the lamina propria
  - On occasion, ciliated epithelium or endometrial-type glands are seen, particularly in lower third of vagina
  - Long-standing lesions that become replaced by squamous metaplasia; obliterated glands or mucin droplets may be identified in these lesions

Special Stains and Immunohistochemistry

  - Noncontributory

Other Techniques for Diagnosis

  - Noncontributory

Differential Diagnosis

▌ Metastatic adenocarcinoma
  - Cytologic atypia
  - Clinical history

Pearls

  - DES was prescribed to women in the 1940s and 1950s to prevent miscarriages
  - History of exposure to DES is important
  - Vaginal adenosis usually regresses spontaneously
  - No treatment is required

Selected References

McCluggage WG: Recent developments in vulvovaginal pathology. Histopathology 54:156-173, 2009.

Robboy SJ, Anderson MC, Russell P: Pathology of the female reproductive tract. London, Churchill Livingstone, 2002.

Kurman R, Norris H, Wilkinson E: Atlas of Tumor Pathology: Tumors of the Cervix, Vagina, and Vulva, 3rd Series, Fascicle 4. Washington DC, Armed Forces Institute of Pathology, pp 146-152, 1992.

Robboy SJ, Hill EC, Sandberg EC, Czernobilsky B: Vaginal adenosis in women born prior to the diethylstilbestrol era. Hum Pathol 17:488-492, 1986.

Robboy SJ, Szyfelbein WM, Goellner JR, et al: Dysplasia and cytologic findings in 4,589 young women enrolled in diethylstilbestrol-adenosis (DESAD) project. Am J Obstet Gynecol 140:579-586, 1981.

Clear Cell Adenocarcinoma

Clinical Features

- Often but not always associated with in utero exposure to DES
- Occurs in less than 0.2% of women exposed to DES
- Generally occurs in women about 20 years of age
- Often presents with vaginal bleeding and discharge
- May be asymptomatic

Gross Pathology

- Occurs anywhere in the vagina
- Polypoid or nodular mass
- Less commonly flat or ulcerated

Histopathology

- Tubulocystic and solid are the most common patterns
- Papillary, tubular, and trabecular patterns may also be seen
- Tumor cells are polyhedral with round, atypical nuclei and clear cytoplasm containing glycogen
- Hobnail cell is a characteristic finding (cell with a nucleus that protrudes beyond the boundaries of the cell into a luminal, tubular, or cystic space)
- Less commonly, the epithelial cells are flattened, cuboidal, oxyphilic, or signet ring
- Adenosis is usually identified adjacent to tumor
- Intracellular hyaline structures and psammoma bodies are common

Special Stains and Immunohistochemistry

- Cytokeratin positive
- PAS positive (intracytoplasmic glycogen)
- PAS with diastase negative
- Mucin negative intracytoplasmic (may be positive in glandular lumina)

Other Techniques for Diagnosis

- Noncontributory

Differential Diagnosis

- ▉ Metastatic clear cell carcinoma from the ovary
  - Clinical history is essential
- ▉ Metastatic renal cell or adrenal carcinoma
  - Clinical history is important
  - Centrally located nuclei with prominent nucleoli
  - Absent gland formation
  - Absent hobnail cells
  - Prominent vascularity

Pearls

- Associated with in utero exposure to DES
- Adenosis believed to be a precursor lesion
- High risk for nodal metastasis if depth of invasion is greater than 3 mm
- More aggressive than squamous cell carcinoma
- Treatment of early-stage disease: vaginectomy with radical hysterectomy and lymphadenectomy to prevent recurrence
- Radiation therapy indicated for advanced disease

Selected References

Robboy SJ, Anderson MC, Russell P: Pathology of the female reproductive tract. London, Churchill Livingstone, 2002, pp 92-97.

Herbst AL, Anderson S, Hubby MM, et al: Risk factors for the development of diethylstilbestrol associated clear cell adenocarcinoma: A case-control study. Am J Obstet Gynecol 154:814-822, 1986.

Sander R, Nuss RC, Rhatigan RM: Diethylstilbestrol-associated vaginal adenosis followed by clear cell adenocarcinoma. Int J Gynecol Pathol 5:362-370, 1986.

Rhabdomyoma

Clinical Features

- Rare; occurs in middle-aged women
- Does not occur in children

Gross Pathology

- Polypoid mass, less commonly flat or ulcerated

Histopathology

- Bland skeletal muscle cells with fetal or adult-type appearance
- Cells are spindle to oval with plump oval nuclei without atypia or mitosis
- Cells are surrounded by a fibrous stroma
- Classic intracytoplasmic fibers with cross-striations

Special stains and Immunohistochemistry

- Noncontributory

Other Techniques for Diagnosis

- Noncontributory

Figure 12-18. Clear cell adenocarcinoma, papillary pattern. The papillae are lined by large pleomorphic cells showing clear cytoplasm. Focal necrosis is present.

Differential Diagnosis

▊ Embryonal rhabdomyosarcoma (sarcoma botryoides)
- Presence of cambium layer
- Pleomorphic strap cells with mitosis

Pearls

- Fewer than 25 cases reported
- Unremarkable overlying squamous mucosa
- Benign behavior

Selected References

López Varela C, López de la Riva M, La Cruz Pelea C: Vaginal rhabdomyomas. Int J Gynaecol Obstet 47:169-170, 1994.

López JI, Brouard I, Eizaguirre B: Rhabdomyoma of the vagina. Eur J Obstet Gynecol Reprod Biol 45:147-148, 1992.

Embryonal Rhabdomyosarcoma (Sarcoma Botryoides)

Clinical Features

- Most common vaginal sarcoma
- Occurs in infants and girls younger than 5 years
- Aggressive tumor
- Classically presents as a mass of small translucent nodules protruding from the vagina
- May present with bleeding and discharge and extension to bladder and rectum
- Metastasis to lung or bone usually presents later in the course of the disease

Gross Pathology

- Classic appearance is a sessile or pedunculated tumor of numerous translucent gray, grapelike, polypoid masses
- Hemorrhagic areas
- Most common location is anterior vaginal wall

Histopathology

- Tumor is organized histologically in layers
  — Superficial attenuated layer of squamous epithelium
  — Underlying cambium layer composed of small, round to spindled, primitive blue cells with dense hyperchromatic nuclei and minimal cytoplasm
    ◆ Cells may invade the overlying epithelium
  — Underlying sparsely cellular region with scattered small round blue cells as above in an edematous or myxoid stroma
    ◆ Rhabdomyoblasts are found in this region
      ◇ Large irregular, elongated, or "strap" cells with prominent eosinophilic cytoplasm
      ◇ Cross-striations may be seen but are not required to make the diagnosis
      ◇ Cells may appear to condense around blood vessels

Figure 12-19. Sarcoma botryoides (embryonal rhabdomyosarcoma). **A,** Low-power view demonstrates a proliferation of pleomorphic tumor cells beneath the vaginal epithelium. **B,** High-power view demonstrates myxoid stroma containing round to spindled tumor cells.

◆ Brisk mitotic activity
◆ Absence of heterologous elements (e.g., bone, cartilage)

Special Stains and Immunohistochemistry

- Desmin and muscle-specific actin (MSA) positive
- Myoglobin: more specific but less sensitive than above stains and therefore may be negative
- Vimentin positive in small and large tumor cells
- Cytokeratin negative (positive in benign overlying layer of attenuated epithelium)

Other Techniques for Diagnosis

- Noncontributory

Differential Diagnosis

▊ Müllerian papilloma
- In the differential not because of histologic similarity, but rather because of its similar clinical presentation in infants and young girls
- Papillary tumor with broad fibrovascular cores lined by cuboidal or mucinous epithelium
- Absence of cytologic atypia and mitotic activity

■ Benign polyp (mesodermal stromal polyp)
- Usually arises in adult women
- Essentially a fibroepithelial polyp as seen histologically in other sites
- Polypoid (as opposed to grapelike) mass
- Edematous fibrous tissue covered by squamous epithelium
- Lymphocytes may be present in the fibrous stroma
- No cambium layer
- Absent small round undifferentiated blue cells and rhabdomyoblasts
- Negative for desmin, MSA, and myoglobin

■ Rhabdomyoma
- Usually occurs in middle-aged women
- Numerous well-developed rhabdomyoblasts
- No nuclear atypia or mitotic figures
- Absence of cambium layer
- Absent small round undifferentiated blue cells

Pearls

- Aggressive tumor with rapid local invasion and high rate of local recurrence
- Survival has been significantly improved by treatment plan of surgical excision (vaginectomy plus hysterectomy with sparing of bladder and rectum) followed by new multiagent chemotherapeutic regimens

Selected References

Ferguson SE, Gerald W, Barakat RR, et al: Clinicopathologic features of rhabdomyosarcoma of gynecologic origin in adults. Am J Surg Pathol 31:382-389, 2007.

Nucci MR, Fletcher CD: Vulvovaginal soft tissue tumours: Update and review. Histopathology 36:97-99, 2000.

Copeland LJ, Gershenson DM, Saul PB, et al: Sarcoma botryoides of the female genital tract. Obstet Gynecol 66:262-266, 1985.

Copeland LJ, Sneige N, Stringer CA, et al: Alveolar rhabdomyosarcoma of the female genitalia. Cancer 56:849-855, 1985.

Other Sarcomas

- Leiomyosarcoma, epithelioid sarcoma, and malignant fibrous histiocytoma may also present as primary sarcomas of the vagina
- Refer to Chapter 17 for detailed discussion

Selected References

Kurman R, Norris H, Wilkinson E: Atlas of Tumor Pathology: Tumors of the Cervix, Vagina, and Vulva, 3rd Series, Fascicle 4. Washington DC, Armed Forces Institute of Pathology, 1992, pp 161-163.

Peters WAD, Kumar NB, Andersen WA, Morley GW: Primary sarcoma of the adult vagina: A clinicopathologic study. Obstet Gynecol 65:699-704, 1985.

Cervix

Endocervical Polyp

Clinical Features

- Most common new growth of the cervix
- Multigravidas during the fourth to sixth decades are the typical patients with polyps
- May present with leukorrhea or abnormal bleeding

Gross Pathology

- Rounded or elongated with a smooth or lobulated surface
- Most commonly single
- May measure from millimeters to a few centimeters

Histopathology

- Variety of patterns
- Varying amounts of squamous or endocervical epithelium depending on proximity to cervical os
- Stroma consists of dense fibroconnective tissue with thin and thick-walled vessels

Special Stains and Immunohistochemistry

- Noncontributory

Other Techniques for Diagnosis

- Noncontributory

Differential Diagnosis

■ Microglandular hyperplasia
- Tightly packed glands in a relatively ordered distribution
- Neutrophils are commonly present in the glandular lumina
- Acute and chronic inflammation in the stroma

Figure 12-20. Endocervical polyp. Polypoid lesion composed of endocervical mucous glands.

▌ Papillary adenofibroma
- Extremely rare and benign
- Leaflike pattern of glandular epithelium compressed by a dense fibrous stroma

Pearls

- Most common new growth of the cervix
- Characterized by dense fibrous stroma with thick-walled vessels

Selected References

Wright TC, Ferenczy A: Benign diseases of the cervix. In Kurman R (ed): Blaustein's Pathology of the Female Genital Tract, 5th ed. New York, Springer, 2002, pp 225-252.

Kurman R, Norris H, Wilkinson E: Atlas of Tumor Pathology: Tumors of the Cervix, Vagina, and Vulva, 3rd Series, Fascicle 4. Washington DC, Armed Forces Institute of Pathology, 1992, pp 77-78.

Microglandular Hyperplasia

Clinical Features

- Incidental finding in cervical specimens mostly in women of reproductive age
- May present with postcoital spotting or bleeding
- Associated with history of oral contraceptive use, pregnancy, or postpartum condition

Gross Pathology

- Single or multiple polypoid lesions resembling small cervical polyps

Histopathology

- Single or multiple foci of crowded glands have variable amounts of mucin
- Variably sized glands include rare mitotic figures (1 mitotic figure/10 hpf)

Figure 12-21. Microglandular hyperplasia. Tightly packed variously sized glandular structures lined by flattened to cuboidal cells.

- Uniform small round nuclei have even chromatin and some signet ring cells
- Focal squamous metaplasia may be present
- Neutrophils are commonly present in the glandular lumina
- Stroma separating the glands shows acute and chronic inflammatory cells

Special Stains and Immunohistochemistry

- CEA generally negative
- Mucin positive

Other Techniques for Diagnosis

- Noncontributory

Differential Diagnosis

▌ Clear cell and classic cervical adenocarcinoma
- Papillary and glandular patterns
- Irregular infiltration of cervical stroma by markedly atypical cells with nuclear pleomorphism
- Brisk mitotic rate
- Clear cytoplasm contains mostly glycogen rather than mucin

Pearls

- Commonly associated with oral contraceptive use
- Usually polypoid lesions
- Tightly packed benign endocervical glands

Selected References

Witkiewicz AK, Hecht JL, Cviko A, et al: Microglandular hyperplasia: A model for the de novo emergence and evolution of endocervical reserve cells. Hum Pathol 36:154-161, 2005.

Greeley C, Schroeder S, Silverberg SG: Microglandular hyperplasia of the cervix: A true "pill" lesion? Int J Gynecol Pathol 14:50-54, 1995.

Young RH, Scully RE: Atypical forms of microglandular hyperplasia of the cervix simulating carcinoma. Am J Surg Pathol 13:50-56, 1989.

Condyloma Acuminatum

Clinical Features

- Benign neoplasm uncommon in the cervix
- Spread by sexual contact
- HPV-6 and HPV-11 are the most common associated types
- When moderate to severe atypia is present, the lesion is classified as high-grade squamous intraepithelial lesion (HGSIL; cervical intraepithelial neoplasia [CIN] grade 2 or 3)
- If the condyloma shows HGSIL, it is almost always associated with HPV-16
- White upon application of 3% to 5% acetic acid under colposcopic examination
- Usually asymptomatic

Figure 12-22. Cervical condyloma (cervical intraepithelial neoplasia 1 with human papillomavirus). Thickened epithelium with irregular cytoplasmic halos and enlarged, binucleate, pyknotic nuclei.

Gross Pathology

- Similar to vulvar condyloma
- May show surface ulceration

Histopathology

- Koilocytes (HPV effect) in superficial epithelial cells
- Identical to vulvar condyloma
- Cytologic atypia is rarely present at the base of the lesion

Special Stains and Immunohistochemistry

- p16 INK4a positive

Other Techniques for Diagnosis

- PCR or ISH: specific identification of HPV type, usually 6 or 11

Differential Diagnosis

▎ Squamous intraepithelial lesion (SIL)
- Most flat lesions display koilocytic changes
- Abnormal mitosis may be present
- Cytologic atypia is seen at the base of the lesion in low-grade lesions
- Nuclear pleomorphism and hyperchromasia
- High nuclear-to-cytoplasmic ratio

▎ Squamous papilloma
- Thick fibrovascular core
- Lacks hyperkeratosis and koilocytosis

Pearls

- HPV-6 is the type most commonly associated with condyloma acuminatum
- Most lesions regress
- Progression to SIL and even squamous cell carcinoma has been reported
- Much more common in the vulva

Selected References

Redman R, Rufforny I, Liu C, et al: The utility of p16(Ink4a) in discriminating between cervical intraepithelial neoplasia 1 and nonneoplastic equivocal lesions of the cervix. Arch Pathol Lab Med 132:795-799, 2008.

Stoler MH: ASC, TBS, and the power of ALTS. Am J Clin Pathol 127:489-491, 2007.

Nordenvall C, Chang ET, Adami HO, Ye W: Cancer risk among patients with condylomata acuminata. Int J Cancer 119:888-893, 2006.

Sano T, Oyama T, Kashiwabara K, et al: Expression status of p16 protein is associated with human papillomavirus oncogenic potential in cervical and genital lesions. Am J Pathol 153:1741-1748, 1998.

Ostor AG: Natural history of cervical intraepithelial neoplasia: a critical review. Int J Gynaecol Pathol 12:186, 1993.

Squamous Intraepithelial Lesion or Cervical Intraepithelial Neoplasia and Carcinoma In Situ

Clinical Features

- Most common in premenopausal women
- Discolored raised plaques, often white after application of acetic acid (3% to 5%), at colposcopy
- High-grade lesions (HGSIL and carcinoma in situ [CIS]) may have a mosaic or cobblestone appearance
- Variety of risk factors, including high number of sexual partners, early age at initiation of sexual activity, and unprotected sex
- Smoking is a cofactor
- Greater than 95% of cervical dysplasias are related to HPV infection

Gross Pathology

- Flat or papular discolored lesions, often white or red

Histopathology

▎ Low-grade squamous intraepithelial lesion (LGSIL; CIN 1)
- Nuclear pleomorphism and hyperchromasia involving the lower third of the epithelium
- Irregular chromatin with inconspicuous nucleoli
- Increased mitotic activity in the lower third
- Most display HPV effect
- Flat condylomata acuminata are considered LGSIL

▎ HGSIL (CIN 2 or 3) and CIS
- Nuclear pleomorphism and hyperchromasia involving the lower two thirds (HGSIL; CIN 2) or the entire thickness of the epithelium (HGSIL; CIN 3; CIS)
- Irregular chromatin with inconspicuous nucleoli
- High nuclear-to-cytoplasmic ratio and atypical mitotic figures are identifiable

Figure 12-23. **A, Low-grade squamous intraepithelial lesion (cervical intraepithelial neoplasia grade 1 [CIN 1]).** Dysplastic cells occupy the lower third of the epithelium. The upper two thirds shows koilocytosis. **B, High-grade squamous intraepithelial lesion (CIN 2).** Squamous mucosa featuring dysplastic cells that involve the endocervical gland. **C, High-grade squamous intraepithelial lesion (CIN 3).** Squamous mucosa with atypical cells and mitotic figures involving the full thickness of the epithelium. **D, High-grade squamous intraepithelial lesion (carcinoma in situ):** p63 stain showing strong positivity in the dysplastic epithelium.

- Binucleate and multinucleate cells are often present but less than in LGSIL
- HPV is occasionally present within the lesion, more commonly adjacent to the lesion
- Involvement of underlying endocervical glands may be seen and should not be confused with microinvasive carcinoma

Special Stains and Immunohistochemistry

- p16 INKa positive
- Mib-1/Ki-67 index high

Other Techniques for Diagnosis

- PCR and ISH: HPV-16 is commonly identified in dysplastic lesions
- Ploidy: dysplastic lesions usually contain an aneuploid population of cells

Differential Diagnosis

▌ Atrophy
- Preserved polarity
- Basal cells in the full thickness of the epithelium
- No nuclear pleomorphism or mitotic figures

- Resolves after a 2-week course of locally applied estrogen therapy
▪ Immature squamous metaplasia
  - Retains cellular polarity
  - Clearly defined cell membranes
  - Absent nuclear atypia and atypical mitoses
  - Residual mucin may be seen
▪ Reactive atypia
  - Associated with inflammation
  - Prominent nucleoli
  - Retained polarity and nuclear-to-cytoplasmic ratio
  - No atypical mitoses
  - Changes more pronounced at the base
  - Halos mimicking koilocytosis may be present
▪ Microinvasive carcinoma versus HGSIL (CIN 3/CIS) with gland involvement
  - No basement membrane around invasive foci
  - Irregular infiltration of stroma instead of rounded nests
  - Stromal reaction, either desmoplastic or inflammatory

Pearls

- SIL is usually multifocal and most often associated with HPV-16
- SIL, particularly low-grade lesions (CIN 1), may spontaneously regress, especially in young or pregnant women
- LGSIL may be followed clinically, while HGSIL CIN (2 or 3) and CIS are generally followed by loop electrocautery excision procedure (LEEP) or cold knife cone and endocervical curetting to determine the extent of dysplasia
- Because of the above statement, it is essential to distinguish between LGSIL (CIN 1) and HGSIL (CIN 2-3) and not advisable to diagnose LGSIL and HGSIL. If both low- and high-grade lesions are present, a diagnosis of HGSIL is appropriate
- Vaccination for HPV is effective in about 60% to 70% of patients

Selected References

Waxman AG, Zsemlye MM: Preventing cervical cancer: The Pap test and the HPV vaccine. Med Clin North Am 92:1059-1082, 2008.

Fadare O, Rodriguez R: Squamous dysplasia of the uterine cervix: Tissue sampling-related diagnostic considerations in 600 consecutive biopsies. Int J Gynecol Pathol 26:469-474, 2007.

Focchi GR, Silva ID, Nogueira-de-Souza NC, et al: Immunohisto-chemical expression of p16(INK4A) in normal uterine cervix, nonneoplastic epithelial lesions, and low-grade squamous intraepithelial lesions. J Low Genit Tract Dis 11:98-104, 2007.

Song SH, Lee JK, Oh MJ, et al: Risk factors for the progression or persistence of untreated mild dysplasia of the uterine cervix. Int J Gynecol Cancer 16:1608-1613, 2006.

Klaes R, Benner A, Friedrich T, et al: p16INK4a immunohisto-chemistry improves interobserver agreement in the diagnosis of cervical intraepithelial neoplasia. Am J Surg Pathol 26:1389-1399, 2002.

Kurman R (ed): Blaustein's Pathology of the Female Genital Tract, 5th ed. Springer, New York, 2002; pp 253-276.

zur Hausen H: Papillomavirus infections: A major cause of human cancers. Biochim Biophys Acta 1288:F55-78, 1996.

Squamous Cell Carcinoma (Invasive)

Clinical Features

- Young women with history of smoking and concomitant HPV-associated lesions
- Microinvasive or invasive
- Microinvasive tumors rarely metastasize

Gross Pathology

- Microinvasive: red papule, white plaque, or irregular ulcerated lesion
- Invasive: exophytic papillary mass or endophytic ulcer, usually solitary

Histopathology

- Usually associated with high-grade dysplasia or CIS
  - Full-thickness involvement of epithelium or cervical glands by pleomorphic cells with high nuclear-to-cytoplasmic ratio and mitotic activity
- Atypical mitotic figures are often readily identifiable
- Variable degree of squamous differentiation, including keratin pearl formation
  - GOG grading as described under "Vulva"
- Desmoplastic reaction is a helpful finding associated with invasion
- Microinvasive
  - Tumor depth less than 3 mm as measured from basal layer of overlying surface epithelium to the point of deepest invasion by the tumor
  - If invasion is present only adjacent to an involved gland, the measurement is from the top of the gland to the point of deepest invasion by tumor
  - Tumor diameter is less than 7 mm
  - Vascular space invasion is not present in microinvasive carcinoma
- Invasive
  - Greater than 3 mm in depth of invasion
  - Generally greater than 7 mm in diameter
- Types of squamous cell carcinoma of cervix
  - Keratinizing
    ◆ Nests, cords, or single malignant polygonal epithelial cells with high nuclear-to-cytoplasmic ratio, nuclear pleomorphism with irregular chromatin, and eosinophilic cytoplasm
    ◆ Atypical mitoses
    ◆ Variable degree of necrosis
    ◆ Keratin pearl formation or individual cell keratinization

Figure 12-24. A, Invasive squamous cell carcinoma of the cervix (gross photograph). Endocervix with endophytic, deeply invasive white to tan ill-defined tumor involving the cervical wall. **B, Invasive squamous cell carcinoma, keratinizing type.** Irregular nests of pleomorphic squamous cells with dyskeratosis infiltrating reactive stroma inflammatory cells. **C, Squamous metaplasia.** In contrast to invasive squamous cell carcinoma, the sheets of metaplastic cells show rounded borders as they involve endocervical glands. The nuclear-to-cytoplasmic ratio is not altered, and desmosomes are obvious. **D, Nonkeratinizing squamous cell carcinoma (invasive).** Continuous sheets of malignant cells with no discernible intercellular bridges adjacent to an unremarkable endocervical gland (grade 3).

Continued

— Nonkeratinizing
  ◆ Usually rounded nests, as above
  ◆ Absent keratin pearl formation
— Verrucous
  ◆ Well-differentiated squamous cell carcinoma with minimal cytologic atypia
  ◆ Exophytic, often bulky tumor
  ◆ Hyperkeratosis at surface
  ◆ Characterized by a bulbous pushing border rather than a truly invasive border
  ◆ Rarely metastasizes
  ◆ Associated with HPV-6 and its subtypes
— Warty (condylomatous)
  ◆ Papillary exophytic growth
  ◆ Fibrovascular fronds
  ◆ Squamous differentiation

  ◆ Numerous koilocytes
  ◆ Irregularly outlined nests of invasive tumor at base
— Papillary (transitional)
  ◆ Rare variant with papillary architecture
  ◆ Papillae are lined by several layers of cytologically atypical spindled cells with frequent mitotic activity
  ◆ Squamous differentiation may be focally present
  ◆ Resembles transitional cell carcinoma of the genitourinary tract histologically
— Lymphoepithelioma-like carcinoma
  ◆ Well-circumscribed tumor
  ◆ Discrete nests of nonkeratinizing epithelial cells with vesicular nuclei and abundant cytoplasm

Figure 12-24, cont'd. E, Warty (condylomatous) squamous cell carcinoma. Low-power view demonstrates frondlike papillae with marked keratinization. Stromal invasion is present. **F, Warty (condylomatous) squamous cell carcinoma.** High-power view demonstrates classic epithelial papillae with condylomatous changes. **G, Lymphoepithelioma-like carcinoma.** Large pleomorphic neoplastic cells with abundant eosinophilic cytoplasm, irregular nuclei, and prominent nucleoli. Notice the marked lymphoplasmacytic infiltrate in the background.

♦ Prominent lymphoplasmacytic inflammatory infiltrate between and around nests
♦ Negative for Epstein-Barr virus (EBV)

Special Stains and Immunohistochemistry

• Cytokeratin and p63 positive
• CEA focally positive
• Mucin negative

Other Techniques for Diagnosis

• PCR and ISH
— HPV-16, -18, -31, -35, and other types have been detected in greater than 95% of tumors, especially in younger women with history of CIN
— HPV-16 has been detected in about 75% of tumors
• Ploidy: most carcinomas are aneuploid
• *Ras* oncogene product p21 overexpression: detected by PCR or ISH; associated with poor prognosis in large cell keratinizing and nonkeratinizing carcinomas

Differential Diagnosis

❚ Squamous metaplasia with gland involvement
• Nuclear atypia absent
• Rare mitotic figures
• Metaplastic glands rounded
• No stromal reaction
❚ Glassy cell carcinoma
• High mitotic activity
• Distinct cell borders
• Prominent nucleoli
• Ground-glass cytoplasm
❚ Small cell carcinoma
• Neuroendocrine patterns (e.g., round nests, trabeculae, ribbons, and rosettes)
• Hyperchromatic smudged chromatin
• No nucleoli
• Neuroendocrine differentiation by immunohistochemistry (neuron-specific enolase [NSE], chromogranin, synaptophysin positive) or electron microscopy (dense neurosecretory granules)

▌ Amelanotic malignant melanoma
  - Negative for cytokeratin
  - Positive for S-100 protein and HMB-45
  - No keratinization and squamous pearl formation
▌ Metastatic squamous cell carcinoma
  - Clinical history is important
  - Generally, metastatic tumor is present deep in the mucosa

Pearls

- Important prognostic indicators are tumor thickness, depth of invasion, tumor diameter, and vascular space invasion
- The invasive component is often much better differentiated than the intraepithelial component
- Microinvasive carcinoma may be treated with cervical cone (cold knife) and endocervical curettage if the cone shows focal microinvasion and free margins
- If curettage is positive, hysterectomy may be indicated
- Invasive carcinomas are treated by radical hysterectomy with or without adjuvant therapy depending on stage of tumor

Selected References

Horn LC, Hentschel B, Braumann UD: Malignancy grading, pattern of invasion, and juxtatumoral stromal response (desmoplastic change) in squamous cell carcinoma of the uterine cervix. Int J Gynecol Pathol 27:606-607, 2008.

Hsu KF, Huang SC, Shiau AL, et al: Increased expression level of squamous cell carcinoma antigen 2 and 1 ratio is associated with poor prognosis in early-stage uterine cervical cancer. Int J Gynecol Cancer 17:174-181, 2007.

Kokka F, Verma M, Singh N, et al: Papillary squamotransitional cell carcinoma of the uterine cervix: Report of three cases and review of the literature. Pathology 38:584-586, 2006.

Papanikolaou A, Kalogiannidis I, Misailidou D, et al: Results on the treatment of uterine cervix cancer: ten years experience. Eur J Gynaecol Oncol 27:607-610, 2006.

Chao A, Wang TH, Lee YS, et al: Molecular characterization of adenocarcinoma and squamous carcinoma of the uterine cervix using microarray analysis of gene expression. Int J Cancer 119:91-98, 2006.

Adenocarcinoma In Situ

Clinical Features

- Occurs in women in third and fourth decades
- Usually asymptomatic
- Often diagnosed incidentally during workup of abnormal Papanicolaou (Pap) test or cervical dysplasia
- Increasing incidence (related to improved detection in Pap smears collected with the current endocervical brush)
- Associated with HPV infection

Figure 12-25. Adenocarcinoma in situ of the cervix. Irregular glands with hyperchromatic nuclei and mitosis and no stromal invasion.

- Risk factors include obesity, hypertension, and oral contraceptives with progesterone content
- Thirty percent to 50% of cases are associated with CIN and invasive squamous cell carcinoma of the cervix

Gross Pathology

- Usually above the squamocolumnar junction
- Often multifocal
- Rarely visible colposcopically

Histopathology

- Normally located glands with malignant epithelial cell lining
- High nuclear-to-cytoplasmic ratio
- Irregular chromatin and inconspicuous nucleoli
- Cellular stratification
- Mitotic activity
- Endocervical (most common), intestinal, and endometrioid types
- Absent stromal desmoplasia

Special Stains and Immunohistochemistry

- CEA usually positive
- Vimentin generally negative
- Mucin positive

Other Techniques for Diagnosis

- PCR or ISH often positive for HPV

Differential Diagnosis

▌ Reactive glandular atypia
  - Prominent nucleoli
  - No stratification
  - Associated with inflammation

■ Microinvasive adenocarcinoma
  ● Adenocarcinoma infiltrates less than 5 mm of the cervical stroma and is less than 7 mm wide
  ● The measurement is from the basement membrane of the overlying endocervical or ectocervical surface
  ● Rare lymph node metastasis
  ● Conservative therapy
■ Invasive adenocarcinoma
  ● Infiltration of the stroma by malignant glands
  ● Glands present deep in the wall of the cervix
  ● Glands may show budding, papillary growth, or cribriforming
  ● Stromal response includes inflammatory cells and desmoplasia
■ Microglandular hyperplasia
  ● Small polypoid lesion
  ● Lobular arrangement
  ● Dense concentration of benign glands
■ Tubal metaplasia
  ● Few glands involved
  ● Nuclear atypia absent
  ● Ciliated epithelium
■ Endometriosis
  ● Endometrial glands and stroma are seen in cervical tissue
  ● Hemosiderin-laden macrophages may also be present

Pearls

● Associated with HPV infection
● Increasingly detected in Pap smears as a result of the use of the endocervical brush, which reaches higher into the endocervical canal than does the spatula
● Treatment is cervical cone with free surgical margins or hysterectomy
● Recurrence may follow second conization because of residual adenocarcinoma in situ at the endocervical canal or lower uterine segment or hysterectomy
● Greater than 30% of cases coexist with CIN

Selected References

Ceballos KM, Shaw D, Daya D: Microinvasive cervical adenocarcinoma (FIGO stage 1A tumors): Results of surgical staging and outcome analysis. Am J Surg Pathol 30:370-374, 2006.

Yap OW, Hendrickson MR, Teng NN, Kapp DS: Mesonephric adenocarcinoma of the cervix: A case report and review of the literature. Gynecol Oncol 103:1155-1158, 2006.

Colgan TJ, Lickrish GM: The topography and invasive potential of cervical adenocarcinoma in situ, with and without associated squamous dysplasia. Gynecol Oncol 36:246-249, 1990.

Tase T, Okagaki T, Clark BA, et al: Human papillomavirus DNA in adenocarcinoma in situ, microinvasive adenocarcinoma of the uterine cervix, and coexisting cervical squamous intraepithelial neoplasia. Int J Gynecol Pathol 8:8-17, 1989.

Adenocarcinoma (Invasive)

Clinical Features

● Increased incidence
● Affected patients are slightly older (fourth and fifth decades) than patients with squamous cell carcinoma
● Associated with HPV infection
● Risk factors include obesity, hypertension, and oral contraceptives with progesterone content
● More than 40% of cases are associated with SIL and invasive squamous cell carcinoma of the cervix
● May present with a watery discharge

Gross Pathology

● Generally exophytic, polypoid, nodular, or papillary

Histopathology

● Variable combinations of cell types
● Mixed cell type if any two or more of the types listed below represent more than 10% of the total tumor volume
● Mucinous endocervical
  — Resembles normal endocervical epithelium
  — Occasionally papillary
● Mucinous intestinal
  — Pseudostratified columnar epithelium with goblet cells
● Mucinous signet ring cell
  — Compressed nucleus with abundant intracytoplasmic mucin
  — Usually not a prominent component
● Endometrioid
  — Stratified epithelial cells with minimal granular cytoplasm resembling malignant endometrial glands
  — Intracytoplasmic mucin absent
● Minimal deviation adenocarcinoma (adenoma malignum)
  — Cytologically bland glands, usually mucinous endocervical type
  — Irregular, branching glands of variable sizes
  — Increased numbers of glands at surface and extending deep into the wall of the cervix (>5 mm)
  — Stromal desmoplasia may be present
  — Cervical biopsy may not be deep enough to permit the diagnosis
● Well-differentiated papillary villoglandular
  — Patients generally in third or fourth decade
  — May be deeply invasive
  — Complex branching papillary architecture
  — Stratified columnar lining: endocervical, endometrioid, or intestinal type
  — Minimal cytologic atypia
  — Minimal mucin

Figure 12-26. A, Moderately differentiated invasive adenocarcinoma of the cervix. Crowded glands and nuclear pleomorphism. **B, Mucinous adenocarcinoma of the cervix.** Clusters of neoplastic mucinous epithelium in lakes of extracellular mucin. **C, Well-differentiated endometrioid adenocarcinoma of the cervix.** Confluent glandular pattern with minimal desmoplastic stroma identical to uterine corpus endometrioid adenocarcinoma. **D, Minimal deviation adenocarcinoma (adenoma malignum).** Low-power view demonstrates irregular neoplastic endocervical glands associated with desmoplasia. **E, Clear cell carcinoma of the cervix.** Solid proliferation of neoplastic cells with clear cytoplasm. **F, Glassy cell carcinoma of the cervix.** Large neoplastic cells with finely granular ground-glass cytoplasm, prominent nuclei, and nucleoli. The stroma contains inflammatory cells, including eosinophils.

- Clear cell
  — Often associated with DES exposure
  — Tubulocystic and solid are the most common patterns
  — Papillary, tubular, and trabecular patterns may also be seen

  — Tumor cells are polyhedral with round, atypical nuclei and clear cytoplasm containing glycogen
  — The hobnail cell is a common and characteristic finding: cell in which the nucleus protrudes beyond the boundaries of the cell into the luminal, tubular, or cystic space

— Less commonly, the epithelial cells are flattened, cuboidal, oxyphilic, or signet ring
— Psammoma bodies or intracellular hyaline bodies may be seen
- Adenocarcinoma with features of carcinoid tumor
  — Occasionally an adenocarcinoma may contain areas of neuroendocrine carcinoma positive for neuroendocrine markers
  — Paraendocrine syndromes are rare
  — Not responsive to the usual treatment modalities
- Grading (not as definitive as corpus cancer)
  — Well-differentiated: more than 50% glands
  — Moderately differentiated: 10% to 50% glands
  — Poorly differentiated: less than 10% glands
- Depth of invasion is measured from the surface

Special Stains and Immunohistochemistry

- CEA usually positive in mucinous adenocarcinomas and negative in normal endocervical glands

Other Techniques for Diagnosis

- HPV often detected by PCR or ISH

Differential Diagnosis

▌ Microglandular hyperplasia
- Polypoid lesion
- Lobular arrangement
- Dense concentration of benign glands
- CEA negative

▌ Adenocarcinoma in situ
- Glands are not present deep in the wall of cervix
- Minimal glandular budding, papillary growth, or cribriforming
- Absence of stromal response (or desmoplasia)

▌ Metastatic adenocarcinoma
- Clinical history essential
- Surface involvement is generally absent
- Extensive lymphatic invasion

▌ Direct extension of endometrial adenocarcinoma
- Clinical history of endometrial carcinoma
- Absence of endocervical glandular or in situ adenocarcinoma
- Negative for HPV infection
- The distinction may be difficult
- Mucinous endometrial adenocarcinoma is also positive for CEA and negative for vimentin

Pearls

- Associated with HPV infection
- Increasingly detected in Pap smears as a result of the use of the endocervical brush, which reaches higher into the endocervix than does the spatula
- Standard treatment is radical hysterectomy with pelvic lymphadenectomy
- Radiation therapy is preferred for tumors that are larger than 5 cm at the time of diagnosis

- Generally tumors smaller than 1 cm do not metastasize to lymph nodes
- Prognosis correlates with stage

Selected References

Wang SS, Sherman ME, Silverberg SG, et al: Pathological characteristics of cervical adenocarcinoma in a multi-center US-based study. Gynecol Oncol 103:541-546, 2006.

Zaino RJ: Symposium part I: Adenocarcinoma in situ, glandular dysplasia, and early invasive adenocarcinoma of the uterine cervix. Int J Gynecol Pathol 21:314-326, 2002.

Kurman R, Norris H, Wilkinson E: Atlas of Tumor Pathology: Tumors of the Cervix, Vagina, and Vulva, 3rd Series, Fascicle 4. Washington DC, Armed Forces Institute of Pathology, 1992, pp 79-95.

Gilks CB, Young RH, Aguirre P, et al: Adenoma malignum (minimal deviation adenocarcinoma) of the uterine cervix: A clinicopathological and immunohistochemical analysis of 26 cases. Am J Surg Pathol 13:717-729, 1989.

Adenosquamous Carcinoma

Clinical Features

- Occurs in women of all ages
- Risk factors as in squamous cell carcinoma: smoking, multiple sexual partners, and low socioeconomic status
- Less common than adenocarcinoma

Gross Pathology

- Polypoid endocervical mass

Histopathology

- Poorly differentiated squamous cell carcinoma intermingled with high-grade adenocarcinoma
- Intracytoplasmic and luminal mucin usually present in the glandular component

Special Stains and Immunohistochemistry

- CEA may be positive in adenocarcinoma
- Mucin positive if mucin is present

Other Techniques for Diagnosis

- Noncontributory

Differential Diagnosis

▌ Direct extension of adenocarcinoma of endometrium
- Bulky tumor in the endometrium
- Usually less squamous differentiation
- More likely endometrioid than mucinous adenocarcinoma
- Precursor lesion in the uterine corpus (i.e., endometrial hyperplasia) is helpful

▌ Endocervical carcinoma with synchronous squamous cell carcinoma
- Separate tumors with no intermingling
- Endometrial or endocervical precursor lesions (i.e., hyperplasia or dysplasia [CIN], respectively) are helpful

Pearls

- Mixed carcinoma
- Occurs in women of any age
- Treatment and prognosis as for other invasive cervical carcinomas

Selected Reference

Bethwaite P, Yeong ML, Holloway L: The prognosis of adenosquamous carcinoma of the uterine cervix. Br J Obstet Gynecol 99:745-750, 1992.

Poorly Differentiated Adenosquamous Carcinoma (Glassy Cell Carcinoma)

Clinical Features

- Rare and unique variant
- Reported in women in third and fourth decades
- In some series, associated with pregnancy
- Worse prognosis than squamous cell carcinoma, stage for stage

Gross Pathology

- Voluminous exophytic mass

Histopathology

- Invasive sheets and nests of cells with thin intervening fibrovascular septa
- Large polygonal uniform cells with distinct borders
- Large nuclei with prominent nucleoli
- Finely granular eosinophilic ground-glass cytoplasm
- Minimal keratinization, if any
- Rare gland lumens and intracytoplasmic mucin
- High mitotic activity
- Prominent eosinophilic and lymphoplasmacytic inflammatory response

Special Stains and Immunohistochemistry

- Mucin may be focally positive
- CEA may be focally positive

Other Techniques for Diagnosis

- Noncontributory

Differential Diagnosis

▌Poorly differentiated, nonkeratinizing squamous cell carcinoma
- Syncytial growth; less distinct cell borders
- Coarse chromatin with less prominent nucleoli
- Lower mitotic activity
- Less granular cytoplasm

Pearls

- Stage for stage, prognosis is worse than for squamous cell carcinomas

- Glassy cytoplasm is due to dilated endoplasmic reticulum and abundant tonofilaments as seen by electron microscopy
- Currently listed as adenosquamous carcinoma grade 3 (glassy cell)

Selected References

Kurman R, Norris H, Wilkinson E: Atlas of Tumor Pathology: Tumors of the Cervix, Vagina, and Vulva, 3rd Series, Fascicle 4. Washington DC, Armed Forces Institute of Pathology, 1992, pp 95-106.

Pak HY, Yokota SB, Paladugu RR, Agliozzo CM: Glassy cell carcinoma of the cervix: Cytologic and clinicopathologic analysis. Cancer 52:307-312, 1983.

Maier RC, Norris HJ: Glassy cell carcinoma of the cervix. Obstet Gynecol 60:219-224, 1982.

Poorly Differentiated Neuroendocrine Carcinoma (Small Cell Carcinoma)

Clinical Features

- Uncommon
- Occurs in women in third and fourth decades
- Aggressive tumor
- Paraendocrine syndromes may manifest

Gross Pathology

- Often ulcerating tumors

Histopathology

- Highly cellular
- Sheets of tightly packed small cells with minimal cytoplasm and round to spindled nuclei
- Smudged chromatin with inconspicuous nucleoli
- Few scattered larger pleomorphic cells
- Brisk mitotic rate is often present

Figure 12-27. Small cell carcinoma of the cervix. Low-power view demonstrates a solid proliferation of small uniform neoplastic cells mimicking a malignant lymphoma.

- Vascular space invasion is frequently identified
- Squamous or glandular differentiation makes up less than 10% of tumor volume
- Similar to pulmonary small cell carcinoma

Special Stains and Immunohistochemistry

- Cytokeratin positive
- Chromogranin positive in about 50% of tumors
- Synaptophysin and NSE positive in a significant number of tumors
- Serotonin and somatostatin rarely positive

Other Techniques for Diagnosis

- PCR, ISH: HPV-18 has been detected; less commonly HPV-16

Differential Diagnosis

▌ Poorly differentiated, nonkeratinizing squamous cell carcinoma
  - May be difficult to distinguish if cells are small
  - No neuroendocrine differentiation
▌ Poorly differentiated adenocarcinoma
  - Gland formation makes up more than 10% of tumor volume
  - Neuroendocrine differentiation is absent
▌ Lymphoma
  - Cells less tightly packed
  - Positive for CD45 (leukocyte common antigen)
  - No neuroendocrine differentiation

Pearls

- Treatment is radical hysterectomy with bilateral pelvic and periaortic lymph node dissection
- Adjuvant radiation therapy if lymph node metastases are present
- Aggressive tumor with frequent recurrence and poor survival
- Distant metastases common

Selected References

Pirog EC, Kleter B, Olgac S, et al: Prevalence of human papillomavirus DNA in different histological subtypes of cervical adenocarcinoma. Am J Pathol 157:1055-1062, 2000.

Ambros RA, Park JS, Shah KV, Kurman RJ: Evaluation of histologic, morphometric, and immunohistochemical criteria in the differential diagnosis of small cell carcinomas of the cervix with particular reference to human papillomavirus types 16 and 18. Mod Pathol 4:586-593, 1991.

Stoler MH, Mills SE, Gersell DJ, Walker AN: Small-cell neuroendocrine carcinoma of the cervix: A human papillomavirus type-18 associated tumor. Am J Surg Pathol 15:28-32, 1991.

Werness BA, Levine AJ, Howley PM: Association of human papillomavirus types 16 and 18 E6 proteins with p53. Science 248:76-79, 1990.

Munger K, Phelps WC, Bubb V, et al: The E6 and E7 genes of the human papillomavirus type 16 together are necessary and sufficient for transformation of primary human keratinocytes. J Virol 63:4417-4421, 1989.

Gersell DJ, Mazoujian G, Mutch DG, Rudloff MA: Small-cell undifferentiated carcinoma of the cervix: A clinicopathologic, ultrastructural, and immunocytochemical study of 15 cases. Am J Surg Pathol 12:684-698, 1988.

Metastatic Adenocarcinoma

Clinical Features

- Ovarian carcinoma is the most common tumor metastatic to the cervix
- Breast is the most common extragenital source of tumor metastatic to the cervix
- Endometrial carcinomas may spread by direct extension; this occurrence increases the stage of the corpus cancer (II versus I)
- Metastases may present with vaginal bleeding

Gross Pathology

- Generally tumors metastasize to the outer surface
- Direct extension from the endometrium may be seen within the endocervical canal

Histopathology

- As per the primary tumor
- Tumors from the endometrium may be difficult to distinguish from primary cervical tumors, which may arise simultaneously
- The absence of CIN in the presence of subepithelial infiltrates or prominent lymphatic permeation suggests metastatic disease

Special Stains and Immunohistochemistry

- As per the primary tumor

Other Techniques for Diagnosis

- CEA is generally positive in cervical adenocarcinoma, whereas vimentin is positive in endometrial tumors
- CEA is generally negative in endometrial tumors, whereas vimentin is positive in cervical adenocarcinoma
- Generally, p16 is positive in cervical adenocarcinomas

Differential Diagnosis

▌ Metastatic carcinoma versus primary cervical carcinoma
  - The absence of CIN and adenocarcinoma in situ in the presence of subepithelial infiltrates or prominent lymphatic permeation suggests metastatic disease
  - Endometrial and cervical adenocarcinomas may be synchronous and indistinguishable
  - Clinical history is essential

Pearls

- The absence of CIN in the overlying epithelium suggests metastatic disease
- Clinical history is essential

Selected References

Kurman R (ed): Blaustein's Pathology of the Female Genital Tract, 5th ed. New York, Springer, 2002, pp 371-372.

Lemoine NR, Hall PA: Epithelial tumors metastatic to the uterine cervix: A study of 33 cases and review of the literature. Cancer 57:2002-2005, 1986.

Uterus

Endometrium

Acute Endometritis

Clinical Features

- Most often associated with pelvic inflammatory disease (PID)
- May be associated with pregnancy
- Elevated temperature, leukocytosis, discomfort, and pain

Gross Pathology

- When secondary to PID, presents with a tubo-ovarian complex with fibrous adhesions, fibrinous exudate, congestion, and edema
- Associated with intrauterine device (IUD) use and may be seen in compressed endometrium overlying large leiomyomas

Histopathology

- Numerous neutrophils in the stroma and several glands
- Ectatic blood vessels
- Fibrin exudate
- Hemorrhage

Special Stains and Immunohistochemistry

- Straightforward hematoxylin and eosin (H&E) diagnosis

Other Techniques for Diagnosis

- Noncontributory

Differential Diagnosis

▋ Menstruation
  - Vacuoles in the distended glands
  - Decidual change in the stroma

Pearls

- Clinical history is important, particularly as it relates to the menstrual cycle
- Aseptic abortion is a possibility in some locations
- Patient may present with acute abdomen

Chronic Endometritis

Clinical Features

- Common condition
- May be asymptomatic, although may present with pelvic pain when associated with menstrual irregularities
- Associated with IUD use and may be identified in compressed endometrium overlying large leiomyomas

Gross Pathology

- Generally the findings are nonspecific

Histopathology

- Plasma cells must be identified in the endometrial stroma
- Endometrium is difficult to date (i.e., glands appear variable in terms of phase [early, mid, and late secretory endometrium or proliferative])
- Focal crowding mimicking hyperplasia
- Glandular epithelium may show mild cytologic atypia and focal or diffuse spindled stroma

Special Stains and Immunohistochemistry

- Straightforward H&E diagnosis

Other Techniques for Diagnosis

- Noncontributory

Differential Diagnosis

▋ Endometrial hyperplasia
  - Stromal plasma cells are unusual
  - Diffuse process
▋ Endometrial adenocarcinoma
  - Confluent or cribriform glandular architecture with cytologic atypia
  - Stromal desmoplasia or necrosis may be present

Figure 12-28. Chronic endometritis. Endometrial glands and stroma in which plasma cells are present.

Pearls

- Lymphocytes are normally present in the endometrium, as are neutrophils in the late secretory and early proliferative phases; therefore, the diagnosis of chronic endometritis requires plasma cells
- In the presence of chronic endometritis, the diagnosis of hyperplasia should be made with caution

Selected References

Kiviat NB, Eschenbach DA, Paavonen JA, et al: Endometrial histopathology in patients with culture-proved upper genital tract infection and laparoscopically diagnosed acute salpingitis. Am J Surg Pathol 14:167-175, 1990.

Rotterdam H: Chronic endometritis: A clinicopathologic study. Pathol Annu 13:209-231, 1978.

Endometrial Polyp

Clinical Features

- Common
- Most often seen in middle-aged and postmenopausal women
- Often presents with abnormal bleeding
- Tamoxifen effect

Gross Pathology

- Usually solitary and highly variable in size
- Most commonly arises in the fundus
- Broad based and sessile, pedunculated or slender stalk

Histopathology

- Irregularly outlined glands that may be out of phase with the endometrium
- Fibrovascular stalk or fibrous stroma with several thick-walled vessels
- Metaplastic epithelium, particularly squamous, may be present
- Polyps in the lower uterine segment may contain endocervical as well as endometrial glands
- If the stroma contains abundant muscle, the polyp may be referred to as *adenomyomatous polyp*
- Absence of cytologic atypia, usually with epithelial lining on three sides
- Hyperplasia might be present and confined to the polyp

Special Stains and Immunohistochemistry

- Noncontributory

Other Techniques for Diagnosis

- Noncontributory

Differential Diagnosis

- Endometrial hyperplasia
  - Diffuse process involving the entire endometrium or, if curetted, most of the fragments

Figure 12-29. Endometrial polyp. A, Cross section of the uterus shows an endometrial polyp filling the endometrial cavity. **B,** Atrophic glandular epithelium is visible. The cystic dilated glands are lined by low columnar to cuboidal epithelium. **C,** The endometrial cavity shows a broad-based polypoid lesion. The external surface is smooth, tan, and glistening.

- Crowded glands with or without cytologic atypia
- Generally thick-walled vessels absent in hyperplasia
- Polypoid adenocarcinoma
  - Malignant epithelial cells lining back-to-back glands
  - Absence of fibrous stroma and thick-walled vessels

- Adenofibroma
  - Extremely rare and benign
  - Lobulated polypoid mass with small cystic spaces and fibrous stroma
  - Spaces lined by müllerian epithelium
- Adenosarcoma
  - Stromal cells are cytologically atypical with mitosis
  - Cells are generally packed tightly around nonmalignant glands
  - Characteristic leaflike pattern reminiscent of phyllodes tumor of breast

Pearls

- Less than 0.5% of otherwise benign polyps show focal adenocarcinoma confined to the polyp; excision of the polyp might be curative in these cases
- Polyps arise from the basalis layer of the endometrium
- Inversion of chromosome 6 has recently been identified as a nonrandom mutation in endometrial polyp

Selected References

Mittal K, Da Costa D: Endometrial hyperplasia and carcinoma in endometrial polyps: Clinicopathologic and follow-up findings. Int J Gynecol Pathol 27:45-48, 2008.

Le Donne M, Lentini M, De Meo L, et al: Uterine pathologies in patients undergoing tamoxifen therapy for breast cancer: ultrasonographic, hysteroscopic and histological findings. Eur J Gynaecol Oncol 26:623-626, 2005.

Shushan A, Revel A, Rojansky N: How often are endometrial polyps malignant? Gynecol Obstet Invest 58:212-215, 2004.

Kim KR, Peng R, Ro JY, Robboy SJ: A diagnostically useful histopathologic feature of endometrial polyp: The long axis of endometrial glands arranged parallel to surface epithelium. Am J Surg Pathol 28:1057-1062, 2004.

Deligdisch L, Kalir T, Cohen CJ, et al: Endometrial histopathology in 700 patients treated with tamoxifen for breast cancer. Gynecol Oncol 78:181-186, 2000.

Endometrial Hyperplasia

Clinical Features

- Can arise at any age, but most common in middle-aged to postmenopausal women
- Usually presents with abnormal bleeding
- Risk factors include obesity, nulliparity, increased endogenous estrogen (i.e., estrogen-producing ovarian tumors and exogenous estrogen; common denominator is continuous exposure to unopposed estrogen)
- Endometrium may be thickened on ultrasound, and uterus may be enlarged on clinical examination
- Inactivation of *PTEN* tumor suppressor gene is associated with the development of hyperplasia and related cancers

Gross Pathology

- Endometrium appears thickened and increased in volume
- May appear diffusely polypoid; more commonly, appears normal and has a soft, velvety surface

Histopathology

- Glands are increased in number and crowded with an increased amount of stroma
- Ratio of glands to stroma is elevated
- Generally the diagnosis is made in proliferative-phase endometrium, as glands normally appear crowded in secretory endometrium
- In simple hyperplasia, the glands are crowded but generally round
- In complex hyperplasia, the glands show irregular branching but no cribriforming pattern
- In both simple and complex patterns, stromal tissue is present between all glands
- Both simple and complex hyperplasia may show normal or atypical cytology
- Atypia may be focal and is characterized by cells featuring increased nuclear-to-cytoplasmic ratios, large hyperchromatic pleomorphic rounded nuclei with hyperchromasia, and prominent nucleoli
- Both architecture and cytology are taken into consideration, but normal versus atypical cytology is more clinically relevant than simple versus complex architecture
- Various types of metaplasia, particularly squamous, may be present

Special Stains and Immunohistochemistry

- Noncontributory

Other Techniques for Diagnosis

- Cytogenetics: atypical hyperplasias are more likely to be aneuploid and more commonly have mutations shared with carcinomas of the endometrium

Differential Diagnosis

- Proliferative endometrium
  - Even distribution of glands without cellular atypia
  - Glands are generally similarly oriented from the base to the surface
- Endometrial polyp
  - Focal process
  - Fibrotic stroma, numerous thick-walled vessels, and epithelial lining on three sides
- Cystic atrophy
  - Atrophic glands lined by a single layer of often flattened epithelium
  - Number of glands is generally less, and stroma is atrophic
- Chronic endometritis
  - May resemble hyperplasia; however, plasma cell infiltrate in the stroma is diagnostic

Figure 12-30. A, Simple endometrial hyperplasia without atypia. Crowded endometrial glands lacking cytologic atypia and surrounded by abundant endometrial stroma. **B, Simple endometrial hyperplasia with squamous metaplasia.** The squamous and glandular components lack cytologic atypia. **C, Complex endometrial hyperplasia without atypia.** Marked glandular crowding is present, whereas only minimal endometrial stroma is identified. **D, Complex endometrial hyperplasia with atypia.** Endometrial curettage displaying haphazardly arranged glands lined by cells with atypical nuclei surrounded by minimal stroma.

▌ Endometrial adenocarcinoma
  - Distinction may be based on architectural pattern, as the cytologic atypia may not be more pronounced than in atypical hyperplasia
  - Cribriforming and back-to-back glands without intervening stroma are features of adenocarcinoma
  - Desmoplastic stromal reaction to infiltrating glands

Pearls
  - Hyperplasia may respond to a course of progestin therapy; adenocarcinoma (grade I) rarely does
  - If hyperplasia is persistent the treatment is hysterectomy to prevent subsequent progression to adenocarcinoma
  - Endometrial adenocarcinoma has been identified in up to 25% of uteri removed for atypical hyperplasia when using the criteria described in 1982

  - The term *endometrial intraepithelial neoplasia* (EIN) is occasionally used to refer to precursor lesions of endometrial carcinoma; however, its relevance is yet to be determined

Selected References

Zaino RJ, Kauderer J, Trimble CL, et al: Reproducibility of the diagnosis of atypical endometrial hyperplasia: A Gynecologic Oncology Group study. Cancer 106:804-811, 2006.

Marchesoni D, Driul L, Fabiani G, et al: Endometrial histologic changes in post-menopausal breast cancer patients using tamoxifen. Int J Gynaecol Obstet 75:257-262, 2001.

Silverberg SG: Problems in the differential diagnosis of endometrial hyperplasia and carcinoma. Mod Pathol 13:309-327, 2000.

Mutter GL: Endometrial intraepithelial neoplasia (EIN): Will it bring order to chaos? The Endometrial Collaborative Group. Gynecol Oncol 76:287-290, 2000.

Zaino RJ, Kurman R, Herbold D, et al: The significance of squamous differentiation in endometrial carcinoma—Data from a Gynecologic Oncology Group study. Cancer 68:2293-2302, 1991.

Silverberg SG: Hyperplasia and carcinoma of the endometrium. Semin Diagn Pathol 5:135-153, 1988.

Kurman RJ, Kaminski PF, Norris HJ: The behavior of endometrial hyperplasia: A long-term study of "untreated" hyperplasia in 170 patients. Cancer 56:403-412, 1985.

Kurman RJ, Norris HJ: Evaluation of criteria for distinguishing atypical endometrial hyperplasia from well-differentiated carcinoma. Cancer 49:2457-2549, 1982.

Endometrial Adenocarcinoma

Two generally accepted types are endometrial adenocarcinoma preceded by hyperplasia (type I) and endometrial adenocarcinoma preceded by endometrial intraepithelial carcinoma (EIC) with or without atrophy (type II).

Clinical Features

- Risk factors include obesity, nulliparity, late menopause, estrogen-producing ovarian tumors (generally stomal), and exogenous estrogen (generally type I)
- Common denominator is continuous exposure to unopposed estrogen (type I)
- Commonly preceded by hyperplasia (type I)
- Usually presents with abnormal vaginal bleeding (types I and II)
- Ultrasound or computed tomography scan findings range from thickened endometrium to extensive tumor (types I and II)

Figure 12-31. A, Endometrial adenocarcinoma. An ill-defined tan to yellow mass with hemorrhage fills the entire endometrial cavity and extends to the endocervix. **B, Well-differentiated endometrial adenocarcinoma, endometrioid type (grade 1).** Back-to-back glands and no solid component. **C, Moderately differentiated endometrial adenocarcinoma, endometrioid type (grade 2),** with nuclear pleomorphism. Cribriform glands and solid foci represent 25% of the tumor volume. **D, Poorly differentiated endometrial adenocarcinoma, endometrioid type.** Minimal gland formation and marked nuclear pleomorphism are seen.

Continued

Figure 12-31, cont'd. E, Endometrioid adenocarcinoma with squamous differentiation. F, Endometrial intraepithelial carcinoma. Section of endomyometrium lined by a single layer of endometrium showing marked nuclear pleomorphism and stratification. The morphology is characteristic of serous differentiation. **G, Serous carcinoma of the endometrium.** Exophytic tan to pink tumor with focal necrosis and superficial invasion of the myometrium. **H, Serous carcinoma of the endometrium.** Papillary structures lined by pleomorphic cells and invading the surrounding desmoplastic stroma. **I, Clear cell carcinoma of the endometrium.** The tumor is composed of sheets of large cells with abundant clear cytoplasm. **J, Mucinous carcinoma of the endometrium.** Neoplastic glands with a papillary configuration. The glands are lined by uniform columnar cells with minimal stratification. Lakes of extracellular mucinous material are evident.

Gross Pathology

- Uterus may be grossly enlarged
- Tumor usually arises in the corpus
- Often single dominant mass; mostly soft, tan to white, and friable
- Endometrium may be diffusely thickened
- Cut surface through endomyometrium is compulsory to show depth of invasion

Histopathology

- Endometrioid
  - Most common type
  - Crowded, complex branching glands with cribriform architecture and back-to back glands without intervening stroma
  - Loss of polarity and cytologic atypia: large, round nuclei with prominent nucleoli, nuclear membrane condensation
  - Glands may infiltrate into the myometrium, inducing a desmoplastic response
  - Grading is based on the degree of glandular differentiation versus solid areas
    - Grade 1: less than 5% of the tumor is composed of solid areas
    - Grade 2: 5% to 50% of the tumor is composed of solid areas
    - Grade 3: greater than 50% of the tumor is composed of solid areas
  - Prominent nuclear atypia and mitotic figures increase the grade by one (i.e., grade 1 tumors with marked atypia should be classified as grade 2)
- Adenocarcinoma with squamous differentiation
  - Malignant glands with benign or malignant squamous foci (squamous differentiation)
  - Areas of squamous differentiation are not regarded as solid areas in the grading
  - Grade of the tumor is based on the morphologic features of the glandular component exclusively
  - Squamous differentiation is characterized by intercellular bridges, sharp cell borders, opaque eosinophilic cytoplasm, and squamous pearl formation or keratinization
- Villoglandular adenocarcinoma
  - Common variant of endometrioid adenocarcinoma
  - Short blunt papillae lined by cells, as described under "Adenocarcinoma (Invasive)"
  - Generally, the cytologic atypia is low grade
  - Papillary carcinoma showing high-grade cytology should be classified as serous
- Secretory adenocarcinoma
  - Commonly associated with hormonal therapy and generally low grade
  - Well-differentiated glands that resemble secretory endometrium; generally grade 1
  - Malignant clear cells with glycogen-filled cytoplasm and secretions in the glandular lumens

- Ciliated carcinoma
  - Endometrioid adenocarcinoma with ciliated cells
  - This variant is usually low grade (grade 1)
- Serous carcinoma
  - Generally presents in women in their 60s
  - Usually preceded by atrophic endometrium or EIC (type II)
  - Thick and thin papillae with marked nuclear pleomorphism
  - Cellular stratification, apoptotic bodies, and tumor necrosis
  - Psammoma bodies may be present (>30% of cases)
  - By definition, a high-grade tumor with poor prognosis (grade 2 or 3)
- Clear cell carcinoma
  - Usually preceded by atrophic endometrium (type II)
  - By definition, a high-grade tumor (grade 2 or 3)
  - Architecture may be papillary, glandular, solid, or mixed
  - Cells are those of a high-grade endometrioid adenocarcinoma but contain abundant clear cytoplasm filled with glycogen
  - Clear cells feature pleomorphic nuclei and hobnail cells (nuclei of atypical cells protrude into the glandular lumens)
- Other rare variants, including mucinous adenocarcinoma and squamous cell carcinoma
  - Mucinous adenocarcinoma is diagnosed when more than 50% of the tumor cells demonstrate mucinous differentiation
  - Squamous cell carcinoma is a rare primary tumor of the endometrium and should be diagnosed only in the absence of a cervical squamous cell carcinoma
  - Associated with ichthyosis uteri (squamous metaplasia of endometrial lining)
- Mixed carcinoma
  - Two or more of the above cell types with a minimum volume of 10% per type
- Undifferentiated carcinomas
  - Several variable phenotypes, which include small cell (neuroendocrine differentiation), giant cell, and spindle cell types

Special Stains and Immunohistochemistry

- Cytokeratin positive in all types
- Vimentin often positive; useful in distinguishing primary endometrial carcinomas from endocervical adenocarcinomas
- CEA often negative
- Mucicarmine positive in mucinous type; may be positive in endometrioid type; essentially negative in clear cell type
- PAS positive in clear cell, negative with diastase digestion

Other Techniques for Diagnosis

- Endometrial carcinomas, particularly endometrioid type, express estrogen and progesterone receptors
- Clear cell and serous carcinomas are mostly negative for estrogen and progesterone receptors, p53 positive, and often aneuploid with *c-myc* gene amplification

Differential Diagnosis

▮ Endometrial hyperplasia
- Stroma between glands, lacks cribriforming and a back-to-back glandular pattern
- Absence of complex papilloglandular areas with cellular atypia, desmoplasia

▮ Metastatic adenocarcinoma
- Usually infiltrates from the serosal surface into the myometrium
- Rarely present in the endometrium
- Clinical history important

▮ Atypical polypoid adenomyoma
- Randomly arranged glands in smooth muscle stroma without desmoplasia
- Slightly atypical cells with loss of polarity but not outright malignant pattern: lack cribriforming or back-to-back arrangement
- Squamous morulas usually present

Pearls

- Depth of myometrial invasion is an important prognostic parameter; therefore, a well-oriented section (or sections if necessary) from endometrium to serosa is imperative
- Endometrioid pattern is the most common
- Presence of squamous differentiation is not prognostically significant
- Villoglandular type is generally low grade
- Serous and clear cell carcinomas (type II) are by definition high grade (grade 2 or 3)

Selected References

Silverberg SG, Kurman RJ, Nogales F, et al: Tumors of the uterine corpus: Epithelial tumours and related lesions. In Travassoli FA, Devilee P (eds): World Health Organization Classification of Tumours: Pathology and Genetics: Tumours of the Breast and Female Genital Organs. Lyon, IARC Press, 2003, pp 221-232.

Clement PB, Young RH: Endometrioid carcinoma of the uterine corpus: A review of its pathology with emphasis on recent advances and problematic aspects. Adv Anat Pathol 9:145-184, 2002.

Sherman ME: Theories of endometrial carcinogenesis: A multidisciplinary approach. Mod Pathol 13:295-308, 2000.

Lax SF, Kurman RJ, Pizer ES, et al: A binary architectural grading system for uterine endometrial endometrioid carcinoma has superior reproducibility compared with FIGO grading and identifies subsets of advance-stage tumors with favorable and unfavorable prognosis. Am J Surg Pathol 24:1202-1208, 2000.

Sherman ME, Bur ME, Kurman RJ: P53 in endometrial cancer and its putative precursors: Evidence for diverse pathways of tumorigenesis. Hum Pathol 26:1268-1274, 1995.

Sherman ME, Bitterman P, Rosenshein NB, et al: Uterine serous carcinoma: A morphologically diverse neoplasm with unifying clinicopathologic features. Am J Surg Pathol 16:600-610, 1992.

Atypical Polypoid Adenomyoma

Clinical Features

- Most common in women in the late reproductive years
- Usually presents with abnormal bleeding
- Benign clinical course; curettage alone may be curative

Gross Pathology

- Solitary polypoid mass that often involves the lower uterine segment

Histopathology

- Random arrangement of numerous glands with irregular outlines in a smooth muscle stroma consisting of small fascicles generally without mitosis
- Epithelial cells are atypical with loss of polarity but no outright pleomorphism
- Squamous metaplasia and morulas with occasional central necrosis are common

Special Stains and Immunohistochemistry

- Noncontributory

Other Techniques for Diagnosis

- Noncontributory

Figure 12-32. Atypical polypoid adenomyoma. Low-power view demonstrates a polypoid lesion composed of a proliferation of compact irregular glands without invasion of the stroma or desmoplasia.

Differential Diagnosis

▌ Endometrial hyperplasia
- Diffuse process, not necessarily polypoid, and without smooth muscle stroma

▌ Infiltrating carcinoma
- Reactive fibrous stroma and absence of short bundles of smooth muscle stroma
- Marked architectural and cytologic atypia including cribriforming of glands

▌ Metaplastic carcinoma (carcinosarcoma)
- Epithelial component as endometrial adenocarcinoma
- Malignant spindle component of highly atypical cells with dense cellularity and cytologic pleomorphism plus a high mitotic rate with atypical forms

Pearls

- This lesion is distinguished by short smooth muscle bundles
- Location of the lesion and age of the patient are helpful for differential diagnosis

Selected References

Heatley MK: Atypical polypoid adenomyoma: A systematic review of the English literature. Histopathology 48:609-610, 2006.

Mazur MT: Atypical polypoid adenomyomas of the endometrium. Am J Surg Pathol 5:473-482, 1981.

Adenofibroma

Clinical Features

- Extremely rare and benign
- Arises in perimenopausal and postmenopausal women
- Commonly presents with abnormal vaginal bleeding

Figure 12-33. Adenofibroma. Cleftlike space lined by cuboidal cells surrounded by hypocellular collagenous stroma.

Gross Pathology

- Lobulated polyploid neoplasm of variable size confined to endometrium
- Tan-brown, focally hemorrhagic cut surface
- Commonly, cut surface shows numerous small cysts

Histopathology

- Consists of fibrous stroma without atypia and rare mitosis (<4 mitotic figures/10 hpf)
- Often contains numerous cystic spaces and papillary projections lined by unremarkable cuboidal, columnar, tubal, or other epithelial cells

Special Stains and Immunohistochemistry

- Noncontributory

Other Techniques for Diagnosis

- Noncontributory

Differential Diagnosis

▌ Adenosarcoma
- Markedly atypical stromal cells and a mitotic index of more than 5 mitotic figures/10 hpf

Pearls

- Hysterectomy is the treatment of choice to prevent recurrence and to exclude more aggressive lesions, such as adenosarcoma

Selected References

Bettaieb I, Mekni A, Bellil K, et al: Endometrial adenofibroma: a rare entity. Arch Gynecol Obstet 275:191-193, 2007.

Clement PB, Scully RE: Müllerian adenofibroma of the uterus with invasion of myometrium and pelvic veins. Int J Gynecol Pathol 9:363-371, 1990.

Vellios F, Ng AB, Reagen JW: Papillary adenofibroma of the uterus: A benign mesodermal mixed tumor of Müllerian origin. Am J Clin Pathol 60:543-551, 1973.

Adenosarcoma

Clinical Features

- May occur at any age and usually presents with abnormal bleeding
- Arises in the endometrium and rarely in the cervix

Gross Pathology

- Solitary sessile polypoid mass that often fills the entire endometrial cavity
- Cut surface is tan-gray with small cysts and focal hemorrhage and necrosis

Histopathology

- Leaflike glandular pattern featuring epithelial-lined broad papillary fronds with a cellular mesenchymal stroma cuffing cystlike spaces and clefts (reminiscent of phyllodes tumor of breast)

Figure 12-34. Adenosarcoma. Characteristic polypoid tumor with malignant stroma featuring pleomorphic spindle cells with mitotic figures and nonmalignant but atypical epithelium.

- Stroma is atypical, particularly dense in periepithelial regions, with mitosis ranging from 4 or 5 to 20 mitotic figures/10 hpf
- Epithelial lining is most often endometrioid but may also be mucinous, serous, squamous, or clear cell
- Sex cord–like elements: plump epithelioid cells with foamy cytoplasm arranged in a trabecular, insular, or tubular pattern are present in about 5% of tumors
- Mesenchymal stroma is usually homologous (e.g., fibrous sarcoma); heterologous elements include rhabdomyosarcoma more commonly than chondrosarcoma

Special Stains and Immunohistochemistry

- Cytokeratin positive in the epithelial component
- Vimentin positive in stromal component
- Desmin, MSA may be positive in heterologous rhabdomyosarcomatous component
- MIB-1 index: high proliferative index around glands and cysts

Other Techniques for Diagnosis

- Noncontributory

Differential Diagnosis

▌ Adenofibroma
- Bland fibrotic stroma with cystic spaces, glands, and papillary projections without cytologic atypia
- Fibrous stroma is cellular, but cells are not atypical
- Stromal mitotic activity is less than 4 mitotic figures/10 hpf

▌ Carcinosarcoma
- Presence of malignant epithelial and spindle cell components

▌ Homologous sarcoma
- Absence of leaflike pattern and absence of epithelial structures

Pearls

- Benign epithelial component and malignant mesenchymal component
- Periepithelial stromal cellularity is highly characteristic of adenosarcoma
- Myometrial invasion in about 20% of cases
- Sarcomatous overgrowth, deep myometrial invasion, and extrauterine involvement at time of diagnosis are associated with increased risk for recurrence and metastasis
- About 25% to 40% recur, and 5% metastasize (typically sarcomatous)

Selected References

Soslow RA, Ali A, Oliva E: Müllerian adenosarcomas: An immunophenotypic analysis of 35 cases. Am J Surg Pathol 32:1013-1021, 2008.

Lyle P, Evans R, Jarboe E, et al: Biphasic tumors of the female genital tract. Oncology 19:1178-1190, 2005.

Clement PB, Scully RE: Müllerian adenosarcoma of the uterus: A clinicopathologic analysis of 100 cases with a review of the literature. Hum Pathol 21:363-381, 1990.

Clement PB, Scully RE: Müllerian adenosarcomas of the uterus with sex cord-like elements: A clinicopathologic analysis of eight cases. Am J Clin Pathol 91:664-672, 1989.

Metaplastic Carcinoma (Carcinosarcoma, Malignant Mixed Mesodermal Tumor)

Clinical Features

- Associated with history of pelvic radiation therapy
- Usually arises in postmenopausal women
- Presents with abnormal bleeding and often abdominal or pelvic pain
- Bulky tumors that are often visible protruding through cervical os

Gross Pathology

- Large friable polypoid mass
- Often the tumor fills the entire endometrial cavity, invading deeply into the myometrium and extending out through the cervical os
- Variegated cut surface with hemorrhage and necrosis
- Hard foci may be present owing to heterologous elements such as bone or cartilage

Histopathology

- Intimate admixture of malignant glands (endometrial adenocarcinoma) and malignant spindle cells (sarcoma)
- Adenocarcinoma may be any type of endometrial adenocarcinoma

Figure 12-35. Metaplastic carcinoma. A, Large nodular exophytic tumor mass is filling the entire endometrial cavity. **B,** Biphasic morphology displaying malignant glands and markedly pleomorphic spindle cell component with mitotic figures. **C,** Heterologous metaplastic carcinoma. Numerous rhabdomyoblasts are evident. **D,** Heterologous metaplastic carcinoma. The neoplasm shows chondroid and osseous differentiation.

- Malignant spindle cell component may be
  — Homologous: often high-grade, spindled, round, or giant cells sometimes resembling fibrosarcoma, leiomyosarcoma., or stromal sarcoma
  — Heterologous: rhabdomyosarcoma (most common), chondrosarcoma, osteosarcoma, or mixture; less common are liposarcoma or neuroectodermal differentiation
- Scattered cells in each tumor display hybrid features, mixture of spindle and epithelial

Special Stains and Immunohistochemistry

- Vimentin: both epithelial and spindle cell components positive
- Cytokeratin 8/18: epithelial component diffusely positive; spindle cell components focally positive
- Myoglobin: rhabdomyomatous component positive
- S-100 protein: chondrosarcoma or liposarcoma positive
- CD 10: positive in stromal sarcoma component

Other Techniques for Diagnosis

- Electron microscopy is rarely used

Differential Diagnosis

▮ Poorly differentiated endometrial carcinoma
  - Lacks biphasic population of cells
  - Diffusely positive for cytokeratin
▮ Adenosarcoma
  - Lacks malignant epithelial component

Pearls

- Malignant epithelial and spindle cell components
- In endometrial curettage, often only the carcinomatous component is identified
- Early metastases are epithelial
- Late metastases are both epithelial and spindle cell or exclusively spindle cell (sarcomatous overgrowth)
- Lungs are a common site of metastasis
- Prognosis is poor

Selected References

Cimbaluk D, Rotmensch J, Scudiere J, et al: Uterine carcinosarcoma: Immunohistochemical studies on tissue microarrays with focus on potential therapeutic targets. Gynecol Oncol 105:138-144, 2007.

McCluggage WG: Uterine carcinosarcomas (malignant mixed müllerian tumors) are metaplastic carcinomas. Int J Gynecol Cancer 12:687-690, 2002.

Bitterman P, Chun B, Kurman RJ: The significance of epithelial differentiation in mixed mesodermal tumors of the uterus: A clinicopathologic and immunohistochemical study. Am J Surg Pathol 14:317-328, 1990.

Silverberg SG, Major FJ, Blessing JA, et al: Carcinosarcoma (malignant mixed mesodermal tumor) of the uterus. A Gynecologic Oncology Group pathologic study of 203 cases. Int J Gynecol Pathol 9:1-19, 1990.

Stromal Nodule

Clinical Features

- Rare, benign tumor
- Occurs at any age, but generally in older, postmenopausal women
- Usually presents with abnormal bleeding
- Uterus may be palpably enlarged

Gross Pathology

- Well-circumscribed, solid, soft, tan-gray mass
- Unencapsulated with pushing margins

Histopathology

- Small uniform oval to spindled cells resembling endometrial stromal cells
- Minimal cytologic atypia and generally less than 10 mitotic figures/10 hpf
- Numerous thin-walled vessels evenly spaced among stromal cells and resembling spiral arterioles
- Rare small foci of necrosis, cystic degeneration, foam cells, calcification, decidualization, and sex cord–like structures

Special Stains and Immunohistochemistry

- CD10 positive
- Vimentin positive
- Reticulin positive surrounding individual cells
- Cytokeratin negative, except in sex cord elements
- SMA, desmin mostly negative except for stromal myoma
- Epithelial membrane antigen (EMA) negative

Other Techniques for Diagnosis

- Noncontributory

Differential Diagnosis

▌ Leiomyoma
- Unevenly spaced, thick-walled vessels
- Spindled cells and interlacing fascicles
- Positive for SMA, desmin, smooth muscle myosin (SMMS), heavy chains

Figure 12-36. A, Endometrial stromal nodule. The neoplastic cells are uniform in size and shape, and they have minimal cytologic atypia and no mitotic figures. **B, Low-grade endometrial stromal sarcoma.** Round to spindled cells with bland nuclei, no mitotic figures, and small plexiform blood vessels. **C, High-grade endometrial stromal sarcoma.** High mitotic activity and nuclear pleomorphism are evident.

▌ Low-grade stromal sarcoma
- More infiltrative margins
- Prominent lymphovascular invasion

▌ Hemangiopericytoma
- Extremely rare in the uterus
- Large branching staghorn vessels

- Definitively diagnosed by immunohistochemistry demonstrating neoplastic cells with pericytic differentiation

Pearls

- Benign without recurrence even if excised without hysterectomy
- Usually expresses estrogen and progesterone receptors

Selected References

Baker P, Oliva E: Endometrial stromal tumours of the uterus: A practical approach using conventional morphology and ancillary techniques. J Clin Pathol 60:235-243, 2007.

Kempson RL, Hendrickson MR: Pure mesenchymal neoplasms of the uterine corpus: Selected problems. Semin Diagn Pathol 5:172-198, 1988.

Chang KL, Crabtree GS, Lim-Tan SK, et al: Primary uterine endometrial stromal neoplasms: A clinicopathologic study of 117 cases. Am J Surg Pathol 14:415-438, 1990.

Low-Grade Endometrial Stromal Sarcoma

Clinical Features

- Rare tumor that usually presents with abnormal vaginal bleeding
- Occurs at any age, but most common in older premenopausal or postmenopausal women
- Uterus is often palpably enlarged

Gross Pathology

- Well-circumscribed mass, diffusely infiltrative mass, or multiple confluent masses
- Wormlike masses within myometrium (gross manifestation of lymphovascular invasion)
- Foci of hemorrhage, necrosis, or cystic degeneration
- Gross extrauterine extension in about 30% of cases at time of diagnosis

Histopathology

- Extensively infiltrative margins
- Plugs of tumor within lymphovascular spaces and myometrium (hence older term *endolymphatic stromal myosis*)
- Variable numbers of mitotic figures, generally 10 to 20 mitotic figures/10 hpf
- Cells with minimal atypia resembling endometrial stromal cells
- Foci of epithelioid differentiation appearing as glandular or sex cord–like elements
- Foci of hemorrhage and necrosis are occasionally present
- Calcification, decidualization, cystic degeneration, and foam cells may be identified

Special Stains and Immunohistochemistry

- CD10, vimentin positive
- Cytokeratin occasionally focally positive
- EMA negative
- SMA, desmin: mostly negative (useful in distinguishing from smooth muscle tumors)

Other Techniques for Diagnosis

- Noncontributory

Differential Diagnosis

- Stromal nodule
  - Lack of lymphovascular invasion
  - Noninfiltrating (pushing) margins
- High-grade stromal sarcoma
  - Marked cytologic atypia
  - Atypical mitotic figures and necrosis
- Hemangiopericytoma
  - Rare in uterus
  - Large, branching staghorn vessels
- Intravenous leiomyomatosis
  - Purely smooth muscle with irregularly spaced thick-walled vessels
  - Uncommon admixture of stromal cells or, rarely, epithelial components
  - More abundant cytoplasm
  - Intracytoplasmic myofibrils demonstrated by trichrome or electron microscopy
  - Positive for SMA, MSA, desmin
- Metaplastic carcinoma versus low-grade endometrial stromal sarcoma with prominent epithelioid elements
  - Metaplastic carcinoma has glands that are outright malignant
  - Generally does not show plugging of lymphovascular spaces
- Adenosarcoma
  - Papillary folds with slitlike or dilated glands composed of cells with nuclei that are epithelial, not stromal
  - Generally demarcated from surrounding stroma

Pearls

- Mitotic activity is not predictive of aggressive behavior
- Distinction from high-grade stromal sarcoma is based on absence of marked cytologic atypia, only minimal necrosis, and atypical mitotic figures
- Treatment is usually total abdominal hysterectomy with bilateral salpingo-oophorectomy with debulking of extrauterine tumor
- Recurrence is common even after several years

Selected References

Czernobilsky B: Uterine tumors resembling ovarian sex cord tumors: An update. Int J Gynecol Pathol 27:229-235, 2008.

McCluggage WG, Sumathi VP, Maxwell P: CD10 is a sensitive and diagnostically useful immunohistochemical marker of normal endometrial stroma and of endometrial stromal neoplasms. Histopathology 39:273-278, 2001.

Chang KL, Crabtree GS, Lim-Tan SK, et al: Primary uterine endometrial stromal neoplasms: A clinicopathologic study of 117 cases. Am J Surg Pathol 14:415-438, 1990.

Fekete PS, Vellios F: The clinical and histologic spectrum of endometrial stromal neoplasms: A report of 41 cases. Int J Gynecol Pathol 3:198-212, 1984.

High-Grade Endometrial Stromal Sarcoma

Clinical Features

- Rare tumor that generally occurs in postmenopausal women
- Usually presents with abnormal bleeding or pelvic pain
- Aggressive tumor, with less than 50% 5-year survival rate

Gross Pathology

- Grossly infiltrative masses, confluent mass, or diffuse infiltration of myometrium
- Endometrial involvement, hemorrhage, and necrosis are common
- Wormlike infiltration of myometrium is usually absent

Histopathology

- Pronounced cytologic atypia; however, cells may still resemble endometrial stromal cells
- Mitotic activity is generally more than 10 mitotic figures/10 hpf with atypical forms
- Uneven distribution of thin-walled vascular spaces
- There may be areas composed of undifferentiated bizarre or giant sarcoma cells
- Heterologous elements, including rhabdomyosarcoma or chondrosarcoma
- Epithelioid foci and wormlike plugs are generally absent
- Frequent lymphovascular invasion
- May be morphologically indistinguishable from other uterine sarcomas (leiomyosarcoma)

Special Stains and Immunohistochemistry

- Vimentin positive
- Cytokeratin focally positive
- EMA negative
- SMA generally negative (useful in distinguishing from leiomyosarcoma)
- S-100 protein positive if chondrosarcomatous component present

Other Techniques for Diagnosis

- Noncontributory

Differential Diagnosis

- Low-grade stromal sarcoma
  - Minimal cytologic atypia
  - Evenly spaced vessels
  - Wormlike projections of tumor
  - May have epithelioid elements
- Undifferentiated endometrial sarcoma
  - Lacks endometrial stromal differentiation
- Metaplastic carcinoma
  - Malignant epithelial component is present
- Leiomyosarcoma
  - Evidence of smooth muscle differentiation by H&E or immunohistochemistry
  - Whorling pattern of plump, atypical spindle cells as opposed to more random streaming distribution of cells in stromal sarcoma
- Adenosarcoma
  - Benign glandular epithelium
- Other sarcomas (e.g., malignant fibrous histiocytoma, rhabdomyosarcoma, osteosarcoma)
  - All of these are rare as primary tumors in the uterine corpus
  - These lack cell populations that resemble endometrial stromal cells
- Poorly differentiated endometrial carcinoma
  - Positive for cytokeratin

Pearls

- Cytologic atypia has proved more accurate than mitotic count in distinguishing low-grade from high-grade stromal sarcomas as well as in predicting behavior
- Necrosis is generally present, and epithelioid elements and wormlike endolymphatic stromal projections are generally absent
- Treatment is total abdominal hysterectomy with bilateral salpingo-oophorectomy and tumor debulking
- Distinction from leiomyosarcoma has no clinical significance

Selected References

Nucci MR, O'Connell JT, Huettner PC, et al: H-caldesmon expression effectively distinguishes endometrial stromal tumors from uterine smooth muscle tumors. Am J Surg Pathol 24:455-463, 2001.

Oliva E, Clement PB, Young RH: Endometrial stromal tumors: An update on a group of tumors with a protean phenotype. Adv Anat Pathol 7:257-281, 2000.

Oliva E, Clement PB, Young RH, Scully RE: Mixed endometrial stromal and smooth muscle tumors of the uterus: A clinicopathologic study of 15 cases. Am J Surg Pathol 22:997-1005, 1998.

Farhood AI, Abrams J: Immunohistochemistry of endometrial stromal sarcoma. Hum Pathol 22:224-230, 1991.

Chang KL, Crabtree GS, Lim-Tan SK, et al: Primary uterine endometrial stromal neoplasms: A clinicopathologic study of 117 cases. Am J Surg Pathol 14:415-438, 1990.

Myometrium

Adenomyosis

Clinical Features

- Non-neoplastic and most common in adult women
- Presents with a palpably enlarged uterus and abnormal bleeding or dysmenorrhea; often associated with leiomyomas
- Commonly an incidental finding in hysterectomy specimen

Gross Pathology

- Thickened myometrium with focal soft, discolored areas or small cysts

Histopathology

- Islands of endometrial glands surrounded by endometrial stroma within the myometrium, or endometrial stroma exclusively
- Often the glands appear inactive, and hemosiderin is generally absent
- Endometrial glands in the myometrium are more than 2 to 2.5 mm away from the basalis in a properly oriented section

Special Stains and Immunohistochemistry

- CD10 positive, confirming endometrial stroma rather than smooth muscle

Other Techniques for Diagnosis

- Noncontributory

Differential Diagnosis

- Normal endometrium that is cut tangentially
  - Deeper levels may demonstrate that the glands in question are actually continuous with the endometrium

Figure 12-37. Adenomyosis. Endometrial glands in the myometrial smooth muscle surrounded by endometrial stroma and adjacent blood vessels.

- Endometrial carcinoma involving adenomyosis
  - Malignant glands, perhaps with cribriforming surrounded by endometrial stroma
- Invasive adenocarcinoma
  - Malignant glands and desmoplastic or inflammatory stromal response
- Stromal tumor
  - Tumor mass composed of stromal cells with or without lymphatic or vascular space invasion and no glands
- Adenomatoid tumor
  - Flat cuboidal epithelial lining glandular spaces as opposed to endometrial glands
  - Mesothelial origin
  - No endometrial stroma
  - Uncommon

Pearls

- It is important to have a properly oriented histologic section because tangential sections may mimic adenomyosis

Selected Reference

Parrott E, Butterworth M, Green A, et al: Adenomyosis: A result of disordered stromal differentiation. Am J Pathol 159:623-630, 2001.

Leiomyoma

Clinical Features

- Benign neoplasm, more commonly referred to as *fibroid*
- Most common tumor in women as well as in the uterus
- Rare in women before 20 years of age and increasingly common in women older than 30 years
- Small tumors may be asymptomatic
- Larger tumors may cause pain, dysmenorrhea, urinary difficulties, changes in bowel habits, and, in extreme cases, infertility; often diagnosed on pelvic examination
- Tumors may be more specifically localized by ultrasound

Gross Pathology

- Often multiple
- Discrete, well-circumscribed masses with firm, whorled, tan-white cut surfaces
- Cystic degeneration is often present in larger tumors
- Hyalinization and calcification may be extensive
- Hemorrhage and necrosis are not prominent findings
- Three types
  - Subserosal: located immediately beneath the serosa; may be pedunculated
  - Intramural: within myometrium
  - Submucosal: located immediately beneath the endometrium

Figure 12-38. A, Pedunculated leiomyoma. Solid tan mass protruding into the cervical canal. **B, Cellular leiomyoma.** The tumor is composed of densely cellular fascicles of smooth muscle cells with minimal intervening collagen. **C, Epithelioid leiomyoma.** The tumor is composed of round to polygonal cells. Focally the tumor cells show clear cytoplasm. **D, Bizarre (symplastic) leiomyoma.** Large atypical cells show hyperchromatic nuclei with chromatin smudging. **E, Leiomyosarcoma.** Uterine cavity displaying a soft, ill-defined tan mass with necrosis and hemorrhage filling the endometrial cavity and infiltrating the myometrium. **F, Leiomyosarcoma.** Interlacing bundles of pleomorphic spindle cells with large nuclei, prominent nucleoli, and mitotic figures.

Histopathology

- Interlacing fascicles of bland monomorphic spindle (smooth muscle) cells
- Well-circumscribed borders with mitotic activity of less than 5 mitotic figures/10 hpf

- Pseudocapsuled; hyalinized areas and calcifications may be present
- Occasionally, the entire leiomyoma may be hyalinized, suggesting an infarcted neoplasm

- Endometritis may be present in the overlying endometrium if compressed by leiomyoma
- Variants
  — Cellular leiomyoma
    - Densely cellular
    - Mitotic activity is less than 5 mitotic figures/10 hpf
    - No coagulative necrosis or cellular pleomorphism
  — Epithelioid leiomyoma
    - Round polygonal (epithelioid) cells
    - Leiomyoblastoma: cells with eccentric nuclei and granular eosinophilic cytoplasm, hyalinization
    - Clear cell: round polygonal cells with abundant clear cytoplasm
    - Plexiform: rows and columns of round polygonal cells separated by fibrous stroma
    - Mitotic activity of less than 5 mitotic figures/10 hpf in all variants
  — Bizarre leiomyoma (also referred to as *symplastic, pleomorphic,* or *atypical*)
    - Bizarre giant cells grouped focally or scattered in an otherwise typical leiomyoma
    - Mitotic activity of less than 5 mitotic figures/10 hpf and no coagulative necrosis
  — Lipoleiomyoma
    - Mostly composed of benign adipocytes with occasional smooth muscle cells
  — Mitotically active leiomyoma
    - Occurs in women younger than 35 years
    - Cytologic atypia and necrosis are absent
    - Mitotic activity more than 5 mitotic figures/10 hpf, perhaps up to 20 mitotic figures/10 hpf
  — Intravenous leiomyomatosis (IVL)
    - Rare condition characterized by leiomyomas that extend into myometrial veins and continue beyond uterus
    - Intravenous leiomyomatosis shows no tendency to metastasize
  — Benign metastasizing leiomyoma
    - Rare condition characterized by leiomyoma in distant sites such as lungs
    - Metastasis may occur years after the diagnosis of typical uterine leiomyoma

Special Stains and Immunohistochemistry

- Vimentin positive
- Desmin, caldesmin, SMA positive
- Cytokeratin negative (rare positive cells)
- Estrogen and progesterone receptors often positive

Other Techniques for Diagnosis

- Electron microscopy demonstrates actin filaments with associated dense bodies as well as incomplete basal lamina (features characteristic of smooth muscle cells)

Differential Diagnosis

- Leiomyosarcoma
  - Cellular neoplasm with moderate to severe cytologic pleomorphism
  - Hemorrhage and coagulative necrosis
  - Mitotic activity generally greater than 5 to 10 mitotic figures/hpf
  - Infiltrating borders, and perhaps metastatic at time of presentation
- Stromal nodule
  - Smaller bland spindled cells resembling endometrial stroma
  - Positive for CD10 with occasional cells positive for SMA
- Low-grade stromal sarcoma
  - Wormlike masses representing lymphatic invasion may be seen grossly within the myometrium
  - Smaller, bland spindled cells with minimal cytoplasm resembling endometrial stroma
  - May find admixture of stromal and epithelioid glandular or sex cord–like components
  - CD10 is positive

Pearls

- Leiomyomas are hormonally responsive; that is, most shrink after menopause
- The following variants are regarded as atypical or of uncertain malignant potential
  — Epithelioid, bizarre, and intravenous leiomyomatosis
  — Tumors in women older than 35 years that show mild cytologic atypia and more than 5 mitotic figures/10 hpf

Selected References

Lee HJ, Choi J, Kim KR: Pulmonary benign metastasizing leiomyoma associated with intravenous leiomyomatosis of the uterus: Clinical behavior and genomic changes supporting a transportation theory. Int J Gynecol Pathol 27:340-345, 2008.

Toledo G, Oliva E: Smooth muscle tumors of the uterus: a practical approach. Arch Pathol Lab Med 132:595-605, 2008.

Leitao MM, Soslow RA, Nonaka D, et al: Tissue microarray immunohistochemical expression of estrogen, progesterone, and androgen receptors in uterine leiomyomata and leiomyosarcoma. Cancer 101:1455-1462, 2004.

Giuntoli RL 2nd, Metzinger DS, DiMarco CS, et al: Retrospective review of 208 patients with leiomyosarcoma of the uterus: Prognostic indicators, surgical management, and adjuvant therapy. Gynecol Oncol 89:460-469, 2003.

O'Connor DM, Norris HJ: Mitotically active leiomyomas of the uterus. Hum Pathol 21:223-227, 1990.

Clement PB, Young RH, Scully RE: Intravenous leiomyomatosis of the uterus: A clinicopathological analysis of 16 cases with unusual histologic features. Am J Surg Pathol 12:932-934, 1988.

Leiomyosarcoma

Clinical Features

- Rapidly growing tumor that usually arises in postmenopausal women
- Large tumor that may cause pain, dysmenorrhea, urinary difficulties, changes in bowel habits, and, in extreme cases, infertility
- Often diagnosed on pelvic examination and specifically localized by ultrasound
- Commonly has spread into the pelvic cavity by the time of presentation
- Often detected as an incidental finding in hysterectomy specimens
- Distant metastases may occur months or years later, often in the lungs
- Treatment is total abdominal hysterectomy with salpingo-oophorectomy and tumor debulking, and radiation; chemotherapeutic agents have not proved effective
- Prognosis is variable depending on stage and grade

Gross Pathology

- Usually solitary
- Large, poorly circumscribed mass, often extending beyond the uterine serosa
- Soft, fleshy, variegated cut surface showing hemorrhage and necrosis

Histopathology

- Densely cellular tumor composed of interlacing fascicles of pleomorphic spindled cells
- Coagulative necrosis is often present
- Mitoses are generally greater than 10 to 20 mitotic figures/hpf in areas with highest mitotic activity (viewed with a 40× objective)
- Infiltrative margins with occasional vascular invasion
- Variants
  - Epithelioid
    - Rounded, highly atypical polygonal cells with necrosis and increased mitosis
  - Myxoid
    - Myxoid matrix that makes tumor appear less cellular and mitotically active
    - Infiltrates myometrium and vessels

Special Stains and Immunohistochemistry

- Vimentin positive
- SMA, desmin, and other muscle markers positive
- Estrogen and progesterone receptors positive in better differentiated areas
- Cytokeratin negative

Other Techniques for Diagnosis

- Noncontributory

Differential Diagnosis

- Mitotically active leiomyoma
  - Women younger than 35 years
  - Smaller and well circumscribed
  - Absence of necrosis, cytologic atypia, and vascular invasion
- High-grade stromal sarcoma
  - Numerous evenly distributed small blood vessels
  - Absence of interlacing fascicular pattern
  - Originates in endometrium and extends down into myometrium
  - Negative or only focally positive for SMA and other muscle markers
- Metaplastic carcinoma (carcinosarcoma)
  - Malignant glands admixed with malignant spindle cell component

Pearls

- Much less common than leiomyomas
- Characterized by hypercellularity, cytologic atypia, and mitotic activity generally greater than 10 mitotic figures/10 hpf
- Coagulative necrosis, hypercellularity with atypia, nuclear pleomorphism, and increased mitosis (>10 to 20 mitotic figures/10 hpf) are diagnostic of leiomyosarcoma
- Tumors with high mitotic activity (>5 to 10 mitotic figures/hpf) but lacking significant cytologic atypia and necrosis should be classified as smooth muscle tumors of uncertain malignant potential (STUMP), or atypical leiomyomas
- Myxoid leiomyosarcoma: mitotic count should be performed in more cellular areas

Selected References

Toledo G, Oliva E: Smooth muscle tumors of the uterus: A practical approach. Arch Pathol Lab Med 132:595-605, 2008.

Prayson RA, Goldblum JR, Hart WR: Epithelioid smooth-muscle tumors of the uterus: A clinicopathologic study of 18 patients. Am J Surg Pathol 21:383-391, 1997.

Berchuck A, Rubin SC, Hoskins WJ, et al: Treatment of uterine leiomyosarcoma. Obstet Gynecol 71:845-850, 1988.

King ME, Dickersin GR, Scully RE: Myxoid leiomyosarcoma of the uterus: A report of six cases. Am J Surg Pathol 6:589-598, 1982.

Adenomatoid Tumor

Clinical Features

- Uncommon tumor that generally affects adult women
- Often asymptomatic, with benign behavior

Gross Pathology

- Poorly circumscribed soft mass within myometrium near the serosal surface
- May involve the endometrium when large

Figure 12-39. Adenomatoid tumor. Spaces lined by cuboidal cells surrounded by a stroma rich in collagen and smooth muscle.

Histopathology

- Adenomatoid or glandular pattern is the most common
- Solid and cystic patterns are less common
- Cell lining composed of single layer of flattened cuboidal cells
- Luminal spaces may contain acid mucin

Special Stains and Immunohistochemistry

- Cytokeratin, vimentin, EMA positive
- CEA negative

Other Techniques for Diagnosis

- Electron microscopy: features of mesothelial cells, including long and slender microvilli, intracellular lumens, and intracytoplasmic filaments in bundles

Differential Diagnosis

- Lymphangioma
  - Negative for cytokeratin
- Invasive primary uterine adenocarcinoma
  - Originates in endometrium and extends downward into myometrium
  - Cytologic atypia, desmoplasia, or inflammatory response to invasive tumor
- Metastatic adenocarcinoma
  - Prominent cytologic atypia with desmoplastic or inflammatory response to tumor
  - Brisk mitotic rate; may be positive for mucicarmine or CEA

Pearls

- This tumor arises from the serosal mesothelium and is essentially a benign mesothelioma

Selected Reference

Nogales FF, Isaac MA, Hardisson D, et al: Adenomatoid tumors of the uterus: An analysis of 60 cases. Int J Gynecol Pathol 21:34-40, 2002.

Ovary

Inflammatory conditions of the ovary are uncommon and generally associated with PID or systemic infections such as tuberculosis. Immune oophoritis is a rare condition, and most commonly a diagnosis of exclusion. Neoplasms of the ovary represent most of the pathology.

Miscellaneous Conditions

Follicular Cyst and Corpus Luteum Cyst

Clinical Features

- Follicular cysts
  - Common; they occur at any age, but often in the reproductive years
  - Occasionally associated with McCune-Albright syndrome
    — Polyostotic fibrous dysplasia, irregular patches of pigmented skin, and endocrine dysfunction, especially precocious puberty in girls
- Corpus luteum cysts
  - Occur frequently during the reproductive years
  - Usually an incidental finding
  - May present as a palpable mass with endocrine manifestations like increased estrogen production and menstrual irregularities
  - Rupture and bleeding into the peritoneum is relatively common

Gross Pathology

- Follicular cysts are typically unilocular with a thin wall and smooth inner surface, usually smaller than 10 cm in diameter, and filled with serous fluid
- Corpus luteum cysts are larger than 2 cm, have a smooth yellow lining, and have bloody fluid

Histopathology

- Follicular cyst
  - Inner layer of granulosa cells separated by the basement membrane from outer layer of theca interna cells; both are often luteinized
  - Granulosa cells
    — Small and round with scanty cytoplasm
    — Hyperchromatic nuclei with occasional grooves
  - Theca interna cells
    — Larger with abundant cytoplasm and mixed with vessels
- Corpus luteum cyst
  - Thin inner layer of connective tissue
  - Outer layer of luteinized, large vacuolated granulosa cells and smaller theca interna cells

Special Stains and Immunohistochemistry

- Reticulin stain: highlights reticular network around theca interna cell layer in a follicular cyst

Figure 12-40. A, Follicular cyst. Cross section shows a thin-walled unilocular cyst. **B, Follicular cyst.** The cyst wall is lined by an inner layer of granulosa cells and an outer layer of theca interna cells. **C, Endometrioma.** Cystic ovary filled with blood and with a glistening external surface. **D, Corpus luteum cyst.** Low-power view shows a classic convoluted cyst wall.

Other Techniques for Diagnosis

- Noncontributory

Differential Diagnosis

- Serous cystadenoma versus follicular cyst
  — Presence of a theca interna layer points toward follicular cyst
  — May be diagnosed as a simple cyst if unclear
- Corpus luteum versus corpus luteum cyst
  — Corpus luteum contains a cavity that is usually filled with blood, versus corpus luteum cyst
  — Cyst is greater than 2 cm in diameter and has a smooth rather than a folded contour
- Endometriosis versus hemorrhagic corpus luteum cyst
  — Peripheral theca interna cells are present, and organized blood clot is more typical of cysts
  — Endometriosis must show endometrial glands, stroma, or hemosiderin pigment; two of the three is diagnostic

Pearls

- Most regress spontaneously within 2 months
- The large, solitary, luteinized follicular cyst of pregnancy and puerperium is usually an incidental finding during cesarean section or physical examination, with a median diameter of 25 cm; it consists of a lining of luteinized cells with hyperchromatic, pleomorphic nuclei

Selected References

Kurman R (ed): Blaustein's Pathology of the Female Genital Tract, 5th ed. New York, Springer, 2002, pp 686-710.

Adashi EY, Hennebold JD, Higgins RV, et al: Comparison of fine-needle aspiration cytologic findings of ovarian cysts with ovarian histologic findings. Am J Obstet Gynecol 180:550-553, 1999.

Scully RE, Young RH, Clement PB: Atlas of Tumor Pathology: Tumors of the Ovary, Maldeveloped Gonads, Fallopian Tube, and Broad Ligament, 3rd Series, Fascicle 23. Washington, DC, Armed Forces Institute of Pathology, 1998, pp 409-410.

Hyperreactio Luteinalis

Clinical Features

- Associated with conditions in which high levels of human chorionic gonadotropin (HCG) are secreted, such as pregnancy and gestational trophoblastic disease (GTD)
- Usually asymptomatic, but may present as a palpable mass or abdominal pain related to hemorrhage, torsion, or rupture

Gross Pathology

- Large ovary with multiple bilateral, thin-walled cysts filled with serous or bloody fluid resulting in massive ovarian enlargement

Histopathology

- Large cysts lined by enlarged, luteinized theca interna cells, and sometimes luteinized granulosa and stromal cells
- Ovarian stroma and the theca interna layer may be noticeably edematous

Special Stains and Immunohistochemistry

- Noncontributory

Other Techniques for Diagnosis

- Noncontributory

Differential Diagnosis

❚ Large, solitary luteinized follicle cyst of pregnancy and puerperium
  - Ovaries in hyperreactio luteinalis contain multiple cysts

Pearls

- Present in about 10% to 45% of women with GTD; the cysts regress after removal of the trophoblastic elements
- Rarely coexists with a pregnancy luteoma

Selected References

Schenker JG: Clinical aspects of ovarian hyperstimulation syndrome. Eur J Obstet Gynecol Reprod Biol 85:13-20, 1999.

Jacobs HS, Agrawal R: Complications of ovarian stimulation. Baillieres Clin Obstet Gynaecol 12:565-579, 1998.

Scully RE, Young RH, Clement PB: Atlas of Tumor Pathology: Tumors of the Ovary, Maldeveloped Gonads, Fallopian Tube, and Broad Ligament, 3rd Series, Fascicle 23. Washington, DC, Armed Forces Institute of Pathology, 1998, pp 424-426.

Polycystic Ovarian Syndrome

Clinical Features

- Characterized by numerous follicular cysts in both ovaries, anovulation, infertility, hirsutism, oligo-menorrhea, and obesity

Figure 12-41. Polycystic ovary. A, Cross sections of both ovaries show cortical fibrosis and multiple cystic follicles. **B,** Expanded ovarian cortex exhibits focal nodular luteinization.

- Also known as Stein-Leventhal syndrome; affects 3.5% to 7.0% of females, usually in the third decade
- Most cases show increased luteinizing hormone (LH): follicle-stimulating hormone (FSH) ratio, whereas occasional cases show hyperprolactinemia

Gross Pathology

- Both ovaries are round and usually 2 to 5 times the normal size
- Many small, superficial cysts visible under a smooth, thick, gray-white outer cortex
- Central homogeneous stroma lacking corpora lutea or albicantia

Histopathology

- Superficial cortex is thickened, hypocellular, and collagenous, frequently with thick-walled blood vessels
- Multiple follicular cysts lined by an inner nonluteinized granulosa and an outer hyperplastic luteinized theca interna (follicular hyperthecosis)
- Corpora lutea are usually absent

Special Stains and Immunohistochemistry

- Noncontributory

Other Techniques for Diagnosis

- Noncontributory

Differential Diagnosis

▌ Pregnancy
- Luteinization of both granulosa and theca interna
▌ Stromal hyperthecosis
- Polycystic ovaries show stromal hyperthecosis, but stromal hyperthecosis, as an entity, is idiopathic

Pearls

- Pelvic ultrasound may help in diagnosis
- Hyperandrogenemia, with increased conversion of androstenedione to estrone
- Endometrium may show hyperplasia or adenocarcinoma in some cases
- Virilism is rarely present
- HAIR-AN syndrome may be associated and includes insulin resistance, acanthosis nigricans, and hyperandrogenism

Selected References

Gordon CM: Menstrual disorders in adolescents: Excess androgens and the polycystic ovary syndrome. Pediatr Clin N Am 46:519-543, 1999.

Guzick D: Polycystic ovary syndrome: Symptomatology, pathophysiology, and epidemiology. Am J Obstet Gynecol 179:S89-S93, 1998.

Scully RE, Young RH, Clement PB: Atlas of Tumor Pathology: Tumors of the Ovary, Maldeveloped Gonads, Fallopian Tube, and Broad Ligament, 3rd Series, Fascicle 23. Washington, DC, Armed Forces Institute of Pathology 1998, pp 410-413.

Taylor AE: Understanding the underlying metabolic abnormalities of polycystic ovary syndrome and their implications. Am J Obstet Gynecol 179:S94-S100, 1998.

Stromal Hyperplasia and Hyperthecosis

Clinical Features

- Patients with stromal hyperthecosis are usually in their sixth to ninth decades; occasional familial cases
- Stromal hyperthecosis in the premenopausal patient may present as virilization, obesity, hypertension, and glucose intolerance. Less often, it may resemble polycystic ovarian syndrome; some cases show endometrial hyperplasia or adenocarcinoma
- Stromal hyperplasia typically presents in the sixth or seventh decade and may be associated with androgen hypersecretion, endometrial adenocarcinoma, obesity, hypertension, and decreased glucose tolerance

Gross Pathology

- Bilateral involvement with or without ovarian enlargement

Figure 12-42. Stromal hyperthecosis. Foci of luteinized stromal cells are present within the ovarian stroma.

- White or yellow tissue occupies a variable percentage of each ovary
- Nodular hyperthecosis may appear as multiple yellow nodules

Histopathology

- Stromal hyperthecosis exhibits luteinization of stromal cells not attached to the follicles, arranged singly and in clusters. Rarely as nodules, with a typical background of stromal hyperplasia
  — Luteinized stromal cells are oval or round with eosinophilic or vacuolated cytoplasm and round, plump nuclei
- Stromal hyperplasia displays minimal collagen production, a diffuse or vaguely nodular proliferation of small stromal cells; the nodules commonly coalesce

Special Stains and Immunohistochemistry

- Oil red O stain: may highlight lipid in vacuolated luteinized cells in stromal hyperthecosis

Other Techniques for Diagnosis

- Noncontributory

Differential Diagnosis

▌ Luteinized thecoma versus stromal hyperthecosis
- Most thecomas are unilateral and form a distinct nodule or tumor
- The pockets or collections of lutein cells in stromal hyperthecosis are surrounded by small hyperplastic stromal cells with minimal collagen production
▌ Fibroma versus stromal hyperplasia
- Fibroma is composed of cells with larger nuclei and characteristic production of large amounts of collagen; typically measures greater than 3 cm in diameter

- Low-grade endometrial stromal sarcoma versus stromal hyperplasia
  - Endometrial stromal sarcoma, which is rare, shows significant ovarian enlargement, marked cellularity, mitotic activity, and regularly distributed arterioles

Pearls

- Stromal hyperthecosis, with additional edema and fibrosis, may accompany the HAIR-AN syndrome, which is characterized by hyperandrogenism, insulin resistance, and acanthosis nigricans

Selected References

Scully RE, Young RH, Clement PB: Atlas of Tumor Pathology: Tumors of the Ovary, Maldeveloped Gonads, Fallopian Tube, and Broad Ligament, 3rd Series, Fascicle 23. Washington, DC, Armed Forces Institute of Pathology, 1998, pp 413-416.

Sluijmer AV, Heineman MJ, Koudstaal J, et al: Relationship between ovarian production of estrone, estradiol, testosterone, and androstenedione and the ovarian degree of stromal hyperplasia in postmenopausal women. Menopause 5:207-210, 1998.

Schwartz ID, Mou SM, Zwick DL, Gilbert-Barness E: Pathological case of the month: Ovarian stromal hyperthecosis. Am J Dis Child 147:591-592, 1993.

Massive Edema and Fibromatosis

Clinical Features

- Enlargement of one or both ovaries with peak incidence in the second decade
- Presents with abdominal pain
- Abnormal menstruation and androgenic manifestations may be present

Gross Pathology

- Usually unilateral, sometimes with torsion of the ovarian pedicle
- Massive edema
  - Pearly-white ovarian surface with seeping fluid
  - Cut section reveals watery or gelatinous tissue with numerous cystic follicles under the capsule
  - Averages 12 cm in diameter, often with hemorrhage
- Fibromatosis
  - Smooth or lobulated ovarian surface, sometimes with cysts; averages about 11 cm in diameter

Histopathology

- Massive edema
  - Pale, edematous, hypocellular stroma; spared outer cortex
  - Follicles widely separated with venous congestion and lymphatic dilation
  - Clusters of lutein cells and foci of fibromatosis may be present

- Fibromatosis
  - Proliferating spindle cells and collagen production enveloping occasional follicles
  - Clusters of lutein cells and foci of edema may be present

Special Stains and Immunohistochemistry

- Noncontributory

Other Techniques for Diagnosis

- Noncontributory

Differential Diagnosis

- Edematous fibroma versus massive edema
  - Follicles and their derivatives are present in massive edema
- Fibroma versus fibromatosis
  - Follicles and their derivatives are present in fibromatosis

Pearls

- Cortical stromal hyperplasia and hyperthecosis are often associated

Selected References

Scully RE, Young RH, Clement PB: Atlas of Tumor Pathology: Tumors of the Ovary, Maldeveloped Gonads, Fallopian Tube, and Broad Ligament, 3rd Series, Fascicle 23. Washington, DC, Armed Forces Institute of Pathology, 1998, pp 416-420.

Nielsen GP, Young RH: Fibromatosis of soft tissue type involving the female genital tract: A report of two cases. Int J Gynecol Pathol 16:383-386, 1997.

Lee AR, Kim KH, Lee BH, Chin SY: Massive edema of the ovary: Imaging findings. AJR Am J Roentgenol 161:343-344, 1993.

Pregnancy Luteoma

Clinical Features

- Ovarian enlargement during pregnancy related to HCG stimulation
- Most patients are black and multiparous; peak incidence in third and fourth decades
- May present with hirsutism or virilization; infants born to such mothers frequently show virilism

Gross Pathology

- Multiple in one half of cases, and bilateral in one third
- Small to large nodules ranging from a few millimeters to 20 cm in diameter
- Soft, well-circumscribed, yellow-brown, or gray on cut surface with areas of hemorrhage

Histopathology

- Well-circumscribed nodules composed of solid proliferations of uniform polygonal cells with abundant eosinophilic, granular cytoplasm

Figure 12-43. Pregnancy luteoma. Solid proliferation of polygonal luteinized cells with abundant eosinophilic granular cytoplasm.

- Nuclei are round and relatively large; may be hyperchromatic with moderate mitotic activity, in a sparse intercellular stroma divided by reticulin fibers into clusters

Special Stains and Immunohistochemistry
- Noncontributory

Other Techniques for Diagnosis
- Noncontributory

Differential Diagnosis
▮ Luteinized thecoma
  - Unilateral and unrelated to pregnancy in most cases
  - Contains moderate to large amounts of lipid, as opposed to little or no lipid in pregnancy luteoma
  - Background of fibroma or typical thecoma with thin reticulin-positive fibers surrounding individual cells rather than clusters

▮ Lipid-poor steroid cell tumor
  - Both may be virilizing
  - Rarely bilateral; if mitotic activity is brisk, more likely to show nuclear atypia

Pearls
- Usually an incidental finding
- After delivery, the ovaries regress and return to normal size within a few weeks

Selected References
Cronje HS, Niemand I, Bam RH, Woodruff JD: Review of the granulosa-theca cell tumors from the Emil Novak ovarian tumor registry. Am J Obstet Gynecol 180:323-327, 1999.

Rodriguez M, Harrison TA, Nowacki MR, Saltzman AK: Luteoma of pregnancy presenting with massive ascites and markedly elevated CA 125. Obstet Gynecol 94:854, 1999.

Scully RE, Young RH, Clement PB: Atlas of Tumor Pathology: Tumors of the Ovary, Maldeveloped Gonads, Fallopian Tube, and Broad Ligament, 3rd Series, Fascicle 23. Washington, DC, Armed Forces Institute of Pathology, 1998, pp 422-424.

Endometriosis

Clinical Features
- Common in women of childbearing age
- Defined as the presence of endometrial tissue outside the uterine corpus
- Complications include rupture or hemorrhage
- May occur in any organ system and mimic a neoplasm

Gross Pathology
- Red, blue, or dark-brown nodules or cysts with a raised or puckered appearance, often with fibrous adhesions on involved serosal surfaces
- "Powder burns" refer to ecchymotic or brown areas

Figure 12-44. Corpus luteum cyst. A, Multiple well-demarcated cysts displaying a yellow rim and intraluminal blood. **B,** Cyst lined by cuboidal epithelium associated with endometrial stroma and hemosiderin-laden macrophages. Adjacent ovarian stroma can be seen.

- Endometriotic cysts frequently involve the ovaries, are often bilateral, and are usually less than 10 cm in diameter
- Cyst lining is ragged and dark-brown to yellow and contains thick chocolate-colored material (chocolate cyst)

Histopathology

- Characterized by epithelium and stroma reminiscent endometrium
- Hemosiderin-laden macrophages are also usually present
- Appearance varies with hormonal fluctuations of the menstrual cycle
- Menstruation may cause hemorrhage into the glands and stroma with a consequent inflammatory reaction consisting predominantly of histiocytes
- Pseudoxanthoma cells are histiocytes that have transformed the red blood cells into glycolipid, hemofuscin, and hemosiderin pigment
- Postmenopausal women show atrophic glands similar to the endometrium
- Extensive fibrosis may be present

Special Stains and Immunohistochemistry

- CD10 highlights the endometrial stroma

Other Techniques for Diagnosis

- Noncontributory

Differential Diagnosis

▌ Endometrioid cystadenoma
- Extremely rare and lined by stratified endometrial type epithelium
- Does not contain endometrial-like stroma or pseudoxanthoma cells

▌ Hemorrhagic corpus luteum cyst versus endometriosis
- Presence of peripheral theca interna cells and organized blood clot are more typical of a corpus luteum cyst
- Endometriosis requires the presence of endometrial glands, stroma, or hemosiderin pigment

Pearls

- Hyperplastic and atypically proliferating changes similar to those seen in the endometrium may be present (i.e., hyperplasia, metaplasia)
- About 0.5% of cases have a malignant neoplasm arising from the endometriotic lesion; associated with a hyperestrogenic state
- Endometrioid and clear cell adenocarcinoma are most frequent associations

Selected References

Miyakoshi K, Tanaka M, Gabionza D, et al: Decidualized ovarian endometriosis mimicking malignancy. AJR Am J Roentgenol 171:1625-1626, 1998.

Scully RE, Young RH, Clement PB: Atlas of Tumor Pathology: Tumors of the Ovary, Maldeveloped Gonads, Fallopian Tube, and Broad Ligament, 3rd Series, Fascicle 23. Washington, DC, Armed Forces Institute of Pathology, 1998, pp 430-434.

Brinton LA, Gridley G, Person I, et al: Cancer risk after a hospital discharge diagnosis of endometriosis. Am J Obstet Gynecol 176:572-579, 1997.

Brosens IA: Endometriosis: A disease because it is characterized by bleeding. Am J Obstet Gynecol 176:263-267, 1997.

Surface Epithelial-Stromal Tumors

These are the most common tumors of the ovary. Table 12-1 shows the pathogenesis of ovarian cancer.

Benign Serous Tumor

Clinical Features

- Common ovarian neoplasm with a peak incidence in the fifth decade
- Makes up about 70% of all serous tumors
- One of the two most common ovarian neoplasms seen in pregnancy

Gross Pathology

- Bilateral in about 10% of cases
- Cystadenomas: usually one (sometimes more) smooth, glistening, thin-walled cyst(s) filled with clear, watery, serous (occasionally mucinous or hemorrhagic) fluid
- Papillary cystadenomas: inner lining with small polypoid excrescences and an underlying cystic component

Table 12-1. Pathogenesis of Ovarian Cancer

Type I

- Low grade with a precursor lesion in a stepwise fashion
  —Represented by cystadenomas and borderline tumors
  —Most often presents at stage I; slow growing, indolent
  —Generally remains low grade but can progress to high grade
  —*K-ras/BRAF* mutations in 65%, and *TP53* mutation in 8%
- Includes
  —Serous carcinoma (grade 1)
  —Mucinous, endometrioid, and clear cell carcinomas and transitional cell carcinoma (Brenner and non-Brenner)

Type II

- High grade, arises de novo, and most often presents at high stage
- Rapidly growing, aggressive
- About 70% have *p53* mutation, whereas *K-ras/BRAF* mutation is rare (1%)
- Includes
  —Serous carcinoma (grade 2 or 3)
  —Malignant mixed müllerian tumor (carcinosarcoma)

Figure 12-45. A, Benign serous tumor. The external surface of the cyst is smooth and glistening with a marked vascular pattern. **B, Benign serous tumor.** Papillary lesion lined by a single layer of cuboidal epithelium. **C, Borderline serous tumor.** Cystic ovary showing tan to yellow papillary excrescences. **D, Invasive implant of serous borderline tumor.** Papillary tumor clusters with bland cytologic features in cleftlike spaces.

- Surface papillomas: coarse papillary projections on the outer surface of the ovary without a cystic cavity
- Adenofibromas and cystadenofibromas are predominantly solid fibrous tumors with a variable number of fluid-filled glands or cysts and firm papillary excrescences

Histopathology

- In general, serous neoplasms mimic the epithelium of the fallopian tube
- Cysts, papillae, and glands are lined mainly by a single layer of cuboidal to low-columnar ciliated cells without significant nuclear atypia; they may also be lined by nonciliated cuboidal to columnar secretory cells
- Epithelium may be flattened by accumulated serous fluid
- Stroma varies from dense and fibrous to distinctly edematous

- Rarely, psammoma bodies may be present
- Variants include cystadenoma and papillary cystadenoma, surface papilloma, and adenofibroma and cystadenofibroma

Special Stains and Immunohistochemistry

- Noncontributory

Other Techniques for Diagnosis

- Noncontributory

Differential Diagnosis

▮ Epithelial inclusion cyst versus small serous cystadenoma
- Epithelial inclusion cyst is less than 1 cm in diameter
▮ Follicle cyst versus serous cystadenoma
- Both may have an atrophic lining, but the presence of a theca interna layer points toward follicle cyst

Figure 12-45, cont'd. E, Papillary serous carcinoma. Cut surface shows a solid tumor with focal cystic changes. **F, Papillary serous carcinoma.** Moderately differentiated tumor composed of crowded papillae lined by pleomorphic cells. **G, Papillary serous carcinoma.** Poorly differentiated tumor invading into the surrounding stroma. Several psammoma bodies are evident. **H, Serous carcinoma of the ovary.** WT-1 stain is strongly positive, confirming the serous differentiation. Coexpression of *p53* is also characteristic of ovarian serous carcinoma.

- May be diagnosed as simple cyst if the morphology of the lining is unclear
▌ Struma ovarii versus serous cystadenoma
- Struma ovarii always contains small colloid-filled cysts
- Histologically identical to thyroid tissue
- Positive for thyroglobulin immunohistochemical stain
▌ Rete cystadenoma versus serous cystadenoma
- Rete cystadenomas are very rare tumors arising in the rete ovarii (ovarian hilus)
- Lined by nonciliated epithelium, showing crevices along their inner surfaces
- Smooth muscle and hilus cells commonly present in their walls

Pearls

- Cystectomy, or oophorectomy is curative

Selected Reference

Scully RE, Young RH, Clement PB: Atlas of Tumor Pathology: Tumors of the Ovary, Maldeveloped Gonads, Fallopian Tube, and Broad Ligament, 3rd Series, Fascicle 23. Washington, DC, Armed Forces Institute of Pathology, 1998, pp 51-79.

Borderline Serous Tumor

Clinical Features

- Peak incidence between 30 and 60 years of age
- Makes up 5% to 10% of all serous tumors

Gross Pathology

- Bilateral in 25% to 30% of cases
- Gross is similar to that of benign tumors or with excrescences on the surface

- Cysts lined by abundant, fine, somewhat firm papillary projections

Histopathology

- Complex, branching papillae with small papillary projections on the surface lined by epithelium showing cellular buds and nuclear stratification
- No destructive stromal invasion
- Cells generally have scant cytoplasm and bland nuclei but may have moderate to abundant eosinophilic cytoplasm with round hyperchromatic nuclei and obvious nucleoli
- Psammoma bodies may be seen
- Variants are similar to those listed in benign serous tumors

Special Stains and Immunohistochemistry

- Weak or negative *p53* essentially excludes high-grade serous carcinoma
- WT-1 positive

Other Techniques for Diagnosis

- Noncontributory

Differential Diagnosis

- ▌ Endocervical-like borderline mucinous tumor versus mucin-secreting borderline serous tumor
  - Borderline mucinous tumor cells are mucin filled, whereas serous tumors contain merely apical mucin
- ▌ Retiform Sertoli-Leydig cell tumor (SLCT)
  - Peak incidence in first decade, sometimes presenting with androgenic manifestations
  - Tubular and cystic structures lined by one or more layers of cells with round, regular nuclei and scanty cytoplasm

Pearls

- Surgical excision of tumors confined to the ovaries results in survival without recurrence in the majority (>95%) of patients
- Postoperative recurrences can occur many years later

Selected References

Yemelyanova A, Mao TL, Nakayama N, et al: Low-grade serous carcinoma of the ovary displaying a macropapillary pattern of invasion. Am J Surg Pathol 32:1800-1806, 2008.

Kurman RJ, Shih IM: Pathogenesis of ovarian cancer: Lessons from morphology and molecular biology and their clinical implications. Int J Gynecol Pathol 27:151-160, 2008.

Hart WR: Borderline epithelial tumors of the ovary. Mod Pathol 18(Suppl 2):S33-S50, 2005.

Burks RT, Kurman RJ, Seidman JD, Shih IM: Serous borderline tumours of the ovary. Histopathology 47:310-315, 2005.

Gershenson DM, Silva EG, Tortolero-Luna G, et al: Serous borderline tumors of the ovary with noninvasive peritoneal implants. Cancer 83:2157-2163, 1998.

Czernobilsky B: What's new in ovarian serous borderline tumors. Pathol Res Pract 193:735-739, 1997.

Seidman JD, Kurman RJ: Subclassification of serous borderline tumors of the ovary into benign and malignant types: A clinicopathologic study of 65 advanced stage cases. Am J Surg Pathol 20:1331-1345, 1996.

Malignant Serous Tumor

Clinical Features

- Most common malignant ovarian neoplasm, with a peak incidence between 40 and 70 years of age and constituting about 20% to 25% of all serous tumors
- Serum shows elevated level of CA-125 (not specific for serous tumors or malignancy)

Gross Pathology

- Bilateral in about 65% of cases
- Well-differentiated forms are partly solid, but mostly cystic, papillary tumors
- Surface serous carcinomas include large hemorrhagic papillary excrescences on the surface of the ovary
- Poorly differentiated tumors show solid areas of friable, necrotic, and hemorrhagic tissue with few recognizable papillae
- Tumor adhesion to adjacent structures is common

Histopathology

- Cellular tumor with obvious invasion of the connective tissue stroma (desmoplasia)
- High-grade tumors (grade 2 or 3) may contain few papillae, which are generally thick, but the tumors are mostly composed of solid sheets of cells with pleomorphic nuclei
- Hyperchromatic nuclei and atypical mitoses are characteristic of high-grade tumors along with cellular budding and stratification
- Well-differentiated low-grade tumor (micropapillary is the most common pattern)
  — Grade 1 tumor featuring large, edematous bulbous papillae from which emanate smaller papillae with nonhierarchical branching of fine lacelike pattern with low-grade nuclei
  — Psammoma bodies are present in most well-differentiated papillary tumors, and if very prominent, the tumor may be designated a psammocarcinoma (grade 1)
- Variants include cystadenocarcinoma, surface carcinoma, and carcinoma arising in adenofibroma

Special Stains and Immunohistochemistry

- Vimentin positive
- CA-125 positive
- More than 60% of high-grade tumors and less than 10% of low-grade tumors positive for p53
- WT-1 positive

Other Techniques for Diagnosis

- Noncontributory

Differential Diagnosis

▪ Papillary clear cell carcinoma versus papillary serous carcinoma
  • Clear cell carcinoma displays plump hobnail cells with large nuclei, cells with clear cytoplasm, or oxyphilic cells
  • Papillae are more regular and may have hyalinized cores
▪ Endometrioid carcinoma versus poorly differentiated serous carcinoma
  • Papillae and glands in endometrioid carcinoma are larger and more regular (villoglandular), without cellular budding
  • Squamous differentiation is commonly associated with endometrioid carcinoma and rarely with serous carcinoma
  • Psammoma bodies are rare in endometrioid carcinomas
▪ Adult granulosa cell tumor (AGCT) versus solid serous carcinoma
  • Cell necrosis in serous carcinoma may be confused for Call-Exner bodies
  • Serous carcinomas are positive for EMA and diffusely positive for keratin 8/18, whereas EMA is negative in AGCT, and keratin 8/18 shows focal positivity only
  • Inhibin is positive in AGCT and generally negative in serous carcinoma; likewise with calretinin
▪ Retiform SLCT
  • Rare tumor with a peak incidence in first decade, sometimes presenting with androgenic manifestations
  • Tubular and cystic structures; tubules lined by one or more layers of cells with round, regular nuclei and scanty cytoplasm; most retiform tumors are seen with other SLCT subtypes

Pearls

  • Most high-grade tumors show extensive intraperitoneal dissemination at diagnosis

Selected References

Kurman RJ, Shih IM: Pathogenesis of ovarian cancer: Lessons from morphology and molecular biology and their clinical implications. Int J Gynecol Pathol 27:151-160, 2008.

Dehari R, Kurman RJ, Logani S, Shih IM: The development of high-grade serous carcinoma from atypical proliferative (borderline) serous tumors and low-grade micropapillary serous carcinoma: A morphologic and molecular genetic analysis. Am J Surg Pathol 31:1007-1012, 2007.

Mutter G, Nogales F, Kurman R, et al: Endometrial cancer. In Tavassoli FA, Stratton MR (eds): World Health Organization Classification of Tumours: Pathology and Genetics: Tumours of the Breast and Female Genital Organs. Lyon, IARC Press, 2003.

Brandenberger AW, Tee MK, Jaffe RB: Estrogen receptor alpha (ER-alpha) and beta (ER-beta) mRNAs in normal ovary, ovarian serous cystadenocarcinoma and ovarian cancer cell lines: Down-regulation of ER-beta in neoplastic tissues. J Clin Endocrinol Metab 83:1025-1028, 1998.

Scully RE, Young RH, Clement PB: Atlas of Tumor Pathology: Tumors of the Ovary, Maldeveloped Gonads, Fallopian Tube, and Broad Ligament, 3rd Series, Fascicle 23. Washington, DC, Armed Forces Institute of Pathology, 1998, pp 51-79.

Burks RT, Sherman ME, Kurman RJ: Micropapillary serous carcinoma of the ovary: A distinctive low-grade carcinoma of the ovary. A distinctive low-grade carcinoma related to serous borderline tumors. Am J Surg Pathol 20:319-330, 1996.

Benign Mucinous Tumor

Clinical Features

  • Makes up about 75% to 85% of all mucinous tumors
  • Peak incidence in fourth and fifth decades
  • Most common epithelial tumor in pregnancy
  • Signs and symptoms may be related to acute torsion

Gross Pathology

  • Bilateral in 2% to 4% of cases
  • Large, mucin-filled, multiloculated tumor with a smooth inner lining
  • Stromal component of adenofibroma is firm and fibrous

Histopathology

  • In general, mucinous tumors mimic endocervical and intestinal epithelium
  • Cysts, papillary structures, and cryptlike structures are lined by a single layer of columnar cells with clear, apical mucin and small basally located nuclei (picket-fence–like) or intestinal-type epithelium with goblet cells
  • Fibrocollagenous walls and stroma
  • Mucinous tumors may have argyrophil and Paneth cells
  • Variants include cystadenoma and adenofibroma or cystadenofibroma

Special Stains and Immunohistochemistry

  • PAS highlights mucinous material
  • Cytokeratin 7 is generally positive

Other Techniques for Diagnosis

  • Noncontributory

Differential Diagnosis

▪ Serous cystadenoma
  • Mucinous cystadenomas may have a cuboidal epithelium similar to serous cystadenoma, but with intracytoplasmic mucin and without ciliated cells
▪ Heterologous SLCT
  • Contains glands and cysts lined by mucinous epithelium that may be similar to the lining in benign mucinous tumors

Figure 12-46. A, Mucinous cystadenoma. Cut surface shows a multiloculated cystic tumor. **B, Mucinous cystadenoma.** The cyst wall is lined by a single layer of tall columnar cells with basally arranged nuclei, reminiscent of cervical glandular epithelium. **C, Borderline mucinous tumor.** Cut surface shows a multiloculated tumor with focal solid areas. **D, Borderline mucinous tumor.** The neoplasm shows stratified mucinous epithelium, nuclear enlargement, and hyperchromasia. **E, Malignant mucinous tumor.** Cut surface shows a cystic tumor with a large solid component.

- Foci of SLCT of intermediate differentiation are characterized by cords of darkly staining Sertoli cells separated by a stroma containing Leydig cells with abundant eosinophilic cytoplasm
- Areas of immature skeletal muscle, cartilage, or both may be seen

▌ Mucinous carcinoid tumor versus mucinous tumor
- Mucinous carcinoid tumors are mostly solid and only rarely predominantly cystic on gross examination
- Argyrophil and argentaffin cells may be present in mucinous carcinoid tumors but are less abundant

Figure 12-46. cont'd. F, Malignant mucinous tumor. High-power view shows glandlike structures lined by stratified tall, columnar, mucin-producing cells. Stromal invasion is evident. **G, Metastatic mucinous adenocarcinoma.** Atypical glands with nuclear pleomorphism and associated mucin infiltrate the omentum. An ovarian primary is unlikely.

Pearls

- Mucinous tumors are associated with dermoid cysts in 3% to 5% of cases, along with appendiceal mucoceles and pseudomyxoma peritonei
- Mucinous cystadenomas are associated with benign transitional cell tumors (Brenner)
- Pseudomyxoma peritonei: condition featuring extensive mucinous ascites, cystic epithelial implants on the peritoneal surfaces, and adhesions most commonly in association with an appendiceal lesion (e.g., mucocele) or, less likely, mucinous ovarian tumor
- Treatment consists of surgical excision of the tumor
- Important to thoroughly sample tumor to exclude areas of borderline or malignant tumor

Selected References

Yemelyanova AV, Vang R, Judson K, et al: Distinction of primary and metastatic mucinous tumors involving the ovary: Analysis of size and laterality data by primary site with reevaluation of an algorithm for tumor classification. Am J Surg Pathol 32:128-138, 2008.

Hristov AC, Young RH, Vang R, et al: Ovarian metastases of appendiceal tumors with goblet cell carcinoidlike and signet ring cell patterns: A report of 30 cases. Am J Surg Pathol 31:1502-1511, 2007.

Hart WR: Mucinous tumors of the ovary: A review. Int J Gynecol Pathol 24:4-25, 2005.

Scully RE, Young RH, Clement PB: Atlas of Tumor Pathology: Tumors of the Ovary, Maldeveloped Gonads, Fallopian Tube, and Broad Ligament, 3rd Series, Fascicle 23. Washington, DC, Armed Forces Institute of Pathology, 1998, pp 81-105.

Raab SS, Robinson RA, Jensen CS, et al: Mucinous tumors of the ovary: Interobserver diagnostic variability and utility of sectioning protocols. Arch Pathol Lab Med 121:1192-1198, 1997.

Shiohara S, Shiozawa T, Shimizu M, et al: Histochemical analysis of estrogen and progesterone receptors and gastric-type mucin in mucinous ovarian tumors with reference to their pathogenesis. Cancer 80:908-916, 1997.

Borderline Mucinous Tumor

Clinical Features

- Makes up about 10% to 15% of all mucinous tumors
- Peak incidence in third to fifth decades with intestinal-type tumors, presenting slightly later than endocervical-like tumors
- Tumors consisting of mostly intestinal-type cells are more common
- Occasional cases show elevation in serum inhibin

Gross Pathology

- Bilateral in about 7% of intestinal-type tumors and 40% of endocervical-like tumors; both types are the largest ovarian epithelial tumors
- Averages 15 to 20 cm in diameter
- Similar to benign mucinous tumor in gross appearance, but the cyst lining shows bulging masses and papillary projections more often
- Intestinal-type tumors are usually larger and more loculated

Histopathology

- Increased crowding of cysts, glands, and papillae, with areas of glandular budding, nuclear atypia, and stratification, but lacking destructive stromal invasion
- Tumor cells are usually mucin filled and have irregular nuclei, large nucleoli, and increased mitotic activity
- Most show mixed mucinous differentiation (endocervical and intestinal)
- Tumors made up of predominantly endocervical-like cells are less common and are often associated with infiltration by acute inflammatory cells

- Foreign-body giant cells may be seen in association with mucin from ruptured cysts
- Variants include mucinous adenofibroma

Special Stains and Immunohistochemistry

- Noncontributory

Other Techniques for Diagnosis

- Noncontributory

Differential Diagnosis

▪ Heterologous SLCT
- Contains glands and cysts lined by areas of mucinous epithelium, which may be similar to a borderline mucinous tumor
- Foci of SLCT of intermediate differentiation also seen, with cords of darkly staining Sertoli cells separated by a stroma containing Leydig cells with abundant eosinophilic cytoplasm
- Areas of immature skeletal muscle, cartilage, or both may be seen

Pearls

- Intestinal-type tumors may be associated with pseudomyxoma peritonei but are less likely to have associated endometriosis than endocervical-like tumors
- Surgical excision of tumors confined to the ovaries may occasionally be associated with recurrence, spread, and rarely death
- Important to thoroughly sample tumor to exclude areas of invasive malignant tumor

Selected References

Szych C, Staebler A, Connolly DC, et al: Molecular genetic evidence supporting the clonality and appendiceal origin of pseudomyxoma peritonei in women. Am J Pathol 154:1849-1855, 1999.

Ronnett BM, Shmookler BM, Sugarbaker PH, Kurman RJ: Pseudomyxoma peritonei: New concepts in diagnosis, origin, nomenclature, and relationship to mucinous borderline (low malignant potential) tumors of the ovary. Anat Pathol 2:197-226, 1997.

Ronnett BM, Kurman RJ, Zahn CM, et al: Pseudomyxoma peritonei in women: A clinicopathologic study of 30 cases with emphasis on site of origin, prognosis and relationship to ovarian mucinous tumors of low malignant potential. Hum Pathol 56:509-524, 1995.

Seidman JD, Elsayed AM, Sobin LH, Tavassoli FA: Association of mucinous tumors of the ovary and appendix: A clinicopathologic study of 25 cases. Am J Surg Pathol 17:22-34, 1993.

Malignant Mucinous Tumor

Clinical Features

- Makes up about 10% of all mucinous tumors
- Peak incidence in fourth to seventh decades
- Some patients show elevated levels of CEA, CA-19-9, inhibin, and CA-125

Gross Pathology

- Bilateral in 15% to 20% of cases
- Cystic spaces with papillae mixed with solid masses; sometimes the tumor is completely solid
- Hemorrhage and necrosis have been reported

Histopathology

- Cellular tumor containing crowded glands, cysts, papillae, or solid sheets of stratified mucinous cells, with stromal invasion by single or small groups of cells or glands, displaying a desmoplastic stromal response
- Cells with hyperchromatic nuclei, atypical mitoses with eosinophilic cytoplasm, and abundant mucin, sometimes with signet ring forms
- Large pools of extracellular mucin with associated histiocytes and less often a foreign-body giant cell reaction
- Variants include mucinous carcinoma arising in mucinous adenofibroma

Special Stains and Immunohistochemistry

- Vimentin negative
- Cytokeratin 7 and 20 positive
- CEA: positive cytoplasmic staining

Other Techniques for Diagnosis

- Noncontributory

Differential Diagnosis

▪ Serous and endometrioid adenocarcinomas
- May contain abundant luminal mucin but minimal intracytoplasmic mucin
- WT-1 positive in serous, negative in endometrioid
- CEA positive in mucinous, negative in serous and endometrioid

▪ Heterologous SLCT
- Contains glands and cysts lined by areas of mucinous epithelium, which may be similar to a malignant mucinous tumor
- Foci of SLCT of intermediate differentiation showing cords of darkly staining Sertoli cells separated by stroma containing Leydig cells with abundant eosinophilic cytoplasm
- Areas of immature skeletal muscle, cartilage, or both may be seen

▪ Krukenberg tumor
- Metastatic mucin-secreting adenocarcinoma with signet ring cells originating from an extragenital source
- Breast and gastrointestinal tract are the most common primary sites
- Contains goblet cells in the stroma and is usually bilateral

Pearls

- Treatment consists of surgery, sometimes with chemotherapy depending on the stage and grade of the tumor
- About 40% 5-year survival rate, with recurrences often occurring in the lungs

Selected References

Seidman JD, Kurman RJ, Ronnett BM: Primary and metastatic mucinous adenocarcinomas in the ovaries: Incidence in routine practice with a new approach to improve intraoperative diagnosis. Am J Surg Pathol 27:985-993, 2003.

Scully RE, Young RH, Clement PB: Atlas of Tumor Pathology: Tumors of the Ovary, Maldeveloped Gonads, Fallopian Tube, and Broad Ligament, 3rd Series, Fascicle 23. Washington, DC, Armed Forces Institute of Pathology, 1998, pp 81-105.

Raab SS, Robinson RA, Jensen CS, et al: Mucinous tumors of the ovary: Interobserver diagnostic variability and utility of sectioning protocols. Arch Pathol Lab Med 121:1192-1198, 1997.

Shiohara S, Shiozawa T, Shimizu M, et al: Histochemical analysis of estrogen and progesterone receptors and gastric-type mucin in mucinous ovarian tumors with reference to their pathogenesis. Cancer 80:908-916, 1997.

Endometrioid Tumors

Clinical Features

- Most are malignant; benign and borderline variants rare
- Peak incidence in fifth decade; women with endometrioid carcinoma and endometriosis in the same ovary are 5 to 10 years younger on average
- May be associated with ovarian or pelvic endometriosis and endometrial carcinoma; serum CA-125 is elevated in most cases

Figure 12-47. Endometrioid carcinoma of ovary. Endometrial-like glands and areas of squamous differentiation.

Gross Pathology

- Most tumors are unilateral; about 30% of malignant tumors are bilateral
- Similar in gross appearance to previously mentioned tumors but may contain obvious foci of endometriosis
- Carcinomas measure up to 20 cm in diameter, are predominantly solid, but may contain papillae; some contain cysts filled with bloody or mucinous fluid

Histopathology

- In general, endometrioid tumors mimic the epithelium of the endometrium, containing cells with basophilic cytoplasm, elongated nuclei, and obvious nucleoli
- Benign (rare)
  — Usually have an adenofibromatous pattern with mature glands in a fibrous stroma
- Borderline (no stromal invasion)
  — Usually have an adenofibromatous pattern with fibrous stroma and squamous morulas
- Carcinoma
  — Characterized by stromal invasion, which includes cribriforming
  — Often displays squamous differentiation
  — Graded as other epithelial tumors

Special Stains and Immunohistochemistry

- Vimentin positive in malignant tumors

Other Techniques for Diagnosis

- Noncontributory

Differential Diagnosis

▌ Poorly differentiated serous carcinoma versus endometrioid carcinoma
- Serous carcinoma contains irregular, slitlike glands, with smaller, more complex papillae, cellular budding, and frequent psammoma bodies
- Squamous differentiation points toward endometrioid carcinoma

▌ Mucinous carcinoma versus endometrioid carcinoma
- Mucinous carcinoma contains abundant luminal mucin and goblet cells with mucin-rich cytoplasm
- Vimentin negative and CEA positive

▌ SLCT versus endometrioid carcinoma
- SLCT has well-differentiated epithelium that is more abundant, has smaller tubules, and has only small amounts of intraluminal mucin
- SLCT does not contain an adenofibromatous component or squamous differentiation

▌ Malignant mixed müllerian tumor (carcinosarcoma) versus endometrioid adenocarcinoma
- Endometrioid adenocarcinoma may contain prominent foci of spindled epithelial cells, but they are less atypical than both the epithelial and mesenchymal components of a malignant mixed mesodermal tumor

Pearls

- Borderline tumors typically have a relatively benign course
- Endometrioid carcinomas are associated with the same risk factors as endometrial carcinomas
- Endometrioid and clear cell carcinomas are the most common tumors arising adjacent to or within endometriosis

Selected References

Garg PP, Kerlikowske K, Subak L, Grady D: Hormone replacement therapy and the risk of epithelial ovarian carcinoma: a meta-analysis. Obstet Gynecol 92:472-479, 1998.

Scully RE, Young RH, Clement PB: Atlas of Tumor Pathology: Tumors of the Ovary, Maldeveloped Gonads, Fallopian Tube, and Broad Ligament, 3rd Series, Fascicle 23. Washington, DC, Armed Forces Institute of Pathology, 1998, pp 107-128.

Duska LR, Chang YC, Flynn CE, et al: Epithelial ovarian carcinoma in the reproductive age group. Cancer 85:2623-2629, 1995.

Heaps JM, Nieberg RK, Berek JS: Malignant neoplasms arising in endometriosis. Obstet Gynecol 75:1023-1028, 1990.

Malignant Mixed Müllerian Tumor (Carcinosarcoma)

Clinical Features

- Classified in the endometrioid category
- Rare tumor occurring in postmenopausal women; peak incidence in sixth decade
- Poor prognosis

Gross Pathology

- Typically large, averaging 15 to 20 cm in diameter
- Most are unilateral
- Solid, or partly cystic, with areas of necrosis and hemorrhage

Figure 12-48. Malignant mixed mesodermal tumor (carcinosarcoma). Malignant epithelial and mesenchymal components are evident.

- Yellow to brown cut surface
- Bone or cartilage may be palpated on occasion

Histopathology

- Epithelial-stromal variant of endometrioid tumor containing malignant epithelial elements (carcinoma) and mesenchymal elements (sarcoma)
- Epithelial elements
  - These include serous or endometrioid carcinoma
  - Squamous cell, clear cell, or mucinous differentiation may be seen
  - Bizarre cells with hyperchromatic nuclei and cells with intracytoplasmic hyaline bodies may be present
- Mesenchymal elements are homologous (native to the female genital tract), such as stromal sarcoma, fibrosarcoma, or leiomyosarcoma; or heterologous (foreign tissue), including chondrosarcoma (most common), rhabdomyosarcoma, or osteosarcoma

Special Stains and Immunohistochemistry

- Reticulin stain highlights areas of undifferentiated carcinoma
- Cytokeratin and EMA highlight areas of undifferentiated carcinoma
- Vimentin highlights areas of sarcoma, although carcinoma may be focally positive

Other Techniques for Diagnosis

- Noncontributory

Differential Diagnosis

▌ Immature teratoma
  - Occurs in younger women, peak incidence in first and second decades; rare in women older than 50 years of age
  - Contains elements of all three germ cell layers, particularly neuroectodermal tissue
  - Lacks a malignant component of müllerian type
  - Cartilage has an embryonic or fetal appearance, rather than that of chondrosarcoma

▌ SLCT
  - May contain islands of cartilage or rhabdomyoblasts but also shows characteristic Leydig cells, sex cord formations, tubules, or endodermal tissues
  - May lead to virilization
  - Inhibin positive; rarely EMA positive

▌ Adenosarcoma
  - Rare tumor showing nonmalignant endometrioid epithelium, sometimes with pseudostratification, and a malignant hypercellular stroma with nuclear atypia
  - Peak incidence in fifth decade

Pearls

- Spreads beyond the ovary in more than half of cases at surgery

- Epithelial or sarcomatous components metastasize early to the omentum, pelvic organs, and liver; poor prognosis with rapid progression

Selected References

Wang P, Lee R, Lin G, et al: Malignant mixed mesodermal tumors of the ovary: Preoperative diagnosis. Gynecol Obstet Invest 47:69-72, 1999.

Kounelis S, Jones MW, Papadaki H, et al: Carcinosarcomas (malignant mixed müllerian tumors) of the female genital tract: Comparative molecular analysis of epithelial and mesenchymal components. Hum Pathol 29:82-87, 1998.

Scully RE, Young RH, Clement PB: Atlas of Tumor Pathology: Tumors of the Ovary, Maldeveloped Gonads, Fallopian Tube, and Broad Ligament, 3rd Series, Fascicle 23. Washington, DC, Armed Forces Institute of Pathology, 1998, pp 128-131.

Abeln EC, Smit VT, Wessels JW, et al: Molecular genetic evidence for the conversion hypothesis of the origin of malignant mixed müllerian tumours. J Pathol 183:424-431, 1997.

Clear Cell Tumors

Clinical Features

- Most are malignant, with rare benign and borderline variants
- Malignant tumors often occur in nulliparous women; peak incidence in fifth decade
- Commonly associated with endometriosis

Gross Pathology

- Most tumors are cystic with solid areas, but some are predominantly solid; often bilateral
- Focal hemorrhage and necrosis may be present
- Clear cell carcinomas average 15 cm in diameter, often have surface adhesions; typically consist of thick-walled unilocular, sometimes multilocular, cysts with white or yellow-tan solid papillary or nodular protrusions into the lumen

Figure 12-49. Clear cell carcinoma. Low-power view demonstrates a papillary pattern with hobnail-shaped and pleomorphic clear cells.

Histopathology

❚ Benign
- Usually have an adenofibromatous pattern with mature glands in a fibrous stroma

❚ Borderline
- Usually an adenofibromatous pattern with atypical glands in a fibrous stroma

❚ Carcinoma
- May show papillary, tubulocystic, solid, or mixed patterns with stromal invasion
- Polyhedral, glycogen-rich clear cells containing round or angular atypical nuclei with frequent abnormal mitoses
- Cells line papillae (which usually have hyalinized cores), tubules, and cysts or may be arranged in nests
- Nucleoli are generally not present, and hyaline globules are common
- Hobnail cells have plump hyperchromatic nuclei and line papillae, tubules, and cysts
- Less often cells are cuboidal, flat, oxyphilic, or mucin-containing signet ring cells

Special Stains and Immunohistochemistry

- PAS highlights abundant glycogen in clear cells
- Mucin negative
- α-Fetoprotein (AFP) rarely stains positive
- Cytokeratin positive

Other Techniques for Diagnosis

- Noncontributory

Differential Diagnosis

❚ Dysgerminoma
- Peak incidence in second and third decades
- Dysgerminoma cell is large and round with smooth edges; it contains a central nucleus with one or more prominent nucleoli
- Dysgerminoma has thin fibrous bands within an almost pure lymphocytic infiltrate

❚ Yolk sac tumor (YST)
- Peak incidence in first and second decades
- YST and clear cell tumors may have a loose edematous pattern
- YST displays primitive nuclei and may demonstrate simple papillae arranged around a single central vessel (Schiller-Duval bodies) typical of the endodermal sinus tumor
- YST may show several other patterns or may be admixed with other forms of germ cell tumor (mixed germ cell tumor)
- YSTs are AFP positive and on occasion show focal positivity for Leu-M1
- Clear cell carcinoma may be admixed with other types of carcinoma, often endometrioid, or with endometriosis

Pearls

- Clear cell and endometrioid carcinomas are associated with ovarian and pelvic endometriosis

Selected References

Cathro HP, Stoler MH: The utility of calretinin, inhibin, and WT1 immunohistochemical staining in the differential diagnosis of ovarian tumors. Hum Pathol 36:195-201, 2005.

Shimizu M, Nikaido T, Toki T, et al: Clear cell carcinoma has an expression pattern of cell cycle regulatory molecules that is unique among ovarian adenocarcinomas. Cancer 85:669-677, 1999.

Scully RE, Young RH, Clement PB: Atlas of Tumor Pathology: Tumors of the Ovary, Maldeveloped Gonads, Fallopian Tube, and Broad Ligament, 3rd Series, Fascicle 23. Washington, DC, Armed Forces Institute of Pathology, 1998, pp 141-151.

Matias-Guiu X, Lerma E, Prat J: Clear cell tumors of the female genital tract. Semin Diagn Pathol 14:233-239, 1997.

Heaps JM, Nieberg RK, Berek JS: Malignant neoplasms arising in endometriosis. Obstet Gynecol 75:1023-1028, 1990.

Transitional Cell Tumors

Clinical Features

- Most are benign Brenner tumors (transitional); peak incidence in fifth decade
- Borderline and transitional cell carcinomas usually occur in seventh decade
- May be associated with estrogenic or, less often, androgenic manifestations

Gross Pathology

- Most benign transitional cell tumors (Brenner) are small (<2 cm in diameter), lobulated, white to yellow, and sharply circumscribed
- Small to large cystic spaces are not uncommon
- Borderline: rare, may be solid or cystic with papillae or nodular projections
- Transitional cell carcinomas are more often bilateral (15%) and appear both solid and cystic
- If a benign component is present, the tumors may be classified as *ex-Brenner*

Histopathology

- In general, transitional cell tumors mimic the urothelium
▌ Brenner tumors
  - Well-defined solid or partially cystic nests and trabeculae of transitional cells with pale cytoplasm and oval, often grooved nuclei
  - Cysts are lined by mucinous or other glandular epithelium and filled with eosinophilic material
  - Stroma is dense and fibrotic, sometimes with calcifications

Figure 12-50. A, Brenner tumor. Solid nests of epithelial cells with grooved nuclei surrounded by a stroma composed of tightly packed, spindle-shaped cells. **B, Brenner tumor associated with mucinous cystadenoma.** Low-power view demonstrates both components. **C, Borderline transitional cell tumor** featuring solid proliferation of epithelial cells with nuclear atypia. There is no invasion of the stroma.

▌ Borderline transitional cell tumor
  - Atypical urothelial-like cells in poorly defined nests with no stromal invasion
  - Focal necrosis and mitotic figures are occasionally present

■ Transitional cell carcinoma
  ● Destructive stromal invasion with desmoplasia and occasional necrosis
  ● Pleomorphic urothelial single and nests of cells with mitotic figures and an intracystic papillary pattern, sometimes with small pools of mucin

Special Stains and Immunohistochemistry

● Cytokeratin 8/18 positive
● Cytokeratin 20 negative

Other Techniques for Diagnosis

● Noncontributory

Differential Diagnosis

■ Mucinous cystadenoma
  ● Benign Brenner tumors may contain large mucinous cysts but have foci of transitional cells at the periphery of the mucinous cells
■ Poorly differentiated and undifferentiated surface epithelial carcinoma
  ● Surface epithelial carcinomas usually grow in diffuse masses; may have a pattern simulating papillary transitional cell carcinoma, but this is usually due to pseudopapillae resulting from central necrosis with dropout of necrotic cellular debris

Pearls

● Occasionally Brenner tumors are associated with a dermoid cyst, or less often with struma ovarii, carcinoid tumor, or mucinous cystadenomas
● Transitional cell carcinoma has a poor prognosis, unless confined to one ovary, with an overall 5-year survival rate of 35%

Selected References

McCluggage WG, Bissonnette JP, Young RH: Primary malignant melanoma of the ovary: A report of 9 definite or probable cases with emphasis on their morphologic diversity and mimicry of other primary and secondary ovarian neoplasms. Int J Gynecol Pathol 25:321-329, 2006.

Ogawa K, Johansson SL, Cohen SM: Immunohistochemical analysis of uroplakins, urothelial specific proteins, in ovarian Brenner tumors, normal tissues, and benign and neoplastic lesions of the female genital tract. Am J Surg Pathol 155:1047-1050, 1999.

Scully RE, Young RH, Clement PB: Atlas of Tumor Pathology: Tumors of the Ovary, Maldeveloped Gonads, Fallopian Tube, and Broad Ligament, 3rd Series, Fascicle 23. Washington, DC, Armed Forces Institute of Pathology, 1998, pp 153-162.

Costa MJ, Hansen C, Dickerman A, Scudder SA: Clinicopathologic significance of transitional cell carcinoma pattern in nonlocalized ovarian epithelial tumors (stages 2-4). Am J Clin Pathol 109:173-180, 1998.

Gersell DJ: Primary ovarian transitional cell carcinoma: Diagnostic and prognostic considerations. Am J Clin Pathol 93:586-588, 1990.

Sex Cord–Stromal Tumors

Fibroma

Clinical Features

● Most common sex cord–stromal tumor
● Nonfunctioning tumor with peak incidence in fourth decade
● Occasionally occurs as a component of Meigs syndrome: ascites, hydrothorax (usually right sided), and ovarian fibroma; other solid ovarian tumors have been reported with Meigs syndrome
● May be associated with basal cell nevus syndrome (Gorlin syndrome), an autosomal dominant disorder consisting of numerous basal cell carcinomas beginning in early life, odontogenic keratocysts, erythematous pitting of the palms and soles, calcification of the cerebral falx, frequent skeletal anomalies, and other abnormalities, including bilateral ovarian fibromas

Figure 12-51. Ovarian fibroma. A, Cross section shows a well-circumscribed, chalky-white, solid tumor mass. **B,** This particular lesion shows a prominent hyalinized fibrous stroma with a scanty spindle cell component.

Gross Pathology

- Greater than 90% bilateral and larger than 3 cm in diameter (averages 5 to 6 cm)
- If less than 1 cm, classified as fibromatous nodule
- Hard, chalky-white, whorled appearance on cut section, often with areas of edema; occasionally hemorrhagic with sporadic calcifications

Histopathology

- Intersecting bundles of spindle cells, often in a storiform pattern
- Moderately cellular without nuclear atypia and infrequent mitotic figures (fewer than 4 mitotic figures/10 hpf)
- Diffuse intercellular edema is common
- Minor sex cord elements (tubules) may occasionally be identified

Special Stains and Immunohistochemistry

- Inhibin may be focally positive
- Vimentin positive

Other Techniques for Diagnosis

- Noncontributory

Differential Diagnosis

▌ Thecoma
- Spectrum exists between fibroma and thecoma (fibrothecoma)
- Thecomas display large cells with abundant pale cytoplasm
- Typically estrogenic, contain intracytoplasmic lipids, and are inhibin positive

▌ Massive edema and fibromatosis
- Edema: usually unilateral with marked intercellular edema, which is characteristic
- Fibromatosis shows stromal cell proliferation with abundant dense collagen
- Envelops rather than displaces follicles, corpora lutea, and corpora albicantia

Pearls

- Considered benign unless nuclear pleomorphism and mitotic figures are present (i.e., fibrosarcoma)

Selected References

Irving JA, Alkushi A, Young RH, Clement PB: Cellular fibromas of the ovary: A study of 75 cases including 40 mitotically active tumors emphasizing their distinction from fibrosarcoma. Am J Surg Pathol 30:929-938, 2006.

Abad A, Cazorla E, Ruiz F, et al: Meigs' syndrome with elevated CA125: Case report and review of the literature. Eur J Obstet Gynecol Reprod Biol 82:97-99, 1999.

Scully RE, Young RH, Clement PB: Atlas of Tumor Pathology: Tumors of the Ovary, Maldeveloped Gonads, Fallopian Tube, and Broad Ligament, 3rd Series, Fascicle 23. Washington, DC, Armed Forces Institute of Pathology, 1998.

Thecoma

Clinical Features

- Usually occurs in postmenopausal women; peak incidence in sixth decade
- In younger patients, luteinized thecomas are much more common than the classic type; they are typically estrogenic and often present with uterine bleeding
- This causes an increased incidence of endometrial hyperplasia and carcinoma

Gross Pathology

- Most are unilateral and measure up to 10 cm in diameter
- Lobulated, solid, yellow tumor sometimes with cystic change, hemorrhage, and necrosis
- Foci of calcification may be seen

Figure 12-52. Thecoma. A, Cut surface shows a well-circumscribed, tan-yellow, solid tumor mass replacing the ovary. **B,** The tumor is composed predominantly of plump spindle cells with pale cytoplasm. Focally, the tumor cells have vacuolated cytoplasm.

Histopathology

- Typical and luteinized variants
- Typical thecoma is composed of sheets and bundles of swollen, lipid-laden, theca-like cells and a variable fibrous component with less than 10% granulosa cells
- Nuclei are round to spindled and have mild atypia and infrequent mitoses
- Stroma may show obvious hyaline plaques and focal calcification
- Luteinized thecomas show luteinized stromal cells and luteinized theca-like cells, with abundant clear or eosinophilic cytoplasm and central, round nuclei

Special Stains and Immunohistochemistry

- Reticulin highlights reticulin fibers surrounding individual tumor cells
- Inhibin positive
- Oil red O positive on fresh tissue (frozen section)

Other Techniques for Diagnosis

- Noncontributory

Differential Diagnosis

❚ Fibroma
- Spectrum exists between fibroma and thecoma (fibrothecoma)
- Large cells with abundant pale cytoplasm; lipid-laden cells are absent
- Fibromas are not associated with steroid hormone production

❚ Steroid cell tumor
- Steroid cell tumors may show extensive luteinization and a fibromatous component
- Fibromatous component accounts for less than 10% of the tumor
- Typically androgenic, does not show hyaline plaques, and is often malignant

❚ Stromal hyperthecosis
- Almost always bilateral
- Lutein cells are mixed with small hyperplastic stromal cells with minimal collagen production

❚ Pregnancy luteoma
- Multiple in about 50% of cases
- Contain little or no lipid
- Lacks intersecting bundles of spindle cells

Pearls

- Most tumors are benign and treated with surgical resection

Selected References

Staats PN, McCluggage WG, Clement PB, Young RH: Luteinized thecomas (thecomatosis) of the type typically associated with sclerosing peritonitis: A clinical, histopathologic, and immunohistochemical analysis of 27 cases. Am J Surg Pathol 32(9):1273-1299, 2008.

Nocito AL, Sarancone S, Bacchi C, Tellez T: Ovarian thecoma: Clinicopathological analysis of 50 cases. Ann Diagn Pathol 12:12-16, 2008.

Adult Granulosa Cell Tumor

Clinical Features

- Represents 1% to 2% of ovarian tumors
- Occurs in middle-aged and older women
- Most women are postmenopausal, with a peak incidence in the fifth decade
- May secrete estrogen, resulting in endometrial hyperplasia and, in less than 5% of cases, endometrial carcinoma
- Endocrine manifestations include irregular excessive uterine bleeding sometimes preceded by amenorrhea in reproductive-age women and uterine bleeding in postmenopausal women
- May present with a palpable mass, abdominal pain, or swelling; occasionally acute abdominal symptoms due to rupture and bleeding into the peritoneum

Figure 12-53. Adult granulosa cell tumor. A, Cut surface of the tumor showing a variegated tan appearance with hemorrhage and yellow foci. **B,** Characteristic round to oval nuclei with grooves, inconspicuous nucleoli, and Call-Exner body.

Gross Pathology

- Usually unilateral and averages 12 cm in diameter
- Solid, soft, yellow-tan or gray tumor with cystic areas and hemorrhage
- Sometimes blood-filled cysts predominate, mixed with solid areas

Histopathology

- The amount of granulosa cells varies; they are mixed with stromal theca cells and fibroblasts
- Microfollicular pattern
  - Groups of granulosa cells forming Call-Exner bodies: small, round cystic spaces containing eosinophilic material or pyknotic nuclei
  - Cells are round to oval and contain scanty cytoplasm with pale, angular to round, often grooved nuclei, with variable mitotic activity
  - AGCT occasionally contains a component of luteinized granulosa cells, with abundant eosinophilic cytoplasm or cells with enlarged, hyperchromatic nuclei, including multinucleate forms
- Trabecular pattern consists of cords of cells
- Insular pattern
  - Made up of islands of cells separated by fibrous stroma
- Macrofollicular pattern
  - Displays large cysts lined by granulosa cells
- Water silk pattern
  - Cells arranged in undulated rows
- Gyriform pattern is characterized by zigzag cords of cells
- Diffuse and sarcomatoid patterns are less differentiated; shows increased nuclear pleomorphism, spindle cells, mitotic activity, and prominent nucleoli
- Call-Exner bodies are rare

Special Stains and Immunohistochemistry

- Reticulin stain: highlights sparse reticulin surrounding aggregates of granulosa cells
- Vimentin, inhibin, and calretinin positive
- EMA, cytokeratin 7, desmin negative

Other Techniques for Diagnosis

- Noncontributory

Differential Diagnosis

- ▌ Undifferentiated carcinoma and adenocarcinoma
  - Carcinomas are bilateral in more than 25% of cases; often spread beyond the ovary and may be necrotic
  - Cells are large and hyperchromatic, with pleomorphic nuclei, many mitosis, and psammoma bodies if serous; stroma is fibrous and often desmoplastic
- ▌ Thecoma, cellular fibroma, and fibrosarcoma
  - Classic AGCT cellular patterns are absent; reticulin stain is diffuse

- AGCT is rarely composed exclusively of spindle cells
- ▌ Carcinoid tumor
  - Glands with regular margins and eosinophilic secretions; nuclei are round, uniform, and coarsely stippled with rare mitotic figures
  - Abundant eosinophilic cytoplasm separates the nuclei from the lumen of glands
  - Neuroendocrine and several keratin immunohistochemical markers are positive
- ▌ Hypercalcemic small cell carcinoma
  - Hypercalcemia and a higher rate of extraovarian spread favor the diagnosis
  - Hyperchromatic, somewhat pleomorphic, nongrooved nuclei with frequent mitoses reminiscent of small cell carcinoma of the lung
  - No evidence of estrogen excess and occasional mucinous epithelium
- ▌ Endometrial stromal sarcoma
  - Large, yellow to tan tumor, often with foci of hemorrhage and necrosis; solid, partially cystic, or rarely predominantly cystic
  - Diffuse arrangement of small, oval to spindle-shaped cells with scanty cytoplasm; small arteries distributed throughout tumor
  - May have areas of sex cord–like patterns, and endometriosis is not unusual
  - High-grade tumor: mitotic rate is brisk; tumor is at an advanced stage and frequently bilateral
  - Reticulin stain highlights individual cells surrounded by fibrils

Pearls

- Spread is largely within the pelvis and lower abdomen
- May recur decades later: 10-year survival rate ranges from 60% to 90%

Selected References

Leuverink EM, Brennan BA, Crook ML, et al: Prognostic value of mitotic counts and Ki-67 immunoreactivity in adult-type granulosa cell tumour of the ovary. J Clin Pathol 61:914-919, 2008.

Ranganath R, Sridevi V, Shirley SS, Shantha V: Clinical and pathologic prognostic factors in adult granulosa cell tumors of the ovary. Int J Gynecol Cancer 18:929-933, 2008.

Roth LM: Recent advances in the pathology and classification of ovarian sex cord-stromal tumors. Int J Gynecol Pathol 25:199-215, 2006.

Schneider DT, Calaminus G, Harms D, et al: Ovarian sex cord-stromal tumors in children and adolescents. J Reprod Med 50:439-446, 2005.

Scully RE, Young RH, Clement PB: Atlas of Tumor Pathology: Tumors of the Ovary, Maldeveloped Gonads, Fallopian Tube, and Broad Ligament, 3rd Series, Fascicle 23. Washington, DC, Armed Forces Institute of Pathology, 1998, pp 169-180.

Fontanelli R, Stefanon B, Raspagliesi F, et al: Adult granulosa cell tumor of the ovary: A clinicopathologic study of 35 cases. Tumori 84:60-64, 1998.

Juvenile Granulosa Cell Tumor

Clinical Features

- Juvenile granulosa cell tumor (JGCT) occurs in children and young adults in first three decades
- Most prepubertal children present with a palpable mass and estrogenic effects, including isosexual pseudoprecocity and irregular uterine bleeding
- Postpubertal patients present with a mass, abdominal pain or swelling, menstrual irregularities, and occasionally rupture and ascites

Gross Pathology

- Similar to adult granulose cell tumor, with an average diameter of 12.5 cm
- Most are unilateral, yellow-tan, or gray solid tumors
- Cysts, sometimes with bloody fluid, are common, as are necrosis and hemorrhage

Histopathology

- Features solid sheets of cells mixed with small immature follicles of varying sizes and shapes containing secretions; nuclear atypia and many mitoses may be present
- The cells line the follicles, blending into diffusely cellular areas, commonly mixed with theca interna cells in the stroma
- Granulosa cells have round, hyperchromatic, ungrooved nuclei with abundant eosinophilic or clear, vacuolated cytoplasm; luteinization is frequent

Special Stains and Immunohistochemistry

- Reticulin highlights sparse reticulin fibrils surrounding aggregates of granulosa cells
- Mucicarmine usually highlights follicular secretions
- Inhibin and vimentin positive
- EMA negative

Other Techniques for Diagnosis

- Noncontributory

Differential Diagnosis

▮ Adult granulosa cell tumor
- Follicles are more regular in size and shape and contain eosinophilic basement membrane material with degenerating nuclei
- Cells have scanty cytoplasm, and extensive luteinization is absent
- Nuclei are pale, angular to round, and often grooved, with variable mitotic activity

▮ YST, embryonal carcinoma
- Affects children and young adults; peak incidence in first decade
- Associated with endocrine manifestations, such as isosexual precocious puberty (elevated HCG) in embryonal carcinoma; YST is positive for AFP
- Follicular pattern is absent, and nuclei appear primitive

▮ Thecoma
- Infrequent before 30 years of age, shows rare mitotic activity
- JGCT may contain areas lacking follicles and occasionally shows a predominance of theca cells, causing confusion with thecoma
- Thorough sampling of JGCT to demonstrate follicles, along with reticulin stain, helps to establish the diagnosis JGCT

▮ Hypercalcemic small cell carcinoma
- Hypercalcemia and a higher rate of extraovarian spread favor the diagnosis
- Small cell carcinoma displays numerous mitotic figures and necrosis
- Evidence of estrogen excess and mucinous epithelium favors AGCT
- Follicles typically contain eosinophilic, rather than mucicarminophilic, fluid

Pearls

- Most tumors are benign; surgical resection usually is curative
- Most recurrences are within 3 postoperative years

Selected References

Schneider DT, Calaminus G, Harms D, et al: Ovarian sex cord-stromal tumors in children and adolescents. J Reprod Med 50:439-446, 2005.

McCluggage WG: Immunoreactivity of ovarian juvenile granulosa cell tumours with epithelial membrane antigen. Histopathology 46:235-236, 2005.

Ligtenberg MJ, Siers M, Themmen AP, et al: Analysis of mutations in genes of the follicle-stimulating hormone receptor signaling pathway in ovarian granulosa cell tumors. J Clin Endocrinol Metab 84:2233-2234, 1999.

Cronjé HS, Niemand I, Bam RH, Woodruff JD: Granulosa and theca cell tumors in children: A report of 17 cases and literature review. Obstet Gynecol Surv 53:240-247, 1998.

Scully RE, Young RH, Clement PB: Atlas of Tumor Pathology: Tumors of the Ovary, Maldeveloped Gonads, Fallopian Tube, and Broad Ligament, 3rd Series, Fascicle 23. Washington, DC, Armed Forces Institute of Pathology, 1998, pp 180-186.

Hildebrandt RH, Rouse RV, Longacre TA: Value of inhibin in the identification of granulosa cell tumors of the ovary. Hum Pathol 28:1387-1395, 1997.

Sclerosing Stromal Tumor

Clinical Features

- Rare, benign, occurring mostly in first three decades, with a peak incidence in second decade

Figure 12-54. Sclerosing stromal tumor. Pseudolobular pattern with edematous connective tissue and prominent thin-walled vessels.

Gross Pathology

- Unilateral, solid, discrete, white tumor that is sharply demarcated
- Frequently with foci of edema, cyst formation, and yellow discoloration

Histopathology

- Moderately cellular pseudolobules with numerous thin-walled vessels
- Pseudotubules are composed of fibroblasts and lipid-laden, vacuolated cells separated by edematous connective tissue or dense collagenous stroma
- Sclerosis is present within the nodules, but mitoses are identified only rarely

Special Stains and Immunohistochemistry

- Inhibin positive
- CD34, CD31 positive

Other Techniques for Diagnosis

- Noncontributory

Differential Diagnosis

▌ Thecoma versus fibroma
- Thecoma is typically an estrogenic tumor with peak incidence in sixth decade; shows characteristic and distinct lutein cells
- Fibroma is a nonfunctioning tumor with peak incidence in fourth decade; may have diffuse edema
- Hyaline plaques may be a noticeable feature, especially with thecoma

Pearls

- Rarely forms a unilocular cyst
- Scarce association with estrogen secretion

Selected References

Kostopoulou E, Moulla A, Giakoustidis D, Leontsini M: Sclerosing stromal tumors of the ovary: A clinicopathologic, immunohistochemical and cytogenetic analysis of three cases. Eur J Gynaecol Oncol 25:257-260, 2004.

Tiltman AJ, Haffajee Z: Sclerosing stromal tumors, thecomas, and fibromas of the ovary: An immunohistochemical profile. Int J Gynecol Pathol 18:254-258, 1999.

Matsubayashi R, Matsuo Y, Doi J, et al: Sclerosing stromal tumor of the ovary: Radiologic findings. Eur Radiol 9:1335-1338, 1999.

Kawauchi S, Tsuji T, Kaku T, et al: Sclerosing stromal tumor of the ovary: A clinicopathologic, immunohistochemical, ultrastructural, and cytogenetic analysis with special reference to its vasculature. Am J Surg Pathol 22:83-92, 1998.

Scully RE, Young RH, Clement PB: Atlas of Tumor Pathology: Tumors of the Ovary, Maldeveloped Gonads, Fallopian Tube, and Broad Ligament, 3rd Series, Fascicle 23. Washington, DC, Armed Forces Institute of Pathology, 1998, pp 197-200.

Sertoli Cell Tumor

Clinical Features

- Rare tumor best regarded as low-grade malignancy
- Mostly affects women of childbearing age; peak incidence in second decade
- Usually nonfunctioning but may be estrogenic or occasionally androgenic

Gross Pathology

- Unilateral, solid, lobulated tumor averaging 9 cm in diameter
- Yellow or brown cut surface

Histopathology

- Well-differentiated Sertoli cell tumor contains round or elongated hollow or solid tubules separated by fibrous stroma devoid of Leydig cells

Figure 12-55. Sertoli cell tumor. The tumor is composed of closely packed tubules lined by cuboidal to columnar epithelial cells. Notice the lack of nuclear atypia.

- Hollow tubules are lined by cuboidal, columnar cells with moderate to abundant pale, occasionally eosinophilic, cytoplasm, and rare to absent nuclear atypia and mitoses
- Solid tubules may be closely packed with small nuclei and scanty cytoplasm or large cells with abundant cytoplasmic lipid (lipid-rich Sertoli cell tumor)
- Stroma may be hyalinized and focally replace the tubules

Special Stains and Immunohistochemistry

- Cytokeratin and inhibin positive
- EMA negative

Other Techniques for Diagnosis

- Noncontributory

Differential Diagnosis

▌ SLCT
- Presence of several clusters of Leydig cells or their spindle cell precursors
▌ Carcinoid tumor
- May rarely have a solid tubular pattern
- Distinguished with immunohistochemical stains for neuroendocrine markers (chromogranin, synaptophysin) and by diffuse cytokeratin positivity

Pearls

- Excellent prognosis

Selected References

Oliva E, Alvarez T, Young RH: Sertoli cell tumors of the ovary: A clinicopathologic and immunohistochemical study of 54 cases. Am J Surg Pathol 29:143-156, 2005.

Scully RE, Young RH, Clement PB: Atlas of Tumor Pathology: Tumors of the Ovary, Maldeveloped Gonads, Fallopian Tube, and Broad Ligament, 3rd Series, Fascicle 23. Washington, DC, Armed Forces Institute of Pathology, 1998, pp 203-204.

Costa MJ, Ames PF, Walls J, Roth LM: Inhibin immunohistochemistry applied to ovarian neoplasms: A novel, effective, diagnostic tool. Hum Pathol 28:1247-1254, 1997.

Rishi M, Howard LN, Bratthauer GL, Tavassoli FA: Use of monoclonal antibody against human inhibin as a marker for sex cord-stromal tumors of the ovary. Am J Surg Pathol 21:583-589, 1997.

Sertoli–Leydig Cell Tumor

Clinical Features

- Androgen-secreting tumor that may occur at any age; peak incidence in the second decade; patients with the retiform subtype are 10 years younger on average
- Plasma testosterone, androstenedione, and other androgen levels may be high; androgenic manifestations may occur with virilization or hirsutism
- Half of patients have no endocrine symptoms, but rather abdominal swelling or pain

Figure 12-56. Sertoli–Leydig cell tumor of intermediate differentiation. Sheets of immature Sertoli cells and clusters of Leydig cells with abundant eosinophilic cytoplasm are present at the center of the photomicrograph.

Gross Pathology

- Most are unilateral, confined to the ovary, and average 10 cm in diameter
- Solid, lobulated, yellow-tan to reddish-brown masses, but may have a cystic component, especially with heterologous or retiform tumors
- Poorly differentiated tumors are larger and show more hemorrhage and necrosis

Histopathology

- Differentiation
  — Well differentiated
    ◆ Hollow or solid tubular pattern with round, oval, elongated, or irregular tubules in a fibrous stroma mixed with clusters of Leydig cells
  — Intermediate differentiation
    ◆ Nodular appearance with dense cellular areas showing occasional mitoses separated by hypocellular fibrous or edematous stroma
    ◆ Cellular areas contain less-differentiated tubules, clusters, and cords of immature Sertoli cells that have small hyperchromatic nuclei and sparse cytoplasm
    ◆ Sertoli cells separated by stromal cells and Leydig cells with abundant pale cytoplasm and round nuclei with prominent nucleoli with or without heterologous elements
  — Poorly differentiated
    ◆ Diffuse pattern of densely packed pleomorphic spindle-shaped cells with frequent mitotic figures
- Heterologous elements
  — Benign mucinous epithelium of gastrointestinal type, with goblet, argentaffin, and argyrophil cells often present is the most common component,

seen in about 15% to 20% of SLCTs, except in the well-differentiated subtype
  — Immature skeletal muscle, cartilage, or both may be identified
- Retiform
  — Significant proportion of cells akin to rete epithelial cells with patterns similar to rete testis, including tubular and cystic structures
  — Morphology of the tubules is identical to tubules in well-differentiated SLCT
  — Most retiform tumors exhibit other SLCT subtypes

Special Stains and Immunohistochemistry

- Inhibin positive

Other Techniques for Diagnosis

- Noncontributory

Differential Diagnosis

❚ Mucinous tumors
- Cysts and glands lined by benign, proliferating, or malignant mucinous cells resembling intestinal or endometrioid epithelium without SLCT elements

❚ Endometrioid carcinoma
- Endometrioid glands, squamous differentiation, occasional adenofibromatous component; may show intraluminal mucin in the glands

❚ Malignant mixed müllerian tumor (carcinosarcoma)
- May contain heterologous elements, including cartilage or rhabdomyoblasts, but lacks Sertoli or Leydig cells and other components
- High-grade malignant epithelial cells with müllerian (e.g., serous, clear) differentiation, but no androgenic secretions
- Cytokeratin and EMA highlight carcinoma, whereas inhibin is negative

Pearls

- Occasional association with androgenic manifestations
- Androgen secretion may result in erythrocytosis
- Rarely associated with sarcoma botryoides of the cervix, thyroid disease, and rare familial occurrence

Selected References

Roth LM: Recent advances in the pathology and classification of ovarian sex cord-stromal tumors. Int J Gynecol Pathol 25:199-215, 2006.

Lantzsch T, Stoerer S, Lawrenz K, et al: Sertoli-Leydig cell tumors. Arch Gynecol Obstet 264:206-208, 2001.

Mooney EE, Man YG, Bratthauer GL, Tavassoli FA: Evidence that Leydig cells in Sertoli-Leydig cell tumors have a reactive rather than a neoplastic profile. Cancer 86:2312-2317, 1999.

Scully RE, Young RH, Clement PB: Atlas of Tumor Pathology: Tumors of the Ovary, Maldeveloped Gonads, Fallopian Tube, and Broad Ligament, 3rd Series, Fascicle 23. Washington, DC, Armed Forces Institute of Pathology, 1998, pp 205-219.

Sex Cord Tumor with Annular Tubules

Clinical Features

- Sex cord tumor with annular tubulus (SCTAT) is a relatively rare tumor; most patients are of childbearing age
- One third of cases are associated with Peutz-Jeghers syndrome (PJS)
- Estrogenic manifestations may be present, including menstrual irregularities and isosexual precocious puberty

Gross Pathology

- Tumors associated with PJS are usually small, multifocal, bilateral, and focally calcified; tumors not associated with PJS are relatively large, solid, and yellow
- Cysts may be seen in both types

Histopathology

- SCTAT is characterized by simple and complex annular tubules encircling hyaline material; simple tubules are shaped like a ring
- Complex tubules are more numerous and form intercommunicating rings; if associated with PJS, calcification of the tubules may be present
- Rings are lined by epithelial cells that have abundant pale cytoplasm oriented toward the center of the ring and a peripheral nucleus

Special Stains and Immunohistochemistry

- Noncontributory

Other Techniques for Diagnosis

- Noncontributory

Differential Diagnosis

❚ Gonadoblastoma
- Stromal and germ cell tumor components must be present; not associated with PJS
- Almost always occurs in phenotypic women with underlying gonadal disorders

Pearls

- Benign, incidental finding at autopsy or surgery when seen in patients with PJS
- Malignant in one fourth of cases; characteristically spreads through lymphatics
- Considered a specific sex cord–stromal tumor with a potential for bidirectional differentiation toward granulosa cell or Sertoli cell tumors

Selected References

Connolly DC, Katabuchi H, Cliby WA, Cho KR: Somatic mutations in the STK11/LKB1 gene are uncommon in rare gynecological tumor types associated with Peutz-Jeghers syndrome. Am J Pathol 156:339-345, 2000.

Hirschman SA, Dottino P, Deligdisch L, Szporn A: Cytology of sex cord tumor with annular tubules: a case report. Diagn Cytopathol 18:362-364, 1998.

Scully RE, Young RH, Clement PB: Atlas of Tumor Pathology: Tumors of the Ovary, Maldeveloped Gonads, Fallopian Tube, and Broad Ligament, 3rd Series, Fascicle 23. Washington, DC, Armed Forces Institute of Pathology, 1998, pp 219-223.

Gynandroblastoma

Clinical Features

- Extremely rare tumor that usually presents in young adults but may occur at any age
- May have androgenic or estrogenic manifestations

Gross Pathology

- Solid, pale tumor less than 6 cm in diameter

Histopathology

- Well-differentiated with granulosa and Sertoli cell components
- Tumors should contain more than 10% of the minor component to warrant the diagnosis

Special Stains and Immunohistochemistry

- Noncontributory

Other Techniques for Diagnosis

- Noncontributory

Differential Diagnosis

▮ Granulosa cell tumor
- If Sertoli cells are present, they represent less than 10% of the total tumor volume
▮ Sertoli tumor or Sertoli-Leydig tumor
- If granulosa cells are present, they represent less than 10% of the total tumor volume
▮ Sex cord tumor with annular tubules
- Simple and complex annular tubules forming intercommunicating rings and encircling hyaline material often associated with PJS

Pearls

- Extremely rare tumor
- Almost always benign

Selected References

Kalir T, Friedman F Jr: Gynandroblastoma in pregnancy: Case report and review of literature. Mt Sinai J Med 65:292-295, 1998.

Scully RE, Young RH, Clement PB: Atlas of Tumor Pathology: Tumors of the Ovary, Maldeveloped Gonads, Fallopian Tube, and Broad Ligament, 3rd Series, Fascicle 23. Washington, DC, Armed Forces Institute of Pathology, 1998, pp 219-222.

Jaworski RC, Fryatt JJ, Turner TB, Osborn RA: Gynandroblastoma of the ovary. Pathology 18:348-351, 1986.

Stromal Luteoma

Clinical Features

- Small benign steroid cell tumor
- Usually develops in postmenopausal women; peak incidence in fifth decade
- Frequently estrogenic with abnormal vaginal bleeding; occasionally androgenic

Gross Pathology

- Solitary, unilateral, well-circumscribed solid tumor, at least 5 mm in diameter, but almost always less than 3 cm
- Gray-white or yellow in most cases with occasional brown-red foci

Histopathology

- Round nodules of lutein cells that, by definition, are confined within ovarian stroma
- Stroma is usually sparse and sometimes focally fibrotic
- Luteinized cells arranged diffusely or in nests and cords, containing eosinophilic cytoplasm with little lipid; nuclei are small and round with one prominent nucleolus and rare mitoses
- Sometimes degeneration produces irregular spaces that may simulate glands or vessels

Special Stains and Immunohistochemistry

- Noncontributory

Other Techniques for Diagnosis

- Noncontributory

Differential Diagnosis

▮ Stromal hyperthecosis
- Microscopic nests of lutein cells may develop (nodular hyperthecosis) but are less than 5 mm in diameter; the nodules are typically multiple

Pearls

- Presumably arises from the ovarian stroma
- Stromal hyperthecosis is present in the ipsilateral or contralateral ovary in most cases

Selected References

Outwater EK, Wagner BJ, Mannion C, et al: Sex cord-stromal and steroid cell tumors of the ovary. Radiographics 18:1523-1546, 1998.

Scully RE, Young RH, Clement PB: Atlas of Tumor Pathology: Tumors of the Ovary, Maldeveloped Gonads, Fallopian Tube, and Broad Ligament, 3rd Series, Fascicle 23. Washington, DC, Armed Forces Institute of Pathology, 1998, pp 227-228.

Rao BR, Slotman BJ: Ovarian tumors with endocrine manifestations. Curr Therapy Endocrinol Metab 6:260-262, 1997.

Leydig Cell Tumor

Clinical Features

- Rare, benign steroid cell, known as a *hilus cell tumor*; peak incidence in fifth decade
- Androgenic manifestations are classic, including hirsutism and virilization
- Occasionally, estrogenic manifestations are present

Gross Pathology

- Unilateral, well-circumscribed, solid, usually less than 5 cm in diameter located near the hilum with hemorrhage frequently present
- Usually red-brown to yellow, or dark brown to black

Histopathology

- Sheets, cords, or clusters of polyhedral cells with abundant eosinophilic, finely granular cytoplasm, which may contain small lipid vacuoles

Figure 12-57. Leydig cell tumor. A, Cross section shows a well-circumscribed, reddish-brown tumor. **B,** Diffuse pattern with a homogeneous population of eosinophilic cells with a low nuclear-to-cytoplasmic ratio, nuclei with noticeable chromatin, and discrete nucleoli.

- By definition, elongated eosinophilic crystals of Reinke are present in the cytoplasm; however, these may not be obvious
- Large, centrally located hyperchromatic nuclei often with one or more prominent nucleoli and rare mitoses; fibrinoid degeneration of vessels walls is common
- Anuclear eosinophilic zones separate cellular areas and surround blood vessels

Special Stains and Immunohistochemistry

- Inhibin positive

Other Techniques for Diagnosis

- Electron microscopy highlights rod-shaped crystals of Reinke, which are hexagonal in cross section

Differential Diagnosis

▌SLCT
- Tubular pattern, Sertoli cells plus Leydig cells characterize the tumor
- Mixed population of different types of cells

Pearls

- Originate most often in the hilus but may arise from the ovarian stroma (nonhilar type)

Selected References

Takeuchi S, Ishihara N, Ohbayashi C, et al: Stromal Leydig cell tumor of the ovary: Case report and literature review. Int J Gynecol Pathol 18:178-182, 1999.

Scully RE, Young RH, Clement PB: Atlas of Tumor Pathology: Tumors of the Ovary, Maldeveloped Gonads, Fallopian Tube, and Broad Ligament, 3rd Series, Fascicle 23. Washington, DC, Armed Forces Institute of Pathology, 1998, pp 228-232.

Baiocchi G, Manci N, Angeletti G, et al: Pure Leydig cell tumour (hilus cell) of the ovary: A rare cause of virilization after menopause. Gynecol Obstet Invest 44:141-144, 1997.

Germ Cell Tumors

Mature Cystic Teratoma (Dermoid Cyst)

Clinical Features

- Dermoid cyst is one of the most common ovarian tumors
- Occurs most commonly in adult women during the reproductive years
- Often asymptomatic, but patients may present with pain, swelling, or uterine bleeding

Gross Pathology

- Bilateral in about 15% of cases, smaller than 15 cm, and may be multiple in one ovary
- Combination solid and cystic mass with white to gray external surface

Figure 12-58. Mature cystic teratoma (dermoid cyst). A, Cut surface shows a cystic lesion containing sebaceous material and teeth. **B,** The cavity of the cyst is lined by keratinized squamous epithelium with underlying cutaneous structures.

- Opened cysts may contain visible hair, cheeselike sebaceous material, skin, bone, cartilage, fat, thyroid tissue, brain tissue, and teeth

Histopathology

- Mature (adult-type) tissues, typically representing all three germ layers
- Often consists of ectodermal tissues with a cyst lined by mature epidermis and its appendages and rare (if any) mitoses
- Neuroectodermal elements: glial, peripheral nervous tissue, cerebrum, and cerebellum are common
- Mesodermal elements like smooth muscle, bone, teeth, cartilage, and fat may be present
- Endodermal elements include respiratory and gastrointestinal epithelium, and thyroid tissue

Special Stains and Immunohistochemistry

- Stains correspond to tissues present

Other Techniques for Diagnosis

- Noncontributory

Differential Diagnosis

▌ Immature teratoma
- Contains immature elements, most commonly glial; on occasion, cartilage and others

Pearls

- Dermoid cysts are lined by keratinizing squamous epithelium with skin appendages
- Skin may be admixed with struma ovarii, carcinoid tumor, or solid teratoma; a foreign-body giant cell reaction may occur with rupture
- Dermoid cysts may be present in the contralateral ovary in patients with yolk sac tumor or immature teratoma about 5% to 10% of the time
- Treatment: cystectomy
- Malignant transformation—usually to squamous cell carcinoma—is rare (<3%)
- Primary carcinoid tumors of the ovary are associated with other teratomatous elements in 85% to 90% of cases

Selected References

Vang R, Gown AM, Zhao C, et al: Ovarian mucinous tumors associated with mature cystic teratomas: Morphologic and immunohistochemical analysis identifies a subset of potential teratomatous origin that shares features of lower gastrointestinal tract mucinous tumors more commonly encountered as secondary tumors in the ovary. Am J Surg Pathol 31:854-869, 2007.

Hurwitz JL, Fenton A, McCluggage WG, McKenna S: Squamous cell carcinoma arising in a dermoid cyst of the ovary: A case series. BJOG 114:1283-1287, 2007.

Iwasa A, Oda Y, Kaneki E, et al: Squamous cell carcinoma arising in mature cystic teratoma of the ovary: an immunohistochemical analysis of its tumorigenesis. Histopathology 1:98-104, 2007.

Mature Solid Teratoma

Clinical Features

- Slow-growing, benign tumor with peak incidence in first and second decades
- Uncommon and asymptomatic until large

Gross Pathology

- Unilateral large, mostly solid tumor with minimal hemorrhage or necrosis

Histopathology

- Solid tumor with morphologic features resembling mature cystic teratoma
- Composed exclusively of mature elements: endoderm, mesoderm, and ectoderm
- Neural tissue sometimes predominates; only rare mitoses are identified
- Important to thoroughly sample the tumor to exclude immature teratoma

Figure 12-59. Mature solid teratoma. The lesion is composed of cartilage, glandular epithelium, and fibrous tissue.

Special Stains and Immunohistochemistry

- Noncontributory

Other Techniques for Diagnosis

- Noncontributory

Differential Diagnosis

▌ Immature teratoma
  - Characterized by the presence of immature elements, most commonly glial

Pearls

- Surgical resection is curative if immature teratoma has been ruled out
- Rarely associated with mature glial peritoneal implants, but prognosis is still excellent

Selected References

Scully RE, Young RH, Clement PB: Atlas of Tumor Pathology: Tumors of the Ovary, Maldeveloped Gonads, Fallopian Tube, and Broad Ligament, 3rd Series, Fascicle 23. Washington, DC, Armed Forces Institute of Pathology, 1998, pp 272-273.

Calame JJ, Schaberg A: Solid teratomas and mixed müllerian tumors of the ovary: A clinical, histological, and immunocytochemical comparative study. Gynecol Oncol 33:212-221, 1989.

Dysgerminoma

Clinical Features

- Most common malignant germ cell tumor; more frequent in women with ovarian dysgenesis; one of the two most common ovarian neoplasms seen in pregnancy
- Pure or mixed with other malignant germ cell components
- Primarily affects young women; peak incidence in second and third decades

Figure 12-60. Dysgerminoma. A, Twenty-centimeter ovary with a solid tan lobulated appearance on cut surface. **B,** Sheets of large germ cells with prominent nucleoli and fibrous bands with plasma cells and lymphocytes.

- Most patients have elevated serum lactic dehydrogenase and isoenzyme-1, which can be used as tumor markers
- Occasionally produces HCG, manifesting with isosexual precocious puberty and menstrual irregularities
- One of the two most common ovarian neoplasms seen in pregnancy

Gross Pathology

- Mostly a unilateral solid, soft tumor with a median diameter of 15 cm
- More often bilateral in patients with gonadal dysgenesis
- External surface is smooth and gray-white; cut surface is lobulated, gray-white, with hemorrhage or necrotic areas giving it a yellow, pink, or tan color
- Important to sample tumor extensively to exclude other germ cell elements (especially variegated and cystic areas)

Histopathology

- Uniform clusters, nests, and cords of large, round cells with abundant, clear, glycogen-rich cytoplasm, separated by lymphocyte-infiltrated fibrous stroma
- Nuclei are centrally located, large, round, and vesicular, with clumped chromatin and one to several prominent nucleoli; frequent mitoses, necrosis, and hemorrhage
- Noncaseating granulomas and multinucleate syncytiotrophoblastic giant cells may be seen
- Frequently dysgerminomas are combined with other germ cell neoplasms, forming mixed tumors; calcifications suggests the presence of a gonadoblastoma

Special Stains and Immunohistochemistry

- Placental alkaline phosphatase (PLAP) and vimentin positive
- Cytokeratin is usually negative and EMA is negative
- PAS highlights glycogen-rich cytoplasm of tumor cells

Other Techniques for Diagnosis

- Noncontributory

Differential Diagnosis

▌ Solid yolk sac tumor
  - Solid tumor with increased nuclear variation, hyaline bodies, and rare stromal lymphocytes
  - AFP positive
▌ Embryonal carcinoma
  - Composed of larger cells with larger markedly hyperchromatic nuclei without lymphocytic infiltration of the stroma
  - Most contain syncytiotrophoblastic giant cells and stain positively for cytokeratin
▌ Diffuse clear cell carcinoma
  - Polygonal cells with eccentric, hyperchromatic nuclei, usually without prominent nucleoli and glycogen-filled cytoplasm; plasma cells may be prominent
  - Less often positive for PLAP, but almost always positive for cytokeratin and EMA
▌ Lymphoma
  - Often bilateral
  - Cells lack cytoplasmic glycogen; stain positively for CD45 and negatively for PLAP

Pearls

- Most patients do not have menstrual abnormalities and are capable of bearing children
- Treated with surgery and radiation; recurrences treated with chemotherapy
- Metastatic spread late in the course of the disease, first through lymphatics and later hematogenously to the liver, lungs, and bones

- Five-year survival rate for a pure tumor in stage I ranges from 90% to 95%
- Sampling is of utmost importance to exclude a mixed germ cell tumor

Selected References

Guillem V, Poveda A: Germ cell tumours of the ovary. Clin Transl Oncol 9:237-243, 2007.

Sever M, Jones TD, Roth LM, et al: Expression of CD117 (c-kit) receptor in dysgerminoma of the ovary: Diagnostic and therapeutic implications. Mod Pathol 18:1411-1416, 2005.

Scully RE, Young RH, Clement PB: Atlas of Tumor Pathology: Tumors of the Ovary, Maldeveloped Gonads, Fallopian Tube, and Broad Ligament, 3rd Series, Fascicle 23. Washington, DC, Armed Forces Institute of Pathology, 1998, pp 239-245.

Reddy KB, Ahuja VK, Kannan V, et al: Dysgerminoma of the ovary: A retrospective study. Australas Radiol 41:262-265, 1997.

Merino MJ, Jaffe G: Age contrast in ovarian pathology. Cancer 71(2 Suppl):537-544, 1993.

Yolk Sac Tumor

Clinical Features

- Malignant tumor also referred to as *endodermal sinus tumor*, which is a common subtype
- Peak incidence in second and third decades; rare after age 40 years
- Presents with abdominal pain associated with a mass
- Elevated serum AFP; levels may be useful in monitoring therapy

Gross Pathology

- Unilateral, large tumor averaging 15 cm in diameter with a smooth external surface
- Soft, solid, gray-yellow mass on cut section, often containing cysts
- Frequent areas of hemorrhage and necrosis
- Several morphologic variants

Histopathology

- Reticular pattern of small cystic spaces lined by cells with clear cytoplasm containing glycogen or lipid.
- Hyperchromatic, irregular, and large nuclei with prominent nucleoli; frequent mitoses, and loose connective tissue stroma
- Schiller-Duval bodies are characteristic, particularly in the endodermal sinus tumor subtype
  — Glomeruloid, epithelial-lined space containing a polypoid projection covered by cuboidal to columnar cells with a single central vessel
- Frequent globular hyaline bodies
- Other structural variants include polyvesicular, hepatoid, glandular, papillary, myxomatous, macrocystic, and solid
  — Polyvesicular-vitelline shows many small cysts, giving a honeycomb appearance; background of

Figure 12-61. **Yolk sac tumor (endodermal sinus tumor). A,** Formalin-fixed firm, smooth, gray-yellow tumor mass with occasional cysts. **B,** Low-power view shows the classic microcystic pattern. **C,** This image shows the classic perivascular distribution of the tumor cells (Schiller-Duval bodies).

dense cellular stroma lined by columnar, cuboidal, or flat epithelium
— Hepatoid (usually a minor component); mimics hepatocellular carcinoma
  ◆ Composed of groups of polygonal cells with abundant eosinophilic cytoplasm and a central nucleus with single nucleolus
  ◆ Abundant hyaline bodies are present

— Glandular (mostly a minor component); may mimic endometrioid adenocarcinoma
  ◆ Intestinal variant contains nests of cells in a cribriform pattern
  ◆ Endometrioid-like variant contains glandular or villoglandular pattern
  ◆ Simple or pseudostratified columnar epithelium may show subnuclear or supranuclear vacuoles
  ◆ Hepatoid cells within gland lumens mimic squamous morulas

Special Stains and Immunohistochemistry

- AFP positive cytoplasmic staining, may be focal or diffuse
- α_1-Antitrypsin positive cytoplasmic staining, may be focal
- Creatine kinase positive cytoplasmic staining
- EMA negative
- PAS highlights hyaline globules and basement membrane material in tumors with parietal differentiation; present in most YSTs

Other Techniques for Diagnosis

- Noncontributory

Differential Diagnosis

▌ Clear cell adenocarcinoma
- Peak incidence in fifth decade
- Can have loose reticular pattern similar to YST
- May show other müllerian differentiation (i.e., endometrioid, serous) or a background of endometriosis
- Polyhedral glycogen-rich clear cells with atypical nuclei and frequent mitoses with occasional nucleoli
- Epidermal growth factor receptor (EGFR) is positive in 25% of cases
- AFP rarely positive

▌ Endometrioid adenocarcinoma
- Peak incidence in fifth decade; may be associated with ovarian or pelvic endometriosis
- AFP negative
- Endometrioid-like YST will show foci of more common YST variants

▌ Hepatoid carcinoma
- Rare tumor, usually in postmenopausal women
- AFP positive
- More nuclear atypia than YST
- Hepatoid YST shows foci of more common YST variants

▌ Dysgerminoma
- Uniform round cells with abundant, clear, glycogen-rich cytoplasm, separated by lymphocyte-infiltrated fibrous stroma
- Cytokeratin is usually negative; AFP negative

Pearls

- Rapidly growing, highly malignant tumor
- Often spreads outside of the ovary to the peritoneum or retroperitoneal lymph nodes
- May be seen in association with endometrioid or mucinous tumors, pregnancy, or gonadal dysgenesis; may be mixed with other germ cell tumors
- Treatment with combination chemotherapy
- Dermoid cyst present in either ovary in about 5% to 15% of cases

Selected References

Dällenbach P, Bonnefoi H, Pelte MF, Vlastos G: Yolk sac tumours of the ovary: An update. Eur J Surg Oncol 32:1063-1075, 2006.

Nawa A, Obata N, Kikkawa F, et al: Prognostic factors of patients with yolk sac tumors of the ovary. Am J Obstet Gynecol 184:1182-1188, 2001.

Tewari K, Cappuccini F, Disaia PJ, et al: Malignant germ cell tumors of the ovary. Obstet Gynecol 95:128-133, 2000.

Scully RE, Young RH, Clement PB: Atlas of Tumor Pathology: Tumors of the Ovary, Maldeveloped Gonads, Fallopian Tube, and Broad Ligament, 3rd Series, Fascicle 23. Washington, DC, Armed Forces Institute of Pathology, 1998, pp 245-255.

Embryonal Carcinoma

Clinical Features

- Rare tumor affecting children and young adults; peak incidence in first decade
- HCG often elevated and may be used as a tumor marker
- Signs and symptoms related to an adnexal mass and sometimes related to endocrine manifestations, including isosexual precocious puberty and irregular bleeding

Gross Pathology

- Unilateral, smooth-surfaced, solid tumor with a median diameter of 17 cm
- Gray-white or yellow with foci of hemorrhage or necrosis
- Variegated pattern may be seen depending on other germ cell elements present

Histopathology

- Solid, papillary, or glandular pattern with sheets and nests of malignant large ovoid or polygonal cells forming syncytiotrophoblastic giant cells in a fibrotic stroma
- Cells display abundant granular, eosinophilic cytoplasm
- Pleomorphic nuclei are centrally located, round, and vesicular with irregular membranes and often contain prominent nucleoli; cleftlike spaces are often present

Figure 12-62. Embryonal carcinoma. A, Cross section shows a lobulated gray-white tumor that is partially cystic and hemorrhagic. **B,** Solid pattern composed of large polygonal cells with poorly defined cytoplasmic borders.

- Frequent, sometimes abnormal, mitoses with foci of necrosis and hemorrhage
- Usually combined with other germ cell elements, most commonly YST

Special Stains and Immunohistochemistry

- Cytokeratin positive
- PLAP positive in syncytiotrophoblasts
- EMA negative

Other Techniques for Diagnosis

- Noncontributory

Differential Diagnosis

❚ Dysgerminoma
  - Consists of relatively smaller, more uniform cells, arranged in clumps and cords, in a fibrous stroma infiltrated with lymphocytes and rare syncytiotrophoblasts
❚ YST
  - Smaller cells with clear, glycogen-rich cytoplasm arranged in a reticular pattern mixed with solid areas
  - Schiller-Duval bodies are classic; rare syncytiotrophoblasts

❚ Juvenile granulosa cell tumor
  ● Focal follicle formation with relatively less nuclear atypia; positive inhibin

Pearls

  ● Treatment: surgery and postoperative chemotherapy

Selected References

Oliver RT: Germ cell cancer. Curr Opin Oncol 11:236-241, 1999.

Scully RE, Young RH, Clement PB: Atlas of Tumor Pathology: Tumors of the Ovary, Maldeveloped Gonads, Fallopian Tube, and Broad Ligament, 3rd Series, Fascicle 23. Washington, DC, Armed Forces Institute of Pathology, 1998, pp 255-257.

Talerman A: Germ cell tumors of the ovary. Curr Opin Obstet Gynecol 9:44-47, 1997.

Polyembryoma

Clinical Features

  ● Rare malignant tumor typically occurring in children and young adults
  ● May have elevation of serum AFP and HCG

Gross Pathology

  ● Typically, a unilateral, solid tumor with areas of hemorrhage and necrosis

Histopathology

  ● Numerous embryoid bodies, resembling early embryos in different stages of development, scattered in a fibrous or edematous stroma
  ● More differentiated embryoid body contains an embryonic disk, amniotic cavity, yolk sac, and extraembryonic mesenchyme
  ● Embryonic disk elements consist of an ectodermal layer of tall columnar cells and an endodermal layer of cuboidal cells
  ● Occasionally chorionic elements, including syncytiotrophoblastic giant cells, are present
  ● Embryoid bodies may appear as a normal early embryo or may appear malformed
  ● Seen in association with other neoplastic germ cell elements, usually mature or immature teratoma

Special Stains and Immunohistochemistry

  ● AFP highlights yolk sac component and hepatic elements
  ● α_1-Antitrypsin may highlight yolk sac component of embryoid bodies and hepatic elements
  ● HCG highlights syncytiotrophoblastic elements

Other Techniques for Diagnosis

  ● Noncontributory

Differential Diagnosis

❚ Retiform SLCT
  ● Peak incidence in first decade, sometimes presenting with androgenic manifestations
  ● Tubular and cystic structures; tubules lined by one or more layers of cells with round, regular nuclei and scanty cytoplasm; most retiform tumors are seen with other SLCT subtypes

Pearls

  ● Embryoid bodies probably arise from multipotential malignant embryonal cells and never appear to develop beyond the 18-day stage
  ● Invasion of adjacent structures and distant metastases usually seen
  ● Treatment consists of surgical excision and chemotherapy

Selected References

Scully RE, Young RH, Clement PB: Atlas of Tumor Pathology: Tumors of the Ovary, Maldeveloped Gonads, Fallopian Tube, and Broad Ligament, 3rd Series, Fascicle 23. Washington, DC, Armed Forces Institute of Pathology, 1998, pp 257-258.

Williams SD: Ovarian germ cell tumors: An update. Semin Oncol 25:407-413, 1998.

Chapman DC, Grover R, Schwartz PE: Conservative management of an ovarian polyembryoma. Obstet Gynecol 83:879-882, 1994.

Choriocarcinoma

Clinical Features

  ● Pure choriocarcinoma is rare; occurs in children and young adults
  ● Presents with an adnexal mass, pain, and sometimes hemoperitoneum

Figure 12-63. Primary ovarian choriocarcinoma. Both components are present: cytotrophoblast and syncytiotrophoblast.

- Serum levels of HCG are elevated, manifesting as isosexual precocious puberty in children and as signs of ectopic pregnancy in adults

Gross Pathology

- Unilateral solid, gray-white hemorrhagic tumor, sometimes with necrosis
- Depends on other germ cell components

Histopathology

- Most are a component of a mixed germ cell tumor and characterized by a mixture of cytotrophoblast and syncytiotrophoblast
- Cytotrophoblastic cells placed centrally within the tumor surrounded by syncytiotrophoblastic cells, frequently with associated hemorrhage
- Mononucleate cytotrophoblasts show clear cytoplasm and obvious cell borders; small, centrally located, round, hyperchromatic vesicular nuclei with prominent nucleoli
- Multinucleate syncytiotrophoblastic cells are large and basophilic with vacuolated cytoplasm and many hyperchromatic nuclei

Special Stains and Immunohistochemistry

- HCG, PLAP highlight syncytiotrophoblastic cells
- Cytokeratin highlights cytotrophoblastic and syncytiotrophoblastic cells
- Human placental lactogen (HPL) highlights syncytiotrophoblastic cells
- HCG highlights cytotrophoblasts

Other Techniques for Diagnosis

- Noncontributory

Differential Diagnosis

▌ Embryonal carcinoma
- Isolated syncytiotrophoblastic cells may be present
- Pleomorphic cells of embryonal carcinoma have large nuclei with irregular chromatin; these cells are positive only for cytokeratin

▌ Dysgerminoma
- Isolated syncytiotrophoblastic cells may be present
- Uniform round cells with abundant clear cytoplasm negative for cytokeratin

▌ YST
- Isolated syncytiotrophoblastic cells may be present
- Small cystic spaces formed by mononuclear cells
- YST cells are positive for AFP
- Hyaline globules and Schiller-Duval bodies may be seen

▌ Poorly differentiated surface epithelial tumors
- Solid carcinomas occurring in older women may show apparent trophoblastic differentiation, with isolated giant cells
- Immunohistochemically, this tumor may be positive for WT-1, EGFR, and cyclooxygenase-2

Pearls

- Highly malignant, spreading locally, intra-abdominally, and through lymphatics and blood vessels
- Treatment consists of surgery with chemotherapy

Selected References

Ezzat A, Raja M, Bakri Y, et al: Malignant ovarian germ cell tumours: A survival and prognostic analysis. Acta Oncol 38:455-460, 1999.

Scully RE, Young RH, Clement PB: Atlas of Tumor Pathology: Tumors of the Ovary, Maldeveloped Gonads, Fallopian Tube, and Broad Ligament, 3rd Series, Fascicle 23. Washington, DC, Armed Forces Institute of Pathology, 1998, pp 258-260.

Immature Teratoma

Clinical Features

- Rare, rapidly growing, malignant tumor presenting in childhood; peak incidence in first and second decades
- Asymptomatic until large, then symptoms are related to an abdominal or pelvic mass
- Serum AFP levels usually elevated

Gross Pathology

- Typically a unilateral tumor with a median diameter of 18 cm, showing capsular perforation in half of cases and adhesions to neighboring structures
- Predominantly solid, but frequently mixed with small fluid-filled cysts
- Sometimes composed of one or more large cysts with solid areas in the wall
- Soft, variegated cut surface often with areas of hemorrhage and necrosis
- Areas of bone, cartilage, or hair may be present

Figure 12-64. Immature teratoma. Small round blue and immature neural cells with rosettes associated with neuropil and mucinous glands.

Histopathology

- Made up of haphazardly arranged immature tissues derived from ectoderm, mesoderm, and endoderm; typically mixed with mature elements
- Ectodermal elements are mostly composed of neural tissue, including neuroepithelial rosettes and tubules, glia, and neuroblastic tissue
- Mesodermal elements include cartilage, muscle, and immature mesenchyme
- Endodermal elements usually consist of tubules lined by columnar epithelium
- Important to sample all teratomas extensively for histologic grading, with neuroectodermal tissue being by far the most common immature tissue identified
  — Grade 0: all tissues mature; no mitotic activity
  — Grade 1: minor foci of abnormally cellular or immature tissue mixed with mature elements; slight mitotic activity
  — Grade 2: moderate quantities of immature tissue mixed with mature elements; moderate mitotic activity
  — Grade 3: large quantities of immature tissue; high mitotic activity
- A two-tier grading system is also used (low versus high)

Stains and Immunohistochemistry

- Neural markers, including chromogranin and synaptophysin; GAFP and S-100 protein highlight neuroectodermal tissue

Other Techniques for Diagnosis

- Noncontributory

Differential Diagnosis

▌ Mature solid teratoma
- Thorough sampling should be performed to exclude immature elements

▌ Malignant mixed mesodermal tumor
- Occurs in postmenopausal women; peak incidence between the ages of 50 and 70 years
- Composed of typical carcinomatous and sarcomatous cells

▌ Primitive neuroectodermal tumor (PNET)
- Resemble PNETs seen in the central nervous system
- Peak incidence in second to fourth decades; hormonal manifestations
- Average diameter 14 cm

Pearls

- Mature cystic teratoma (dermoid cyst) may exist simultaneously in the contralateral ovary
- Spreads most commonly through peritoneal implantation, less commonly through lymphatics to retroperitoneal, para-aortic, and distant lymph nodes, and only rarely hematogenously to lungs, liver, and other organs

- Histologic grading is helpful in determining treatment and prognosis
- Poor prognosis for higher-grade tumors (grade 2 or 3), with treatment consisting of surgery and chemotherapy

Selected References

McCluggage WG: Ovarian neoplasms composed of small round cells: A review. Adv Anat Pathol 11:288-296, 2004.

Ulbright TM: Gonadal teratomas: A review and speculation. Adv Anat Pathol 11:10-23, 2004.

Cushing B, Giller R, Ablin A, et al: Surgical resection alone is effective treatment for ovarian immature teratoma in children and adolescents: A report of the pediatric oncology group and the children's cancer group. Am J Obstet Gynecol 181:353-358, 1999.

Heifetz SA, Cushing B, Giller R, et al: Immature teratomas in children. Pathologic considerations: A report from the combined Pediatric Oncology Group/Children's Cancer Group. Am J Surg Pathol 22:1115-1124, 1998.

Bezuidenhout J, Schneider JW, Hugo F, Wessels G: Teratomas in infancy and childhood at Tygerberg Hospital, South Africa, 1973 to 1992. Arch Pathol Lab Med 121:499-502, 1997.

Kojs Z, Urbanski K, Reinfuss M, et al: Pure immature teratoma of the ovary: Analysis of 22 cases. Eur J Gynaecol Oncol 18:534-536, 1997.

O'Connor DM, Norris HJ: The influence of grade on the outcome of stage I ovarian immature (malignant) teratomas: the reproducibility of grading. Int J Gynecol Pathol 13:283, 1994.

Monodermal Teratomas: Struma Ovarii

Clinical Features

- Occurs most commonly during the reproductive years and is usually asymptomatic
- Some patients may present with a painful mass, swelling, or ascites; uterine bleeding has been reported
- Occasionally associated with thyrotoxicosis and thyroid enlargement

Gross Pathology

- Typically unilateral, less than 10 cm in diameter, and smooth surfaced
- Solid, brown or green-brown, glistening tissue separated by fibrous septa, with or without an associated mature cystic teratoma
- Fluid-filled cysts containing brown to green gelatinous fluid
- Hemorrhage, necrosis, and fibrosis reported

Histopathology

- Composed solely or predominantly of mature thyroid tissue or adenoma with small and large follicles lined by a layer of columnar, cuboidal, or flattened epithelium

Figure 12-65. A, Struma ovarii. The neoplasm shows small papillary projections similar to those in hyperactive thyroid tissue. **B, Carcinoid tumor.** Trabecular pattern composed of long cords of neuroendocrine tumor cells surrounded by dense collagenous stroma.

- Follicles with colloid mixed with solid, cellular areas and sometimes cysts
- Thyroid adenoma includes oxyphilic, clear cell, and solid tubular forms
- May show changes similar to that of the thyroid gland, including hyperplasia, or thyroiditis
- Carcinoma is rare

Special Stains and Immunohistochemistry

- PAS highlights colloid
- Thyroglobulin highlights thyroglobulin in the struma component

Other Techniques for Diagnosis

- Noncontributory

Differential Diagnosis

▌ Mucinous cystic tumor
  - Cyst contents is usually colorless gelatinous material; cystic struma ovarii may contain green-brown gelatinous fluid
  - Cyst is lined by mucinous epithelium with abundant intracytoplasmic mucin

▌ Serous cystadenoma
  - Struma ovarii may rarely take the form of a unilocular, thin-walled cyst containing watery fluid; always contains at least one recognizable thyroid follicle

▌ Steroid cell tumors
  - May be confused with an oxyphilic thyroid adenoma, but no thyroid follicles are present
  - Struma ovarii shows calcium oxalate crystals and immunoreactivity for thyroglobulin

▌ Sertoli cell tumor
  - May be mistaken for a solid tubular adenoma
  - Struma ovarii shows true thyroid follicles and calcium oxalate crystals and immunoreactivity for thyroglobulin

Pearls

- Thyroid tissue is commonly found as a component of mature cystic teratoma
- Regarded as a teratoma with an exclusively or mainly thyroid tissue component
- Generally benign and treated with surgical excision
- Infrequently complicated by ascites, adhesions, or malignant change with metastases

Selected References

Roth LM, Miller AW 3rd, Talerman A: Typical thyroid-type carcinoma arising in struma ovarii: A report of 4 cases and review of the literature. Int J Gynecol Pathol 27:496-506, 2008.

Roth LM, Talerman A: The enigma of struma ovarii. Pathology 39:139-146, 2007.

Papadias K, Kairi-Vassilatou E, Kontogiani-Katsaros K, et al: Teratomas of the ovary: A clinico-pathological evaluation of 87 patients from one institution during a 10-year period. Eur J Gynaecol Oncol 26:446-448, 2005.

Scully RE, Young RH, Clement PB: Atlas of Tumor Pathology: Tumors of the Ovary, Maldeveloped Gonads, Fallopian Tube, and Broad Ligament, 3rd Series, Fascicle 23. Washington, DC, Armed Forces Institute of Pathology, 1998, pp 285-291.

Monodermal Teratomas: Carcinoid Tumor

Clinical Features

- Primary carcinoid tumors of the ovary are associated with other teratomatous elements in 85% to 90% of cases
- Most commonly an insular carcinoid; age range from 30 to 80 years
- Occasional presentation with carcinoid syndrome; more often with older patients
- Carcinoid syndrome consists of flushing, diarrhea, abdominal cramping, and often, cardiac involvement
- Elevated urinary 5-hydroxyindole acetic acid (5-HIAA)

Gross Pathology

- Unilateral yellow-tan, small nodular neoplasm projecting into a dermoid cyst
- Less often found in a mucinous cystic tumor or mature solid teratoma
- Can predominate as a large, firm, homogeneous mass

Histopathology

- Insular carcinoid resembles a midgut carcinoid with discrete groups of small uniform cells separated by fibrous stroma
- Cells are uniform with abundant cytoplasm, nuclei with coarse chromatin, and rare mitoses; most are associated with other teratomatous components
- Variants also include trabecular, strumal, and goblet cell

Special Stains and Immunohistochemistry

- Chromogranin, synaptophysin, and NSE positive

Other Techniques for Diagnosis

- Noncontributory

Differential Diagnosis

▮ Granulosa cell tumor (microfollicular pattern)
- Mimics insular carcinoid showing round to oval cells with pale cytoplasm and round, often grooved nuclei; neuroendocrine markers are negative
- Mitotic activity is generally higher in carcinoid tumors

Pearls

- Tumor usually confined to the ovary
- Strumal carcinoid consists of a combination of thyroid and carcinoid components

Selected References

Athavale RD, Davies-Humphreys JD, Cruickshank DJ: Primary carcinoid tumours of the ovary. J Obstet Gynaecol 24:99-101, 2004.

Soga J, Osaka M, Yakuwa Y: Carcinoids of the ovary: An analysis of 329 reported cases. J Exp Clin Cancer Res 19:271-280, 2000.

Scully RE, Young RH, Clement PB: Atlas of Tumor Pathology: Tumors of the Ovary, Maldeveloped Gonads, Fallopian Tube, and Broad Ligament, 3rd Series, Fascicle 23. Washington, DC, Armed Forces Institute of Pathology, 1998, pp 291-300.

Mixed Malignant Germ Cell Tumors

Clinical Features

- Mixture of two or more germ cell tumors with their characteristic morphologies

Gross Pathology

- Tumor needs to be sampled extensively, especially in hemorrhagic, necrotic areas and distinct-appearing foci, to identify all the components

Figure 12-66. Mixed germ cell tumor. A mixture of choriocarcinoma and embryonal carcinoma components is evident.

Histopathology

- Patterns described for each separate germ cell tumor may be combined in different variations and amounts in one tumor
- Usually two components: most often dysgerminoma and YST, or dysgerminoma combined with other germ cell neoplasms
- Other tumors typically have between three and five types present

Special Stains and Immunohistochemistry

- See specific tumor types

Other Techniques for Diagnosis

- Noncontributory

Differential Diagnosis

▮ Gynandroblastoma
- Extremely rare
- Granulosa cell tumor component present, representing more than 10% of tumor volume

▮ Gonadoblastoma
- Occurs in phenotypic women with gonadal dysgenesis
- Sex cord–stromal tumor elements also present

▮ Metastatic carcinoma
- Clinical history is of extreme importance
- Lacks histologic features of germ cell tumors and is characterized by glands and sheets of malignant epithelial cells
- Negative for AFP, PLAP, HPL, and HCG

Pearls

- Tumor must be sampled extensively; each component and its quantity needs to be mentioned in the diagnosis in descending order of prevalence
- Prognosis may depend on quantity of most aggressive component

Selected References

Tewari K, Cappuccini F, Disaia PJ, et al: Malignant germ cell tumors of the ovary. Obstet Gynecol 95:128-133, 2000.

Akahira J, Ito K, Kosuge S, et al: Ovarian mixed germ cell tumor composed of dysgerminoma, endodermal sinus tumor, choriocarcinoma and mature teratoma in a 44-year-old woman: Case report and literature review. Pathol Int 48:471-474, 1998.

Scully RE, Young RH, Clement PB: Atlas of Tumor Pathology: Tumors of the Ovary, Maldeveloped Gonads, Fallopian Tube, and Broad Ligament, 3rd Series, Fascicle 23. Washington, DC, Armed Forces Institute of Pathology, 1998, pp 260-262.

Other Tumors

Gonadoblastoma

Clinical Features

- Mixed germ cell and sex cord–stromal tumor affect children and young adults
- Almost always found in phenotypic women with an underlying gonadal disorder
  — Usually 46XY pure gonadal dysgenesis or mixed gonadal dysgenesis
  — Often associated with 45X or 46XY karyotype
- Presentation may include signs of virilization
- Can occur in phenotypic male or normal women with a history of pregnancy

Gross Pathology

- Solid, slightly lobulated, and often speckled with calcifications or totally calcified
- Brown, yellow, or gray ranging from a microscopic lesion to 8 cm in diameter, and frequently bilateral
- Large tumors usually show dysgerminoma overgrowth
- Gonad may be of uncertain nature: abdominal or inguinal testis, or a gonadal streak

Figure 12-67. Gonadoblastoma. Low-power view shows solid nests of tumor cells surrounded by thin connective tissue stroma.

Histopathology

- Germ cell or cells of sex cord–stromal differentiation arranged in nests; cells surround amorphous eosinophilic material (hyaline)
- Large germ cells resembling dysgerminoma and seminoma, immature testicular germ cells, or spermatogonia
- Malignant cells contain vesicular nuclei with finely granular chromatin and prominent nucleoli and mitotic activity
- Epithelial cells of sex cord–stromal origin resemble immature Sertoli or granulosa cells: small, uniform, round or elongated cells, with scanty cytoplasm and pale nuclei; mitotically inactive
- Cells resembling lutein or Leydig cells are identified in the stroma between nests
- May show foci of calcification, hyalinization, or overgrowth by a malignant germ cell neoplasm (usually dysgerminoma)

Special Stains and Immunohistochemistry

- Noncontributory

Other Techniques for Diagnosis

- Noncontributory

Differential Diagnosis

▌ Dysgerminoma
- In patients with gonadal dysgenesis and a Y chromosome, gonadoblastoma is always a possibility
- Gonadoblastoma within dysgerminoma may appear as a small focus of calcification or a nest of typical gonadoblastoma

▌ Sex cord tumor with annular tubules
- Steroid cell tumor characterized by simple and complex annular tubules encircling hyaline material with few mitotic figures; lacks a germ cell component
- Tumors associated with PJS may show focal calcification of the tubules

Pearls

- Patient may have a malignant germ cell neoplasm in the contralateral ovary

Selected References

Pauls K, Franke FE, Büttner R, Zhou H: Gonadoblastoma: Evidence for a stepwise progression to dysgerminoma in a dysgenetic ovary. Virchows Arch 447:603-609, 2005.

Gibbons B, Tan SY, Yu CC, et al: Risk of gonadoblastoma in female patients with Y chromosome abnormalities and dysgenetic gonads. J Paediatr Child Health 35:210-213, 1999.

Scully RE, Young RH, Clement PB: Atlas of Tumor Pathology: Tumors of the Ovary, Maldeveloped Gonads, Fallopian Tube, and Broad Ligament, 3rd Series, Fascicle 23. Washington, DC, Armed Forces Institute of Pathology, 1998, pp 307-310.

Iezzoni JC, Von Kap-Herr C, Golden WL, Gaffey MJ: Gonadoblastomas in 45,X/46,XY mosaicism: Analysis of Y chromosome distribution by fluorescence in situ hybridization. Am J Clin Pathol 108:197-201, 1997.

Hypercalcemic Small Cell Carcinoma

Clinical Features

- Hypercalcemic small cell carcinoma (HSCC) is most associated with paraendocrine hypercalcemia
- Occurs predominantly in young patients; peak incidence in second decade

Gross Pathology

- Unilateral, fleshy, solid, cream-colored to pale-yellow–gray tumor
- Frequent hemorrhage and necrosis, cystic degeneration, and focal softening

Histopathology

- Sheets, nests, and cords of small round cells with sparse cytoplasm
- Large cells are often present displaying hyperchromatic nuclei with one or two small nucleoli and abundant eosinophilic cytoplasm
- Brisk mitotic rate, necrosis, and occasional intracytoplasmic eosinophilic globules
- Small follicle-like structures containing eosinophilic material may be present
- Some tumors contain mucinous epithelium or focal mucin production

Special Stains and Immunohistochemistry

- Generally noncontributory
- Undifferentiated tumor negative for neuroendocrine markers, inhibin, and CEA

Other Techniques for Diagnosis

- Noncontributory

Figure 12-68. Small cell carcinoma. Solid proliferation of neoplastic cells with a fine chromatin pattern and scanty cytoplasm.

Differential Diagnosis

▮ Granulosa cell tumor (adult)
- Older age group (AGCT); frequently produces estrogens and not hypercalcemic
- Uniform cells forming Call-Exner bodies with much lower mitotic rate
- Less hyperchromatic cells sometimes with grooved nuclei (AGCT)
- Much lower rate of extraovarian spread

▮ Lymphoma
- Lymphoma with an unusual insular or follicular pattern may mimic
- Diffuse HSCC may resemble malignant lymphoma
- Different immunohistochemical profile (CD45, B-cell markers, or T-cell markers positive)

Pearls

- Rarely familial
- Extraovarian spread often present and poor prognosis

Selected References

Lindboe CF: Large cell neuroendocrine carcinoma of the ovary. APMIS 115:169-176, 2007.

Mebis J, De Raeve H, Baekelandt M, et al: Primary ovarian small cell carcinoma of the pulmonary type: A case report and review of the literature. Eur J Gynaecol Oncol 25:239-241, 2004.

Hamilton S, Beattie GJ, Williams AR: Small cell carcinoma of the ovary: A report of three cases and review of the literature. J Obstet Gynaecol 24:169-172, 2004.

Seidman JD: Small cell carcinoma of the ovary of the hypercalcemic type: p53 protein accumulation and clinicopathologic features. Gynecol Oncol 59:283-287, 1995.

Young RH, Oliva E, Scully RE: Small cell carcinoma of the hypercalcemic type in the ovary. Gynecol Oncol 57:7-8, 1995.

Young RH, Oliva E, Scully RE: Small cell carcinoma of the ovary, hypercalcemic type: A clinicopathological analysis of 150 cases. Am J Surg Pathol 18:1102-1116, 1994.

Metastatic Tumors

Clinical Features

- Ovarian masses are metastatic tumors in less than 10% of cases
- Most common primary sites are gynecologic tract, large intestine, stomach, and breast carcinomas
- *Krukenberg tumor* originally referred to gastric carcinomas metastatic to the ovaries; currently it refers to cancers with signet ring cells of any origin

Gross Pathology

- Ill-defined, occasionally mucinous masses that are bilateral in about 70% of cases
- Hematogenous spread is an important factor, but transcoelomic dissemination, direct extension, and lymphatics also play a role

Figure 12-69. A, Metastatic gastric carcinoma, signet ring cell type. Cut surface shows the tumor replacing almost the entire ovarian stroma. A multinodular gelatinous tumor with cystic change is evident. **B, Krukenberg tumor.** Tumor cells are infiltrating the ovarian stroma. Notice the signet ring nature of the cells.

- Solitary or multiple discrete nodules and surface tumor deposits
- Predominantly solid, but may form one or more cysts

Histopathology

- Tumor on the surface, often with a desmoplastic stroma, multiple nodules, and blood or lymph vessel invasion and morphology different from that of primary ovarian tumors
- Usually adenocarcinoma
- Krukenberg tumors may completely replace the ovarian parenchyma with signet ring cells and glandular structures

Special Stains and Immunohistochemistry

- See specific tumors
- Mucin positive in Krukenberg tumors and other types of mucin-producing carcinomas (e.g., intestinal, pancreatic, and occasionally breast)

Other Techniques for Diagnosis

- See specific tumors

Differential Diagnosis

- Clinical history is most important
- Metastatic tumors usually involve the cortex and the hilum of the ovary
- Histochemical and immunohistochemical stains as per suspected site of origin
- Primary mucinous adenocarcinoma versus Krukenberg tumor
  - Primary mucinous adenocarcinomas are typically unilateral with rare signet ring cells in the stroma, as opposed to Krukenberg tumors, which are bilateral in more than 70% of patients and essentially composed of signet ring cells
  - This differential is often challenging in the absence of clinical history

Pearls

- May also include appendiceal carcinoid and pancreatic tumors as well as small cell carcinoma, malignant melanoma, malignant lymphoma, and leukemia
- Relevant clinical history, search for primary tumor elsewhere, and careful gross and histologic examination are important in the diagnosis of metastatic tumors

Selected References

Khunamornpong S, Lerwill MF, Siriaunkgul S, et al: Carcinoma of extrahepatic bile ducts and gallbladder metastatic to the ovary: A report of 16 cases. Int J Gynecol Pathol 27:366-379, 2008.

Yemelyanova AV, Vang R, Judson K, et al: Distinction of primary and metastatic mucinous tumors involving the ovary: analysis of size and laterality data by primary site with reevaluation of an algorithm for tumor classification. Am J Surg Pathol 32:128-138, 2008.

Young RH: From Krukenberg to today: The ever present problems posed by metastatic tumors in the ovary. Part I. Historical perspective, general principles, mucinous tumors including the Krukenberg tumor. Adv Anat Pathol 13:205-227, 2006.

Hart WR: Diagnostic challenge of secondary (metastatic) ovarian tumors simulating primary endometrioid and mucinous neoplasms. Pathol Int 55:231-243, 2005.

Scully RE, Young RH, Clement PB: Atlas of Tumor Pathology: Tumors of the Ovary, Maldeveloped Gonads, Fallopian Tube, and Broad Ligament, 3rd Series, Fascicle 23. Washington, DC, Armed Forces Institute of Pathology, 1998, pp 335-372.

Fallopian Tube

Tumor-like Lesions

Acute and Chronic Salpingitis

Clinical Features

- Young and middle-aged women who may present with acute abdomen
- Considered an ascending infection that may result in infertility
- Culprits: *Chlamydia* species or *Neisseria gonorrhoeae* followed by polymicrobial infection
- Less commonly associated with curettage or IUD placement
- Granulomatous salpingitis may be caused by tuberculosis, parasitosis, actinomycosis, or even systemic diseases such as Crohn disease and sarcoidosis

Gross Pathology

- Acute: tubal lumen distended by pus and secretions
- Massive hemorrhage may result in hemosalpinx
- Chronic: fibrotic tubal wall with adhesions

Histopathology

- Acute
  - Marked acute inflammation in plicae and tubal wall, fibrinous adhesions with congestion and edema
  - Pyosalpinx: mucosal ulceration with purulent exudate within lumen
  - Hematosalpinx: blood-filled lumen resulting from massive hemorrhage
- Chronic
  - Lymphoplasmacytic infiltrate in plicae and paratubal fibrous adhesions
  - Lymphofollicular hyperplasia suggests chlamydial infection
- Granulomatous
  - Caseating granulomas (tuberculosis) or noncaseating granulomas, such as sarcoidosis
- End stage
  - Hydrosalpinx: thinned wall with clear hypocellular fluid in the lumen

Special Stains and Immunohistochemistry

- Gram stain may identify bacterial organisms
- Fite stain may identify mycobacteria in necrotizing granulomatous salpingitis

Other Techniques for Diagnosis

- Noncontributory

Differential Diagnosis

▌ Ectopic pregnancy
- Particularly when hemosalpinx is present and serum HCG is elevated

Figure 12-70. A, Acute salpingitis. Cross section shows a dilated fallopian tube containing purulent material. **B, Acute salpingitis.** Marked neutrophilic exudate in the tubal mucosa. The lumen also contains inflammatory exudate material. **C, Granulomatous salpingitis (tuberculous salpingitis).** Multiple granulomas and multinucleate giant cells are present (*center*).

- Immature villi or trophoblasts in clotted blood or tubal lumen
- Clinically may present as acute abdomen; clinical differential diagnosis includes PID and acute appendicitis
- May result in infertility

Selected References

Obermair A, Taylor KH, Janda M, et al: Primary fallopian tube carcinoma: The Queensland experience. Int J Gynecol Cancer 11:69-72, 2001.

Aziz S, Kuperstein G, Rosen B, et al: A genetic epidemiological study of carcinoma of the fallopian tube. Gynecol Oncol 80:341-345, 2001.

Endometriosis

Clinical Features

- Tube is frequently involved; other organs may also be affected
- Generally occurs in women of reproductive age and is associated with infertility
- May also occur after tubal ligation (*postsalpingectomy endometriosis*)

Gross Pathology

- Serosal nodules or dark areas of discoloration

Histopathology

- Identical to the morphology previously described in the ovary
- In postsalpingectomy endometriosis, the endometrial glands with stroma extend from the mucosal surface into the wall at the site of the proximal stump

Special Stains and Immunohistochemistry

- CD10 highlights endometrial stroma

Other Techniques for Diagnosis

- Noncontributory

Differential Diagnosis

- Physiologic extension of endometrial tissue into the fallopian tube
  - Endometrial glands with stroma replace mucosa of isthmic portion of tube

Figure 12-71. Endometriosis of the fallopian tube. The tubal wall contains endometrial glands and stroma.

- May fill lumen, resulting in occlusion of tube (endometrial colonization)
- Salpingitis isthmica nodosa
  - Dilated spaces lined by ciliated tubal epithelium (nonendometrial) within the thickened wall of the fallopian tube (similar to colonic diverticula)
- Metastatic adenocarcinoma
  - Glands are malignant
  - Absent endometrial stroma around glands

Pearls

- Fallopian tube is a common site of endometriosis
- Serosal and subserosal process, which also involves other pelvic organs
- Must be differentiated from physiologic extension of endometrium (mucosal replacement)

Selected References

Scully RE, Young RH, Clement PB: Atlas of Tumor Pathology: Tumors of the Ovary, Maldeveloped Gonads, Fallopian Tube, and Broad Ligament, 3rd Series, Fascicle 23. Washington, DC, Armed Forces Institute of Pathology, 1998, pp 477-498.

Fortier KJ, Haney AF: The pathologic spectrum of uterotubal junction obstruction. Obstet Gynecol 65:93-98, 1985.

Salpingitis Isthmica Nodosa

Clinical Features

- Most common in young women in the third or fourth decade
- Predisposes to ectopic pregnancy and is associated with infertility
- Pathogenesis is unclear

Gross Pathology

- Often bilateral
- Fallopian tubes display an intact serosal surface
- Isthmic nodules (1 to 2 cm) in the wall of the fallopian tube

Histopathology

- Outpouchings of tubal epithelium in the thickened muscle wall of the fallopian tube
- Small nests or cysts with tubal epithelium lining spaces surrounded by a muscle coat

Special Stains and Immunohistochemistry

- Noncontributory

Other Techniques for Diagnosis

- Noncontributory

Differential Diagnosis

- Endometriosis
  - Classic microscopic features as previously described in the ovary

- Glands tightly cuffed by endometrial stroma (not muscle coat)
- Generally present over serosal surface; no connection of glands to tubular lumen
▌ Metastatic adenocarcinoma
  - Glands are malignant
  - No ciliated epithelial lining
  - Desmoplastic or inflammatory stromal response dissecting muscle fibers

Pearls

- Salpingitis isthmica nodosa is analogous to adenomyosis in the uterus
- Unclear pathogenesis but associated with infertility and ectopic pregnancy
- Glands have been shown to connect to tubal lumen

Selected References

Scully RE, Young RH, Clement PB: Atlas of Tumor Pathology: Tumors of the Ovary, Maldeveloped Gonads, Fallopian Tube, and Broad Ligament, 3rd Series, Fascicle 23. Washington, DC, Armed Forces Institute of Pathology, 1998, pp 477-498.

Majmudar B, Henderson PH, Semple E: Salpingitis isthmica nodosa: A high-risk factor for tubal pregnancy. Obstet Gynecol 62:73-78, 1983.

Tubal Ectopic Pregnancy

Clinical Features

- 1% to 2% of all conceptions are ectopic; fallopian tube is the most common site
- Number one risk factor is chronic salpingitis (35% to 45% have a history of PID)
- Other risk factors include congenital tubal anomalies, salpingitis isthmica nodosa, and endometriosis
- Often patients present emergently with tubal rupture and hemorrhagic shock
- Elevated serum HCG
- Ultrasound examination may identify the gestational sac

Gross Pathology

- Most commonly ampullary, although it may occur in isthmus or fimbriated end
- Blood-filled dilated lumen with chorionic villi that may be identified grossly
- Most cases contain at least one embryo

Histopathology

- Intermediate trophoblasts in tubal wall and vessels
- Syncytiotrophoblasts are present
- Lamina propria often shows decidual change
- Chorionic villi may invade muscularis and then serosa

Figure 12-72. Tubal pregnancy. A, Cut surface shows a well-formed embryo. **B,** The lamina propria shows decidual changes. **C,** Histologic section of a tubal pregnancy shows a 7- to 10-day-old embryo (*right side*).

- Microscopically identifiable embryo in many cases
- Atherosclerotic changes in tubal vessels
- Uterine curettage shows gestational change, including Arias-Stella reaction and decidualization, but no chorionic villi or trophoblasts

— Arias-Stella reaction: due to gestational-hormonal effect on the endometrium featuring hypersecretory endometrial glands with complex architecture, hobnail cells, and nuclear atypia

Special Stains and Immunohistochemistry

- Cytokeratin positive in trophoblasts
- HPL positive in intermediate trophoblasts
- HCG positive in syncytiotrophoblasts

Other Techniques for Diagnosis

- Noncontributory

Differential Diagnosis

▌ Missed abortion of intrauterine pregnancy
- Absent chorionic villi, trophoblasts, or embryonic tissue
▌ Placental site trophoblastic tumor (PSTT)
- Absent chorionic villi or embryonic tissue

Pearls

- Commonly associated with PID
- Patients often present emergently with hemorrhagic shock after tubal rupture
- Hematosalpinx results from rupture of maternal vessels
- An embryo is often present; the most common outcome is abortion

Selected References

Scully RE, Young RH, Clement PB: Atlas of Tumor Pathology: Tumors of the Ovary, Maldeveloped Gonads, Fallopian Tube, and Broad Ligament, 3rd Series, Fascicle 23. Washington, DC, Armed Forces Institute of Pathology, 1998, pp 493-498.

Jacques SM, Qureshi F, Ramirez NC, Lawrence WD: Retained trophoblastic tissue in fallopian tubes: A consequence of unsuspected ectopic pregnancies. Int J Gynecol Pathol 16:219-224, 1997.

Benign Tumors

Adenomatoid Tumor

Clinical Features

- Most common benign neoplasm of the fallopian tube
- Usually occurs in adult women and often asymptomatic

Gross Pathology

- Well-circumscribed, 1- to 2-cm, firm, yellow-gray nodule within the muscle wall
- Most often unilateral

Histopathology

- As previously described in the uterus
- Adenomatoid and glandular patterns are most common
- Solid and cystic patterns are less common

Figure 12-73. Adenomatoid tumor. Tumor composed of small slitlike spaces lined by cuboidal epithelium.

- Luminal spaces may contain acid mucin
- Hyperplasia of surrounding smooth muscle

Special Stains and Immunohistochemistry

- Cytokeratin, vimentin, EMA positive
- Mucicarmine, CD31, CEA negative
- SMA positive in the surrounding smooth muscle

Other Techniques for Diagnosis

- Electron microscopy: features of mesothelial cells, including long slender microvilli, intracellular lumina, and intracytoplasmic filaments in bundles

Differential Diagnosis

▌ Lymphangioma
- Positive for D2-40, CD31, and factor VIII; negative for cytokeratin
▌ Leiomyoma
- As described in the uterus
▌ Malignant mesothelioma
- Poorly circumscribed tumor with cytologic atypia and mitosis; rare
▌ Metastatic adenocarcinoma
- Most likely from a gynecologic primary; extremely rare from extrapelvic organs
▌ Invasive primary adenocarcinoma
- Rare; tumor originates in the mucosa and extends through the wall

Pearls

- Arises from the peritoneal mesothelium and is essentially a benign mesothelioma
- May represent a nodular reactive mesothelial hyperplasia

Selected Reference

Scully RE, Young RH, Clement PB: Atlas of Tumor Pathology: Tumors of the Ovary, Maldeveloped Gonads, Fallopian Tube, and Broad Ligament, 3rd Series, Fascicle 23. Washington, DC, Armed Forces Institute of Pathology, 1998, pp 477-480.

Other Benign Tumors

Clinical Features

- Mostly incidental findings; the most common is epithelial papilloma
- Most common benign mesenchymal tumor is leiomyoma
- Other epithelial, stromal, or neural tumors are extremely rare

Gross Pathology

- Epithelial tumors: small papillary or cystic mucosal lesions
- Mesenchymal tumors: small, well-circumscribed intramural nodules

Histopathology

- Epithelial papilloma: branching fibrovascular stalk lined by a single layer of benign nonciliated columnar or oncocytic epithelial cells
- Other tumors show identical morphology to their counterparts in other sites

Special Stains and Immunohistochemistry

- Noncontributory

Other Techniques for Diagnosis

- Noncontributory

Differential Diagnosis

❚ Adenomatous hyperplasia
- Rare preneoplastic process showing epithelial cell stratification and crowding with loss of polarity, cytologic atypia, and occasional mitoses
❚ Metastatic adenocarcinoma
- Patients have history of a primary malignant tumor elsewhere

Figure 12-74. Epithelial papilloma. Papillary lesion lined by a single layer of uniform, nonciliated columnar cells.

Pearls

- Generally benign tumors are incidental findings of no clinical significance

Selected References

Bartnik J, Powell WS, Moriber-Katz S, Amenta PS: Metaplastic papillary tumor of the fallopian tube: Case report, immunohistochemical features, and review of the literature. Arch Pathol Lab Med 113:545-547, 1989.

Doleris A, Macrez F: Endosalpingeal papillomas. Gynecology 3:289-308, 1988.

Keeney GL, Thrasher TV: Metaplastic papillary tumor of the fallopian tube: A case report with ultrastructure. Int J Gynecol Pathol 7:86-92, 1988.

Gisser SD: Obstructing fallopian tube papilloma. Int J Gynecol Pathol 5:179-182, 1986.

Malignant Tumors

Carcinoma

Clinical Features

- Rare, occurring in the sixth and seventh decades, and frequently bilateral
- May present with vaginal bleeding, clear discharge, pelvic pain, or pelvic mass
- Almost always invasive at time of diagnosis.
- Serum CA-125 may be elevated

Gross Pathology

- Swollen tube filled and distended by solid and papillary tumor
- Bulk of the tumor is within the tube

Histopathology

- CIS
  - Papillary proliferation of atypical tubal epithelial cells with large, stratified, pleomorphic nuclei, clumped chromatin, irregular nuclear membranes with loss of polarity, and high mitotic activity
  - A transitional area between benign and malignant epithelium may be identified
- Invasive adenocarcinoma
  - Most common type is serous carcinoma histologically identical to ovarian counterpart
  - Less common types include mucinous, endometrioid, and clear cell

Special Stains and Immunohistochemistry

- As per ovarian counterparts

Other Techniques for Diagnosis

- Noncontributory

Differential Diagnosis

❚ Metastatic carcinoma
- Overwhelmingly more common than primary fallopian tube malignancies

Figure 12-75. A, Serous carcinoma of the fallopian tube. Cut surface of an engorged fallopian tube filled with tan to yellow tumor with central hemorrhage and necrosis. Adjacent paratubal cyst and atrophic ovary. **B, Papillary serous carcinoma.** The papillary tumor shows cellular pleomorphism and marked nuclear stratification. Invasion of the lamina propria is present in other areas of the lesion.

- Presence of tubal CIS supports the diagnosis of primary tubal malignancy
- Clinical history is most helpful
▎ Benign tubal epithelial tumors
- Absence of cytologic atypia and mitotic activity

Pearls

- Primary cancers of the fallopian tube are rare and have a poor prognosis
- Morphologically, they resemble their ovarian counterparts
- Serous cancer is the most common
- Dysplastic epithelium adjacent to areas of outright malignancy is helpful

Selected References

Callahan MJ, Crum CP, Medeiros F, et al: Primary fallopian tube malignancies in BRCA-positive women undergoing surgery for ovarian cancer risk reduction. J Clin Oncol 1:3985-3990, 2007.

Medeiros F, Muto MG, Lee Y, et al: The tubal fimbria is a preferred site for early adenocarcinoma in women with familial ovarian cancer syndrome. Am J Surg Pathol 30:230-236, 2006.

Alvarado-Cabrero I, Young R, Vamvakas E, Scully R: Carcinoma of the fallopian tube: A clinicopathological study of 105 cases with observations on staging and prognostic factors. Gynecol Oncol 72:367-379, 1999.

Sarcomas and Mixed Tumors

- Leiomyosarcoma, although rare, is the most common sarcoma of the fallopian tube
- Carcinosarcoma, which is extremely rare, may arise in the fallopian tube

Selected References

Buchwalter CL, Jenison EL, Fromm M, et al: Pure embryonal rhabdomyosarcoma of the fallopian tube. Gynecol Oncol 67:95-101, 1997.

Hellstrom A, Auer G, Silversward C, Pettersson F: Malignant mixed müllerian tumor of the fallopian tube: The Radiumhemmett series, 1923-1993. Int J Gynecol 5(Suppl):68-73, 1995.

Carlson JA, Ackerman BL, Wheeler JE: Malignant mixed müllerian tumor of the fallopian tube. Cancer 71:187-192, 1993.

Metastatic Tumors

- Overwhelmingly more common than primary fallopian tube malignancies
- Tumor metastatic to the fallopian tube usually originates within the pelvis
- Tubal involvement by lymphoma has been reported
- May extend from endometrium to mucosal surface of tube
- May invade the serosal surface by vascular space invasion or direct extension from a pelvic mass
- Presence of squamous differentiation implies metastasis; primary squamous cell carcinoma of the tube is extremely rare
- Presence of tubal in situ carcinoma suggests a diagnosis of primary tubal malignancy
- Synchronous tubal and other gynecologic organ tumors may occur
- Clinical history is essential

Selected Reference

Scully RE, Young RH, Clement PB: Atlas of Tumor Pathology: Tumors of the Ovary, Maldeveloped Gonads, Fallopian Tube, and Broad Ligament, 3rd Series, Fascicle 23. Washington, DC, Armed Forces Institute of Pathology, 1998, pp 482-484.

Gestational Trophoblastic Disease

Exaggerated Placental Site (Exaggerated Implantation Site)

Clinical Features

- Occurs during normal pregnancy or in association with abortion or hydatidiform mole

Gross Pathology

- Gestational endometrium

Histopathology

- Extensive infiltration of myometrium by intermediate trophoblast (IT) (single hyperchromatic nuclei) and some syncytiotrophoblast (ST) (multinucleated)
- Invasion of spiral arterioles by IT may be noted at implantation site; however, mitoses are rare, and chorionic villi may be present

Special Stains and Immunohistochemistry

- Cytokeratin positive
- HPL positive in intermediate trophoblasts
- HCG positive in syncytiotrophoblasts

Other Techniques for Diagnosis

- Noncontributory

Differential Diagnosis

▌ Placental site nodule
- Well-circumscribed and extensively hyalinized

▌ PSTT
- Deeply invades the myometrium
- Composed predominantly of sheets of intermediate trophoblasts with mitotic figures

▌ Choriocarcinoma
- Alternating areas of cytotrophoblasts, IT, and ST
- Vascular invasion may be prominent, and chorionic villi are absent
- May be extensively necrotic or hemorrhagic

▌ Epithelioid trophoblastic tumor
- Extremely rare
- Features markedly atypical mononucleated trophoblastic cells with a striking epithelioid appearance

Pearls

- Formerly referred to as *syncytial endometritis* or *benign chorionic invasion*
- Shows rare mitosis
- Preservation of normal uterine architecture

Selected References

Papadopoulos AJ, Foskett M, Seckl MJ, et al: Twenty-five years' clinical experience with placental site trophoblastic tumors. J Reprod Med 47:460-464, 2002.

Castrillon DH, Sun D, Weremowicz S, et al: Discrimination of complete hydatidiform mole from its mimics by immunohistochemistry of the paternally imprinted gene product p57KIP2. Am J Surg Pathol 25:1225, 2001.

Placental Site Nodule (Placental Site Plaque)

Clinical Features

- Occurs in women of reproductive age
- Often presents with abnormal bleeding or is asymptomatic
- Generally without elevation in serum HCG

Gross Pathology

- Often not grossly visible
- Single or multiple tan-yellow excrescences or nodules may be identified in the endometrium

Histopathology

- Nodules and plaques of IT and rare ST
- Round cells with hyperchromatic nuclei, irregular membranes, and rare mitotic figures
- Abundant amphophilic, eosinophilic, or vacuolated cytoplasm and extensive hyalinization
- Central collapsed vascular lumina (thought to represent hyalinized spiral arterioles)

Special Stains and Immunohistochemistry

- Cytokeratin positive
- HPL focally positive in IT
- HCG rarely positive

Other Techniques for Diagnosis

- Noncontributory

Differential Diagnosis

▌ PSTT
- Larger, poorly circumscribed, minimal hyalinization
- More cellular with brisk mitotic rate and atypical nuclei
- Deeply invades myometrium with necrosis
- Composed predominantly of IT; elevated HCG

Pearls

- Believed to represent unresorbed involuted placental site
- Benign, no treatment required even if diagnosed in curettage specimen

Selected Reference

Silverberg S, Kurman R: Atlas of Tumor Pathology: Tumors of the Uterine Corpus and Gestational Trophoblastic Disease, 3rd Series, Fascicle 3. Washington, DC, Armed Forces Institute of Pathology, 1992, pp 274-277.

Hydatidiform Mole: Complete Mole

Clinical Features

- Complete mole (CM) is the most common form of GTD; presents in second trimester
- Serum HCG continues to rise after 14 weeks of gestation instead of normal drop
- Uterus is disproportionately enlarged
- Vaginal bleeding suggests spontaneous abortion of mole
- Past history of mole increases the risk for future molar pregnancy
- Increased incidence of choriocarcinoma in patients with history of CM
- More common in Asia, Africa, and Latin America

Gross Pathology

- Grapelike clusters of vesicles corresponding to swollen villi microscopically
- Entire specimen appears involved

Histopathology

- All villi are abnormal; most are enlarged and rounded with cystic swelling
- Central cisternae, or empty spaces without vessels in the center of the villi, are readily identified
- Irregular diffuse circumferential proliferation of trophoblasts instead of normal, even, perivillous distribution
- Absence of fetal parts, including nucleated red blood cells

Special Stains and Immunohistochemistry

- HCG diffusely positive
- PLAP positive in syncytiotrophoblast
- HPL positive in intermediate trophoblast
- Positive for p53 in complete moles (owing to proliferation of cytotrophoblast)
- Focally positive for p57

Figure 12-76. A, Complete mole. Gross appearance of the villi showing marked hydropic change reminiscent of bunches of grapes. **B, Complete mole.** Villi show marked stromal edema. Trophoblast proliferation is noted. Hydropic chorionic villi devoid of blood vessels with cisternae and trophoblastic proliferation. **C, Partial mole.** Hydropic villi with cisternae and minimal trophoblast proliferation. **D, Invasive mole.** Within the myometrial wall, there are several enlarged molar villi surrounded by concentric trophoblastic proliferation.

Other Techniques for Diagnosis

- Cytogenetics: usually diploid 46XX
  — All chromosomes derived from sperm (androgenesis), hence absence of fetal parts
  — Less commonly 46XY and rarely triploid

Differential Diagnosis

▌ Partial mole
- Biphasic populations of normal and hydropic villi
- Villi with irregular, scalloped borders with few if any central cisternae
- Fetal parts (e.g., nucleated red blood cells) may be seen
- Less pronounced, more focal trophoblastic proliferation
- Triploid by cytogenetics

▌ Early nonmolar pregnancy
- Edematous villi are not apparent grossly
- Villous edema on microscopic examination is focal and mild
- Polar as opposed to circumferential trophoblastic proliferation, which lacks atypia, and rare to absent cisternae

▌ Choriocarcinoma
- Absent chorionic villi
- Myometrial and vascular invasion with necrosis

▌ PSTT
- Absence of chorionic villi in greater than 98% of cases
- Proliferation of atypical IT rather than cytotrophoblast and syncytiotrophoblast

Pearls

- About 2% of complete molar gestations are followed by choriocarcinoma
- Ten percent to 20% develop persistent GTD
- CM should be distinguished from partial moles because of the higher incidence of persistent GTD and choriocarcinoma in the former
- Therapy is complete evacuation by curettage with follow-up monitoring of serum HCG
  — Levels should be down to normal by day 60
  — If levels continue to rise, chemotherapy may be indicated

Selected References

Silverberg S, Kurman R: Atlas of Tumor Pathology: Tumors of the Uterine Corpus and Gestational Trophoblastic Disease, 3rd Series, Fascicle 3. Washington, DC, Armed Forces Institute of Pathology, 1992, pp 233-238.

Brescia RJ, Kurman RJ, Main CS, et al: Immunocytochemical localization of chorionic gonadotropin, placental lactogen, and placental alkaline phosphatase in the diagnosis of complete and partial hydatidiform moles. Int J Gynecol Pathol 6:213-229, 1987.

Fisher RA, Lawler SD, Ormerod MG, et al: Flow cytometry used to distinguish between complete and partial hydatidiform moles. Placenta 8:249-256, 1987.

Szulman A. Complete hydatidiform mole: Clinico-pathologic features. In Szulman A, Buchsbaum H (eds): Gestational Trophoblastic Disease, vol 7. New York, Springer-Verlag, 1987, pp 27-36.

Smith EB, Szulman AE, Hinshaw W, et al: Human chorionic gonadotropin levels in complete and partial hydatidiform moles and in nonmolar abortuses. Am J Obstet Gynecol 149:129-132, 1984.

Hydatidiform Mole: Partial Mole

Clinical Features

- Partial mole (PM) revealed by abnormal uterine bleeding
- Uterus is often small for gestational age
- Slightly elevated serum HCG level

Gross Pathology

- Few grapelike vesicular villi admixed with normal-appearing villi

Histopathology

- Edematous villi with irregular, scalloped borders admixed with normal-appearing villi
- Trophoblast proliferation is focal, as opposed to circumferential in CM
- Fetal vessels often contain nucleated red blood cells

Special Stains and Immunohistochemistry

- HCG strongly positive
- PLAP weakly positive (less cytotrophoblast proliferation, therefore fewer syncytiotrophoblasts)
- Weaker p53 than in complete mole (less cytotrophoblast proliferation)
- Diffuse p57 positivity

Other Techniques for Diagnosis

- Cytogenetics: most are triploid 69XXX or 69XXY (fertilization of one ovum by two sperm)

Differential Diagnosis

▌ Complete mole
- All villi are abnormal; many are hydropic
- Villi have more rounded borders with frequent central cisternae and more pronounced circumferential trophoblastic proliferation
- Absence of fetal parts
- Diploid by cytogenetics

▌ Early nonmolar pregnancy
- Villous edema is not grossly visible and is microscopically focal and mild
- Focal polar trophoblast proliferation without atypia
- Absence of scalloping of villous borders
- Generally diploid by cytogenetics

Pearls

- Fetal parts, such as nucleated red blood cells, may be identified in villous capillaries
- Less common than complete moles
- Risk for persistent GTD is 5% to 10%
- Lower to negligible risk for subsequent choriocarcinoma (1% to 3%) than for complete mole

Selected References

Genest DR: Partial hydatidiform mole: Clinicopathological features, differential diagnosis, ploidy and molecular studies, and gold standards for diagnosis. Int J Gynecol Pathol 20:315-332, 2001.

Chilosi M, Piazzola E, Lestani M, et al: Differential expression of p57kip2, a maternally imprinted cdk inhibitor, in normal human placenta and gestational trophoblastic disease. Lab Invest 78:269-276, 1998.

Paradinas FJ: The diagnosis and prognosis of molar pregnancy: The experience of the National Referral Centre in London. Int J Gynaecol Obstet 6(Suppl 1):S57-S64, 1998.

Fisher RA, Lawler SD, Ormerod MG, et al: Flow cytometry used to distinguish between complete and partial hydatidiform moles. Placenta 8:249-256, 1987.

Smith EB, Szulman AE, Hinshaw W, et al: Human chorionic gonadotropin levels in complete and partial hydatidiform moles and in nonmolar abortuses. Am J Obstet Gynecol 149:129-132, 1984.

Szulman AE, Surti U: The clinicopathologic profile of the partial hydatidiform mole. Obstet Gynecol 59:597-602, 1982.

Invasive Hydatidiform Mole

Clinical Features

- Presents with vaginal bleeding
- Uterine enlargement
- Persistently elevated HCG
- Most follow complete rather than partial molar pregnancy

Gross Pathology

- Invades the myometrium and shows irregular borders and hemorrhage
- May extend through the serosa and beyond to adnexa

Histopathology

- Abnormal chorionic villi with features of PM or CM penetrate myometrium or myometrial vascular spaces
- Proliferation of cytotrophoblastic and syncytiotrophoblastic cells
- Fetal parts are rarely identified (most arise from complete moles)

Special Stains and Immunohistochemistry

- Generally as per CM
- HCG diffusely positive
- PLAP positive in ST
- HPL positive in IT
- Positive for p53 as in CM (owing to proliferation of cytotrophoblast)

Other Techniques for Diagnosis

- Cytogenetics: usually diploid 46XX as per complete moles; triploid if invasive partial mole

Differential Diagnosis

- ▌ Noninvasive hydatidiform mole
  - Absence of hydropic villi in myometrium or vascular spaces (trophoblast may be present in myometrium as a normal occurrence)
- ▌ Placenta accreta, increta, or percreta
  - Normal villi without molar change
  - Absence of chorionic villi within the myometrium or blood vessels
- ▌ Choriocarcinoma
  - Absence of chorionic villi
  - Dimorphic population of cytotrophoblast and ST

Pearls

- Sequelae of complete moles
- Significant morbidity may result from uterine rupture and hemorrhage
- Responsive to chemotherapy
- Hydropic villi may embolize to lungs and brain but do not grow and usually regress spontaneously
- Differential diagnosis of persistent elevation of serum HCG following curettage of molar pregnancy is invasive mole versus choriocarcinoma, both of which respond to chemotherapy; tissue diagnosis is not often clinically indicated in this situation

Selected References

Genest DR, Dorfman DM, Castrillon DH: Ploidy and imprinting in hydatidiform miles: Complementary use of flow cytometry and immunohistochemistry of the imprinted gene product p57KIP2 to assist molar classification. J Reprod Med 47:342-346, 2002.

Castrillon DH, Sun D, Weremowicz S, et al: Discrimination of complete hydatidiform mole from its mimics by immunohistochemistry of the paternally imprinted gene product p57KIP2. Am J Surg Pathol 25:1225-1230, 2001.

Gaber LW, Redline RW, Mostoufi-Zadeh M, Driscoll SG: Invasive partial mole. Am J Clin Pathol 85:722-724, 1986.

Gestational Choriocarcinoma

Clinical Features

- Often presents with irregular bleeding and discharge of bloody, brown fluid
- High levels of serum HCG
- Complete mole is a risk factor (5% to 6% of cases)
- Older age (>40 years) is also a risk factor

Figure 12-77. Choriocarcinoma. A, Mixed population of neoplastic cells featuring intermediate trophoblast and binucleate and multinucleate neoplastic cells. Cytotrophoblast cells are not readily identified in this picture. **B,** Mixture of cytotrophoblast and syncytiotrophoblast cells is present in this lesion.

- Rapidly invasive and widely metastatic: most commonly to vagina and lungs, followed by brain, bone marrow, and liver
- Highly responsive to chemotherapy (in contrast to nongestational or extrauterine choriocarcinoma)

Gross Pathology

- Usually present within uterine cavity but may also arise in sites of ectopic pregnancy (uncommon)
- Soft, fleshy, tan-white tumor
- Variegated cut surface with large areas of necrosis, cystic degeneration, and hemorrhage

Histopathology

- Purely trophoblastic proliferation: chorionic villi are absent
- Alternating areas of cytotrophoblast and ST or IT
  — Cytotrophoblast
    ◆ Small mononuclear cells with pale granular or clear cytoplasm and distinct cell borders
    ◆ May be mitotically active

— Syncytiotrophoblast
  ◆ Larger multinucleate cells
  ◆ Opaque cytoplasm with vacuoles
— Intermediate trophoblast
  ◆ Medium-sized cells with single nucleus
  ◆ Opaque cytoplasm without vacuoles
  ◆ Irregular cell borders
- Marked nuclear pleomorphism and brisk mitotic rate
- Central necrosis and hemorrhage (owing to rapid growth) and prominent vascular invasion

Special Stains and Immunohistochemistry

- HCG positive in syncytiotrophoblast
- HPL positive in intermediate trophoblast
- Cytokeratin positive in all forms of trophoblast
- CEA may be positive

Other Techniques for Diagnosis

- Noncontributory

Differential Diagnosis

▌ Early nonmolar pregnancy
  - Smaller numbers of randomly arranged trophoblastic cells with or without villi
  - Serum HCG levels will return to normal following curettage or spontaneous abortion
▌ Hydatidiform mole
  - Hydropic villi present grossly and microscopically
▌ Invasive mole
  - Hydropic villi present grossly and microscopically within the myometrium
▌ PSTT
  - Lower serum HCG levels
  - Predominance of IT (HPL much higher than HCG immunohistochemically)
  - Fibrin within and around vessel walls
  - Less hemorrhage and necrosis
▌ Poorly differentiated carcinoma
  - Usually not biphasic
  - Negative HCG and HPL immunohistochemically
  - Negative serum HCG level (unless in pregnant patient)
▌ Epithelioid trophoblastic tumor
  - Pleomorphic mononucleate trophoblastic cells predominate
  - Remarkable epithelioid appearance
  - Less necrosis and hemorrhage than choriocarcinoma

Pearls

- Characteristic biphasic pattern of cytotrophoblast and ST (less commonly, IT and ST)
- There is a variant that is composed of highly atypical intermediate cells in a rich fibrovascular network
- Primary tumor may be so extensively necrotic that in patients with metastatic disease the primary may not be found

- Gestational choriocarcinoma is highly responsive to chemotherapy (cure rate approaches 100%), whereas nongestational and extrauterine choriocarcinomas are significantly more resistant

Selected References

Seckl MJ, Fisher RA, Slerno G, et al: Choriocarcinoma and partial hydatidiform moles. Lancet 356:36-39, 2000.

Duncan DA, Mazur MT: Trophoblastic tumors: Ultrastructural comparison of choriocarcinoma and placental-site trophoblastic tumor. Hum Pathol 20:370-381, 1989.

Mazur MT: Metastatic gestational choriocarcinoma: Unusual pathologic variant following therapy. Cancer 63:1370-1377, 1989.

Heyderman E, Chapman DV, Richardson TC, et al: Human chorionic gonadotropin and human placental lactogen in extragonadal tumors: An immunoperoxidase study of ten non-germ cell neoplasms. Cancer 56:2674-2682, 1985.

Brewer JI, Mazur MT: Gestational choriocarcinoma: Its origin in the placenta during seemingly normal pregnancy. Am J Surg Pathol 5:267-277, 1981.

Placental Site Trophoblastic Tumor

Clinical Features

- Presents with amenorrhea or abnormal bleeding
- Most follow a normal pregnancy or missed abortion (rather than molar pregnancy)
- Uterus is often enlarged, and uterine perforation may occur
- Low but persistently elevated serum HCG level
- Most are considered benign (75% to 85%)

Gross Pathology

- Variable gross pathology: circumscribed or ill-defined borders
- Confined to myometrium, extension into endometrial cavity, or invasion to serosa
- Soft with a tan cut surface with small foci of tumor necrosis

Figure 12-78. Placental site trophoblastic tumor. Intermediate trophoblast surrounds and invades the blood vessel wall.

Histopathology

- Predominance of intermediate trophoblast
  — Medium-sized cells with single nucleus, opaque cytoplasm, and no vacuoles
  — Cells may be atypical and mitotically active with irregular cell borders
- Trophoblast infiltrates and splits the myometrial smooth muscle fibers
- There is vascular invasion from the periphery of the vessel to the lumen with eventual replacement of the entire vessel wall
- Fibrinoid material is deposited in the vessel wall
- Poor prognostic indicators include high cellularity, high mitotic index, marked necrosis, local spread, and distant metastasis (lungs, liver, peritoneal cavity, brain)

Special Stains and Immunohistochemistry

- Cytokeratin positive
- HPL positive diffusely (predominance of intermediate trophoblast)
- HCG positive focally

Other Techniques for Diagnosis

- Cytogenetics: diploid by flow cytometry

Differential Diagnosis

- ▌ Exaggerated placental site
  - Microscopic focus
  - Serum HCG level returns to normal following curettage
- ▌ Placental site nodules and plaques
  - Small and well circumscribed
  - Extensive hyalinization
  - Absence of cytologic atypia and mitoses
  - Serum HCG level returns to normal following curettage
- ▌ Choriocarcinoma
  - High elevation of serum HCG: tens of thousands (mIU/mL)
  - Biphasic trophoblastic population with marked hemorrhage and necrosis
  - Absence of fibrinoid material in and around vessels
- ▌ Epithelioid leiomyosarcoma
  - Normal serum HCG level
  - Lack of fibrinoid material in and around vessels
  - Cytokeratin HCG and HPL are negative
- ▌ Poorly differentiated carcinoma
  - No fibrinoid deposits in vessel walls
  - Negative HCG and HPL immunohistochemically
  - Negative serum HCG level (except in pregnant patients)

Pearls

- These tumors are believed to result from dysregulation of extravillous IT as evidenced by myometrial infiltration and vascular invasion recapitulating implantation site

- Most are benign (10% to 15% are malignant)
- Malignant tumors do not respond to chemotherapy
- May be associated with a renal syndrome of hematuria and proteinuria with eosinophilic deposits in glomerular capillaries
- Treated with hysterectomy

Selected References

Duncan DA, Mazur MT: Placental site trophoblastic tumor: A study of 55 cases and review of the literature emphasizing factors of prognostic significance. Gynecol Oncol 100:511-520, 2006.

Papadopoulos AJ, Foskett M, Seckl MJ, et al: Twenty-five years' clinical experience with placental site trophoblastic tumors. J Reprod Med 47:460-464, 2002.

Martha M. Quezado and Maria J. Merino

Breast

Subareolar Abscess

Clinical Features

- Develops in lactating and nonlactating breasts, usually in nonlactating breasts
- Found in women of any age, typically during reproductive years
- May present as a painful, erythematous, and edematous breast
- Organisms associated with abscess formation include bacteria such as *Staphylococcus, Proteus, Bacteroides,* and *Streptococcus* species
- May have a tendency to recur and to form extended fistulas

Gross Pathology

- Incision and drainage of acute lesion yields purulent drainage

Figure 13-1. Subareolar abscess. Dilated ductal structures lined by metaplastic squamous epithelium are noted. The lumens contain keratinous and cellular debris. Mixed inflammatory cells are seen in the background.

- Chronic lesion may show development of a fistula from the abscess cavity to the overlying skin

Histopathology

- Extensive neutrophilic inflammatory infiltrate associated with surrounding breast ducts
- Involved ducts show extensive squamous metaplasia, with cell debris and keratin plugs in lactiferous ducts
- Foreign-body giant cell reaction may be seen

Special Stains and Immunohistochemistry

- Special stains for microorganisms (Gomori methenamine silver [GMS], periodic acid–Schiff [PAS], and acid-fast bacillus [AFB]) are negative

Other Techniques for Diagnosis

- Noncontributory

Differential Diagnosis

▮ Plasma cell mastitis
- Inflammation consists primarily of plasma cells with admixed lymphocytes rather than neutrophils
▮ Granulomatous lobar mastitis
- Granulomatous inflammation in and around breast lobules

Pearls

- Incision, drainage, and course of antibiotics is first-line treatment
- May require surgical resection of nipple and major duct system if sinus tract develops or in cases that repeatedly recur

Selected References

Li S, Grant CS, Degnim A, et al: Surgical management of recurrent subareolar breast abscesses: Mayo Clinic experience. Am J Surg 192:528-529, 2006.
Versluijs-Ossewaarde FN, Roumen RM, Goris RJ: Subareolar breast abscesses: Characteristics and results of surgical treatment. Breast J 11:179-182, 2005.
Meguid MM, Oler A, Numann PJ, Khan S: Pathogenesis-based treatment of recurring subareolar breast abscess. Surgery 118:775, 1995.

Plasma Cell Mastitis

Clinical Features

- Typically found in women in second to fourth decades
- Usually found several years (average interval, 4 years) after cessation of lactation
- Presents with acute onset of breast tenderness, redness, and nipple discharge
- Following acute episode, a hard, palpable mass often remains

Gross Pathology

- Large, dilated ducts containing thick, tan-yellow secretion

Histopathology

- Extensive lymphoplasmacytic infiltrate in and around ducts and lobules
- Hyperplasia of ductal epithelium often seen
- Areas of necrosis may be present
- Scattered granulomas and histiocytes (xanthomatous reaction) are common

Special Stains and Immunohistochemistry

- Special stains for microorganisms (GMS, PAS, AFB) are negative

Figure 13-2. Plasma cell mastitis. Dense lymphoplasmacytic infiltrate is noted around a lobular unit. Xanthomatous reaction is also evident.

Other Techniques for Diagnosis

- Noncontributory

Differential Diagnosis

▮ Granulomatous lobar mastitis
  - Consists primarily of granulomatous inflammation with a minor component of plasma cells
▮ Tuberculous mastitis
  - Granulomatous inflammation with caseating necrosis
  - May occasionally be positive for AFB

Pearls

- Clinically mimics carcinoma
- May be diagnosed by fine-needle aspiration, but hyperplastic ductal epithelium should not be mistaken for carcinoma
- Excisional biopsy is curative and avoids possible skin ulceration or fistula formation

Selected References

Baslaim MM, Khayat HA, Al-Amoudi SA: Idiopathic granulomatous mastitis: A heterogeneous disease with variable clinical presentation. World J Surg 31:1677-1681, 2007.

Tavassoli FA: Plasma cell mastitis. In Pathology of the Breast, 2nd ed. Stamford, CT, Appleton & Lange, 1999, pp 792-793.

Tournant B: Lymphocytic plasma cell mastitis. Arch Anat Cytol Pathol 43:88-92, 1995.

Granulomatous Lobar Mastitis

Clinical Features

- Etiology unknown, but has been linked to pregnancy, hormonal therapy, infection, and autoimmune disorders
- Appears after pregnancy
- Usually presents about 2 years postpartum; may be seen many years later

Figure 13-3. Granulomatous mastitis. The granulomatous inflammation distorts the lobular unit and shows giant cells.

- Typically presents as a distinct, hard breast mass
- Clinically mimics carcinoma

Gross Pathology

- Firm to hard breast mass, usually located peripherally
- Mass often has a nodular architecture
- Measures up to 8 cm; usually 4 to 6 cm

Histopathology

- Granulomatous inflammation in and around breast lobules (granulomatous lobulitis)
- Inflammatory reaction in lobules consisting of granulomas, multinucleated giant cells, plasma cells, and eosinophils
- Fat necrosis and small abscess formation occasionally present

Special Stains and Immunohistochemistry

- Special stains for microorganisms (GMS, PAS, AFB) are negative
- Cytokeratin or other epithelial markers can help identify or rule out carcinoma obscured by florid granulomatous reaction

Other Techniques for Diagnosis

- Noncontributory

Differential Diagnosis

▮ Plasma cell mastitis
  - Marked plasma cell infiltrate in and around lobules
  - Associated ductal epithelial hyperplasia often seen
▮ Tuberculous mastitis
  - Granulomatous inflammation with caseating necrosis, possibly AFB positive
▮ Breast abscess
  - Well-defined aggregates of acute inflammatory cells (abscess formation)
▮ Sarcoidosis
  - Primary sarcoid of the breast is uncommon
  - Noncaseating, sarcoid-type granulomas typically are diffuse and found between breast lobules
▮ Cat-scratch disease
  - Granulomatous reaction in lymph nodes that may involve intramammary lymph nodes

Pearls

- Appears after pregnancy
- Clinically mimics carcinoma
- Classic histologic picture is an inflammatory reaction in and around lobules with numerous multinucleated giant cells

Selected References

Marriott DA, Russell J, Grebosky J, et al: Idiopathic granulomatous lobular mastitis masquerading as a breast abscess and breast carcinoma. Am J Clin Oncol 30:564-565, 2007.

Khamapirad T, Hennan K, Leonard M Jr, et al: Granulomatous lobular mastitis: Two case reports with focus on radiologic and histopathologic features. Ann Diagn Pathol 11:109-112, 2007.

Bhaskaran CS, Prasad KR, Rao G, et al: Chronic granulomatous mastitis: review of 26 cases with special reference to chronic lobular mastitis. Ind J Pathol Microbiol 35:38-43, 1992.

Fat Necrosis

Clinical Features

- May present with a painless palpable breast mass or with breast tenderness
- May clinically and mammographically mimic carcinoma
- Believed to be related to trauma, most commonly previous breast surgery; other possibly related etiologic factors include cyst aspiration, radiotherapy, warfarin use, breast infection

Gross Pathology

- Typically of small size (<2 cm)
- Single or multiple firm, round or irregular masses
- Tan-yellow streaks and often areas of dense fibrosis
- Areas of hemorrhage may be seen
- Cystic degeneration and calcification may develop

Histopathology

- Abundant lipid-laden and foamy macrophages surrounding small cystic spaces
- Foreign-body giant cells and chronic inflammation (lymphoplasmacytic infiltrate) usually seen
- Fibroblastic proliferation and collagen deposition seen in older lesions
- Scar formation and peripheral calcification are late manifestations

Figure 13-4. Fat necrosis. Fat vacuoles surrounded by chronic inflammatory cells and giant cells.

Special Stains and Immunohistochemistry

- CD68: histiocytes are positive
- S-100 protein negative
- Cytokeratin negative

Other Techniques for Diagnosis

- Noncontributory

Differential Diagnosis

▎ Infiltrating ductal carcinoma
- Neoplastic cells show cytologic atypia and increased mitotic activity and lack vacuolated cytoplasm seen in cells of fat necrosis
- Tumor cells are cytokeratin positive and CD68 negative

▎ Granular cell tumor
- Nests or sheets of polygonal cells with abundant eosinophilic granular cytoplasm
- Lacks associated giant cells and lymphoplasmacytic infiltrate
- Granular cells are S-100 protein positive and CD68 negative

Pearls

- History of trauma found in greater than 50% of cases
- Fat necrosis is almost always found surrounding previous biopsy cavity
- Skin changes that mimic carcinoma may be seen
- Mammographically, peripheral calcification, described as *eggshell calcifications*, may be seen

Selected References

Tan PH, Lai LM, Carrington EV, et al: Fat necrosis of the breast: A review. Breast 15:313-318, 2006.

Miller JA, Festa S, Goldstein M: Benign fat necrosis simulating bilateral breast malignancy after reduction mammoplasty. South Med J 91:765-767, 1998.

Mandrekas AD, Assimakopoulos GI, Mastorakos DP, Pantzalis K: Fat necrosis following breast reduction. Br J Plast Surg 47:560-562, 1994.

Diabetic Mastopathy

Clinical Features

- Most cases found in females with type 1 diabetes mellitus, with exogenous insulin use
- Widely reported in premenopausal women, with broad age distribution (teenage years up to fifth or sixth decade)
- Bilateral in about 50% of cases
- Presenting complaint is usually a hard, nontender, freely mobile breast mass
- Mammographic findings are nonspecific

Gross Pathology

- Hard, homogeneous, white-gray breast tissue
- Typically no distinct tumor is identified

Figure 13-5. Diabetic mastopathy. Atrophic duct surrounded by dense collagenous stroma.

Histopathology

- Dense, collagenous stroma (keloid-like) with proliferation of benign-appearing fibroblasts
- No cytologic atypia
- Lymphocytic infiltrate around small blood vessels, in and around lobules and ducts

Special Stains and Immunohistochemistry

- Lymphocytes are typically CD20 positive (B-cell lineage)

Other Techniques for Diagnosis

- Noncontributory

Differential Diagnosis

▌ Granulomatous lobar mastitis
- Granulomatous inflammation in and around breast lobules

▌ Breast abscess
- Prominent neutrophilic inflammatory infiltrate

▌ Fibrocystic change
- Shows heterogeneous histologic features that may include cyst formation, apocrine metaplasia, adenosis, and ductal epithelial hyperplasia

Pearls

- Contributory factor may be alterations in collagen metabolism that exist in diabetic patients
- Self-limited condition primarily affecting premenopausal women
- Excisional biopsy is adequate treatment; rare cases have recurred

Selected References

Fong D, Lann MA, Finlayson C, et al: Diabetic (lymphocytic) mastopathy with exuberant lymphohistiocytic and granulomatous response: A case report and review of the literature. Am J Surg Pathol 30:1330-1336, 2006.

Hunfeld KP, Bassler R: Lymphocytic mastitis and fibrosis of the breast in long-standing insulin-dependent diabetics: A histopathologic study on diabetic mastopathy and report of ten cases. Gen Diagn Pathol 143:49-58, 1997.

Morgan MC, Weaver MG, Crowe JP, Abdul-Karim FW: Diabetic mastopathy: A clinicopathologic study in palpable and nonpalpable breast lesions. Mod Pathol 8:349-354, 1995.

Tomaszewski JE, Brooks JS, Hicks D, Livolsi VA: Diabetic mastopathy: A distinctive clinicopathologic entity. Hum Pathol 23:780-786, 1992.

Juvenile or Virginal Hypertrophy

Clinical Features

- Typically occurs in young girls (<16 years)
- History of rapid growth of one or both breasts to massive, persistent proportions; overlying skin hyperemia and necrosis can occur
- Benign findings on mammography

Gross Pathology

- Diffuse process involving one or both breasts
- Discrete masses are not seen

Histopathology

- Characterized by proliferation of connective tissue and ductal structures
- Lacks normal lobular development
- May be histologically identical to gynecomastia

Special Stains and Immunohistochemistry

- Noncontributory

Other Techniques for Diagnosis

- Noncontributory

Differential Diagnosis

▌ Juvenile fibroadenoma
- Discrete nodules measuring an average of 2 to 3 cm in diameter that are able to be "shelled out" from surrounding breast tissue

Figure 13-6. Juvenile hypertrophy. Ductal structures surrounded by loose proliferating connective tissue.

- Hypercellular collagenous stroma with proliferation of slitlike, branching ducts

Pearls

- Cases in which each breast weighed more than 17 pounds have been reported
- Histologically resembles gynecomastia of the male breast
- May be related to hypersensitivity of mammary tissue to estrogen stimulation that occurs during puberty
- Usually sporadic, but familial cases have been described; *PTEN* gene mutation has been linked to virginal hypertrophy with increased risk for malignant transformation

Selected References

Koves IH, Zacharin M: Virginal breast hypertrophy of an 11 year old girl. J Pediatr Child Health 43:315-317, 2007.

Govrin-Yehudain J, Kogan L, Cohen HI, Falik-Zaccai F: Familial juvenile hypertrophy of the breast. J Adolesc Health 35:151-155, 2004.

Netscher D, Mosharrafa AM, Laucirica R: Massive asymmetric virginal breast hypertrophy. South Med J 89:434-437, 1996.

Granular Cell Tumor

Clinical Features

- Typically found in premenopausal women
- Presents as a firm, painless, solitary mass more frequently in the upper inner quadrant
- Mimics carcinoma on mammography

Gross Pathology

- Firm, hard mass with well-circumscribed or occasionally infiltrative borders
- Typically measures less than 5 cm
- Gray-white or tan cut surface
- May grossly mimic infiltrating carcinoma

Figure 13-7. Granular cell tumor. Microscopically, the tumor cells infiltrate the breast parenchyma in small nests separated by delicate fibrous bands.

Histopathology

- Composed of nests or sheets of polygonal cells with abundant eosinophilic cytoplasmic granules
- Cells have uniform, round nuclei with open chromatin and prominent nucleoli
- Occasional mitotic figures may be seen
- Infiltrative growth pattern; often surrounds lobules and invades adipose tissue

Special Stains and Immunohistochemistry

- S-100 protein: highlights cytoplasmic granularity with strong cytoplasmic and nuclear staining
- Carcinoembryonic antigen (CEA): diffuse immunoreactivity
- Cytokeratin and epithelial membrane antigen (EMA) negative
- Actin, myoglobin, desmin negative
- Estrogen receptor (ER) and progesterone receptor (PR) negative

Other Techniques for Diagnosis

- Electron microscopy demonstrates myelin figures and numerous lysosomes

Differential Diagnosis

- ∎ Histiocytic lesions, including fat necrosis and mammary duct ectasia
  - Granular cell tumor is usually not immunoreactive with histiocyte-associated antigens, such as α_1-antitrypsin and α_1-antichymotrypsin, but reactivity for CD68 has been described
- ∎ Apocrine carcinoma
  - Tumor cells are large, with pleomorphic nuclei and prominent nucleoli
  - Typically shows an associated intraductal component
  - Positive for cytokeratin
- ∎ Metastatic neoplasms, including oncocytic renal cell carcinoma, melanoma, and alveolar soft part sarcoma
  - Malignant histologic features, along with panel of immunohistochemical stains, including cytokeratin, EMA (positive in renal cancer), MART-1, HMB-45 (positive in melanoma), and myoglobin (positive in alveolar sarcoma), help in the differential diagnosis

Pearls

- Virtually always benign; only rare reports of metastasis
- Eosinophilic cytoplasmic granules are due to abundant lysosomes
- Treated by wide local excision; may recur if not completely resected

Selected References

Adeniran A, Al-Ahmadie H, Mahoney MC, Robinson-Smith TM: Granular cell tumor of the breast: A series of 17 cases and review of the literature. Breast J 10:528-531, 2004.

Sirgi KE, Sneige N, Fanning TV, et al: Fine-needle aspirates of granular cell lesions of the breast: Report of three cases, with emphasis on differential diagnosis and utility of immunostaining for CD68 (KP1). Diagn Cytopathol 15:403-408, 1996.

Damiani S, Koerner FC, Dickersin GR, et al: Granular cell tumour of the breast. Virchows Arch A Pathol Anat Histopathol 420:219-226, 1992.

Fibrocystic Changes

Clinical Features

- Most common condition involving the female breast
- Affects primarily premenopausal women (third to fifth decades)
- Bilateral and multifocal
- Irregular, firm, and nodular breast tissue with discrete lumps
- Breasts often tender
- Breast nodularity typically fluctuates with the menstrual cycle

Gross Pathology

- Irregular, rubbery, fibrotic breast tissue
- Macroscopic cysts containing clear or turbid fluid often seen
- Blue-domed cysts may be present

Histopathology

▌ Cyst formation
- Variably sized cysts lined by flattened or cuboidal epithelial cells

▌ Stromal fibrosis
- Dense periductal and perilobular fibrosis

▌ Apocrine metaplasia
- Cysts lined by large, polygonal cells with abundant granular, eosinophilic cytoplasm and small, hyperchromatic nuclei

Figure 13-8. Fibrocystic changes characterized by cyst formation, stromal fibrosis, and sclerosing adenosis.

Figure 13-9. Fibrocystic changes with columnar cell lesions.
A, Dilated acini showing columnar cell change are lined by two cell layers with occasional apical snouts, luminal secretions, and no atypia. Distended acini showing (**B**) columnar cell change and (**C**) columnar cell hyperplasia with cytologic atypia (flat epithelial atypia) are lined by more than two layers, with occasional papillary formation and cell atypia.

Figure 13-10. A, Apocrine metaplasia. Dilated ducts lined by metaplastic apocrine cells. The cells are columnar and have granular pink cytoplasm. **B, Ductal hyperplasia without atypia.** The ductal spaces are distended by a solid proliferation of hyperplastic ductal cells. Notice prominent fenestrations with variable size of the secondary lumens.

■ Sclerosing adenosis
  ● Multiple well-defined foci are usually present
  ● Proliferation of attenuated ductules with preservation of the lobular configuration
  ● Increased stromal and myoepithelial cells
  ● Microcalcifications are often seen
■ Epithelial hyperplasia without atypia
  ● Proliferation of ductal cells with duct lumens filled with a heterogeneous population of round to oval cells
  ● Irregular, slitlike fenestrations often seen at the periphery of the ducts
■ Columnar cell lesions (CCLs)
  ● Enlarged acini of terminal ductal lobular units (TDLUs) lined by columnar cells with occasional luminal secretions and calcification
    — Columnar cell change (CCC)
      ◆ Distended acini with undulating borders; up to two epithelial layers; ovoid nuclei oriented perpendicular to basement membrane and inconspicuous nucleoli; infrequent mitosis; apical snouts may be seen with occasional luminal secretions and calcification
    — Columnar cell hyperplasia (CCH)
      ◆ More than two cell layers with papillary formation; apical snouts, secretions, and calcifications are common
    — Flat epithelial atypia (CCC and CCH with cytologic atypia)
      ◆ Acini with rigid contours, round nuclei with nucleoli not oriented perpendicular to basement membrane, occasional mitosis; high-grade epithelial atypia *not* a feature

Special Stains and Immunohistochemistry

● ER, PR, BCL-2, cytokeratin 19 positive in CCL
● Negative for p53, C-erb-B2 (HER-2-neu) in CCL

Other Techniques for Diagnosis

● Noncontributory

Differential Diagnosis

■ Fibromatosis
  ● Greater cellularity composed of elongated spindle cells
  ● Lacks cyst formation and other features that characterize fibrocystic changes
■ Atypical ductal hyperplasia (ADH) or ductal carcinoma in situ (DCIS)
  ● Shows greater cytologic atypia and complex architectural changes than CCLs with atypia (flat epithelial atypia)

Pearls

● May clinically mimic carcinoma
● Most common diagnosis made after lumpectomy (>50% of all surgical procedures involving the breast)
● Typically displays several features, including cyst formation, apocrine metaplasia, fibrosis, chronic inflammation, and epithelial hyperplasia without atypia
● CCLs show 16q loss; may represent early lesion of low-grade DCIS
● Believed to be related to hormonal imbalance involving estrogen and progesterone; oral contraceptives decrease risk for fibrocystic changes
● Sclerosing adenosis is associated with a slight (1.5 to 2 times) increased risk for carcinoma
● No increased risk for carcinoma associated with apocrine metaplasia, stromal fibrosis, or mild ductal epithelial hyperplasia without atypia; florid ductal hyperplasia without atypia increases risk for carcinoma slightly (1.5 to 2 times)

Selected References

Santen RJ, Mansel R: Benign breast disorders. N Engl J Med 353:275-285, 2005.

Fiorica JV: Fibrocystic changes. Obstet Gynecol Clin North Am 21:445-452, 1994.

Vorherr H: Fibrocystic breast disease: Pathophysiology, pathomorphology, clinical picture, and management. Am J Obstet Gynecol 154:161-179, 1986.

Adenosis

Clinical Features

- Primarily affects premenopausal women (third and fourth decades)
- Typically found in association with fibrocystic changes
- May be found in biopsy material removed for suspicious or indeterminate microcalcifications

Gross Pathology

- Findings are often those of fibrocystic changes with areas of fibrosis and cyst formation
- Florid adenosis tumors are well circumscribed; sclerotic tumors tend to be less well defined at borders
- Lesions with abundant microcalcifications have a gritty cut surface

Histopathology

- Usually consists of a circumscribed, benign proliferation of ductal structures
- Ducts have an oval or elongated contour
- Well-defined epithelial and myoepithelial layers
- Microcalcifications are often seen
- Increase in cell size, nuclear pleomorphism, normal mitoses, focal necrosis, or infarction can be seen in florid adenosis, especially during pregnancy and lactation
- Sclerosing adenosis can involve nerves
- Several patterns and variants of adenosis exist
  — Sclerosing adenosis (most common variant)
    ◆ Multiple well-defined foci are usually present
    ◆ Proliferation of attenuated ductules with preservation of the lobular configuration
    ◆ Increased stromal and myoepithelial cells
    ◆ Dense stroma surrounding ducts
    ◆ Microcalcifications are often seen
  — Apocrine adenosis
    ◆ Ductule proliferation with extensive apocrine metaplasia
    ◆ Cells with large nucleolus
  — Microglandular adenosis (rare variant)
    ◆ Haphazard arrangement of small, round ductules lacking lobular architecture
    ◆ Background shows hypocellular, collagenous stroma

Figure 13-11. A, Sclerosing adenosis. Well-circumscribed area of closely packed ducts retaining a lobular configuration. **B, Sclerosing adenosis** showing dense collagenous stroma between the proliferating tubules. Notice multiple microcalcifications in the tubules. **C, Microglandular adenosis.** Proliferation of tubules lacking lobular architecture in a dense collagenous background.

- ◆ Proliferating ducts often extend around normal breast ducts and lobules and may extend into adjacent adipose tissue
- ◆ Duct lumens contain a colloid-like eosinophilic, secretory material (PAS positive)

- ◆ Bland cytologic features with cells typically showing clear or vacuolated cytoplasm and rare mitotic figures
- ◆ Atypical microglandular adenosis has foci of both typical adenosis and areas of more complex structure and cytologic atypia
- ◆ Myoepithelial layer is absent (negative for S-100 protein, smooth muscle actin [SMA], smooth muscle myosin heavy-chain, and p63)
- ◆ Usually negative for EMA and ER
- Adenosis tumor: grossly recognized mass formed by numerous adjacent foci of adenosis

Special Stains and Immunohistochemistry

- Cytokeratin, S-100, and cathepsin D highlight epithelial cells of microglandular adenosis
- SMA, S-100, smooth muscle myosin heavy chain, and p63 highlight myoepithelial cell layer
- PAS, laminin, and collagen IV highlight basement membrane of sclerosing adenosis

Other Techniques for Diagnosis

- Noncontributory

Differential Diagnosis

▌Infiltrating tubular carcinoma
- Haphazardly arranged ducts with angulated, open lumens and bridges of epithelial cells
- Absent myoepithelial layer (also absent in microglandular adenosis)
- Lumens lack eosinophilic secretions
- Lining cells have eosinophilic cytoplasm and often show apical snouts
- Reactive, fibroblastic stroma with desmoplasia often seen
- Often associated with an intraductal carcinoma component
- Usually positive for EMA and ER

▌Infiltrating lobular carcinoma
- Classically shows small, uniform, rounded cells infiltrating in single-file lines or alveolar pattern
- Lacks lobular configuration and myoepithelial cell layer (similar to microglandular adenosis)

Pearls

- Classically sclerosing adenosis is a ductule proliferation that maintains a lobular architecture
- Myoepithelial cell proliferation in sclerosing adenosis is helpful to distinguish from carcinoma
- Microglandular adenosis is often difficult to distinguish from tubular carcinoma; best distinguishing features include the shape of the ductules and the stromal characteristics
- Adenosis has been shown to be associated with a slight increased risk for carcinoma (1.5 to 2 times)

Selected References

Salarieh A, Sneige N: Breast carcinoma arising in microglandular adenosis: A review of the literature. Arch Pathol Lab Med 131:1397-1399, 2007.

Seidman JD, Ashton M, Lefkowitz M: Atypical apocrine adenosis of the breast: A clinicopathologic study of 37 patients with 8.7 year follow up. Cancer 77:2529-2537, 1996.

Lee KC, Chan JK, Gwi E: Tubular adenosis of the breast: A distinctive benign lesion mimicking invasive carcinoma. Am J Surg Pathol 20:46-54, 1996.

James BA, Cranor ML, Rosen PP: Carcinoma of the breast arising in microglandular adenosis. Am J Clin Pathol 100:507-513, 1993.

Eusebi V, Foschini MP, Betts CM, et al: Microglandular adenosis, apocrine adenosis, and tubular carcinoma of the breast: An immunohistochemical comparison. Am J Surg Pathol 17:99-109, 1993.

Radial Sclerosing Lesion and Radial Scar

Clinical Features

- Uncommon before 30 years of age
- Typically small and therefore usually nonpalpable
- Usually an incidental finding; associated with adenosis and fibrocystic changes
- Mammographically shows a dense central radiolucent zone with thin, linear densities radiating outward; microcalcifications may be seen
- Can mimic carcinoma on mammography
- In many patients, this lesion is multifocal or bilateral; clustering of scars may occur

Gross Pathology

- Typically of small size, rarely larger than 1 cm (*radial scar* refers to lesions <1 cm; *complex sclerosing lesion* describes lesions ≥1 cm)

Figure 13-12. Radial scar. Central collagenous scar surrounded by proliferating ducts in a radial pattern resembling sclerosing adenosis.

- Shows irregular, stellate, dense fibrotic tissue; may grossly mimic carcinoma

Histopathology

- Pseudoinfiltrative lesions
- Central collagenous scar showing fibrosis and elastosis, with entrapped ducts showing dual epithelial and myoepithelial layer; basement membrane intact
- Epithelial proliferation with stellate or radial arrangement of ductules resembling sclerosing adenosis
- Commonly see fibrocystic changes, including ductal hyperplasia, duct ectasia, adenosis, and papillomatosis surrounding fibrotic zone
- Ducts may show squamous metaplasia
- Perineural infiltration by benign ducts may be seen
- Necrosis is rare, but small areas can be present
- Ducts should not infiltrate into adjacent adipose tissue

Special Stains and Immunohistochemistry

- SMA highlights myoepithelial layer
- S-100 protein highlights myoepithelial layer

Other Techniques for Diagnosis

- Noncontributory

Differential Diagnosis

▌ Tubular carcinoma
- Ducts do not have a myoepithelial cell layer
- Often infiltrates into surrounding fatty tissue

Pearls

- Most commonly seen in association with adenosis
- Can grossly and histologically mimic carcinoma
- Presence of a myoepithelial layer and lack of infiltration are the best distinguishing characteristics
- Carcinoma has been seen to arise in a background of radial scar
- Believed to be benign but associated with atypia and malignancy; radial scar may be an independent risk factor for the development of carcinoma

Selected References

Doyle EM, Banville N, Quinn CM, et al: Radial scars/complex sclerosing lesions and malignancy in a screening programme: Incidence and histological features revisited. Histopathology 50:607-614, 2007.

Sanders ME, Page Dl, Simpson JF, et al: Interdependence of radial scar and proliferative disease with respect to invasive breast carcinoma risk in patients with benign breast biopsies. Cancer 1:1453-1461, 2006.

Jacobs TW, Byrne C, Colditz G, et al: Radial scars in benign breast-biopsy specimens and the risk of breast cancer. N Engl J Med 340:430-436, 1999.

Nielsen M, Christensen L, Andersen J: Radial scars in women with breast cancer. Cancer 59:1019-1025, 1987.

Intraductal Papilloma (Solitary and Multiple)

Clinical Features

▌ Solitary papilloma
- Typically arises from lactiferous ducts in central breast tissue (beneath the areola) and often presents with serous or bloody nipple discharge

Figure 13-13. **Intraductal papilloma. A,** Dilated duct showing papillary proliferation on a sclerotic fibrovascular core. **B,** Distended duct showing a papillary lesion with a delicate fibrovascular core. **C,** Multiple intraductal papillomas. Distended ducts showing multiple papillary lesions.

- Usually found in women in their fifth or sixth decade
▮ Multiple papillomas
  - Multiple papillary masses typically located in peripheral breast tissue in contiguous branches of the ductal system
  - Occurs in younger women (40s and early 50s)
  - Occurs far less frequently than solitary papillomas

Gross Pathology

- Large papillomas may be visible in the lumen of a dilated or cystic duct
- Palpable lesions typically measure 2 to 3 cm, but cystic lesions can be larger than 10 cm

Histopathology

- Organized papillary proliferation of ductal epithelium on a frond-forming fibrovascular core or stroma
- Any degree of epithelial hyperplasia of the usual type may be seen
- Fusion of papillae often results in glandlike spaces or solid areas
- Presence of a myoepithelial cell layer in papillae and around glandular spaces, although it can be focally absent
- Papillomas may show apocrine, squamous, mucinous, clear cell, or sebaceous metaplasia
- Sclerosis of the cores with entrapment of ductal epithelium may occur and may be mistaken for invasive carcinoma
- Infarction associated with torsion of the cores may happen, hindering evaluation of atypia and malignancy
  — Solitary papilloma
    ◆ Papillae with single layer of cuboidal to columnar epithelium; focal epithelial hyperplasia may be seen
    ◆ Typically shows minimal cellular atypia and rare mitotic activity
    ◆ May show extreme distortion and fusion of papillary fronds (solid intraductal papilloma) or marked sclerosis (sclerosing papilloma)
  — Multiple papillomas
    ◆ Multiple papillomas with involvement of more than one duct system or multiple foci within a single duct system
    ◆ Arise in terminal duct lobular units and may extend into terminal
    ◆ May show prominent epithelial hyperplasia
    ◆ Atypia may develop with papillae lined by pseudostratified, elongated epithelial cells
  — Papilloma with atypia (atypical papilloma; papilloma with ADH) and papilloma with DCIS
    ◆ Papillomas with foci of epithelial proliferation with full architectural and cytologic criteria for the diagnosis of ADH or DCIS
      ◇ Papillomas with non–high-grade DCIS when lesion is larger than 3 mm

◇ Papillomas with ADH (atypical papillomas) when lesion is smaller than or equal to 3 mm
◇ DCIS most often of low or intermediate nuclear grade with solid, cribriform, or micropapillary patterns; small necrotic foci may be present
◇ Focal loss or reduction of myoepithelial cells in the ADH and DCIS foci
    ◆ Presence of large atypical or higher-grade lesion foci or necrosis should prompt designation of *carcinoma in situ arising within a papilloma*

Special Stains and Immunohistochemistry

- SMA, calponin, S-100 protein, smooth muscle myosin heavy chain, and p63 highlight myoepithelial cells
- ER stains a variable minority of epithelial cells in papillomas without atypia, with diffuse positivity in ADH and low-grade DCIS foci
- High-molecular-weight cytokeratins (HMWCKs), such as 5/6, 14, and 34βE12, stain epithelial cells in papillomas without atypia, whereas ADH and low-grade DCIS foci are negative
- Combination of ER positivity and HMWCK negativity is a useful indicator of neoplastic population in an intraductal papillary proliferation
- Factor VIII demonstrates vascular endothelial cells within fibrovascular cores (helps distinguish between endothelial and myoepithelial cells)

Other Techniques for Diagnosis

- Noncontributory

Differential Diagnosis

▮ Papillary DCIS
- Prominent neoplastic proliferation of epithelial cells showing papillary architecture and features of intraductal carcinoma characterized by unequivocal comedo, cribriform, solid, or micropapillary architecture; no apocrine metaplasia; necrosis often seen
▮ Encapsulated (intracystic) papillary carcinoma and noninvasive papillary carcinoma
- Papillary proliferation growing within dilated ducts and consisting entirely of papillae lacking a myoepithelial cell layer; recent studies failed to demonstrate myoepithelial cells at the periphery of tumor nodules

Pearls

- Papillomas, solitary and multiple, without atypia have been shown to be associated with an increased risk for malignancy, the risk being greater with multiple lesions
- Women with multiple papillomas with atypia have a particularly high breast cancer risk

- Clinical significance of atypical papillary lesions is uncertain, and complete excision is recommended with careful follow-up
- Deferring the diagnosis of carcinoma to paraffin sections is recommended when diagnosis of an intraductal papilloma is made on frozen section
- Loss of heterozygosity (LOH) at loci 16p13 is identified in papillomas with florid hyperplasia
- Frozen sections are not recommended on papillary lesions
- Most important feature for distinguishing between a benign papilloma and a papillary carcinoma is the presence of a uniform myoepithelial layer in the proliferating papillary intraluminal component
- Presence of apocrine metaplasia within the lesion favors a benign diagnosis

Selected References

Collins LC, Schnitt SJ: Papillary lesions of the breast: Selected diagnostic and management issues. Histopathology 52:20-29, 2008.

Mulligan AM, O'Malley FP: Papillary lesions of the breast: A review. Adv Anat Pathol 14:108-119, 2007.

Cristofano CD, Mrad K, Zavaglia K, et al: Papillary lesions of the breast: A molecular progression? Breast Cancer Res Treat 90:71-76, 2005

Renshaw AA, Derhagopian RP, Tizol-Blanco DM, Gould EW: Papillomas and atypical papillomas in breast core needle biopsy specimens: Risk of carcinoma in subsequent excision. Am J Clin Pathol 122:217-221, 2004.

Ciatto S, Andreoli C, Cirillo A, et al: The risk of breast cancer subsequent to histologic diagnosis of benign intraductal papilloma follow-up study of 339 cases. Tumori 77:41-43, 1991.

Florid Papillomatosis of the Nipple

Clinical Features

- May be seen at any age, typically in middle-aged women (fourth and fifth decades)
- Rarely reported in men
- Frequently presents with serous or bloody nipple discharge
- Pain or itching may be experienced
- Palpable mass is present in most cases

Gross Pathology

- Generally forms a discrete mass
- Nipple frequently shows ulceration, erythema, and scaling

Histopathology

- Characteristic feature is florid ductal hyperplasia with lesions grouped into four subtypes according to their growth pattern: sclerosing papillomatosis, papilloma, adenosis, and mixed proliferative patterns
- Myoepithelial cell hyperplasia is common but in sclerosing lesions may be inconspicuous or absent

Figure 13-14. Florid papillomatosis. A, Distended ducts filled with hyperplastic ductal cells are extending into the upper dermis. **B,** Tubular arrangement with focal ductal hyperplasia and fibrous stroma.

- Foci of necrosis and normal mitosis may be present
- Areas of ADH, DCIS, or invasive carcinoma within papillomatosis may be seen

Special Stains and Immunohistochemistry

- SMA, calponin, S-100 protein, smooth muscle myosin heavy chain, and p63 highlight myoepithelial cells

Other Techniques for Diagnosis

- Noncontributory

Differential Diagnosis

▌ Paget disease
- Identification of neoplastic tumor cells within epidermis of nipple

▌ DCIS or invasive carcinoma
- Often present when florid papillomatosis is found
- May be associated with or be present away from area of papillomatosis
- Intraductal carcinoma should show a cribriform, comedo, solid, or micropapillary architecture and may show necrosis

Pearls

- Benign epithelial tumor arising in the large ducts of the nipple
- Treatment involves complete excision, usually with removal of the nipple
- Associated with concomitant or subsequent carcinoma in 10% of cases; carcinoma may be found anywhere in the breast

Selected References

Rosen PP, Oberman HA: Atlas of Tumor Pathology: Tumors of the Mammary Gland, 3rd Series, Fascicle 7. Washington, DC, Armed Forces Institute of Pathology, 1993.

Rosen PP, Caicco JA: Florid papillomatosis of the nipple: A study of 51 patients, including nine with mammary carcinoma. Am J Surg Pathol 10:87-101, 1986.

Brownstein MH, Phelps RG, Magnin PH: Papillary adenoma of the nipple: Analysis of fifteen new cases. J Am Acad Dermatol 12:707-715, 1985.

Pseudoangiomatous Stromal Hyperplasia

Clinical Features

- Found in women of childbearing age
- Presents as a firm, palpable, nontender, solitary breast mass or area of thickening
- Can be found as an incidental finding in patients undergoing biopsies for other reasons

Gross Pathology

- Well circumscribed and typically encapsulated
- Variable size (typically 3 to 4 cm)
- Cut section demonstrates a fibrous, tan-white, homogeneous tumor

Figure 13-15. Pseudoangiomatous stromal hyperplasia. Complex anastomosing slitlike spaces in a dense collagenous background.

Histopathology

- Characterized by complex, anastomosing, empty slitlike spaces (pseudoangiomas) in a dense collagenous stroma
- Empty spaces lined by monomorphic myofibroblastic spindle cells resembling endothelial cells
- Can form solid foci of prominent spindle cells

Special Stains and Immunohistochemistry (Myofibroblasts)

- Vimentin positive in spindle cells lining pseudoangiomatous spaces
- CD34 positive in most lesions
- CD31 rarely positive
- SMA variably reactive
- Cytokeratin, factor VIII, and *Ulex europaeus* negative

Other Techniques for Diagnosis

- Electron microscopy: pseudoangiomatous spaces lined by cells showing fibroblastic differentiation

Differential Diagnosis

▌ Hemangioma
- Slitlike spaces are vascular channels and often contain blood
- Lining cells are endothelial and show cytokeratin, CD31, factor VIII, and *U. europaeus* positivity

▌ Low-grade angiosarcoma
- Intercommunicating vascular spaces lined by atypical endothelial cells with hyperchromatic nuclei
- Infiltrative architecture typically extending into adjacent breast tissue

Pearls

- Pseudoangiomatous stromal hyperplasia is a benign lesion that must be distinguished from low-grade angiosarcoma
- Treatment is wide local excision; clear margins are necessary to avoid recurrences
- Development may be related to hormonal factors
- Positivity for CD34 supports the diagnosis

Selected References

Ferreira M, Albarracin CT, Resetkova E: Pseudoangiomatous stromal hyperplasia tumor: A clinical, radiologic and pathologic study of 26 cases. Mod Pathol 21:201-207, 2008.

Tan PH, Jayabaskar T, Chuah KL, et al: Phyllodes tumors of the breast: The role of pathologic parameters. Am J Clin Pathol 123:529-540, 2005.

Spitz DJ, Reddy V, Gattuso P: FNA of pseudoangiomatous stromal hyperplasia of breast. Diagn Cytopathol 20:323-324, 1999.

Cohen MA, Morris EA, Rosen PP, et al: Pseudoangiomatous stromal hyperplasia: Mammographic, sonographic, and clinical patterns. Radiology 198:117-120, 1996.

Adenoma

Clinical Features

- Some may represent unusual types of fibroadenomas
- All present as breast masses
- Lactating adenoma is often recognized during pregnancy or while lactating

Gross Pathology

- Well-defined, circumscribed, tan-yellow tumors
- Typically less than 5 cm in greatest diameter
- Lactating adenomas may be multiple

Histopathology

▮ Tubular adenoma
  - Proliferation of benign glands of uniform size and shape
  - Lined by a single layer of epithelial cells showing bland nuclear features
  - Myoepithelial cells surround each gland
▮ Lactating adenoma
  - Proliferation of benign ducts with preservation of a lobular architecture; typically sharply delineated from the surrounding breast tissue
  - Ducts lined by benign-appearing epithelial cells with vacuolated cytoplasm; may show hobnail appearance
  - Duct lumens contain eosinophilic secretions
  - Typically shows increased secretion if removed postpartum, less secretion if removed during pregnancy
  - Prone to infarction during pregnancy
▮ Apocrine adenoma
  - Extremely rare lesions

Figure 13-16. A, Tubular adenoma. Densely packed ductal structures lined by epithelial and myoepithelial cells. **B, Lactating adenoma.** The ducts are lined by vacuolated secretory cells. The lumens contain secretory material.

- Discrete mass, homogeneous throughout, sharply demarcated from surrounding breast tissue and composed of benign breast ducts with apocrine epithelium and minimal supportive stromal component
- Often shows papillary and cystic architecture

Special Stains and Immunohistochemistry

- SMA, S-100, and p63 highlight myoepithelial cell layer
- PAS highlights luminal secretion in lactating adenoma

Other Techniques for Diagnosis

- Noncontributory

Differential Diagnosis

▮ Tubular carcinoma
  - Composed of small angulated ducts with infiltrative growth pattern
  - Lacks myoepithelial cell layer
  - Shows reactive, desmoplastic stroma surrounding proliferating ducts

Pearls

- Tubular adenomas do not recur after excision and show no increased risk for subsequent carcinoma
- Lactating adenomas may infarct, causing significant pain
- Apocrine adenoma is a discrete mass composed of benign breast ducts all showing apocrine epithelium
- Carcinoma can develop in adenomas

Selected References

Sumkin JH, Perrone AM, Harris KM, et al: Lactating adenoma: US features and literature review. Radiology 206:271-274, 1998.

Maiorano E, Albrizio M: Tubular adenoma of the breast: an immunohistochemical study of ten cases. Pathol Res Pract 191:1222-1230, 1995.

O'Hara MF, Page DL: Adenomas of the breast and ectopic breast under lactational influences. Hum Pathol 16:707-712, 1985.

Hertel B, Zaloudek C, Kempson R: Breast adenomas. Cancer 37:2891-2905, 1976.

Fibroadenoma

Clinical Features

- Most common breast tumor in adolescents and young women
- Often develops in transplant recipients receiving cyclosporine
- Presents as discrete, nontender, palpable breast mass
- Typically solitary but can be multifocal or bilateral
- Giant fibroadenomas are larger than 5 cm or weigh more than 500 g

Gross Pathology

- Tan-white to gray, firm to rubbery, round to oval mass
- Well circumscribed and typically encapsulated

Figure 13-17. Fibroadenoma. Delicate capsule surrounds this fibroadenoma. The glandular and stromal components are evident.

- No infiltration into surrounding fatty breast tissue
- Most fibroadenomas measure up to 3 cm

Histopathology

- Benign tumor that arises from lobules and stroma of the terminal duct–lobular unit
- Typically shows a well-defined capsule
- Characteristic features include a collagenous stroma and distorted, slitlike, elongated ducts
- Variable degree of stromal cellularity
- Fibrocystic changes (apocrine metaplasia, adenosis, ductal epithelial hyperplasia) are common associated findings
- Benign multinucleated giant cells may be seen

Special Stains and Immunohistochemistry

- Noncontributory

Other Techniques for Diagnosis

- Noncontributory

Differential Diagnosis

▎ Tubular carcinoma
- Composed of small, angulated ducts with infiltrative growth pattern
- Desmoplastic stromal response surrounding ducts

▎ Phyllodes tumor
- Fibroadenomas are 50 times more common than phyllodes tumor
- Shows an exaggerated intracanalicular growth pattern (leaflike structure) exceeding that which is typical for a fibroadenoma
- Often shows increased cytologic atypia and mitotic activity
- Unequivocal malignant areas may be seen

▎ Tubular adenoma
- Composed of regular benign breast ducts of similar size and shape
- Distinction between these two benign entities is of little importance; they are believed to be related to each other and may occasionally show overlapping histologic features, but neither shows an increased risk for carcinoma

Pearls

- Some use the term *juvenile fibroadenoma* when the tumor is found in young girls; often larger with greater degree of stromal cellularity when compared with typical fibroadenoma
- Most common breast tumor in young women
- Karyotypic abnormalities are detected in about 20% to 30% of fibroadenomas
- No increased risk for malignant transformation or subsequent carcinoma in the setting of noncomplex fibroadenomas and negative family history of breast cancer

- Lobular carcinoma in situ (LCIS) is the most common malignancy found in fibroadenoma
- Rare cases of invasive lobular and ductal carcinoma arising in fibroadenomas have been reported
- Excision biopsy with narrow margins is adequate treatment; rare recurrence if incompletely excised

Selected References

Lerwill MF: Biphasic lesions of the breast. Semin Diagn Pathol 21:48-56, 2004.

Kuijper A, Mommers E, van der Wall E, van Diest PJ: Histopathology of fibroadenoma of the breast. Am J Clin Pathol 115:736-742, 2001.

López-Ferrer P, Jiménez-Heffernan JA, Vicandi B, et al: Fine needle aspiration cytology of breast fibroadenoma: A cytohistologic correlation study of 405 cases. Acta Cytol 43:579-586, 1999.

Takei H, Iino Y, Horiguchi J, et al: Natural history of fibroadenomas based on the correlation between size and patient age. Jpn J Clin Oncol 29:8-10, 1999.

Ciatto S, Bonardi R, Zappa M, Giorgi D: Risk of breast cancer subsequent to histological or clinical diagnosis of fibroadenoma: Retrospective longitudinal study of 3938 cases. Ann Oncol 8:297-300, 1997.

Phyllodes Tumor

Clinical Features

- Rare tumor; about 1% of all breast tumors
- Usually affects adults (fifth and sixth decades); rarely found in pediatric age group
- History of a rapidly growing, discrete, palpable breast mass

Gross Pathology

- Variably sized, discrete, gray-tan mass with firm consistency
- Variegated, lobulated cut surface; cleft formation may be seen
- Areas of necrosis and hemorrhage (more common in malignant lesions)

Histopathology

- Composed of both mesenchymal and epithelial elements
- May be well circumscribed or microscopically invasive
- Adipose tissue within stroma is seen in about one third of phyllodes tumors (in biopsies)
- Epithelial component
  — Elongated, leaflike epithelial proliferation (similar to that seen in fibroadenoma)
  — Squamous metaplasia of ductal epithelium
- Mesenchymal component
  — Increased stromal cellularity typically in periductal regions (greater than seen in fibroadenoma)
  — Cellular atypia or increased mitotic activity may be seen
- Metaplastic change is common in both epithelial and stromal elements
  — Metaplastic bone, cartilage, fat, or muscle can be present in mesenchymal component (more frequent in malignant tumors)
- Classified as benign, borderline, or malignant based on histologic features
  — Malignant phyllodes tumor
    - In general show stromal pleomorphism, overgrowth (×10 field with no epithelium), increased mitotic activity, and infiltrative margins
    - Sarcomatous appearance with increased cellularity and atypia; heterologous mesenchymal differentiation may be seen
    - High mitotic rate (more than 5 mitotic figures/10 high-power fields [hpf])
    - Stromal overgrowth with loss of epithelial component
    - Areas of necrosis
    - Infiltrative tumor margin
  — Benign phyllodes tumor
    - In general, stromal cells are not markedly pleomorphic; mitoses are few (>4) and show well-circumscribed edges
  — Variable cellularity
    - Minimal pleomorphism
    - Low mitotic activity
    - No necrosis
    - Well-defined tumor margin
  — Low-grade malignant or borderline phyllodes tumor
    - Tumors with some but not all of the above features, 2 to 5 mitoses/10 hpf, and moderate stromal cellularity)

Special Stains and Immunohistochemistry

- Cytokeratin highlights epithelial component
- Vimentin stromal cells positive
- Actin, desmin variably positive
- CD34 frequently expressed in stromal cells
- β-Catenin frequently expressed in stromal cells

Other Techniques for Diagnosis

- Electron microscopy: most tumor cells show fibroblastic and myofibroblastic differentiation
- Flow cytometry: most malignant tumors are aneuploid and have a high proliferative index

Differential Diagnosis

▌ Juvenile fibroadenoma
- Lacks the exaggerated intracanalicular growth pattern (leaflike architecture) characteristic of phyllodes tumor

Figure 13-18. Phyllodes tumor. A, Benign phyllodes tumors are variably sized, discrete masses of firm consistency. **B,** The benign neoplasm shows leaflike pattern with mild cellular stroma. **C,** Malignant phyllodes tumors frequently show areas of necrosis and hemorrhage. **D,** The malignant tumor displays a leaflike pattern with highly cellular stroma and cytologic pleomorphism. **E,** This malignant phyllodes tumor shows marked nuclear pleomorphism and mitotic activity of the stromal component.

- Shows uniform stromal cellularity
- No pleomorphism or mitotic activity
▌ Carcinosarcoma
- Rarely found in the breast
- Characterized by malignant epithelial and stromal components that are distinct and separate from each other

Pearls
- Benign phyllodes tumors closely resemble fibroadenomas but are typically more cellular and show an exaggerated intracanalicular growth pattern
- In young girls, surgical approach may be different for fibroadenoma and benign phyllodes tumor; narrow margin is reasonable with fibroadenoma, but because

of possibility of recurrence, phyllodes tumor should be excised with wider margins

- Lymph node dissection is not indicated because malignant tumors spread hematogenously (to lungs, pleura, and bones)
- May recur locally, and malignant variants may metastasize
- Metastases usually contain only sarcomatous component
- ER and PR are not useful to determine prognosis
- Gain of chromosome 1q is common in phyllodes tumors; stromal *p53* gene expression and complex karyotypic abnormalities are more commonly observed in malignant tumors

Selected References

Lee AHS: Recent developments in the histological diagnosis of spindle cell carcinoma, fibromatosis and phyllodes tumor of the breast. Histopathology 52:45-57, 2008.

Lee AH, Hodi Z, Ellis IO, Elston CW: Histological features useful in the distinction of phyllodes tumour and fibroadenoma on needle core biopsy of the breast. Histopathology 51:336-344, 2007.

Jacobs TW, Chen YY, Guinee DG: Fibroepithelial lesions with cellular stroma on breast core needle biopsy: Are there predictors of outcome in surgical excision? Am J Clin Pathol 124:342-354, 2005.

Dietrich CU, Pandis N, Rizou H, et al: Cytogenetic findings in phyllodes tumors of the breast: Karyotypic complexity differentiates between malignant and benign tumors. Hum Pathol 28:1379-1382, 1997.

Reinfuss M, Mitus J, Duda K, et al: The treatment and prognosis of patients with phyllodes tumor of the breast: An analysis of 170 cases. Cancer 77:910-916, 1996.

Atypical Ductal Hyperplasia and Ductal Carcinoma In Situ

Clinical Features

- Age distribution similar to that of invasive mammary carcinomas

Figure 13-19. A, Atypical ductal hyperplasia. Duct involved by a complex proliferation of epithelial cells. Notice the irregularity of the luminal spaces. Scattered small myoepithelial cells can also be seen. **B, Atypical ductal hyperplasia.** Uniform cell proliferation. Notice some cellular overlap and irregularity of secondary lumens. **C, Ductal carcinoma in situ, comedo type.** High-grade ductal carcinoma in situ with central necrosis, large pleomorphic nuclei, and prominent nucleoli. **D, Ductal carcinoma in situ, cribriform type.** Several ducts displaying proliferation of epithelial cells with formation of secondary lumens. Notice that the secondary lumens are round and have clean, punched-out borders. Central necrosis is also noted.

Continued

Figure 13-19. cont'd. E, Ductal carcinoma in situ, cribriform type. The tumor shows sharp, well-demarcated, punched-out lumens. Central necrosis is also noted. **F, Ductal carcinoma in situ, cribriform type.** Distended duct displaying classic cribriform pattern. **G, Ductal carcinoma in situ, solid type.** Several distended ducts demonstrating a solid proliferation of uniform epithelial cells. Central necrosis is seen. **H, Ductal carcinoma in situ, micropapillary type.** Dilated duct containing a proliferation of a monomorphic cell population forming epithelial tufts around the duct.

- Usually not associated with a palpable breast mass
- Mammogram may show suspicious calcifications
- May be an incidental finding in breast biopsy performed for other reasons

Gross Pathology

- Comedo DCIS may show small areas of necrosis within dense fibrotic breast tissue
- ADH and noncomedo-type DCIS usually show no distinct gross pathologic changes

Histopathology

▍ADH
- Epithelial cell proliferation within breast ducts
- Consists of a monotonous cell population similar to that seen in DCIS
- Typically shows more nuclear overlapping and indistinct cell membranes when compared with DCIS

- Secondary lumens show irregular borders with variable size and shape; lack the rounded, punched-out appearance of DCIS
- Does not show necrosis
- Criteria for diagnosis of ADH
  — Diagnosis of ADH is made when cytologic features are typical of DCIS, but the characteristic architecture of DCIS is lacking, or
  — Characteristic cytologic features and architecture of DCIS are seen but only focally present within one or two ducts
▍DCIS (several well-recognized variants exist)
- Comedocarcinoma
  — Ducts showing extensive epithelial cell proliferation with marked pleomorphism and central necrosis
  — Must have high-grade (grade III) nuclei and central necrosis
  — Periductal fibrosis and inflammation
  — May extend into adjacent lobules

— Retrograde cancerization of lobules is often present
- Cribriform type
  — Epithelial cell proliferation with formation of secondary lumens
  — Secondary lumens are round and have a clean, punched-out appearance
  — Areas of necrosis may be seen
  — Cells have round nuclei and distinct cell membranes; no or minimal nuclear overlapping
  — Uniform population of monotonous cells; may show mild to moderate atypia
  — Low mitotic activity
- Solid type
  — Ducts are completely filled and distended with proliferating epithelial cells
  — Round to polygonal cells with distinct cell membranes and no or minimal nuclear overlapping
  — Central necrosis may be seen; high-grade nuclear features seen in comedo variant are not seen
  — Uniform population of monotonous cells; may show mild to moderate atypia
- Micropapillary type (Table 13-1)
  — Uniform epithelial cells forming small papillary tufts extending into the lumen of the duct
  — Papillary projections are regularly spaced around the duct
  — Lining cells usually show minimal cytologic atypia
  — Combination of micropapillary and cribriform types occasionally seen
  — Involves the breast extensively

Special Stains and Immunohistochemistry

- C-erb-B2 (HER-2-neu): more commonly positive in high-grade tumors
- Mib-1 (Ki-67): higher percentage (>20%) of tumor cells positive in high-grade tumors
- ER and PR: lower-grade tumors more frequently positive

Other Techniques for Diagnosis

- Noncontributory

Differential Diagnosis

▌ ADH versus intraductal carcinoma
- Diagnosis of ADH is made when cytologic features are typical of DCIS but the characteristic architecture of DCIS is lacking, or
- Characteristic cytologic features and architecture of DCIS are seen but are only focally present within one or two ducts

▌ Invasive ductal carcinoma
- Shows infiltration of the neoplastic cells outside the basement membrane of the duct
- Immunohistochemical staining for basement membrane proteins, including laminin or type IV collagen, may help identify areas of invasion by showing loss of continuity of the basement membrane

▌ LCIS
- Typically shows small, uniform cells that fill and distend the lobular unit
- Intraductal carcinoma involving lobules shows larger cells with greater nuclear pleomorphism

Pearls

- Occasionally multicentric or bilateral but much less frequently than lobular carcinomas
- Typically treated by excisional biopsy following radiologic needle localization with or without radiation therapy
- Occasionally occult microinvasive carcinoma is found
- Lymph node metastases may be seen in about 3% of comedocarcinomas (these cases are believed to actually have microinvasion that is not identified)
- Aneuploid tumors have been shown to be more likely to recur after excisional biopsy
- Carcinoma risk
  — ADH is associated with a 400% to 500% increased risk for carcinoma
  — ADH is a marker for subsequent invasive carcinoma, which usually develops at the site of disease
  — DCIS (especially comedocarcinoma) shows high likelihood of progression to invasive carcinoma

Selected References

Goldstein NS, Lacerna M, Vicini F: Cancerization of lobules and atypical ductal hyperplasia adjacent to ductal carcinoma in situ of the breast. Am J Clin Pathol 110:357-367, 1998.

Tavassoli FA: Ductal carcinoma in situ: introduction of the concept of ductal intraepithelial neoplasia. Mod Pathol 11:140-152, 1998.

Marshall LM, Hunter DJ, Connolly JL, et al: Risk of breast cancer associated with atypical hyperplasia of lobular and ductal types. Cancer Epidemiol Biomarkers Prev 6:297-301, 1997.

Bocker W, Decker T, Ruhnke M, Schneider W: Ductal hyperplasia and ductal carcinoma in situ: Definition, classification and differential diagnosis. Pathologe 18:3-18, 1997.

Table 13-1. Grading of Intraductal Carcinoma

Grade	Characteristics
High	Marked cytologic atypia and necrosis; high mitotic rate All comedocarcinomas are high grade by definition
Intermediate	Cribriform, solid, or micropapillary types with minimal nuclear pleomorphism and necrosis or moderate nuclear pleomorphism without necrosis
Low	Cribriform, solid, or micropapillary types with minimal nuclear pleomorphism and no necrosis

Raju U, Vertes D: Breast papillomas with atypical ductal hyperplasia: A clinicopathologic study. Hum Pathol 27:1231-1238, 1996.

Atypical Lobular Hyperplasia and Lobular Carcinoma In Situ

Clinical Features

- No palpable lesion is present
- Typically found as an incidental lesion in biopsy performed for a different indication or may be associated with invasive lobular carcinoma
- Mammography not useful in detecting either ALH or LCIS; nonspecific calcifications may be seen
- Multicentric and bilateral disease is often present
- LCIS shows high probability of progressing to invasive lobular carcinoma (about 25% to 35% of cases)

Gross Pathology

- LCIS by itself usually causes no gross pathologic changes
- Extensive LCIS may cause a firm granular cut surface
- Proliferative lesions (fibrocystic changes) are often associated with both ALH and LCIS and are what often prompts biopsy

Histopathology

▌ Atypical lobular hyperplasia (ALH)
- Neoplastic cells are evenly spaced, round to polygonal cells with bland nuclei, scant cytoplasm, and indistinct cell borders; cells usually lack intracytoplasmic mucin droplets and show minimal or no loss of cohesion
- Involved lobules show residual ductule lumens
- Lobules are filled with neoplastic cells, but there is no distention of involved lobular units
- Involvement of only a single lobular unit

▌ LCIS
- Proliferation of evenly spaced, round to polygonal, monotonous cells with small, bland nuclei, clear or eosinophilic cytoplasm, and indistinct cell borders
- Signet ring cells (cells with intracytoplasmic vacuoles containing mucin, which compresses the nucleus to the periphery of the cell) are often seen
- Neoplastic cells causing expansion and distention of lobular unit
- Intervening stroma between involved ductules are typically seen; confluent ductules may be seen when massively distended
- Pagetoid spread of neoplastic cells into adjacent ducts may be seen
- Necrosis is rare
- Pleomorphic LCIS (PLCIS) shows pleomorphic nuclei grade III, with more obvious nucleoli, and is more likely associated with comedo-type necrosis and microcalcifications

Figure 13-20. A, Atypical lobular hyperplasia. Mildly distended lobular unit filled with a small round monomorphic population of epithelial cells. **B, Lobular carcinoma in situ.** Several distended lobular units filled with a monotonous population of small round neoplastic cells. **C, Lobular carcinoma in situ.** Classic histologic features of lobular carcinoma in situ. Notice the small size and uniformity of the neoplastic cells.

Special Stains and Immunohistochemistry

- Mucicarmine or Alcian blue and PAS highlight signet ring cells (intracytoplasmic mucin)
- ER and PR show variable reactivity
- HER-2 and p53, E-cadherin negative

- PLCIS immunohistochemistry profile is often ER, PR negative and C-erb-B2 (HER-2-neu) positive; glycoprotein of cystic breast disease (GCDFP-15) and p53 show increased immunoreactivity

Other Techniques for Diagnosis

- Genetic alterations common to both processes include loss at 19q13.2, 11q13, and 16q21 and gains at 20q13

Differential Diagnosis

▌ DCIS involving lobules
- Typically shows larger cells with greater pleomorphism
- Neoplastic cells show distinct cell borders
- Small ductule formation with rosette-like pattern
- Presence of intracytoplasmic mucin (mucicarmine positivity) favors LCIS
- Mitosis and necrosis may be present

Pearls

- Many investigators believe that no prognostic information is gained by distinguishing between ALH and LCIS; some use the term *lobular neoplasia*, or more recently, *in situ lobular neoplasia*, to encompass both ALH and LCIS
- High probability of multicentricity and bilaterality (up to 50% of cases)
- Follow-up surgical excision is recommended when the diagnosis of AHL or LCIS is made on core needle biopsy
- Loss or down-regulation of E-cadherin (*CDH1*) gene is the most important molecular feature of lobular neoplasias
- Carcinoma risk
  — Eight- to 10-fold risk and 4- to 5-fold risk for developing invasive carcinoma after a diagnosis of LCIS
  — ALH and LCIS are markers for subsequent invasive carcinoma, which may develop at any location within the breast or in the contralateral breast, with greater risk in the ipsilateral breast
  — Recommended treatment includes close follow-up and hormonal therapy
  — Treated LCIS progresses to invasive carcinoma at similar rate to that for untreated DCIS
  — May develop invasive carcinoma of any type, although invasive lobular carcinoma is most common after a diagnosis of ALH or LCIS

Selected References

Karabakhtsian RG, Johnson R, Sumkin J, Dabbs DJ: The clinical significance of lobular neoplasia on core biopsy. Am J Sur Pathol 31(Suppl):717-723, 2007.

Mohsin SK, O'Connel P, Allred DC, Libby AL: Biomarker profile and genetic abnormalities in lobular carcinoma in situ. Breast Cancer Res Treat 90:249-256, 2005.

Page DL, Schuyler PA, Dupont WD, et al: Atypical lobular hyperplasia as a unilateral predictor of breast cancer risk: A retrospective cohort study. Lancet 361;125-129, 2003.

Marshall LM, Hunter DJ, Connolly JL, et al: Risk of breast cancer associated with atypical hyperplasia of lobular and ductal types. Cancer Epidemiol Biomarkers Prev 6:297-301, 1997.

Goldschmidt RA, Victor TA: Lobular carcinoma in situ of the breast. Semin Surg Oncol 12:314-320, 1996.

Infiltrating Ductal Carcinoma

Clinical Features

- Most frequently diagnosed mammary carcinoma
- Wide age distribution; most commonly at 40 to 60 years of age
- Risk factors include positive family history of breast carcinoma, early menstruation, late menopause, and nulliparity
- Often presents as palpable or mammographically detectable mass
- Skin ulceration, dimpling (peau d'orange), or nipple discharge may be seen
- Prognosis depends on numerous factors; most important is lymph node status

Gross Pathology

- Hard, fibrotic mass typically with stellate, infiltrative borders
- Rare tumors appear circumscribed with pushing borders
- Gray-white color with gritty, yellow-white streaks
- Gross evidence of necrosis may be seen
- Wide variation in size depending on duration of growth before treatment

Histopathology

- Infiltrating tumor composed of clusters or sheets of tumor cells together with single or cords of neoplastic cells
- Neoplastic cells often form tubules or glands
- Prominent lymphoplasmacytic response seen in 15% to 20% of cases
- Angiolymphatic or perineural invasion often seen, especially in high-grade lesions
- Most cases show intraductal carcinoma involving adjacent ducts; LCIS involving adjacent lobules may be seen
- Grading determined by cytologic and architectural features (Table 13-2)

Special Stains and Immunohistochemistry

- ER and PR
  — Positive in most grade I and grade II lesions
  — Higher-grade (grade III) tumors are typically ER and PR negative
  — Occasionally ER positive and PR negative (about 10% to 15% of cases)

Figure 13-21. Infiltrating ductal carcinoma. A, Well differentiated (grade I). **B,** Moderately differentiated (grade II). **C,** Poorly differentiated (grade III).

Table 13-2. Grading of Invasive Ductal Carcinoma

Grade	Characteristics
I	Distinct duct formation composing 75% of overall architecture Minimal variation in cell size Minimal pleomorphism with nuclear size equal to that of a normal duct epithelial cell nucleus; inconspicuous nucleoli Rare mitotic activity
II	Less than 75% tubule formation Increased variation in cell size (twofold to threefold variation) Tumor cells with larger nuclei, coarse chromatin, and distinct nucleoli Increased mitotic activity
III	Lacks distinct tubule formation Marked variation in cell size (greater than threefold variation) Marked nuclear pleomorphism with hyperchromatic nuclei showing coarse chromatin and prominent, often multiple nucleoli Numerous mitotic figures; atypical mitoses often seen

Differential Diagnosis

▌ Infiltrating tubular carcinoma
- Composed of small, well-formed, angulated glands with open lumens and minimal pleomorphism

▌ Infiltrating lobular carcinoma
- Neoplastic cells are small and uniform; typically infiltrates in single-file (linear) or alveolar pattern

▌ Radial scar
- Shows central zone of fibrosis and elastosis with stellate or radial arrangement of ductules
- No infiltration into adjacent adipose tissue
- Proliferating ducts show myoepithelial cells

▌ Sclerosing adenosis
- Benign ductule proliferation that retains lobular architecture
- Lacks infiltration into surrounding adipose tissue
- Ductules show a myoepithelial cell layer

Pearls

- Often difficult to distinguish between well-differentiated infiltrating ductal carcinoma (grade I) and tubular carcinoma
- Invasive ductal carcinomas that are associated with a high percentage (>25%) of DCIS show a higher likelihood of recurrence and treatment failure
- Overall survival significantly lower in patients with C-erb-B2 (Her-2-neu)–positive tumors
- Tumors with increased S-phase fraction (SPF) or abnormal ploidy show decreased disease-free survival
- Presence of *p53* mutation is associated with a worse prognosis

- C-erb-B2 (HER-2-neu): more commonly positive in high-grade tumors
- Mib-1 (Ki-67): higher percentage of tumor cells positive in high-grade tumors

Other Techniques for Diagnosis

- Molecular studies
  — Mutation of *ras* proto-oncogene found in about 10% to 30% of breast carcinomas
  — Two to threefold amplification of *C-erb-B2 (HER-2-neu)* reported in up to 30% of breast carcinomas

- Lymph node status appears to be the most predictive prognostic factor
- Sentinel lymph node biopsy is an alternative to axillary lymph node dissection
- Factors associated with increased risk for invasive breast carcinoma
  - Family history of breast cancer, especially in first-degree relatives
  - Patients positive for tumor suppressor genes *BRCA1* (chromosome 17) and *BRCA2* (chromosome 13) show up to an 85% lifetime risk for breast carcinoma
  - Early menarche, late menopause
  - Obesity
  - Delivery of first child after age 30 years
  - Li-Fraumeni syndrome (associated with presence of *p53* tumor suppressor gene)
  - Heterologous carriers of the ataxia-telangiectasia (*ATM*) gene
  - Cowden disease (gastrointestinal polyps, multiple trichilemmomas, and increased risk for thyroid and breast carcinomas); associated with abnormal gene on chromosome 10

Selected References

Dowlatshahi K, Fan M, Bloom KJ, et al: Occult metastases in the sentinel lymph nodes of patients with early breast carcinoma. Cancer 86:990-996, 1999.

Frierson HF Jr, Wilbur DC, Gaffey MJ, et al: Quantitative image cytometry of infiltrating ductal carcinoma: Comparison with prognostic parameters and reproducibility of histological grade. Hum Pathol 27:821-826, 1996.

Zhou D, Battifora H, Yokota J, et al: Association of multiple copies of the c-erb B-2 oncogene with spread of breast cancer. Cancer Res 47:6123-6125, 1987.

Infiltrating Lobular Carcinoma

Clinical Features

- Similar age distribution and risk factors as infiltrating ductal carcinoma
- Accounts for 5% to 14% of all invasive breast carcinomas
- Presents as a mass with poorly defined margins
- High incidence of multifocal or bilateral disease (up to 20%)
- May not be identified on mammograms

Figure 13-22. Infiltrating lobular carcinoma. A, Classic targetoid pattern. **B,** Classic growth pattern of linear or "single-file" infiltration. **C,** Pleomorphic cell variant. **D,** Pleomorphic cell variant. Tumor cells infiltrating stroma are highly pleomorphic, some with signet ring cell morphology.

Gross Pathology

- Variable size (may be of microscopic size to well-defined, large masses to large tumors that are diffusely present throughout the breast)
- Typically forms a hard mass with irregular, infiltrative borders

Histopathology

- Classic growth pattern shows tumor cells in a linear or single-file (Indian filing) pattern in a sclerotic background; cells may show mucin-filled vacuoles sometimes resulting in signet ring cells
- Other common growth patterns and subtypes include
  — Solid: irregular solid nests of tumor cells
  — Tubulolobular: small tubule formation with linear infiltration
  — Alveolar: numerous small round aggregates of tumor cells separated by fibrous tissue
  — Apocrine and histiocytoid subtypes: tumor cells resemble macrophages with copious cytoplasm and prominent nucleoli
  — Pleomorphic subtype: tumors with high-grade nuclei and high mitotic index
- Tumor cells concentrically arranged around ducts (targetoid or bull's-eye pattern)
- Uniform, small bland cells with round nuclei and inconspicuous nucleoli
- Often associated with LCIS

Special Stains and Immunohistochemistry

- Mucicarmine, Alcian blue, and PAS positive in signet ring cells containing intracytoplasmic sialomucin
- Mib-1 (Ki-67): variable reactivity
- ER and PR: variable reactivity
- C-erb-B2 (HER-2-neu): about 30% of tumors show 2+ or 3+ positivity
- E-cadherin negative

Other Techniques for Diagnosis

- Noncontributory

Differential Diagnosis

▪ Sclerosing adenosis
  - Ductule proliferation that retains lobular architecture
  - Lacks infiltration into surrounding adipose tissue
  - Myoepithelial cells present
▪ Infiltrating ductal carcinoma
  - Neoplastic cells often form distinct ducts
  - Typically composed of large, pleomorphic cells with prominent nucleoli and numerous mitotic figures
▪ Malignant lymphoma
  - Small, noncohesive cells
  - Immunohistochemistry negative for cytokeratin and EMA and positive for lymphoid markers

Pearls

- Loss or down-regulation of E-cadherin (*CDH1*) gene is the most important molecular feature of lobular neoplasias
- Most frequent breast carcinoma to be multifocal or bilateral
- Tubulolobular variant may be better categorized with ductal-type carcinomas
- Classic cytogenetic changes of the classic variant are loss of 16q and 1p gain resembling grade I ductal carcinomas
- Cytogenetic profile of pleomorphic variant resembles more grade III ductal carcinoma with overexpression of HER-2-neu (with gene amplification), p53 positivity, and loss of ER and PR expression
- Classic form of invasive lobular carcinoma has better prognosis than other subtypes
- Higher likelihood of metastases to the ovary, bone marrow, serosal surfaces, and cerebrospinal fluid when compared with invasive ductal carcinomas

Selected References

Hanby AM, Hughes TA: In situ and invasive lobular neoplasia of the breast. Histopathology 52:58-66, 2008.

Karabakhtsian RG, Johnson R, Sumkin J, Dabbs DJ: The clinical significance of lobular neoplasia on breast core biopsy. Am J Surg Pathol 31:717-723, 2007.

Dabbs DJ, Bhargava R, Chivukula M: Lobular versus ductal breast neoplasms: the diagnostic utility of p120 catenin. Am J Surg Pathol 31:427-437, 2007.

Palacios J, Sarrió D, García-Macias MC, et al: Frequent E-cadherin gene inactivation by loss of heterozygosity in pleomorphic lobular carcinoma of the breast. Mod Pathol 16:674-678, 2003.

Triple Negative Carcinomas

Clinical Features

- Account for 10% to 17% of all breast carcinomas
- Found more frequently in women younger than 50 years
- More common in premenopausal women
- Behave as biologically aggressive cancers, with most deaths occurring in the first 5 years
- Heterogeneous group of tumors defined by the absent expression of ER, PR, and C-erb-B2 (HER-2-neu) proteins

Gross Pathology

- Tumors are of relatively large size
- Tumors have pushing borders

Histopathology

- Most triple negative breast cancers are of a basal-like phenotype (tumors with basal cytokeratin, myoepithelial, and epidermal growth factor receptor [EGFR] expression) and are high-grade ductal

Figure 13-23. Triple negative breast carcinomas. A, Triple negative breast carcinomas are high-grade neoplasms with high-grade nuclear features. **B,** Cytokeratin 5/6 is positive in most, but these tumors are estrogen receptor, progesterone receptor, and C-erb-B2 negative.

carcinomas of no specific type; many high-grade metaplastic carcinomas and medullary carcinomas exhibit a basal-like immunophenotype
- Triple negative breast cancers have high-grade nuclear features, high mitotic rate, and geographic tumor necrosis
- Areas of squamous metaplasia and differentiation are seen, and spindled and sarcomatoid foci may be present
- Variable lymphocytic inflammatory infiltrate may be seen

Special Stains and Immunohistochemistry

- ER, PR, and C-erb-B2 (HER-2-neu) negative
- Cytokeratins 5/6, 14, 17 positive in most basal-like phenotype tumors
- EGFR positive in most basal-like phenotype tumors
- SMA and p63 positive in most basal-like phenotype tumors

Other Techniques for Diagnosis

- Tissue microarray gene expression profiling identified triple negative breast cancers as tumors that have negativity for hormone receptors and C-erb-B2 (HER-2-neu)

Differential Diagnosis

- Some tumors may mimic large cell lymphomas

Pearls

- *BRCA1* gene–related breast cancers, triple negative breast cancers, and basal-like breast cancers are a closely related group of carcinomas with significant morphologic, phenotypic, and genetic overlap
- Triple negative breast cancers of basal-like morphology favor a hematogenous spread with

metastatic deposits to lungs and brain and less to axillary nodes and bones
- Tumors may show objective response to neoadjuvant chemotherapeutic regimens, but lack of complete pathologic response implies poor prognosis

Selected References

Reis-Filho JS, Tutt ANJ: Triple negative tumours: A critical review. Histopathology 52:108-118, 2008.

Diaz LK, Cryns VL, Symmans WF, Sneige N: Triple negative breast carcinoma and basal phenotype: From expression profiling to clinical practice. Adv Anat Pathol 14:419-430, 2007.

Nielsen TO, Hsu FD, Jensen K, et al: Immunohistochemical and clinical characterization of the basal-like subtype of invasive breast carcinoma. Clin Cancer Res 10:5367-5374, 2004.

Medullary Carcinoma

Clinical Features

- About 3% to 5% of all mammary carcinomas
- Similar age distribution as infiltrating ductal carcinoma, although some reports suggest a younger age (35 years)
- Mammography shows well-circumscribed mass; may mimic fibroadenoma

Gross Pathology

- Firm, discrete mass (typically 2 to 3 cm)
- Noninvasive tumors that are typically well circumscribed; often show distinct capsule
- Faintly nodular, soft, tan-brown or gray tumor

Histopathology

- Poorly differentiated tumor with syncytial pattern (>75% of tumor)

Figure 13-24. Infiltrating medullary carcinoma. Composed of a proliferation of large neoplastic cells with vesicular nuclear chromatin and prominent nucleoli. Syncytial growth pattern is visible. Characteristic lymphoplasmacytic infiltrate is also evident.

- Pleomorphic cells with high nuclear grade and numerous mitoses
- Must show a prominent lymphoplasmacytic response around tumor cells
- No invasion into surrounding adipose tissue
- Well-defined margins with pushing borders
- Glandular or ductal structures should not be seen

Special Stains and Immunohistochemistry

- Cytokeratin 5/6 positive
- ER and PR negative in more than 90% of cases
- C-erb-B2 (HER-2-neu) negative
- EGFR frequently expressed

Other Techniques for Diagnosis

- Flow cytometry: tumor cells typically aneuploid or polypoid

Differential Diagnosis

- Infiltrating ductal carcinoma
  - Typically does not show extensive syncytial pattern
  - Less prominent lymphocytic infiltrate
  - Infiltrative borders

Pearls

- Relatively better prognosis than infiltrating ductal carcinoma
- Patients have decreased likelihood of axillary lymph node metastases
- Designation of atypical medullary carcinoma should be avoided because these lesions have been shown to behave similarly to infiltrating ductal carcinomas
- More commonly associated with *BRCA1* and *BRCA2* gene mutations

Selected References

Khomsi F, Ben Bachouche W, Bouzaiene H, et al: Typical medullary carcinoma of the breast: A retrospective study of about 33 cases. Gynecol Obstet Fertil 35:1117-1122, 2007.

Vincent-Salomon A, Gruel N, Lucchesi C, et al: Identification of typical medullary breast carcinoma as a genomic sub-group of basal-like carcinomas, a heterogeneous new molecular entity. Breast Cancer Res 9(2):R24, 2007.

Bertucci F, Finetti P, Cervera N, et al: Gene expression profiling shows medullary breast cancer is a subgroup of basal breast cancers. Cancer Res 66:4636-4644, 2006.

Vu-Nishino H, Tavassoli FA, Ahrens WA, Haffty BG: Clinicopathologic features and long-term outcome of patients with medullary breast carcinoma managed with breast-conserving therapy (BCT). Int J Radiat Oncol Biol Phys 62:1040-1047, 2005.

Reinfuss M, Stelmach A, Mitus J, et al: Typical medullary carcinoma of the breast: A clinical and pathological analysis of 52 cases. J Surg Oncol 60:89-94, 1995.

Mucinous (Colloid) Carcinoma

Clinical Features

- Constitutes less than 2% of all breast carcinomas
- Typically presents as a discrete mass
- Older women are more commonly affected
- Mammogram shows a well-defined tumor

Gross Pathology

- Well-circumscribed, gelatinous mass

Histopathology

- Clusters of infiltrating tumor cells surrounded by lakes of extracellular mucin
- Extracellular mucin must make up greater than 50% of the tumor
- May have alveolar, cribriform, or papillary configuration or infiltrate as diffuse sheets of cells

Figure 13-25. Mucinous (colloid) carcinoma. Numerous clusters of neoplastic ductal cells surrounded by pools of extracellular mucin material.

- Gland formation is not typically seen
- Intraductal carcinoma often involves peripheral ducts

Special Stains and Immunohistochemistry

- Cytokeratin 7 positive
- Cytokeratin 20 typically negative
- PAS highlights intracellular mucin
- ER and PR: variable reactivity, usually positive
- Neuroendocrine differentiation can be seen in some cases

Other Techniques for Diagnosis

- Electron microscopy: demonstrates intracellular mucin (mucigen granules)
- Flow cytometry: pure mucinous carcinomas are almost always diploid; mixed tumors with areas of invasive ductal carcinoma are more commonly aneuploid

Differential Diagnosis

▌ Mucocele-like tumor
  - Benign epithelial-lined cysts containing mucin
  - No tumor cells floating in the extracellular mucin
  - Extracellular mucin dissecting through fibrous stroma
▌ Mixed mucinous carcinoma
  - Lesions with minimal mucin (<50% of tumor) relative to epithelial component
▌ Metastatic mucinous ovarian or pancreatic carcinoma
  - Exceedingly rare
  - Malignant epithelial cells are positive for cytokeratin 20

Pearls

- Mucinous carcinoma is a variant of invasive ductal carcinoma

- Lymph node metastases are found in fewer than 20% of patients
- Mucinous carcinoma is associated with an excellent prognosis with increased survival compared with infiltrating ductal carcinoma

Selected References

Tan PH, Tse GM, Bay BH: Mucinous breast lesions: Diagnostic challenges. J Clin Pathol 61:11-19, 2008.

Molavi D, Argani P: Distinguishing benign dissecting mucin (stromal mucin pools) from invasive mucinous carcinoma. Adv Anat Pathol 15:1-17, 2008.

Tse GM, Ma TK, Chu WC, et al: Neuroendocrine differentiation in pure type mammary mucinous carcinoma is associated with favorable histologic and immunohistochemical parameters. Mod Pathol 17:568-572, 2004.

Chinyama CN, Davies JD: Mammary mucinous lesions: Congeners, prevalence and important pathological associations. Histopathology 29:533-539, 1996.

Tubular Carcinoma

Clinical Features

- Wide age distribution (second to eighth decades), usually fourth decade
- Pure tubular carcinoma makes up about 5% of all invasive mammary carcinomas
- Presents as a palpable breast mass
- May show skin changes if superficially located

Gross Pathology

- Most lesions are less than 2 cm in diameter
- Firm, stellate, sclerotic appearance

Histopathology

- Infiltrative margins often extending into adjacent adipose tissue

Figure 13-26. Tubular carcinoma. A, Characterized by a proliferation of tubular structures in a background of loose desmoplastic stroma. **B,** The neoplastic tubules have open lumens and are lined by a single layer of epithelial cells.

- Composed of small, angulated tubules with open lumens
- Tubules are haphazardly arranged in dense collagenous stroma showing a desmoplastic response surrounding the neoplastic ducts
- Bland cytologic features, including cells with small nuclei and eosinophilic cytoplasm; rare mitotic activity
- Tubules lack myoepithelial cells
- Pure tubular carcinoma must show virtually 100% tubular architecture
- DCIS is an associated finding in up to 40% of cases; 10% are associated with LCIS
- May have mixed forms; tubulolobular type or ductal carcinoma with tubular features

Special Stains and Immunohistochemistry

- EMA usually positive
- ER positive in most cases
- SMA negative (lack of myoepithelial cells)
- S-100 protein negative (lack of myoepithelial cells)

Other Techniques for Diagnosis

- Noncontributory

Differential Diagnosis

▐ Sclerosing adenosis
- Lobular architecture is maintained
- Tubules are lined by myoepithelial cells
▐ Microglandular adenosis
- Haphazard arrangement of round ductules lacking lobular architecture and stellate configuration (similar to tubular carcinoma)
- Background shows hypocellular, collagenous stroma
- Ductal cells typically show clear or vacuolated cytoplasm
- Usually negative for EMA and ER
- Lumens often contain eosinophilic, PAS-positive secretions
▐ Mixed tumors (tubulolobular or ductal carcinoma with tubular features)
- Tumor is not completely composed of well-formed tubules
- Invasive ductal or lobular carcinoma makes up more than 5% to 25% of tumor

Pearls

- Highly differentiated form of invasive ductal carcinoma
- Rare perineural, vascular, or lymphatic invasion
- Axillary lymph node involvement is seen in less than 10% of cases
- Associated microcalcifications are present in more than 50% of cases
- Relatively good prognosis compared with infiltrating ductal carcinoma

Selected References

Abdel-Fatah TM, Powe DG, Hodi Z, et al: High frequency of coexistence of columnar cell lesions, lobular neoplasia, and low grade ductal carcinoma in situ with invasive tubular carcinoma and invasive lobular carcinoma. Am J Surg Pathol 31:417-426, 2007.

Marchiò C, Sapino A, Arisio R, Bussolati G: A new vision of tubular and tubulo-lobular carcinomas of the breast, as revealed by 3-D modelling. Histopathology 48:556-562, 2006.

Fernández-Aguilar S, Simon P, Buxant F, et al: Tubular carcinoma of the breast and associated intra-epithelial lesions: A comparative study with invasive low-grade ductal carcinomas. Virchows Arch 447:683-687, 2005.

Mitnick JS, Gianutsos R, Pollack AH, et al: Tubular carcinoma of the breast: Sensitivity of diagnostic techniques and correlation with histopathology. AJR Am J Roentgenol 172:319-323, 1999.

Winchester DJ, Sahin AA, Tucker SL, Singletary SE: Tubular carcinoma of the breast: Predicting axillary nodal metastases and recurrence. Ann Surg 223:342-347, 1996.

Papillary Carcinoma (Intraductal, Intracystic, Encapsulated, and Invasive)

Clinical Features

- Rare breast tumor makes up 1% to 2% of mammary carcinomas
- Age distribution is similar to that of other mammary carcinomas; patients are older than those with solitary intraductal papillomas
- Most patients have a palpable mass
- Associated with higher likelihood of nipple discharge (often hemorrhagic) and nipple retraction
- Rounded, circumscribed mass with rare microcalcifications on mammography

Gross Pathology

- Usually well-circumscribed mass with pushing borders
- Tan-gray tumor; may be focally hemorrhagic
- Typically cystic with obvious papilla formation

Histopathology

- Papillary lesions composed of numerous complex epithelial fronds proliferating into a distended duct lumen
- Must demonstrate papillae with absence of myoepithelial cell layer; in addition, recent studies failed to demonstrate myoepithelial cells at the periphery of tumor nodules
- Apocrine metaplasia is not a feature
- Diagnosis of invasive papillary carcinoma should be made only with identification of unequivocal stromal invasion (tumor should be clearly present beyond the capsule of the lesion)

Figure 13-27. A, Intracystic papillary carcinoma. Distended duct with highly complex proliferating epithelial fronds with absence of a myoepithelial cell layer are the hallmark of encapsulated, intracystic, and intraductal papillary carcinoma. **B, Intracystic papillary carcinoma** with non–high-grade ductal carcinoma in situ. **C, Infiltrating papillary carcinoma.** Stromal invasion is evident in the left lower corner.

Special Stains and Immunohistochemistry

- SMA, calponin, S-100 protein, smooth muscle myosin heavy chain, and p63 demonstrate focal or complete lack of myoepithelial cell layer
- ER and PR stains typically positive
- C-erb-B2 (HER-2-neu) negative
- HMWCK (5/6, 14, 34βE12) stains are negative in neoplastic cells

- CEA positive in 85% of papillary carcinomas and negative in benign papillary lesions

Other Techniques for Diagnosis

- LOH on chromosome 16q23 appears to be limited to papillary carcinomas
- LOH at *TP53* locus significantly associated with malignant papillary lesions
- Flow cytometry: tumor cells may be diploid or occasionally aneuploid (of little help in distinguishing benign papillomas from papillary carcinoma)

Differential Diagnosis

▌ Benign papilloma versus intraductal papillary carcinoma
  - Myoepithelial cell layer must be demonstrated in benign lesions and is absent in papillary carcinoma
  - Degree of cytologic atypia and complexity is typically not helpful in distinguishing benign papillomas from intraductal papillary carcinoma
  - Apocrine metaplasia is present in benign lesions
  - Papillary carcinoma is typically CEA positive, is diffusely ER/PR positive, and lacks HMWCK expression
▌ Invasive papillary carcinoma
  - Complex papillary proliferation with unequivocal stromal invasion

Pearls

- Intraductal (intracystic, encapsulated) papillary carcinoma, long considered a variant of intraductal carcinoma, may represent a form of low-grade carcinoma, being part of a spectrum of progression from in situ to invasive disease
- Patients with intraductal papillary carcinoma are typically good candidates for breast-conserving surgery
- Invasive papillary carcinoma rarely shows nodal metastases

Selected References

Collins LC, Schnitt SJ: Papillary lesions of the breast: Selected diagnostic and management issues. Histopathology 52:20-29, 2008.

Mulligan AM, O'Malley FP: Papillary lesions of the breast: A review. Adv Anat Pathol 14:108-119, 2007.

Tse GM, Tan PH, Lui PC, et al: The role of immunohistochemistry for smooth-muscle actin, p63, CD10 and cytokeratin 14 in the differential diagnosis of papillary lesions of the breast. J Clin Pathol 60:315-320, 2007.

Collins LC, Carlo VP, Hwang H, et al: Intracystic papillary carcinomas of the breast: A reevaluation using a panel of myoepithelial cell markers. Am J Surg Pathol 30:1002-1007, 2006.

Carder PJ, Garvican J, Haigh I, Liston JC: Needle core biopsy can reliably distinguish between benign and malignant papillary lesions of the breast. Histopathology 46:320-327, 2005.

Metaplastic Carcinoma

Clinical Features

- Uncommon, occurring in less than 5% of breast cancer patients
- Typically presents as palpable breast mass
- Rapid growth is common
- Mammogram shows a well-defined tumor

Gross Pathology

- Distinct, firm mass with circumscribed margins
- Nodular or cystic areas can be seen

Histopathology

- Heterogenous group of lesions, simply designated as biphasic (mixed carcinomatous and sarcomatoid components) or monophasic (sarcomatoid elements only)
- Carcinomatous component is usually high grade and typically a poorly differentiated ductal carcinoma with glandular and tubular formation or the presence of intracellular or extracellular mucin production; additional subtypes include squamous component with intercellular bridges with or without keratin pearl formation
- Spindle cell proliferation or sarcomatous component is usually high grade with occasional heterologous elements, including bone or cartilage; recently described fibromatosis-like metaplastic carcinoma appears to be a low-grade variant
- Metaplastic changes include squamous metaplasia with or without keratin formation, chondroid metaplasia, or metaplastic bone
- Spindle cell proliferation or sarcomatous appearance may be seen
- Metastases from metaplastic carcinoma may consist of metaplastic elements, adenocarcinoma, or both

- Focal metaplastic changes in other invasive tumor subtypes (tubular, medullary, and lobular) may be seen

Special Stains and Immunohistochemistry

- Cytokeratin (AE1/AE3; CAM5.2): epithelial component positive; spindle cell component focally positive
- EMA: epithelial component positive; may be focally positive in mesenchymal areas
- Vimentin: typically positive in both epithelial and mesenchymal components
- ER and PR usually negative
- C-erb-B2 (HER-2-neu) usually negative
- Positive for p63 in the spindle and sarcomatous component
- EGFR overexpressed and amplified

Other Techniques for Diagnosis

- Noncontributory

Differential Diagnosis

▮ Infiltrating ductal carcinoma
- Lacks metaplastic elements

▮ Adenosquamous carcinoma
- Rare variant of metaplastic carcinoma
- Mixture of malignant glandular and epidermoid elements in dense fibrous stroma

▮ Squamous cell carcinoma
- Composed entirely of neoplastic, typically keratinizing squamous cells

Pearls

- Most common metaplastic change is squamous metaplasia
- Squamous metaplasia has little impact on prognosis; chondroid or osteoid metaplasia has a negative impact on prognosis

Selected References

Luini A, Aguilar M, Gatti G, et al: Metaplastic carcinoma of the breast, an unusual disease with worse prognosis: The experience of the European Institute of Oncology and review of the literature. Breast Cancer Res Treat 101:349-353, 2007.

Tse GM, Tan PH, Putti TC, et al: Metaplastic carcinoma of the breast: A clinicopathological review. J Clin Pathol 59:1079-1083, 2006.

Carter MR, Hornick JL, Lester S, Fletcher CD: Spindle cell (sarcomatoid) carcinoma of the breast: A clinicopathologic and immunohistochemical analysis of 29 cases. Am J Surg Pathol 30:300-309, 2006.

Barnes PJ, Boutilier R, Chiasson D, Rayson D: Metaplastic breast carcinoma: Clinical-pathologic characteristics and HER2/neu expression. Breast Cancer Res Treat 91:173-178, 2005.

Wargotz ES, Norris HJ: Metaplastic carcinomas of the breast: A matrix-producing carcinoma. Hum Pathol 20:628-635, 1989.

Figure 13-28. Metaplastic carcinoma. High-grade ductal carcinoma is seen in the lower portion of the photomicrograph. Notice metaplastic cartilaginous tissue in the upper area.

Oberman HA: Metaplastic carcinoma of the breast: A clinicopathologic study of 29 patients. Am J Surg Pathol 11:918-929, 1987.

Secretory Carcinoma

Clinical Features

- Affects women of any age; increased incidence in children and young adults (mean age, 25 years)
- Patients present with distinct painless breast mass

Gross Pathology

- Well-defined, circumscribed, nodular mass
- Cut surface shows gray-white or tan tumor
- Variable size (0.6 to 12 cm); larger lesions typically found in older women

Histopathology

- Proliferation of variably sized ducts with loss of the normal lobular architecture
- Tumor forms cystic spaces filled with abundant pale-pink secretion
- Both intracellular and extracellular secretory material
- Neoplastic ductal epithelial cells are small with bland nuclei and abundant pale, eosinophilic, granular, and vacuolated cytoplasm; rare mitotic activity
- Ducts lack a myoepithelial layer
- Often shows an intraductal component, which may be papillary, cribriform, solid, or comedo-type

Special Stains and Immunohistochemistry

- Mucicarmine- and diastase-resistant PAS: luminal secretion positive
- CEA (polyclonal), EMA, S-100, and α-lactalbumin positive
- ER and PR show variable reactivity

Figure 13-29. Secretory carcinoma. Secretory material in the neoplastic lumens. Notice the uniformity of the nuclei.

Other Techniques for Diagnosis

- Electron microscopy: cytoplasm shows numerous membrane-bound secretory vacuoles lined by microvilli

Differential Diagnosis

- Lactating adenoma
  - Typically presents during pregnancy or while lactating
  - Sharply circumscribed mass
  - Myoepithelial cell layer is present (SMA and S-100 protein positive)
- Secretory changes
  - Lobulocentric hypersecretory changes
  - Occur in nonparous breast
  - Associated with hormonal and other drug intake

Pearls

- Good prognosis compared with other invasive carcinomas (age related), especially in patients younger than 20 years
- Axillary lymph node metastasis can rarely be seen; increased incidence of axillary node metastases in patients older than 20 years; distant metastases are extremely rare
- Radiation and chemotherapy not usually part of treatment
- Increased incidence in young women; occasionally found in pediatric age group
- ETV6-NTRK3 fusion gene, the product of t(12;15)(p13;q25) translocation, is expressed in secretory carcinomas

Selected References

Diallo R, Schaefer K-L, Bankfalvi A, et al: Secretory carcinoma of the breast: A distinct variant of invasive ductal carcinoma assessed by comparative genomic hybridization and immunohistochemistry. Hum Pathol 34:1299-1305, 2003.

Tognon C, Knezevich SR, Huntsman D, et al: Expression of the ETV6-NTRK3 gene fusion as a primary event in human secretory breast carcinoma. Cancer Cell 2:367-376, 2002.

Lamovec J, Bracko M: Secretory carcinoma of the breast: Light microscopic, immunohistochemical and flow cytometric study. Mod Pathol 7:475-479, 1994.

Rosen PP, Cranor ML: Secretory carcinoma of the breast. Arch Pathol Lab Med 115:141-144, 1991.

Apocrine Carcinoma

Clinical Features

- Uncommon breast tumor; incidence of pure apocrine carcinoma varies from less than 1% to 4%
- Presents as a firm, distinct breast mass (similar to other breast carcinomas)
- Age distribution similar to that of other breast carcinomas

Figure 13-30. Infiltrating apocrine carcinoma. A, Classic histologic features include a large amount of pink granular cytoplasm and prominent nucleoli. **B,** Notice the pink granular cytoplasm and the prominent nucleoli.

- Mammographic findings similar to those of typical infiltrating ductal carcinoma

Gross Pathology

- Firm, tan-brown tumor with infiltrative or well-defined margins
- Focal cyst formation may be seen

Histopathology

- Tumor composed of nests or sheets of neoplastic apocrine cells showing large pleomorphic nuclei with prominent and often multiple nucleoli
- Cells show abundant eosinophilic cytoplasm; may be granular and vacuolated
- Gland formation often with apocrine snouts may be seen
- Intraductal apocrine carcinoma may have solid, cribriform, micropapillary, or comedo architecture
- Apocrine carcinoma must be composed almost completely of apocrine cells

Special Stains and Immunohistochemistry

- Diastase-resistant PAS: cytoplasmic granules positive
- CEA positive in most cases
- Cytokeratin and GCDFP-15 positive
- Androgen receptor (AR) positive in many cases
- ER and PR show variable positivity
- S-100 protein negative

Other Techniques for Diagnosis

- Recent molecular studies suggest that apocrine carcinomas are characterized by overexpression of the AR and metabolism-related genes
- Electron microscopy: apocrine cells contain numerous mitochondria, empty vesicles, and osmiophilic membrane-bound secretory granules

Differential Diagnosis

▌ Sclerosing adenosis with apocrine metaplasia
- Typically has lobular arrangement without infiltrative pattern
- Benign-appearing apocrine cells without pleomorphic nuclei and prominent nucleoli

Pearls

- Apocrine metaplasia is a common finding and is associated with benign proliferative conditions (fibrocystic changes)
- Malignant tumors with focal apocrine differentiation should not be called apocrine carcinoma; must be nearly completely composed of apocrine cells
- Apocrine differentiation within invasive or in situ tumors plays little role in determining prognosis or treatment
- Similar natural history to that of nonapocrine-infiltrating ductal carcinoma

Selected References

Farmer P, Bonnefoi H, Becette V, et al: Identification of molecular apocrine breast tumours by microarray analysis. Oncogene 24:4660-4671, 2005.

Honma, N, Takubo K, Akiyama F: Expression of GCDFP-15 and AR decreases in larger or node-positive apocrine carcinomas of the breast. Histopathology 47:195-201, 2005.

Japaze H, Emina J, Diaz C: "Pure" invasive apocrine carcinoma of the breast: A new clinicopathologic entity? Breast 14:3-10, 2005.

Tavassoli FA, Norris HJ: Intraductal apocrine carcinoma: A clinicopathologic study of 37 cases. Mod Pathol 7:813-818, 1994.

Gilles R, Lesnik A, Guinebretiere JM, et al: Apocrine carcinom Clinical and mammographic features. Radiology 190:495 497, 1994.

Adenoid Cystic Carcinoma

Clinical Features

- Rare lesion accounting for less than 0.5% of all breast carcinomas
- Found in the same age distribution as other mammary carcinomas
- Presents as a palpable breast mass, typically periareolar or subareolar
- Patients may have nipple discharge
- Mammographic findings are often nonspecific

Gross Pathology

- Variable size (0.7 to 12 cm); most measure less than 3 cm
- Firm, well-circumscribed, pale, tan-gray tumor
- Nodular architecture is common
- Small cyst formation occasionally seen

Histopathology

- Tumor composed of epithelial and myoepithelial cells
- Invasive tumor forming distinct islands and cords of neoplastic cells
- Characteristically shows proliferating glands (adenoid component) and abundant eosinophilic basement membrane–like material or hyaline globules
- Solid, cribriform, tubular, or trabecular architecture may be seen
- Tumor composed of two distinct cell types: basal cell population (believed to be related to myoepithelial cells) and cells with bright eosinophilic cytoplasm
- Areas of squamous differentiation and sebaceous features may be seen
- Divided into grades I, II, and III
  - Grade I: composed of glandular and cystic areas; no solid zones
  - Grade II: solid areas make up less than 30% of the tumor
  - Grade III: solid areas make up more than 30% of the tumor

Special Stains and Immunohistochemistry

- S-100 protein, cytokeratin 14, calponin, p63: basaloid cells positive
- SMA: basaloid cells positive
- Cytokeratin 7: highlight eosinophilic cell population
- Laminin: basement membrane–like material positive
- ER and PR typically negative

Other Techniques for Diagnosis

- Electron microscopy
  - Basaloid cells show few organelles with cytoplasmic projections and well-developed desmosomes
  - Eosinophilic cells are spindled or cuboid with microvilli at the luminal border and abundant tonofilaments

Differential Diagnosis

- Invasive cribriform carcinoma
  - Rare breast tumor, composed entirely of cribriform pattern
  - Lacks dual cell population
  - Lacks eosinophilic basement membrane–like material
  - Negative for S-100 protein and SMA
- Cylindroma
  - Benign skin tumor overlying the breast

Pearls

- Much less aggressive than other mammary carcinomas
- Salivary gland adenoid cystic is much more aggressive than its breast counterpart
- No evidence of perineural invasion
- Rarely metastasizes to axillary lymph nodes
- May occasionally recur or metastasize (usually to lungs) many years after treatment
- Alterations of chromosome 6q present (similar to related salivary gland tumors)

Selected References

Page DL: Adenoid cystic carcinoma of breast, a special histopathologic type with excellent prognosis. Breast Cancer Res Treat 93:189-190, 2005.

Acs G, Simpson JF, Bleiweiss IJ, et al: Microglandular adenosis with transition into adenoid cystic carcinoma of the breast. Am J Surg Pathol 27:1052-1060, 2003.

Pia-Foschini M, Reis-Filho JS, Eusebi V, Lakhani SR: Salivary glandlike tumours of the breast: Surgical and molecular pathology. J Clin Pathol 56:497-506, 2003.

Kleer CG, Oberman HA: Adenoid cystic carcinoma of the breast: Value of histologic grading and proliferative activity. Am J Surg Pathol 22:569-575, 1998.

Figure 13-31. Adenoid cystic carcinoma. Classic cribriform pattern of adenoid cystic carcinoma. Notice the eosinophilic basement membrane–like material.

Inflammatory Carcinoma

Clinical Features

- Represents about 1% to 5% of all breast cancers and is the most aggressive form
- Typically presents as swelling and diffuse induration of the mammary skin along with rapid enlargement of the breast
- Often associated with skin retraction and dimpling (peau d'orange)
- Palpable mass often present
- May present with enlarged axillary lymph nodes

Gross Pathology

- Mammary skin is erythematous and thickened
- Must be associated with an invasive mammary carcinoma

Histopathology

- Usually associated with an infiltrating ductal carcinoma (typically high grade or poorly differentiated)
- Must have tumor present in dilated dermal lymphatic channels
- Lymphoplasmacytic infiltrate seen around involved lymphatic spaces
- Tumor emboli usually seen throughout breast tissue

Special Stains and Immunohistochemistry

- ER and PR usually negative
- Usually positive for p53

- C-erb-B2 (HER-2-neu) usually positive
- E-cadherin usually positive

Other Techniques for Diagnosis

- Noncontributory

Differential Diagnosis

▌ Metastatic carcinoma
  - Lacks underlying invasive mammary carcinoma, which is needed for diagnosis of inflammatory carcinoma

Pearls

- Must have an invasive breast cancer and tumor in dermal lymphatics to make diagnosis
- Associated with amplified expression of *C-erb-B2 (HER-2-neu)* proto-oncogene
- Treatment combination of neoadjuvant chemotherapy, mastectomy, and radiotherapy results in local control in about 80% of patients; axillary dissection is not typically performed; recurrence is seen in about 20% of patients
- Poor prognosis; less than 40% 5-year survival rate
- Overexpression of RhoC oncoprotein and loss of *LIBC/WISP3* gene has been associated with inflammatory breast cancer, highly invasive phenotype

Selected References

Cristofanilli M, Valero V, Buzdar AU, et al: Inflammatory breast cancer (IBC) and patterns of recurrence: Understanding the biology of a unique disease. Cancer 110:1436-1444, 2007.

Hance KW, Anderson WF, Devesa SS, et al: Trends in inflammatory breast carcinoma incidence and survival: The surveillance, epidemiology, and end results program at the National Cancer Institute. J Natl Cancer Inst 97:966-975, 2005.

Merajver SD, Wu M: Molecular biology of inflammatory breast cancer: Applications to diagnosis, prognosis, and therapy. Breast Dis 22:25-34, 2005/2006.

Noguchi S, Miyauchi K, Nishizawa Y, et al: Management of inflammatory carcinoma of the breast with combined modality therapy including intra-arterial infusion chemotherapy as an induction therapy: Long-term follow-up results of 28 patients. Cancer 61:1483-1491, 1988.

Paget Disease of the Nipple

Clinical Features

- More frequent in postmenopausal women (sixth decade)
- Usually unilateral lesion with nipple pain or irritation
- Nipple erythema, ulceration, or discharge may be present
- About 50% of patients have a palpable, hard, underlying breast mass

Figure 13-32. Inflammatory carcinoma. Dermal and lymphatic spread of tumor cells, which is characteristic of inflammatory carcinoma.

Figure 13-33. Paget disease. Classic histologic features of this entity, including large pleomorphic cells with vacuolated cytoplasm involving the epidermis.

- May have no clinical abnormality; found on routine histologic section of nipple
- Overall found in 1% to 2% of women with breast carcinoma

Gross Pathology

- Dilated ducts in subareolar breast tissue may be seen
- Many patients have an obvious invasive mammary carcinoma
- Rarely, no carcinoma is found in mastectomy specimen

Histopathology

- Characteristic finding is Paget cell in the epidermis of the nipple
- Paget cells are large, round cells with large nuclei, prominent nucleoli, and abundant pale vacuolated cytoplasm
- Cytoplasm may contain mucin (about 50% to 60% of cases)
- Paget cells may occur in small clusters, with occasional glandlike structures with a lumen, or singly within the epidermis
- Associated carcinoma almost always seen with Paget disease
- Associated lesion is usually intraductal carcinoma (solid and comedo form), often with an infiltrating component
- Paget disease rarely occurs without associated mammary carcinoma (<5% of cases)

Special Stains and Immunohistochemistry

- Mucicarmine and PAS positive in about 50% to 60% of cases
- Cytokeratin 7, EMA, CEA, GCDFP-15 positive
- HMWCK negative
- C-erb-B2 (HER-2-neu) and p53 positive in more than 90% of cases
- ER often positive
- S-100 protein typically negative
- AR positive

Other Techniques for Diagnosis

- Noncontributory

Differential Diagnosis

- Malignant melanoma
  - Not associated with intraductal or invasive mammary carcinoma
  - Immunohistochemical staining pattern is characteristic
    — Positive for S-100 and HMB-45
    — Typically negative for CEA, EMA, and C-erb-B2 (HER-2-neu)
- Bowen disease (squamous cell carcinoma in situ)
  - Not associated with intraductal or invasive mammary carcinoma
- Clear cell change of keratinocytes
  - Large cells with small nuclei
  - Vacuolated, empty cytoplasm; no cytoplasmic mucin

Pearls

- Immunohistochemical stains are helpful in confirming the diagnosis of Paget disease
- Typically results from superficial spread of underlying intraductal or invasive carcinoma
- Prognosis is based on extent of underlying carcinoma
- Treatment is usually mastectomy with lymph node excision regardless of whether obvious breast mass is identified
- Adjuvant chemotherapy (tamoxifen) may be an option for premenopausal women with positive nodes

Selected References

Kanitakis J: Mammary and extra-mammary Paget's disease. J Eur Acad Dermatol Venereol 21:581-590, 2007.

Chen CY, Sun LM, Anderson BO: Paget disease of the breast: Changing patterns of incidence, clinical presentation, and treatment in the U.S. Cancer 107:1448-1458, 2006.

Bianco MK, Vasef MA: *HER-2* gene amplification in Paget disease of the nipple and extramammary site: A chromogenic in situ hybridization study. Diagn Mol Pathol 15:131-135, 2006.

Sakorafas GH, Blanchrad K, Sarr MG, Farley DR: Paget's disease of the breast. Cancer Treat Rev 27:9-18, 2001.

Kollmorgen DR, Varanasi JS, Edge SB, Carson WE 3rd: Paget's disease of the breast: A 33 year experience. J Am Coll Surg 187:171-177, 1998.

Yim JH, Wick MR, Philpott GW, et al: Underlying pathology in mammary Paget's disease. Ann Surg Oncol 4:287-292, 1997.

Hemangioma

Clinical Features

- Often presents as a palpable breast lesion or as a suspicious lesion on mammogram
- May be an incidental finding in mastectomy performed for carcinoma

Gross Pathology

- Typically less than 2 cm
- Firm, well-defined hemorrhagic mass within breast parenchyma

Histopathology

- Typically found in perilobular region
- Tumor composed of dilated, congested vascular channels
- Vascular spaces lined by benign-appearing endothelial cells
- Vessels surrounded by fibrous stroma
- Cavernous hemangiomas are the most common form
- No evidence of mitosis or necrosis

Special Stains and Immunohistochemistry

- CD31, factor VIII, CD34: endothelial cells positive
- Mib-1 shows low values

Other Techniques for Diagnosis

- Noncontributory

Figure 13-34. Hemangioma. The neoplasm is composed of well-spaced vascular channels lined by flat endothelial cells.

Differential Diagnosis

- Low-grade angiosarcoma
  - Typically several centimeters larger than hemangiomas
  - Poorly defined with infiltrative margins
  - Composed of complex anastomosing vascular spaces
  - Endothelial cells show atypical features with hyperchromatic nuclei; occasional mitotic activity may be seen
  - Often shows thrombi, necrosis, and hemorrhage
- Pseudoangiomatous stromal hyperplasia (PASH)
  - Composed of anastomosing, empty, slitlike spaces, lined by myofibroblasts with endothelial-like nuclei
  - Lining cells (myofibroblasts) are variably reactive for CD34 and SMA, negative for factor VIII, and rarely positive for CD31

Pearls

- Complete excision is recommended to render an accurate diagnosis
- No recurrences or malignant transformations have been documented
- Infantile hemangiomas have been associated with decreased *Hox-A5* gene expression and immunopositivity for GLUT1
- Immunohistochemistry for Ki-67 may assist in the differentiation between hemangioma and low-grade angiosarcoma

Selected References

Shin SJ, Lesser M, Rosen PP: Hemangiomas and angiosarcomas of the breast: Diagnostic utility of cell cycle markers with emphasis on Ki-67. Arch Pathol Lab Med 131:538-544, 2007.

Hoda SA, Cranor ML, Rosen PP: Hemangiomas of the breast with atypical histological features: Further analysis of histological subtypes confirming their benign character. Am J Surg Pathol 16:553-560, 1992.

Rosen PP: Vascular tumors of the breast. V. Nonparenchymal hemangiomas of mammary subcutaneous tissues. Am J Surg Pathol 9:723-729, 1985.

Rosen PP: Vascular tumors of the breast III. Angiomatosis. Am J Surg Pathol 9:652-658, 1985.

Jozefczyk MA, Rosen PP: Vascular tumors of the breast II. Perilobular hemangiomas and hemangiomas. Am J Surg Pathol 9:491-503, 1985.

Angiosarcoma

Clinical Features

- Overall rare breast tumor
- May be found in women of all ages; mean age, between 30 and 40 years
- Presents as a rapidly growing typically painless mass; often causes red-blue discoloration of the overlying skin
- More commonly found in irradiated breasts
- Cases of primary angiosarcoma arising in pregnant women are well documented

Figure 13-35. Angiosarcoma. A, Grossly, angiosacromas are friable, spongy hemorrhagic masses. **B,** Under light microscopy, they can be low grade with minimal atypia. **C,** Section shows frankly malignant spindle cell neoplasm with marked cytologic pleomorphism. **D,** Frequent mitotic figures including atypical ones can be seen.

Gross Pathology

- Variably sized mass ranging from 1 to 20 cm, average size of 4 to 5.5 cm
- Typically have infiltrative margins
- Cut surface shows an ill-defined, friable, spongy, and hemorrhagic mass
- Cystic degeneration and necrosis often seen in higher-grade lesions

Histopathology

- Divided into three grades depending on histologic findings (low grade, intermediate grade, and high grade)
    — Low grade (grade I)
    - Tumor consists of open, irregular vascular channels
    - Tumor characteristically infiltrates into adjacent breast lobules
    - Hyperchromatic nuclei may be seen, but nuclei lack significant pleomorphism
    - Mitotic activity is rare to absent
    - Endothelial tufting is minimal
    - Papillary formations, solid and spindle cell areas, blood lakes, and necrosis are absent
    - May appear deceptively benign
    — Intermediate grade (grade II)
    - Shows irregular vascular channels with focal areas of increased cellularity due to endothelial tufting and papillary fronds that project into the vascular lumens
    - Degree of cellularity is used to distinguish low-grade from intermediate-grade tumors
    - Tumor cells are hyperchromatic and show a moderate degree of pleomorphism
    - Show infiltration into adjacent breast lobules
    - Mitotic activity and solid and spindle cell areas are infrequent
    - Blood lakes and necrosis are absent
    — High grade (grade III)
    - Highly cellular lesion with endothelial tufting and increased degree of papillary formation
    - Tumor cells show marked pleomorphism
    - High mitotic rate often with atypical mitotic figures
    - Typically extensive hemorrhage with blood lake formation
    - Necrosis is typically present
    - Solid or spindle cell areas resembling fibrosarcoma or malignant fibrous histiocytoma may be seen

Special Stains and Immunohistochemistry

- Factor VIII: endothelial cells positive
- CD31 and CD34: endothelial cells positive (>90% of cases)
- Cytokeratin negative in most cases, but epithelioid areas may be positive in up to 35% of cases

Other Techniques for Diagnosis

- Electron microscopy: features associated with endothelial cells are seen, including Weibel-Palade bodies, intermediate filaments, and pinocytotic vesicles

Differential Diagnosis

▌ Hemangioma
- Typically smaller and better defined than angiosarcoma

Figure 13-36. Postradiation angiosarcoma. A, Hemorrhagic focus on the skin surface is noted. **B,** Microscopically, there is a proliferation of vascular spaces lined by pleomorphic cells with frequent mitotic figures.

- Lacks malignant cytologic features
- Does not infiltrate breast lobules
- Usually located in perilobular region
▌ PASH
  - Well-circumscribed lesions with a tan-white, homogeneous cut surface
  - Composed of anastomosing, slitlike spaces in a dense collagenous stroma
  - Lining cells are negative for CD31 and factor VIII

Pearls

- Correlation between patient age and clinical outcome is significant; high-grade lesions are more common in younger patients and have a worse prognosis
- Tumor grade is the most important prognostic factor
- High-grade (grade III) lesions have a poor prognosis
- Low- and intermediate-grade tumors (grades I and II) have increased disease-free and overall survival rates
- Treatment includes total mastectomy; axillary dissection is not indicated because these tumors rarely metastasize to axillary lymph nodes
- The role of adjuvant chemotherapy remains unclear, but chemotherapy for patients with high-grade lesions should be considered

Selected References

Brodie C, Provenzano E: Vascular proliferations of the breast. Histopathology 52:30-44, 2008.

Billings SD, McKenney JK, Folpe AL, et al: Cutaneous angiosarcoma following breast-conserving surgery and radiation: an analysis of 27 cases. Am J Clin Pathol 28:781-788, 2004.

Christodoulakis M, Gontikakis E, Giannikaki E, et al: Primary angiosarcoma of the breast. Eur J Surg Oncol 24:76-78, 1998.

Strobbe LJ, Peterse HL, Van Tinteren H, et al: Angiosarcoma of the breast after conservative therapy for invasive cancer, the incidence and outcome: An unforeseen sequela. Breast Cancer Res Treat 47:101-109, 1998.

Postmastectomy Angiosarcoma (Stewart-Treves Syndrome)

Clinical Features

- Arises in a lymphedematous upper extremity after mastectomy, with or without radiotherapy; in irradiated patients, it arises outside of the treated field
- Associated with chronic lymphedema, but pathogenesis is unknown
- Occurs in less than 0.45% of postmastectomy patients
- Typically presents about 10 years after mastectomy
- Presents as subtle, blue-purple discoloration of skin and can progress into large nodules and superficial vesicles that contain hemorrhagic fluid

Gross Pathology

- Early lesions appear as hemorrhagic foci on the skin surface and are confined to the superficial soft tissue
- Advanced disease presents as multiple hemorrhagic tumor nodules involving deeper soft tissue and muscle

Histopathology

- Proliferation of irregular, variably sized interconnecting vascular spaces lined by large endothelial cells with hyperchromatic, atypical nuclei
- Highly atypical endothelial cells with large pleomorphic nuclei showing prominent nucleoli and numerous mitotic figures
- Papillary structures may be seen within neoplastic vessels
- Dense collagenous background
- Infiltrative borders with involvement of surrounding fibroadipose tissue

- Typically, changes of chronic lymphedema are seen, including hyperplasia of the epidermis, subcutaneous edema, fibrosis, mild chronic inflammation, and small-vessel proliferation with reactive endothelial cells

Special Stains and Immunohistochemistry
- CD34, CD31, and factor VIII: endothelial cells are positive
- Cytokeratin negative

Other Techniques for Diagnosis
- Electron microscopy: features associated with endothelial cells are seen, including Weibel-Palade bodies, intermediate filaments, and pinocytotic vesicles

Differential Diagnosis
▌ Postirradiation angiosarcoma
- Develops in field of radiation, not in area of chronic lymphedema
- Typically develops within 5 years after irradiation
▌ Kaposi sarcoma
- May be difficult to differentiate from early findings in angiosarcoma
- Typically lacks pleomorphism that is commonly seen in angiosarcoma
- Found in immunocompromised hosts
▌ Reactive vascular proliferation associated with chronic lymphedema
- Lacks pleomorphism and mitotic activity seen in angiosarcoma

Pearls
- First reported by Stewart-Treves in 1948
- Why angiosarcoma develops in a background of chronic lymphedema is unknown
- Special stains for vascular endothelium do not distinguish benign from malignant vascular tumors; need to distinguish these entities based on morphology
- Amputation and systemic chemotherapy is best treatment
- Most patients die from this disease within 2 years; few long-term survivors

Selected References

Clements WD, Kirk SJ, Spence RA: A rare late complication of breast cancer treatment. Br J Clin Pract 47:219-220, 1993.

Kindblom LG, Stenman G, Angervall L: Morphological and cytogenetic studies of angiosarcoma in Stewart-Treves syndrome. Virchows Arch 419:439-445, 1991.

Tomita K, Yokogawa A, Oda Y, Terahata S: Lymphangiosarcoma in postmastectomy lymphedema (Stewart-Treves syndrome): Ultrastructural and immunohistologic characteristics. J Surg Oncol 38:275-282, 1988.

Gynecomastia

Clinical Features
- Most common physiologic and pathologic change in male breast
- Typically presents as diffuse mammary enlargement, with pain and tenderness
- Both breasts are commonly affected (clinically bilateral in about half of patients)
- Associated with many medical conditions, including cirrhosis, renal failure, chronic pulmonary disease, Klinefelter disease, and various tumors, including Leydig cell, Sertoli cell, and human chorionic gonadotropin–secreting tumors (gonadal and extragonadal germ cell tumors, large cell lung carcinoma, and some gastric and kidney cancers)
- Pathogenesis has been linked to an imbalance between free estrogen and free androgen actions in breast tissues, which can result from multiple mechanisms
- Several drugs can be associated with development of gynecomastia, including herbal products, protease inhibitors, cimetidine, spironolactone, digitalis, alcohol, heroin, anabolic steroids, and alkylating agents

Gross Pathology
- Appears as a firm and rubbery gray-white mass or as ill-defined fibrotic tissue around the nipple-areolar complex

Histopathology
- Ducts show epithelial and myoepithelial cells with varying degrees of hyperplasia that is irregularly distributed
- Lobule formation is usually not seen
- Micropapillary or cribriform pattern is typical

Figure 13-37. Gynecomastia. Proliferation of loose connective tissue around ductal structures.

- Increased amount and cellularity of stroma with prominent vessels, edema, and mononuclear infiltrate in initial phase; stromal fibrosis follows
- Epithelial cells may show some atypia with hyperchromatic nuclei
- PASH may develop

Special Stains and Immunohistochemistry

- Noncontributory

Other Techniques for Diagnosis

- Electron microscopy: demonstrates proliferating epithelial and myoepithelial cells

Differential Diagnosis

▌ Intraductal carcinoma
- Epithelial proliferation is more regular and organized
- May show intraductal necrosis

Pearls

- No increased risk for carcinoma is associated with this lesion
- Regression occurs with treatment of underlying condition
- Tamoxifen use during acute stages has been shown to result in partial or complete regression of gynecomastia
- Surgical therapy might be indicated in cases that fail to respond to medical therapy

Selected References

Braustein GD: Gynecomastia. N Engl J Med 357:1229-1237, 2007.

Cakan N, Kamat D: Gynecomastia: Evaluation and treatment recommendations for primary care providers. Clin Pediatr (Phila) 46:487-490, 2007.

Janes SE, Lengyel JA, Singh S, et al: Needle core biopsy for the assessment of unilateral breast masses in men. Breast 15:273-275, 2006.

Volpe CM, Raffetto JD, Collure DW, et al: Unilateral male breast masses: Cancer risk and their evaluation and management. Am Surg 65:250-253, 1999.

Milanezi MF, Saggioro FP, Zanati SG, et al: Pseudoangiomatous hyperplasia of mammary stroma associated with gynecomastia. J Clin Pathol 51:204-206, 1998.

Male Breast Carcinoma

Clinical Features

- About 1000 new cases each year, with about 300 deaths
- Represents less than 1% of all mammary carcinomas
- Risk factors include mutations in high-penetrance genes (more common in *BRCA2* than in *BRCA1* families), Klinefelter syndrome, hyperthyroidism, obesity, liver or testicular damage, and radiation or trauma to chest wall

Figure 13-38. Infiltrating ductal carcinoma, grade I (male breast). Tubular structures surrounded by desmoplastic stroma.

- Wide age distribution (peak age frequency at 71 years)
- Presents as painless, well-defined, distinct breast mass
- Occasionally patients present with bloody nipple discharge, retraction, or ulceration

Gross Pathology

- Similar features to those seen in female breasts
- Tumors are typically less than 3 cm at time of diagnosis

Histopathology

- Most male breast carcinoma is infiltrating ductal carcinoma
- Typically shows infiltrating tumor with variable degree of gland formation
- Neoplastic cells are pleomorphic and have nuclei showing vesicular, coarse chromatin and distinct nucleoli
- Angiolymphatic or perineural invasion is often present
- Rarely associated DCIS (most are papillary type, of low to intermediate grade)
- Tumor grading is based on same architectural and cytologic features as infiltrating ductal carcinoma in female breasts
- All carcinoma variants identified in female breasts can be seen in male breasts; lobular neoplasia is exceedingly rare in males

Special Stains and Immunohistochemistry

- ER and PR: variable reactivity, usually positive
- AR: variably positive
- C-erb-B2 (HER-2-neu): more frequently positive in high-grade lesions; overall, 2+ or 3+ positivity in 25% to 30% of cases

Other Techniques for Diagnosis

- Noncontributory

Differential Diagnosis

❚ Metastatic prostate carcinoma
- Immunostain for prostate-specific antigen (PSA) is positive
- Presence of bilateral or multifocal disease suggests metastasis

Pearls

- No increased risk for carcinoma following diagnosis of gynecomastia
- About 50% of cases have axillary node metastases at time of presentation
- *BRCA2* gene (not *BRCA1* gene) is strongly associated with male breast carcinoma
- Common sites of metastasis include lung, bone, and central nervous system
- Initial treatment involves limited surgical excision and chest wall irradiation
- Overall 5-year survival rate estimates are about 40% to 65%; prognosis in age-matched, stage-matched breast cancer is the same for men and women
- Recent studies reveal benefits for the use of adjuvant hormonal therapy and chemotherapy for men in intermediate or high-risk categories (as determined by tumor grade, axillary nodal status, and tumor markers)

Selected References

Nahleh Z, Girnius S: Male breast cancer: A gender issue. Natl Clin Pract Oncol 3:428-437, 2006.

Fentiman IS, Fourquet A, Hortobagyi GN: Male breast cancer. Lancet 367:595-604, 2006.

Joseph A, Mokbel K: Male breast cancer. Int J Fertil Womens Med 49:198-199, 2004.

Goss PE, Reid C, Pintilie M, et al: Male breast carcinoma. A review of 229 patients who presented to the Princess Margaret Hospital during 40 years: 1955-1996. Cancer 85:629-639, 1999.

Wick MR, Sayadi H, Ritter JH, et al: Low-stage carcinoma of the male breast: A histologic, immunohistochemical, and flow cytometric comparison with localized female breast carcinoma. Am J Clin Pathol 111:59-69, 1999.

Metastatic Tumors

Clinical Features

- Metastases to the breast are uncommon in both sexes but are much more common in women
- Most common metastatic carcinoma of the female breast is metastatic tumor from the opposite breast
- Other common metastatic tumors to the breast are malignant melanoma; carcinomas of the lung, ovary, stomach, cervix, kidney, and prostate; and carcinoid tumors
- Most common metastatic tumor of the male breast is metastatic prostate carcinoma
- Secondary lymphomas of the breast are rare; however, they are much more common than primary breast lymphomas, which comprise 0.38% to 0.7% of all non-Hodgkin lymphomas
- Presentation may be similar to primary breast carcinoma with a rapidly growing, painless, firm, palpable mass usually lacking nipple discharge or skin changes
- Bilateral tumors may be the initial clinical manifestation

Gross Pathology

- Well-defined tumors without calcification and spiculation

Histopathology

- Sharply demarcated from adjacent breast tissue
- Infiltrating tumor with the presence of adjacent intraductal carcinoma or LCIS is convincing evidence of a primary breast tumor
- Elastosis is common in primary breast cancer but rare in metastatic tumors
- Calcification is common in primary breast cancer but rare in metastatic tumors, except for metastatic serous papillary carcinoma of the ovary or peritoneum

Figure 13-39. Metastasis to the breast. Common metastatic tumors to the breast include melanoma **(A)** and renal cell carcinoma **(B)**.

- Cytoplasmic pigment, intranuclear inclusions, and spindle cells are useful clues to a diagnosis of metastatic melanoma
- Signet ring, mucin-secreting cells suggest gastric origin
- Clear cell changes and prominent delicate vascularization suggest kidney origin

Special Stains and Immunohistochemistry

- Immunohistochemistry profile should be used in conjunction with clinical history and hematoxylin and eosin stain morphology
- Positivity for S-100 protein, HMB-45, melan-A, microphthalmia transcription factor, and tyrosinase; negativity for EMA and cytokeratin supports a diagnosis of malignant melanoma; melanomas can show aberrant expression of cytokeratins and EMA; breast carcinomas can express S-100
- Expression of Wilms tumor 1, CA-125, and mesothelin, along with negativity for GCDFP-15, favors a diagnosis of metastatic ovarian carcinoma over primary breast cancer
- Expression of thyroid transcription factor-1, along with negativity for GCDFP-15 and ER, favors a diagnosis of metastatic lung cancer
- PSA and prostatic acid phosphatase are excellent markers of prostatic carcinomas; ER, GCDFP-15, and cytokeratin 7 expression are uncommon in prostate carcinoma
- CDX2 and cytokeratin 20 expressions favor a diagnosis of metastatic gastric cancer over breast cancer primary

Other Techniques for Diagnosis

- Noncontributory

Differential Diagnosis

▌ Clinical history is important
▌ Gastric signet ring cell carcinoma
- May mimic primary signet ring cell carcinoma of breast

- Well-defined mass without infiltrating margins
- No in situ component

▌ Ovarian carcinoma
- Serous papillary carcinoma is the most common type
- Lacks infiltrating margins
- No in situ component
- May grow within ducts and lobules, making distinction from a primary breast carcinoma difficult
- Papillary architecture is not typical for most invasive breast cancers, aside from invasive micropapillary carcinoma
- May be bilateral

Pearls

- Identification of metastasis to the breast is usually an indication of widespread disease, and survival is typically less than 2 years
- Identification of in situ carcinoma is helpful to diagnose a primary breast lesion
- Treatment typically consists of wide excision with radiotherapy; systemic treatment suitable for the primary lesion is most important

Selected References

Lee AH: The histological diagnosis of metastases to the breast from extramammary malignancies. J Clin Pathol 60:1333-1341, 2007.

Topalovski M, Domnita C, Mattson JC: Lymphoma of the breast: A clinicopathologic study of primary and secondary cases. Arch Pathol Lab Med 123:1208-1218, 1999.

Yamasaki H, Saw D, Zdanowitz J, et al: Ovarian carcinoma metastasis to the breast: Case report and review of the literature. Am J Surg Pathol 17:193-197, 1993.

DiBonito L, Luchi M, Giarelli L, et al: Metastatic tumors to the female breast: An autopsy study of 12 cases. Pathol Res Pract 187:432-436, 1991.

Jerome M. Loew and William R. Macon

14

Lymph Nodes

Reactive, Predominantly Follicular Hyperplasias

Nonspecific Follicular Hyperplasia

Clinical Features

- Affects patients of any age, more common in children and young adults
- Localized or regional lymphadenopathy; nodes are firm and mobile; may be tender
- Patient may be febrile

Gross Pathology

- Usually less than 3 cm with smooth thin capsule and soft, uniform, pale to creamy-tan parenchyma

Histopathology

- Nodal capsule is usually intact, and sinuses remain patent
- Prominent, uniformly spaced but enlarged germinal centers under the capsule
- Germinal centers are sharply demarcated from surrounding mantle zones
- Follicle center B cells are polarized into a light zone (centrocyte-rich) and a dark zone (centroblast-rich); other cell types include follicular dendritic cells (large cells with regular round or oval nuclei, stippled chromatin, single prominent central eosinophilic nucleolus, and inconspicuous cytoplasm), tingible (stainable) body macrophages, and follicular T-helper cells; mitoses are often prominent
- Germinal centers contain
  — Numerous mitoses and apoptotic cells
  — Tingible body macrophages containing phagocytosed nuclear debris

Special Stains and Immunohistochemistry

- Reticulin, CD21, or CD23 highlight germinal centers
- CD20-positive B cells in germinal centers and mantle zone
- CD3-positive T cells in paracortex and few in germinal centers
- Kappa and lambda stains demonstrate a polytypic plasma cell population
- Follicle center B cells are negative for bcl-2 protein
- Numerous Ki-67–positive cells in germinal centers, may show gradation from dark to light zones

Figure 14-1. Nonspecific follicular hyperplasia. A, Evenly spaced, well-defined, pale germinal centers surrounded by darker mantle zones. **B,** Germinal center with a polymorphous cell population, mitotic figures, and tingible body macrophages. Adjacent mantle zone with annular arrangement of small lymphocytes. **C,** bcl-2–Negative germinal center cells contrast with bcl-2–positive mantle zones. This pattern may help distinguish follicular hyperplasia from follicular lymphoma.

Other Techniques for Diagnosis

- Flow cytometry or gene rearrangements show no clonal population

Differential Diagnosis

- Follicular lymphoma
  - Most patients are older than 40 years of age
  - Ill-defined and crowded follicles without normal zoning pattern of follicular B cells and fewer mitoses
  - Follicle center B cells are CD10 positive and often bcl-2 positive
  - t(14;18)(q32;q21) chromosomal abnormality present in most cases
- Nodular sclerosis–type Hodgkin lymphoma
  - Sclerotic bands usually separate cellular nodules
  - Eosinophils, plasma cells, and neutrophils usually easy to find
  - Hodgkin cells, Reed-Sternberg cells, or lacunar cells are characteristic
- Human immunodeficiency virus (HIV)-associated lymphadenopathy
  - Lymphadenopathy more likely to be generalized
  - Follicles more likely to show regressive changes
  - Paracortex is usually atrophic with decreased numbers of lymphocytes
- Syphilis (luetic lymphadenitis)
  - Capsule is usually thickened and fibrotic with plasma cell vasculitis
- Infectious mononucleosis
  - Follicular and paracortical hyperplasia with atypical immunoblasts
  - Adolescent or young adult with fever, malaise, pharyngitis, and hepatosplenomegaly
  - Diagnosis usually made on serology; biopsy is rarely performed
- Autoimmune lymphoproliferative syndrome (ALPS)
  - Patients have recurrent or chronic lymphadenopathy
  - Autoantibodies and often autoimmune cytopenias
  - Paracortical expansion including immunoblasts in paracortex
  - Increased population of CD4 and CD8 double-negative T cells by flow cytometry
- *Toxoplasma* lymphadenitis
  - Usually posterior cervical or supraclavicular lymphadenopathy in adolescents and young adults
  - Follicular lymphoid hyperplasia
  - Clusters of epithelioid cells throughout the node, including mantle zones and follicles
  - Monocytoid B-cell aggregates prominent

Pearls

- Generalized lymphadenopathy suggests systemic disease or occult malignancy
- Most often seen in biopsies of cervical, supraclavicular, or axillary nodes
- Sclerosis more common in iliac and inguinal nodes (below bifurcation of aorta)
- Immunohistochemical panel and flow cytometry (if available) for occult lymphoma recommended if patient is older than 65 years

Selected References

Bryant RJ, Banks PM, O'Malley DP: Ki67 staining pattern as a diagnostic tool in the evaluation of lymphoproliferative disorders. Histopathology 48:505-515, 2006.

Hartsock RJ: Reactive lesions in lymph nodes. In Rebuck JW, Berard CW (eds): The Reticuloendothelial System. International Academy of Pathology Monograph #16. Baltimore, Williams & Wilkins, 1975, pp 153-183.

Human Immunodeficiency Virus–Associated Lymphadenopathy

Clinical Features

- Most patients are younger than 40 years
- Homosexual males, parenteral drug users, and their partners are most commonly affected
- Persistent generalized lymphadenopathy
- Fever and wasting are commonly seen

Gross Pathology

- Usually less than 3 cm with smooth thin capsule and uniform, pale- to creamy-tan, soft parenchyma

Histopathology

- Enlarged, hyperplastic germinal centers that are irregular, serpentine, or dumbbell shaped
- May have follicle lysis with ratty edges of germinal centers and infiltration of germinal centers by small lymphocytes
- Interfollicular areas (paracortex) are almost always relatively atrophic and show numerous plasma cells and macrophages
- Vascular proliferation may be seen
- Granulomas, if present, are poorly developed

Figure 14-2. HIV-associated lymphadenopathy. Follicular hyperplasia with mantle zones that are focally indistinct and discontinuous, and a thin hypocellular paracortex.

- Collections of monocytoid B cells near sinuses
- Erythrophagocytosis may rarely be seen
- In later stages of HIV disease, lymph nodes may show follicular involution and rare atypical patterns
- Look for occult neoplasms, especially Kaposi sarcoma

Special Stains and Immunohistochemistry

- Stains for organisms (acid-fast, fungal stains) indicated when there is follicle lysis or follicular involution
- Immunohistochemistry for T cells shows decreased cellularity in paracortex
- Reticulin or CD21 stain highlights irregular outlines of germinal centers

Other Techniques for Diagnosis

- HIV serology; typically high viral load if HIV positive
- CD4/CD8 ratio reduced, parallels peripheral blood

Differential Diagnosis

- Follicular hyperplasia in HIV-negative patient
  - More uniform size and spacing of germinal centers
  - Smoother outlines of germinal centers (follicle lysis and follicular involution less commonly seen)
  - Paracortex is more expanded and more cellular
- Syphilis (luetic lymphadenitis)
  - Plasma cell vasculitis
  - Not mutually exclusive; this is more common in HIV-infected patients
- Infectious mononucleosis
  - Germinal centers may contain atypical cells
  - Paracortex expanded with immunoblasts, mitotic cells, Reed-Sternberg–like cells; may obscure germinal centers
  - Typically no follicle lysis in acute phase; may be present in convalescent stage
  - Hepatosplenomegaly is common
  - History and serology for Epstein-Barr virus (EBV) and HIV may be necessary for differentiation
- Follicular lymphoma
  - Most patients are older than 40 years
  - Ill-defined and crowded follicles without normal zoning pattern of follicular B cells and fewer mitoses
  - Follicle center B-cells are CD10 positive and often bcl-2 positive
  - t(14;18)(q32;q21) chromosomal abnormality present in most cases
- Progressive transformation of germinal centers (PTGC)
  - Lymphadenopathy is usually localized
  - Process is focal within lymph node
  - Enlarged germinal centers are ill-defined but round, not serpentine
  - Uninvolved germinal centers are uniform in size
  - HIV serology negative
- ALPS
  - Patients with ALPS are usually children and may have positive family history

- Autoimmune cytopenias are common in both HIV and ALPS
- Hepatosplenomegaly is common to both conditions
- Histology may be similar
- HIV testing essential
- Flow cytometric phenotyping for double-negative CD4 and CD8 T-cell population may be necessary

Pearls

- Centers with extensive clinical experience in treating HIV patients rarely request lymph node biopsies for adenopathy in early disease
- None of the histologic features are specific; clinical history and serology are needed for definitive diagnosis
- Suspect this in children with persistent generalized lymphadenopathy
- Opportunistic infections are rare when the histology shows follicular hyperplasia without regressive changes

Selected References

Quijano G, Siminovich M, Drut R: Histopathologic findings in the lymphoid and reticuloendothelial system in pediatric HIV infection: A postmortem study. Pediatr Pathol Lab Med 17:845-856, 1997.

Baroni CD, Uccini S: The lymphadenopathy of HIV infection. Am J Clin Pathol 99:397-401, 1993.

Wood GS: The immunohistology of lymph nodes in HIV infection: A review. Prog AIDS Pathol 2:25-32, 1990.

Infectious Mononucleosis

Clinical Features

- Primarily affects adolescents and young adults
- Patients have fever, malaise, and pharyngitis
- May have generalized lymphadenopathy and hepatosplenomegaly
- Caused by primary infection with EBV

Gross Pathology

- Fleshy, pink to pale, creamy lymph node parenchyma, which may be very soft

Histopathology

- Distortion of lymph node architecture secondary to intense follicular hyperplasia with irregular germinal centers
- Paracortical hyperplasia and expansion secondary to numerous immunoblasts, small lymphocytes, and plasma cells; some atypical immunoblasts may resemble Reed-Sternberg cells
- Paracortical expansion may obscure the germinal centers, but the latter are uniformly spaced
- Lymphoid infiltration of the nodal capsule and perinodal tissues may be seen
- Subcapsular and peritrabecular sinuses may contain large, pleomorphic lymphocytes

Figure 14-3. Infectious mononucleosis. A, Marked paracortical expansion and pallor and small germinal centers are typical features. **B,** High magnification of the paracortex. Immunoblasts, mitotic figures, plasmacytoid cells, and apoptotic cells can make mononucleosis difficult to distinguish from an aggressive lymphoma.

Special Stains and Immunohistochemistry

- Caveat: CD30-positive large atypical cells will be present; some may resemble Hodgkin or Reed-Sternberg cells morphologically
- Ki-67–positive proliferating cells may be present in the interfollicular regions

Other Techniques for Diagnosis

- Monospot or other screening test positive in infected patients
- Anti-EBV immunoglobulin M (IgM) positive in acute infection
- In situ hybridization for EBV-encoded RNA (EBER)

Differential Diagnosis

▌ HIV-associated lymphadenopathy
- May have follicular involution
- Paracortex is thin rather than expanded

- Patient usually has longer duration of symptoms
- Peak age slightly older (20s to 40s)

▌ Cytomegalovirus (CMV) mononucleosis
- Clinical presentation may be identical
- CMV inclusions appear in lymph node
- Serology indicates acute CMV rather than EBV infection
- Viral detection by culture or polymerase chain reaction (PCR) may also differentiate

▌ Cat-scratch disease
- Early phase shows capsulitis with abscesses near germinal centers
- Granulomas develop in later stages
- Organisms may be seen (silver stain) in early disease
- Hepatosplenomegaly is rare

▌ *Toxoplasma* lymphadenitis
- Follicular lymphoid hyperplasia
- Prominent monocytoid B cells
- Clusters of epithelioid cells throughout the node
- Hepatosplenomegaly, pharyngitis, and severe systemic symptoms uncommon

▌ Phenytoin (Dilantin) adenopathy
- Patients have lymphadenopathy and possibly gingival hyperplasia, not generally febrile
- Slower onset
- History of seizure disorder with phenytoin use
- Usually more follicular hyperplasia and less prominent paracortical atypia

▌ ALPS
- See "Differential Diagnosis" under "Human Immunodeficiency Virus–Associated Lymphadenopathy"

▌ Hodgkin lymphoma
- Low-power examination shows at least focal destruction of normal nodal architecture
- Eosinophils, neutrophils, and plasma cells are usually numerous in all except nodular lymphocyte–predominant and lymphocyte-rich classic subtypes
- Lymphocytes are less activated and less pleomorphic
- Atypical cells (Reed-Sternberg cells) are positive for both CD15 and CD30 and negative for CD45
- Hepatosplenomegaly is uncommon in younger patients with Hodgkin lymphoma
- Symptomatic patients usually have more gradual onset of symptoms

▌ Large cell lymphoma or Burkitt lymphoma
- Complete effacement of lymph node architecture
- Diffuse infiltrate of medium-sized or large lymphocytes

▌ Follicular lymphoma
- See "Differential Diagnosis" under "Human Immunodeficiency Virus–Associated Lymphadenopathy"

Pearls

- Usually diagnosed by clinical symptoms and serologic tests; patients are rarely subjected to lymph node biopsy

- CMV can produce an identical picture
- Typically self-limited but transmissible
- Numerous immunoblasts can be confused with an aggressive non-Hodgkin lymphoma; however, preserved follicles are present in mononucleosis but rare in nodes diffusely infiltrated by an aggressive lymphoma
- Germinal centers may be present when a lymphoma partially involves a lymph node or infiltrates in an interfollicular pattern; in these situations, the spacing of the germinal centers is usually not uniform
- Reed-Sternberg–like cells may be present; these cells may express CD30, so carefully evaluate nodal architecture at low power to avoid misdiagnosis
- Unlike those with Hodgkin lymphoma, infectious mononucleosis patients usually have acute onset of fever, pharyngitis, and systemic symptoms
- Circulating atypical CD8-positive T cells that are activated by the infected B-cells are often seen in peripheral blood

Selected References

Kojima M, Sugiura I, Itoh H, et al: Histological varieties of Epstein-Barr virus-related lymph node lesion resembling autoimmune disease-like clinicopathological findings in middle-aged and elderly patients: A study of six cases. Pathol Res Pract 202:609-615, 2006.

Kojima M, Nakamura S, Shimizu K, et al: Reactive lymphoid hyperplasia of the lymph nodes with giant follicles: A clinicopathologic study of 14 Japanese cases, with special reference to Epstein-Barr virus infection. Int J Surg Pathol 13:267-272, 2005.

Reynolds DJ, Banks PM, Gulley ML: New characterization of infectious mononucleosis and a phenotypic comparison with Hodgkin's disease. Am J Pathol 146:379-388, 1995.

Syphilis (Luetic Lymphadenitis)

Clinical Features

- Most commonly affects adolescents and adults
- Inguinal and cervical nodes are most commonly involved
- Mucosal lesions are often inconspicuous

Gross Pathology

- Lymph node capsule is often thickened
- Other gross features are the same as for nonspecific follicular hyperplasia

Histopathology

- Follicular hyperplasia with large secondary follicles
- Capsule is often thickened, and capsulitis is typically seen
- Interfollicular and intrafollicular plasma cell vasculitis (plasma cells within walls of blood vessels)

Figure 14-4. Syphilitic lymphadenitis. Vasculitis with plasma cells.

Special Stains and Immunohistochemistry

- Warthin-Starry or other silver impregnation stains for spirochetes may be positive (most numerous in endothelial cells of small blood vessels)

Other Techniques for Diagnosis

- Serology for syphilis is typically positive

Differential Diagnosis

- Nonspecific follicular hyperplasia
  - Thin nodal capsule and no plasma cell vasculitis
- Rheumatoid arthritis
  - Follicular hyperplasia is present but lacks plasma cell vasculitis
- HIV-associated lymphadenopathy
  - May coexist with syphilitic lymphadenitis; both are sexually transmitted
  - Lacks plasma cell vasculitis
- Castleman disease
  - In the hyaline-vascular type, germinal centers are small with a distinctive concentric onion-skin pattern of mantle cells
  - Plasma cells are predominantly interfollicular, not in vessel walls or in the lymph node capsule
- Capsular fibrosis in inguinal lymph nodes
  - Hyalinization of the capsule and acellular to hypocellular hyaline fibrous bands within the node
  - No plasma cell vasculitis

Pearls

- Ask patient's physician about skin and mucosal lesions
- Silver stains for spirochetes are difficult to perform and interpret; serologic confirmation is needed anyway, so recommend serologic studies if this diagnosis is a serious histologic consideration
- HIV-positive patients have a higher than average incidence of syphilitic infection, but the lymph node histology is not altered in these patients

Selected References

Farhi DC, Wells SJ, Siegel RJ: Syphilitic lymphadenopathy: Histology and human immunodeficiency virus status. Am J Clin Pathol 112:330-334, 1999.

Singh AE, Romanowski B: Syphilis: Review with emphasis on clinical, epidemiologic, and some biologic features. Clin Microbiol Rev 12:187-209, 1999.

Toxoplasma Lymphadenitis

Clinical Features

- Most commonly affects children and young adults
- Patients usually have asymptomatic posterior cervical or supraclavicular lymphadenopathy
- Caused by a protozoan, *Toxoplasma gondii*, acquired from cats, sheep, or goats

Gross Pathology

- Nonspecific features; tan, fleshy nodal parenchyma

Figure 14-5. Toxoplasmosis in a lymph node. A, Irregular but hyperplastic germinal centers, pale collections of monocytoid B cells in and around sinuses, and eosinophilic aggregates of epithelioid cells in mantle zones and at the periphery of germinal centers constitute a characteristic and highly specific histologic triad. **B,** Higher magnification of epithelioid cells near a somewhat irregularly outlined germinal center.

Histopathology

- Classic histologic triad is highly specific and consists of
  — Follicular hyperplasia
  — Large numbers of pale monocytoid B cells near nodal sinuses
  — Small clusters of epithelioid histiocytes throughout the node, including within mantle zones and sometimes in germinal centers

Special Stains and Immunohistochemistry

- Immunohistochemistry for *Toxoplasma* species most effective special stain

Other Techniques for Diagnosis

- Serology: elevated *Toxoplasma* species titer

Differential Diagnosis

▌ Nonspecific follicular hyperplasia
- Monocytoid B cells are rarely as prominent
- Lacks clusters of epithelioid cells

▌ HIV-associated lymphadenopathy
- Germinal centers may have regressive changes
- Interfollicular zones show numerous plasma cells
- Macrophages if numerous are usually loosely distributed and do not form tight clusters; they are rarely epithelioid
- Lymphadenopathy is more likely to be generalized

▌ Sarcoidosis
- Granulomas are larger and better circumscribed
- Germinal centers are inconspicuous to atrophic
- Granulomas are not seen in germinal centers or mantle zones
- Patients are somewhat older on average

▌ Histiocytic necrotizing lymphadenitis (Kikuchi-Fujimoto disease)
- Higher incidence in young adult women
- Pattern of zonal paracortical necrosis in which there are histiocytes with twisted nuclei surrounded by immunoblasts
- No clusters of epithelioid cells or neutrophils

▌ Foreign-body granulomas
- Giant cells are usually prominent
- Epithelioid cells are concentrated near sinuses, not seen in mantle zones or germinal centers
- Foreign material is seen in giant cells (may be polarizable)

Pearls

- Classic histologic triad allows a specific etiologic diagnosis with excellent correlation with serology, even without histologic demonstration of the organisms, which are hard to demonstrate
- Self-limited disease in immunocompetent adults
- May cause devastating damage to the fetus or patients with acquired immunodeficiency syndrome (AIDS)

Selected References

Lin MH, Kuo TT: Specificity of the histopathological triad for the diagnosis of toxoplasmic lymphadenitis: Polymerase chain reaction study. Pathol Int 51:619-623, 2001.

Rose I: Morphology and diagnostics of human toxoplasmosis. Gen Diagn Pathol 142:257-270, 1997.

Dorfman RF, Remington JS: Value of lymph node biopsy in the diagnosis of acute acquired toxoplasmosis. N Engl J Med 298:878-881, 1973.

Dermatopathic Lymphadenopathy

Clinical Features

- Primarily seen in adults ages 20 to 60 years
- Found in lymph nodes draining an inflammatory dermatitis
- More common in axillary and inguinal lymph nodes
- Should not be seen in biopsies from deep-seated intra-abdominal or mediastinal lymph nodes
- Usually firm, rubbery, and mobile

Gross Pathology

- Color varies from pale-tan to brown depending on amount of pigment present
- Usually smaller than 3 cm, with smooth, thin capsule

Histopathology

- Follicular hyperplasia
- Paracortical expansion with immunoblasts and dendritic cells creating a mottled appearance
- Cerebriform lymphocytes possibly found
- Pigmented macrophages in sinuses and paracortex

Special Stains and Immunohistochemistry

- Pigment is positive with Fontana-Masson or other argentaffin stain; negative with iron stain

Figure 14-6. Dermatopathic lymphadenopathy. High magnification showing polymorphous background with lymphocytes, plasma cells, and pigment-laden macrophages.

- Macrophages express MAC387, CD68, and other macrophage markers
- Negative for HMB-45 and melan-A

Other Techniques for Diagnosis

- A clonal T-cell receptor gene rearrangement may indicate involvement by mycosis fungoides or other T-cell neoplasm

Differential Diagnosis

- Metastatic melanoma
  - Abnormal melanocytes that are often less pigmented than the macrophages
  - Positive for S-100 protein and HMB-45
- Hemolysis with hemosiderosis
  - Pigment is coarse, more golden brown, and more refractile than melanin
  - Iron stain is positive, Fontana-Masson (argentaffin) is negative
- Foreign pigment or tattoo ink
  - History and physical examination
  - Pigment may be birefringent or refractile; cannot be bleached
  - Iron and Fontana-Masson (argentaffin) stains are usually negative
- Metastatic mycosis fungoides
  - May have pigment and cerebriform lymphocytes in paracortex
  - History of mycosis fungoides
  - Flow cytometry or gene rearrangement studies identify abnormal T-cell population
- Langerhans cell histiocytosis
  - Neoplastic Langerhans cells preferentially infiltrate lymph node sinuses
  - Paracortex is not expanded and usually lacks follicular hyperplasia
  - Eosinophils prominent

Pearls

- May be seen with any exfoliative dermatitis
- Dermatitis is not always active

Selected Reference

Winter LK, Spiegel JH, King T: Dermatopathic lymphadenitis of the head and neck. J Cutan Pathol 34:195-197, 2007.

Progressive Transformation of Germinal Centers

Clinical Features

- Rare
- Most patients are asymptomatic adolescents or young adults with one or a few enlarged lymph nodes, most often cervical

Gross Pathology

- Nonspecific features; tan, fleshy nodal parenchyma

Figure 14-7. Progressive transformation of germinal centers (PTGC). A, The transformed germinal centers are several times the size of the adjacent, more normal reactive germinal centers. Two of the PTGCs are ill-defined. **B,** High magnification of one transformed germinal center showing intermixture of small lymphocytes with large centroblastic cells.

Histopathology

- Background of follicular hyperplasia
- One or a few germinal centers several times the size of the others, with an indistinct border between the germinal center and mantle zone
- At high magnification, germinal center cells are intermixed with small lymphocytes

Special Stains and Immunohistochemistry

- Germinal centers are infiltrated by clusters of mantle zone lymphocytes, which express CD20, CD23, and bcl-2
- Relatively few CD10-positive cells in transformed follicles

Other Techniques for Diagnosis

- Noncontributory

Differential Diagnosis

- Nonspecific follicular hyperplasia
  - Germinal centers are more uniform in size
  - Larger germinal centers are more sharply demarcated from the mantle zones
  - Most of the cells in the germinal centers are bcl-2 negative
- Follicle lysis within follicular hyperplasia
  - Infiltrates of small lymphocytes are geographically distinct areas within the follicles
  - Small lymphocytes within the follicles in follicle lysis are CD3-positive T lymphocytes
  - Small lymphocytes within the follicles in PTGC are a mixture of follicular B cells and T cells and mantle cells
- HIV adenopathy
  - Enlarged germinal centers are serpentine and extremely reactive
  - Intermixture of small lymphocytes within germinal centers is patchy, owing to follicle lysis, not uniform
  - HIV serology positive
- Hodgkin lymphoma, nodular lymphocyte predominant
  - Generally replaces normal germinal centers in all or a large part of the lymph node
  - Nodules contain lymphocyte and histiocyte (L&H) type of Hodgkin cells in a background of small reactive lymphocytes
  - CD20-positive large cells scattered among many small lymphocytes, which are a mixture of CD3-positive T cells and CD20-positive small B cells
- Hodgkin lymphoma, nodular sclerosis type
  - Normal follicular architecture are usually effaced
  - Sclerosis
  - Pleomorphic background population of lymphocytes, eosinophils, and plasma cells
  - Diagnostic Reed-Sternberg cells and lacunar cells should always be present but may be rare
- Follicular lymphoma
  - See "Differential Diagnosis" under "Nonspecific Follicular Hyperplasia"

Pearls

- Patients with multiple foci of PTGC have a slightly increased risk for developing nodular lymphocyte–predominant Hodgkin lymphoma (NLPHL)
- PTGC is also more common in patients who have a history of or concurrent NLPHL

Selected References

Chang CC, Osipov V, Wheaton S, et al: Follicular hyperplasia, follicular lysis, and progressive transformation of germinal centers: A sequential spectrum of morphologic evolution in lymphoid hyperplasia. Am J Clin Pathol 120:322-326, 2003.

Nguyen PL, Ferry JA, Harris NL: Progressive transformation of germinal centers and nodular lymphocyte predominance Hodgkin's disease: A comparative immunohistochemical study. Am J Surg Pathol 23:27-33, 1999.

Autoimmune Lymphoproliferative Syndrome

Clinical Features

- Onset in infancy or childhood
- Familial: autosomal dominant with varied expression within families
- Autoimmune disorders, particularly autoimmune anemia and thrombocytopenia
- Autoantibodies are present in all patients with immune cytopenias and in most other patients
- Lymphadenopathy and hepatosplenomegaly

Gross Pathology

- Enlarged, fleshy pale lymph nodes

Histopathology

- Florid paracortical hyperplasia with immunoblasts and plasmacytosis and small to only occasionally hyperplastic lymphoid follicles
- Spleen has expanded marginal zones and periarteriolar lymphoid sheaths

Special Stains and Immunohistochemistry

- Phenotypic abnormalities are best detected by flow cytometry
- Increased numbers of double-negative T cells, expressing neither CD4 nor CD8
- These cells do express CD45RA and CD57
- T cells are negative for CD45RO and CD56

Other Techniques for Diagnosis

- Testing for mutations in the *Fas-l* or caspase 8 and 10 genes

Differential Diagnosis

▌ Nonspecific follicular hyperplasia
  - Usually localized or regional, acute onset
  - Hepatosplenomegaly rare
  - No abnormal T-cell population by flow cytometry
▌ Systemic lupus erythematosus (SLE)
  - Onset usually in adolescence or adult years
  - Histology may be similar
  - Flow cytometry may be useful
▌ Syphilitic lymphadenitis
  - Onset usually in late adolescent or adult years
  - Plasma cells are mostly in the capsule, with a plasmacytic vasculitis
  - Serologic tests and special stains show evidence of *Treponema pallidum* infection
  - No abnormal T-cell population by flow cytometry
▌ Infectious mononucleosis
  - Acute onset of systemic illness with fever and pharyngitis
  - EBV serology positive
  - No abnormal T-cell population by flow cytometry
▌ *Toxoplasma* lymphadenitis
  - Most often in posterior cervical nodes
  - Hepatosplenomegaly uncommon
  - Not associated with autoimmune cytopenias
  - Small clusters of epithelioid cells in mantle zones and germinal centers
  - Aggregates of monocytoid B cells around sinuses
  - Paracortex otherwise unremarkable; usually does not have the marked expansion or immunoblasts seen in ALPS
  - Serology for *Toxoplasma* species positive
  - No abnormal T-cell population by flow cytometry
▌ HIV-related adenopathy
  - Onset usually later than for ALPS
  - HIV serology positive
  - Paracortex is thin and depleted of lymphocytes, not expanded
  - There is depletion of CD4-positive cells with a relative increase in CD8-positive cells

Figure 14-8. Autoimmune lymphoproliferative syndrome. A, Active germinal center with expanded paracortex with a polymorphous cell population including large cells, giving a mottled appearance. **B,** High magnification of interfollicular area showing sheets of plasma cells, including one with intracellular immunoglobulin inclusions.

■ Peripheral T-cell lymphoma
- ALPS may present with lymphadenopathy in early childhood; peripheral T-cell lymphoma is usually a disease of adults
- Diffuse effacement of nodal architecture, including effacement of follicles
- There is usually a dominant population with an abnormal T-cell phenotype
- CD4 and CD8 double-negative T-cell phenotype is rare in T-cell lymphomas except precursor T-lymphoblastic lymphoma and leukemia

Pearls

- This disease is due to mutations in either the *Fas-l* (Fas ligand) gene or downstream caspase genes; these result in defective lymphocyte apoptosis, and lymphocytes do not undergo apoptosis when antigen stimulation is withdrawn
- Patients have infections that are rarely life threatening
- Patients with HIV, SLE, or peripheral T-cell lymphoma may have autoimmune cytopenias, as do most patients with ALPS
- The lifetime risk for lymphoma, either Hodgkin or non-Hodgkin, is much higher than normal
- This entity has been relatively recently recognized; not all kindred have been identified
- It may be worthwhile to mention this diagnosis if a child has had multiple lymph node biopsies with compatible histology

Selected References

Worth A, Thrasher AJ, Gaspar HB: Autoimmune lymphoproliferative syndrome: Molecular basis of disease and clinical phenotype. Br J Haematol 133:124-140, 2006.

Poppema S: Autoimmune lymphoproliferative syndrome. USCAP, 2004. Available at: http://www.uscap.org/site~/93rd/companion21h6.htm.

Reactive Processes with Necrosis

Cat-Scratch Disease

Clinical Features

- Most frequent in children but can occur at any age
- Axillary, epitrochlear, or cervical nodes most often involved
- Erythema of overlying skin
- Lymphadenopathy typically appears 3 weeks after exposure
- Caused by a zoonotic bacterium, *Bartonella henselae*, usually transmitted by cats
- Initially, there is a persistent pustule or erythematous papule at the cutaneous inoculation site, which is usually on the extremities; lymphadenopathy develops in draining nodes

Figure 14-9. Cat-scratch disease. A, Two granulomas with central necrotic areas and surrounding palisaded epithelioid cells, near germinal centers. **B,** Higher magnification of an earlier lesion showing numerous neutrophils surrounded by epithelioid macrophages.

- Patient may have fever or malaise; rarely, a mild encephalitic picture
- Disease is typically self-limited

Gross Pathology

- Nonspecific features; tan, fleshy nodal parenchyma

Histopathology

- Early phase
  - Capsulitis
  - Follicular hyperplasia
  - Abscesses near germinal centers that may be stellate and confluent
  - Prominent endothelial cell swelling with organisms, sometimes numerous, in endothelial cells
- Later stage
  - Abscesses become granulomas with palisaded epithelioid cells
  - Organisms rarely seen

Special Stains and Immunohistochemistry

- Warthin-Starry or similar silver impregnation stain helps visualize the organisms, which are short pleomorphic bacilli

Other Techniques for Diagnosis

- Culture (requires special media)
- PCR for bacterial nucleic acids
- Serology for *B. henselae*

Differential Diagnosis

▌ Lymphogranuloma venereum
- Occurs in sexually active, mostly older patients
- Usually involves inguinal nodes
- Histology is identical to that of cat-scratch disease
- Caused by *Chlamydia*; tests for *Bartonella* species are negative

▌ Tularemia
- Patients usually systemically ill
- Cortical necrosis
- Histiocytic rim around lesions absent

▌ Histiocytic necrotizing lymphadenitis (Kikuchi-Fujimoto disease)
- Skin lesions unusual
- Adults, female predominance, more common in patients of South Asian ancestry
- Necrotic foci may be surrounded by immunoblasts, which are CD8 positive
- Macrophages with twisted nuclei amidst nuclear debris, but neutrophils usually are not present

▌ Tuberculous lymphadenitis
- Skin lesions are rare
- Granulomas are larger and more necrotizing
- Etiologic agent (*Mycobacterium tuberculosis*) identified by acid-fast stain, culture, PCR, or skin test

▌ Suppurative lymphadenitis
- Abscesses are often larger; nodes may be clinically fluctuant
- Pyogenic bacteria identified on routine Gram stain or microbial culture

▌ Foreign-body granulomas
- Usually closer to lymph node sinuses
- Contains foreign material (typically refractile under polarized light)

Pearls

- Self-limited disease
- *Bartonella* species may cause disseminated visceral infection in patients with acquired immunodeficiency syndrome (bacillary angiomatosis)

Selected References

Qian X, Jin L, Hayden RT, et al: Diagnosis of cat scratch disease with *Bartonella henselae* infection in formalin-fixed paraffin-embedded tissues by two different PCR assays. Diagn Mol Pathol 14:146-151, 2005.

Lamps LW, Scott MA: Cat-scratch disease: Historic, clinical, and pathologic perspectives. Am J Clin Pathol 121(Suppl):S71-S80, 2004.

Miller-Catchpole R, Variakojis D, Vardiman JW, et al: Cat scratch disease: Identification of bacteria in seven cases of lymphadenitis. Am J Surg Pathol 10:276-281, 1986.

Cytomegalovirus and Herpes Lymphadenitis

Clinical Features

- Two clinical pictures
  — CMV may mimic EBV mononucleosis clinically
  — Necrotizing lymphadenitis
- More common in immunocompromised or immunosuppressed patients
- Patients usually systemically ill
- Patients with herpes may have mucosal or cutaneous lesions
- The infection may be lethal or leave long-term sequelae

Gross Pathology

- Foci of necrosis or hemorrhage may be visible on cut surface

Histopathology

- Foci of hemorrhage and necrosis with neutrophilic infiltrate and macrophages with debris
- Viral inclusions in cells at the periphery of the necrotic area
- CMV lymphadenitis may have prominent follicular hyperplasia and monocytoid B-cell hyperplasia

Special Stains and Immunohistochemistry

- The viruses may be detected by immunohisto-chemistry or in situ hybridization
- Immunohistochemical stains for herpes can be useful but are not specific for the herpesvirus type

Other Techniques for Diagnosis

- Viral culture may detect the virus
- Rapid PCR techniques have also been developed

Differential Diagnosis

▌ Histiocytic necrotizing lymphadenitis (Kikuchi-Fujimoto disease)
- Patients usually have a subacute rather than a catastrophic illness
- Necrotic foci are surrounded by frequent immunoblasts
- Neutrophils characteristically are absent and hemorrhage is not common

▌ Bacterial lymphadenitis
- More commonly a localized illness
- Neutrophils usually common
- Viral inclusions not evident
- Bacteria may be detected by Gram stain or culture

▌ Cat-scratch disease
- Onset usually subacute
- Skin lesions, if present, are localized
- Early lesions are neutrophilic but not necrotizing
- Later lesions are granulomatous, usually without necrosis

Pearls

- Distinguishing degenerating cells from cells with viral inclusions may be difficult
- In CMV, only a small proportion of the infected cells have visible viral inclusions
- CMV infects many cell types, especially endothelial cells
- Herpes inclusions may be easier to find in epithelial or mucosal lesions
- A Tzanck preparation from a mucosal or skin lesion in a patient with herpes may provide a rapid noninvasive diagnosis

Selected References

Joseph L, Scott MA, Schichman SA, Zent CS: Localized herpes simplex lymphadenitis mimicking large-cell (Richter's) transformation of chronic lymphocytic leukemia/small lymphocytic lymphoma. Am J Hematol 68:287-291, 2001.

Gaffey MJ, Ben-Ezra JM, Weiss LM: Herpes simplex lymphadenitis. Am J Clin Pathol 95:709-714, 1991.

Histiocytic Necrotizing Lymphadenitis (Kikuchi-Fujimoto Disease)

Clinical Features

- Found predominantly in cervical lymph nodes of younger adults, particularly females
- Prevalence is higher in persons from India and other southern Asian countries
- Patients may have asymptomatic or painful lymphadenopathy, fever, and malaise
- Disease is self-limited but may last several months

Gross Pathology

- Nonspecific features; soft, tan to fleshy nodal parenchyma

Histopathology

- Zonal process involving part of a node in a background of follicular hyperplasia
- Abnormal areas are centered in but not limited to the paracortex
- One or more large, well-defined foci of necrosis containing macrophages with twisted nuclei amidst abundant karyorrhectic debris and few neutrophils
- Immunoblasts and plasmacytoid monocytes at the periphery of the necrotic zones

Special Stains and Immunohistochemistry

- Immunoblasts at periphery of lesions are predominantly CD8-positive T cells that may express CD30; plasmacytoid monocytes are positive for CD4 and CD123
- Histiocytes express both CD68 and myeloperoxidase
- Stains for microorganisms are negative

Figure 14-10. Necrotizing lymphadenitis (Kikuchi-Fujimoto disease). A, Low magnification demonstrating a localized area of pale cells and apoptotic cells; normal lymphoid tissue is adjacent to this area. **B,** Higher magnification of the affected area. Large cells with apoptotic cells and macrophages containing karyorrhectic debris. Note lack of neutrophils.

Other Techniques for Diagnosis

- Culture for microorganisms is negative
- Southern blot does not show a clonal lymphocyte population

Differential Diagnosis

- Lupus lymphadenitis
  - Histologic features overlap considerably
  - Clinical and serologic evidence of systemic lupus, including skin lesions, arthralgias, and renal disease
  - Some authors have postulated that histiocytic necrotizing lymphadenitis may be a forme fruste of SLE
- Bacterial lymphadenitis
  - Necrotic foci typically contain numerous neutrophils
  - Bacteria grow on culture
- Necrotizing CMV or herpes lymphadenitis
  - Patients usually immunocompromised or immunosuppressed

- Patients typically have an acute, severe systemic illness
- Infected lymph nodes are often grossly hemorrhagic
- Neutrophils are usually seen
- Necrotic foci may be surrounded by macrophages or granulation tissue but not by frequent immunoblasts
- Cells at the periphery of the necrotic areas may contain viral inclusions
- Immunohistochemistry, in situ hybridization, PCR, or viral culture should reveal the etiologic virus
- Fungal lymphadenitis
  - Multinucleated giant cells are often prominent
  - Gomori methenamine silver (GMS) or other fungal stains help identify organisms; culture positive
- Tuberculous lymphadenitis
  - Necrosis, if present, is caseous
  - Granulomas contain macrophages and multinucleated cells, including Langhans-type giant cells
  - Acid-fast stains, PCR, and cultures positive
- Cat-scratch disease
  - Common in children
  - Early involvement manifests with follicular hyperplasia, capsulitis, and abscess formation
  - Later lesions are granulomatous with epithelioid macrophages
  - Lesions are usually multifocal within the lymph node
  - Warthin-Starry or similar stains for spirochetes may show organisms in early lesions
- Diffuse large B-cell lymphoma (DLBCL)
  - Diffuse effacement of lymph node architecture
  - Consists of sheets of large CD20-positive B cells with vesicular nuclei, distinct nucleoli, and high mitotic rate
  - Foci of necrosis may be present, but the abundant karyorrhectic debris seen in macrophages of Kikuchi-Fujimoto disease is less frequently found
  - Immunohistochemistry, flow cytometric phenotyping, or gene rearrangement studies show a clonal population and may be necessary for differentiation
- Peripheral T-cell lymphoma (PTCL)
  - Diffuse effacement of lymph node architecture
  - Most node-based PTCLs contain a mixture of small, medium-sized, and large T cells rather than monotonous large cells at the periphery of necrotic foci
  - Foci of necrosis may be present, but the abundant karyorrhectic debris seen in macrophages of Kikuchi-Fujimoto disease is rarely found
  - Immunohistochemistry, flow cytometric phenotyping, or gene rearrangement studies to detect a clonal population may be necessary
- Hodgkin lymphoma, nodular sclerosis type
  - Sclerosis is typical
  - Polymorphous background with eosinophils, plasma cells, macrophages, and lymphocytes

- Areas of necrosis, if present, usually contain numerous eosinophils and neutrophils
- Lacunar or Reed-Sternberg cells are characteristic

Pearls

- Initially described in young Asian women; now recognized in all parts of the world
- Skin lesions are relatively common
- May be related to systemic lupus erythematosus; this is still controversial

Selected References

Bosch X, Guilabert A, Miquel R, Campo E: Enigmatic Kikuchi-Fujimoto disease: A comprehensive review. Am J Clin Pathol 122:141-152, 2004.

Onciu M, Medeiros LJ: Kikuchi-Fujimoto lymphadenitis. Adv Anat Pathol 10:204-211, 2003.

Other Reactive Conditions

Nonspecific Paracortical Hyperplasia

Clinical Features

- Any age may be affected
- Usually a short clinical history of an enlarged lymph node, no specific site
- Occurs early in the course of an infection (particularly viral) or immune response
- Patients may have symptoms of a viral illness

Gross Pathology

- Nonspecific features; tan, fleshy nodal parenchyma

Histopathology

- Paracortex is expanded
- Germinal centers are inconspicuous and may be difficult to see, particularly if the section is of poor quality

Figure 14-11. Paracortical hyperplasia of lymph node. Paracortex with prominent capillaries and with numerous dendritic cells creating a mottled appearance.

- Vasculature is prominent with thick endothelial cells
- Sinuses are usually preserved
- Mostly small lymphocytes with scattered large pale cells (dendritic reticulum cells)

Special Stains and Immunohistochemistry

- Immunohistochemical stains for T and B lymphocytes show a normal distribution; paracortex has predominantly mature T cells
- Stains for B cells or follicular dendritic cells (CD21 or CD35) may reveal germinal centers not identified on routine stains

Other Techniques for Diagnosis

- Flow cytometric phenotyping shows normal mature T and B cells
- Gene rearrangement studies do not show a clonal lymphocyte population

Differential Diagnosis

- Small lymphocytic lymphoma (SLL) and chronic lymphocytic leukemia (CLL)
  - Usually affect elderly patients
  - Lymphadenopathy is generally widespread, not localized
  - Patients typically have lymphocytosis (peripheral blood involvement)
  - May have ill-defined proliferation centers consisting of larger lymphocytes (prolymphocytes and paraimmunoblasts)
  - Interfollicular cells are B cells expressing CD19, CD20, CD23, and CD5
- Mantle cell lymphoma
  - Most patients are older than 40 years of age; male predominance
  - Lymphadenopathy is widespread; rarely localized disease
  - Extranodal disease is common; may have hepatosplenomegaly
  - Diffuse or vaguely nodular B-cell proliferation
  - Infiltrate involves mantle zones and expands out into paracortex with "naked" germinal centers
  - Small to medium-sized lymphocytes with few to no large lymphocytes; cells are round, but careful high-power examination shows irregular nuclear contours
  - Infiltrate may obliterate sinuses
  - Positive for CD5, CD20, and cyclin D1; negative for CD23
  - Characteristic t(11;14)(q13;q32) chromosomal abnormality
- Lymphoblastic lymphoma and leukemia
  - Patients usually have a mass elsewhere or history of acute leukemia
  - Cells have open, finely dispersed chromatin
  - Apoptotic bodies present
  - Flow cytometry or immunohistochemistry needed for subclassification

- Metastatic small cell carcinoma
  - Tumor cells appear molded to each other and have angulated rather than round nuclei
  - Nuclei have salt-and-pepper granular chromatin rather than clumpy chromatin of lymphocytes; crush artifact is typically present
  - Necrosis is almost always present (except for well-differentiated tumors)
  - Positive for low-molecular-weight cytokeratins
- NLPHL
  - Large, ill-defined follicular areas
  - Large L&H or "popcorn" cells
  - Does not have the mottled appearance of paracortical hyperplasia
  - Large cells are phenotypically B cells, positive for CD20 and PAX5; these may have a collar of CD57-positive cells
  - Small cells are predominantly B cells

Pearls

- Paracortical hyperplasia may be accompanied by follicular hyperplasia
- Immunohistochemistry to evaluate the nodal architecture is useful in some cases

Selected References

Willard-Mack CL: Normal structure, function, and histology of lymph nodes. Toxicol Pathol 34:409-424, 2006.

Ghirardelli ML, Jemos V, Gobbi PG: Diagnostic approach to lymph node enlargement. Haematologica 84:242-247, 1999.

Angiofollicular Hyperplasia (Castleman Disease)

Clinical Features

- Three forms
  - Hyaline-vascular type
    - Most common type, any age group or gender may be affected
    - Typically presents as a mediastinal mass in asymptomatic patients
    - Usually involves a single node
  - Plasma cell type
    - Much less common
    - Relatively more frequent in extranodal sites outside of the chest
    - Usually involves multiple nodes or forms several masses
  - Multicentric type
    - Patients are older with slight male predominance
    - Often seen in patients with HIV infection
    - Systemic symptoms are common at presentation
    - Hepatosplenomegaly is common
    - Increased incidence of development of a malignant neoplasm (carcinoma, lymphoma)

Figure 14-12. Castleman disease. A, Hyaline-vascular type. Onion-skin pattern of mantle cells surrounding affected germinal center. The germinal center contains mostly follicular dendritic cells with few lymphocytes. **B, Plasma cell type.** Interfollicular area populated mostly by plasma cells.

◆ Laboratory abnormalities are frequently present: cytopenias, proteinuria, and hypoalbuminemia

Gross Pathology

- Nonspecific features; tan, fleshy nodal parenchyma

Histopathology

- Hyaline-vascular type
  - Follicles are numerous and may contain multiple germinal centers
  - Germinal centers are small and regressively transformed ("burnt-out" or "atretic") with few centroblasts; look like Hassall corpuscles but consist mostly of follicular dendritic cells rather than epithelial cells
  - Some germinal centers may be penetrated by a hyalinized blood vessel

  - Germinal centers are often surrounded by concentrically arranged small lymphocytes, looking like an expanded mantle zone and creating an onion-skin appearance
  - Interfollicular areas are extremely vascular and contain small lymphocytes and plasma cells
  - Perivascular fibrosis around some vessels
- Plasma cell and multicentric types
  - Follicles are hyperplastic and expanded as in nonspecific follicular hyperplasia
  - A few hypocellular follicles similar to the hyaline-vascular type are usually present
  - Interfollicular areas are expanded; almost all of the cells are plasma cells

Special Stains and Immunohistochemistry

- Kappa and lambda stains: usually a polyclonal plasma cell population, but lambda light chain–restricted plasma cells may be found in some plasma cell or multicentric variants

Other Techniques for Diagnosis

- Multicentric type may express human herpesvirus-8 (HHV-8; Kaposi sarcoma–associated herpesvirus)

Differential Diagnosis

▌ Nonspecific follicular hyperplasia
- Follicles are hyperplastic without onion-skin pattern of mantle cells
- Paracortex contains small lymphocytes and immunoblasts
- Plasma cells are usually not prominent but may be so in patients with rheumatologic diseases

▌ HIV-associated lymphadenopathy
- Many patients with multicentric Castleman disease are HIV positive; history is important
- Follicles are often hyperplastic with atypical shapes
- Paracortex may contain plasma cells but is usually depleted, with few lymphocytes

▌ B-cell lymphoma with plasmacytic differentiation
- Nodal architecture is generally effaced
- Immunophenotypic studies show a major clonal population of B cells

Pearls

- Hyaline-vascular type is commonly cured by surgical removal of the mass
- Occasional regressively transformed germinal centers can be seen in lymph nodes in a variety of reactive or neoplastic conditions
- Plasma cell type commonly involves more than one lymph node
- Diagnosis of the plasma cell type requires exclusion of other causes of a reactive plasmacytosis
- Multicentric type may be stable or progressive
- Multicentric type is often seen in patients with HIV infection and is strongly associated with HHV-8

- HIV-positive patients have a high incidence of Kaposi sarcoma and lymphoma
- Abnormal interleukin-6 expression is involved in the pathogenesis of plasma cell and multicentric types

Selected References

McClain KL, Natkunam Y, Swerdlow SH: Atypical cellular disorders. Hematol Am Soc Hematol Educ Prog 1:283-296, 2004.

Frizzera G: Castleman's disease and related disorders. Semin Diagn Pathol 5:346-364, 1988.

Keller AR, Hochholzer L, Castleman B: Hyaline-vascular and plasma cell types of giant lymph node hyperplasia of mediastinum and other locations. Cancer 29:670-683, 1972.

Mast Cell Disease (Mastocytosis)

Clinical Features

- Mast cell disease includes a clinical spectrum including
  - Localized cutaneous disease
  - Systemic mastocytosis
  - Mastocytosis associated with other hematologic neoplasms
  - Mast cell leukemia
  - Mast cell sarcoma
- Systemic symptoms include fatigue, weakness, weight loss, fever, and night sweats
- Peptic ulcer disease and other gastrointestinal symptoms are common
- Osteoporosis is common
- Physical findings: skin lesions, hepatomegaly, and splenomegaly

Gross Pathology

- Nonspecific; involved lymph nodes may be normal or fibrotic

Histopathology

- Lymph node infiltration may be sinusoidal or diffuse
- Lymph nodes may be fibrotic
- Features of neoplastic mast cell infiltrates
  - Sheets or masses of mast cells
  - Predominance of spindle-shaped mast cells
  - Mast cells with bilobed or multilobed nuclei
  - Mast cell sarcoma
  - Infiltrative and invasive tumor
  - Mast cells are often spindle shaped or have bilobed nuclei
  - High nuclear-to-cytoplasmic ratio, distinct nucleoli, hypogranular cytoplasm

Special Stains and Immunohistochemistry

- Romanovsky stains such as Wright or Giemsa stain the cytoplasmic granules; hematoxylin and eosin (H&E) stain does not

Figure 14-13. Mast cell disease. A, Stellate focus in a section of spleen contains mast cells in a fibrous background. Lymph node involvement has a similar pattern. **B,** Mast cells are inconspicuous amid the fibroblasts and eosinophils. In hematoxylin and eosin–stained sections, mast cells resemble plasma cells.

- Metachromatic stains such as toluidine blue or even Ziehl-Neelsen acid-fast stain highlight the granules
- Mast cells are positive with specific (chloracetate) esterase stain
- Immunohistochemical stains (CD117 or mast cell tryptase) are both more sensitive and more specific than histochemical stains and also stain degranulated cells
- Neoplastic mast cells may express CD25 and CD2

Other Techniques for Diagnosis

- Serum tryptase levels greater than 20 ng/mL support the diagnosis of mast cell disease
- *C-kit* mutation analysis may be confirmatory

Differential Diagnosis

▋ Peripheral T-cell lymphoma
- Diffuse infiltrate
- May have eosinophils and mast cells

- Mast cells should be scattered, round cells without predominant nuclear abnormalities
- Lymphocytes are mostly T cells; flow cytometry or genetic studies establish T-cell clonality
- Neoplastic T cells may express CD2 and CD25, but not mast cell tryptase

▋ Nodal marginal zone lymphoma with monocytoid features
- Sclerosis is less common
- Tumor cells do not stain with metachromatic stains
- Tumor cells do not have cytoplasmic granules on Romanowsky stains
- The monocytoid cells will express CD20 and other B-cell antigens, not CD117, mast cell tryptase, or CD2

▋ Langerhans cell histiocytosis
- Clinical features may overlap mastocytosis
- Eosinophilia and fibrosis may occur in either
- Langerhans cells express S-100, CD1a; they do not have metachromatic granules and do not express CD117 or mast cell tryptase

▋ Follicular lymphoma
- Ill-defined follicles
- Mixture of centrocytes and centroblasts replace normal follicular B cells in germinal centers
- Sclerosis is less common
- Tumor cells do not stain with metachromatic stains or chloracetate esterase
- Tumor cells express CD20, bcl-6, and bcl-2, but not mast cell tryptase or CD117

▋ Classical Hodgkin lymphoma
- Sclerosis and mixed inflammatory cell background typical of Hodgkin lymphoma may be present in mastocytosis
- Large Hodgkin and Reed-Sternberg cells not seen in mast cell disease
- Sheets of mast cells not seen in Hodgkin lymphoma

▋ Dendritic cell sarcoma
- Rare tumors
- Histologic features may overlap with mast cell disease
- Tumors obviously malignant with mitotic activity and necrosis
- No metachromatic granules
- Tumor cells express CD21 or CD35, but not mast cell tryptase or CD117

Pearls

- Symptoms may be caused either by tumor infiltration or by effects of mast cell–derived inflammatory mediators
- Fibrosis in infiltrated tissues is caused by mediators released by the neoplastic cells
- Mast cell granules do not stain with H&E, and in routine sections, mast cells resemble plasma cells
- Mast cell disease in patients with myeloproliferative disorders or myelodysplastic syndromes may represent either a second hematologic neoplasm or a

line of differentiation in a disorder arising from a pluripotent stem cell
- Degranulated or hypogranulated mast cells may be neoplastic, but these changes can also result from manipulation of biopsy tissue
- *C-kit* mutations in mast cell disease cause gain of function, mimicking the effects of stem cell factor
- Mast cell sarcoma in lymph nodes is extremely rare

Selected References

Gupta R, Bain BJ, Knight CL: Cytogenetic and molecular genetic abnormalities in systemic mastocytosis. Acta Haematol 107:123-128, 2002.

Horny H-P, Akin C, Metcalfe DD, et al: Mastocytosis. In Swerdlow SH, Campo E, Harris NL, et al (eds): World Health Organization: Classification of Tumours: Pathology and Genetics of Tumours of Haematopoietic and Lymphoid Tissues. Lyon, IARC, 2008, pp 54-63.

Bain BJ: Systemic mastocytosis and other mast cell neoplasms. Br J Haematol 106:9-17, 1999.

Amyloidosis

Clinical Features

- Occurs in older adults
- Most often seen in systemic disease with illness related to infiltration of heart, kidneys, or other vital organs
- Seen in patients with plasma cell or related neoplasms or with chronic inflammatory conditions
- Also reported in patients with Castleman disease
- Caused by tissue deposition of protein in a β pleated-sheet configuration

Gross Pathology

- With massive infiltration, the tissue may be translucent and waxy
- More commonly, infiltration is not evident on gross inspection

Figure 14-14. Amyloidosis. Amyloid deposits may elicit a foreign-body giant cell response, as in this image.

Histopathology

- Amorphous eosinophilic material is present, usually within or surrounding blood vessel walls
- With massive infiltration, amorphous eosinophilic material can compress and replace normal lymph node tissue

Special Stains and Immunohistochemistry

- Congo red stain birefringence or thioflavine T fluorescence

Other Techniques for Diagnosis

- Immunohistochemistry for immunoglobulin light chains, or amyloid A protein
- Amyloid P protein is present in all types of amyloid and can be identified with immunohistochemistry
- Electron microscopy shows characteristic fibrils

Differential Diagnosis

▎ Amorphous eosinophilic material in lymph node
- Usually in follicles, not perivascular
- Not birefringent with Congo red

▎ Sclerosis in inguinal nodes
- Can be present in lymph nodes below the bifurcation of the aorta
- Forms bands in the lymph node rather than localizing around blood vessels
- Fibrillar when examined at high magnification
- Stains as collagen with Congo red

▎ Lymph node scarring
- Usually thickens the lymph node capsule, not vessel walls
- Not birefringent with Congo red (stains like collagen)

Pearls

- Many patients with amyloidosis in a lymph node also have a B-cell lymphoma or plasma cell neoplasm; examine the morphology carefully; immunohistochemistry is often indicated
- Light chain amyloid (AL) is most common; λ light chains more common than κ light chains
- AA amyloid occurs in patients with chronic inflammatory processes; the precursor is SAA protein, an acute-phase reactant
- Significant lymph node infiltration in other forms of amyloidosis is rare
- P protein is found in all types of amyloid
- The terms *primary amyloidosis* and *secondary amyloidosis* are useless; amyloidosis should be identified by the origin of the amyloid protein

Selected References

Cohen AD, Zhou P, Xiao Q, et al: Systemic AL amyloidosis due to non-Hodgkin's lymphoma: An unusual clinicopathologic association. Br J Haematol 124:309-314, 2004.

Kutlay S, Hasan T, Keven K, et al: Primary amyloidosis presenting with massive generalized lymphadenopathy. Leuk Lymph 43:1501-1503, 2002.

Sinus Histiocytosis

Sinus Histiocytosis with Massive Lymphadenopathy (Rosai-Dorfman Disease)

Clinical Features

- Most common in children and young adults but can occur at any age
- Less frequent in patients of Asian ancestry
- Slight male predominance
- Despite the name, it is not limited to lymph nodes and has been reported in almost every organ in the body
- Patients typically present with localized lymphadenopathy, often in the cervical region
- Most common sites of extranodal disease include skin, upper respiratory tract, and bone
- Persists or recurs in many patients; minority have progressive disease with fatal outcome

Figure 14-15. Sinus histiocytosis with massive lymphadenopathy (Rosai-Dorfman disease). A, Dilated sinuses, with sheets of histiocytes. **B,** Higher magnification shows large macrophages, some of which contain lymphocytes within their cytoplasm (emperipolesis).

- Almost all patients have polyclonal hypergammaglobulinemia; erythrocyte sedimentation rate is usually elevated
- Autoimmune hemolytic anemia is common

Gross Pathology

- Enlarged, pale, tan to creamy lymph nodes; may be nodular or diffuse
- Often thickened, fibrotic capsule

Histopathology

- Nodal architecture is preserved but usually distorted; fibrotic capsule
- Sinuses are massively distended because of numerous large histocytes
- Histiocytes have vesicular nuclei, distinct nucleoli, and abundant pale cytoplasm
- Cytologic atypia is rarely seen, and mitotic activity is minimal to absent
- Characteristic feature is the presence of other blood cells within the histiocytes (emperipolesis)
- Lymphocytes are usual; intracytoplasmic red blood cells, neutrophils, and plasma cells may also be seen
- Many plasma cells are seen in the medulla
- In extranodal sites, the histiocytes are in the lymphatics rather than in the sinuses, giving a striped appearance

Special Stains and Immunohistochemistry

- Histiocytes are positive for S-100 protein, α_1-antitrypsin, and periodic acid–Schiff (PAS); also positive for CD68, CD31, CD15, MAC387, and fascin
- May be positive or negative for CD30; negative for CD1a, CD21, and CD35

Other Techniques for Diagnosis

- Electron microscopy: cytoplasm shows lipid vacuoles and lysosomes; no Birbeck granules

Differential Diagnosis

- Nonspecific sinus histiocytosis
  - Rarely causes massive lymphadenopathy
  - Commonly associated with follicular hyperplasia
  - Little or no emperipolesis; erythrophagocytosis may occur
- Histoplasmosis
  - Small punctate organisms in macrophages
  - Emperipolesis absent or rare
  - GMS or other fungal stain shows intracellular yeasts
- Mycobacteriosis
  - Emperipolesis is absent to rare
  - In immunocompetent hosts, granulomas are usually present; caseating necrosis is classic
  - A neutrophilic response may be seen with infection by atypical rapid-growing organisms

- Large numbers of macrophages with grayish cytoplasm may be present in *Mycobacterium avium-intracellulare* infection in AIDS patients
- Langerhans cell histiocytosis
  - Prominent eosinophilia
  - Langerhans cells distinct from phagocytic macrophages
  - Little or no emperipolesis
  - Cells are smaller, with bean-shaped or grooved nuclei
  - Positive for S-100, CD1a, and CD31; usually negative for CD15 and CD68
  - Birbeck granules on electron microscopy
- Classical Hodgkin lymphoma
  - Nodal architecture is effaced
  - Infiltrate centered in parenchyma rather than sinuses
  - Sinuses, if preserved, usually do not contain abnormal cells
  - The atypical cells stand out at lower magnification because of their nuclei with prominent nucleoli rather than cytoplasmic contents
  - Macrophages may be prominent but rarely contain much karyorrhectic debris
  - The neoplastic cells do not express macrophage antigens such as CD31, MAC387, or CD68 (PGM1 clone)
- Metastatic melanoma
  - Usually found in adults
  - History of melanocytic skin lesion is helpful
  - Infiltrate of atypical, large cells with large vesicular nuclei and prominent nucleoli
  - Positive for vimentin, S-100 protein, melan-A, and usually HMB-45
  - May be positive for CD30 but negative for MAC387 and CD15
- Metastatic carcinoma
  - Usually found in older adults
  - Typically cohesive clusters of malignant cells; often found in subcapsular sinus
  - Cells may have intercellular bridges, form glands, or display nuclear molding
  - Stromal response is most likely desmoplastic
  - Positive for cytokeratin, negative for CD45; may express CD68, but not other macrophage markers
- Anaplastic large cell lymphoma
  - More common in older children and adults
  - Can also have sinusoidal growth pattern
  - Cells are pleomorphic and have vesicular nuclei with prominent nucleoli
  - High mitotic rate
  - Positive for CD30 and often positive for T-cell antigens but negative for S-100 protein

Pearls

- Considered an idiopathic histiocytic proliferation
- May be related to infection with HHV-6 or EBV

- Patients with localized lymph node involvement are considered to have benign disease; often spontaneously regresses
- Patients with widespread disease have a poor prognosis
- Emperipolesis in extranodal sites may be subtle; a high index of suspicion is needed to make the diagnosis

Selected References

McClain KL, Natkunam Y, Swerdlow SH: Atypical cellular disorders. Hematol Am Soc Hematol Educ Prog 1:283-296, 2004.

Slone SP, Fleming DR, Buchino JJ: Sinus histiocytosis with massive lymphadenopathy and Langerhans cell histiocytosis express the cellular adhesion molecule CD31. Arch Pathol Lab Med 127:341-344, 2003.

Foucar E, Rosai J, Dorfman R: Sinus histiocytosis with massive lymphadenopathy (Rosai-Dorfman disease): Review of the entity. Semin Diagn Pathol 7:19-73, 1990.

Langerhans Cell Histiocytosis

Clinical Features

- Typically affects infants or young adults
- More common in persons of European ancestry
- No gender predilection
- Three classic clinical syndromes
  - Eosinophilic granuloma
    - Most common form, seen in children and adults
    - Most commonly in the lung or bone and usually localized
    - Favorable prognosis in most patients, although some patients with lung involvement develop progressive pulmonary fibrosis

  - Letterer-Siwe (systemic) form
    - Seen in infants
    - Patients present with a skin rash, organomegaly, and multiorgan involvement
    - Prognosis is poor
  - Hand-Schüller-Christian disease
    - Extremely rare
    - Found in somewhat older children than Letterer-Siwe type
    - Diabetes insipidus is often present
    - Lytic skull lesions are common
    - Somewhat better prognosis
    - Overlaps with localized and systemic forms
    - Lymph node involvement is most often secondary to skin or visceral involvement but may be the only site evident

Gross Pathology

- Pale and creamy, nodal parenchyma

Histopathology

- Nodal architecture may be retained or effaced
- If architecture is retained, the infiltrate is in the nodal sinuses
- Langerhans cells are generally mononuclear and medium sized (12 to 15 μm), with pale, eosinophilic cytoplasm and bland, bean-shaped nuclei
- Mitotic activity is minimal to absent
- Eosinophils may be numerous; lymphocytes and macrophages are also present
- Plasma cells are present in long-standing lesions
- Macrophages may become foamy (xanthomatous)
- Long-standing lesions tend to become fibrotic

Special Stains and Immunohistochemistry

- Typically positive for CD45; some cases may be CD45 negative
- Positive for S-100 protein, CD1a, CD31, HLA-DR, CD11b, CD11c, CD14, CD25, and CD71
- May be weakly positive for CD68
- CD15 generally negative without neuraminidase treatment
- Vimentin positive and cytokeratin negative

Other Techniques for Diagnosis

- Electron microscopy: demonstrates Birbeck granules (diagnostic structures)

Differential Diagnosis

- Nonspecific sinus histiocytosis
  - More often associated with local trauma or a storage disease
  - Nuclei are round rather than bean shaped
  - Eosinophils and plasma cells are not usually numerous
  - Phagocytic macrophages are negative for S-100 protein and CD1a

Figure 14-16. Langerhans cell histiocytosis. The large cells are Langerhans cells. They have abundant pale-staining cytoplasm and large oval to bean-shaped pale nuclei, sometimes with a cleft. Lymphocytes are scattered through the lesion but are concentrated at one corner. Eosinophils are also present.

■ Sinus histiocytosis with massive lymphadenopathy (Rosai-Dorfman disease)
  ● Eosinophils are rare
  ● Large macrophages with emperipolesis
  ● Positive for CD68 and S-100 protein but not CD1a
■ Anaplastic large cell lymphoma
  ● See "Differential Diagnosis" under "Sinus Histiocytosis with Massive Lymphadenopathy"
■ Metastatic melanoma
  ● See "Differential Diagnosis" under "Sinus Histiocytosis with Massive Lymphadenopathy"
■ Metastatic carcinoma
  ● See "Differential Diagnosis" under "Sinus Histiocytosis with Massive Lymphadenopathy"

Pearls

● Langerhans cells are antigen-presenting cells of the skin
● The cells of Langerhans cell histiocytosis are functionally immature; numerous cytokines are present, which may inhibit maturation
● Treatment, when necessary, includes combination of surgery, radiation, and chemotherapy
● Prognosis is most dependent on the extent of organ involvement; histologic features are of little value in determining prognosis

Selected References

Avram MM, Gobel V, Sepehr A: Case records of the Massachusetts General Hospital. Case 30-2007. A newborn girl with skin lesions. N Engl J Med 357:1327-1335, 2007.

McClain KL, Natkunam Y, Swerdlow SH: Atypical cellular disorders. Hematol Am Soc Hematol Educ Prog 1:283-296, 2004.

Herzog KM, Tubbs RR: Langerhans cell histiocytosis. Adv Anat Pathol 5:347-358, 1998.

Granulomatous Reactions

Tuberculous Lymphadenitis

Clinical Features

● Three common clinical settings
  — Children with primary tuberculosis (TB)
  — Elderly patients with reactivation of old TB
  — Immunocompromised patients, especially those infected with HIV
● Most often involves pulmonary hilar or mediastinal nodes
● Cervical nodes are the superficial lymph nodes most commonly involved
● Chest radiograph usually shows evidence of pulmonary tuberculosis
● *Mycobacterium* species: *M. tuberculosis*, *M. bovis*, *M. kansasii*, and *M. avium-intracellulare* (in HIV-positive patients) are etiologic agents

Figure 14-17. Tuberculosis in lymph node. A, Granulomas with central Langhans-type giant cells. This field does not show caseous necrosis. **B,** High-magnification view of an organism, Ziehl-Neelsen stain.

Gross Pathology

● Irregular serpentine, whitish areas in the lymph node or confluent areas of yellow-gray, chalky, caseous necrosis

Histopathology

● Irregular granulomas with central areas of caseous necrosis and giant cells
● Old lesions may be sclerotic and calcified

Special Stains and Immunohistochemistry

● Acid-fast and fluorescent stains help identify organisms

Other Techniques for Diagnosis

● Microbial culture
● PCR for mycobacterial genes is commercially available and rapid

Differential Diagnosis

■ Necrotizing sarcoidosis
  ● Granulomas are smaller and more uniform
  ● Acid-fast stain negative

- Fungal granulomas
  - Necrosis, if present, is usually coagulative rather than caseous
  - Necrosis may be due to vascular invasion and thrombosis
  - Acid-fast stain is negative; positive for fungal stains (GMS, PAS)
- Foreign-body granulomas
  - Necrosis is rare
  - Giant cells are usually more numerous and not of Langhans type
  - Foreign material is often identified
  - Acid-fast stain and microbial cultures negative
- Histiocytic necrotizing lymphadenitis (Kikuchi-Fujimoto disease)
  - Coagulative necrosis without giant cells
  - Abundant karyorrhectic debris in macrophages; few neutrophils
  - Large lymphocytes (immunoblasts) at the periphery of the necrotic areas
  - Not calcified
- Lymphoma with necrosis
  - No giant cells (except Hodgkin lymphoma or anaplastic large cell lymphoma)
  - Abnormal lymphoid cells present in preserved areas
  - Stains for organisms are negative
  - Monoclonal lymphoid population (except in Hodgkin lymphoma)

Pearls

- Many cases of TB in the United States are now found in immunocompromised hosts, in whom organisms are numerous and readily found
- Organisms are rare in immunocompetent hosts, and careful search is needed
- Mycobacterial infections in immunocompromised patients look different
  — Granulomas are smaller, ill-formed, indistinct; usually lack well-defined necrosis
  — Fewer giant cells and more histiocytes (macrophages)
  — Organisms are more numerous
  — In patients with AIDS, *M. avium-intracellulare* may cause lymph node enlargement due to massive infiltration of the node by macrophages stuffed with organisms; differential diagnosis includes histiocytosis or large cell lymphoma
- Organisms can be grown from snap-frozen tissue if necessary

Selected References

Lazarus AA, Thilagar B: Tuberculous lymphadenitis. Dis Mon 53:10-15, 2007.

Polesky A, Grove W, Bhatia G: Peripheral tuberculous lymphadenitis: Epidemiology, diagnosis, treatment, and outcome. Medicine (Baltimore) 84:350-362, 2005.

Brugge WR, Mueller PR, Misdraji J: Case records of the Massachusetts General Hospital. Weekly clinicopathological exercises. Case 8-2004. A 28-year-old man with abdominal pain, fever, and a mass in the region of the pancreas. N Engl J Med 350:1131-1138, 2004.

Woods GL: Molecular methods in the detection and identification of mycobacterial infections. Arch Pathol Lab Med 123:1002-1006, 1999.

Yan JJ, Chen FF, Jin YT, et al: Differentiation of BCG-induced lymphadenitis from tuberculosis in lymph node biopsy specimens by molecular analyses of *pncA* and *oxyR*. J Pathol 184:96-102, 1998.

Sarcoidosis

Clinical Features

- Classic presentation is interstitial pulmonary disease with hilar lymphadenopathy in a patient with pulmonary symptoms, but the disease may involve almost any organ system
- Female predominance; more common in African Americans

Figure 14-18. Sarcoidosis. A, Small round granulomas with fibrous capsules, composed predominantly of epithelioid cells. Germinal centers are not seen. **B,** High-power view of a granuloma. Note the content of epithelioid cells and giant cells, and surrounding fibrous capsule.

- Typically affects patients aged 20 to 50 years
- Peripheral lymphadenopathy present in most patients

Gross Pathology

- Nonspecific features; tan, fleshy nodal parenchyma

Histopathology

- Multiple small, circumscribed, compact granulomas without necrosis
- Granulomas are composed mostly of epithelioid cells and Langhans-type giant cells
- Germinal centers are inconspicuous or absent
- May have Schaumann bodies or asteroid bodies; however, these structures are not diagnostic
- There is a rare necrotizing variant of sarcoidosis that has granulomas with necrosis

Special Stains and Immunohistochemistry

- Stains for acid-fast organisms and fungi (PAS, GMS) are negative

Other Techniques for Diagnosis

- Elevated levels of serum angiotensin-converting enzyme (ACE)
- No pathogenic fungi or acid-fast organisms on culture of involved tissue

Differential Diagnosis

▎ Tuberculous lymphadenitis
- Granulomas with caseating necrosis
- Granulomas are ill-defined; may be stellate and confluent
- Granulomas often may be larger than typical of sarcoid
- Acid-fast stains, PCR, or culture positive

▎ Fungal infection (blastomycosis, coccidioidomycosis, histoplasmosis)
- Granulomatous infiltrate typically with necrosis
- Special stains (GMS, PAS) or culture helps identify specific organisms

▎ Cat-scratch disease
- Primarily affects younger patients
- Pulmonary lesions are uncommon; usually involves axillary or cervical nodes
- Early lesions show capsulitis, follicular hyperplasia, and abscess formation
- Later lesions consist of ill-defined granulomas
- Serologic or molecular evidence of *Bartonella henselae* infection

▎ Foreign-body granulomas
- Giant cells are prominent
- Foreign material typically seen within giant cells

Pearls

- Diagnosis requires exclusion of an infectious cause

- Treatment is steroid therapy, which is dangerous for patients with tuberculosis or a disseminated fungal infection
- Etiology remains unknown; however, many investigators believe it is probably caused by an organism that is yet to be cultured

Selected References

Rosen Y: Pathology of sarcoidosis. Semin Respir Crit Care Med 28:36-52, 2007.

Zissel G, Prasse A, Muller-Quernheim J: Sarcoidosis: Immunopathogenetic concepts. Semin Respir Crit Care Med 28:3-14, 2007.

Lymphomas with a Follicular Pattern

Follicular Lymphoma

Clinical Features

- Most patients are older than 40 years; incidence increases with age
- Most patients have widespread lymphadenopathy at presentation; at least half have bone marrow involvement
- Involvement of the splenic white pulp and hepatic portal tracts is frequently seen
- Represent about 25% of all lymphoma cases in the United States

Gross Pathology

- Nodes are soft and pinkish-tan
- Nodules are rarely apparent on cut surface; may get a hint of nodularity on gross inspection of stained touch prep slides

Histopathology

- Normal nodal architecture is partially or completely replaced by ill-defined nodules (follicles); diffuse growth pattern may be seen in part of the lymph node
- Infiltrate may extend outside the lymph node capsule into adjacent tissue
- Follicles are variably sized, variably shaped, and closely spaced; may be confluent
- Follicles contain varying proportions of centrocytes and centroblasts
- Centrocytes are usually small (nuclear diameter less than that of a histiocyte or nonactivated endothelial cell) with angulated nuclei, condensed chromatin, inconspicuous nucleoli, and scant cytoplasm (also called *small cleaved cells*); large centrocytes (also called *large cleaved cells*) have elongated nuclei, clumpy chromatin, inconspicuous nucleoli, and scant cytoplasm
- Centroblasts are usually large (nuclear diameter greater than that of a histiocyte or nonactivated endothelial cell) with irregular round nuclei,

Figure 14-19. Follicular lymphoma. A, Numerous indistinct, partially confluent follicles throughout the node, effacing normal tissue. Cracking around the follicles is a common useful artifact. **B,** Grade I. Most of the cells are centrocytes with elongated nuclei and nuclear indentations.

dispersed chromatin, multiple nuclei that often abut the nuclear membrane, and modest amounts of cytoplasm
- Blood vessels are displaced and typically wrap around the follicles
- Sclerotic bands may be present between follicles
- Subclassification is based on the number of centroblasts in the follicles, but this varies in a given patient over time, between sites of involvement, and even within different parts of one involved node
  — Aggressiveness of a follicular lymphoma correlates with the proportion of centroblasts; in general, the more centroblasts, the more aggressive (subclassification affects therapy and prognosis)
  — World Health Organization classification provides semiquantitative criteria for grading
    ◆ Grade I: 5 or fewer centroblasts/high power field (hpf) in follicles

- ◆ Grade II: 6-15 centroblasts/hpf in follicles
- ◆ Grade III: more than 15 centroblasts/hpf in follicles
- Less mitotic activity and apoptosis in follicular lymphomas than in the germinal centers of follicular hyperplasia

Special Stains and Immunohistochemistry

- Immunohistochemistry may highlight follicles that are not apparent on H&E
- Cells in follicles express CD19, CD20, CD79a, CD10 (often weakly), bcl-2, bcl-6, and surface immunoglobulin (sIg); CD23 may be expressed; negative for CD5 and CD43
- Interfollicular CD10+ lymphoid cells (not stromal cells) may help in the differentiation from reactive follicular hyperplasia when the cells are bcl-2 negative

Other Techniques for Diagnosis

- Touch preps do not show the nuclear elongation as much as tissue sections, but nuclear indentations can be seen
- Flow cytometry phenotyping shows positivity for CD10, CD19, CD20, HLA-DR, and sIg
- t(14;18)(q32;q21) chromosome abnormality detected by cytogenetics, PCR, or fluorescent in situ hybridization (FISH) in about 85% of cases; translocation involves immunoglobulin heavy-chain gene locus on chromosome 14 and *bcl-2* gene locus on chromosome 18
- Clonal immunoglobulin gene rearrangements

Differential Diagnosis

▌ Follicular hyperplasia
- Most patients are younger than 60 years
- Lymph node architecture is preserved
- Reactive germinal centers are usually uniformly well spaced from one another
- Germinal centers are sharply demarcated from mantle zones
- Zoning of centroblasts and centrocytes in germinal centers
- The bcl-2 stain is negative in the follicle center B cells but positive in the intrafollicular T cells and mantle zones
- No clonal B-cell population

▌ SLL with pseudofollicles
- Patients are likely to have peripheral blood involvement or full-blown CLL
- Pseudofollicles (proliferation centers) are usually subtle and indistinct
- Lymphocytes are small, round, and uniform
- Cells express CD19 and CD20 (often faint), but also CD5 and CD23
- Negative for CD10, bcl-6, and cyclin D1

▌ Mantle cell lymphoma, mantle zone pattern
- Well-defined, normal-appearing germinal centers

- Infiltrate blurs the border between mantle zone and paracortex
- Infiltrate consists of small to medium-sized uniform, round cells with hyperchromatic, irregularly contoured nuclei
- Cells express CD19, CD20, sIg, and bcl-1 (cyclin D1)
- Positive for CD5, but negative for CD10 and CD23
- t(11;14)(q13;q32) chromosomal abnormality is characteristic; can be detected by a FISH probe for *IgH-CCND1* fusion

■ Hodgkin lymphoma, nodular sclerosis
  - More common in younger patients
  - Mediastinal mass is common
  - Sclerotic bands are present between nodules
  - Polymorphic reactive cell background in the nodules, with lymphocytes, macrophages, eosinophils, neutrophils, and plasma cells; lymphocytes are reactive T cells
  - Hodgkin cells, Reed-Sternberg cells, or lacunar cells are always present
  - Large cells positive for CD15 and CD30; negative for CD20 and CD45

■ Hodgkin lymphoma, nodular lymphocyte predominant
  - Most patients are younger than 40 years
  - Usually involves cervical or axillary nodes
  - Indistinct macrofollicles with small round lymphocytes and scattered large cells, including L&H Reed-Sternberg cell variants
  - Small lymphocytes in the nodules are usually a mixture of B and T cells

■ Nodal marginal zone lymphoma
  - This may have a follicular pattern owing to colonization of germinal centers
  - The colonized germinal centers contain a mixture of small and large lymphocytes, but not a large population of centrocytes
  - Monocytoid areas may be present
  - Clonal B-cell population by flow cytometry
  - Tumor cells express B-cell markers and bcl-2, but not bcl-6 or CD10

Pearls

- Follicular lymphomas with many large cells are more likely to have diffuse areas
  — Follicles are paler
  — The bcl-2 staining may be weak to absent in these cases
- Bone marrow involvement usually takes the form of paratrabecular lymphoid aggregates
- Low-grade follicular lymphomas may be extremely indolent but are not curable
- Median survival is longer than 7 years in many series
- Transformation to a DLBCL occurs in up to 60% of 10-year survivors
- Grading requires excellent histology to distinguish centroblasts from follicular dendritic cells or artifactual changes in centrocytes

Selected References

Isaacson PG: Hematopathology practice: The commonest problems encountered in a consultation practice. Histopathology 50:821-834, 2007.

Cerhan JR, Wang S, Maurer MJ, et al: Prognostic significance of host immune gene polymorphisms in follicular lymphoma survival. Blood 109:5439-5446, 2007.

de Jong D: Molecular pathogenesis of follicular lymphoma: A cross talk of genetic and immunologic factors. J Clin Oncol 23:6358-6363, 2005.

Dave SS, Wright G, Tan B, et al: Prediction of survival in follicular lymphoma based on molecular features of tumor-infiltrating immune cells. N Engl J Med 351:2159-2169, 2004.

Harris NL, Nathwani BN, Swerdlow SH, et al: Follicular lymphoma. In Swerdlow SH, Campo E, Harris NL, et al (eds): World Health Organization: Classification of Tumours: Pathology and Genetics of Tumours of Haematopoietic and Lymphoid Tissues. Lyon, IARC, 2008, pp 220-226.

Hodgkin Lymphoma, Nodular Sclerosis Type

Clinical Features

- Peak incidence in adolescents and young adults (aged 15 to 40 years); second peak at ages 55 to 75 years; may occur at any age
- Slight female predominance, especially at younger ages
- Most common type of Hodgkin lymphoma (60% to 80% of cases)
- Most patients present with lymphadenopathy: cervical in 70% to 80% of cases, axillary in 15%, inguinal in 10%; rare patients present with a chest wall mass
- Mediastinal involvement common at presentation
- Extranodal presentation except by extension from involved nodes is rare
- Systemic symptoms occur in about 25% of patients and include fever, night sweats, weight loss, and pruritus; alcohol intolerance often mentioned but rarely seen

Gross Pathology

- Involved nodes vary from fleshy and creamy-tan to hard, white, and fibrotic
- Capsule shows variable degree of thickening
- Nodules and sclerotic bands may be visible grossly

Histopathology

- Thickened nodal capsule with fibrous bands separating nodules of a cellular, pleomorphic lymphoid infiltrate; fibrous bands have central arterioles with perivascular sclerosis of abnormally refractile, birefringent collagen
- Cellular infiltrate includes classic Reed-Sternberg cells and lacunar cells

Figure 14-20. Hodgkin lymphoma, nodular sclerosis type. A, Sclerotic bands surround cellular nodules at the lower left and a necrotic focus to the right. **B,** High-magnification view showing numerous eosinophils, Reed-Sternberg cells, a few mononuclear Hodgkin cells, lymphocytes, and macrophages. *Inset,* High-magnification view showing a lacunar cell.

- Background reactive cells are polymorphic and include small lymphocytes, eosinophils, macrophages, and plasma cells; may be predominantly lymphocytes or may be depleted of lymphocytes
- Lacunar cell
  — Artifact of formalin fixation, not seen in sections fixed in hardening fixatives
  — These are variant Hodgkin cells with multilobated nuclei and pale cytoplasm that shrinks during fixation and processing, leaving the appearance of a small cell tethered in the middle of a large, otherwise empty space
- Variants
  - Interfollicular Hodgkin lymphoma
    — Residual germinal centers and mantle zones are surrounded by an infiltrate of Hodgkin cells

— Normal nodal structures and germinal centers are generally partially replaced or displaced by the infiltrate
— Usually little sclerosis; this may represent early involvement of the lymph node
- Cellular phase
  — This is basically nodular sclerosis Hodgkin lymphoma without the sclerosis; lacunar cells are key to the diagnosis
- Syncytial Hodgkin lymphoma
  — Confluent sheets of Hodgkin cells or Reed-Sternberg cells are present at least focally in the node, but generally do not replace the entire node

Special Stains and Immunohistochemistry

- Neoplastic cells are highly altered B lymphocytes, usually negative for CD45, T-cell antigens (CD3, CD5), and epithelial membrane antigen (EMA)
- Positive for CD15 and CD30; typically demonstrate a cytoplasmic membrane and perinuclear (Golgi) staining pattern
- PAX5 positive (confirms B-cell lineage of the tumor cells); CD20 may be weakly expressed in a subset of tumor cells
- Tumor cells express fascin

Other Techniques for Diagnosis

- Generally noncontributory

Differential Diagnosis

▌ Hodgkin lymphoma, nodular lymphocyte predominant
- Almost always affects adolescents or young adults, who present with cervical lymphadenopathy
- Classic Reed-Sternberg cells are rare; variant Hodgkin cells (L&H or popcorn cells) typically seen
- Background consists of an infiltrate of small non-neoplastic lymphocytes
- Neoplastic cells express CD20, CD45, and EMA; negative for CD15 and CD30
▌ T-cell–rich large B-cell lymphoma (TCRLBCL) variant of DLBCL
- Diffuse infiltrate without sclerosis or nodularity
- Scattered large, mononuclear neoplastic cells in a background of small reactive lymphocytes that are almost all T cells
- Large neoplastic cells are positive for CD45 and CD20, negative for CD15 and CD30
- Tumor cells do not express fascin
▌ Follicular lymphoma
- Patients are usually older than 40 years
- Variable mixture of centrocytes and centroblasts without polymorphic reactive cell background
- Reed-Sternberg–like cells rarely present; sclerosis is incidental

- Both small and large cells are CD20-positive B cells; may express CD10, usually express bcl-6
- Clonal B-cell population usually detectable by flow cytometry
- Characteristic t(14;18)(q32;q21) chromosomal abnormality

■ Anaplastic large cell lymphoma
- Large cells are usually predominant and often resemble a large cell lymphoma or metastatic carcinoma
- If the infiltrate is focal, it tends to be in nodal sinuses
- Fibrosis, if present, is fine and diffuse rather than nodular
- Reed-Sternberg–like cells may be numerous
- Abnormal large cells are positive for CD30; usually T cells but may not express common T-cell antigens or CD45
- Tumor cells are typically positive for EMA and often anaplastic lymphoma kinase (ALK-1)
- Negative for CD15, PAX5, and fascin

■ Peripheral T-cell lymphoma with sclerosis
- Fine compartmentalizing sclerosis rather than nodular sclerosis is typically seen
- Eosinophils and plasma cells may be prominent
- Reed-Sternberg–like cells may be present and even "too easy to find" compared with typical Hodgkin lymphoma; these cells lack the perinucleolar clearing and coarse nuclear membranes of true Reed-Sternberg cells
- Background composed of variably sized lymphocytes (spectrum from small to large cells) without distinct populations
- Tumor cells express common T-cell antigens (CD2, CD3, CD5, and CD7), have clonal T-cell antigen receptor gene rearrangement, and are CD15 negative and either positive or negative for CD30
- Tumor cells do not express PAX5 or fascin

■ Infectious mononucleosis
- Rapid clinical onset with systemic symptoms and disseminated disease
- Follicular hyperplasia with interfollicular expansion
- Background of small lymphocytes and immunoblasts
- Reed-Sternberg–like cells may be present, often express CD30; do not express CD15

Pearls
- Be certain immunohistochemical studies show staining of the neoplastic cells, not adjacent small lymphocytes
- Classic Reed-Sternberg cells are needed for a definitive diagnosis; however, many other diseases can have cells that look similar; the reactive cell background must be consistent with Hodgkin lymphoma

- In addition to eosinophils, nodular sclerosis Hodgkin lymphoma can have neutrophilic abscesses or areas of necrosis; Hodgkin cells and Reed-Sternberg cells are typically concentrated at the periphery of these areas
- Granulomas or eosinophils in spleen or bone marrow of patients with nodular sclerosis Hodgkin lymphoma do not necessarily indicate that these tissues contain tumor
- Neoplastic cells are EBV positive in about half of cases

Selected References
Bakshi NA, Finn WG, Schnitzer B, et al: Fascin expression in diffuse large B-cell lymphoma, anaplastic large cell lymphoma, and classical Hodgkin lymphoma. Arch Pathol Lab Med 131:742-747, 2007.

Brauninger A, Schmitz R, Bechtel D, et al: Molecular biology of Hodgkin's and Reed/Sternberg cells in Hodgkin's lymphoma. Int J Cancer 118:1853-1861, 2006.

Stein H, von Wasielewski R, Poppema S, et al: Nodular sclerosis classical Hodgkin lymphoma. In Swerdlow SH, Campo E, Harris NL, et al (eds): World Health Organization: Classification of Tumours: Pathology and Genetics of Tumours of Haematopoietic and Lymphoid Tissues. Lyon, IARC, 2008, p 330.

Hodgkin Lymphoma, Nodular Lymphocyte Predominant

Clinical Features
- Uncommon variant of Hodgkin lymphoma, accounting for about 5% of cases in the United States
- Most common in adolescents and young adults
- "B" symptoms are less common than with classical Hodgkin lymphoma
- Mediastinal mass is rare
- Usually stage I or II at presentation with cervical or axillary lymphadenopathy

Gross Pathology
- Nonspecific, soft, tan lymph nodes
- Nodularity typically not evident grossly

Histopathology
- Normal nodal architecture is totally or at least partially effaced by macrofollicular proliferation, imparting a nodular configuration
- Nodules contain numerous small lymphocytes and a variable number of variant Hodgkin cells (L&H or popcorn cells) that are large cells with folded or lobulated nuclei, vesicular chromatin, and small basophilic nucleoli
- Plasma cells and eosinophils are not part of the infiltrate
- Classical Hodgkin cells and diagnostic Reed-Sternberg cells are extremely rare

Figure 14-21. Nodular lymphocyte–predominant Hodgkin lymphoma. A, The nodularity is usually subtle, requiring careful examination at low-power magnification. **B,** High-magnification view showing several of the lymphocyte and histiocyte or "popcorn" cells. (Courtesy of C. H. Koo, Kaiser-Permanente.)

Special Stains and Immunohistochemistry

- Neoplastic cells (popcorn cells) express CD45 and CD20 but are usually negative for CD15 and CD30
- Surrounding small lymphocytes are a mixture of B cells and T cells; the former often predominate
- In about 25% of cases, the neoplastic cells are surrounded by a collar of CD57-positive and CD279-positive small T cells

Other Techniques for Diagnosis

- Gene rearrangement studies are negative by Southern blot; may be positive by PCR

Differential Diagnosis

▮ Lymphocyte-rich classical Hodgkin lymphoma
- Usually has a diffuse growth pattern
- In the rare cases with a nodular pattern, the tumor tends to arise in mantle zones and displace germinal centers rather than replacing them
- Background is mostly small lymphocytes, as in lymphocyte-predominant Hodgkin lymphoma
- Classic Reed-Sternberg cells are more readily found

- Neoplastic Hodgkin cells are positive for CD15 and CD30 but usually negative for CD20 and CD45
- The neoplastic cells in this entity *and* in lymphocyte-predominant Hodgkin lymphoma express PAX5
- Neoplastic cells in classical Hodgkin lymphoma express fascin
- Most cases have a higher percentage of T lymphocytes in the background than is seen in lymphocyte-predominant Hodgkin lymphoma

▮ SLL
- Usually affects elderly patients
- See other features in "Differential Diagnosis" under "Follicular Lymphoma"

▮ TCRLBCL variant of DLBCL
- Diffuse infiltrate
- "B" symptoms are more common
- Large lymphocytes are typically centroblasts
- Small lymphocytes are almost all CD3-positive T cells
- Large cells are CD20-positive B cells (may also be CD30 positive)
- Aggressive clinical course

▮ Metastatic carcinoma
- Infiltrate may be diffuse or consist of small cohesive clusters of neoplastic cells; often present in subcapsular sinus
- Often have a sclerotic (desmoplastic) reaction
- Neoplastic cells are smaller with a higher nuclear-to-cytoplasmic ratio and form cohesive clusters; multinucleated cells are less common
- Tumor cells are positive for cytokeratin, negative for CD45

Pearls

- NLPHL may coexist with, precede, or rarely follow PTGC
- Phenotypically this is a B-cell lymphoma
- NLPHL differs phenotypically and cytologically from classical Hodgkin lymphoma, but the orderly pattern of spread and response to therapy are similar to other types of Hodgkin lymphoma
- NLPHL responds well to chemotherapy but may have a proportionately greater incidence of late relapse than classical Hodgkin lymphoma
- May transform to a DLBCL
- Differentiation from classical Hodgkin lymphoma and other mimics is important; treatment is different for NLPHL than for classical Hodgkin lymphoma

Selected References

Nogova L, Rudiger T, Engert A: Biology, clinical course and management of nodular lymphocyte-predominant Hodgkin lymphoma. Hematol Am Soc Hematol Educ Prog 1:266-272, 2006.

Poppema S, Swerdlow SH, Delsol G, et al: Nodular lymphocyte predominant Hodgkin lymphoma. In Swerdlow SH, Campo E, Harris NL, et al (eds): World Health Organization:

Classification of Tumours: Pathology and Genetics of Tumours of Haematopoietic and Lymphoid Tissues. Lyon, IARC, 2008, pp 323-325.

Diffuse Lymphomas Resembling Small Mature Lymphocytes

Small Lymphocytic Lymphoma/Chronic Lymphocytic Leukemia

Clinical Features

- Most patients are older than 65 years
- Most patients present with asymptomatic generalized lymphadenopathy, which is often extensive; most patients present with Ann Arbor stage III or IV disease
- Splenomegaly or hepatosplenomegaly is frequent
- Many have peripheral blood lymphocytosis characteristic of CLL

Figure 14-22. **A, Chronic lymphocytic leukemia involving a lymph node.** Infiltrate with numerous indistinct pale pseudofollicles. **B, Small lymphocytic lymphoma.** Uniform small cells with plasmacytoid peripheral chromatin distribution.

Gross Pathology

- Diffuse, fleshy, creamy, tan to fish-flesh nodal parenchyma

Histopathology

- Diffuse infiltrate with complete effacement of nodal architecture
- Pseudofollicular pattern with rounded, ill-defined, paler areas may be present
- Infiltrate may extend through capsule and involve surrounding soft tissue
- Predominant cells are small lymphocytes, which may have plasmacytoid features
- Pseudofollicles (proliferation centers) contain prolymphocytes, paraimmunoblasts, and mitotic figures

Special Stains and Immunohistochemistry

- Positive for CD19, CD20, CD5, and CD23; negative for bcl-6
- Weak positivity for sIg

Other Techniques for Diagnosis

- Touch preps may show plasmacytoid features
- Prognostic chromosomal abnormalities for CLL are more frequently found by FISH studies than by conventional karyotype
- Quantitation of CD38 or ZAP-70 expression for CLL may predict prognosis and need for treatment
- Mutation status of the rearranged immunoglobulin gene is predictive of prognosis for CLL and need for treatment
- Flow cytometry is used for phenotyping; PCR or Southern blot for gene rearrangement

Differential Diagnosis

▌ Paracortical hyperplasia
  - Consists of small lymphocytes and occasional large reticulum cells but no prolymphocytes
  - No pseudofollicular pattern; however, preserved germinal centers are usually at least focally present
  - Infiltrate generally does not extend beyond nodal capsule
  - Most of the cells are T cells positive for both CD3 and CD5, no clonal B-cell population
▌ Follicular lymphoma
  - Prominent follicular pattern
  - Follicles contain varying mixture of centrocytes and centroblasts
  - Follicular B cells express bcl-2, CD19, CD20, and often CD10; strong positivity for sIg, negative for CD5 and cyclin D1 (bcl-1)
  - Chromosomal abnormalities include t(14;18)(q32;q21)
  - *IgH-bcl-2* rearrangement detectable by FISH or PCR

- Mantle cell lymphoma
  - Variable patterns: mantle zone pattern with expanded, confluent mantle zones with preserved germinal centers and diffuse pattern
  - Infiltrate consists of small to medium-sized lymphocytes with an irregular nuclear envelope; no large cells and no proliferation centers
  - Cells express CD5, CD19, CD20, and cyclin D1 (bcl-1); negative for CD23
  - Characteristic t(11;14)(q13;q32); *IgH-CCND1* rearrangement detectable by FISH
- Hodgkin lymphoma, nodular lymphocyte predominant
  - See "Differential Diagnosis" under "Follicular Lymphoma"
  - No prolymphocytes or immunoblasts; no pseudofollicles (proliferation centers)
- Lymphoplasmacytic lymphoma
  - Plasma cells may be a minor population and are clonal
  - IgM paraprotein may be detectable in either, but levels are higher in lymphoplasmacytic lymphoma
  - Symptoms due to the paraprotein and hyperviscosity are common
  - Tumor cells generally do not express CD5 or CD23
- Marginal zone lymphoma
  - May infiltrate spleen, bone marrow, blood, or lymph nodes
  - Monocytoid cells with abundant cytoplasm are typical, occasionally mimic pseudofollicles (proliferation centers)
  - Tumor cells generally do not express CD5 or CD23

Pearls

- SLL and CLL form a continuous disease spectrum; phenotype is virtually identical
- Transformation to DLBCL (Richter syndrome) is seen in about 10% of patients
- Genetic and immunophenotypic tests are important prognostic indicators in CLL
- Patients whose tumors have unmutated immunoglobulin genes have more aggressive disease than those with mutated immunoglobulin genes
- High expression of CD38 or ZAP-70 by tumor cells is also correlated with more aggressive disease and is more readily detected
- Deletion of 11q or 17p is associated with poor overall survival; del(11q) is also associated with lymphadenopathy
- Trisomy 12/12q has uncertain effect on survival, similar to normal karyotype
- The only cytogenetic abnormality associated with better survival than normal cytogenetics is del(13q)
- Tumors with t(11;14)(q13;q32) should be classified as mantle cell lymphoma, not SLL
- FISH probes detect chromosomal abnormalities more often than conventional cytogenetics

- Treatment paradigms are changing to risk-adjusted therapy based on clinical and biologic assessment of the patient and the tumor, to aim for long-term control for younger, healthier patients

Selected References

Thieblemont C, Nasser V, Felman P, et al: Small lymphocytic lymphoma, marginal zone B-cell lymphoma, and mantle cell lymphoma exhibit distinct gene-expression profiles allowing molecular diagnosis. Blood 103:2727-2737, 2004.

Müller-Hermelink HK, Montserrat E, Catovsky D, et al: Chronic lymphocytic leukemia/small lymphocytic lymphoma. In Swerdlow SH, Campo E, Harris NL, et al (eds): World Health Organization: Classification of Tumours: Pathology and Genetics of Tumours of Haematopoietic and Lymphoid Tissues. Lyon, IARC, 2008, pp 180-182.

Chen CC, Raikow RB, Sonmez-Alpan E, Swerdlow SH: Classification of small B-cell lymphoid neoplasms using a paraffin section immunohistochemical panel. Appl Immunohistochem Mol Morphol 8:1-11, 2000.

Mantle Cell Lymphoma

Clinical Features

- Most patients are older than 40 years; male predominance
- Present with localized or generalized lymphadenopathy
- Hepatosplenomegaly is frequent
- Most patients have bone marrow involvement
- May have lymphocytosis with peripheral blood involvement
- Intestinal and other extranodal involvement is common

Gross Pathology

- Nonspecific features; soft, fleshy nodal parenchyma

Histopathology

- Generally have effacement of entire nodal architecture
- Infiltrate may extend through nodal capsule into adjacent soft tissue
- Several patterns
  - Mantle zone pattern
    - "Naked" preserved germinal centers surrounded by expanded, focally confluent mantle zones replacing the paracortex
  - Diffuse pattern
  - Vague follicular pattern
- Infiltrate consists of a proliferation of small to medium-sized uniform, round cells with hyperchromatic nuclei with irregular contours
- Large cells are typically absent; no proliferation centers
- Mitoses are usually relatively uncommon
- Blastoid variant: cells may resemble lymphoblastic lymphoma or a DLBCL; genetic and phenotypic studies are needed for differentiation

Figure 14-23. Mantle cell lymphoma. A, Mantle zone pattern. "Naked" germinal centers surrounded by the neoplastic infiltrate, replacing mantle zones and interfollicular areas. **B,** Uniform small to medium-sized cells with overall round nuclear shape. Some cells have nuclear clefts. The few large cells are probably dendritic cells. Note the absence of large lymphoid cells, unlike small lymphocytic lymphoma and follicular lymphoma. *Inset,* Immunohistochemical stain for cyclin D1 showing nuclear staining of the tumor cells.

Special Stains and Immunohistochemistry

- Positive for CD19, CD20, CD5, and CD43; negative for CD23
- Positive for sIg and cyclin D1 (bcl-1)

Other Techniques for Diagnosis

- Flow cytometric phenotyping: CD19, CD20, FMC7, CD5 positive; CD23 negative
- Immunoglobulin gene rearrangement identifies a clonal population
- Cytogenetics: t(11;14)(q13;q32) chromosomal abnormality; immunoglobulin heavy-chain gene locus on chromosome 14 and the *bcl-1* gene locus on chromosome 11

- FISH for the *IgH-CCND1* translocation, which is the basis for the t(11;14) detected by cytogenetics

Differential Diagnosis

- Paracortical hyperplasia
  - See "Differential Diagnosis" under "Small Lymphocytic Lymphoma"
- SLL
  - See "Differential Diagnosis" under "Follicular Lymphoma"
- Follicular lymphoma
  - See "Differential Diagnosis" under "Small Lymphocytic Lymphoma"
- Hodgkin lymphoma, nodular lymphocyte predominant
  - See "Differential Diagnosis" under "Follicular Lymphoma"
- Precursor B-lymphoblastic lymphoma (versus blastoid variant of mantle cell lymphoma)
  - CD20 negative to only weakly positive, CD5 negative
  - Cyclin D1 not expressed; t(11;14)(q13;q32) chromosomal abnormality not detected
  - Terminal deoxynucleotidyl transferase (TdT) usually positive and bcl-2 negative
- DLBCL (versus blastoid variant of mantle cell lymphoma)
  - CD5 usually negative; CD10 may be expressed
  - Cyclin D1 not expressed; t(11;14)(q13;q32) chromosomal abnormality absent

Pearls

- Mantle cell lymphomas are cytologically bland but clinically aggressive
- More aggressive than low-grade B cell lymphomas; median survival less than 3 years
- Like low-grade B cell lymphomas, no proven curative treatment
- Bone marrow involvement usually takes the form of nonparatrabecular and paratrabecular lymphoid aggregates
- Gene expression profiling may distinguish more aggressive from less aggressive cases

Selected References

Leoncini L, Delsol G, Gascoyne RD, et al: Aggressive B-cell lymphomas: A review based on the workshop of the XI Meeting of the European Association for Haematopathology. Histopathology 46:241-255, 2005.

Rosenwald A, Wright G, Wiestner A, et al: The proliferation gene expression signature is a quantitative integrator of oncogenic events that predicts survival in mantle cell lymphoma. Cancer Cell 3:185-197, 2003.

Swerdlow SH, Campo E, Seto M, et al: Mantle cell lymphoma. In Swerdlow SH, Campo E, Harris NL, et al (eds): World Health Organization: Classification of Tumours: Pathology and Genetics of Tumours of Haematopoietic and Lymphoid Tissues. Lyon, IARC, 2008, pp 229-232.

Nodal Marginal Zone Lymphoma

Clinical Features

- Rare lymphoma, about 2% of all lymphomas
- Less common than extranodal marginal zone lymphomas of mucosa-associated lymphoid tissue (MALT)
- Mostly in middle-aged adults
- Most patients are asymptomatic but have widespread disease at diagnosis, Ann Arbor stage III or IV

Gross Pathology

- Nonspecific with diffuse fleshy enlargement of lymph nodes

Histopathology

- Patterns of involvement vary—may be diffuse, perifollicular, or vaguely nodular
- Partially involved nodes or regions of nodes may have preserved follicles with confluence of marginal zones
- Follicular colonization by tumor cells is common; the colonizing cells may be large cells, but unlike true follicle center B cells, they are negative for CD10 and bcl-6
- Cellular composition varies; there are always a variety of cell types
- Monocytoid B cells are rarely predominant but often present focally
- Small lymphocytes or cells resembling mantle cells are always present
- Plasmacytoid or plasmacytic differentiation may be present
- Large cells may be present
- Peripheral blood may contain tumor cells

Special Stains and Immunohistochemistry

- Positive for CD20 and usually bcl-2
- Negative for CD5, CD10, CD23, and cyclin D1
- Large cells may have partial expression of bcl-6
- Plasma cells express MUM-1

Other Techniques for Diagnosis

- Flow cytometry
- Cytogenetic abnormalities include trisomies of chromosomes 3, 18, 7, and 12, and t(3;14)

Differential Diagnosis

- ▌Small lymphocytic lymphoma
  - See "Differential Diagnosis" under "Follicular Lymphoma"
- ▌Mantle cell lymphoma
  - See "Differential Diagnosis" under "Small Lymphocytic Lymphoma"
- ▌DLBCL
  - Mostly large cells
  - Extensive plasmacytic or monocytoid differentiation not seen

- Greater cellular proliferation; Ki-67 usually expressed in more than 50% of the tumor cells
- ▌Lymphoplasmacytic lymphoma
  - See "Differential Diagnosis" under "Small Lymphocytic Lymphoma"
- ▌Nodular lymphocyte-predominant Hodgkin lymphoma
  - See "Differential Diagnosis" under "Follicular Lymphoma"
- ▌Marginal zone differentiation of follicular lymphoma
  - Usually produces a targetoid pattern of a pale zone around neoplastic follicles
  - Rarely massive, obscuring the follicular pattern
  - Typically shows centrocytes in the follicles
  - Tumor cells express bcl-6 and CD10
  - *IgH-bcl-2* translocation on FISH; t(14;18) (q32;q21) on karyotype

Pearls

- Good histology and thorough examination are essential to see the varied cell types
- Node-based marginal zone lymphoma is somewhat more aggressive than extranodal marginal zone MALT lymphomas
- No established association with an infectious agent; some studies report association with hepatitis C
- The morphology and phenotype are similar to extranodal marginal zone lymphomas, but the node-based tumors are cytogenetically distinct
- Node-based tumors do not have translocations involving the *MALT1* gene on chromosome 18 that are common in extranodal marginal zone lymphomas

Selected References

Traverse-Glehen A, Felman P, Callet-Bauchu E, et al: A clinicopathological study of nodal marginal zone B-cell lymphoma: A report on 21 cases. Histopathology 48:162-173, 2006.

Campo E, Pileri SA, Jaffe ES, et al: Nodal marginal zone lymphoma. In Swerdlow SH, Campo E, Harris NL, et al (eds): World Health Organization: Classification of Tumours: Pathology and Genetics of Tumours of Haematopoietic and Lymphoid Tissues. Lyon, IARC, 2008, pp 218-219.

Remstein ED, James CD, Kurtin PJ: Incidence and subtype specificity of API2-MALT1 fusion translocations in extranodal, nodal, and splenic marginal zone lymphomas. Am J Pathol 156:1183-1188, 2000

Diffuse Neoplasms, "Aggressive" Histology

Diffuse Large B-Cell Lymphoma

Clinical Features

- Most common type of lymphoma
- Most often in adults but may occur at any age; mean age is about 60 years

Figure 14-24. Diffuse large B-cell lymphoma. A, Normal lymph node architecture is effaced. It is replaced by a diffuse, pleomorphic infiltrate, mostly large cells. **B,** High magnification showing the pleomorphic large tumor cells with vesicular nuclei and prominent nucleoli. Cytoplasm is more abundant than in most indolent lymphomas. The tumor cells are several times the size of the scattered small lymphocytes.

- Slight male predominance
- Patients may present with localized or extensive disease and may have nodal or extranodal presentation
- Common extranodal locations include the gastrointestinal tract, spleen, skin, bone, brain, or oropharyngeal lymphoid tissue
- May present with asymptomatic nodal enlargement or with systemic symptoms such as fever, malaise, weight loss, or organ dysfunction
- May arise in the setting of immunodeficiency, including HIV infection, congenital immunodeficiency, or Sjögren syndrome or other autoimmune disorders, or after allogeneic bone marrow or solid organ transplantation (immunodeficiency-associated large B-cell lymphoma)

Gross Pathology

- Soft, pinkish-tan fish-flesh masses

Histopathology

- Diffuse growth pattern with effacement of nodal architecture
- Infiltrate consists predominantly of noncohesive large cells with round to oval, vesicular nuclei showing distinct nucleoli and a moderate amount of pale to basophilic cytoplasm
- Nuclei are at least as large as macrophage nuclei
- A minority of small lymphocytes are often seen in the background
- Mitoses are often numerous; apoptotic bodies or areas of necrosis are common
- Infiltrate may extend into or primarily involve extranodal soft tissue
- Variants
  — Primary effusion lymphoma
    ◆ Arises as malignant pleural or ascitic effusions
    ◆ Most patients have advanced HIV infection
    ◆ Tumor cells are infected with HHV-8
  — TCRLBCL
    ◆ Neoplastic large B cells are a distinct minority (<10%) of cells, and reactive small T cells markedly predominate (>90%); small B cells are few in number
    ◆ May be difficult to detect light-chain restricted B cells by flow cytometry because of paucity of tumor cells
    ◆ PCR demonstrates clonal immunoglobulin gene rearrangements characteristic of the presence of monoclonal B cells; the T cells are polyclonal
    ◆ Some TCRLBCLs have pathologic features that overlap with nodular lymphocyte-predominant Hodgkin lymphoma; these may represent different parts of a disease spectrum rather than separate diseases
    ◆ Patients with TCRLBCL have aggressive disease similar to typical DLBCL but are more likely to have splenic and bone marrow involvement

Special Stains and Immunohistochemistry

- Typically positive for CD45
- CD19, CD20, and sIg expressed; small population of T cells may be seen
- Variable expression of CD10, CD23, bcl-2, bcl-6, and MUM-1; CD5 expression is uncommon, negative for TdT
- Positive for vimentin; negative for cytokeratin

Other Techniques for Diagnosis

- Flow cytometric phenotyping; some laboratories have poor recovery of larger lymphoid cells, yielding false-negative results
- Immunoglobulin gene rearrangement

- May have t(14;18)(q32;q21) chromosomal abnormality if of follicular origin (about 30% of cases)
- DNA microarrays allow identification of three types of DLBCL
  — One type resembles germinal center B cells
  — The second type is similar to activated peripheral blood B cells and has a worse prognosis
  — The third type more closely resembles Hodgkin lymphoma, and most of these are mediastinal large B-cell lymphomas

Differential Diagnosis

▌Paracortical hyperplasia
- See "Differential Diagnosis" for "Small Lymphocytic Lymphoma"

▌Metastatic carcinoma
- If the node is partially involved, involvement is usually mostly in nodal sinuses
- Positive for cytokeratin; negative for CD45

▌Clear cell sarcoma
- Usually presents in soft tissue
- Cells have abundant clear cytoplasm and are more cohesive than in lymphoma
- Positive for vimentin, S-100 protein, and melan-A; negative for HMB-45 and CD45

▌Ewing sarcoma
- Usually found in adolescents or young adults
- Tumor cells are usually small (small round blue cell tumor)
- Cells are positive for glycogen and vimentin; negative for CD45
- Variable weak expression of S-100 protein, synaptophysin, and muscle markers
- CD99 and Fli-1, typical of Ewing sarcoma, also expressed in hematopoietic cells
- FISH for *EWS* gene rearrangement but no immunoglobulin gene rearrangement

▌Dysgerminoma and seminoma
- Primarily affects young adults
- Cells have small nuclei (low nuclear-to-cytoplasmic ratio) and clear cytoplasm ("fried-egg" appearance); distinct vascular stroma with prominent lymphocytic infiltrate
- Typically presents with a gonadal or mediastinal mass
- Positive for placental alkaline phosphatase (PLAP) and vimentin; negative for CD45

▌Lymphoblastic lymphoma and acute leukemia
- Usually occurs in children through young adults
- Mediastinal mass is common for precursor T-cell type
- Medium-sized cells with large nuclei and fine "blastic" chromatin; high nuclear-to-cytoplasmic ratio
- Expresses CD34, CD10, and TdT

▌Acute myeloid leukemia (myeloblastoma, myeloid sarcoma, granulocytic sarcoma)

- Careful examination of Wright- or Giemsa-stained touch preps may reveal myeloid granules or diagnostic Auer rods
- Careful review of H&E sections may also show maturing myeloid cells
- Positive for chloracetate esterase, myeloperoxidase, CD13, and CD33
- Cells usually express CD34; generally negative for CD20 and other B-cell antigens

▌Peripheral T-cell lymphoma
- Node-based T-cell lymphomas consisting mostly of large cells are rare; most have a mixture of small, medium-sized, and large cells
- Acute T-cell leukemia-lymphoma (ATLL) is rare in North America and Europe; most common in southern Japan but occurs worldwide
  — Patients often have skin lesions, peripheral blood involvement, hypercalcemia
  — Tumor cells express CD2, CD3, CD4, and CD5 but not B-cell antigens
  — Positive for human T-cell lymphotrophic virus type 1 (HTLV-1)

▌Anaplastic large cell lymphoma (ALCL)
- Large wreath-shaped or embryoid hallmark cells are characteristic
- Tumor cells express CD30 with variable loss of T-cell antigens and CD45; negative for CD20 and other B-cell antigens

Pearls

- Unlike most other entities in the current classification of lymphoma, DLBCL contains several biologically distinct types of lymphoma unified by cell size and B-cell lineage
- CD30 expression in a B-cell large cell lymphoma does not change classification or prognosis
- Natural history is aggressive (rapidly fatal if untreated), but these tumors may be curable with multiagent chemotherapy
- Immunohistochemical detection of many proteins has correlated with outcome for patients with DLBCL; CD10-positive or bcl-6-positive and MUM-1-negative phenotype indicates germinal center cell origin; prognostic significance of most other markers is still controversial and yet to be confirmed in multivariate studies
- The recent addition of rituximab to therapy may alter prognostic significance of some phenotypic markers; it may overcome the poor prognosis associated with bcl-2 protein expression in DLBCL
- The outcome of patients whose tumors do not express bcl-6 may not be improved by adding rituximab
- There is as yet no evidence that detection of CD20 by immunohistochemistry on tissue sections predicts response to rituximab in DLBCL; the antibody usually used in immunohistochemistry (L26) recognizes a different epitope than does rituximab

Selected References

Shivakumar L, Armitage JO: *Bcl-2* gene expression as a predictor of outcome in diffuse large B-cell lymphoma. Clin Lymphoma Myeloma 6:455-457, 2006.

Winter JN, Weller EA, Horning SJ, et al: Prognostic significance of Bcl-6 protein expression in DLBCL treated with CHOP or R-CHOP: A prospective correlative study. Blood 107:4207-4213, 2006.

Stein H, Warnke RA, Chan WC, et al: Diffuse large B-cell lymphoma, not otherwise specified. In Swerdlow SH, Campo E, Harris NL, et al (eds): World Health Organization: Classification of Tumours: Pathology and Genetics of Tumours of Haematopoietic and Lymphoid Tissues. Lyon, IARC, 2008, pp 233-237.

Alizadeh AA, Eisen MB, Davis RE, et al: Distinct types of diffuse large B-cell lymphoma identified by gene expression profiling. Nature 403:503-511, 2000.

Precursor B-Cell and T-Cell Lymphoblastic Lymphoma and Leukemia

Clinical Features

- Peak incidence in childhood through young adulthood (<30 years old)

Figure 14-25. Precursor B-lymphoblastic lymphoma. A, Diffuse cellular infiltrate with starry-sky pattern. **B,** High magnification shows sheets of uniform cells with convoluted nuclei, inconspicuous nucleoli, and scant cytoplasm. Mitoses are numerous.

- Most patients have bone marrow involvement and often have peripheral blood involvement (leukemia)
- Skin lesions are commonly present in patients with precursor B-cell lymphoblastic lymphoma
- Mediastinal mass is commonly present in patients with precursor T-cell lymphoblastic lymphoma

Gross Pathology

- Soft, fleshy (fish-flesh) masses

Histopathology

- Diffuse infiltrate
- Uniform, medium-sized to large cells with round to convoluted nuclei; blastic, finely dispersed chromatin; and inconspicuous nucleoli
- High nuclear-to-cytoplasmic ratio; cytoplasm is scant and typically appears blue on Wright stain
- Numerous tingible body macrophages creating a starry-sky pattern

Special Stains and Immunohistochemistry

- Immunophenotyping is essential; precursor B-cell and precursor T-cell types are morphologically indistinguishable
- Precursor B cells positive for CD10, CD19, PAX5, TdT, and CD34; may express CD22; CD20 negative to only weakly positive; sIg negative
- Precursor T cells: variable expression of pan T-cell antigens (CD2, CD3, CD5, and CD7), may coexpress CD4 and CD8 or lack one or both, are TdT positive and CD34 negative, and express CD10 in a minority of cases (25%)

Other Techniques for Diagnosis

- Immunoglobulin gene rearrangement (precursor B cells)
- T-cell receptor gene rearrangement (precursor T cells)
- Flow cytometric phenotyping

Differential Diagnosis

▌ Myeloid sarcoma (chloroma)
- More common in older adults
- Cytoplasm is paler on Wright stain
- Wright or Giemsa stain of touch preps may show granules or diagnostic Auer rods
- Specific and nonspecific esterases may be positive on touch preps
- Myeloperoxidase is positive on touch preps by histochemistry or on tissue sections by immunohistochemistry
- Myeloid, but not lymphocyte-specific markers, present on flow cytometry
- May be positive for one or more T-cell–associated antigens, most often CD4 or CD7
- CD43 and CD45 may be positive

- Burkitt lymphoma
  - More often presents as an abdominal mass
  - Monotonous cells with round to oval nuclei, multiple nucleoli, and dark blue, vacuolated cytoplasm
  - B-cell phenotype (positive for CD10, CD19, CD20, and bcl-6) with expression of sIg; negative for CD34 and TdT
  - Characteristic t(8;14)(q24;q32) chromosomal abnormality
  - FISH shows *c-myc* translocation
- DLBCL
  - Cells are larger and have nuclei with vesicular chromatin (not blastic) and more prominent nucleoli
  - Nuclear-to-cytoplasmic ratio tends to be lower
  - Mature B-cell phenotype; cells do not express CD34 or TdT
- Neuroblastoma
  - Predominantly in younger children
  - Cells are smaller and more uniform; may be spindled but typically show nuclear molding; may have ganglionic differentiation or Homer-Wright pseudorosettes
  - Positive for chromogranin, synaptophysin, and neuron-specific enolase (NSE)
  - Negative for CD45, CD10, CD19, CD22, and TdT
- Metastatic alveolar rhabdomyosarcoma
  - Mediastinal mass is unlikely; typically presents as a soft tissue mass
  - Alveolar architecture; cells are spindled to blunt-ended rather than round
  - Necrosis rather than apoptosis typically seen
  - Positive for muscle-specific actin (MSA), desmin, and myoD1, myogenin, or both
  - Negative for CD45, CD10, CD19, CD22, and TdT
- Metastatic Ewing sarcoma
  - Patients typically present with skeletal or soft tissue disease; mediastinal mass is uncommon
  - Both lymphoblastic neoplasms and tumors of the Ewing and peripheral neuroectodermal tumor (PNET) family express CD99 and Fli-1
  - Tumor cells are negative for lymphoid antigens (CD45, CD3, CD4, CD8, CD19, and CD20)
  - PAS highlights cytoplasmic glycogen
  - Characteristic t(11;22); *EWS* gene translocation may be detected by FISH

Pearls

- Starry-sky pattern is not diagnostic of Burkitt lymphoma
- Lymphoblastic lymphoma and lymphoblastic leukemia are part of a disease spectrum rather than distinct diseases; the morphology and phenotype overlap
- Current treatment regimens are intense and prolonged, but the outcome is good

Selected References

Borowitz M, Chan JKC: B lymphoblastic leukaemia/lymphoma, not otherwise specified. In Swerdlow SH, Campo E, Harris NL, et al (eds): World Health Classification: Classification of Tumours of Haematopoietic and Lymphoid Tissues. Lyon, IARC, 2008, pp 168-170.

Soslow RA, Baergen RN, Warnke RA: B-lineage lymphoblastic lymphoma is a clinicopathologic entity distinct from other histologically similar aggressive lymphomas with blastic morphology. Cancer 85:2648-2654, 1999.

Yeh KH, Cheng AL, Su IJ, et al: Prognostic significance of immunophenotypes in adult lymphoblastic lymphomas. Anticancer Res 17:2269-2272, 1997.

Anaplastic Large Cell Lymphoma, Systemic

Clinical Features

- Uncommon (3% of non-Hodgkin lymphomas in adults)
- Bimodal age distribution: large peak in children and young adults; small peak in older adults
- Presentation: lymphadenopathy or extranodal masses and B symptoms; secondary skin, bone, soft tissue, lung, and liver involvement not uncommon
- Aggressive disease with prognosis closely related to ALK-1 expression

Gross Pathology

- Fleshy, creamy to tan enlarged lymph nodes
- Violaceous skin nodules

Histopathology

- Preferential infiltration of lymph node sinuses by tumor cells that extend into paracortex, often sparing lymphoid follicles
- Tumor cells in sinuses may appear cohesive, mimicking metastatic carcinoma
- Common type (70% of cases): monomorphic to pleomorphic large lymphocytes with prominent nucleoli and abundant eosinophilic cytoplasm; frequent multinucleate large cells with horseshoe- or doughnut-shaped nuclei (hallmark cells) that sometimes resemble Reed-Sternberg cells of classical Hodgkin lymphoma
- Lymphohistiocytic variant (10% of cases): numerous irregular small lymphocytes admixed with frequent histiocytes and few hallmark cells
- Small cell variant (10% of cases): numerous irregular small lymphocytes with only occasional perivascular hallmark cells
- Other variants (10% of cases): Hodgkin-like, giant cell, sarcomatous, and neutrophil-rich are uncommon

Special Stains and Immunohistochemistry

- Tumor cells are always CD30 positive and typically have cytoplasmic membrane and paranuclear (Golgi zone) staining pattern

Figure 14-26. Anaplastic large cell lymphoma. A, Tumor cells are large and pleomorphic with abundant cytoplasm. There is a hallmark cell in the center of the field. The tumor cells are several times the size of the intermixed small lymphocytes. **B,** Most tumor cells are CD30 positive and show the characteristic cytoplasmic membrane and Golgi zone staining pattern.

- T-cell phenotype (80% to 90% of cases): generally incomplete with loss of multiple T-cell antigens
- Null cell phenotype (10% to 20% of cases): do not express lymphocyte lineage–associated antigens but generally have clonal T-cell receptor (*TCR*) gene rearrangements
- Most cases CD45 positive, but 20% to 40% negative to only focally weakly positive
- EMA frequently positive (60% of cases)
- PAX5, a B-cell transcription factor, is always negative
- ALK-1 positive in most cases (70% to 80%); CD15 occasionally positive (15% to 25%)

Other Techniques for Diagnosis

- Clonal *TCR* gene rearrangements in 90% of cases
- Classic t(2;5)(p23;q35) chromosomal abnormality fuses *ALK* and nucleophosmin (*NPM*) genes, resulting

in a unique NPM-ALK fusion protein (60% of cases); variant *ALK* translocations in 10% to 20% of cases
- No *ALK* translocations in 20% to 30% of cases
- Translocations may be detected by classic cytogenetics or FISH
- Abnormal ALK fusion proteins detectable by immunohistochemistry
- ALK-2 positive in most cases (70% to 80%): mostly diffuse cytoplasmic and nuclear staining pattern corresponding to classic *ALK/NPM* translocation; subset of cases with only cytoplasmic staining have variant *ALK* translocations
- ALK positive ALCL: 80% 5-year overall survival rate
- ALK negative ALCL: 40% 5-year overall survival rate

Differential Diagnosis

▮ Hodgkin lymphoma, classical type
  - Reed-Sternberg cells are typically not abundant and are scattered in a polymorphic reactive cell background consisting of small lymphocytes, plasma cells, eosinophils, and histiocytes
  - Reed-Sternberg cells express CD30, PAX5, and usually CD15; negative for CD45, EMA, and ALK-1
▮ DLBCL
  - Tumor cells may have pleomorphic cytologic features and express CD30 in a few cases
  - One or more B-cell antigens are expressed, including PAX5
▮ Peripheral T-cell lymphoma, unspecified
  - Tumor cells may have pleomorphic cytologic features and express CD30 in a few cases
  - Unlike ALCL, there is not uniform strong staining of nearly all tumor cells for CD30, and T-cell antigen expression is more complete
▮ Histiocytic sarcoma
  - Pleomorphic large cells fill lymph node sinuses
  - Tumor cells are generally CD30 negative and express antigens characteristic of histiocytes (CD68, CD163, and lysozyme)
▮ Metastatic carcinoma or melanoma
  - Large cells fill sinuses and often appear cohesive
  - Look for gland formation, keratinization, or other "epithelial" structures for carcinomas; melanin pigment for melanomas
  - Cytokeratin positive for carcinomas; S-100, HMB-45, or melan-A positive for melanomas

Pearls

- CD30 expression is not exclusive to ALCL
- CD30 is an activation antigen and is expressed in a variable number of immunoblasts in reactive lymph nodes, such as in EBV infection (infectious mononucleosis)
- CD30 expression is present on tumor cells of most classical Hodgkin lymphomas and in some DLBCLs; these tumors are PAX5 positive, whereas ALCL is not

- CD30 expression is characteristic of large lymphocytes in primary cutaneous CD30 positive lymphoproliferative disorders (e.g., lymphomatoid papulosis and primary cutaneous ALCL), which have far less aggressive behavior than systemic ALCL and are classified separately
- Some carcinomas (e.g., embryonal and pancreatic) are CD30 positive
- Do not make a diagnosis of metastatic carcinoma based on EMA positive and CD45-negative phenotype because up to 40% of systemic ALCLs have this phenotype; cytokeratin staining is needed for confirmation

Selected References

Amin HM, Lai R: Pathobiology of ALK+ anaplastic large-cell lymphoma. Blood 110:2259-2267, 2007.

Kinney MC, Kadin ME: The pathologic and clinical spectrum of anaplastic large cell lymphoma and correlation with ALK gene dysregulation. Am J Clin Pathol 111:S56-S67, 1999.

Benharroch D, Meguerian-Bodoyan Z, Lamant L, et al: ALK-positive lymphoma: A single disease with a broad spectrum of morphology. Blood 91:2076-2084, 1998.

Burkitt Lymphoma

Clinical Features

- Sporadic type
  - Primarily seen in children or patients with AIDS; does occur rarely in HIV-negative adults
  - Male predominance
  - Rapidly progressive disease; patients often have extranodal disease
  - Gastrointestinal involvement is common

Gross Pathology

- Fleshy, creamy lymph nodes

Histopathology

- Nodal architecture is effaced with a diffuse or nodular infiltrate
- Tumor cells are medium sized and uniform, with scant cytoplasm, clumpy chromatin, and multiple small nucleoli; numerous mitotic figures
- Many apoptotic bodies and tingible body macrophages with phagocytosed nuclear debris create a starry-sky pattern
- Wright-stained touch preps show cells with scant basophilic cytoplasm and clear vacuoles in the cytoplasm and overlying the nucleus

Special Stains and Immunohistochemistry

- B-cell phenotype (positive for CD10, CD19, CD20, PAX5, and bcl-6); expresses sIg
- Negative for TdT and CD34, bcl-2, CD5, CD21, and CD23
- Ki-67 positive in almost 100% of cells

Figure 14-27. Burkitt lymphoma. A, Diffuse cellular infiltrate with starry-sky pattern. **B,** Higher-power magnification showing uniform round cells with clumpy chromatin, small nucleoli, and numerous mitotic figures. Scattered cells with nuclear debris create the starry-sky pattern.

Other Techniques for Diagnosis

- Cytogenetics often detects a translocation involving the *c-myc* gene on chromosome 8; characteristic t(8;14)(q24;q32)
- FISH for *c-myc* gene rearrangement; PCR for immunoglobulin gene rearrangement
- In situ hybridization for EBV

Differential Diagnosis

▌ DLBCL
- More common in older adults
- Cells are larger and more pleomorphic and have paler cytoplasm, vesicular nuclei, and fewer nucleoli
- Mitoses are usually fewer; lacks starry-sky pattern
- Usually CD10 negative
- Rearrangement of *c-myc* gene, when present, is usually one of many cytogenetic abnormalities
- Additional immunohistochemistry or gene expression studies may aid in differentiation

▌ Lymphoblastic lymphoma
- Peak incidence in adolescents and young adults
- Precursor B cells and precursor T cells have inconspicuous to absent nucleoli

- Positive for TdT; precursor B cells also express CD34
- No *c-myc* gene rearrangement
◗ Acute leukemia in lymph node
- Presentation with bulky nodal or soft tissue mass extremely uncommon
- Typically found in patients with end-stage disease
- Precursor B cells or precursor T cells with features similar to corresponding lymphoblastic lymphoma
- Acute myeloid leukemia: positive for myeloperoxidase; negative for CD19 and CD20; phenotype depends on subtype
◗ Small cell carcinoma
- Typically occurs in older adults
- Bulky nodal disease is rare
- Tumor cells are small to medium-sized and have high nuclear-to-cytoplasmic ratio and prominent nuclear molding
- Zonal necrosis in larger biopsies, crush artifact typical of small biopsies
- Positive for cytokeratin (especially 8 and 18), negative for CD19, CD20, and CD45
◗ Alveolar rhabdomyosarcoma
- Typically presents as a soft tissue mass without nodal involvement
- Tumor usually has an alveolar architecture; starry-sky pattern is rare
- Positive for MSA, myogenin, myoD1; negative for CD10, CD19, and CD20
- Immunoglobulin gene rearrangement absent
- Electron microscopy may be helpful
- FISH study shows *FKHR* gene rearrangement but not *c-myc* translocation
◗ Ewing sarcoma and PNET
- Usually affects older children through younger adults
- Patients typically present with skeletal or soft tissue mass
- Cells typically have more abundant cytoplasm
- Positive for CD99 and Fli-1; negative for CD19 and CD20
- PAS stain highlights cytoplasmic glycogen
- Characteristic t(11;22); *c-myc* gene not rearranged
- FISH may detect *EWS-1* gene translocation
◗ Neuroblastoma
- Most frequent in infants and preschool-aged children
- Patients usually have primary disease in the adrenal gland or paraganglia
- Calcification often present on radiography
- Tumor cells are smaller and more uniform; may be spindled and typically show nuclear molding, often have Homer-Wright pseudorosettes
- Positive for chromogranin, synaptophysin, and NSE; negative for CD19, CD20, and CD22

Pearls

- Burkitt lymphoma is the most rapidly proliferating human tumor

- Review diagnosis carefully if Ki-67 on well-preserved tissue is obviously below 100%
- Endemic Burkitt lymphoma in Africa and other tropical areas is consistently associated with EBV and malaria and often presents in the jaw, orbit, or ovary
- Nonendemic (sporadic) Burkitt lymphoma is not associated with malaria and only sporadically with EBV; intestinal presentation is more common
- Both endemic and sporadic types have translocation involving *c-myc* gene on chromosome 8 and an immunoglobulin gene (heavy or light chain)
- Endemic and sporadic types have slightly different break points for the translocation
- Endemic type has somewhat better response to therapy

Selected References

Harris NL, Horning SJ: Burkitt's lymphoma: The message from microarrays. N Engl J Med 354:2495-2498, 2006.

Hummel M, Bentink S, Berger H, et al: A biologic definition of Burkitt's lymphoma from transcriptional and genomic profiling. N Engl J Med 354:2419-2430, 2006.

McClure RF, Remstein ED, Macon WR, et al: Adult B-cell lymphomas with Burkitt-like morphology are phenotypically and genotypically heterogeneous with aggressive clinical behaviour. Am J Surg Pathol 29:1652-1660, 2005.

Peripheral T-Cell Lymphoma, Unspecified

Clinical Features

- Uncommon, but represent nearly half of T-cell lymphomas
- Most patients are older than 50 years
- Presentation: generalized lymphadenopathy and B symptoms
- Aggressive disease with poor prognosis (25% overall survival rate)

Figure 14-28. Peripheral T-cell lymphoma, unspecified. The proportions of large and small lymphocytes can vary in this entity. There are scattered eosinophils and plasma cells. Fine sclerosis separating clusters of tumor cells (compartmentalizing sclerosis) is characteristic.

Gross Pathology

- Diffusely enlarged, fleshy, white-tan lymph nodes

Histopathology

- Partial to complete effacement of nodal architecture by diffuse lymphoid infiltrate
- Tumor cells vary in size (small, intermediate, and large) in same case and have mildly atypical to pleomorphic cytologic features; large cells have irregular to hyperlobate nuclei, vesicular chromatin pattern, prominent nucleoli, and pale eosinophilic or clear cytoplasm and may resemble Reed-Sternberg cells
- Polymorphic reactive cell background resembling that in classical Hodgkin lymphoma often present; epithelioid histiocytes may form prominent clusters
- Fine compartmentalizing sclerosis may be present, separating small groups of tumor cells
- High endothelial venules are discernible but not exceedingly prominent
- T-zone lymphoma variant: atypical small lymphocytes with clear cytoplasm have interfollicular growth pattern sparing or infiltrating residual hyperplastic secondary lymphoid follicles
- Lymphoepithelioid cell (Lennert) lymphoma variant: atypical small lymphocytes infiltrate between numerous evenly dispersed clusters of epithelioid histiocytes

Special Stains and Immunohistochemistry

- T-cell antigen expression often aberrant; loss of surface CD3 and CD7 most commonly observed
- More CD4 positive cases than CD8 positive cases

Other Techniques for Diagnosis

- Clonal *TCR* gene rearrangements detectable in most cases
- Translocation t(5;9)(q33;q22) chromosomal abnormality that fuses *ITK* and *SYK* in rare cases in which CD4-, CD10-, and bcl-6-positive tumor cells are preferentially localized in lymphoid follicles

Differential Diagnosis

▮ Paracortical lymphoid hyperplasia (PLH)
- Nodal architecture preserved with secondary lymphoid follicles
- Paracortex expanded by small lymphocytes with no significant cytologic atypia accompanied by scattered immunoblasts and other reactive cells in nonspecific PLH
- Immunoblasts may be a much more frequent constituent of paracortex in virus-associated lymphadenopathies, which are more common in children and adolescents, who often have an acute febrile illness
- No aberrant T-cell antigen expression

▮ Anaplastic large cell lymphoma
- Pleomorphic large cells preferentially infiltrate lymph node sinuses
- Uniform strong CD30 staining of nearly all tumor cells; T-cell antigen expression is incomplete
▮ Angioimmunoblastic T-cell lymphoma
- Pronounced hypervascularity with branching high endothelial venules
- Perivascular clusters of clear cell immunoblasts; small lymphocytes generally not cytologically atypical
- Amorphous eosinophilic intercellular material on H&E-stained slides that corresponds to disrupted and proliferated follicular dendritic cell (FDC) networks
- Clear cell immunoblasts are CD4, CD10, CD279, and CXCL13 positive
- FDC networks are CD21, CD23, CD35, and clusterin positive
▮ Hodgkin lymphoma, classical type
- Lymphocytes are dichotomous: large Reed-Sternberg cells and small reactive lymphocytes with no significant cytologic atypia
- RS cells are CD45 negative and PAX5 positive and do not express T-cell antigens
▮ DLBCL
- Neoplastic large cells usually have little cytologic variability and are not often pleomorphic; cytoplasm is amphophilic to basophilic rather than clear
- Small lymphocytes generally are not cytologically atypical
- Reactive cell background is not as polymorphic
- Large tumor cells express B cell antigens

Pearls

- This category is a "wastebasket" for T-cell lymphomas that are not yet well defined as distinct entities
- Prognosis is similar to that for ALK-negative ALCL, and some recommend reclassifying the latter as PTCL, unspecified
- Prognosis is worse than for DLBCL and is not related to extent of large cell component
- Prognosis is worse than for Hodgkin lymphoma, classical type, and peripheral T-cell lymphoma; requires more intensive chemotherapy, necessitating correct distinction

Selected References

Attygalle AD, Chuang S-S, Diss TC, et al: Distinguishing angioimmunoblastic T-cell lymphoma from peripheral T-cell lymphoma, unspecified, using morphology, immunophenotype and molecular genetics. Histopathology 50:498-508, 2007.

Streubel B, Vinatzer U, Willheim M, et al: Novel t(5;9) (q33;q22) fuses ITK to SYK in unspecified peripheral T-cell lymphoma. Leukemia 20:313-318, 2006.

ten Berge RL, de Bruin PC, Oudejans JJ, et al: ALK-negative anaplastic large-cell lymphoma demonstrates similar poor prognosis to peripheral T-cell lymphoma, unspecified. Histopathology 43:462-469, 2003.

Chan JK: Peripheral T-cell and NK-cell neoplasms: an integrated approach to diagnosis. Mod Pathol 12:177-199, 1999.

Angioimmunoblastic T-Cell Lymphoma

Clinical Features

- Uncommon (1% to 2% of all non-Hodgkin lymphomas, but 15% to 20% of T-cell lymphomas)
- Most patients are middle-aged to elderly
- Presentation: generalized lymphadenopathy, hepatosplenomegaly, skin rash, polyclonal hypergammaglobulinemia, autoimmune hemolytic anemia, and B symptoms
- Aggressive disease with 1- to 2-year median survival

Figure 14-29. Angioimmunoblastic T-cell lymphoma. A, Cellular composition of these tumors can vary. **B,** There is a cluster of plasma cells in the center of the field, surrounded by lymphocytes of varying size with abundant clear cytoplasm.

Gross Pathology

- Enlarged fleshy, white-tan lymph nodes

Histopathology

- Partial to complete effacement of nodal architecture by diffuse lymphoid infiltrate that often extends beyond the capsule into perinodal soft tissue; regressively transformed ("burnt-out" or "atretic") germinal centers may be seen
- Neoplastic large cells with round to oval nuclei, vesicular chromatin, prominent nucleoli, and abundant clear cytoplasm (clear cell immunoblasts) form small perivascular clusters; small lymphocytes generally not cytologically atypical
- Polymorphic reactive cell background resembling that in Hodgkin lymphoma often present; epithelioid histiocytes may form prominent clusters
- Pronounced hypervascularity with branching ("arborizing") high endothelial venules
- Amorphous intercellular eosinophilic material

Special Stains and Immunohistochemistry

- Clear cell immunoblasts are CD4, CD10, CD279, and CXCL13 positive and often have loss of some T-cell antigens
- Reactive small lymphocytes are mostly CD4- or CD8-positive T cells; small CD20-positive B cells are mainly peripheralized to outer cortex; scattered CD20-positive B-cell immunoblasts, often CD30 positive, are intermixed among the reactive and neoplastic T cells
- Plasma cells, often numerous, have polytypic κ and λ immunoglobulin light-chain expression
- Disrupted and proliferated follicular dendritic cell (FDC) networks, corresponding to the amorphous intercellular eosinophilic material, are CD21, CD23, CD35, and clusterin positive

Other Techniques for Diagnosis

- In situ hybridization for EBV-encoded RNA shows EBV-positive immunoblasts in a similar number and distribution as the B-cell immunoblasts
- Clonal *TCR* gene rearrangements in 75% of cases
- Clonal immunoglobulin gene rearrangements detectable in a small number of cases
- No recurring chromosomal translocations, but trisomies 3 and 5, an additional X chromosome, and 1p alterations common

Differential Diagnosis

▌ PLH
- See "Differential Diagnosis" under "Peripheral T-Cell Lymphoma, Unspecified"

▌ Hodgkin lymphoma, classical type
- Reed-Sternberg cells are present in varying numbers, but multinucleate large cells resembling Reed-Sternberg cells are not seen in angioimmunoblastic T-cell lymphoma (AITL)

- Less vascular than AITL
- Reed-Sternberg cells are CD30 and PAX5 positive and lack staining for T-cell antigens, CD10, CD45, and CXCL13

■ DLBCL
- Most cases not difficult to distinguish from AITL because of sheetlike proliferation of neoplastic large cells, rather than focal perivascular clusters of clear cell immunoblasts
- TCRLBCL variant of DLBCL may be difficult to distinguish from AITL because a pattern of singly distributed, neoplastic, large CD20-positive B cells among numerous reactive small T cells in TCRLBCL resembles the pattern of B-cell immunoblasts among numerous reactive small T cells in AITL
- TCRLBCL generally has fewer eosinophils and no disrupted or proliferated FDC networks compared with AITL
- Neoplastic large cells in TCRLBCL have κ or λ immunoglobulin light-chain restriction, whereas B-cell immunoblasts in AITL are generally polytypic

Pearls

- Cases described in the 1970s as angioimmunoblastic lymphadenopathy with dysproteinemia (AILD) and immunoblastic lymphadenopathy (IBL) are now regarded as AITL; AILD and IBL are no longer diagnosed
- The neoplastic clear cell immunoblasts are a minor cellular constituent in AITL (5% to 30% of cells), and the clonally rearranged *TCR* genes are confined to these cells
- The detection of a CD10-positive lymphocyte population that is CD19 and CD20 negative by flow cytometry may be a diagnostic clue for AITL
- The expression of CD4, CD10, CD279, and CXCL13 by the clear cell immunoblasts and their association with disrupted or proliferated FDC networks suggest that these neoplastic T cells are derived from follicular T-helper cells
- EBV-positive DLBCLs can arise in patients with AITL, presumably from a subset of the cases with clonal immunoglobulin gene rearrangements

Selected References

Willenbrock K, Bräuninger A, Hansmann M-L: Frequent occurrence of B-cell lymphomas in angioimmunoblastic T-cell lymphoma and proliferation of Epstein-Barr virus-infected cells in early cases. Br J Haematol 138:733-739, 2007.

Grogg KL, Attygalle AD, Macon WR, et al: Expression of CXCL13, a chemokine highly upregulated in germinal center T-helper cells, distinguishes angioimmunoblastic T-cell lymphoma from peripheral T-cell lymphoma, unspecified. Mod Pathol 19:1101-1107, 2006.

Dogan A, Attygalle AD, Kyriakou C: Angioimmunoblastic T-cell lymphoma. Br J Haematol 121:681-691, 2003.

Attygalle A, Al-Jehani R, Diss TC, et al: Neoplastic T-cells in angioimmunoblastic T-cell lymphoma express CD10. Blood 99:627-633, 2002.

Hodgkin Lymphoma, Mixed Cellularity

Clinical Features

- Second most common subtype of Hodgkin lymphoma; represents about 25% of cases
- Occurs at all ages; relatively more common in patients older than 40 years
- Mediastinal mass at presentation is uncommon

Gross Pathology

- Nonspecific; white to pale-tan lymph nodes without gross nodularity

Histopathology

- Nodal architecture is diffusely effaced and lacks nodularity
- Mixture of cell types: classic Reed-Sternberg cells and mononuclear Hodgkin cells are readily found, in a polymorphic reactive cell background of lymphocytes, plasma cells, eosinophils, and macrophages
- Lymph node capsule is not usually thickened
- Sclerosis, when present, is fine and uniform
- Lacunar cells are not present

Special Stains and Immunohistochemistry

- Neoplastic cells are highly altered B lymphocytes, usually negative for CD45, T-cell antigens (CD3, CD5), and EMA
- Positive for CD15 and CD30; typically with a cytoplasmic membrane and perinuclear (Golgi) staining pattern; positive for PAX5 and fascin
- CD20 may be expressed but is usually faint and on only a few of the tumor cells

Figure 14-30. Mixed-cellularity Hodgkin lymphoma. Pleomorphic infiltrate of lymphocytes, eosinophils, and plasma cells. *Inset,* Higher magnification, Reed-Sternberg cell.

Other Techniques for Diagnosis
- Generally noncontributory

Differential Diagnosis
- Hodgkin lymphoma, nodular sclerosis type
  - Patients are more likely to have a mediastinal mass
  - May have bandlike sclerosis or thickening of the nodal capsule
  - Lacunar cells present
- TCRLBCL
  - Large lymphocytes are typically centroblasts
  - Small lymphocytes are almost all CD3-positive T cells
  - Large cells are CD20-positive B cells (may also be CD30 positive)
  - Eosinophils and plasma cells are typically sparse
  - Aggressive clinical course
- Angioimmunoblastic T-cell lymphoma
  - Prominent vascularity contrasts with Hodgkin lymphoma, which tends to be hypovascular
  - Lymphoid cells are more pleomorphic than in Hodgkin lymphoma
  - Both small and large cells are T lymphocytes, negative for CD15
  - Tumor cells do not express PAX5
- Anaplastic large cell lymphoma
  - Common in children
  - When the lymph node is partially involved, it is commonly in a sinus pattern, mimicking metastatic carcinoma or melanoma
  - Multinucleated cells are present and may have a wreathlike arrangement of nuclei
  - Tumor cells with indented (horseshoe or embryoid) nuclei are characteristic
  - Tumor cells form large sheets with intermixed small lymphocytes rather than the pattern of scattered tumor cells among reactive cells typical of Hodgkin lymphoma
  - Eosinophils are rarely numerous
  - Neoplastic cells are positive for CD30 but also express T-cell antigens (CD3, CD5, CD43, and CD45RO) and often EMA and ALK-1; may express fascin
  - Neoplastic cells do not express PAX5 or other B-cell antigens
  - *TCR* gene rearrangement positive
- Viral lymphadenopathy
  - More common in children and adolescents
  - Patients usually have acute onset of a febrile illness with systemic symptoms
  - Nodal architecture usually distorted but not effaced
  - Paracortex may be expanded, but follicles are usually uniformly spaced
  - Reed-Sternberg–like cells and atypical immunoblasts may be present, especially with EBV infection, but are not associated with a polymorphic reactive cell background
  - Viral titers may be helpful

- Metastatic carcinoma or melanoma
  - When only a few tumor cells are present, nodal architecture is usually preserved
  - Focal infiltration is most likely to be in the subcapsular sinuses
  - With extensive replacement of the node, tumor cells form sheets with few lymphocytes or other cells
  - Eosinophils are rarely numerous
  - Carcinomas are positive for cytokeratin (but may express CD15 and CD30)
  - Melanoma is negative for CD15 but expresses S-100 protein, HMB-45, and melan-A

Pearls
- Adenocarcinomas may express CD15
- Metastatic carcinoma and melanoma can contain a few CD30-positive cells
- CD30 is a lymphoid activation antigen and may be seen in cells in normal and reactive lymph nodes

Selected References
Brauninger A, Schmitz R, Bechtel D, et al: Molecular biology of Hodgkin's and Reed/Sternberg cells in Hodgkin's lymphoma. Int J Cancer 118:1853-1861, 2006.

Tzankov A, Dirnhofer S: Pathobiology of classical Hodgkin lymphoma. Pathobiology 73:107-125, 2006.

Weiss LM, von Wasielewski R, Delsol G, et al: Mixed cellularity classical Hodgkin lymphoma. In Swerdlow SH, Campo E, Harris NL, et al (eds): World Health Organization: Classification of Tumours: Pathology and Genetics of Tumours of Haematopoietic and Lymphoid Tissues. Lyon, IARC, 2008, p 331.

Myeloid Sarcoma

Clinical Features
- Occurs at any age
- More common in skin, soft tissue, viscera, or gingiva than in lymph node
- This may precede the onset of clinically evident acute myeloid leukemia, appear at the same time as the development of clinically evident leukemia, or be a manifestation of relapse or progressive disease in a patient with known acute myeloid leukemia
- Almost all patients have acute myeloid leukemia or develop the leukemia within 3 years
- Most frequent in patients with acute monocytic or monoblastic leukemia, or acute leukemia associated with t(8;21)(q22;q22) chromosomal abnormality
- Usually localized

Gross Pathology
- Soft fleshy mass; the fresh cut surface may have a greenish color before exposure to air (chloroma)

Histopathology
- Diffuse effacement of nodal architecture by blastic cells

Figure 14-31. Myeloid sarcoma in lymph node. A, Interfollicular infiltrate surrounds germinal centers and mantle zones. At this magnification, this is indistinguishable from a diffuse lymphoma. **B,** Touch prep stained with Wright or Diff-Quik may show immature myeloid cells and blasts.

- Varied mitotic rate; necrosis and apoptotic bodies common
- Scant to moderate cytoplasm, may be finely granular
- Nuclei have fine blastic chromatin, may be lobated; nucleoli typically present to prominent

Special Stains and Immunohistochemistry

- Wright stain on touch prep may reveal the presence of myeloid granules or pathognomonic Auer rods
- Histochemical stains on touch preps may be useful; myeloperoxidase, Sudan black, chloracetate (specific) esterase, or nonspecific esterase may be positive
- Chloracetate esterase stain works in formalin-fixed tissue
- Cells typically express myeloperoxidase, CD34, CD45, CD117, and CD33
- Cells may express CD4 and CD7 but not CD3
- CD13 and CD33 detected by flow cytometry

Other Techniques for Diagnosis

- Flow cytometry for myeloid antigens
- Cytogenetics

Differential Diagnosis

▌ DLBCL
- Much more common
- Patients are likely to have widespread lymphadenopathy or organomegaly
- Cells lack myeloid granules or Auer rods
- Cells do not express myeloperoxidase, specific esterase, CD34, or other myeloid antigens on flow
- Cells express CD20, PAX5, and other B-cell antigens

▌ Lymphoblastic lymphoma (pre-B or pre-T)
- Most common in children, adolescents, and young adults
- Patients usually have widespread disease
- Bone marrow involvement is common in this disease, as it is in myeloid sarcoma
- Tumor cells do not have myeloid granules or Auer rods
- Cells may express CD34; CD10 typically positive
- Typically positive for TdT and early B-cell antigens (CD19) or T-cell antigens (CD3), but not myeloid antigens

▌ Metastatic carcinoma
- Typically in older adults
- Cells form cohesive epithelial sheets, glands, or cords
- Touch prep morphology is often useful
- Express keratins and EMA; negative for CD45, myeloperoxidase, and specific esterase
- Cells are cohesive; flow cytometry usually not informative

Pearls

- Almost all patients with myeloid sarcoma have acute myeloid leukemia when they present with the sarcoma, or develop it within 1 to 3 years; exceptions are rare
- Touch prep cytology can be extremely useful in diagnosing this process
- Think of myeloid sarcoma when a tumor that looks like a large cell or other aggressive lymphoma does not have the expected lymphoid phenotype
- Get tissue for karyotyping when possible; it can support the diagnosis and correlates with the prognosis

Selected References

Paydas S, Zorludemir S, Ergin M: Granulocytic sarcoma: 32 Cases and review of the literature. Leuk Lymphoma 47:2527-2541, 2006.

Kojima M, Nakamura S, Shimizu K, et al: Granulocytic sarcoma presenting with lymph node infarction at disease onset. APMIS 111:1133-1136, 2003.

Attilio Orazi and Magdalena Czader

15

Spleen

Non-neoplastic Diseases Involving the Splenic White Pulp

Reactive Follicular Hyperplasia

Clinical Features

- Occurs at any age; more common in children and younger adults
- Caused by a variety of both acute and chronic immunologic stimuli (e.g., bacterial infections, autoimmune diseases including hemolytic processes)
- May represent an incidental finding

Gross Pathology

- May present with splenomegaly
- Prominent white pulp nodularity may be grossly visible

Histopathology

- Tripartite germinal centers with well-defined marginal and mantle zones
- Marginal zones may be expanded in chronic cases
- Polarized (dark and light zones) germinal centers with abundant mitoses and tingible body macrophages
- Increased number of plasma cells and small plasma cell aggregates in red pulp

Special Stains and Immunohistochemistry

- Immunohistochemistry can be useful in differential diagnosis from lymphomatous infiltration
- Germinal centers are positive for CD20, CD10, bcl-6, and bcl-2

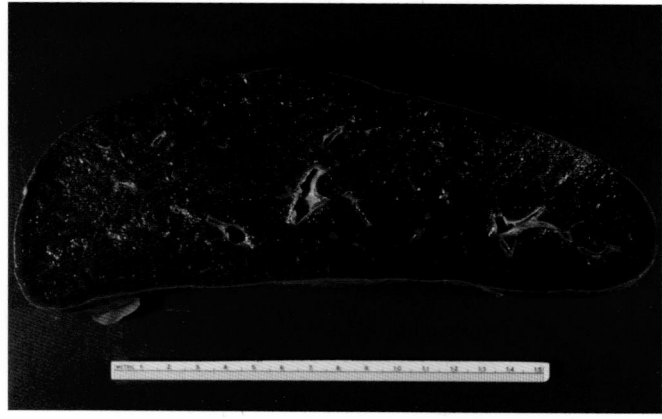

Figure 15-1. Follicular white pulp hyperplasia, gross photograph. The spleen is enlarged. Small indistinct pale foci of hyperplastic white pulp are seen on the cut surface and under the capsule.

- Mantle cells are positive for CD20, CD5, and bcl-2 and negative for CD43 and cyclin D1

Other Techniques for Diagnosis

- Evaluation of light-chain expression by flow cytometry may be complicated by high nonspecific binding; nevertheless, polyclonal pattern is always seen supporting the diagnosis of reactive hyperplasia

Differential Diagnosis

∎ Follicular, mantle cell, and marginal zone lymphomas
   - Neoplastic follicles may vary in size, are less sharply defined, and may coalesce

Figure 15-2. Primary (nonfollicular) white pulp hyperplasia. Heterogeneous lymphoid population including immunoblasts with open chromatin pattern.

Figure 15-3. Marginal zone hyperplasia.

- Reactive follicles have well-defined marginal and mantle zones with polarized germinal centers, tingible body macrophages, and mitotic figures
- Neoplastic lymphoid infiltrates may be abnormally located and present in red pulp as well as in white pulp
- Immunophenotypic features are dependent on the lymphoma subtype

Pearls

- Causes and histologic features similar to those of nodal reactive follicular hyperplasia
- Well-developed germinal centers are considered a normal finding in children and young adults
- Uncommon in elderly individuals; differential diagnosis includes follicular lymphoma
- Localized (nodular) reactive lymphoid hyperplasia may grossly simulate lymphoma; histologically, it

presents as an aggregation of hyperplastic follicles with typical reactive features
- Prominent marginal zone expansion seen in chronic antigenic simulation may resemble marginal zone lymphoma
- Common in patients with systemic lupus erythematosus and rheumatoid arthritis (Felty syndrome: rheumatoid arthritis, splenomegaly with follicular hyperplasia, plasmacytosis, and red pulp expansion including proliferation of CD3-, CD8-, and CD57-positive cytotoxic T cells, neutropenia, and leg ulcers)

Selected References

Burks EJ, Loughran TP Jr: Pathogenesis of neutropenia in large granular lymphocyte leukemia and Felty syndrome. Blood Rev 20:245-266, 2006.

Neiman RS, Orazi A: Reactive lymphoid hyperplasia. In Disorders of the Spleen, 2nd ed. Philadelphia, WB Saunders, 1999, pp 67-84.

Burke JS, Osborne BM: Localized reactive lymphoid hyperplasia of the spleen simulating malignant lymphoma: A report of seven cases. Am J Surg Pathol 7:373-380, 1983.

Reactive Lymphoid Hyperplasia without Germinal Center Formation

Clinical Features

- Occurs in any age group
- Most common pattern encountered in viral infections (infectious mononucleosis, herpes simplex virus), transplant recipients, and immunosuppressed individuals (e.g., steroid-treated immune thrombocytopenic purpura, patients with rheumatoid arthritis on methotrexate) and in functional immunodeficiencies encountered in infants and elderly individuals

Gross Pathology

- Modest splenomegaly
- Cut surface may be grossly unremarkable

Histopathology

- White pulp shows a heterogeneous lymphoid population
- Numerous immunoblasts with open chromatin pattern and prominent nucleoli are seen
- Tingible body macrophages may be prominent
- Similar proliferation is seen surrounding splenic arterioles
- Transformed lymphocytes may infiltrate splenic trabeculae, predisposing to splenic rupture

Special Stains and Immunohistochemistry

- Immunohistochemistry can be useful in differential diagnosis from lymphomatous infiltration, such as immunoblastic lymphoma

- Immunohistochemical stains and in situ hybridization studies to exclude viral infection may be helpful

Other Techniques for Diagnosis

- Evaluation of light-chain expression by flow cytometry shows polyclonal B-cell population

Differential Diagnosis

▌ Diffuse large B-cell lymphoma (DLBCL), immunoblastic variant
- Uniform expansive sheets of immunoblasts favor the diagnosis of DLBCL
- Correlation of histologic findings with clinical history and immunohistochemistry is of value

▌ Hodgkin lymphoma
- Immunoblastic proliferation in infectious mononucleosis may contain Reed-Sternberg–like cells
- Immunoblasts are positive for B- or T-cell markers and CD45, may be positive for CD30 antigen; however, in contrast to classical Hodgkin lymphoma, are negative for CD15 antigen

Pearls

- Careful examination of the histologic sections with a high-power objective is mandatory; on low-power examination, nonfollicular lymphoid hyperplasia may appear as unremarkable unstimulated spleen

Selected Reference

Neiman RS, Orazi A: Reactive lymphoid hyperplasia. In Disorders of the Spleen, 2nd ed. Philadelphia, WB Saunders, 1999, pp 67-84.

Smith EB, Custer RP: Rupture of the spleen in infectious mononucleosis. A clinicopathologic report of seven cases. Blood 61:317-333, 1994.

Castleman Disease (Angiofollicular Hyperplasia)

Clinical Features

- Splenic involvement occurs most frequently in multicentric Castleman disease, usually of plasma cell type
- Patients with multicentric Castleman disease present with constitutional symptoms such as fever and frequently show a host of hematologic and immunologic abnormalities (anemia, hypergamma-globulinemia)
- Plasmablastic type of multicentric Castleman disease is a variant associated with human herpesvirus type 8 (HHV-8) seen in HIV-positive patients and in about 40% of HIV-negative cases
- Splenic involvement by Castleman disease of hyaline-vascular type is rarely seen

Gross Pathology

- Modest to moderate splenomegaly

Figure 15-4. Castleman disease (mixed type).

Histopathology

▌ Hyaline-vascular type (see Chapter 14)
▌ Multicentric Castleman disease
- Plasma cell type
  - Hyperplastic or regressively transformed follicles
  - Significant red pulp plasmacytosis
- Plasmablastic type
  - Spectrum of hyperplastic and regressively transformed follicles surrounded by a band of fibrosis with large number of plasma cells
  - Mantle zone with increased number of large lymphoid cells with plasmablastic and immunoblastic features
  - Red pulp is unremarkable
  - Rarely, confluent aggregates of HHV-8–positive plasmablasts are seen, a finding termed *microlymphoma*

Special Stains and Immunohistochemistry

- Plasma cells are usually polyclonal; however may be monotypic (lambda restricted)
- Plasmablasts of plasmablastic type of multicentric Castleman disease are positive for CD20, IgM, lambda light chain, and HHV-8 and are negative for CD30 antigen

Other Techniques for Diagnosis

- Noncontributory

Differential Diagnosis

▌ Reactive lymphoid hyperplasia
- Hyalinization may be present; however, hyaline-vascular changes associated with follicles characteristic of hyaline-vascular type are not seen
▌ Rheumatoid arthritis versus Castleman disease, plasma cell type
- Germinal centers in the white pulp may be hyperplastic
- Polyclonal plasmacytosis of red pulp may be prominent
- Clinical history and serologic tests are important

Pearls

- Interleukin-6 (IL-6) is important in the pathogenesis of the multicentric type of Castleman disease (check serum IL-6 level)
- Multicentric Castleman disease occurs relatively frequently in individuals with immune defects such as HIV infection or elderly patients with Kaposi sarcoma
- There is an increased incidence of overt plasmablastic lymphoma in cases of plasmablastic Castleman disease

Selected References

Dupin N, Diss TL, Kellam P, et al: HHV-8 is associated with a plasmablastic variant of Castleman disease that is linked to HHV-8-positive plasmablastic lymphoma. Blood 95:1406-1412, 2000.

Frizzera G: Castleman's disease and related disorders. Semin Diagn Pathol 5:346-364, 1998.

Cesarman E, Knowles DM: Kaposi's sarcoma-associated herpesvirus: A lymphotropic human herpesvirus associated with Kaposi's sarcoma, primary effusion lymphoma, and multicentric Castleman's disease. Semin Diagn Pathol 14:54-56, 1997.

Menke DM, Tiemann M, Camariano JK, et al: Diagnosis of Castleman's disease by identification of an immunophenotypically aberrant population of mantle zone B lymphocytes in paraffin-embedded lymph node biopsies. Am J Clin Pathol 105:268-276, 1996.

Weisenburger DD: Multicentric angiofollicular lymph node hyperplasia: Pathology of the spleen. Am J Surg Pathol 12:176-181, 1988.

Keller AR, Hochholzer L, Castleman B: Hyaline-vascular and plasma-cell types of giant lymph node hyperplasia of mediastinum and other locations. Cancer 29:670-683, 1972.

Common Variable Immunodeficiency

Clinical Features

- Presentation in childhood or in an adult patient
- Recurrent infections
- Clinical history necessary for adequate interpretation
- Increased risk for lymphoma

Gross Pathology

- Spleen normal sized to enlarged
- May be grossly unremarkable

Histopathology

- Variable histologic features dependent on the primary pathogenetic deficiency in lymphoid stimulatory molecules (inducible costimulator, transmembrane activator, and CAML interactor or CD19 deficiencies)
- Follicular atrophy to hyperplasia
- Atypical follicular hyperplasia may occur
- Granulomas may be prominent
- Immunoblastic proliferation and atypical cells resembling Hodgkin or Reed-Sternberg cells may be present
- There may be lymphoid hyperplasia in the red pulp

Special Stains and Immunohistochemistry

- Most cases are positive for Epstein-Barr virus–encoded latent membrane protein (EBV-LMP) immunostain or Epstein-Barr virus–encoded RNA (EBER) in situ hybridization
- Stains for T cells and B cells will show a mixed population (B and T cells present in variable proportions)
- Polyclonal B-cell population

Other Techniques for Diagnosis

- Noncontributory

Differential Diagnosis

▮ Nonspecific follicular hyperplasia
- Detailed clinical history of immunodeficiency; immunologic and genetic studies

▮ Lymphoproliferative disorders
- Careful clinical history of immunodeficiency has to be obtained to avoid misinterpretation of significant immunoblastic proliferation associated with common variable immunodeficiency (CVID) as malignant lymphoma
- Often necessary to establish clonality for the diagnosis of malignant lymphoma

Pearls

- Histologic features are variable and nonspecific
- Include special stains for microorganisms in cases with granulomatous presentation

Selected References

Salzer U, Grimbacher B: Common variable immunodeficiency: The power of co-stimulation. Semin Immunol 18:337-346, 2006.

Wang J, Rodriguez-Davalos M, Levi G, et al: Common variable immunodeficiency presenting with a large abdominal mass. J Allergy Clin Immunol 115:1318-1320, 2005.

Cunningham-Rundles C, Bodian C: Common variable immunodeficiency: Clinical and immunological features of 248 patients. Clin Immunol 92:34-48, 1999.

Spickett GP, Farrant J, North ME, et al: Common variable immunodeficiency: How many diseases? Immunol Today 18:325-328, 1997.

Case records of the Massachusetts General Hospital. N Engl J Med 332:663-671, 1995.

Huber J, Zegers BJ, Schuurman H-J: Pathology of congenital immunodeficiencies. Semin Diagn Pathol 9:31-62, 1992.

Autoimmune Lymphoproliferative Syndrome

Clinical Features

- Rare heritable lymphoproliferative syndrome due to mutations in *Fas* (CD95), *Fas ligand*, *caspase 8*, or *caspase 10* genes
- Presents in early childhood, usually in patients younger than 2 years

Figure 15-5. Autoimmune lymphoproliferative syndrome. Mixed population of small T cells, T-cell immunoblasts, and polyclonal plasma cells.

- Generalized lymphadenopathy, splenomegaly, and autoimmunity
- Increased risk for development of non-Hodgkin and Hodgkin lymphoma

Gross Pathology
- Massive splenomegaly

Histopathology
- Prominent white pulp with follicular hyperplasia and expansion of marginal zones
- Marked expansion of periarteriolar lymphoid sheath (PALS) and red pulp due to the infiltration by a mixed population of small T cells, T-cell immunoblasts, and polyclonal plasma cells

Special Stains and Immunohistochemistry
- Double negative T cells (CD4 and CD8 negative) are the hallmark of the disease and can be predominantly found in the red pulp
- Splenic T cells are also negative for CD25

Other Techniques for Diagnosis
- Noncontributory

Differential Diagnosis
▌ Lymphoproliferative disorder
  - Correlation with clinical history and the presence of splenomegaly in infancy are critical to avoid interpretation of an abnormal T-cell population in the spleen as a T-cell lymphoproliferative disorder

Selected References

Worth A, Thrasher AJ, Gaspar HB: Autoimmune lymphoproliferative syndrome: Molecular basis of disease and clinical phenotype. Br J Haematol 133:134-140, 2006.

Lim MS, Straus SE, Dale JK, et al: Pathological findings in human autoimmune lymphoproliferative syndrome. Am J Pathol 153:1541-1550, 1998.

Neoplastic Diseases Involving the Splenic White Pulp

Splenic Marginal Zone Lymphoma with or without Villous Lymphocytes

Clinical Features
- Most common in middle-aged to elderly patients, with a slight male predominance
- Presentation with left upper quadrant pain, anemia, and weight loss
- Most common type of lymphoma to present with massive splenomegaly
- Peripheral blood, bone marrow, and liver involvement are common at presentation
- Usually no lymphadenopathy

Figure 15-6. Splenic marginal zone lymphoma. A, Histologic section shows expanded marginal zone replaced by tumor cells. **B,** High-power view shows tumor cells with round nuclei and abundant clear cytoplasm and numerous plasma cells.

- Association with hepatitis C, cryoglobulinemia, and autoimmunity
- Splenectomy may produce long-term remission

Gross Pathology

- Prominent lymphoid follicles (malpighian corpuscles): miliary pattern of white pulp expansion

Histopathology

- Malignant lymphoid cells may form expanded marginal zones or more often show colonization of germinal centers with attenuated mantle zones (Table 15-1)
- An "indolent" variant, which simulates marginal zone hyperplasia, has been reported
- The lymphoid proliferation may infiltrate the red pulp and PALS
- Lymphoma cells are medium-sized with round to oval nuclei and abundant clear cytoplasm
- Larger lymphoid cells are usually seen at the periphery of neoplastic nodules

- A subset of splenic marginal zone lymphoma (SMZL) presents with a predominant diffuse red pulp involvement and an atrophic white pulp

Special Stains and Immunohistochemistry

- SMZLs express the B-cell markers (CD20, CD79a); CD5, cyclin D1, bcl-6, and CD10 antigens are absent
- Because no specific routine markers are expressed by SMZL, the diagnosis is based on the absence of immunophenotypic features specific for other lymphoma subtypes

Other Techniques for Diagnosis

- By flow cytometry, the expression of B-cell markers (CD19, CD20, and CD22) and clonal surface light chains is seen; SMZL with red pulp involvement is positive for B-cell markers and dim CD103 and is negative for annexin-1
- Immunoglobulin heavy-chain gene shows clonal rearrangements
- The *bcl-1* and *bcl-2* genes are not rearranged

Table 15-1. Morphologic and Immunophenotypic Features of Non-Hodgkin Lymphomas with Prominent Spleen Involvement

Type of Lymphomas	Morphologic and Immunophenotypic Features			
	Architectural Features	Cytologic Features	Immunophenotype Cytogenetics	Cell of Origin
Chronic lymphocytic leukemia/small lymphocytic lymphoma	White and red pulp involvement; occasional growth centers	Small lymphoid cells with interspersed prolymphocytes and paraimmunoblasts, with or without growth centers	CD20, CD19, CD5, and CD23 positive	Naive or memory B cell
Mantle cell lymphoma	White pulp involvement; nodular or mantle zone pattern	Monotonous population of medium-sized lymphocytes with irregular nuclei; blastlike or pleomorphic cells in blastoid variant	CD20, CD19, CD5, FMC7, and cyclin D1 positive; t(11;14)	Mantle zone cell
Follicular lymphoma	White pulp involvement; follicular pattern	Medium-sized lymphocytes with indented nuclei and variable admixture of large lymphoid cells	CD20, CD19, CD10, BCL-6, and BCL-2 positive; t(14;18)	Germinal center cell
Splenic marginal zone lymphoma	Predominantly white pulp involvement; red pulp infiltrates with scattered cells and nodules of lymphoma cells; a variant with predominant diffuse red pulp involvement	Medium-sized lymphocytes with clear cytoplasm, indented nuclei, and large lymphoid cells scattered at the periphery of the nodules	CD20 and CD19 positive, CD43 positive or negative	Marginal zone cell
Hairy cell leukemia	Predominantly red pulp with pseudosinuses	Medium-sized cells with abundant cytoplasm and cytoplasmic projections	CD20, CD19, CD103, and CD11c positive, CD25 positive or negative	Suggested origin: post–germinal center memory B cell
Hepatosplenic T-cell lymphoma	Diffuse involvement of red pulp with infiltrate in cords and sinuses, frequently atrophic white pulp	Small to medium-sized lymphoid cells	CD3 and CD2 positive, CD7 positive or negative, CD5, CD4, and CD8 negative; most commonly γδ T-cell receptor	Cytotoxic γδ T cells

Differential Diagnosis

▌ Hairy cell leukemia
- Predominantly a red pulp infiltrate with blood lakes
- Cells with fine, hairlike cytoplasmic processes may be seen in peripheral blood
- Diffuse pattern of bone marrow involvement (versus nodular in SMZL)
- Distinct immunophenotype: B cells positive for tartrate-resistant acid phosphatase (TRAP), DBA.44, CD25, CD11c, and CD103

▌ T-cell large granular lymphocytic leukemia
- Predominantly a red pulp infiltrate
- Distinct T-cell immunophenotype with varying degrees of loss or decreased density of CD7, CD2, and CD3; CD8 and CD57 positive in most cases; aberrant expression of natural killer receptors for class I major histocompatibility complex molecules (of killer cell immunoglobulin-like receptor type, CD158 antigens, and C-type lectin type, CD94 and NKG2 molecules); a minority of cases express CD56, CD16, or both

▌ Hepatosplenic T-cell lymphoma
- More common in young men
- May occur in the post-transplantation setting
- Typically presents with significant hepatomegaly and splenomegaly, abnormal liver function tests, and cytopenias
- Diffuse red pulp infiltration by slightly irregular medium-sized lymphocytes
- T-cell immunophenotype with surface CD3 and associated γδ T-cell receptor (TCR), and absent CD5, CD4, and CD8 antigens; CD56 and CD16 are expressed in some cases

Pearls

- Thorough examination of splenectomy specimens with clinical correlation and, if appropriate, with immunohistochemical and molecular analysis is mandatory because rare cases of minimal involvement by splenic marginal zone lymphoma have been reported, such as in cases of refractory idiopathic thrombocytopenic purpura (ITP)
- Early cases of splenic marginal cell lymphoma may resemble marginal zone hyperplasia; however, in the latter, mantle zones are preserved, a feature invariably missing in lymphoma cases.
- Subtle lymphomatous infiltrate is also present in the red pulp
- Bone marrow involvement is common, often subtle, and intrasinusoidal; sinusoidal infiltrate is best visualized by immunohistochemistry on the marrow core biopsy

Selected References

Traverse-Glehen A, Baseggio L, Callet-Bauchu E, et al: Splenic red pulp lymphoma with numerous basophilic villous lymphocytes: A distinct clinico-pathological and molecular entity? Blood 111:2253-2260, 2008.

Traverse-Glehen A, Verney A, Baseggio L, et al: Analysis of BCL-6, CD95, PIM1, RHO/TTF and PAX5 mutations in splenic and nodal marginal zone B-cell lymphomas suggests a particular B-cell origin. Leukemia 21:1821-1824, 2007.

Saadoun D, Suarez F, Lefrere F, et al: Splenic lymphoma with villous lymphocytes, associated with type II cryoglobulinemia and HCV infection: A new entity? Blood 105:74-76, 2005.

Delsol G, Diebold J, Isaacson PG, et al: Pathology of the spleen: Report of the workshop of the VIIIth Meeting of the European Association for Haematopathology, Paris 1996. Histopathology 32:172-179, 1998.

Rosso R, Neiman RS, Paulli M, et al: Splenic marginal zone cell lymphoma: Report of an indolent variant without massive splenomegaly presumably representing an early phase of the disease. Hum Pathol 26:39-46, 1995.

Isaacson PG, Norton AJ: Extranodal Lymphomas. Edinburgh, Churchill Livingstone, 1994, pp 253-259.

Fend F, Kraus-Hounder B, Müller-Hermelink HK, Feller AC: Monocytoid B cell lymphoma: Its relationship to and possible cellular origin from marginal zone cells. Hum Pathol 24:336-339, 1993.

Ngan BY, Warnke RA, Wilson M, et al: Monocytoid B cell lymphoma: A study of 36 cases. Hum Pathol 22:409-421, 1991.

Chronic Lymphocytic Leukemia/Small Lymphocytic Lymphoma

Clinical Features

- Occur predominantly in elderly individuals
- Patients present with varying degrees of spleen, peripheral blood, and bone marrow involvement

Gross Pathology

- Variable splenomegaly with prominent white pulp (miliary pattern) or more homogeneous diffuse involvement in advanced stages

Figure 15-7. Chronic lymphocytic leukemia/small lymphocytic lymphoma. Histologic section shows a neoplasm composed of small uniform lymphoid cells with dense chromatin pattern and scant cytoplasm.

Histopathology

- Diffuse infiltrate of both red and white pulp; no residual germinal centers are present
- Neoplastic lymphoid cells are small with a coarse chromatin pattern, inconspicuous nucleoli, and scant cytoplasm
- Prolymphocytes and paraimmunoblasts can be intermingled with small lymphoid cells or form ill-defined aggregates (pseudofollicles, proliferation centers) but are less common than in lymph nodes or bone marrow
- Epithelioid granulomas may be seen in rare cases

Special Stains and Immunohistochemistry

- Neoplastic cells express CD20, CD5, CD23, and CD43

Other Techniques for Diagnosis

- Neoplastic cells express CD19, CD5, CD23, CD43, and low-density clonal surface light chain and are weakly positive for CD20
- Clonal immunoglobulin gene rearrangement is present
- Chronic lymphocytic leukemia (CLL)/small lymphocytic lymphoma (SLL) are derived from recirculating CD5 and from immunoglobulin M (IgM) positive and IgD positive or negative B cells normally present in the peripheral blood
- Two groups of CLL/SLL are recognized; this subclassification roughly corresponds to the expression of ZAP-70 and CD38 molecules, which can be quantified by flow cytometry
  - One type corresponding to the pregerminal center phenotype (naive, showing no mutations in the variable region of immunoglobulin heavy-chain [V_H] gene)
  - A second type derived from memory B cells (postgerminal center, mutated V_H gene)

Differential Diagnosis

- ▌ Splenic marginal zone lymphoma
  - Predominantly white pulp infiltrate, frequently with marginal zone pattern
  - Cells are strongly positive for CD20 and surface light chain (flow cytometry) and negative for CD5 and CD23
- ▌ Follicular lymphoma
  - Principally a white pulp infiltrate with minimal red pulp involvement
  - Infiltrate is composed of a mixture of medium-sized centrocytes and large centroblasts
  - Cells are positive for CD19, CD20, CD22, CD10, and bcl-2 [t(14;18)] and negative for CD43, CD5, and CD23
- ▌ Mantle cell lymphoma
  - Predominantly white pulp involvement with expansion into the red pulp
  - Uniform small to medium-sized cells with irregular nuclear outlines
  - Neoplastic cells are positive for CD20, CD19, CD5, CD43, cyclin D1 [t(11;14)], and FMC7 (flow cytometry) and negative for CD23
- ▌ Waldenström macroglobulinemia
  - The defining feature is the demonstration of monoclonal IgM protein in the serum, frequently with symptoms related to hyperviscosity
  - Prominent plasmacytic component or a mixture of plasma cells and plasmacytoid lymphocytes
  - B-cell–associated antigens, including CD19, CD20, and CD22, are consistently expressed; the surface IgM expression can be demonstrated in all cases, most cases show dim CD25; coexpression of CD5, CD23, and FMC7 have been reported; a minute monoclonal plasma cell component can be identified by flow cytometry in most cases
- ▌ Prolymphocytic leukemia
  - In contrast to small lymphoid cells of CLL/SLL, prolymphocytes are medium-sized cells with vesicular nuclei and prominent nucleoli
  - Patients typically present with high white blood cell counts
  - Splenomegaly may be massive
  - CD20 and surface immunoglobulin (sIg) density are stronger than in typical cases of CLL/SLL; CD5 expression is variable
  - Cyclin D1 is positive in 20% cases; these cases are currently considered a splenomegalic form of mantle cell lymphoma

Pearls

- White and red pulp infiltrate is composed of uniform small lymphoid cells
- Modest splenic enlargement occurs
- Most patients whose disease is dominated by massive splenomegaly have mantle zone lymphoma or SMZL rather than SLL/CLL
- Richter transformation may present in the spleen; this appears as fleshy, cream-colored tumor nodules similar to the involvement by DLBCL

Selected References

Hollema H, Visser L, Poppema S: Small lymphocytic lymphomas with predominant splenomegaly: A comparison of immunophenotypes with cases of predominant lymphadenopathy. Mod Pathol 4:712-717, 1991.

Van Krieken JH, Feller AC, te Velde J: The distribution of non-Hodgkin's lymphoma in the lymphoid compartments of the human spleen. Am J Surg Pathol 13:757-765, 1989.

Pangalis GA, Nathwani BN, Rappaport H: Malignant lymphoma, well-differentiated lymphocytic: Its relationship with chronic lymphocytic leukemia and macroglobulinemias of Waldenström. Cancer 39:999-1010, 1977.

Prolymphocytic Leukemia

Clinical Features

- Presentation in elderly patients, with male predominance
- Marked lymphocytosis (often greater than $100 \times 10^9/L$) with more than 55% prolymphocytes
- Massive splenomegaly with hypersplenism and resulting cytopenias and the absence of lymphadenopathy are common features

Gross Pathology

- Massive splenomegaly
- Diffuse red pulp infiltration with variable prominence of white pulp

Histopathology

- Diffuse red pulp infiltration associated with involvement of the white pulp in most cases
- Heterogeneous population of lymphoid cells with a predominance of prolymphocytes characterized by a medium-sized, abundant cytoplasm and prominent nucleoli

Special Stains and Immunohistochemistry

- Eighty percent of prolymphocytic leukemia cases are of B-cell immunophenotype and are positive for CD20, with variable coexpression of CD5 and CD23
- Twenty percent of cases show T-cell immunophenotype (T-cell prolymphocytic leukemia) with a predominant expression of CD3, CD5, and CD4; loss of T-cell antigens may be seen

Other Techniques for Diagnosis

- By flow cytometry, a strong expression of CD20, CD19, FMC7, and clonal surface immunoglobulin is seen in most cases

Differential Diagnosis

- CLL/SLL
  - Massive splenomegaly is relatively uncommon
  - Homogeneous population of small lymphoid cells with scant cytoplasm; prolymphocytes are rare
  - Weaker expression of sIg and CD20, positive for CD5 and CD23, negative for FMC7
- Splenic marginal zone lymphoma
  - Significant peripheral lymphocytosis is uncommon
  - Neoplastic B-cells usually do not have prominent nucleoli

Pearls

- Prolymphocytic leukemia occurs predominantly in elderly males
- Massive splenomegaly with significant lymphocytosis and absence of peripheral lymphadenopathy
- Characterized by increased numbers of prolymphocytes (large to medium-sized cells with prominent nucleoli) admixed with the small round lymphocytes
- Usually B-cell phenotype
- Variable expression of CD5 and CD23 (both positive in CLL/SLL)

Selected References

Ruchlemer R, Parry-Jones N, Brito-Babapulle V, et al: B-prolymphocytic leukaemia with t(11;14) revisited: A splenomegalic form of mantle cell lymphoma evolving with leukaemia. Br J Haematol 125:330-336, 2004.

Lampert I, Catovsky D, Marsh GW, et al: The histopathology of prolymphocytic leukemia with particular reference to the spleen: A comparison with chronic lymphocytic leukemia. Histopathology 4:3-19, 1980.

Bearman RM, Pangalis GA, Rappaport H: Prolymphocytic leukemia: Clinical, histopathological and cytochemical observations. Cancer 42:2360-2372, 1978.

Mantle Cell Lymphoma

Clinical Features

- Most patients present with widespread peripheral lymphadenopathy and bone marrow involvement
- A splenomegalic variant of mantle cell lymphoma with leukemic peripheral blood involvement and with no appreciable lymphadenopathy has been reported

Gross Pathology

- Prominent white pulp in an enlarged spleen
- Massive splenomegaly may be seen (>1000 g)

Figure 15-8. Prolymphocytic leukemia. The infiltrate is composed of a heterogeneous population of lymphoid cells, many of which have large nuclei and prominent nucleoli.

Histopathology

- Nodular expansion of white pulp with or without a mantle zone pattern (i.e., lymphoid proliferation surrounding residual germinal centers)
- A pure mantle zone lymphomatous pattern is rarely seen
- Homogeneous population of medium-sized lymphoid cells with irregular nuclear outlines
- Blastoid variant of mantle cell lymphoma is composed of blastlike lymphoid cells (lymphoblastoid variant) or of large pleomorphic cells resembling those of DLBCL

Special Stains and Immunohistochemistry

- Neoplastic cells are positive for CD20, CD5, and cyclin D1 [t(11;14)] and negative for CD23
- See Chapter 14 for more detailed information

Other Techniques for Diagnosis

- By flow cytometry, the neoplastic cells are positive for CD20 (bright expression), CD19, CD5, and FMC7 and negative for CD23
- The defining feature of mantle cell lymphoma is the presence of t(11;14), the translocation of proto-oncogene cyclin D1 (*bcl-1*; involved in the regulation of G_1- to S-phase progression) to the immunoglobulin heavy-chain gene locus

Differential Diagnosis

▌ CLL/SLL
  - Diffuse red pulp infiltration is prominent
  - Small lymphocytes with some large cells (prolymphocytes and paraimmunoblasts)
  - Low-density sIg and CD20 positivity; positive for both CD5 and CD23
  - Generally cyclin D1 is not present; cyclin D1 can be expressed in scattered cells of CLL/SLL
▌ Splenic marginal zone lymphoma
  - Present with massive splenomegaly without peripheral lymphadenopathy
  - Expanded, confluent marginal zones can be difficult to distinguish from expanded mantle zones
  - Neoplastic population composed of medium-sized lymphoid cells with rare admixed large cells
  - Neoplastic cells do not express CD5 or cyclin D1

Pearls

- Mantle cell lymphoma can present with leukemic peripheral blood involvement and massive splenomegaly
- Blastoid mantle cell lymphoma may mimic lymphoblast proliferation or DLBCL

Selected References

Angelopoulou MK, Siakantariz MP, Vassilakopoulous TP, et al: The splenic form of mantle cell lymphoma. Eur J Haematol 68:12-21, 2002.

Molina TJ, Delmer A, Cymbalista F, et al: Mantle cell lymphoma, in leukaemic phase with prominent splenomegaly: A report of eight cases with similar clinical presentation and aggressive outcome. Virchows Arch 437:591-598, 2000.

Banks PM, Chan J, Cleary ML, et al: Mantle cell lymphoma: A proposal for unification of morphologic, immunologic and molecular data. Am J Surg Pathol 16:637-640, 1992.

Follicular Lymphoma

Clinical Features

- Patients typically present with multifocal lymphadenopathy and bone marrow involvement (stage IV)
- About half of patients show splenic involvement, often detected only at the microscopic level

Gross Pathology

- Uniform expansion of the white pulp nodules (miliary pattern)

Histopathology

- Uniform multifocal involvement of the white pulp, frequently with small aggregates of lymphoma cells within red pulp
- In grades 1 and 2 follicular lymphoma, neoplastic follicles are composed predominantly of medium-sized cleaved centrocytes with a variable admixture of large atypical lymphoid cells with vesicular nuclei and multiple nucleoli mostly attached to the nuclear membrane (centroblasts)
- In grade 3 follicular lymphoma, centroblasts predominate

Special Stains and Immunohistochemistry

- The immunophenotype reflects the follicle center cell origin of follicular lymphoma

Figure 15-9. Follicular lymphoma. Low-power view shows multiple white pulp tumor nodules.

- B-cell marker CD20 is positive, along with the coexpression of antigens characteristic for germinal center cells, such as CD10 and bcl-6
- Antiapoptotic protein bcl-2 is positive
- See Chapter 14 for more detailed information

Other Techniques for Diagnosis

- By flow cytometry, pan B-cell markers (CD19, CD20) and clonal surface immunoglobulin are present along with the coexpression of CD10 antigen in most cases
- By flow cytometry, the coexpression of CD10, similar in density to that seen in reactive follicular hyperplasia, in association with a relatively low-density CD19, is a characteristic feature of follicular lymphoma
- Expression of bcl-2 is due to the t(14;18)(q32;q21), which places the *bcl-2* gene under a promoter of the immunoglobulin heavy-chain gene

Differential Diagnosis

- Reactive follicular hyperplasia
  - Well-defined follicles with distinct marginal and mantle zones, polarization of germinal center into dark and light zones, tingible body macrophages, and mitotic figures
  - Germinal centers negative for bcl-2
- Castleman disease
  - Expanded mantle zones
  - White pulp follicles are variably hyalinized and expanded
  - Red pulp is expanded with large numbers of polyclonal plasma cells
- Mantle cell lymphoma
  - Uniform population of small to medium-sized lymphocytes without centroblasts
  - Cells express CD5 and are generally CD10 negative
  - Overexpression of cyclin D1
  - Expression of bcl-2 is not useful in the differential diagnosis
- Splenic marginal zone lymphoma
  - More prominent involvement of red pulp
  - The expression of markers associated with germinal center origin is not seen

Pearls

- Expression of bcl-2 is seen in most types of indolent B-cell lymphomas; however, when seen in nodular proliferation showing germinal center cell immunophenotype, bcl-2 is diagnostic of follicular lymphoma
- About 20% of follicular lymphomas are negative for bcl-2 antigen; in a proportion of these cases, molecular studies (polymerase chain reaction [PCR] or fluorescent in situ hybridization [FISH] based) may demonstrate the presence of t(14;18) or bcl-6 rearrangement
- Predominantly white pulp involvement, but discrete invasion of red pulp is common

Selected References

Horsman DE, Okamoto I, Ludkovski O, et al: Follicular lymphoma lacking the t(14;18)(q32;q21): identification of two disease subtypes. Br J Haematol 120:424-433, 2003.

Gauland P, D'Agay MF, Peuchmar M, et al: Expression of the bcl-2 gene product in follicular lymphoma. Am J Pathol 140:1089-1095, 1992.

Kim H, Dorfman RF: Morphological studies of 84 untreated patients subjected to laparotomy for the staging of non-Hodgkin's lymphoma. Cancer 33:647-674, 1974.

Diffuse Large B-Cell Lymphoma

Clinical Features

- Less likely than small cell lymphomas to involve the spleen at presentation
- Accounts for about one third of lymphomas localized to the spleen at presentation
- May arise de novo or represent transformation of low-grade lymphoma

Gross Pathology

- Typically presents as large tumor nodules that may coalesce into larger masses randomly distributed in the splenic parenchyma
- May show large areas of necrosis
- Usually involves also hilar and retroperitoneal lymph nodes

Histopathology

- Focal aggregates and sheets of large atypical lymphoid cells with variable cytologic features (centroblasts, immunoblasts)
- Involves both white and red pulp, effacing the normal splenic architecture

Figure 15-10. Intravascular large B-cell lymphoma. The tumor cells are large with round nuclei, vesicular chromatin, prominent nucleoli, and abundant cytoplasm.

Special Stains and Immunohistochemistry

- DLBCLs express CD20 and CD79a; as in lymph nodes, they may express other antigens, such as bcl-6 and CD10, suggesting origin from germinal center, and MUM-1 or CD5 antigen
- See Chapter 14 for more detailed information

Other Techniques for Diagnosis

- By flow cytometry, DLBCLs express CD19, CD20, and CD22; most commonly, there is a clonal surface light chain; rare cases are negative for sIg
- Immunoglobulin gene rearrangement analysis can be useful (see Chapter 14 for more detailed information)

Differential Diagnosis

- ▌ Hodgkin lymphoma
  - Patients almost always have nodal Hodgkin lymphoma
  - Typical heterogeneous cellular background composed of small lymphocytes, plasma cells, eosinophils, neutrophils, and macrophages with large pleomorphic Reed-Sternberg cells and their variants
  - Neoplastic cells are typically negative for CD20, CD45, and CD3 but express CD15 and CD30 antigens
- ▌ Inflammatory pseudotumor (IPT)
  - Usually a single, well-demarcated whitish mass
  - Histology shows a polymorphous collection of bland spindle cells and inflammatory cells

Pearls

- Large tumor nodules often with foci of necrosis
- Tumor usually involves hilar and retroperitoneal lymph nodes with or without peripheral lymphadenopathy

Selected References

Kobrich U, Falk S, Middeke B, et al: Primary large cell lymphoma of the splenic sinuses: A variant of angiotropic B-cell lymphoma (neoplastic angioendotheliomatosis)? Hum Pathol 23:1184-1187, 1992.

Falk S, Stutte HJ: Primary malignant lymphomas of the spleen: A morphologic and immunohistochemical analysis of 17 cases. Cancer 66:2612-2619, 1990.

Kraemer BB, Osborne BM, Butler JJ: Primary splenic presentation of malignant lymphoma and related disorders: A study of 49 cases. Cancer 54:1606-1619, 1984.

Hodgkin Lymphoma

Clinical Features

- Splenic involvement is common in cases of nodal-based classical Hodgkin lymphoma
- True primary splenic Hodgkin lymphoma is exceedingly rare
- Lymphocyte-predominant Hodgkin lymphoma rarely involves spleen

Figure 15-11. Hodgkin lymphoma. A, Low-power view shows multiple distinct white pulp tumor nodules. **B,** The nodules consist of a polymorphous infiltrate, which includes Hodgkin cells, lymphocytes, eosinophils, and epithelioid histiocytes.

Gross Pathology

- Focal nodules scattered in spleen parenchyma, often with apparent fibrosis
- Occasionally nodules are small, visible only on thin sectioning of the organ

Histopathology

- Early lesions are found in the T-cell zones of white pulp, periarteriolar lymphoid sheaths, or marginal zones
- Characteristic cell population corresponds to the subtype diagnosed
- Classical Hodgkin lymphoma: Reed-Sternberg cells in a heterogeneous background of T cells, histiocytes, and eosinophils

- Lymphocyte-predominant Hodgkin lymphoma: "popcorn" cells characterized by large size and multilobated nucleus with delicate chromatin, in a background of small lymphocytes
- Accompanying fibrosis may be prominent
- Epithelioid granulomas may be present

Special Stains and Immunohistochemistry

- Small lymphocytes are a mixture of CD3-positive T cells (predominantly helper, CD4-positive) and CD20-positive B cells; the former usually predominate
- Reed-Sternberg cells and their variants are positive for CD30 and CD15 and negative for CD45RB (leukocyte common antigen [LCA]) and CD3; CD20 is usually negative but can be seen in a proportion of neoplastic cells
- Popcorn cells of lymphocyte-predominant Hodgkin lymphoma are positive for CD20 and CD45RB (LCA) and can be surrounded by CD57-positive T cells

Other Techniques for Diagnosis

- Noncontributory

Differential Diagnosis

▌ DLBCL
  - Similarly, random distribution of tumor nodules
  - Composed predominantly of large lymphoid cells
  - In most cases, neoplastic cells are positive for CD20 and CD45 and negative for CD15
  - Rare cases of Hodgkin lymphoma may be "combined" with DLBCL (composite lymphoma) or more often, in lymphocyte-predominant Hodgkin lymphoma, show transformation to DLBCL
▌ Anaplastic large cell lymphoma
  - May form tumor masses or diffusely infiltrate the spleen
  - Pleomorphic multinucleated large cells with prominent nucleoli may resemble Reed-Sternberg cells; however, heterogeneous background typical for Hodgkin lymphoma is absent
  - Neoplastic cells of anaplastic large cell lymphoma express CD30 and anaplastic lymphoma kinase (ALK-1) but are usually negative for CD15
▌ IPT
  - Usually a solitary mass with whitish cut surface
  - Tumor localized to the spleen; no lymphadenopathy
  - Mixture of bland spindle cells, lymphocytes, and plasma cells
  - Reed-Sternberg cells are not identified
▌ Splenic hamartoma
  - Usually presents as solitary mass with reddish cut surface
  - Does not involve tissues other than the spleen
▌ Metastatic carcinoma or melanoma
  - Almost always a previous history of primary tumor
  - Single or multiple randomly distributed tumor nodules
  - Microscopy shows sheets of large nonhematopoietic cells (negative for lymphoid antigens)

Pearls

- True primary Hodgkin lymphoma of the spleen is rare (<3% of cases)
- Modern radiologic imaging techniques have virtually replaced splenectomy for staging of Hodgkin lymphoma; splenectomy, however, remains the single most effective method for documenting Hodgkin lymphoma involvement

Selected References

Burke JS, Osborne BM: Localized reactive lymphoid hyperplasia of the spleen simulating malignant lymphoma: A report of seven cases. Am J Surg Pathol 7:373-380, 1983.

Farrer-Brown G, Bennett MH, Harrison CV, et al: The diagnosis of Hodgkin's disease in surgically excised spleens. J Clin Pathol 25:294-300, 1972.

Lukes RJ: Criteria for involvement of lymph nodes, bone marrow, spleen and liver in Hodgkin's disease. Cancer Res 31:1755-1767, 1971.

Non-neoplastic Diseases Involving the Splenic Red Pulp

Gaucher Disease and Other Storage Disorders

Clinical Features

- Gaucher disease has two major forms: infantile and adult
  — Infantile form: hepatosplenomegaly and mental deterioration in the first year of life, death in infancy or early childhood

Figure 15-12. Gaucher disease. Gaucher cells occupy the cords of the red pulp. They have abundant cytoplasm and round to oval pale nuclei with uniform nucleoli. This must be distinguished from Langerhans cell histiocytosis, in which the cells are smaller with bean-shaped nuclei. Rarely, macrophages engorged with *Mycobacterium avium* may resemble Gaucher cells.

Figure 15-13. Niemann-Pick disease. A, Low-power magnification. The histiocytes occupy the cords of the red pulp and surround a splenic follicle. **B,** High-power magnification. The histiocytes have abundant clear multivacuolated cytoplasm and round to oval pale nuclei with uniform nucleoli.

— Adult (later-onset) form
  ◆ Most common form
  ◆ Highest incidence in Ashkenazi Jews
  ◆ Most common lysosomal storage disease
  ◆ Insidious onset in late childhood or adulthood
  ◆ No mental retardation
  ◆ Pancytopenia may be the presenting symptom
  ◆ Hepatomegaly, splenomegaly, and adrenal involvement
  ◆ Bone lesions include pathologic fractures, lytic lesions, and avascular necrosis of the femoral head

● Most other inherited metabolic storage diseases have onset in infancy or childhood; all are extremely rare
● Non-neuronopathic cases of Niemann-Pick disease may also present in adulthood with clinically significant hypersplenism
● Features and differential diagnosis are summarized in Table 15-2

Gross Pathology

● Diffuse enlargement of the spleen with a pale, dry appearance on its cut surface

Table 15-2. Differential Diagnosis of Storage Diseases with Special Stains and Additional Techniques

	Storage Diseases			
Stain or Technique	Gaucher Disease	Niemann-Pick Disease	Mucopolysaccharidoses	Glycogen Storage Diseases
Enzyme defect	Glucocerebrosidase (β-glucosidase)	Sphingomyelinase	Varies; multiple types known	Varies; 10 types
Storage product	Glucocerebroside	Sphingomyelin	Varies	Glycogen
Other organs affected	Liver, adrenals, lung, bone; central nervous system in infantile form	Brain, liver, lungs, bone marrow	Central nervous system, tongue, skeleton, liver, cornea, heart valves	Liver, muscle, heart (dependent on type)
Hematoxylin and eosin stain	"Wrinkled silk"	Yellow-green	Clear	Clear
Wright-Giemsa stain	Colorless	Blue-green		
Periodic acid–Schiff stain	Positive	Variable	Weakly positive	Positive
Periodic acid–Schiff with diastase stain	Positive	Variable		Negative
Iron	Positive	Negative		Negative
Acid-fast	Negative	Positive		
Electron microscopy	Lysosomes with twisted helical tubules	Variably sized residual bodies	Membrane-bound vacuoles with lamellar inclusions	Glycogen granules

Histopathology

- Expansion of the red pulp and distention of splenic cords by large macrophages
- Gaucher cells have a characteristic "wrinkled-silk" cytoplasm and should be distinguished from Niemann-Pick cells, which are also large macrophages, but their cytoplasms appear foamy or bubbly owing to the presence of numerous small vacuoles
- Another important distinction is with the sea-blue histiocytes encountered in cases of ceroid histiocytosis (e.g., in patients Hermansky-Pudlak syndrome)
- Ceroid histiocytes are smaller, are faintly yellow-brown (blue-green in Wright-Giemsa stain), and have a distinctive cytoplasmic granularity

Special Stains and Immunohistochemistry

- See Table 15-2

Other Techniques for Diagnosis

- Biochemical analysis of the storage product and determination of the activity of the relevant enzyme in fresh tissue samples are the gold standards for definitive diagnosis
- Detection of the specific gene mutations in patients at risk in affected families is possible in an increasing number of metabolic diseases

Differential Diagnosis

- See Table 15-2

Pearls

- Pancytopenia may be the presenting clinical feature; it may result from hypersplenism and marrow infiltration by the Gaucher cells

- Diagnoses in these diseases are made biochemically from peripheral blood, bone marrow, or other tissues
- Patients most often have an established diagnosis by the time the pathologist sees the spleen at autopsy or surgery; thus, the need of clinical correlation cannot be overemphasized

Selected References

Barranger JA, Ginns EI: Glucosylceramide lipidoses: Gaucher disease. In Scriver CR, Beaudet AL, Sly WS, et al (eds): The Metabolic Basis of Inherited Diseases, 6th ed. New York, McGraw-Hill, 1989.

Elleder M: Niemann-Pick disease. Pathol Res Pract 185:293-328, 1989.

Lee RE, Peters SP, Glew RH: Gaucher's disease: Clinical, morphologic and pathogenetic considerations. Pathol Ann 12:309-339, 1977.

Hematologic Diseases

Extramedullary Hematopoiesis

Clinical Features

- Extramedullary hematopoiesis (EMH) refers to the accumulation of hematopoietic precursor cells in the spleen
- EMH may be divided into two types
  - A non-neoplastic EMH refers to the accumulation in the splenic red pulp of nonclonal hematopoietic precursor cells
  - A neoplastic form refers to the secondary "spread" to the spleen of a hematologic malignancy capable of manifesting itself as EMH

Figure 15-14. Extramedullary hematopoiesis. A, The red pulp and the vascular sinuses contain trilinear hematopoietic cells with a predominance of erythroblasts and megakaryocytes. **B,** Extramedullary hematopoiesis in myelofibrosis. Numerous neutrophils accompany abnormal megakaryocyte morphologically similar to those that characterize the bone marrow in cases of primary myelofibrosis with myeloid metaplasia.

- Non-neoplastic EMH
  - Usually an incidental finding in a spleen removed for some other cause
  - Typically seen in patients with severe anemia (e.g., thalassemia major) or a disease that replaces the bone marrow (lymphoma, myeloma, metastatic malignancy)
  - Normal in the fetus and premature infant
- Neoplastic EMH
  - Often associated with a more marked degree of splenomegaly, and splenectomy is most often performed to relieve pain associated with the presence of a large spleen or to ameliorate cytopenia due to hypersplenism
  - Typically occurs in patients with the classic myeloproliferative disorders, particularly chronic idiopathic myelofibrosis (primary myelofibrosis), in which EMH is one of the major manifestations of that disease
  - Also seen in other myeloproliferative disorders with "secondary myelofibrosis," such as polycythemia vera and, rarely, essential thrombocythemia
  - Less frequently, can also be seen in patients with myelodysplastic/myeloproliferative diseases (e.g., chronic myelomonocytic leukemia) or in myelodysplastic syndromes
- In all patients with myeloid neoplasms, splenic EMH needs to be distinguished from extramedullary (splenic) acute leukemia; when the latter is found superimposed on an EMH background, it may represent disease transformation

Gross Pathology

- Usually an incidental finding without gross features
- May cause diffuse expansion of the red pulp
- Rarely causes multiple soft, bulging, dark-red to brown berry-like nodules; these are most often seen in patients with late stages of chronic idiopathic myelofibrosis or polycythemia vera (after polycythemic myeloid metaplasia)

Histopathology

- Cellular infiltrates are seen in red pulp cords or within red pulp sinuses
- Small clusters of normoblasts are easiest to identify; this is the predominant cell type found in nonclonal EMH
- Identification of megakaryocytes and granulocytic precursors may be facilitated by immunohisto-chemistry (e.g., myeloperoxidase)
- Trilineage EMH is most commonly seen in patients with chronic myeloproliferative disorders
- Clusters of large pleomorphic megakaryocytes displaying abnormally clumped nuclear chromatin suggest a diagnosis of EMH associated with chronic idiopathic myelofibrosis (or secondary myelofibrosis after polycythemia vera)

Special Stains and Immunohistochemistry

- Wright stains (e.g., touch preparations)
- Antihemoglobin (or glycophorin A) immunostaining to highlight the presence of erythroid precursors (erythroblasts)
- Antibodies reactive with myeloperoxidase or lysozyme can be used to highlight myeloid cells
- Antibodies reactive with platelet glycoproteins such as CD42b or CD61 may facilitate the identification of megakaryocytes
- CD34 and other paraffin reactive antibodies, which are commonly used to type hematologic malignancies in tissue sections, can also be useful in selected cases, such as to identify accumulations of blasts, which may indicate transformation to extramedullary acute leukemia

Other Techniques for Diagnosis

- Usually not necessary; flow cytometry and cytogenetic techniques may be useful to confirm evolution to acute leukemia

Differential Diagnosis

▌ Lymphoid infiltrate in red pulp
- Cells are more pleomorphic; nuclei are not as round as normoblasts and have less dense chromatin (that is, have a more visible chromatin pattern) than normoblasts
- Cell borders are indistinct

▌ Acute leukemia
- Rapid onset usually with severe cytopenias
- Blasts have high nuclear-to-cytoplasmic ratio and display fine chromatin and scant indistinct cytoplasm; however, monoblasts and megakaryoblasts may have more abundant cytoplasm

Pearls

- The formerly used term *myeloid metaplasia* to indicate EMH is a misnomer; the phenomenon results from entrapment in the spleen (filtration theory) of circulating immature hematopoietic cells
- The identification of early extramedullary (splenic) blastic transformation may be challenging, and immunohistochemistry may be invaluable in these cases

Selected References

O'Malley DP, Kim YS, Perkins SL, et al: Morphologic and immunohistochemical evaluation of splenic hematopoietic proliferations in neoplastic and benign disorders. Mod Pathol 18:1550-1561, 2005.

Neiman RS, Orazi A: Functions of the spleen. In Disorders of the Spleen, 2nd ed. Philadelphia, WB Saunders, 1999, pp 26-38.

Wilkins BS, Green A, Wild AE, Jones DB: Extramedullary haemopoiesis in fetal and adult human spleen: A quantitative immunohistological study. Histopathology 24:241-247, 1994.

Hereditary Spherocytosis

Clinical Features

- Patients have familial history of hemolytic anemia (autosomal dominant)
- Splenectomy in this condition is most often performed in late childhood or early adult years
- Autosomal dominant inheritance

Gross Pathology

- Splenomegaly; usually of moderate degree
- Red pulp shows intense congestion
- Attenuation of the normal white pulp nodularity

Histopathology

- White pulp is normal to atrophic
- Red pulp cords are distended and the sinuses appear empty
- Increased cordal macrophages and hypertrophy of sinus-lining cells
- Erythrophagocytosis is hard to see, and hemosiderin deposition is minimal
- Extramedullary hematopoiesis is not seen

Special Stains and Immunohistochemistry

- Noncontributory

Other Techniques for Diagnosis

- Osmotic fragility test on patient's red cells
- Polyacrylamide gel electrophoresis for molecular subtyping

Differential Diagnosis

▌ Autoimmune hemolytic anemia
- No family history
- Acquired disease
- Spleen is of normal size to slightly enlarged

Figure 15-15. Hereditary spherocytosis. High-power magnification shows that the splenic cords are distended with red cells, the sinuses relatively empty.

- If untreated, the spleen shows significant white pulp hyperplasia and red pulp plasmacytosis
- Cords are not as distended, and it is easier to detect erythrophagocytosis both in cordal and in sinus macrophages
- Hemosiderin deposition and extramedullary erythropoiesis may be prominent
- Coombs test positive

▌ Sickle cell disease and variants
- Usually autosplenectomy due to multiple infarctions by age 7 years (hemoglobin S [HbSS])
- Splenomegaly may be seen in adults with sickle cell variants (e.g., sickle cell and hemoglobin C disease)
- Infarcts much more common
- Stacked, sickled cells in red pulp
- History is important, including ancestry (more common in people of African or Arab ancestry)

▌ Fibrocongestive splenomegaly
- Patients usually have liver disease, often with ascites
- Red pulp shows a combination of congestion (due to blood stasis) and fibrosis

Pearls

- Rarely, areas of marked red pulp congestion may superficially resemble capillary hemangiomas or even a splenic hamartoma; however, the latter two conditions are usually more demarcated focal lesions; additionally, hemangiomas show abnormal vascular channels
- In hereditary spherocytosis, hemolysis and anemia are relieved by splenectomy, but the underlying red cell defect remains
- At a molecular level this disease is heterogeneous; caused by a variety of mutations involving any of several red cell membrane proteins

Selected References

Iolascon A, Miraglia del Giudice E, Perrotta S, et al: Hereditary spherocytosis: From clinical to molecular defects. Haematologica 83:240-257, 1998.

Chang CS, Li CY, Liang YH, Cha SS: Clinical features and splenic pathologic changes in patients with autoimmune hemolytic anemia and congenital hemolytic anemia. Mayo Clin Proc 68:757-762, 1993.

Sickle Cell Disease and Variants

Clinical Features

- Inherited hemolytic anemia
- Predominantly in patients of African or Arab ancestry
- Children may have impaired growth
- Disease course is punctuated by various crises
  — Painful (infarcts)
  — Hemolytic crisis
  — Aplastic crisis
  — Splenic sequestration (in young children or in older patients with variant sickling disorders)

Figure 15-16. A, Hemoglobin SC disease, adult patient with hemolytic crisis, gross photograph. Enlarged spleen with a central round infarct and small peripheral infarcts. **B, Classic sickle cell disease (hemoglobin SS).** Normal red pulp morphology is lost; there are masses of stacked, sickled red cells and pigment-laden macrophages. Evaluation of red cell morphology on tissue sections is not reliable, but the appearance of stacked masses of sickled cells is characteristic of this disease. **C, Classic sickle cell disease, Gamna-Gandy body**. An old organized microinfarct is encrusted by iron and focally calcified.

— Hand-foot syndrome
— Acute chest syndrome
- Patients with homozygous HbSS become functionally asplenic in childhood and are at risk for sepsis from *Haemophilus influenza, Staphylococcus pneumoniae,* and *Neisseria meningitidis*
- Patients may be jaundiced
- Gallstones can develop at an early age
- Increased incidence of *Salmonella* osteomyelitis

Gross Pathology

- HbSS disease: by age 7 years, the spleen has become a small greenish-brown fibrotic nubbin (autosplenectomy)
- With hemoglobin C disease and other variants, the spleen may be enlarged with red pulp congestion; infarcts may occur, but the spleen does not usually totally infarct

Histopathology

- Sickling causes stasis and hypoxia, which in turn result in hemorrhagic infarcts; infarcts result in the formation of Gamna-Gandy bodies, that is, fibrotic foci with hemosiderin deposits and calcification; these are not, however, unique to this disease
- HbSS: splenic architecture is progressively destroyed; in the initial stage of the disease, there is a loss of marginal zones due to preferential sickling in this area; this is followed by a progressive loss of all splenic tissue; what remains is fibrous tissue with hemosiderin and other pigment deposits and variable numbers of macrophages
- Other sickling diseases
  — Red pulp congestion
  — Sickled red cells in cords and sinuses
  — Increased macrophages with phagocytosed red cells and hemosiderin

Special Stains and Immunohistochemistry

- Noncontributory

Other Techniques for Diagnosis

- Hemoglobin electrophoresis

Differential Diagnosis

▌ Splenic infarcts
- Extensive loss of splenic parenchyma is rare, especially in children
- Typically subcapsular, wedge-shaped lesions
- Normal hemoglobin electrophoresis
- No sickled red cells

▌ Hereditary spherocytosis
- Family history
- Patients usually not of African ancestry
- Splenic enlargement in both children and adults
- Normal hemoglobin electrophoresis

- Red cells spherocytic, not sickled
- Splenic infarcts uncommon
▌ Malaria
  - Acquired disease, usually after residence in or travel to an endemic area
  - Periodic fever
  - Intermittent hemolysis
  - Organisms detectable in peripheral blood
  - Sickled cells usually not present
  - Hemoglobin electrophoresis usually normal; sickle hemoglobin provides some protection against severe malaria

Pearls

- Formalin fixation distorts red cell morphology, but presence of numerous tactoids and stacked red cells is usually diagnostic
- Splenic sequestration crises are an indication for splenectomy; this is done for preventing recurrence; these specimens account for most spleens with sickle cell disease seen in pathology
- Patients of Arab ancestry with HbSS typically have a higher percentage of hemoglobin F and milder disease

Selected References

Dover GH, Platt OS: Sickle cell disease. In Nathan DG, Orkin SH (eds): Nathan and Oski's Hematology of Infancy and Childhood, 5th ed. Philadelphia, WB Saunders, 1998, pp 762-809.

Bunn HF: Pathogenesis and treatment of sickle cell disease. N Engl J Med 337:762-769, 1997.

Autoimmune Hemolytic Anemia

Clinical Features

- Most common in adults
- Female predominance
- May occur as a primary disorder or may coexist with another disease, such as systemic lupus, lymphoid neoplasms (e.g., chronic lymphocytic leukemia), or solid tumors, or may be drug induced
- Increased reticulocytes
- Coombs test positive

Gross Pathology

- Spleen normal to moderately enlarged
- Diffuse process without focal lesions
- White pulp normal to hyperplastic
- Red pulp expanded and congested

Histopathology

- Follicular hyperplasia in white pulp
- Variably expanded red pulp
- Increased plasma cells
- Erythrophagocytosis detectable both in cordal and sinus macrophages
- Hemosiderin deposition and extramedullary erythropoiesis may be prominent
- Cords congested; sinuses may appear empty (like in congenital spherocytosis)

Special Stains and Immunohistochemistry

- Noncontributory

Other Techniques for Diagnosis

- Coombs test on blood

Differential Diagnosis

- History and Coombs test critical for all differential diagnoses
▌ ITP
  - Patients have thrombocytopenia but are usually not anemic

Figure 15-17. Autoimmune hemolytic anemia. A, Intravascular hemophagocytosis of antibody-covered erythrocytes. **B,** Iron overload. It can be massive and simulate other diseases with severe iron overload (e.g., thalassemia).

- The coexistence of ITP and hemolytic anemia is called *Evans syndrome*
- Antiplatelet antibodies are present in plasma and on patient's platelets
- Histologically, "dirty cords" are due to phagocytosis of platelets (best seen in touch preparations), but there is no evident erythrophagocytosis
- Congestive splenomegaly
  - Patients have portal hypertension and usually have liver disease
  - Spleen shows an increased stroma content (fibrocongestive splenomegaly)
  - Coombs test negative
- Hereditary spherocytosis
  - Family history
  - Lifelong hemolytic anemia
  - Abnormal red blood cell morphology
  - Coombs test negative

Pearls

- Most common in women
- Check clinical history and Coombs test result

Selected References

Chang CS, Li CY, Liang YH, Cha SS: Clinical features and splenic pathologic changes in patients with autoimmune hemolytic anemia and congenital hemolytic anemia. Mayo Clin Proc 68:757-762, 1993.

Sokol RJ, Booker DJ, Stamps R: The pathology of autoimmune haemolytic anaemia. J Clin Pathol 45:1047-1052, 1992.

Idiopathic Thrombocytopenic Purpura (Autoimmune Thrombocytopenic Purpura)

Clinical Features

- Seen at any age
- Acute condition more common in children

Figure 15-18. Idiopathic (autoimmune) thrombocytopenic purpura (ITP). This photomicrograph shows pale-red pulp with many pale-staining macrophages in the cords. Most patients who undergo splenectomy for ITP have been treated with other modalities first, and thus these features are rarely seen.

- Chronic condition most common in middle-aged adults
- Female predominance
- Common in HIV infection; the cause of thrombocytopenia is usually multifactorial in these patients

Gross Pathology

- Spleen is usually of normal size
- White pulp may be enlarged

Histopathology

- Follicular hyperplasia in white pulp
- Increased plasma cells
- Granular, dirty appearance of the cordal macrophages (periodic acid–Schiff stain–positive debris in cytoplasm)
- Foamy macrophages in red pulp
- Increased number of neutrophils in red pulp
- Only minimal extramedullary hematopoiesis
- Bone marrow aspirate and biopsy show normal to increased number of megakaryocytes

Special Stains and Immunohistochemistry

- Noncontributory

Other Techniques for Diagnosis

- Tests for antiplatelet antibodies

Differential Diagnosis

- Nonspecific follicular hyperplasia
  - History and clinical manifestations important
  - Complete blood count
  - Antiplatelet antibody test negative

Pearls

- One of the most common indications for splenectomy
- The spleen in these patients is an important site of both platelet destruction and the production of antiplatelet antibodies
- Splenectomy is performed only in patients refractory to steroids and other treatment; resected spleens from steroid treated patients rarely show most of the features listed previously

Selected References

Sandier SG: The spleen and splenectomy in immune (idiopathic) thrombocytopenic purpura. Semin Hematol 37(1 Suppl 1):10-12, 2000.

McMillan R: The pathogenesis of chronic immune (idiopathic) thrombocytopenic purpura. Semin Hematol 37(1 Suppl 1):5-9, 2000.

Hassan NM, Neiman RS: The pathology of the spleen in steroid-treated immune thrombocytopenic purpura. Am J Clin Pathol 84:433-438, 1985.

Neoplastic Diseases Involving the Splenic Red Pulp

Hairy Cell Leukemia

Clinical Features

- Occurs in middle age with marked male predominance
- Splenomegaly, anemia, and infections
- Lymphadenopathy is absent
- Hairy cells are not always found in the blood or marrow aspirate smear
- Monocytopenia is almost always present in the peripheral blood
- Bone marrow is involved in more than 95% of patients; diagnosis is often confirmed by flow cytometry; the most specific marker is CD103
- Bone marrow biopsy shows the characteristic cellular infiltrates associated with fibrosis; in some cases, however, the infiltration might be subtle, and its identification may be greatly facilitated by immunohistology of the bone marrow biopsy (e.g., with DBA.44 and anti-TRAP antibodies)

Gross Pathology

- Marked splenomegaly
- Diffuse enlargement with uniform firm, dark-red appearance
- Infarcts may be observed
- Bone marrow fibrosis (dry tap)

Histopathology

- Infiltrate is extremely homogeneous and diffusely expands the red pulp

- The cells are found both within the cords and intrasinusoidally
- Cells have oval nuclei and abundant pale eosinophilic cytoplasm
- Hairlike cytoplasmic projections may be seen on touch preparations or peripheral blood and bone marrow smears
- White pulp may be atrophic or totally obliterated by the expanded red pulp
- Virtually lack mitotic activity
- Red cell lakes (pseudosinuses) lined by hairy cells
- Erythrophagocytosis and extramedullary hematopoiesis are usually absent
- In rare cases, the presence of marked congestion of the red pulp with dispersal of hairy cells can make their recognition difficult (immunohistology beneficial)
- Rare hairy cell leukemia variants characterized by larger cells or cells with blastic morphology have been reported; in these cases, the diagnosis relies on a hairy cell–like pattern of tissue involvement and an immunophenotypic profile, both consistent with hairy cell leukemia

Special Stains and Immunohistochemistry

- Reticulin: branching network of reticulin that surrounds individual cells
- Hairy cell leukemia is a low-grade B-cell lymphoid neoplasm; the cells are strongly positive with CD20
- TRAP positive in hairy cells
- DBA.44 and annexin A1: hairy cells positive

Other Techniques for Diagnosis

- Flow cytometry: hairy cells express CD103, CD19, CD20, CD11c, CD25, FMC7, and sIg
- Electron microscopy: ribosome-lamellar complexes are characteristic of but not specific to this tumor

Differential Diagnosis

- Marginal zone B-cell lymphoma
  - Predominant infiltration of white pulp as opposed to the diffuse red pulp expansion in hairy cell leukemia
  - Cells are usually negative for CD103, CD11c, CD25, TRAP, and annexin A1
  - Pattern of bone marrow infiltration is different (usually multinodular)
- CLL/SLL
  - Cells with less cytoplasm
  - Weakly positive for CD20 and sIg
  - Positive for CD5, CD23, and often CD38
  - Negative for TRAP, CD103, and annexin A1
- Mast cell disease
  - Morphologic features are only superficially similar
  - Mastocytosis has usually more fibrosis
  - Capsular, trabecular, and perifollicular distribution
  - Different cytochemistry and immunophenotype results

Figure 15-19. Hairy cell leukemia. Monomorphous infiltrate is seen in the red pulp. Notice a poorly demarcated red cell lake.

■ Myeloid leukemias
  ● Blastic proliferation and high mitotic activity in acute myeloid leukemia and myeloid sarcoma
  ● Polymorphism and maturation to neutrophils in chronic myeloid leukemias (e.g., chronic myelomonocytic leukemia)
  ● Different peripheral blood and bone marrow findings
  ● Different cytochemistry and immunophenotype results

Pearls

● Seen predominantly in older males
● Associated with blood lakes (peliosis)
● Characteristic flow cytometric and immunohistologic profile
● One of the most successfully treatable indolent lymphoproliferative diseases
● Splenectomy is now rarely needed for either diagnosis or therapy

Selected References

Burke JS, Rappaport H: The diagnosis and differential diagnosis of hairy cell leukemia in bone marrow and spleen. Semin Oncol 11:334-346, 1984.

Bearman RM, Kjeldsberg CR, Pangalis GA, Rappaport H: Chronic monocytic leukemia in adults. Cancer 48:2239-2255, 1981.

Hepatosplenic T-Cell Lymphoma

Clinical Features

● Occurs in young adults, with male predominance
● May be associated with long-term immunosuppressive therapy (e.g., after transplantation)
● Presents with severe hepatosplenomegaly, cytopenias, and B symptoms
● Usually no lymphadenopathy is seen at presentation
● Bone marrow involvement is a constant feature

Gross Pathology

● Massive splenomegaly
● Homogeneous cut surface with loss of white pulp

Histopathology

● Diffuse expansion of the red pulp cords and sinuses
● Sinuses filled with sheets of neoplastic cells are commonly seen
● Loss of the white pulp

Special Stains and Immunohistochemistry

● Neoplastic cells express CD3 and CD56 and are negative for CD4, CD8, CD5, and frequently, for CD7

Other Techniques for Diagnosis

● $\gamma\delta$ TCR can be demonstrated by flow cytometry
● Rare $\alpha\beta$ TCR–positive cases have been reported
● Isochromosome 7q is a defining cytogenetic abnormality in hepatosplenic T-cell lymphoma

Differential Diagnosis

■ CLL/SLL
  ● Involve both white and red pulp
  ● Cells weakly positive for CD20 and sIg
■ Hairy cell leukemia
  ● Predominantly a red pulp infiltrate with blood lakes
  ● Cells with fine, hairlike cytoplasmic processes may be seen in peripheral blood
  ● Distinct immunophenotype: B-cells positive for TRAP, DBA.44, CD25, CD11c, and CD103
■ Prolymphocytic leukemia
  ● Prolymphocytes are medium-sized cells with vesicular nuclei and prominent nucleoli

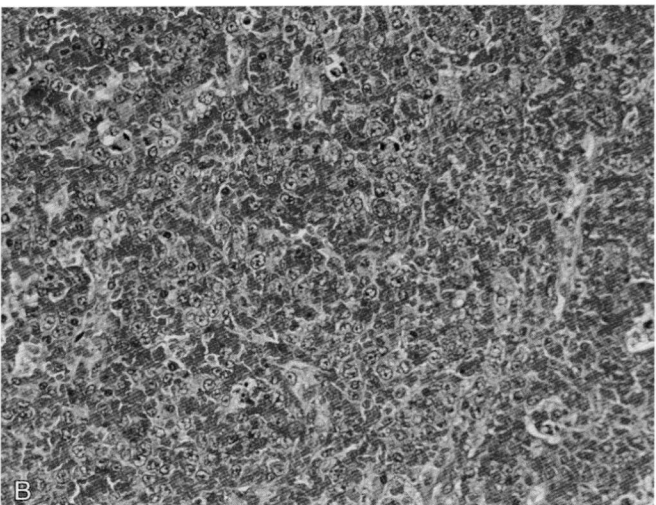

Figure 15-20. Hepatosplenic T-cell lymphoma. A, Numerous neoplastic T cells distending splenic sinuses. **B,** Large neoplastic T cells can be seen in cases of hepatosplenic T-cell lymphoma, particularly at the time of disease progression.

- Patients typically present with high white blood cell counts
- B-cell immunophenotype is seen: high-density CD20, CD19, CD22, and sIg
▮ Large granular lymphocytic leukemia
  - Cells may occasionally look similar in fixed tissue, and both involve red pulp
  - No fibrosis
  - CD3, CD8, CD57, CD16, and CD56 are variably positive

Pearls

- Massive hepatosplenomegaly in a solid organ transplant recipient on immunosuppression is not an uncommon presentation of hepatosplenic T-cell lymphoma
- Bone marrow involvement is common; the typical intravascular infiltration is best visualized using immunohistochemical stains (e.g., for CD3)

Selected References

Vega F, Medeiros LJ, Gaulard P: Hepatosplenic and other γδ T-cell lymphomas. Am J Clin Pathol 127:869-880, 2007.

Neiman RS, Orazi A: Lymphomas of the spleen. In Disorders of the Spleen, 2nd ed. Philadelphia, WB Saunders, 1999, pp 109-136.

Systemic Mastocytosis

Clinical Features

- Rare disorder
- Spleen is often involved, and most patients have palpable splenomegaly
- Most patients have urticaria pigmentosa or other systemic manifestations of mast cell activity at diagnosis

Gross Pathology

- Splenomegaly
- Thickened splenic capsule
- Multifocal ill-defined nodules with associated fibrosis and sclerosis; calcification may be present

Histopathology

- Mast cells form aggregates and nodules associated with a variable degree of fibrosis, often associated with eosinophils, which are more numerous at the periphery of the aggregates
- The nodules are often perivascular; they may also display peritrabecular and perifollicular distribution
- In routine hematoxylin and eosin (H&E)-stained sections, mast cells have mature indented nuclei and abundant cytoplasm with well-defined borders (fried-egg appearance)
- The mast cells may, however, resemble monocytes, monocytoid B cells, or hairy cells, particularly because in routine H&E-stained sections, their granules are difficult to detect
- Splenic hilar lymph nodes may also be involved
- Bone marrow is usually involved

Special Stains and Immunohistochemistry

- Mast cells can be detected with specific esterase stain, Giemsa, toluidine blue, or other metachromatic stains, or by immunostains for tryptase, chymase, or CD117

Other Techniques for Diagnosis

- Immunoreactivity with tryptase and CD25 (and often CD2), whose aberrant expression is limited to neoplastic mast cells, is usually sufficient to confirm the diagnosis

Figure 15-21. Mastocytosis. A, Low power. Aggregates of mast cells within the red pulp. The neoplastic cells have abundant cytoplasm. Note the presence of peritrabecular and perivascular fibrosis. **B,** High power. Perifollicular localization is also characteristically seen.

- Serum tryptase persistently elevated (>20 ng/mL)
- Detection of activating *c-kit* mutation D816V

Differential Diagnosis

▌ Hairy cell leukemia
- Hairy cells form red cell lakes and lack significant fibrosis
- Mastocytosis has associated fibrosis, which may be diffuse or around the infiltrates
- Lineages are different, myeloid versus lymphoid, demonstrable by immunostains (hairy cells express lymphoid antigens and are negative for tryptase), flow cytometry, or molecular diagnostic techniques

▌ Large granular lymphocytic leukemia
- Cells may occasionally look similar in fixed tissue, and both involve red pulp
- No fibrosis
- CD3, CD8, CD57, CD16, and CD56 are variably positive
- Mast cell tryptase and CD117 are negative

Pearls

- Splenomegaly is common
- Histologically, the mast cells may superficially resemble monocytes, hairy cells, or monocytoid B cells; the low-power appearance with fibrotic nodules and eosinophils is seen only in mastocytosis
- Mast cells have a distinctive immunophenotype

Selected References

Horny HP, Sotlar K, Valent P: Mastocytosis: State of the art. Pathobiology 74:121-132, 2007.

Horny HP, Ruck MT, Kaiserling E: Spleen findings in generalized mastocytosis: A clinicopathologic study. Cancer 70:459-468, 1992.

Brunning RD, McKenna RW, Rosai J, et al: Systemic mastocytosis: Extracutaneous manifestations. Am J Surg Pathol 7:425-438, 1983.

Chronic Myelogenous Leukemia

Clinical Features

- Patients usually present with leukocytosis with significant neutrophilia and a variable proportion of immature myeloid cells and basophilia
- Splenomegaly common at presentation

Gross Pathology

- Solid, deep-red, homogeneous appearance
- No malpighian corpuscles visible

Histopathology

- White pulp is usually obliterated
- Red pulp cords and sinuses show a polymorphic infiltration by myeloid cells at all stages of maturation with a predominance of mature granulocytes

Figure 15-22. Chronic myelogenous leukemia, blastic phase. Diffuse infiltration of the red pulp by leukemic blasts. Acute transformation may manifest itself in the spleen (extramedullary transformation).

- Occasionally blastic transformation is first identified in the spleen
- Bone marrow is always involved

Special Stains and Immunohistochemistry

- Naphthol-AS-D chloracetate esterase stain and antibodies such as myeloperoxidase or lysozyme can be used to facilitate the identification of myeloid cells
- Decreased neutrophil alkaline phosphatase (NAP)
- A combination of blastic reactive markers such as CD34, CD117, and TdT can be used to confirm extramedullary (splenic) blastic transformation, and a panel of lineage-specific antibodies (e.g., MPO, lysozyme, CD79a, PAX5, CD3) is valuable in characterizing its type (e.g., myeloid transformation versus lymphoid or megakaryocytic)

Other Techniques for Diagnosis

- Identification of Philadelphia chromosome translocation t(9;22) by karyotype analysis, PCR, or FISH in blood, marrow, or splenic tissue is necessary to confirm a diagnosis of chronic myelogenous leukemia
- Some patients with the disease are initially negative for Philadelphia chromosome by cytogenetics but are subsequently found to positive for *bcr-abl* translocation by PCR or FISH
- In cases of blastic transformation, flow cytometry is useful to confirm the presence of blast and evaluate their lineage

Differential Diagnosis

- The histologic features are classic, particularly in view of the peripheral blood findings
- In selected cases, cytochemistry for naphthyl butyrate esterase or reactivity with antibody to histiocytic

markers may be helpful in separating extramedullary chronic myelogenous leukemia from chronic myelomonocytic leukemia or other types of Ph'-negative myeloid neoplasms

- **Reactive splenic red pulp hyperplasia**
  - Usually part of a nonspecific stress response process, which may be associated with a leukemoid reaction in the blood, or related to chronic congestive hypersplenism
  - Basophilia is uncommon
  - Elevated NAP
  - Normal cytogenetics
- **Acute leukemia**
  - Differential diagnosis is with blast crisis of chronic myelogenous leukemia
  - History of chronic phase disease or cytogenetic demonstration of t(9;22) is needed

Pearls

- Associated with the Philadelphia chromosome t(9;22) or *bcr-abl* gene translocation
- Prominent splenomegaly with predominant involvement of red pulp
- Almost all patients eventually undergo a blastic transformation, which is associated with a poor outcome
- In pediatric patients, chronic myelogenous leukemia, adult type, needs to be distinguished from juvenile myelomonocytic leukemia; in spleen sections, however, the two conditions largely overlap

Selected References

Pinkus GS, Pinkus JL: Myeloperoxidase: A specific marker for myeloid cells in paraffin sections. Mod Pathol 4:733-741, 1991.

Shepherd PC, Ganesan TS, Galton DA: Haematological classification of the chronic myeloid leukaemias. Baillieres Clin Haematol 1:877-906, 1987.

Burke JS: Surgical pathology of the spleen: An approach to the differential diagnosis of splenic lymphomas and leukemias. Part II. Diseases of the red pulp. Am J Surg Pathol 5:681-694, 1981.

Langerhans Cell Histiocytosis

Clinical Features

- Splenic involvement occurs in infants and young children with the disseminated form of the disease (Letterer-Siwe disease)
- Presenting symptoms include fever and skin lesions

Gross Pathology

- Splenomegaly with diffuse red pulp enlargement

Histopathology

- Langerhans cell infiltration of the red pulp may be diffuse or multinodular (loose aggregates are granuloma-like), or rarely has large discrete tumor masses
- Cells have typical pale, bean-shaped nuclei and pale cytoplasm
- Eosinophils and plasma cells are usually also present, although are much less numerous than in the localized form of the disease

Special Stains and Immunohistochemistry

- CD1a, S-100 protein, and CD68 (KP-1) positive
- CD68R (PG-M1) negative

Other Techniques for Diagnosis

- Electron microscopy to demonstrate Birbeck granules

Differential Diagnosis

- **Disseminated juvenile xanthogranuloma (JXG)**
  - Nuclei not bean shaped
  - The characteristic Touton giant cell may be either absent or present in reduced numbers in the various extracutaneous lesions when compared with JXG in the skin
  - Immunohistochemistry: the histiocytic cells are positive for CD68 and factor XIIIa and negative for S-100 protein and CD1a
- **Gaucher disease (and other lysosomal storage diseases)**
  - Infants present with neurologic deterioration and organomegaly; skin is not involved
  - Absence of eosinophils
  - Nuclei not bean shaped
  - Cells usually larger than Langerhans cells
  - Cytoplasm abundant, with wrinkled-silk pattern in Gaucher disease
  - Cells PAS positive in most cases; S-100 protein and CD1a negative
- **Hemophagocytic syndromes**
  - Patients are systemically ill with cytopenias (similar to Letterer-Siwe disease)
  - Cells contain red cells, leukocytes, and iron
  - CD68 positive; S-100 protein and CD1a negative
- ***Mycobacterium avium-intracellulare***
  - Extremely rare in infants
  - Patients usually have evidence of immune deficiency
  - Special stains for acid-fast bacilli, PAS, and Gomori methenamine silver (GMS) reveal organisms in the cells
- **Hairy cell leukemia**
  - Not reported in children
  - Cells with abundant cytoplasm, forming pseudosinuses
  - Eosinophils rare
  - CD20, TRAP, DBA.44, and CD103 positive; S-100 protein and CD1a negative
- **Acute myeloid leukemia, particularly acute monoblastic leukemia**
  - Presents with cytopenias and peripheral blood or bone marrow involvement

Figure 15-23. Hemophagocytic syndrome in a pediatric patient. Marked hyperplasia of cordal and intravascular macrophages. A similar appearance may be seen in patients with hemolytic anemia or those that were hypertransfused.

- Blasts have large nuclei with finely dispersed chromatin and scanty to variably abundant cytoplasm depending on the acute myeloid leukemia subtype
- Mitoses more numerous than in Langerhans cell histiocytosis

▌ Malignant histiocytosis
- Patients are seriously ill with profound cytopenias
- Bone marrow usually shows diffuse involvement
- Rarely presents as isolated splenomegaly
- Red pulp infiltration may be associated with prominent necrosis
- Highly atypical cells with pleomorphic nuclei, which can be bean shaped and eccentric with prominent nucleoli and irregularly clumped chromatin; giant cells may resemble Reed-Sternberg cells

- Mitoses much more numerous than in Langerhans cell histiocytosis
- Erythrophagocytosis is seen in reactive macrophages and rarely in the tumor cells
- May express S-100 protein but is always CD1a negative; expresses histiocytic markers (e.g., CD68, CD163)

Pearls
- Patients usually have skin, liver, and lymph node involvement
- Diagnosis is more readily made from bone marrow biopsy
- Splenic involvement is more likely to be seen at autopsy than in a surgical specimen

Selected References

Pileri SA, Grogan TM, Harris NL, et al: Tumours of histiocytes and accessory dendritic cells: An immunohistochemical approach to classification from the International Lymphoma Study Group based on 61 cases. Histopathology 41:1-29, 2002.

Herzog KM, Tubbs RR: Langerhans cell histiocytosis. Adv Anat Pathol 5:347-358, 1998.

Vardiman JW, Byrne GE Jr, Rappaport H: Malignant histiocytosis with massive splenomegaly in asymptomatic patients: A possible chronic form of the disease. Cancer 36:419-427, 1975.

Vascular Tumors

Splenic Hemangioma

Clinical Features
- Most frequent in young to middle-aged adults with no sex predilection
- Usually asymptomatic

Figure 15-24. Hemangioma. A, Cut surface. In addition to the dilated vessels and cystic spaces, there are pale, spongy tumor nodules around dilated vessels. The intervening parenchyma looks normal. **B,** Photomicrograph. The dilated blood vessels of the tumor are surrounded by red pulp cordal macrophages.

- Symptoms and abnormalities reported include
  — Abdominal discomfort
  — Hypersplenism with cytopenias
  — Consumption coagulopathy (disseminated intravascular coagulation)

Gross Pathology

- Single, sometimes multiple masses
- Spleen normal to moderately enlarged
- Masses are well circumscribed but not encapsulated
- Reddish-purple and spongy
- Secondary changes may include infarct or fibrosis
- Angiomatosis is diffuse replacement of the spleen by angiomatous tissue

Histopathology

- Most are cavernous hemangiomas
- Interconnected vascular channels of varying size
- Channels may be thrombosed with focal infarction
- Endothelium is usually flattened but may be plump; no endothelial tufting
- Mitoses are usually absent (except in children)
- No cellular pleomorphism or hyperchromasia

Special Stains and Immunohistochemistry

- CD34, CD31, and factor VIII positive
- CD8, CD68, and Ki-67 negative

Other Techniques for Diagnosis

- Noncontributory

Differential Diagnosis

- ▌ Hematoma
  - Few or no blood vessels inside the mass
- ▌ Peliosis
  - Often associated with hepatic peliosis
  - More often multifocal or diffuse
  - Dilated sinuses with attenuated lining cells
  - Sinus lining cells CD8 and CD68 positive
  - Concentrated at the periphery of white pulp follicles (not a diffuse red pulp lesion)
- ▌ Littoral cell angioma
  - More often multifocal
  - Endothelial cells plumper than in hemangiomas
  - Endothelial cells are CD68 and CD163 positive and CD34 negative; in contrast with normal littoral cells, they are negative for CD8; CD21 and S-100 protein have also been reported
- ▌ Hemangioendothelioma
  - Greater cytologic atypia, for example, plump endothelial cells with hyperchromatic nuclei
  - Epithelioid and spindle cell variants
  - Endothelial cell forming papillary projections protruding into vascular spaces
  - Low to absent mitotic activity and lack of necrosis and invasive growth

- ▌ Angiosarcoma
  - Splenomegaly in elderly patients with fatigue, fever, weight loss, and abdominal pain
  - Poorly delineated, often necrotic large masses that may involve the entire organ
  - Papillary cell proliferation producing tufts and partially filling vascular spaces
  - Anastomosing vascular channels may be alternating with solid poorly differentiated areas
  - Nuclear pleomorphism, hyperchromasia, and atypia
  - Frequent mitoses
  - Infiltrative growth pattern
  - CD31 is the best marker; expression of other endothelial antigens is variable
- ▌ Splenic hamartoma
  - Usually a single mass that is bulging and fleshy
  - Color similar to splenic red pulp
  - Contains both cords and sinus structures (the latter CD8 positive)
  - Endothelia are positive with CD8 and negative for CD68 and CD21
  - A hamartoma variant termed *cordal hamartoma* is morphologically similar to cases of capillary hemangiomas with sclerosis and may represent the same entity
  - Another lesion related to hamartoma is myoid angioendothelioma, a rare benign tumor of the spleen, which is morphologically characterized by a composite of vascular spaces and stromal cells with myoid features
- ▌ Lymphangioma
  - Mostly occurs in children
  - Grossly indistinguishable
  - Gross cyst formation is common
  - Spaces contain proteinaceous material, lymph, and cholesterol clefts (not blood)
  - D2-40, CD31, and factor VIII positive; CD34 usually negative

Pearls

- Microangiopathic hemolytic anemia and platelet consumption have been reported with large lesions

Selected Reference

Arber DA, Strickler JG, Chen YY, Weiss LM: Splenic vascular tumors: A histologic, immunophenotypic, and virologic study. Am J Surg Pathol 21:827-835, 1997.

Littoral Cell Angioma

Clinical Features

- Rare
- Occurs at any age and in either sex
- May cause splenomegaly and hypersplenism

Figure 15-25. Littoral cell angioma. A, Rarely the whole spleen can be replaced by a spongy hemorrhagic, vaguely nodular proliferation. This may raise the possibility of an angiosarcoma. **B,** At this magnification, the larger size and more cuboidal to hobnail pattern of the cells lining the vascular spaces is apparent. These cells do not have the nuclear pleomorphism, atypia, or mitotic activity seen in more aggressive vascular tumors.

Gross Pathology

- Single or multiple spongy, purplish-black, well-circumscribed nodules
- Rarely may replace the whole organ
- Sometimes is only vaguely multinodular; in other cases, it may appear subdivided into lobules by bands of fibrosis

Histopathology

- Pleomorphic vascular spaces: from slitlike to dilated and cystic
- Lined by tall endothelial cells with large vesicular nuclei
- Papillary projections protruding into the vascular spaces
- Tumor cells can exfoliate into the lumen
- No significant cellular atypia, and mitotic activity is low
- Lacks solid areas and necrosis

Special Stains and Immunohistochemistry

- Reticulin: annular fibers around vascular spaces
- Occasional PAS-positive cytoplasmic globules
- Distinctive phenotype: CD31, CD68, and CD68R (both KP-1 and PG-M1), CD21, and CD163 positive; negative for CD8 and CD34; may also express S-100 protein

Other Techniques for Diagnosis

- Noncontributory

Differential Diagnosis

▌ Hairy cell leukemia
  - Diffuse red pulp infiltrate
  - Bone marrow almost always involved
  - Abnormal cells may be present in peripheral blood
  - CD20, CD25, TRAP, and DBA.44 positive; CD31 and CD68 negative

▌ Hemangioma
  - No irregular anastomosing channels
  - More often single
  - Vascular spaces lined by flattened cells
  - CD68 negative
▌ Splenic hamartoma
  - Usually a single mass that is bulging and fleshy
  - Color similar to splenic red pulp
  - Contains both cords and sinus structures (the latter CD8 positive)
  - Endothelia are positive for CD8 and negative for CD68 and CD21
▌ Hemangioendothelioma
  - Patients may have disease outside the spleen
  - Endothelial cells have hyperchromatic nuclei
  - Epithelioid or spindle-shaped endothelia
  - Endothelial cells are more often negative for CD68
▌ Angiosarcoma
  - Elderly patients
  - Greater splenic enlargement
  - Necrosis
  - Infiltrative growth pattern
  - Papillary cell proliferation producing tufts and partially filling vascular spaces
  - More mitoses
  - Nuclear pleomorphism, atypia, and hyperchromasia
  - Endothelial cells are more often negative for CD68
  - Metastases are not uncommon

Pearls

- Littoral cell angioma is benign despite multifocality
- No counterpart outside the spleen
- Extremely rare aggressive counterparts have been described (littoral cell angioendothelioma and littoral cell angiosarcoma)

Selected References

Arber DA, Strickler JG, Chen YY, Weiss LM: Splenic vascular tumors: A histologic, immunophenotypic, and virologic study. Am J Surg Pathol 21:827-835, 1997.

Rosso R, Paulli M, Gianelli U, et al: Littoral cell angiosarcoma of the spleen: Case report with immunohistochemical and ultrastructural analysis. Am J Surg Pathol 19:1203-1208, 1995.

Falk S, Stutte HJ, Frizzera G: Littoral cell angioma: A novel splenic vascular lesion demonstrating histiocytic differentiation. Am J Surg Pathol 15:1023-1033, 1991.

Splenic Angiosarcoma

Clinical Features

- Although it can occur at any age, it is most common in elderly patients; no sex predominance

Figure 15-26. Splenic angiosarcoma. A, In this case of splenic angiosarcoma, most of the organ is replaced by a neoplastic proliferation characterized by a mixture of spongy and solid areas with extensive necrosis and hemorrhages. **B,** Pleomorphic neoplastic endothelial cells with a high nuclear-to-cytoplasmic ratio and hyperchromatic nuclei lining the vascular spaces. Some of the cells appear to be floating free in the vascular spaces. Mitotic figures could be found easily. Outside the obvious vascular spaces are solid areas composed of cells similar to those lining the larger vascular spaces. Red cells are present in the vascular lumina.

- Not associated with vinyl chloride or thorium dioxide (Thorotrast) exposure
- Can cause splenic rupture
- Fatigue, fever, weight loss, and abdominal pain
- Cytopenias have been reported
- Prognosis is poor: hematogenous metastases to liver and lung

Gross Pathology

- Splenomegaly, often marked (weight > 1000 g common)
- Single or multiple hemorrhagic and necrotic masses
- Sometimes diffuse infiltration, blending with splenic red pulp

Histopathology

- Cellular appearances, degree of differentiation and proliferation vary within and between tumors
- Irregular anastomosing vascular channels or solid masses partially or largely occluding vascular spaces
- Cells may be flattened, spindled, polygonal, epithelioid, or small and poorly differentiated; may form papillary projections that protrude into vascular spaces
- Cytologic atypia varies from slightly prominent endothelial cells with slight hyperplasia, pleomorphism, and occasional mitoses to anaplastic cells with numerous mitoses, associated with areas of hemorrhage and necrosis
- Extramedullary hematopoiesis and erythrophagocytosis can both be found in some cases

Special Stains and Immunohistochemistry

- Expression of common endothelial cell antigens is variable but CD31 and *Ulex* lectin are usually positive
- CD34 and factor VIII are usually detected in better differentiated areas only; CD163 is negative
- Positivity for CD68 and CD8 suggests a littoral cell derivation (littoral cell angiosarcoma)
- Expression of D2-40, a marker of differentiation along the lymphatic endothelial lineage, has been reported in some cases; these cases could be classified as lymphangiosarcomas

Other Techniques for Diagnosis

- Electron microscopy: Weibel-Palade bodies

Differential Diagnosis

▮ Hemangioma
- Lacks pleomorphism, mitoses, atypia, and necrosis
- Vascular channels lined by a single layer of uniform cells
- These may thrombose, but otherwise there is no necrosis

▮ Hemangioendothelioma
- Differentiation from angiosarcoma may be subtle
- No necrosis

- Less prominent papillary formation
- Less pleomorphism, less atypia, fewer mitoses, and less nuclear hyperchromasia

▌ Hemangiopericytoma (see Chapter 17)
- Staghorn vascular channels
- No necrosis
- Usually few mitoses
- Little or no cellular pleomorphism
- Endothelial cells lining the vascular spaces are a single layer of flattened cells with no atypia
- The proliferating spindle cells surround rather than form the vascular spaces
- Proliferating cells have smooth muscle differentiation (α-smooth muscle actin (α-SMA), muscle-specific actin positive)
- Reticulin, CD34, and CD31 are often helpful
- It may correspond to myopericytoma (see "Pearls")

▌ Kaposi sarcoma
- Elderly men of Mediterranean ancestry or patients with acquired immunodeficiency syndrome (AIDS)
- Usually forms small nodules
- Composed of spindle cells without papillary formation or vascular channels (except for vessels at the periphery of the nodules)
- No necrosis or hemorrhage
- Slitlike vascular spaces with eosinophilic globules
- Hemosiderin (can also be present in angiosarcoma)
- Immunohistochemistry positivity for D2-40, CD34, and HHV-8

▌ Bacillary angiomatosis
- Typically younger individuals; increased incidence in AIDS patients
- No anastomosing vascular channels
- Few mitoses, little or no pleomorphism
- Grayish interstitial material
- Bacteria identified using Warthin-Starry stain
- HHV-8 negative

▌ Metastatic melanoma
- Patients usually have a history of melanoma elsewhere
- Pigment may be melanin
- No vascular channels
- CD34, CD31, and factor VIII negative
- S-100 protein, HMB-45, and melan-A positive
- Electron microscopy can show melanosomes

▌ Malignant fibrous histiocytoma
- Rarely primary in spleen
- No anastomosing vascular channels
- Multinucleated giant cells may be present
- Vimentin, α$_1$-antichymotrypsin, α$_1$-antitrypsin, and CD68 positive; CD31 and factor VIII negative

Pearls
- The existence of hemangiopericytoma as a separate entity has been questioned because a number of neoplasms of different lines of differentiation are characterized by a hemangiopericytoma-like vascular growth pattern
- Myopericytoma represents a recently delineated entity showing a hemangiopericytoma-like vascular pattern; it is likely that at least a proportion of cases that have been previously termed *splenic hemangiopericytoma* may represent examples of myopericytoma
- Most cases of myopericytoma behave in a benign fashion, but local recurrences and rarely metastases have been reported; more recently, a malignant variant has also been described

Selected References

Granter SR, Badizadegan K, Fletcher CD: Myofibromatosis in adults, glomangiopericytoma, and myopericytoma: A spectrum of tumors showing perivascular myoid differentiation. Am J Surg Pathol 22:513-525, 1998.

Falk S, Krishnan J, Meis JM: Primary angiosarcoma of the spleen: A clinicopathologic study of 40 cases. Am J Surg Pathol 17:959-970, 1993.

Cysts and Pseudotumoral Lesions

Epidermoid Cyst (True Cysts)

Clinical Features
- Occurs in children to young adults; no gender predominance
- Unrelated to trauma
- Most likely of mesothelial derivation

Gross Pathology
- Single or, rarely, multiple lesions
- Cyst has a trabeculated appearance covered by a shiny lining
- Fluid clear to turbid and yellowish; can contain cholesterol crystals

Figure 15-27. Epidermoid splenic cyst. The wall is thicker, and its trabeculation may be reminiscent of the endocardial surface of the ventricular cavities. The cyst contained clear fluid.

Histopathology

- Thin, fibrous wall with epithelial lining
- Epithelium may be attenuated or denuded
- Epithelium can be squamous, transitional, or columnar

Special Stains and Immunohistochemistry

- Cytokeratin stains highlight the epithelium

Other Techniques for Diagnosis

- Noncontributory

Differential Diagnosis

▌ Pseudocyst
- No epithelial lining
▌ Parasitic (echinococcal) cyst
- Adults are most commonly affected
- Resident in areas of the world where the parasite is endemic (e.g., Greece); in the United States, the disease is rare, but it has been reported in several states (see also "Parasitic [Echinococcal] Cyst")
- Usually requires significant exposure to animal vectors
- Cyst is often multilocular
- Hepatic or peritoneal cysts commonly present
- Granular wall with small granules in cyst contents
- Scolices in wall or secondary cysts

Pearls

- Usually asymptomatic unless infected
- Not known if these are congenital developmental abnormalities or the result of abdominal trauma with mesothelial entrapment in the spleen

Pseudocyst

Clinical Features

- Four times as common as epithelial cyst
- Clinical presentation identical to that of epithelial cyst
- Believed to result from degradation of a splenic hematoma of post-traumatic origin or to be a consequence of cystic degeneration of a splenic infarct or hemangioma

Gross Pathology

- Same as for epithelial cyst, but fluid is usually darker reddish-brown

Histopathology

- Smooth internal surface (rather than trabeculated)
- Fibrous wall *without* epithelial lining
- Calcification in wall
- Cholesterol clefts can be present

Special Stains and Immunohistochemistry

- Cytokeratin negative

Other Techniques for Diagnosis

- Noncontributory

Differential Diagnosis

▌ Epithelioid cyst
- Epithelial lining present
▌ Parasitic cyst
- See "Parasitic (Echinococcal) Cyst"

Pearls

- Usually asymptomatic unless infected
- Large cysts can rupture; resection is recommended
- Can also be drained under radiologic guidance but are more likely to recur
- Thought to be related to splenic trauma and organizing hematoma

Parasitic (Echinococcal) Cyst

Clinical Features

- Occurs in residents of areas of the world where the parasite is endemic (e.g., Greece); in the United States, the disease is rare but has been reported in California, Arizona, New Mexico, and Utah
- Adults are most commonly affected; patients usually have significant exposure to animal vectors; risk factors include exposure to cattle, sheep, pigs, or deer or exposure to the feces of dogs, wolves, or coyotes
- Cysticercosis can produce grossly similar cysts, differing in the nature of the parasite

Gross Pathology

- Often multilocular
- Hepatic or peritoneal cysts commonly present
- Granular wall with small granules in cyst contents

Histopathology

- Fibrous wall
- Daughter cysts or brood capsules contain parasites with scolices
- Inflammatory reaction is present

Special Stains and Immunohistochemistry

- Noncontributory

Other Techniques for Diagnosis

- Smears of fluid or touch preparations of cyst wall reveal scolices
- Scolices are acid fast

Differential Diagnosis

▌ Epithelioid cyst (see "Epidermoid Cyst [True Cysts])
- No inflammation
- No scolices
- Epithelial lining

■ Pseudocyst (see "Pseudocyst")
- No inflammation
- No scolices

Pearls

- Intraoperative rupture of the cyst with leakage of cyst contents can cause peritoneal dissemination of the disease and can be fatal

Selected References

Hulzebos CV, Leemans R, Halma C, de Vries TW: Splenic epithelial cysts and splenomegaly: Diagnosis and management. Neth J Med 53:80-84, 1998.

Garvin DF, King FM: Cysts and nonlymphomatous tumors of the spleen. Pathol Ann 16:61-80, 1981.

Splenic Hamartoma (Splenoma)

Clinical Features

- Occurs at any age
- Usually asymptomatic
- Rarely causes abdominal pain or thrombocytopenia

Gross Pathology

- Usually single nodule
- Size ranges from less than 1 cm to about 10 cm
- Color usually resembles splenic red pulp
- Bulging from cut surface
- Fleshy consistency
- Well circumscribed but not encapsulated
- Can have foci of infarction and fibrosis

Figure 15-28. A, Splenic hamartoma (splenoma), gross photograph. Hamartoma presents as a well-demarcated, bulging lesion displaying a characteristic "red pulp only" appearance. **B, Splenic hamartoma.** Flattened endothelial cells line irregular vascular spaces, which are surrounded by disorganized red pulp tissue. Unlike a hemangioma, both the blood vessels and other red pulp spaces are disorganized. **C, Splenic hamartoma (splenoma), cordal variant.** A predominance of cordal macrophages is noted. Occasionally, this may resemble an inflammatory pseudotumor.

Histopathology

- A tumor-like lesion composed of structurally disorganized splenic red pulp tissue
- Resembles normal red pulp with no "organized" white pulp within the lesion; may, however, contain scattered lymphocytes
- Consists of both cordal and sinus-like structures
- Compressed red pulp at the periphery, but no true capsule
- Can have foci of infarction and fibrosis, sometimes with hemosiderin deposition
- May contain immature hematopoietic cells and eosinophils
- May show fibrosis
- Cases of "sclerosing" capillary hemangioma may represent the same entity; these have been termed *cordal hamartomas*
- A histiocyte-rich variant has also been described

Special Stains and Immunohistochemistry

- Endothelia are positive for CD8 and negative for CD68 and CD21
- Reticulin stain shows a disorganized sinusoidal wall with partial loss of ring fibers

Other Techniques for Diagnosis

- Noncontributory

Differential Diagnosis

▌ Hemangioma
- Hemorrhagic, not fleshy or bulging
- Darker than red pulp
- Vascular endothelial differentiation only, no sinus-like structures
- CD34 positive; CD68 and CD8 negative

▌ Littoral cell angioma
- Often multifocal
- Dark, purplish-black, spongy
- Irregular vascular spaces all of one type
- Mostly polygonal to tall lining cells
- CD68 and CD21 positive

▌ IPT
- Usually paler than surrounding parenchyma
- Lacks sinus structures
- Numerous plasma cells and lymphocytes
- Prominent spindle cell component

Pearls

- There is still controversy about whether this is a true neoplasm or a hamartoma
- Always benign
- Occurs only in spleen

Selected References

Krishnan J, Frizzera G: Two splenic lesions in need of clarification: Hamartoma and inflammatory pseudotumor. Semin Diagn Pathol 20:94-104, 2003.

Hayes TC, Britton HA, Mewborne EB, et al: Symptomatic splenic hamartoma: Case report and literature review. Pediatrics 101:E10, 1998.

Inflammatory Pseudotumor of the Spleen

- This condition is also referred to as *plasma cell pseudotumor* and *inflammatory myofibroblastic tumor*, among many other terms

Clinical Features

- Occurs at any adult age
- Can be asymptomatic or present with fever, weight loss, or abdominal pain

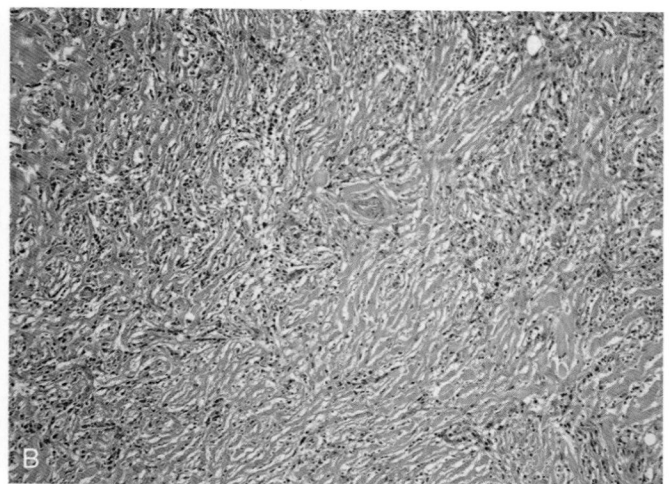

Figure 15-29. A, True inflammatory pseudotumor. Macrophages and relatively rare myofibroblasts are found associated with numerous inflammatory cells, particularly plasma cells. **B, Inflammatory pseudotumor (inflammatory myofibroblastic tumor).** The lesion has a predominance of spindle cells, mostly myofibroblasts, and resembles mesenchymal soft tissue tumor.

- Less common in spleen than in lung
- Rarely present in more than one organ in a given patient

Gross Pathology

- Size ranges from less than 1 cm up to 10 cm
- Usually single but can be multiple; multiple lesions are usually small
- Well circumscribed, pale to white, and bulging

Histopathology

- Splenic IPT includes at least three variants
  - A "truly inflammatory" IPT most commonly seen in older individuals
  - Inflammatory myofibroblastic tumor, which is in fact a neoplastic process that often harbors balanced chromosomal translocations involving the *ALK* gene that result in expression of ALK by immunohistochemistry
  - A rare form of IPT containing follicular dendritic cells (FDCs), termed *hepatosplenic IPT-like FDC tumor*, which consistently harbors clonal EBV DNA
- Irregularly oriented, bland spindle cells intermixed with variable numbers of lymphocytes, plasma cells, macrophages (which can be foamy), and neutrophils
- Eosinophils uncommon
- No proliferative activity or cellular atypia
- Occasional features: sclerosis, hemorrhage, necrosis, calcification, and hemosiderin deposits

Special Stains and Immunohistochemistry

- Spindle cells have smooth muscle differentiation: muscle-specific actin, SMA, sometimes desmin positive
- Clear-cut myofibroblastic differentiation is only seen in IPT of inflammatory myofibroblastic tumor type; a proportion of these cases are ALK positive
- In true inflammatory IPT, the epithelioid and spindle cells are positive for vimentin and CD68 but lack expression of follicular dendritic cell markers and actin
- IPT-like follicular dendritic cell tumor of the spleen shows positivity for CD21 (and CD35) and evidence of EBV infection by EBV-LMP immunostaining or EBV-RNA by in situ hybridization
- Lymphocytes are mostly T cells
- Plasma cells are polyclonal

Other Techniques for Diagnosis

- Gene rearrangement studies
- EBER in situ hybridization

Differential Diagnosis

▌ Splenic hamartoma
  - Nodules red and fleshy rather than pale
  - Contains sinus-like structures, no solid areas except in foci of fibrosis

- Less inflamed cellular background with fewer lymphocytes and plasma cells

▌ Castleman disease
  - More often multifocal; patients usually have lymph node involvement
  - Distinct germinal centers (hyalinized or hyperplastic) in the lesion
  - Spindle cells not prominent
  - Sheets of plasma cells present in plasma cell and multicentric type

▌ Hodgkin lymphoma
  - Patients have Hodgkin lymphoma elsewhere
  - Eosinophils more numerous
  - Hodgkin cells or classic Reed-Sternberg cells present

▌ Plasmacytoma
  - Occurs in older adults
  - Patients usually have known multiple myeloma
  - Sclerosis is rare (exception: an osteosclerotic variant associated with hepatosplenomegaly known as POEMS syndrome [polyneuropathy, organomegaly, endocrinopathy, monoclonal paraprotein, and skin hyperpigmentation])
  - Plasma cells are monoclonal

▌ Follicular dendritic cell sarcoma (versus IPT-like follicular dendritic cell tumor of the spleen)
  - Sheets of plump spindle cells
  - Infiltrative growth pattern
  - Cells are CD21 and CD35 positive and SMA negative
  - A small proportion of cases have been associated with Castleman disease of the hyaline-vascular type, and others with EBV infection

▌ Mycobacterial pseudotumor
  - Patients with AIDS
  - Most have mycobacteriosis elsewhere
  - Few spindle cells (exception is the rare mycobacterial spindle cell pseudotumor, a lesion seen in immunocompromised patients, composed of proliferative spindle cells admixed with histiocytes and inflammatory cells associated with the presence of *Mycobacterium avium-intracellulare*)
  - Consists of sheets of large macrophages with abundant gray cytoplasm, not foamy cells
  - Acid-fast stain positive
  - Culture for mycobacteria positive

▌ Bacillary angiomatosis
  - AIDS patients
  - Vascular proliferation
  - Gray interstitial material
  - Bacteria in interstitial material positive with Warthin-Starry stain
  - HHV-8 negative

Pearls

- IPT is not a single entity
- Its precise characterization relies on a combination of morphology and immunohistochemistry

Selected References

Brittig F, Ajtay E, Jakso P, Kelenyi G: Follicular dendritic reticulum cell tumor mimicking inflammatory pseudotumor of the spleen. Pathol Oncol Res 10:57-60, 2004.

Horiguchi H, Matsui-Horiguchi M, Sakata H, et al: Inflammatory pseudotumor-like follicular dendritic cell tumor of the spleen. Pathol Int 54:124-131, 2004.

Lewis JT, Gaffney RL, Casey MB, et al: Inflammatory pseudotumor of the spleen associated with a clonal Epstein-Barr virus genome: Case report and review of the literature. Am J Clin Pathol 120:56-61, 2003.

Sarker A, An C, Davis M, et al: Inflammatory pseudotumor of the spleen in a 6-year-old child: A clinicopathologic study. Arch Pathol Lab Med 127:e127-130, 2003.

Neiman RS, Orazi A: Splenic cysts, nonhematopoietic tumors, and tumorlike lesions. In Disorders of the Spleen, 2nd ed. Philadelphia, WB Saunders, 1999, pp 249-285.

Arber DA, Weiss LM, Chang KL: Detection of Epstein-Barr virus in inflammatory pseudotumor. Semin Diagn Pathol 15:155-160, 1998.

Thomas RM, Jaffe ES, Zarate-Osorno A, Medeiros LJ: Inflammatory pseudotumor of the spleen: A clinicopathologic and immunophenotypic study of eight cases. Arch Pathol Lab Med 117:921-926, 1993.

Circulatory Abnormalities

Congestive Splenomegaly

Clinical Features

- Occurs in patients with cirrhosis causing portal hypertension
- Occurs in patients with splenic vein thrombosis (e.g., in paroxysmal nocturnal hemoglobinuria or polycythemia vera)

Gross Pathology

- Moderate, diffuse splenic enlargement; weight usually less than 1 kg
- White pulp inconspicuous
- Red pulp dark, may be firm
- Small infarcts common in larger spleens

Histopathology

- White pulp histology is variable
- Diffuse expansion of the red pulp
- In early stages, the red pulp is more cellular, becomes fibrotic later
- Increased number of hemosiderin-laden macrophages
- Long-standing cases
  — Fibrosis with excess reticulin deposition in long-standing cases
  — The sinuses may become dilated (pulled open by the fibrosis)
  — It may resemble a capillary hemangioma with sclerosis or a hamartoma
  — Gamna-Gandy bodies can occur (for definition of Gamna-Gandy bodies, see "Sickle Cell Disease and Variants")

Special Stains and Immunohistochemistry

- Reticulin to show increased fibrosis throughout the red pulp
- Increased expression of SMA (splenic myoid cells)

Other Techniques for Diagnosis

- Noncontributory

Figure 15-30. Fibrocongestive splenomegaly (chronic passive congestion). A, High-power magnification of red pulp. Both cords and sinuses are distended and are surrounded by an increased amount of stroma, which imparts a rigid appearance to the red pulp. **B,** Increased expression of smooth muscle actin due to a reactive hyperplasia of splenic myoid cells is a characteristic finding seen in spleen with chronic passive congestion.

Differential Diagnosis

▌ Leukemic infiltration
  - Red pulp is diffusely infiltrated by blasts, small lymphocytes, or hairy cells depending on the type of leukemia
  - Immunohistochemistry to confirm the diagnosis of leukemia
▌ Lymphoma
  - Subtypes of lymphoid neoplasms involving the red pulp (e.g., hepatosplenic T-cell lymphoma, intravascular large B-cell lymphoma)
  - Intrasinusoidal lymphocytosis with cytologic atypia
  - Immunohistochemistry to confirm the diagnosis of lymphoma
▌ Myelofibrosis or other myeloproliferative disorders
  - Lesions are more discrete
  - Prominent extramedullary hematopoiesis, usually trilineage
  - Atypical megakaryocytes often present in chronic idiopathic myelofibrosis (primary myelofibrosis)
  - Cellularity often increased
▌ Peliosis
  - Lesions are more discrete
  - Dilated sinuses concentrated near white pulp follicles
  - Sinuses appear open, but there is no fibrosis

Pearls

- Congestive splenomegaly can cause hypersplenism in patients with liver cirrhosis
- Consider additional causes if spleen weight is greater than 1 kg
- Coagulation abnormalities in these patients are more commonly the result of liver disease

Selected References

Neiman RS, Orazi A: Chronic passive congestion. In Disorders of the Spleen, 2nd ed. Philadelphia, WB Saunders, 1999, pp 238-239.
O'Reilly RA: Splenomegaly in 2,505 patients at a large university medical center from 1913 to 1995. 1963 to 1995: 449 patients. West J Med 169:88-97, 1998.
Sheth SG, Amarapurkar DN, Chopra KB, et al: Evaluation of splenomegaly in portal hypertension. J Clin Gastroenterol 22:28-30, 1996.

Vasculitides

Polyarteritis Nodosa, Hypersensitivity Angiitis (Churg-Strauss Disease), Systemic Lupus Erythematosus, Rheumatoid Arthritis, and Thrombotic Thrombocytopenic Purpura

Clinical Features

- Rarely limited to the spleen; more commonly part of a systemic vasculitis

Figure 15-31. Vasculitis in a splenic vessel. The section shows fibrinoid necrosis.

Figure 15-32. Systemic lupus erythematosus. Small artery with concentric collagen formation around a vessel. This is also termed *onion-skinning.*

- Seen in patients with
  — Polyarteritis nodosa
  — Systemic lupus erythematosus
  — Rheumatoid arthritis
  — Thrombotic thrombocytopenic purpura
  — Hypersensitivity angiitis

Gross Pathology

- Multiple infarcts, which can be confluent
- Splenic rupture has been reported

Histopathology

- Vasculitis similar to the manifestation of the basic disease in other organs
- Infarcts can be present
▌ Polyarteritis nodosa
  - Small arteries
  - Fibrinoid necrosis

- Neutrophils and eosinophils in vessel walls
- Splenic rupture has been reported
▪ Hypersensitivity angiitis (Churg-Strauss disease)
  - Leukocytoclastic vasculitis in arterioles
  - Fibrinoid necrosis in small vessels
  - Eosinophils in infiltrate
▪ Systemic lupus erythematosus
  - Leukocytoclastic vasculitis in arterioles
  - Fibrinoid necrosis in small vessels
  - Onion-skin appearance in arterioles owing to concentric perivascular fibrosis
  - Plasmacytosis in red pulp
▪ Rheumatoid arthritis
  - Leukocytoclastic vasculitis in arterioles
  - Fibrinoid necrosis in small vessels
  - Splenomegaly in Felty syndrome
  - Follicular hyperplasia in white pulp
  - Lacks concentric perivascular fibrosis
▪ Thrombotic thrombocytopenic purpura
  - Platelet-fibrin thrombi in small vessels
  - Subendothelial PAS-positive hyaline deposits
  - Onion-skin periarteriolar fibrosis may occasionally be observed

Special Stains and Immunohistochemistry

- Elastic stains for vascular damage

Other Techniques for Diagnosis

- Direct immunofluorescence for fibrinogen, immunoglobulin, and complement deposits
- Serologic studies
- Antinuclear antibody test and other anti-DNA tests for lupus
- Rheumatoid factor in rheumatoid arthritis

Differential Diagnosis

- The differential diagnosis in cases of vasculitis includes each of the entities listed previously; additional diseases to consider include
▪ Thromboemboli
  - Patients usually have severe atherosclerotic cardiac disease, or left-sided endocarditis
  - Thromboembolic or atheroembolic material in arterioles
  - True vasculitis only with septic emboli and endocarditis
  - Elastic stain may be useful
▪ Postmortem clot
  - No lines of Zahn
  - No true vasculitis
  - No changes in splenic parenchyma
▪ Amyloidosis
  - Patients usually have systemic amyloidosis
  - Eosinophilic deposits around small blood vessels
  - No vasculitis
  - Congo red or thioflavin T stains positive

Pearls

- Splenic involvement in systemic vasculitis is rarely clinically significant
- In lupus and other autoimmune disorders, the changes previously described may have been substantially modified by antecedent therapy (e.g., steroids)
- Atypical lymphoid hyperplasia and rarely lymphoma may occur in patient treated with methotrexate for rheumatoid arthritis (methotrexate-associated lymphoproliferative disorders)
- Immunohistology for EBV may be helpful to confirm an immunosuppression associated etiology

Selected References

D'Cruz D: Vasculitis in systemic lupus erythematosus. Lupus 7:270-274, 1998.

Lhote F, Cohen P, Guillevin L: Polyarteritis nodosa, microscopic polyangiitis and Churg-Strauss syndrome. Lupus 7:238-258, 1998.

Danning CL, Illei GG, Boumpas DT: Vasculitis associated with primary rheumatologic diseases. Curr Opin Rheumatol 10:58-65, 1998.

Drenkard C, Villa AR, Reyes E, et al: Vasculitis in systemic lupus erythematosus. Lupus 6:235-242, 1997.

Nguyen VD: A rare cause of splenic infarct and fleeting pulmonary infiltrates: Polyarteritis nodosa. Comput Med Imaging Graph 15:61-65, 1991.

Viral and Other Nongranulomatous Infections

Infectious Mononucleosis

Clinical Features

- Most commonly affecting adolescents and young adults
- Patients have fever, malaise, and pharyngitis
- May have generalized lymphadenopathy and hepatosplenomegaly
- Caused by primary infection with EBV

Gross Pathology

- Mild to moderate splenomegaly with red pulp congestion and hyperplastic white pulp; rarely, massive spleen enlargement
- Spleen susceptible to spontaneous rupture

Histopathology

- Borders between red and white pulp are blurred
- Variable degree of follicular hyperplasia in white pulp
- Red pulp is expanded by a polymorphic cellular population, which includes pleomorphic lymphocytes, immunoblasts, and plasma cells
- PALS may be infiltrated by lymphoid cells, including immunoblasts

Figure 15-33. Infectious mononucleosis. High-power magnification shows a heterogeneous lymphoid population with numerous immunoblasts.

- Splenic trabeculae, capsule, and vessels are often infiltrated by lymphoid cells

Special Stains and Immunohistochemistry

- Immunohistochemical stains: large immunoblasts are positive for EBV, CD20, and often CD30
- Activated lymphoid population consists of mixed B-cells and T-lymphocytes with a predominance of CD8-positive cytotoxic T cells

Other Techniques for Diagnosis

- In situ hybridization for EBER is positive

Differential Diagnosis

▌ Large cell lymphoma or T-cell/histiocyte-rich large B-cell lymphoma
  - These generally form discrete masses in splenic parenchyma
  - Homogeneous population or B or T cells in large cell lymphomas; in T-cell/histiocyte-rich large B-cell lymphoma, the neoplastic B cells are scattered within a background of small T lymphocytes
▌ Hodgkin lymphoma
  - Usually forms discrete, grossly visible nodules rather than causing diffuse splenic enlargement
  - Neoplastic Hodgkin and Reed-Sternberg cells are scattered within lymphohistiocytic nodules; splenic follicles are normal or reactive
  - Eosinophils and plasma cells may be numerous in Hodgkin lymphoma and are rare in infectious mononucleosis
▌ Reactive lymphoid hyperplasia not related to EBV infection
  - May present similar histologic findings

- Immunohistochemical stains to exclude the presence of other viruses (e.g., cytomegalovirus [CMV]) and correlation with viral serology are necessary for definitive diagnosis

Pearls

- Patients with acute infectious mononucleosis may have acute splenomegaly and are at risk for spontaneous splenic rupture
- Infectious mononucleosis may be misinterpreted as malignant lymphoma or Hodgkin lymphoma owing to the massive immunoblastic proliferation, which may include Reed-Sternberg-like cells
- Detailed clinical history, EBV serology, and appropriate immunostains are helpful in the differential diagnosis

Selected References

Knobel B, Melamud E, Nofech-Moses S, et al: [Follicular splenic lymphoid hyperplasia associated with EBV infection]. Harefuah 137:449-451, 511, 1999.

Neiman RS, Orazi A: Reactive lymphoid hyperplasia. In Disorders of the Spleen, 2nd ed. Philadelphia, WB Saunders, 1999, pp 67-84.

Asgari MM, Begos DG: Spontaneous splenic rupture in infectious mononucleosis: A review. Yale J Biol Med 70:175-182, 1997.

Reynolds DJ, Banks PM, Gulley ML: New characterization of infectious mononucleosis and a phenotypic comparison with Hodgkin's disease. Am J Pathol 146:379-388, 1995.

Gowing NFC: Infectious mononucleosis: Histopathologic aspects. Pathol Ann 1:1-20, 1975.

Cytomegalovirus Infection

Clinical Features

- Uncommon
- Occurs most commonly in immunocompromised patients
- Virus-associated hemophagocytic syndrome is a rare complication in early CMV infection; these patients present with general malaise, fever, chills, and leukopenia associated with thrombocytopenia

Gross Pathology

- Congested red pulp
- White pulp usually inconspicuous
- May have small, variably shaped red to pale foci of necrosis

Histopathology

- Necrotic foci with cells with viral inclusions are typically found at the periphery of the lesions
- Scattered neutrophils may be present, but there are usually fewer than in bacterial infections

Special Stains and Immunohistochemistry

- Immunohistochemical stains for CMV

Other Techniques for Diagnosis

- In situ hybridization for CMV
- Viral cultures

Differential Diagnosis

▌ Abscess
- Often lacks viral inclusions, but degenerating cells at the periphery can resemble Cowdry (i.e., owl-eye inclusion bodies) type A inclusions
- Neutrophils more numerous
- Bacteria or fungi may be present on appropriate stains or culture

▌ Infarct
- Peripheral location under capsule and wedge shape
- No viral inclusions

Pearls

- Rarely seen in surgical pathology material
- Occurs predominantly in immunocompromised patients

Selected Reference

Neiman RS, Orazi A: Reactive lymphoid hyperplasia. In Disorders of the Spleen, 2nd ed. Philadelphia, WB Saunders, 1999, pp 67-84.

Mycobacterium avium-intracellulare

Clinical Features

- Occurs in patients with AIDS
- Most patients present with generalized wasting, hepatosplenomegaly, and lymphadenopathy; anemia is the most common laboratory abnormality

Gross Pathology

- Variable degree of splenomegaly
- White pulp variable, atrophic to hyperplastic
- Diffuse, firm expansion of the red pulp

Figure 15-34. *Mycobacterium avium-intracellulare.* Numerous intracellular organisms on periodic acid–Schiff stain.

Histopathology

- Diffuse expansion of red pulp by numerous large macrophages with abundant pale-gray–staining cytoplasm
- Erythrophagocytosis may be present

Special Stains and Immunohistochemistry

- Acid-fast, Fite, and PAS stain acid-fast bacilli in the macrophages
- Wright- or Papanicolaou-stained touch preparations reveal negative images in macrophage cytoplasm

Other Techniques for Diagnosis

- Cultures

Differential Diagnosis

▌ Lepromatous leprosy
- Involvement is most intense in skin, nerves, and extremities; peripheral disease predominates clinically
- History of residence in area where leprosy is endemic
- Spleen may contain clusters of macrophages filled with acid-fast organisms (lepra cells)
- Splenic involvement consists of small clusters of macrophages rather than diffuse tumorous infiltration
- Fite stain necessary to demonstrate organisms

▌ Histoplasmosis
- Most common in Ohio River Valley and upper Mississippi River areas and adjacent Midwestern states
- GMS and PAS stains demonstrate fungi in macrophages

▌ Gaucher disease (and other metabolic storage diseases)
- Bone, liver, and joints involved (depending on disease type)
- HIV negative
- Gaucher cells have wrinkled-silk appearance
- Stains for organisms negative, but storage products may be PAS positive or acid fast

▌ Langerhans cell histiocytosis
- Usually occurs in young children
- Cells have pale pink cytoplasm and bean-shaped nuclei
- Eosinophils are usually prominent
- Acid-fast stain and microbiologic studies negative
- Cells are S-100 protein and CD1a positive

▌ *Pneumocystis carinii*
- Extracellular foamy exudate
- GMS or immunohistochemical stain highlight the organisms

▌ Malaria
- History of travel or residence in endemic area
- Patients are anemic with intermittent fevers
- Spleen is black with malarial pigment
- Macrophages contain red cells, malarial pigment, or both
- Stains for organisms may be difficult to interpret because of malarial pigment, but acid-fast stain is negative

Pearls

- History is important
- Look for additional diseases in AIDS patients, including
  — Other infections
  — Aggressive lymphoma
  — Kaposi sarcoma

Selected References

Brettle RP: Mycobacterium avium intracellulare infection in patients with HIV or AIDS. J Antimicrob Chemother 40:156-160, 1997.

Horsburgh R Jr: The pathophysiology of disseminated *Mycobacterium avium* complex disease in AIDS. J Infect Dis 179(Suppl 3):S461-S465, 1999.

Malaria

Clinical Features

- Affects children and young adults living in endemic areas
- History of travel or residence in an area where malaria is endemic
- Episodic, recurrent fevers
- Hemolytic anemia
- Hemoglobinuria
- Most common cause of splenic rupture worldwide

Gross Pathology

- Splenomegaly, most prominent in *Plasmodium vivax* infection
- Acute phase: splenomegaly with dark-red parenchyma due to congestion and deposition of malarial pigment; splenic rupture most frequent in acute phase
- Chronic phase: marked splenomegaly, gray discoloration with areas of fibrosis and scarring
- White pulp normal to hyperplastic
- Rarely, development of splenic pseudocyst due to cystic degeneration of hematoma or hemorrhagic infarct

Histopathology

- Acute phase
  - Venous sinuses engorged with parasitized red cells
  - Proliferation of cordal macrophages and desquamation of sinus lining cells containing phagocytosed erythrocytes
  - Increase in small lymphocytes (γδ T cells) in red pulp
  - Macrophages lining the sinuses contain hemosiderin, red cell debris, and malarial pigment
  - Erythrocytes containing parasites can be seen in the sinuses in falciparum malaria
  - Sinus lining cells may contain malarial organisms
- Chronic phase
  - Fibrosis and scarring
  - Macrophages with malarial pigment concentrated around periarteriolar lymphoid sheaths

- Syndrome of hyperactive malarial splenomegaly
  — Common presentation of chronic infection in endemic areas
  — Sinusoidal and reticuloendothelial hyperplasia
  — Intense splenic sequestration and phagocytosis of erythrocytes

Special Stains and Immunohistochemistry

- Malarial pigment
  — Refractile
  — Birefringent
  — Not melanin
  — Negative on iron stain (although macrophages will also contain hemosiderin)
- Thick film of peripheral blood stained to look for organisms

Other Techniques for Diagnosis

- Noncontributory

Differential Diagnosis

- Leishmaniasis
  - No malarial pigment in macrophages
  - Amastigotes of *Leishmania* species can be detected with Wright-Giemsa staining
  - Splenic histology otherwise identical
- Hemochromatosis
  - Prolonged history of dark bronzed skin, arthralgias, and involvement of pancreas, liver, and heart
  - Symptoms associated with malaria such as anemia and fevers are not present
  - Abundant iron in tissues
- Formalin pigment
  - Artifact of prolonged fixation in unbuffered formalin
  - Histologically similar to malarial pigment
  - Clinical manifestations of malaria are lacking

Pearls

- Diagnosis should be supported by clinical history and peripheral blood smear findings

Selected References

Herwaldt BL: Leishmaniasis. Lancet 354:1191-1199, 1999.

Neiman RS, Orazi A: Non-neoplastic disorders of erythrocytes, granulocytes and platelets. In Disorders of the Spleen, 2nd ed. Philadelphia, WB Saunders, 1999, pp 67-84.

Zingman BS, Viner BL: Splenic complications in malaria: Case report and review. Clin Infect Dis 16:223-232, 1993.

Edington GM: Pathology of malaria in West Africa. Br Med J 1:715-718, 1967.

Pyogenic Bacterial Infections (Abscess)

Clinical Features

- Occurs in patients with acute systemic bacterial infections with hematogenous dissemination (e.g., patients with bacterial endocarditis)

- Most often gram-positive organisms, particularly *Staphylococcus* species

Gross Pathology

- Follicular hyperplasia with enlarged prominent white pulp follicles; not always present in immunocompromised or clinically septic patients
- Abscesses are localized to white pulp and variably sized, soft to liquid, cream-colored to greenish
- May be surrounded by a thin rim of hyperemic tissue

Histopathology

- Septic emboli produce infarcts as well as abscesses
- Abscesses contain neutrophils and necrotic debris; older abscesses may be surrounded by granulation tissue or fibrous tissue

Special Stains and Immunohistochemistry

- Gram stain or fungal stains for organisms

Other Techniques for Diagnosis

- Microbiologic cultures for organisms

Differential Diagnosis

▍ Splenic infarct
- Usually larger than abscess
- Peripherally located and wedge shaped rather than round
- Examine arteries carefully for thrombi or emboli
- Infarcts are pale but firm, not liquid
- Inflammation, if present, is most intense at the periphery of the infarct

▍ Hodgkin lymphoma
- Necrotic nodules of Hodgkin lymphoma; these are usually better circumscribed, firm to fibrotic, and elevated above the cut surface of the spleen, but may also form tumorous lumps under the splenic capsule
- Nodules of Hodgkin lymphoma contain lymphocytes, Reed-Sternberg or Hodgkin cells, eosinophils, and plasma cells

▍ Extramedullary hematopoiesis
- Rarely forms grossly evident nodules
- Clusters of erythroid precursors are usually evident on microscopic examination and are often the predominant cell type; also look for myeloid cells and megakaryocytes

Pearls

- Splenic abscesses are seen more often on autopsy than in surgically resected spleens
- When seen in a surgical specimen removed for other indications, consider the possibility of splenic embolization with infarcts

Selected Reference

Neiman RS, Orazi A: Reactive lymphoid hyperplasia. In Disorders of the Spleen, 2nd ed. Philadelphia, WB Saunders, 1999, pp 67-84.

Granulomatous Diseases

Sarcoidosis, Miliary Tuberculosis, Histoplasmosis, Coccidioidomycosis, and Lipogranulomas

Clinical Features

▍ Sarcoidosis
- See Chapter 4
- Patients usually have hilar adenopathy, pulmonary symptoms, or other sites of involvement
- Most common in African Americans; female predominance
- Schaumann bodies and asteroid bodies may be present but are not diagnostic
- Small foci of necrosis may be present
- Stains and culture for infectious agents are negative

▍ Miliary tuberculosis
- Occurs most often in elderly patients with history of tuberculosis and in immunocompromised patients

▍ Histoplasmosis
- Occurs at any age
- Clinical spectrum ranging from asymptomatic infection to disseminated disease
- Splenic involvement more common in elderly and immunocompromised patients

Figure 15-35. Miliary tuberculosis. In this gross photograph, notice the multiple whitish granulomas with necrosis. In patients with miliary tuberculosis, especially immunocompromised patients, the granulomas are often less well formed and lack grossly visible necrosis.

- Histoplasmosis is most common in the upper Midwest, upper Mississippi River, and Ohio River regions
- Organism found in soil
- Pigeons are common vectors; exposure to pigeon droppings can lead to infection

▮ Coccidioidomycosis
  - Occurs at any age
  - Splenic involvement is uncommon but can occur in elderly and immunocompromised patients
  - Occurs in California in the San Joaquin and Central valleys (valley fever) and in southwestern United States
  - Clinical spectrum ranging from asymptomatic infection to disseminated disease

▮ Lipogranulomas
  - *Lipogranulomatosis* refers to the presence, in lymph nodes and spleen, of lipid material arising from endogenous sources, such as tumors, hematomas, cholesterol deposits, fat embolism, and fat necrosis
  - Common in the spleen (seen in 20% of splenectomy specimens and 62% of autopsy specimens; incidence increases with age)
  - Usually is an incidental finding without a clear etiology in spleens examined for other indications

Gross Pathology

▮ Sarcoidosis
  - Often not seen grossly; white pulp inconspicuous
  - Occasionally show multiple small, round, well-circumscribed nodules

▮ Miliary tuberculosis
  - Modest splenomegaly
  - Small 1- to 2-mm diameter, whitish nodules resembling white pulp follicles; miliary pattern
  - Larger confluent granulomas with dry, caseous to calcified material are uncommon

▮ Histoplasmosis
  - May present with splenomegaly and hypersplenism
  - Spherical yellow to white calcified granules, 1 to 2 mm in diameter
  - May present as a miliary pattern

▮ Coccidioidomycosis
  - Spherical yellow to white granules, 1 to 2 mm in diameter
  - May present as a miliary pattern

▮ Lipogranulomas
  - Not seen on gross examination

Histopathology

▮ Sarcoidosis
  - More commonly localizes to white pulp
  - Small epithelioid granulomas similar to those seen in lung and lymph nodes
  - Schaumann bodies and asteroid bodies may be present but are not diagnostic
  - Small foci of necrosis can be seen

▮ Miliary tuberculosis
  - Scattered randomly in the white and red pulp, may be more frequent in the latter
  - Granulomas with central caseous necrosis
  - Multinucleated Langhans giant cells are characteristic
  - Epithelioid cells and lymphocytes also are present
  - Lesions may calcify

▮ Histoplasmosis
  - Scattered randomly in the white and red pulp, may be more frequent in the latter
  - In the acute phase, the infection often does not form distinct granulomas, but manifests as small collections of histiocytes containing fungal forms, with an infiltrate of plasma cells and lymphocytes
  - Neutrophils are usually not seen
  - Old inactive lesions are more common; these are partially calcified fibrous nodules with a few lymphocytes at the periphery
  - Histiocytes are generally not seen
  - Organisms can be detected with GMS stain

▮ Coccidioidomycosis
  - Scattered randomly in the white and red pulp, may be more frequent in the latter
  - Granulomas may have central necrosis, and fungal forms may be seen on H&E, GMS, and PAS stains

▮ Lipogranulomas
  - Localized in the white pulp in the vicinity of arterioles
  - Small, ill-defined aggregates of macrophages with single large or numerous small lipid vacuoles

Special Stains and Immunohistochemistry

- GMS, PAS, and acid-fast stains for organisms required in all cases
- Additional techniques
  — Acid-fast and fungal culture recommended; these organisms can survive snap-freezing

Other Techniques for Diagnosis

- Noncontributory

Differential Diagnosis

- See all Granulomatous Diseases

Pearls

- Special stains for microorganisms are essential when granulomas are present in the spleen sample
- Correlation with results of culture or other microbiology studies from spleen or other source (e.g., blood) is helpful

Selected Reference

Neiman RS, Orazi A: Granulomatous disorders. In Disorders of the Spleen, 2nd ed. Philadelphia, WB Saunders, 1999, pp 85-96.

Other Conditions

Amyloidosis

Clinical Features

- Most occur in older adults
- Occur in patients with systemic amyloidosis
- AL-type amyloid in patients with plasma cell dyscrasia
- AA-type amyloid found in patients with tuberculosis, rheumatoid arthritis, or other chronic inflammatory processes

Gross Pathology

- Three patterns; these do not correlate with amyloid protein type
  - Incidental: seen only on microscopic examination
  - Sago spleen: grayish-white, small, multiple nodules resembling exaggerated white pulp
  - Lardaceous spleen: enlarged spleen with diffuse infiltration; dark, firm, rubbery

Histopathology

- Amyloid is a bright-pink (eosinophilic) amorphous hyaline-like material
- Incidental type: amyloid deposits around small vessels
- Sago spleen: deposits surround cells in the white pulp, eventually with replacement and atrophy of the white pulp
- Lardaceous spleen: deposits in the red pulp adjacent to sinus walls and around small vessels; may become confluent and replace the red pulp

Figure 15-36. Amyloidosis. Masses of amorphous eosinophilic extracellular material (amyloid) replace normal splenic tissue. A few sinuses and blood vessels remain.

Special Stains and Immunohistochemistry

- Congo red (apple-green staining at polarizing microscope) or thioflavin T stain (fluorescent microscope)
- Immunohistochemistry for amyloid chain type and immunoglobulin light chains

Other Techniques for Diagnosis

- Electron microscopy: shows fibrils (generally not needed)

Differential Diagnosis

▮ Castleman disease, hyaline-vascular type
  - Rare in spleen
  - Hyalinized follicular centers with penetrating arterioles, no perivascular hyaline deposits
▮ Infarct
  - Grossly irregular, wedge shaped
  - Peripheral location, rarely diffuse
  - Microscopy shows coagulative necrosis
▮ Granulomas
  - Cores contain necrotic material or epithelioid giant cells (no amorphous uniform material); however, old granulomas can be extensively hyalinized
▮ Hyalinosis
  - A common, usually incidental microscopic finding occurring at any age after early childhood
  - Eosinophilic hyaline thickening of small arteries and arterioles in the spleen
  - Looks like early amyloid
  - Deposits are composed of plasma proteins
  - Congo red or thioflavin T stains negative

Pearls

- Classification of amyloid is based on the protein type; 23 different fibril proteins are described in human amyloidosis and are associated with variable clinical features
- AL amyloid is derived from immunoglobulin light chains, more often λ than κ, and is associated with plasma cell dyscrasias or B-cell lymphoproliferative disorders
- AA amyloid is derived from SAA protein, an acute-phase reactant; accumulates in chronic inflammatory processes
- Amyloid is also present in patients with familial Mediterranean fever (FMF), a febrile disease characterized by acute, spontaneously resolving episodes of fever and pain caused by serosal inflammation and associated with mutations in the FMF gene, *MEFV*

Selected References

Westermark P: The pathogenesis of amyloidosis: Understanding general principles. Am J Pathol 152:1125-1127, 1998.

Falk RH, Comenzo RL, Skinner M: The systemic amyloidoses. N Engl J Med 337:898-909, 1997.

Hematoma and Traumatic Rupture

Clinical Features

- Hematoma usually follows blunt trauma to the abdomen
- Hematoma results from an internal tear without capsular rupture
- Rupture may follow blunt abdominal trauma or penetrating injury
- Rupture can occur without abdominal trauma in patients with
  — Infections: malaria, infectious mononucleosis
  — Tumors: leukemia, lymphoma, angiosarcoma
  — Congestion
- Rupture can occur "spontaneously" in a patient with a normal spleen (owing to cough, vomiting)

Gross Pathology

- Hematoma
  - Spleen is expanded by an irregularly shaped soft, dark mass of blood
  - Capsule is intact
  - Parenchyma otherwise grossly normal
- Rupture
  - Capsular tear with adherent blood clot
  - Weigh spleen after removal of blood clot and gross examination to exclude spontaneous rupture from underlying splenic pathology

Histopathology

- Hematoma
  - Mass of clotted blood
  - Older lesions may have granulation tissue at the periphery and progressive fibrosis
  - May be followed by a splenic pseudocyst
- Rupture
  - Similar to hematoma but with capsular tear
  - Splenic parenchyma is usually normal

Special Stains and Immunohistochemistry

- Noncontributory

Other Techniques for Diagnosis

- Noncontributory

Differential Diagnosis

- Spontaneous rupture
  - Spleen normal or enlarged
  - No history of abdominal trauma, or minimal abdominal trauma
  - Histologic features depend on cause
- Infarct
  - Lesion shows coagulative necrosis
  - Wedge-shaped, peripheral focal lesions
  - Usually does not cause splenomegaly
- Splenic cyst
  - Contents usually clear to turbid liquid (not hemorrhagic)
  - Fibrous wall
  - Epithelial lining may or may not be present
- Hemangioma and other vascular tumors
  - No granulation tissue at periphery
  - Proliferated blood vessels throughout the lesion

Pearls

- Splenic hyalinosis has been reported to be more common in ruptured spleens; however, hyalinosis is present in most spleens, including those of children

Selected References

Pratt DB, Andersen RC, Hitchcock CR: Splenic rupture: A review of 114 cases. Minn Med 54:177-184, 1971.

Rawsthorne GB, Cole TP, Kyle J: Spontaneous rupture of the spleen in infectious mononucleosis. Br J Surg 57:396-398, 1970.

Orloff MJ, Peskin GW: Spontaneous rupture of the normal spleen: A surgical enigma. Int Abstr Surg 106:1-11, 1958.

Byron E. Crawford

16 Bones and Joints

Osteoid Tumors

Osteoma

Clinical Features

- Male predominance (2:1 to 3:1)
- Age ranges from second decade to elderly, with most cases occurring in fourth and fifth decades
- Occurs most commonly in skull bones, including mandible, maxilla, frontal sinuses, ethmoid sinuses, paranasal sinuses, orbital bones, and calvarium; rarely involves the clavicles and long bones
- May be asymptomatic, or if in sinuses, may present with signs of obstruction, including sinusitis and nasal discharges
- Orbital tumors may produce diplopia, exophthalmos, and blindness

Radiographic Findings

- Radiodense, circumscribed surface or intramedullary mass usually without destructive features

Gross Pathology

- Nodular or dome-shaped, dense cortical bone

Histopathology

- Consists of dense lamellar bone with or without haversian canals and usually without a medullary component

- When a medullary component is present, it is represented by hematopoietic tissue or fibroadipose tissue; the process extends up to uninvolved bone and does not blend in with the adjacent normal bone

Special Stains and Immunohistochemistry

- Noncontributory

Other Techniques for Diagnosis

- Noncontributory

Differential Diagnosis

▌ Osteoblastoma
- Lamellar bone with prominent osteoblastic rimming
- Osteoma may have focal areas of reactive bone with similar features

▌ Parosteal osteosarcoma
- Tumor osteoid is arranged in parallel arrays and separated by a hypocellular fibroblastic stroma

Pearls

- Asymptomatic, nodular, radiodense tumor involving craniofacial bones and composed of mature osteoid is typically an osteoma
- Gardner syndrome (colonic polyposis, fibromatoses, osteomas, and epidermal cysts of skin) should be considered in the presence of multiple osteomas or osteomas of long bones
- If surgically removed, recurrences rarely develop; no reported cases of malignant transformation

Selected References

Larrea-Oyarbide N, Valmaseda-Castellon E, Berini-Aytes L, Gay-Escoda C: Osteomas of the craniofacial region: Review of 106 cases. J Oral Pathol Med 37:38-42, 2008.

Unni KK: Dahlin's Bone Tumors. General Aspects and Data on 11,087 Cases. Philadelphia, Lippincott-Raven, 1996, pp 117-120.

Osteoid Osteoma

Clinical Features

- Male-to-female ratio of 3:1
- Usually occurs in second or third decade
- Most commonly occurs in the leg, usually in the proximal femur
- May involve tibia, vertebra (arch more so than body), and small bones of foot and hand

Figure 16-1. Osteoma. Histologic section shows dense lamellar bone.

Figure 16-2. Osteoid osteoma. Histologic section shows a central nidus of thin bony trabeculae with prominent benign osteoblastic rimming.

- Typically are intracortical tumors
- Classic clinical presentation includes progressive pain that is greater at night and is relieved by aspirin
- Depending on the site, other symptoms may develop
  — Vertebrae: peripheral nerve compression and painful scoliosis owing to muscle spasms (symptoms of intravertebral disk disease)
  — Upper and lower extremities: peritumoral muscular atrophy
  — Epiphyseal tumors: skeletal asymmetry, arthritis, and joint effusions

Radiographic Findings
- Routine radiographs reveal a small, round, central area of radiolucency (nidus) surrounded by sclerosis
- Nidus is usually cortical in location and may exhibit central ossification
- When plain radiographs fail to reveal the tumor (about 25%), tomograms, bone scans, computed tomography (CT), or magnetic resonance imaging (MRI) may be necessary

Gross Pathology
- Dense sclerotic bone surrounds a central nidus that is round, red, soft, and friable; nidus may be granular if ossified
- Typically less than 1 cm

Histopathology
- Central nidus is composed of interlacing thin bone trabeculae or woven bone with variable degrees of mineralization
- Trabeculae may vary in thickness
- Prominent benign osteoblastic rimming of the trabeculae and multinucleated osteoclast-like giant cells are present within intervening fibrovascular stroma

- Outside the nidus is an abrupt zone of fibrovascular tissue surrounded by sclerotic compact lamellar bone
- No cartilage in the tumor unless there has been a fracture at the tumor site
- No hematopoietic tissue or adipose tissue within the tumor

Special Stains and Immunohistochemistry
- Noncontributory

Other Techniques for Diagnosis
- Preoperative tetracycline allows osteoblastic incorporation in the nidus, which is fluorescent under ultraviolet light
- Preoperative intravenous technetium-99m with specimen autoradiography is another technique that may be used to identify a small nidus when curettage is used
- May express *c-fos* and *c-jun* by immunohistochemical analysis; some cases have demonstrated partial deletion of the long arm of chromosome 22

Differential Diagnosis
▌Osteomyelitis and bone abscesses
- Lack a central nidus
- Prominent acute inflammatory cell infiltrate

▌Osteoblastoma
- Pain is usually not as severe
- Tumor size is usually much greater, and there is evidence of progressive growth
- Lacks a peripheral rim of fibrovascular tissue
- Exhibits variable mineralization and thickness of woven osteoid trabeculae, whereas the nidus of an osteoid osteoma shows a pattern of central maturation toward a more calcified and thicker woven osteoid trabecula

▌Osteosarcoma
- Lacks the fibrovascular stroma and osteoblastic rimming of osteoid osteoma
- May exhibit chondroid or fibrous differentiation

▌Stress fracture
- Zonal pattern with central, more mature, denser bone and peripheral woven bone
- Cartilage with endochondral ossification may be present

Pearls
- Pain is related to presence of unmyelinated nerve fibers in the fibrovascular stroma of the nidus, production of prostaglandin E$_2$, and production of prostacyclin
- Clinical pain may precede radiographic evidence of osteoid osteoma
- When osteoid osteoma is present in the small bones of the hands and feet, patients are typically treated for an inflammatory process (osteomyelitis, arthritis) first

- Intra-articular tumors may produce chronic villous synovitis similar to rheumatoid arthritis
- Prostaglandin receptors have been identified within bone, and it has been postulated that prostaglandins may also contribute to the formation of osteoid osteoma
- Few reports of spontaneous regression of osteoid osteomas
- Treatment is surgical removal

Selected References

Unni KK, Inwards CY, Bridge J, et al: Tumors of the Bones and Joints, 4th Series, Fascicle 2. Washington, DC, Armed Forces Institute of Pathology, 2005, pp 119-126.

Baruffi MR, Volpon JB, Neto JB, Casartelli C: Osteoid osteomas with chromosome alterations involving 22q. Cancer Genet Cytogenet 124:127-131, 2001.

Franchi A, Calzolari A, Zampi G: Immunohistochemical detection of c-fos and c-jun expression in osseous and cartilaginous tumors of the skeleton. Virchows Arch [B] 432:515-519, 1998.

Sim FH, Dahlin DC, Beabout JW: Osteoid-osteoma: Diagnostic problems. J Bone Joint Surg 57A:154-159, 1975.

Freiberger RH, Loitman BS, Helpern M, Thompson TC: Osteoid osteoma: A report on 80 cases. AJR Am J Roentgenol 82:194-205, 1959.

Osteoblastoma

Clinical Features

- Male predominance, with a male-to-female ratio of 2:1 to 3:1
- Occurs in first through fourth decades, with most occurring in second and third decades
- Predilection for the vertebral column (arch) and sacrum followed by the mandible and craniofacial bones; the next most common sites are the extremities, where it follows a distribution similar to that of osteoid osteoma
- Typically intramedullary

Figure 16-3. Osteoblastoma. Histologic section shows an irregular interlacing network of osteoid with prominent osteoblastic rimming.

- Localized pain may be present, but not with the intensity of an osteoid osteoma
- Vertebral tumors may produce scoliosis, muscle atrophy, and neurologic deficits

Radiographic Features

- Round, well-demarcated, expansile, radiolucent zone with a peripheral rim of sclerosis (sclerosis may not be as extensive as in osteoid osteoma)
- Central radiolucent zone (nidus) is greater than 1.5 cm; central stippled calcifications may be present
- Tumor may be surrounded by an area of new bone formation
- About one fourth may exhibit cortical destruction with periosteal new bone formation, suggesting a malignant tumor (osteosarcoma)
- Secondary aneurysmal cyst formation may be present

Gross Pathology

- Features similar to osteoid osteoma; however, these tumors are larger (>1.5 cm)
- Central nidus is red, soft, and friable; if calcified, the nidus may be yellow and gritty
- Cortical bone may be destroyed or thin, and there may be hemorrhagic cysts within the nidus, representing secondary aneurysmal cyst formation

Histopathology

- Irregular interlacing network of osteoid with prominent osteoblastic rimming and features of woven bone
- Osteoid may be fine and lacelike with variable mineralization
- Osteoblasts have benign cytologic features
- Osteoblasts may exhibit abundant mitotic activity but no atypical forms
- Osteoid is separated by fibrovascular stroma containing multinucleated osteoclast-like giant cells
- Appears well circumscribed, with tumor osteoid merging with adjacent uninvolved bone
- Large blood lakes representing secondary aneurysmal cystic changes may be seen
- Cartilage is usually not present in the tumor
- Osteoblasts may have epithelioid features represented by large cells with abundant eosinophilic cytoplasm and enlarged nuclei containing large nucleoli
  — When epithelioid cells exceed 75% of the osteoblast population, the diagnosis of aggressive osteoblastoma should be made, which denotes an increased risk for recurrence, although no cases of metastases are reported
- Rare tumors may contain bizarre, cytologically atypical multinucleated giant cells without mitotic activity (these tumors may be designated *bizarre osteoblastoma* or *pseudomalignant osteoblastoma*)

Special Stains and Immunohistochemistry

● Noncontributory

Other Techniques for Diagnosis

● Noncontributory

Differential Diagnosis

▌ Osteoid osteoma
  ● Usually smaller than 1 cm; clinically, the pain is of greater intensity
  ● Periphery of tumor contains a fibrovascular rim
  ● Nidus exhibits a more zonal pattern with central maturation and less variability in the thickness and degree of mineralization of the osteoid
  ● No evidence of progressive growth
▌ Giant cell tumor
  ● Usually involves the epiphyses of long bones
  ● Rare in vertebrae, but when they occur in a vertebra, the body and not the arch is usually involved
  ● Giant cells in giant cell tumors are larger and contain more nuclei
  ● Often composed of sheets of giant cells
  ● Giant cell tumors contain mononuclear stromal cells
▌ Aneurysmal bone cyst
  ● Both processes may have similar presentations and radiographic findings and tend to involve the vertebra
  ● Small foci of reactive osteoid may be present in aneurysmal bone cysts, which should not be confused with osteoblastoma
▌ Osteoblastic osteosarcoma
  ● Radiographically, osteosarcoma is poorly circumscribed with cortical destruction and evidence of periosteal reactive bone
  ● Permeative pattern of growth at the periphery
  ● Stroma of osteosarcoma is sarcomatoid with cytologic atypia and atypical mitoses
  ● Sheets or aggregates of atypical osteoblasts are present in osteosarcoma, in contrast to a single rim of osteoblasts around osteoid in osteoid osteoma

Pearls

● About one fourth of the cases of osteoblastoma will exhibit radiographic evidence suggesting a malignant tumor (osteosarcoma); differentiation from an osteoblastic osteosarcoma can be difficult (see "Differential Diagnosis")

Selected References

De Oliveira CR, Mendonca BB, de Camargo OP, et al: Classical osteoblastoma, atypical osteoblastoma, and osteosarcoma: A comparative study based on clinical, histological, and biological parameters. Clinics 62:167-174, 2007.

Jones AC, Prihoda TJ, Kacher JE, et al: Osteoblastoma of the maxilla and mandible: A report of 24 cases, review of the literature, and discussion of its relationship to osteoid osteoma of the jaws. Oral Surg Oral Med Oral Pathol Oral Radiol Endod 102:639-650, 2006.

Unni KK, Inwards CY, Bridge J, et al: Tumors of the Bones and Joints, 4th Series, Fascicle 2. Washington, DC, Armed Forces Institute of Pathology, 2005, pp 126-135.

Vigorita VJ: Orthopaedic Pathology. Philadelphia, Lippincott Williams & Wilkins, 1999, pp 322-325.

Conventional Intramedullary Osteosarcoma

Clinical Features

● Slight male predominance, with a male-to-female ratio of 1.5:1
● Bimodal age distribution, with most cases occurring in second decade; a second, smaller peak occurs in patients older than 50 years
● Patients with hereditary retinoblastoma are at increased risk for developing an osteosarcoma
● Other conditions that may be associated with the development of osteosarcoma: Li-Fraumeni syndrome, Ollier disease, osteoblastoma, fibrous dysplasia, Paget

Figure 16-4. Conventional osteosarcoma. A, Gross photograph showing distal femur with destructive tumor mass with medullary and cortical involvement and extension into the surrounding soft tissue. **B,** Histologic section shows a neoplasm composed of sarcomatous stromal cells embedded in a background of osteoid.

disease of bone, hereditary multiple exostosis, previous radiation or chemotherapy, hypoplastic or aplasia of thumbs, Werner syndrome, and Rothmund-Thomson syndrome
- Occurs in parts of the skeleton with the highest growth rates
- Predilection for the distal femur, proximal tibia, and proximal humerus
- Typically presents with a history of short-term (several weeks to several months), mild, intermittent pain
- Affected area may be swollen and tender to palpation, and the overlying skin may exhibit telangiectasia and be warm
- Serum alkaline phosphatase may be elevated

Radiographic Features

- Classically shows a large lytic, sclerotic, or mixed lytic-sclerotic mass arising in medullary bone of the metaphysis that extends through the cortex and creates a soft tissue mass
- Variable mineralization within the tumor, which causes cloudy opacities
- Outer cortical surface exhibits prominent periosteal reaction represented by Codman triangle, sunbursts, or onion-skinning
- CT and MRI are used for staging (intramedullary involvement, presence of skip lesions in marrow, and soft tissue involvement)

Gross Pathology

- Resected specimens exhibit an intramedullary metaphyseal mass that has usually penetrated through the cortex and invades into soft tissue
- Marrow extension of the tumor proximally is usually seen, and there may be skip lesions in which normal marrow separates islands of tumor
- Gross characteristics of the tumor are heterogeneous and variable, depending on the stromal component
  - Highly ossified areas are yellow to white and hard
  - Chondroid areas are lobulated, translucent, and light gray to white
  - Osteoblastic areas are firm, white to yellow, and sometimes gritty
  - Fibroblastic areas are soft and fleshy
  - Tumor may contain areas of necrosis, hemorrhage, and cystic changes

Histopathology

- Microscopic features may vary considerably in different areas of a tumor
  - Tumor is basically composed of sarcomatous, spindle-shaped cells exhibiting evidence of tumor osteoid production
  - Sarcomatous stroma is hypercellular and may exhibit osteoblastic, chondroblastic, fibroblastic, or malignant fibrous histiocytoma-like differentiation

- Cells usually have obvious cytologic malignant features, including brisk mitotic activity with atypical forms
  - Some cells may exhibit epithelioid features
- Tumor osteoid is represented by eosinophilic, amorphous, fibrillary deposits between individual tumor cells or small aggregates of tumor cells
- Early tumor osteoid forms a lacelike pattern around tumor cells, whereas the more advanced type is mineralized and has the appearance of woven tumor bone
- As tumor cells become incorporated with tumor osteoid, they tend to become smaller; this feature is regarded as *normalization*
- Some tumors exhibit prominent chondroblastic differentiation requiring careful search for tumor osteoid
- Fibroblastic areas may exhibit a herringbone pattern; diligent search for tumor osteoid is sometimes required
- Some tumors may have large numbers of osteoclast-like giant cells and are designated as *giant cell rich osteosarcoma*
- Some tumors may contain foci rich in vascular structures that imitate hemangiopericytoma
- Small cell variant
  - May have features suggestive of Ewing sarcoma, mesenchymal chondrosarcoma, and lymphoma and require immunohistochemistry for differentiation
  - Presence of tumor osteoid
  - Rare cases of small cell variant share genetic features of Ewing sarcoma
- Preoperative chemotherapy may result in tumor necrosis represented by acellular tumor osteoid, acellular chondroid tissue, fibrosis, or hyalinized vascular stroma; preoperative chemotherapy is considered effective when greater than 90% of the tumor is necrotic

Special Stains and Immunohistochemistry

- Noncontributory, except in the small cell variant (see "Differential Diagnosis")

Other Techniques for Diagnosis

- DNA ploidy analysis usually shows prominent aneuploid clones
  - Conversion from pretreatment aneuploidy to predominant diploidy after chemotherapy correlates with subtotal or total necrosis of the tumor
- Small cell variant may demonstrate chromosome translocation 11/22
- Hereditary form shows a loss of function of the *RB* gene; in nonhereditary form, there may be mutation of the *TP53* gene

Differential Diagnosis

▌ Fracture callus
  - Callus woven bone or osteoid exhibits a parallel pattern with prominent osteoblastic rimming
  - Absence of nuclear atypia and abnormal mitoses in callus
  - Cartilage with endochondral ossification is present in callus

▌ Osteomyelitis
  - Radiographic findings may mimic osteosarcoma
  - Readily differentiated using histologic features

▌ Osteoblastoma
  - Lacks atypical mitoses, infiltrative pattern, and destructive growth pattern

▌ Giant cell tumor
  - Giant cell tumors usually affect skeletally mature patients with closed epiphyses
  - Usually involves the epiphyses and extends toward the articular cartilage
  - Mononuclear stromal cells without atypia or abnormal mitotic activity
  - Radiographic findings can help in differentiating these two entities

▌ Chondrosarcoma
  - Low-grade chondrosarcoma with areas of ossification may mimic osteosarcoma, whereas chondroblastic osteosarcoma usually contains a high-grade cartilaginous component
  - Dedifferentiated chondrosarcoma contains an osteoblastic osteosarcoma component but retains low-grade chondrosarcoma foci
  - Clear cell chondrosarcomas may produce bone, thus imitating osteosarcoma
  - Presence of clear cells and typical epiphyseal location of clear cell chondrosarcoma help differentiate these two entities

▌ Malignant fibrous histiocytoma
  - Typically occurs in older patients
  - Lacks tumor osteoid formation

▌ Fibrosarcoma
  - No production of tumor osteoid

▌ Small cell tumors (Ewing sarcoma, lymphoma, mesenchymal chondrosarcoma)
  - Small cell variant of osteosarcoma will have tumor osteoid
  - Immunohistochemistry may be helpful in differentiating these tumors (leukocyte common antigen is positive in lymphoma, S-100 protein is positive in mesenchymal chondrosarcoma, CD99 is positive in Ewing sarcoma)

▌ Metastatic carcinoma
  - Prostate and mammary carcinomas can elicit a prominent osteoblastic reaction
  - Epithelial markers and specific tumor markers by immunohistochemistry can help differentiate metastatic carcinoma

Pearls

- Osteosarcoma is the fourth most common malignant tumor found in adolescents; the three most common ones in descending order are leukemia, brain tumors, and lymphoma
- If pain has been present for more than 1 year, the diagnosis of osteosarcoma is unlikely
- About half of cases of primary osteosarcomas of bone occur in the knee region; osteosarcomas of the hands and feet are rare
- Initial clinical presentation of osteosarcoma as a pathologic fracture is rare
- Elevated serum alkaline phosphatase levels typically occur in tumors with prominent osteoblastic patterns but may also be elevated in other conditions such as osteoblastoma, osteomyelitis, and callus; post-therapy increase in serum alkaline phosphatase suggests metastatic disease or recurrence
- Most osteosarcomas exhibit diagnostic features on routine radiographs, whereas occasionally, they may exhibit deceptively benign radiographic features
- Rare cases of epiphyseal osteosarcoma may exhibit radiographic features of clear cell chondrosarcoma or chondroblastoma
- A radiologically malignant metaphyseal tumor in 10- to 30-year-olds is most likely osteosarcoma
- Rare osteosarcomas contain cytologically benign-appearing stromal giant cells that hide the sarcomatous component; careful search is necessary to identify the sarcomatous component and tumor osteoid, which is usually found in a perivascular location
- Osteosarcomas of craniofacial bones, ribs, and vertebrae are usually related to Paget disease or radiation and typically occur in older individuals

Selected References

Unni KK, Inwards CY, Bridge J, et al: Tumors of the Bones and Joints, 4th Series, Fascicle 2. Washington, DC, Armed Forces Institute of Pathology, 2005, pp 136-170.

Dorfman HD, Czerniak B: Bone Tumors. St. Louis, Mosby, 1998, pp 128-194.

Glasser DB, Lane JM, Huvos AG, et al: Survival, prognosis, and therapeutic response in osteogenic sarcoma. The Memorial Hospital experience. Cancer 69:698-708, 1992.

Benedict WF, Fung YK, Murphree AL: The gene responsible for retinoblastoma and osteosarcoma. Cancer 62:1691-1694, 1988.

Telangiectatic Osteosarcoma

Clinical Features

- Male-to-female ratio is 2:1
- Most occur in second decade
- Accounts for about 4% of all osteosarcomas
- Similar distribution as conventional intramedullary osteosarcoma

Figure 16-5. Telangiectatic osteosarcoma. Histologic section shows cystlike spaces surrounded by atypical stromal cells and osteoid.

- Predominantly affects distal femur, proximal tibia, and proximal humerus
- Similar symptoms to conventional osteosarcoma, except it is more likely to present as a pathologic fracture (25% of cases)

Radiographic Findings

- Recognizable as a completely lytic lesion involving the metaphysis with infiltrating destructive margins
- May cause cortical expansion of the bone
- Periosteal new bone formation may be represented by onion-skinning or Codman triangle
- Some cases may exhibit benign features and mimic an aneurysmal bone cyst

Gross Pathology

- Hemorrhagic mass that may be multicystic and necrotic
- No areas of fleshy, sarcoma-like tissue or sclerotic areas

Histopathology

- Multiple cystlike spaces resembling an aneurysmal bone cyst, except that the septa of the cysts contain stromal cells (mononuclear and multinucleated) with cytologically malignant features intermixed with benign osteoclast-like giant cells
- Mitotic features are present, including atypical forms
- Sometimes the malignant stromal cells are floating in the center of the hemorrhagic cysts; identification of the stromal cells may be difficult, requiring multiple sections
- Tumor osteoid can be difficult to identify; usually focal and found in a delicate lacelike pattern

Special Stains and Immunohistochemistry

- Noncontributory

Other Techniques for Diagnosis

- Noncontributory

Differential Diagnosis

- Aneurysmal bone cyst
  - Stroma may be cellular but typically lacks cytologic atypia and atypical mitoses; may contain reactive bone with atypical osteoblasts
  - Definitive cytologic malignant features and atypical mitoses are absent
- Conventional osteosarcoma
  - Radiographically, these tumors are not purely lytic
  - Intramedullary osteosarcoma may contain focal telangiectatic areas, which should not be overinterpreted

Pearls

- Telangiectatic osteosarcoma is frequently the type of osteosarcoma associated with long-term Paget disease
- Better prognosis than conventional intramedullary osteosarcoma
- If the diagnosis of aneurysmal bone cyst is being considered, all tissue should be evaluated histologically for evidence of malignant stroma to rule out telangiectatic osteosarcoma

Selected References

Weiss A, Khoury JD, Hoffer FA, et al: Telangiectatic osteosarcoma: The St. Jude Children's Research Hospital's experience. Cancer 109:1627-1637, 2007.

Unni KK, Inwards CY, Bridge J, et al: Tumors of the Bones and Joints, 4th Series, Fascicle 2. Washington, DC, Armed Forces Institute of Pathology, 2005, pp 155-158.

McCarthy EF: Differential Diagnosis in Pathology: Bone and Joint Disorders. New York, Igaku-Shoin, 1996, pp 44-51, 82-85.

Ruiter DJ, Cornelisse CJ, van Rijssel TG, van der Velde EA: Aneurysmal bone cyst and telangiectasia osteosarcoma: A histopathological and morphometric study. Virchows Arch IV A 373:311-325, 1977.

Parosteal Osteosarcoma

Clinical Features

- Slight female predominance, with a male-to-female ratio of 1:1.5
- Occurs predominantly in third decade
- About three fourths of cases involve the distal posterior femur, with the proximal tibia as the second most common site
- Clinically presents as a painless mass of long duration; pain may occur late in the course of this tumor but is not typical initially

Radiographic Features

- Radiodense, bosselated, or mushroom-shaped mass arising on the surface of a bone; in long-term lesions, tumor may encircle the bone

Figure 16-6. Parosteal osteosarcoma. Histologic section shows parallel arrangement of tumor osteoid separated by fibroblastic stroma with only minimal atypia.

- A separate lucent zone between the tumor and the cortex known as a *string sign* may be seen
- No evidence of periosteal bone reaction
- Peripheral lucent areas may represent a cartilaginous cap
- Central lucent areas may represent high-grade sarcoma or dedifferentiated tumors
- CT or MRI may be necessary to visualize lucent areas

Gross Pathology

- Well-ossified mass that appears attached to the cortical surface of the bone
- Cartilaginous cap may be present and there may be soft foci, which should be sampled; these foci may represent high-grade sarcomatous regions or dedifferentiated tumor

Histopathology

- Tumor osteoid is arranged in parallel arrays and separated by a hypocellular fibroblastic stroma that exhibits minimal cytologic atypia and minimal mitotic activity without atypical forms
- Islands of cartilaginous tissue and a cartilaginous cap may be present
  — Chondrocytes are atypical and do not exhibit orderly arrangement
  — Atypia is mild and reminiscent of chondrocytic atypia seen in enchondromas
- No evidence of periosteal new bone formation
- Areas of dedifferentiated high-grade sarcoma may be seen

Special Stains and Immunohistochemistry

- Noncontributory

Other Techniques in Diagnosis

- Cytogenetic studies: a ring chromosome may be seen

Differential Diagnosis

- Osteochondroma
  - Medullary spaces contain adipose tissue or marrow hematopoietic tissue
- Myositis ossificans
  - Maturation toward lamellar bone and marrow adipose tissue begins peripherally and extends centrally in this proliferative process, which is the reverse in parosteal osteosarcoma
- High-grade surface osteosarcoma
  - These tumors are cytologically high grade and lack residual low-grade areas
- Periosteal osteosarcoma
  - Abundant cartilage is present
  - Higher-grade osseous component and evidence of periosteal reaction

Pearls

- Symptoms may last up to 10 years
- Typically affects an older age group compared with intramedullary osteosarcoma
- It is not uncommon for these patients to have a history of recurrence of a previously diagnosed osteochondroma
- Radiologic and histologic evidence of periosteal new bone formation is absent
- Central lucent areas identified on CT scan or MRI may represent high-grade sarcomatous areas or regions of dedifferentiation
- Children may exhibit radiographic lesions that mimic parosteal osteosarcoma of the distal femur; histologically, they have features of fibrous cortical defect

Selected References

Han I, Oh JH, Na Yg, et al: Clinical outcome of parosteal osteosarcoma. J Surg Oncol 97:146-149, 2008.

Hoshi M, Matsumoto S, Manabe J, et al: Oncologic outcome of parosteal osteosarcoma. Int J Clin Oncol 11:120-126, 2006.

Unni KK, Inwards CY, Bridge J, et al: Tumors of the Bones and Joints, 4th Series, Fascicle 2. Washington, DC, Armed Forces Institute of Pathology, 2005, pp 170-177.

Sinovic JK, Bridge JA, Neff JR: Ring chromosome in parosteal osteosarcoma: Clinical and diagnostic significance. Cancer Genet Cytogenet 62:50-52, 1992.

Bertoni F, Present D, Hudson T, Enneking WF: The meaning of radiolucencies in parosteal osteosarcoma. J Bone Joint Surg Am 67:901-910, 1985.

Periosteal Osteosarcoma

Clinical Features

- Slight male predominance, with a male-to-female ratio of 1.7:1
- Typically occurs in second to third decades (older than conventional osteosarcoma appears and younger than parosteal osteosarcoma appears)

- Most occur in the diaphysis and metaphysis of the tibia and femur
- Patients present with pain, swelling, and tenderness; symptoms often present for less than 1 year

Radiographic Findings

- Represented by a surface radiolucent tumor containing a spiculated pattern of calcifications that are oriented perpendicular to the long axis of the primary bone
- May see cortical thickening or erosion
- Periosteal reaction may be present
- No medullary involvement

Gross Pathology

- Lobulated surface mass having a cartilaginous appearance
- Cortical erosion may be seen, but the tumor does not extend into the medullary cavity

Histopathology

- Malignant osteoid must be present, but the predominant pattern of tumor is represented by lobulated chondromatous tissue with cytologic features of grade 2 or 3 chondrosarcoma
- Tumor is located on the surface of the bone and may extend into soft tissue
- High-grade anaplastic sarcomatous spindle cell component may separate lobules of the malignant chondroid component
- Periosteal bone formation may be present, and there may be cortical erosion, but the tumor does not involve the medullary cavity

Special Stains and Immunohistochemistry

- Noncontributory

Other Techniques for Diagnosis

- Noncontributory

Differential Diagnosis

- ▌ Periosteal chondroma
  - Usually smaller and better defined
  - Composed of benign chondroid tissue; does not contain malignant tumor osteoid
- ▌ Periosteal chondrosarcoma
  - Radiographically, it contains "popcorn" calcifications
  - Histologically, it is a low-grade chondrosarcoma containing no tumor osteoid
- ▌ Parosteal osteosarcoma
  - Radiographically, these tumors are more radiodense
  - Histologically, this is a low-grade malignant fibro-osseous tumor without chondroid differentiation
- ▌ Conventional intramedullary osteosarcoma
  - This is a higher-grade osteosarcoma involving the medullary cavity

- Periosteal osteosarcoma does not involve the medullary cavity
- ▌ High-grade surface osteosarcoma
  - Lacks cartilaginous differentiation
  - Osteoid component is pleomorphic and high grade

Pearls

- By definition, periosteal osteosarcoma does not involve the medullary cavity
- CT scan or MRI may be necessary to rule out medullary involvement

Selected References

Rose PS, Dickey ID, Wenger DE, et al: Periosteal osteosarcoma: Long-term outcome and risk of late recurrence. Clin Orthop 453:314-317, 2006.

Grimer RJ, Bielack S, Flege S, et al; European Musculo Skeletal Oncology Society. Periosteal osteosarcoma: A European review of outcome. Eur J Cancer 41:2806-2811, 2005.

Unni KK, Inwards CY, Bridge J, et al: Tumors of the Bones and Joints, 4th Series, Fascicle 2. Washington, DC, Armed Forces Institute of Pathology, 2005, pp 178-182.

Murphy MD, Jelinek JS, Temple HT, et al: Imaging of periosteal osteosarcoma: Radiologic-pathologic comparison. Radiology 233:129-138, 2004.

High-Grade Surface Osteosarcoma

Clinical Features

- Rare tumor with male-to-female ratio of about 3:1
- Occurs predominantly in third and fourth decades
- Distal and mid-femur, proximal humerus, and proximal fibula are most common sites
- Pain and swelling are most common symptoms, with duration from less than a year to many years

Radiographic Features

- Exhibits a surface mass with features similar to those of periosteal osteosarcoma, except the mineralization pattern is similar to that of conventional osteosarcoma, revealing a fluffy, cumulus cloud appearance
- May be cortical destruction, periosteal reaction, and focal medullary involvement

Gross Pathology

- Large, lobulated surface mass with variable consistency ranging from soft to firm
- Should not significantly involve the medullary region
- May be hemorrhagic

Histopathology

- Histologically high-grade osteosarcoma with features similar to those of conventional intramedullary osteosarcoma, but lacks significant medullary involvement

Special Stains and Immunohistochemistry

- Noncontributory

Other Techniques for Diagnosis

- Noncontributory

Differential Diagnosis

▋ Dedifferentiated parosteal osteosarcoma
- Usually has residual low-grade malignant fibroblastic stromal component

▋ Parosteal osteosarcoma
- Lacks high-grade anaplastic appearance

▋ Conventional intramedullary osteosarcoma
- Significant medullary component (minimal medullary component in a high-grade surface osteosarcoma)

Pearls

- Radiographically mimics periosteal osteosarcoma, except it has cumulus cloud–like patterns of mineralization
- Of all the types of surface osteosarcomas, this has the least favorable prognosis (similar to conventional intramedullary osteosarcoma)

Selected References

Staals EL, Bacchini P, Bertoni F: High-grade surface osteosarcoma: A review of 25 cases from the Rizzoli Institute. Cancer 112:1592-1599, 2008.

Okada K, Unni KK, Swee RG, Sim FH: High grade surface osteosarcoma: A clinicopathologic study of 46 cases. Cancer 85:1044-1054, 1999.

Wold LE, Unni KK, Beabout JW, Pritchard DJ: High grade surface osteosarcomas. Am J Surg Pathol 8:181-186, 1984.

Low-Grade Central Osteosarcoma

Clinical Features

- Male-to-female ratio is about 1:1
- Most cases occur in third and fourth decades; this variant of osteosarcoma can occur in older age groups
- Patients present with a history of pain for many months up to several years; usually no complaint of swelling
- Most common sites include mid- and distal femur and proximal and mid-tibia
- Some patients may have been previously diagnosed with fibrous dysplasia

Radiographic Features

- Large, poorly marginated intramedullary mass that either is sclerotic or exhibits trabeculations
- Usually no evidence of periosteal reaction
- Medullary tumor may extend along the length of the bone to the subarticular bone
- May have cortical destruction with formation of a soft tissue mass

Gross Pathology

- Tumors are gritty, gray, medullary masses that may have fibrous and fleshy areas
- Cortical destruction may be seen, and the tumor may extend the length of the bone with poor demarcation between tumor and uninvolved medullary bone

Histopathology

- Similar to parosteal osteosarcoma and can also mimic fibrous dysplasia
- Well-differentiated intramedullary fibro-osseous process represented by irregular bony trabeculae separated by fibrous spindly stroma
- Spindle cells are fibroblastic-like and have elongated nuclei with nucleoli
- Nuclei exhibit minimal atypia and infrequent mitoses; atypical mitoses are rare to absent
- Rare chondroid foci may be seen

Special Stains and Immunohistochemistry

- Noncontributory

Other Techniques for Diagnosis

- Noncontributory

Differential Diagnosis

▋ Fibrous dysplasia
- Benign nonaggressive radiographic features
- Histologically, the woven bone in fibrous dysplasia is delicate and curved, in contrast to the coarse tumor osteoid in low-grade central osteosarcoma
- Fibrous dysplasia lacks nuclear atypia and mitotic activity

▋ Desmoplastic fibroma
- No radiographic evidence of matrix formation
- Histologically, the central portion of desmoplastic fibroma will not contain any tumor osteoid

▋ Osteoblastoma
- Typically has benign radiographic features
- Prominent osteoblastic rimming of bony trabeculae

▋ Conventional intramedullary osteosarcoma, fibroblastic variant
- Nuclear pleomorphism and mitotic activity with atypical forms is greater in this tumor compared with low-grade central osteosarcoma

Pearls

- This variant can affect older patients more often than traditional osteosarcomas can
- Not associated with previous radiation therapy or preexisting Paget disease (typical of osteosarcoma seen in elderly patients)
- A small number of these tumors may be interpreted as benign radiographically
- Histologically similar to parosteal osteosarcoma

Selected References

Andresen KJ, Sundaram M, Unni KK, Sim FH: Imagining features of low-grade central osteosarcoma of the long bones and pelvis. Skeletal Radiol 33:373-379, 2004.

Vigorita VJ: Orthopaedic Pathology. Philadelphia, Lippincott Williams & Wilkins, 1999, pp 340-341.

Choong PF, Pritchard DJ, Rock MG, et al: Low grade central osteogenic sarcoma: A long-term follow-up on 20 patients. Clin Orthop 322:198-206, 1996.

McCarthy EF: Differential Diagnosis in Pathology: Bone and Joint Disorders. New York, Igaku-Shoin, 1996, pp 44-51, 76-81.

Chondroid Tumors

Osteochondroma

Clinical Features

- Male-to-female ratio is about 2:1
- Mostly occur in second and third decades, but can present at any age
- Most occur in distal femur, proximal tibia, and humerus; pelvis is also a relatively common site
- Extremely rare in craniofacial bones, vertebrae, sacrum, and sternum
- Patients present with a long-standing mass that may be painful or asymptomatic
- Some lesions are asymptomatic and are identified on radiographs obtained for other reasons
- Pain may be secondary to impingement of a bursa, fracture, or infarction of the lesion
- May develop after radiation treatment (more than 1 year) for other malignant processes
- Hereditary form (autosomal dominant) is called *osteochondromatosis* (any bone may be involved except craniofacial bones)
- Other hereditary forms with multiple osteochondromas include Langer-Giedion syndrome and DEFECT-11 syndrome

- Fewer than 2% of osteochondromas undergo malignant transformation; clinical features suggestive of malignant transformation include pain, rapid growth, large tumor size (>6 cm), and location (axial skeleton)

Radiographic Findings

- Radiographs reveal a pedunculated mass projecting from the surface of a bone
- Variable smooth or irregular surface and a variable base (narrow to wide); points toward the diaphysis and away from the nearest epiphysis
- Has appearance of mature bone and is continuous with the cortex of the uninvolved adjacent bone
- Surface cap represented by cartilage is not identified with routine radiographs unless calcified; MRI is necessary to evaluate the nonmineralized cartilaginous cap

Gross Pathology

- Pedunculated or broad-based mass containing a smooth, thin (<1 cm) cartilaginous cap
- In older patients, the cartilaginous cap may be attenuated or absent
- Central part of the mass is represented by normal-appearing medullary bone

Histopathology

- Outer surface is covered by a thin layer of periosteal fibrous tissue
- Cap is represented by hyaline cartilage that contains evenly distributed chondrocytes
- Nuclei may exhibit atypia and pleomorphism
- Junction of the cap and bone mimics the epiphyseal plate and contains linear rows or columns of chondrocytes
  — Columns undergo endochondral ossification and form bony trabeculae

Figure 16-7. Osteochondroma. A, Radiograph of the distal femur shows a pedunculated mass. The cortex and medulla at the base of the stock are continuous with those of the femur. **B,** Low-power view shows a cartilaginous cap overlying bony trabeculae.

— Medullary spaces between the trabeculae of bone contain adipose tissue and sometimes hematopoietic tissue

- Chondrocytic atypia must be evaluated with clinicoradiographic features to determine their significance
  — Nuclear enlargement, variation in nuclear shape, multinucleation, and formation of chondrocytic clusters that are irregularly shaped may cause some concern but can be found in osteochondromas
  — Chondrocytic atypia, along with clinical features of malignancy (pain, rapidly enlarging tumor, size > 6 cm) and radiographic features of malignancy (irregular thickened cartilaginous cap > 2 cm, radiolucent areas of the cartilaginous cap, extension through periosteum into soft tissue, and bone destruction), are more ominous
  — High mitotic activity is indicative of malignancy

Special Stains and Immunohistochemistry

- Noncontributory

Other Techniques for Diagnosis

- Chromosome rearrangements of 8q24.1 (EXT1) is found in patients with Langer-Giedion syndrome
- Deletions of chromosomal bands 11p11-12 (EXT2) is seen in patients with DEFECT-11 syndrome

Differential Diagnosis

▎ Parosteal osteochondromatous proliferation (Nora lesion)
- Usually involves small bones of hands and feet
- Occurs in third and fourth decades of life
- Medullary component of lesion is not in continuity with host bone
- Histologically, the cartilage is hypercellular with atypia and multinucleation
- Chondroid nodules are separated by a spindle cell proliferation that exhibits mitotic activity (no atypical mitoses or nuclear atypia)
- Woven bone with deep basophilia may be present

▎ Chondrosarcoma arising in an osteochondroma
- Clinical findings consist of pain and a rapidly enlarging mass
- Radiographic findings consist of thickened (>2 cm), irregular cartilaginous cap, radiolucent zones in cartilaginous cap, extension through periosteum into soft tissue, and evidence of bone destruction
- Histologic findings consist of increased cellularity, nuclear atypia represented by enlarged nuclei with open chromatin pattern, multinucleation, and mitotic activity
- Fibroblastic stroma is present in the medullary spaces instead of fat and hematopoietic tissue
- If a cartilaginous cap is present, it is composed of cytologically low-grade malignant chondrocytes without endochondral ossification

▎ Parosteal osteosarcoma
- Continuity with the medullary component of the parent bone is not present
- Appears to be attached to the surface of the parent bone

Pearls

- Clinical and radiographic findings are important in the evaluation of chondrocytic atypia
- Radiographically, the long axis of the stalk points away from the nearest epiphysis
- Malignant transformation is rare (<2%)

Selected References

Chikhladze R, Nishnianidze T: Clinical-morphological aspects of osteochondroma of long bones. Georgian Med News 152:57-59, 2007.

Altay M, Bayrakci K, Yildiz Y, et al: Secondary chondrosarcoma in cartilage bone tumors: Report of 32 patients. J Orthop Sci 12:415-423, 2007.

Unni KK, Inwards CY, Bridge J, et al: Tumors of the Bones and Joints, 4th Series, Fascicle 2. Washington, DC, Armed Forces Institute of Pathology, 2005, pp 37-46.

Nora FE, Dahlin DC, Beabout JW: Bizarre parosteal osteochondromatous proliferations of the hands and feet. Am J Surg Pathol 7:245-250, 1983.

Enchondroma

Clinical Features

- Male-to-female ratio is about equal; affects all age groups (most occur in second to fifth decades)
- Occurs predominantly in the appendicular skeleton, with most occurring in bones of the hands and feet (hands more often affected than feet)
- Proximal humerus and femur and distal femur are also affected; rarely found in the pelvis, ribs, sternum, and vertebrae (no reported cases in craniofacial bones)
- In general, these tumors are asymptomatic and may be identified on routine radiographs or nuclear scans
- Phalangeal tumor may present as a mass
- Pain may be a presenting feature in association with a pathologic fracture or trauma to the tumor

Radiographic Features

- Well-defined, predominantly lucent medullary mass
- Usually lobulated and sharply demarcated with variable mineralization, stippled, ringlike, or flocculent
- Cortical expansion and thinning may be seen, but the cortex should be intact; rare evidence of periosteal reaction

Gross Pathology

- Curettage produces fragments of blue-gray translucent, glistening chondroid tissue intermixed with fragments containing yellow foci representing calcification

Figure 16-8. Enchondroma. A, Radiograph of the rib shows an expanding radiolucent area with associated calcifications. Gross section of the tumor mass shows a gray-white lesion extending from cortex to cortex. **B,** Low-power view shows a well-circumscribed nodule composed of lobules of mature hyaline cartilage.

- Resected specimens consist of a medullary, confluent, lobulated, cartilaginous mass; periphery of the tumor may be irregular

Histopathology

- Composed of lobulated, mature, hyaline-like cartilage
- Lobules may be separated by marrow hematopoietic tissue or endochondral bone
- Chondrocytic cellularity is low and usually evenly distributed
- Bland cytologic features with small, slightly hyperchromatic nuclei without pleomorphism
- Rare multinucleated forms may be present
- Nuclei with open chromatin patterns and mitoses are generally absent
- Cellularity may be higher in tumors of the hands and feet
- Calcifications and endochondral ossification may be present
- Myxoid areas should arouse suspicion of malignancy except in tumors of the hands and feet

Special Stains and Immunohistochemistry

- Mib-1 (Ki-67): in tumors involving bones other than the hands and feet in which malignancy is suspected clinically or radiologically, Mib-1 may be used to demonstrate proliferative activity
- Proliferative index is low in enchondroma

Other Techniques for Diagnosis

- Enchondromas may exhibit abnormalities of chromosomes 6 and 12
- Molecular studies have shown chromosomal rearrangements involving the *HMGA2* gene localized to 12q15 in some patients with enchondromas

Differential Diagnosis

- **Prominent costochondral cartilage**
  - May clinically mimic enchondroma
  - Composed of histologically benign chondrocytes with an orderly and regular appearance
- **Fibrous dysplasia with chondroid differentiation**
  - Radiographs reveal a ground-glass diaphyseal lesion
  - Fibro-osseous elements are seen (absent in enchondroma)
- **Low-grade chondrosarcoma**
  - Differentiating this tumor from an enchondroma can be extremely difficult and requires clinical, radiographic, and histologic information
  - Pain is usually present in low-grade chondrosarcoma; pain is typically absent in enchondroma unless traumatized or pathologically fractured
  - Radiographic features of low-grade chondrosarcoma include cortical destruction, cortical thickening due to extension of tumor in haversian canals, and a soft tissue mass
  - Increased cellularity and binucleate chondrocytes are more prominent
  - Marrow permeation represented by cellular cartilage surrounding mature bone trabeculae and lobules of cartilage separated by fibrous tissue is seen in low-grade chondrosarcoma
  - Extension of the tumor into haversian canals (not seen in enchondroma)
  - Prominent myxoid features are not typical of enchondromas
  - Immunoperoxidase stains for proliferative activity (Mib-1) reveal nuclear positivity in low-grade chondrosarcomas (generally minimal or no staining in enchondromas except for hand and foot tumors)

Pearls

- Any cartilaginous neoplasm in the pelvis, ribs, sternum, or vertebrae should be considered a potentially aggressive tumor unless exhibiting completely benign clinical features, benign radiographic features, and benign histologic features

- Presence of pain in the absence of trauma or associated pathologic fracture should arouse suspicion of malignancy in a patient with a low-grade chondroid neoplasm
- Myxoid features in an enchondroma should raise suspicion of malignancy
- Significance of atypical cytologic features, atypical cellularity, and myxoid features in an enchondroma increases as the tumor location gets closer to the axial skeleton
- *Ollier disease* (*enchondromatosis*) presents with multiple enchondromas and carries a higher risk for malignant transformation
- *Maffucci syndrome:* congenital syndrome consisting of multiple enchondromas and hemangiomas; increased risk for developing chondrosarcomas and malignant vascular tumors (angiosarcoma)

Selected References

Gajewski DA, Burnette JB, Murphy MD, Temple HT: Differentiating clinical and radiographic features of enchondroma and secondary chondrosarcoma in the foot. Foot Ankle Int 27:240-244, 2006.

Unni KK, Inwards CY, Bridge J, et al: Tumors of the Bones and Joints, 4th Series, Fascicle 2. Washington, DC, Armed Forces Institute of Pathology, 2005, pp 46-52.

Dorfman HD, Czerniak B: Bone Tumors. St. Louis, Mosby, 1998, pp 253-276.

Mirra JM, Gold R, Downs J, Eckardt JJ: A new histologic approach to the differentiation of enchondroma and chondrosarcoma of the bones: A clinicopathologic analysis of 51 cases. Clin Orthop 201:214-237, 1985.

Periosteal Chondroma

Clinical Features

- Male-to-female ratio is 2:1
- Most cases occur in second and third decades

Figure 16-9. Periosteal chondroma. Histologic section shows lobulated cellular hyaline cartilage.

- Proximal humerus, proximal femur, distal femur, and hand bones are most commonly affected
- Usually asymptomatic and often found incidentally on routine radiographs
- Occurs near tendon insertions and thus may cause functional abnormalities and discomfort related to movement
- May occasionally be palpable

Radiographic Features

- Typically a periosteal mass with variable mineralization
- May appear lytic or markedly calcified
- Erodes the outer cortex but does not extend into the medullary cavity
- Periosteal bone formation creating a peripheral buttress causing the tumor to be cup shaped or crater-like

Gross Pathology

- Cortical, subperiosteal, gray-white lobulated chondroid mass with an outer thin layer of periosteum
- Does not extend into the medullary cavity
- Yellow calcifications may be present

Histopathology

- Similar features to those of an enchondroma composed of hyaline cartilage
- May exhibit higher cellularity, increased nuclear atypia, and more multinucleated chondrocytes than enchondromas
- Myxoid change may be present
- Tumor may appear to extend or push into the medullary cavity, but there is a rim of lamellar bone at the junction of the tumor and medullary cavity

Special Stains and Immunohistochemistry

- Tumors express S-100 protein

Other Techniques for Diagnosis

- Noncontributory

Differential Diagnosis

▌ Juxtacortical chondrosarcoma
- Exhibits radiographic features of an aggressive process and does not have buttressing periosteal new bone at the peripheral margins
- May extend into soft tissue and may show variable cytologic atypia

▌ Periosteal osteosarcoma
- Radiographically, this tumor exhibits perpendicular feathery calcifications and lacks peripheral buttressing
- Composed of tumor osteoid and has immature mesenchymal stroma between lobules of cartilage

Pearls

- Periosteal tumor that creates a cup- or crater-shaped mass extending into the superficial cortex but not into the medullary canal
- Composed of hyaline cartilage similar to enchondroma

Selected References

Unni KK, Inwards CY, Bridge J, et al: Tumors of the Bones and Joints, 4th Series, Fascicle 2. Washington, DC, Armed Forces Institute of Pathology, 2005, pp 56-59.

Robinson P, White LM, Sundaram M, et al: Periosteal chondroid tumors: Radiologic evaluation with pathologic correlation. AJR Am J Roentgenol 177:1183-1188, 2001.

Nojima T, Unni KK, McLeod RA, Pritchard DJ: Periosteal chondroma and periosteal chondrosarcoma. Am J Surg Pathol 9:666-667, 1985.

Bauer TW, Dorfman HD, Latham JT: Periosteal chondroma: A clinicopathologic study of 23 cases. Am J Surg Pathol 6:631-637, 1982.

Chondroblastoma

Clinical Features

- Male-to-female ratio is 1.5:1
- Most cases occur in second decade; 95% occur between ages 5 and 25 years
- Predilection for epiphyses of bones
- Typically involves long bones in skeletally immature patients
- Common sites include distal femur, proximal tibia, and proximal humerus
- Other sites include acetabular area, iliac crest of pelvis, ribs, scapulae, spine, tarsal bones, base of skull, and temporal bone
- Usually presents with pain over months to years; may have muscle wasting, arthralgia of the adjacent joint, and joint effusion

Figure 16-10. Chondroblastoma. Histologic section shows a neoplasm composed of immature chondroblasts, multinucleated giant cells, and chondroid matrix.

Radiographic Findings

- Circumscribed, well-demarcated epiphyseal lytic mass with a rim of sclerotic bone
- Calcifications vary from focal stippling to coarse trabecular patterns
- Periosteal reaction is variable, but never to the degree seen in malignant neoplasms

Gross Pathology

- Curettage reveals friable and gritty red tissue with yellow foci of calcifications
- Resected specimens reveal a well-circumscribed, epiphyseal gray mass containing regional calcification, hemorrhage, and cystic changes
- May have bluish-gray areas representing chondroid matrix
- Rim of sclerotic bone surrounds the tumor

Histopathology

- Composed of immature cells with features of fetal chondroblasts (stromal cells), multinucleated giant cells, and chondroid matrix
- Stromal cells are round and have distinct cell membranes
  - Contain predominantly eosinophilic cytoplasm and a centrally placed round nucleus, which gives a fried-egg appearance to the cell
  - Nuclei contain grooves or clefts, and chromatin patterns are finely granular and evenly distributed
  - Infrequent mitotic figures without atypical forms are seen
  - Regional areas where cells do not have well-demarcated borders and form syncytia may be seen
  - Often have areas in which the cells contain larger atypical nuclei
- Multinucleated giant cells containing numerous nuclei (more than 20) are scattered throughout the tumor
- Variable amounts of chondroid matrix, which may contain stromal cells
- Calcification is an important histologic feature and has two patterns
  - Most common pattern is represented by linear calcifications surrounding stromal cells, imparting a chicken-wire appearance
  - Other pattern includes coarse calcifications of the chondroid matrix
- May also have areas of spindle-shaped cells, secondary aneurysmal cystic changes, myxoid changes, and cystic changes containing eosinophilic amorphous material

Special Stains and Immunohistochemistry

- S-100 protein: stromal cells are positive
  - May be helpful for identifying scant numbers of stromal cells in tumors with prominent secondary aneurysmal cystic changes

Other Techniques for Diagnosis

- Noncontributory

Differential Diagnosis

❚ Chondromyxoid fibroma
- Usually involves the metaphyses
- Lacks calcifications and has more prominent lobulated myxoid stroma

❚ Giant cell tumor
- Usually occurs in skeletally mature patients
- Stromal cells with nuclear grooves are absent (negative for S-100 protein)
- Lacks chondroid matrix and calcification

❚ Eosinophilic granuloma
- May radiographically and cytologically (nuclear grooves) mimic chondroblastoma
- Contains eosinophils and lacks chondroid matrix and calcifications

❚ Aneurysmal bone cyst
- Chondroblastoma with prominent secondary aneurysmal bone cyst formation may mimic a primary aneurysmal bone cyst
- S-100 protein may be useful in identifying stromal cells in chondroblastoma

❚ Clear cell chondrosarcoma
- Usually seen in older patients
- Composed of cells with clear-staining cytoplasm
- Contains chondrocytic cells with cytologic malignant features
- Tends to be more heavily calcified than chondroblastoma

❚ Chondroblastic osteosarcoma
- May rarely involve the epiphyses and mimic chondroblastoma
- Contains tumor osteoid

Pearls

- Three common epiphyseal tumors are giant cell tumor, clear cell chondrosarcoma, and chondroblastoma
- Rare cases of metastasizing chondroblastoma have been reported without consistent, definitive, and predictable histopathologic features
- Aneurysmal lesions of tarsal bones may have minute foci of chondroblastic stroma

Selected References

Atalar H, Basarir K, Yildiz Y, et al: Management of chondroblastoma: Retrospective review of 28 patients. J Orthop Sci 12:334-340, 2007.

Unni KK, Inwards CY, Bridge J, et al: Tumors of the Bones and Joints, 4th Series, Fascicle 2. Washington, DC, Armed Forces Institute of Pathology, 2005, pp 61-66.

Vigorita VJ: Orthopaedic Pathology. Philadelphia, Lippincott Williams & Wilkins, 1999, pp 363-367.

Kurt AM, Unni KK, Sim FH, McLeod RA: Chondroblastoma of bone. Hum Pathol 20:965-976, 1989.

Dahlin DC, Ivins JC: Benign chondroblastoma: A study of 125 cases. Cancer 30:401-413, 1972.

Chondromyxoid Fibroma

Clinical Features

- Male-to-female ratio is 1.5:1
- Most cases occur in second and third decades, 80% before the age of 40 years
- Typically occur in the metaphyses of long bones in the lower extremity; most common sites are the distal femur and proximal tibia; may also involve the pelvis or small bones of the feet
- Patients usually present with a long-term history of pain

Radiographic Features

- Eccentric, expansile, lobulated metaphyseal mass that sometimes extends to the epiphysis
- Long axis of the tumor runs parallel to the long axis of the parent bone
- Well-demarcated, completely lytic mass with scalloped margins
- Calcifications on radiographs are rare

Figure 16-11. Chondromyxoid fibroma. A, Histologic section shows a lobulated myxoid neoplasm composed of spindle cells. **B,** Histologic section from another example of chondromyxoid fibroma shows the stellate cells in the stroma.

- Pelvic tumors have a multiloculated soap-bubble appearance
- Secondary aneurysmal bone cystic changes may be present

Gross Pathology

- Sharply circumscribed, lobulated, soft, gray-white tumor
- Hemorrhagic and cystic areas may be present
- Myxoid areas may be seen

Histopathology

- At low magnification, the tumor has a lobulated appearance
- Lobulated areas are myxoid and are composed of spindled or stellate cells
- Cellularity of the lobules is decreased centrally and hypercellular at the periphery
- In the hypercellular peripheral areas, the cells have features of chondroblasts
- In about 30% of cases, bizarre cells with pleomorphic hyperchromatic nuclei are present and may suggest malignancy; however, there is no mitotic activity
- Matrix of the lobules may have chondroid or myxoid characteristics
- Lobules are separated by fibrous tissue containing vessels, multinucleated giant cells, and occasionally osteoid
- Secondary aneurysmal bone cyst changes and foci of necrosis may be seen
- Rare to absent mitotic activity
- Solid cellular areas with features of chondroblastoma may be present
- Although not seen on radiographs, calcifications are extensive histologically and interfere with appreciation of a lobular architecture

Special Stains and Immunohistochemistry

- S-100 protein: to demonstrate the presence of chondroid differentiation
- Smooth muscle actin (SMA) and CD34 positive

Other Techniques for Diagnosis

- Noncontributory

Differential Diagnosis

▌ Chondroblastoma
- Typically involves the epiphyses
- Calcifications seen both radiographically and histologically (chicken-wire appearance)

▌ Medullary chondrosarcoma
- Most occur in older patients and predominantly in the axial skeleton
- Radiographically, these tumors are poorly circumscribed and contain calcifications; may demonstrate cortical thickening or cortical destruction if high grade

- May cause a soft tissue mass
- Demonstrates marrow extension with chondroid tissue surrounding bony trabeculae
- High-grade tumors may mimic chondromyxoid fibroma but exhibit abundant mitotic activity not seen in the latter
- Multinucleated giant cells and aneurysmal bone cyst changes are usually not present in chondrosarcoma

Pearls

- Use low power to appreciate the lobulated or nodular architecture
- In curettage, the fibrous septa may be fragmented and go unnoticed histologically
- Mitotic activity is not prominent and, if present, supports diagnosis of chondrosarcoma

Selected References

Budny AM, Ismail A, Osher L: Chondromyxoid fibroma. J Foot Ankle Surg 47:153-159, 2008.

Unni KK, Inwards CY, Bridge J, et al: Tumors of the Bones and Joints, 4th Series, Fascicle 2. Washington, DC, Armed Forces Institute of Pathology, 2005, pp 68-72.

Rahima A, Beabout JW, Ivins JC, Dahlin DC: Chondromyxoid fibroma: A clinicopathologic study of 76 cases. Cancer 30:726-736, 1972.

Intramedullary Chondrosarcoma (Conventional)

Clinical Features

- Male-to-female ratio is 1.5:1
- Usually seen in older adults; most patients are older than 50 years; rare in patients younger than 45 years
- Predilection for the trunk, with pelvis, ribs, proximal femur, and proximal humerus also affected
- Dull pain at rest that is often worse at night; symptom duration is typically several months to years

Radiographic Features

- Radiolucent mass with variable calcifications ranging from ring-shaped or punctate calcifications to markedly calcified lesions
- Cortex is thin with endosteal scalloping and erosion through the cortex
- Prominent cortical thickening, representing extension into haversian canals, may be seen
- Periosteal reaction is minimal or absent

Gross Pathology

- Nodular mass with blue-gray, glistening, translucent tissue resembling cartilage
- Areas of yellow calcifications at the periphery
- May have foci of necrosis, hemorrhage, or myxoid degeneration
- Presence of fleshy tissue indicates a high-grade tumor

Figure 16-12. Chondrosarcoma. A, Radiograph shows a sacral mass sparsely calcified. Resected specimen shows a smooth, lobulated, gray-white, pearly tumor mass with multiple calcifications. **B,** Histologic section shows a neoplasm composed of chondrocytes with hyperchromatic nuclei and multinucleated forms.

Histopathology

- Significant histologic variation; diagnosis of low-grade tumors requires clinical and radiographic features to correlate with histology
- Large amounts of chondroid matrix with variable cellularity; no tumor osteoid
- Chondrocytes within the matrix form clusters and are swollen as a result of cytoplasmic vacuolization
- Nuclei are mildly pleomorphic, and multinucleated forms are present in variable numbers
- Cells with chondroid differentiation containing nuclei with open chromatin patterns, nucleoli, and mitoses are indicative of malignancy
- The following are criteria for grading based on cellularity and cytology
  - Grade 1: cellularity is low, chondrocytes have small, dark nuclei, and multinucleated forms are rare; no mitotic activity, small foci of necrosis
  - Grade 2: cellularity is increased mainly at the periphery of lobules, myxoid change is present, chondrocytes have more abundant cytoplasm with mildly pleomorphic nuclei, and

multinucleated forms are more common; mitoses are rare, foci of necrosis are present
  - Grade 3: cellularity is increased with sparse chondroid matrix; nuclei are large and pleomorphic and contain nucleoli; mitoses are present, and necrosis may be prominent
- Features suggestive of malignancy (hypercellularity, hyperchromasia, binucleated forms, and myxoid changes) may be seen in benign chondroid processes of the hands and feet; must have clinical and radiologic data before rendering diagnosis

Special Stains and Immunohistochemistry

- S-100 protein positive in grades 1 and 2 tumors; grade 3 tumors may be negative in poorly differentiated areas

Other Techniques for Diagnosis

- DNA ploidy analysis may have prognostic significance
  - Grade 1 tumors are diploid
  - Grade 2 tumors may be diploid or aneuploid
  - Grade 3 tumors are aneuploid

Differential Diagnosis

▌ Enchondroma
- Clinical and radiographic features are needed to differentiate this tumor from grade 1 chondrosarcoma
- Typically not painful
- Radiographically, tumor lacks evidence of an aggressive process (intramedullary lucent lesion without cortical destruction)
- Histologically, tumor may have features similar to those of a grade 1 chondrosarcoma
- Lobules of chondroid tissue are separated by normal hematopoietic tissue, whereas in chondrosarcoma, fibrous tissue separates lobules

▌ Fracture callus
- Clinical and radiographic features do not support the diagnosis of chondrosarcoma
- Composed of benign chondrocytes

▌ Chondroblastic osteosarcoma
- Careful sampling of the tumor identifies tumor osteoid
- Radiographically, this tumor exhibits features of an osteoid-producing tumor; prominent periosteal reaction and cumulus cloud–like mineralization
- Occurs in a younger age group than chondrosarcoma

Pearls

- Presence of endochondral ossification in a malignant chondroid neoplasm is not indicative of osteosarcoma
- About 90% of chondrosarcomas are grade 1 or 2
- Cartilaginous tumors of the hands and feet generally behave as benign lesions, whereas cartilaginous tumors of the axial skeleton are usually aggressive
- Pain is an important clinical feature that may be used to differentiate a benign chondroid process from malignancy

- Chondrosarcomas should be extensively sampled in search of tumor osteoid
- Generally, the smaller amounts of calcium seen on radiographs of a chondrosarcoma, the higher the grade of the tumor
- Chondrosarcomas are half as common as osteosarcomas
- Secondary chondrosarcomas may occur in fibrous dysplasia, enchondromatosis, Maffucci syndrome, and osteochondromas
- *Juxtacortical chondrosarcoma*
  — Rare variant
  — Periosteal location and lacks tumor osteoid
  — May be confused with periosteal chondroma

Selected References

Duarte MP, Maldjian C, Katta US, Kenan S: Conventional intramedullary chondrosarcoma with subarticular involvement. Clin Imaging 32:69-72, 2008.

Unni KK, Inwards CY, Bridge J, et al: Tumors of the Bones and Joints, 4th Series, Fascicle 2. Washington, DC, Armed Forces Institute of Pathology, 2005, pp 73-90.

Marco RA, Gitelis S, Brebach GT, Healey JH: Cartilage tumors: Evaluation and treatment. J Am Acad Orthop Surg 8:292-304, 2000.

Schiller AL: Diagnosis of borderline cartilage lesions of bone. Semin Diagn Pathol 2:42-62, 1985.

Dedifferentiated Chondrosarcoma

Clinical Features

- Male-to-female ratio is equal
- Most patients older than 50 years
- Femur, pelvis, and humerus are the most common sites
- Recent increase in pain associated with rapid growth is typical presentation
- Most patients have a pathologic fracture

Figure 16-13. Dedifferentiated chondrosarcoma. Histologic section shows a relatively well-differentiated chondrosarcoma surrounded by highly malignant stromal cells.

Radiographic Features

- Exhibits two distinct different components
  — Poorly defined lytic area with a second superimposed area of radiodensity containing calcifications characteristic of chondroid differentiation
  — Lytic area is poorly demarcated and exhibits areas of cortical expansion and destruction with formation of a soft tissue mass

Gross Pathology

- As in the radiographs, there are two different components: areas of blue-gray, glistening chondroid tissue admixed with well-demarcated areas of soft, fleshy, tan-yellow tissue with hemorrhagic areas and foci of necrosis

Histopathology

- Cartilaginous component usually has features of a grade 1 chondroid neoplasm (enchondroma or grade 1 chondrosarcoma) and occasionally has features of a grade 2 chondrosarcoma
- Dedifferentiated component is sharply demarcated from the chondroid component, with no transition or intermediate zone
- Dedifferentiated component usually has features of malignant fibrous histiocytoma, fibrosarcoma, or osteosarcoma; rhabdomyoblastic, angiosarcomatous, and smooth muscle differentiation have also been reported

Special Stains and Immunohistochemistry

- S-100 protein: chondroid component is positive
- Dedifferentiated areas of the tumor may express SMA, desmin, myoglobin, CD68, or CD34, depending on dedifferentiated tissue type

Other Techniques for Diagnosis

- DNA ploidy analysis demonstrates a diploid cartilaginous component and an aneuploid dedifferentiated component

Differential Diagnosis

▮ Malignant fibrous histiocytoma and fibrosarcoma
  - Lack cartilaginous component
▮ Mesenchymal chondrosarcoma
  - Typically occurs in a younger age group and exhibits a more gradual transition between the cartilaginous component and the undifferentiated component
▮ High-grade intramedullary chondrosarcoma
  - May contain spindle cell areas suggestive of dedifferentiated chondrosarcoma; however, there is a gradual rather than an abrupt transition between the spindle cell and the chondroid components
▮ Metastatic sarcoma to bone (leiomyosarcoma, angiosarcoma, rhabdomyosarcoma)
  - Lacks cartilaginous component

Pearls

- Dedifferentiated chondrosarcoma is a rare tumor representing about 10% to 11% of chondrosarcomas
- Abrupt and sharply demarcated transition zone between the chondroid and dedifferentiated components is an important histologic feature in the diagnosis of dedifferentiated chondrosarcoma
- Prognosis of primary malignant fibrous histiocytoma is significantly better than prognosis for dedifferentiated chondrosarcoma exhibiting malignant fibrous histiocytoma differentiation
- If a patient has clinical and radiographic features suggestive of dedifferentiated chondrosarcoma, biopsies of the tumor should include areas of calcification seen on the radiographs, which helps in the identification of the cartilaginous component

Selected References

Sopta J, Dordevic A, Tulic G, Mijucic V: Dedifferentiated chondrosarcoma: Our clinico-pathological experience and dilemmas in 25 cases. J Cancer Res Clin Oncol 134:147-152, 2008.

Grimer RJ, Gosheger G, Taminiau A, et al: Dedifferentiated chondrosarcoma: Prognostic factors and outcome from a European group. Eur J Cancer 43:2060-2065, 2007.

Staals EL, Bacchini P, Bertoni F: Dedifferentiated central chondrosarcoma. Cancer 15:2682-2691, 2006.

Unni KK, Inwards CY, Bridge J, et al: Tumors of the Bones and Joints, 4th Series, Fascicle 2. Washington, DC, Armed Forces Institute of Pathology, 2005, pp 91-95.

Mesenchymal Chondrosarcoma

Clinical Features

- Male-to-female ratio is equal
- Most cases occur in second and third decades; 80% of cases occur between ages 10 and 40 years

Figure 16-14. Mesenchymal chondrosarcoma. Histologic section shows a biphasic pattern consisting of islands of cartilage surrounded by cellular areas containing small, primitive-appearing mesenchymal cells arranged around blood vessels.

- Maxilla, mandible, ribs, vertebrae, and pelvis are the most common sites
- Pain and swelling of variable duration are typical presenting symptoms

Radiographic Features

- Presents as a lucent process with variable mineralization
- Cortical destruction and a soft tissue mass may be seen
- Features similar to those of conventional intramedullary chondrosarcoma may be exhibited

Gross Pathology

- Gross features are variable
- Tumor is gray to pink and may exhibit lobulated architecture with sharp delineation from adjacent soft tissue and bone
- Foci of hemorrhage and necrosis may be present

Histopathology

- Biphasic pattern consisting of islands of cytologically benign hyaline cartilage with surrounding hypercellular areas containing small, primitive-appearing round and spindled mesenchymal cells
- Mesenchymal cells have scant cytoplasm, mildly pleomorphic nuclei that exhibit irregular chromatin clumping, and small nucleoli; mitotic activity is variable
- Primitive cells surround delicate branching vessels, imparting a hemangiopericytoma-like appearance on low power
- In some areas, the small cells have a pattern suggestive of Ewing sarcoma or embryonal rhabdomyosarcoma
- Chondroid areas may exhibit calcification or endochondral ossification
- Transition zone is between the chondroid foci and the mesenchymal component (unlike dedifferentiated chondrosarcoma, which shows an abrupt, sharp demarcation between the two components)

Special Stains and Immunohistochemistry

- S-100 protein: tissue with chondroid differentiation is positive
- Neuron-specific enolase (NSE): primitive mesenchymal cells may be focally positive (negative for S-100 protein)
- Desmin and muscle-specific actin (MSA) positive in tumors with rhabdomyoblastic differentiation
- Small cell component of tumor may express CD99

Modern Techniques for Diagnosis

- Cytogenetic studies: some cases show t(11;22) or 13;21 translocation

Differential Diagnosis

▪ Dedifferentiated chondrosarcoma
  - Occurs in older age group and is more likely to affect the appendicular skeleton
  - Exhibits abrupt, sharp margins between the chondroid component and the dedifferentiated component; lacks hemangiopericytoma-like pattern
▪ Ewing sarcoma of bone
  - Lacks chondroid component
  - Positive for CD99
▪ Embryonal rhabdomyosarcoma
  - Lacks chondroid component
  - Expresses muscle markers (desmin, actin, and myoglobin)
▪ Hemangiopericytoma
  - Lacks chondroid component

Pearls

- Rare tumor accounting for less than 2% of chondrosarcomas
- Bimorphic histologic pattern of a chondroid component and a small primitive cell component with hemangiopericytoma or Ewing sarcoma patterns
- Should be considered in patients with malignant bimorphic cartilaginous tumors arising in the mandible or maxilla

Selected References

Dantonello TM, Int-Veen C, Leuschner I, et al: Mesenchymal chondrosarcoma of soft tissues and bone in children, adolescents, and young adults: experiences of the CWS and COSS study groups. Cancer 112:2424-2431, 2008.

Pellitteri PK, Ferlito A, Fagan JJ, et al: Mesenchymal chondrosarcoma of the head and neck. Oral Oncol 43:970-975, 2007.

Cesari M, Bertoni F, Bacchini P, et al: Mesenchymal chondrosarcoma: An analysis of patients treated at a single institution. Tumori 93:423-427, 2007.

Hameed M: Small round cell tumors of bone. Arch Pathol Lab Med 131:192-204, 2007.

Unni KK, Inwards CY, Bridge J, et al: Tumors of the Bones and Joints, 4th Series, Fascicle 2. Washington, DC, Armed Forces Institute of Pathology, 2005, pp 99-104.

Naumann S, Krallman PA, Unni KK, et al: Translocation der(13;21)(q10;q10) in skeletal and extraskeletal mesenchymal chondrosarcoma. Mod Pathol 15:572-576, 2002.

Clear Cell Chondrosarcoma

Clinical Features

- Male-to-female ratio is about 2:1
- Most tumors occur in third and fourth decades
- Predilection for the epiphyses
- More than 50% of these tumors arise in the proximal femur; other common sites include the proximal humerus and distal femur
- Pain of variable duration is the usual presentation; range of motion in the adjacent joint may be limited

Figure 16-15. Clear cell chondrosarcoma. High-power view shows large cells with abundant clear cytoplasm embedded in a chondroid matrix and scattered foci of osteoid.

Radiographic Features

- Patient typically has a lytic lesion in the epiphysis that is sharply demarcated and contains a sclerotic rim
- Cortical expansion may be seen, but the cortex is usually intact
- Secondary aneurysmal bone cyst formation may be present

Gross Pathology

- Soft, gray to red tumor that may contain foci of yellow calcification
- Well circumscribed and may contain foci of hemorrhage and cystic change
- Elements of chondroid tissue may be difficult to identify grossly

Histopathology

- May have a lobular architecture at low power
- Consists of a cellular proliferation of large cells with abundant clear cytoplasm embedded in chondroid matrix
- Cell borders of the clear cells are usually distinct; nuclei are not pleomorphic and contain vesicular chromatin patterns and prominent nucleoli
- Mitotic rate is low
- Multinucleated giant cells may be present
- Scattered bony trabeculae or woven bone is present in the matrix
- May have areas of conventional chondrosarcoma (50% of cases)

Special Stains and Immunohistochemistry

- S-100 protein: clear cells are strongly positive
- Periodic acid–Schiff (PAS) stain with diastase: positive in the clear cells (glycogen)

Modern Techniques for Diagnosis

- Noncontributory

Differential Diagnosis

- **Chondroblastoma**
  - Lacks prominent clear cells and bony trabeculae
- **Osteoblastoma**
  - Lacks chondroid differentiation
- **Aneurysmal bone cyst**
  - Clear cells and cartilaginous differentiation are absent
- **Intramedullary chondrosarcoma**
  - Multinucleated giant cells and reactive bony trabeculae are absent within the malignant cartilage
- **Metastatic renal cell carcinoma**
  - Clear cells in renal cell carcinoma are positive for vimentin and cytokeratin; typically negative for S-100 protein; however, staining may be variable
  - Metastatic renal cell carcinoma has a prominent delicate vascular background surrounding clear cells

Pearls

- Three common epiphyseal tumors include giant cell tumor, clear cell chondrosarcoma, and chondroblastoma
- May mimic chondroblastoma clinically and radiographically; however, histologically, chondroblastoma lacks prominent clear cells and bony trabeculae
- Rare tumor accounting for about 5% of chondrosarcomas

Selected References

Donati D, Yin JQ, Colangeli M, et al: Clear cell chondrosarcoma of bone: Long time follow-up of 18 cases. Arch Orthop Trauma Surg 128:137-142, 2008.

Unni KK, Inwards CY, Bridge J, et al: Tumors of the Bones and Joints, 4th Series, Fascicle 2. Washington, DC, Armed Forces Institute of Pathology, 2005, pp 104-108.

Dorfman HD, Czerniak B: Bone Tumors. St. Louis, Mosby, 1998, pp 410-421.

Bjornsson J, Unni KK, Dahlin DC, et al: Clear cell chondrosarcoma of bone: Observations in 47 cases. Am J Surg Pathol 8:223-230, 1984.

Vascular Tumors

Hemangioma

Clinical Features

- Male-to-female ratio is about 1:1.5
- Most cases diagnosed between fourth and sixth decades
- Most common sites are craniofacial bones (calvarium) and vertebrae
- Often asymptomatic; if symptomatic, pain and swelling are most common complaints

Figure 16-16. Hemangioma. Histologic section shows delicate, thin-walled vessels.

- May produce neurologic deficits such as facial nerve paralysis (temporal bone) and signs of nerve root and spinal cord compression (vertebral); symptoms of vertebral tumors may be accentuated in women during pregnancy

Radiographic Features

- Calvarium tumors are lytic and exhibit a sunburst pattern of reactive bone; bulging of the inner and outer tables (outer greater than inner)
- Multiple tumors may be present
- Vertebral tumors present as intramedullary lytic masses with vertical striations ("corduroy cloth"); CT scan of vertebra demonstrates characteristic polka-dot pattern (striations in cross section)

Gross Pathology

- Well-demarcated, intramedullary mass
- Red and spongy with bony trabeculae

Histopathology

- Composed of a proliferation of delicate, thin-walled vessels lined by flat benign endothelial cells
- Most tumors are of cavernous type or mixed cavernous and capillary
- Pure capillary hemangiomas of bone are rare
- Secondary changes may complicate the diagnosis of these tumors
  - Thrombosis of hemangiomas may result in the development of papillary endothelial hyperplasia, which could cause confusion with angiosarcoma
  - Endothelial cells can undergo epithelioid change, which could lead to a misdiagnosis of epithelioid hemangioendothelioma

Special Stains and Immunohistochemistry

- Vascular endothelial cells express CD31, factor VIII, and CD34

Other Techniques for Diagnosis

- Noncontributory

Differential Diagnosis

▋ Epithelioid hemangioendothelioma
  - Exhibits solid nests of epithelioid endothelial cells that form narrow anastomosing vascular channels
▋ Angiosarcoma
  - Composed of vascular spaces lined by atypical endothelial cells that bridge across vascular lumina or form endothelial tufts

Pearls

- Only rarely do these tumors become symptomatic
- Secondary changes (thrombosis, papillary endothelial hyperplasia, and reactive epithelioid endothelial cells) can be confusing but should still permit the diagnosis of hemangioma
- Cystic angiomatosis is a rare condition that includes multiple hemangiomas (predominantly cavernous) of the skeleton, soft tissue, and internal organs (spleen, lung, and liver)
- Massive osteolysis (phantom bone disease, Gorham disease) is a rare type of aggressive angiomatosis affecting predominantly trunk bones in children and young adults
- Hemangiomas (sometimes lymphangiomas) within bone exhibit osteoclastic reabsorption of trabecular bone at the periphery of the tumor
- Extensive involvement of ribs may rarely lead to pulmonary dysfunction and death

Selected References

Acosta FL Jr, Sanai N, Chi JH, et al: Comprehensive management of symptomatic and aggressive vertebral hemangiomas. Neurosurg Clin N Am 19:17-29, 2008.

López-Gutiérrez JC, Garcia-Miguel P: Skeletal hemangiomas and vascular malformations. J Pediatr Hematol Oncol 28:634, 2006.

Unni KK, Inwards CY, Bridge J, et al: Tumors of the Bones and Joints, 4th Series, Fascicle 2. Washington, DC, Armed Forces Institute of Pathology, 2005, pp 261-264.

Wold LE, Swee RG, Sim FH: Vascular lesions of bone. Pathol Ann 20:101-137, 1985.

Epithelioid Hemangioendothelioma

Clinical Features

- Male-to-female ratio is about 3.5:1
- Most frequently occurs in second and third decades
- Most common sites are the lower extremities, axial skeleton, and skull; most tumors are multifocal within the same bone
- Multicentricity has been reported in 50% to 66% of cases

Figure 16-17. Epithelioid hemangioendothelioma. Histologic section shows a neoplasm composed of cords and nests of epithelioid cells forming irregular vascular channels.

- Synchronous tumors in paired bones (tibia and fibula) is common
- Patients typically present with pain; may have pathologic fractures

Radiographic Features

- Radiographic features are not specific
- Appears as a well-demarcated, lytic lesion with variable peripheral sclerosis
- May see expansion of the bone, cortical erosion, or cortical disruption

Gross Pathology

- Well-demarcated mass with irregular, scalloped peripheral margins
- Soft and bright-red with a hemorrhagic appearance

Histopathology

- Cords and nests of relatively large epithelioid cells that form irregular anastomosing vessels
- Cells are round to polygonal with bland, round nuclei containing small nucleoli and eosinophilic to amphophilic cytoplasm
- Some cells contain intracytoplasmic vacuoles representing primitive vascular lumina; erythrocytes may be present in these structures
- Vacuolization may give the appearance of signet ring cells
- Mitotic activity is rare to absent
- Mixed inflammatory infiltrate is often present, composed of variable numbers of eosinophils, plasma cells, and lymphocytes; sometimes eosinophils predominate
- Foci of myxoid stroma or chondroid-like matrix may be seen

Special Stains and Immunohistochemistry

- Vacuoles are negative for mucin and PAS stains
- Epithelioid cells variably express CD31, CD34, and factor VIII–related antigen

- Some tumors are positive for epithelial membrane antigen (EMA) and cytokeratin (low molecular weight)

Other Techniques for Diagnosis

- Noncontributory

Differential Diagnosis

▌ Angiosarcoma
- Exhibits pleomorphic endothelial cells that bridge across lumina or create intraluminal buds
- Prominent mitotic activity

▌ Metastatic carcinoma
- Clinical history is important
- Negative for vascular markers
- Expression of high-molecular-weight cytokeratin
- Immunostains specific to tumor of origin, that is, prostate-specific antigen (prostate) or thyroid transcription factor-1 (lung)

Pearls

- In biopsy samples of this tumor, chondroid-like matrix with myxoid stroma may suggest that the tumor is of cartilaginous differentiation; however, these areas will not express S-100 protein and will be variably positive for endothelial cell markers
- Considered an indolent, low-grade malignant vascular tumor

Selected References

Bruegel M, Waldt S, Weirich G, et al: Multifocal epithelioid hemangioendothelioma of the phalanges of the hand. Skeletal Radiol 35:787-792, 2006.

Unni KK, Inwards CY, Bridge J, et al: Tumors of the Bones and Joints, 4th Series, Fascicle 2. Washington, DC, Armed Forces Institute of Pathology, 2005, pp 273-276.

Kulkarni KR, Jambhekar NA: Epithelioid hemangioendothelioma of bone: A clinicopathologic and immunohistochemical study of 7 cases. Indian J Pathol Microbiol 46:600-604, 2003.

Evans HL, Raymond AK, Ayala AG: Vascular tumors of bone: A study of 17 cases other than ordinary hemangioma, with an evaluation of the relationship of hemangioendothelioma of bone to epithelioid hemangioma, epithelioid hemangio-endothelioma and high-grade angiosarcoma. Hum Pathol 34:680-689, 2003.

Hemangiopericytoma

Clinical Features

- Male-to-female ratio is 1:1
- Wide variation in age; most occur in fourth and fifth decades
- Pelvis (innominate bone), lower extremities, vertebrae, and mandible are the most common sites
- Usually presents with pain of variable duration
- May be associated with osteomalacia

Figure 16-18. Hemangiopericytoma. Histologic section shows solid areas of spindle cells surrounded by delicate, branching vascular structures.

Radiographic Findings

- Nonspecific radiographic findings
- Consists of an intramedullary lytic mass with variable sharp to ill-defined margins
- Cortical disruption with extension into soft tissue may be seen

Gross Pathology

- Curettage reveals tan to gray, firm tissue

Histopathology

- Solid areas of spindle cells surrounding delicate branching vascular structures lined by benign endothelial cells
- Vascular structures create a deer antler or staghorn pattern
- Variable nuclear atypia, mitotic activity, and necrosis
- Tumors may be graded based on cellularity, presence of nucleoli, nuclear chromatin pattern, mitotic activity, and degree of deer antler pattern; significance of grading has not been determined

Special Stains and Immunohistochemistry

- Reticulin stain highlights reticulin fibers surrounding individual pericytes

Other Techniques for Diagnosis

- Noncontributory

Differential Diagnosis

- Diagnosis of hemangiopericytoma of bone is one of exclusion
  — Metastatic hemangiopericytoma to bone from a soft tissue primary must be ruled out
  — Other tumors, both primary tumors and metastatic tumors to bone with hemangiopericytoma-like vascular pattern,

including mesenchymal chondrosarcoma, small cell osteosarcoma, malignant fibrous histiocytoma, synovial sarcoma, gastrointestinal stromal tumors, and angioblastic meningioma, must be excluded

Pearls

- Extremely rare bone neoplasm
- Diagnosis is one of exclusion
- Biologic behavior is difficult to predict, but it is considered a malignant neoplasm

Selected References

Megdiche Bazarbacha H, Bouchriha M, Sebai R, et al: Hemangiopericytoma of the lumbar spine. Tunis Med 84:509-512, 2006.

Unni KK, Inwards CY, Bridge J, et al: Tumors of the Bones and Joints, 4th Series, Fascicle 2. Washington, DC, Armed Forces Institute of Pathology, 2005, pp 276-278.

Vigorita VJ: Orthopaedic Pathology. Philadelphia, Lippincott Williams & Wilkins, 1999, p 400.

Dorfman HD, Czerniak B: Bone Tumors. St. Louis, Mosby, 1998, pp 797-800.

Tang JS, Gold RH, Mirra JM, Eckardt J: Hemangiopericytoma of bone. Cancer 62:848-859, 1988.

Angiosarcoma

Clinical Features

- Male-to-female ratio is about 1.5:1
- Occurs in all age groups but is rare in patients younger than 30 years
- Most occur in femur, tibia, and humerus; pelvic bones, vertebrae, and ribs are also common sites
- Can present as multicentric tumors, particularly in bones of the lower extremities
- Pain of several months' duration is typical symptom
- May occur in association with previous bone infarct, chronic osteomyelitis, and radiation exposure

Figure 16-19. Angiosarcoma. Histologic section shows a neoplasm composed of irregular vascular channels.

Radiographic Features

- Radiographic features are nonspecific
- Presents as a lytic mass with ill-defined borders
- Cortical erosion and soft tissue extension may be seen
- May be multifocal

Gross Pathology

- Consists of spongy, bloody red tissue containing foci of trabecular bone
- May have solid areas with necrosis

Histopathology

- Only intermediate- and high-grade tumors are considered angiosarcomas
- Tumors contain irregularly shaped vascular structures lined by endothelial cells containing pleomorphic, hyperchromatic nuclei
- Mitotic figures are readily found
- Malignant endothelial cells may be stratified and create intraluminal tufts or papillae
- In poorly differentiated tumors, the malignant endothelial cells are closely packed, and the vascular pattern may not be well appreciated

Special Stains and Immunohistochemistry

- Reticulin stain highlights endothelial pattern by demonstrating clusters of cells surrounded by a network of reticulin
- CD31, CD34, and factor VIII–related antigen: endothelial cells are positive
- Cytokeratin typically negative; epithelioid angiosarcoma may express cytokeratin

Other Techniques for Diagnosis

- Noncontributory

Differential Diagnosis

▮ Epithelioid hemangioendothelioma
  - Lacks nuclear features of malignancy
  - Does not exhibit vascular intraluminal tufting, stratification, or bridging of malignant endothelial cells
▮ Metastatic carcinoma
  - Lacks vascular marker expression and shows positivity for epithelial markers

Pearls

- Rare tumor that may be seen in association with a previous history of radiation exposure, chronic osteomyelitis, and bone infarcts

Selected References

Mittal S, Goswami C, Kanoria N, Bhattacharya A: Post-irradiation angiosarcoma of bone. J Cancer Res Ther 3:96-99, 2007.

Abraham JA, Hornicek FJ, Kaufman AM, et al: Treatment and outcome of 82 patients with angiosarcoma. Ann Surg Oncol 14:1953-1967, 2007.

Unni KK, Inwards CY, Bridge J, et al: Tumors of the Bones and Joints, 4th Series, Fascicle 2. Washington, DC, Armed Forces Institute of Pathology, 2005, pp 266-273.

Fibro-osseous, Histiocytic, and Giant Cell Lesions

Fibrous Dysplasia

Clinical Features

- Male-to-female ratio is about equal
- Three fourths of tumors diagnosed before age 30 years
- In monostotic form, the most common sites of involvement are craniofacial bones, femur, tibia, and ribs
- In polyostotic form, the most common sites are femur, tibia, and pelvis
- Symptoms are variable, depending on whether disease is monostotic or polyostotic and on location of lesions; many lesions are asymptomatic
- In polyostotic disease, symptoms usually develop in childhood with pain and recurrent fractures
- Polyostotic form may also present with café-au-lait skin lesions, hyperfunctioning endocrinopathies such as precocious puberty and hyperthyroidism, and soft tissue myxomas
- Other symptoms are as follows
  - Craniofacial bones: facial deformities
  - Long bones: recurrent fractures with shepherd's crook deformity
  - Lesions of the ribs, which are usually asymptomatic

Figure 16-20. Fibrous dysplasia. Histologic section shows immature woven bone composed of thin and irregularly curved trabeculae surrounded by fibroblastic stroma.

Radiographic Features

- Radiographic features are variable
- Typically an intramedullary metaphyseal or diaphyseal lytic lesion; ground-glass appearance
- Usually symmetrically centered in the medullary canal exhibiting cortical expansion
- If there is cartilaginous differentiation, ringlike and punctate calcifications may be present
- Shepherd's crook deformity may be seen

Gross Pathology

- Intramedullary gritty, gray mass that expands the cortex
- If there is any cartilaginous differentiation, tumor may contain bluish-gray translucent nodules
- May exhibit hemorrhagic foci and cystic regions containing yellow serous fluid

Histopathology

- Spindle cell proliferation with immature woven bone lacking a rim of osteoblasts
- Variably cellular tumor composed of fibroblastic, benign spindle cells arranged in a storiform pattern and a variable amount of fibrocollagenous stroma
- Immature woven bone is represented by trabeculae that are thin and irregularly curved, resembling Chinese letters
  - Lacks osteoblastic rimming
  - May undergo mineralization, and in some cases, the mineralization forms concentric, laminated bodies reminiscent of cementoid bodies; when prominent, the process has been called *fibrous cementoma* or *cementomatous variant of fibrous dysplasia*
- At the periphery of the tumor adjacent to uninvolved bone is a margin of reactive bone with osteoblastic rimming (this should not inhibit the diagnosis of fibrous dysplasia)
- Foci of cartilaginous differentiation are common in fibrous dysplasia; if prominent, the diagnosis should be fibrocartilaginous dysplasia
- Other features include myxoid stroma, giant cell reaction, prominent foamy histiocytes, and cystic changes; more common in rib lesions

Special Stains and Immunohistochemistry

- Noncontributory

Other Techniques for Diagnosis

- *GNAS1* mutations may be seen in fibrous dysplasia

Differential Diagnosis

- Osteofibrous dysplasia
  - Almost universally involves the tibia
  - Occurs in younger children
  - Cortical location
  - Bony trabeculae with osteoblastic rimming

■ Desmoplastic fibroma
  ● May be considered in a small biopsy that does not have woven bone (these tumors do not contain woven bone)
■ Low-grade intramedullary osteosarcoma
  ● Spindle cells in the fibrous stroma are larger and have pleomorphic nuclei with chromatin clumping

Pearls

  ● About 90% of cases of fibrous dysplasia are of the monostotic form
  ● Fibrous dysplasia is a medullary process; rarely it may form an exophytic mass that is attached to or grows on the surface of the bone (fibrous dysplasia protuberans)
  ● In small biopsies, a misdiagnosis of desmoplastic fibroma may be made if no woven bone is present
  ● Presence of woven bone with osteoblastic rimming (reactive bone) at the periphery of the process should not interfere with making the diagnosis of fibrous dysplasia
  ● Regressed lesions of monostotic fibrous dysplasia in females may become reactivated during pregnancy
  ● Albright syndrome consists of polyostotic fibrous dysplasia and hyperfunctional endocrinopathies such as precocious puberty and hyperthyroidism; patients have café-au-lait skin lesions (irregular borders, said to resemble the coast of Maine)
  ● Cherubism is a variant of fibrous dysplasia that primarily affects the jaws; contains prominent giant cells and causes facial deformities
  ● Mazabraud syndrome consists of polyostotic fibrous dysplasia and soft tissue myxomas
  ● Fibrosarcoma, osteosarcoma, chondrosarcoma, and malignant fibrous histiocytoma can arise as a complication of fibrous dysplasia either de novo or after radiation

Selected References

Orcel, P, Chapurlat R: Fibrous dysplasia of bone. Rev Prat 57:1749-1755, 2007.

Riminucci M, Robey PG, Bianco P: The pathology of fibrous dysplasia and the McCune-Albright syndrome. Pediatr Endocrinol Rev 4(Suppl 4):401-411, 2007.

Unni KK, Inwards CY, Bridge J, et al: Tumors of the Bones and Joints, 4th Series, Fascicle 2. Washington, DC, Armed Forces Institute of Pathology, 2005, pp 337-343.

Vigorita VJ: Orthopaedic Pathology. Philadelphia, Lippincott Williams & Wilkins, 1999, pp 300-306.

Reed RJ: Fibrous dysplasia of bone: A review of 25 cases. Arch Pathol 75:480-495, 1963.

Osteofibrous Dysplasia (Ossifying Fibroma of Long Bones)

Clinical Features

  ● Male-to-female ratio is about 1.5:1
  ● Most cases diagnosed before age 5 years

Figure 16-21. Osteofibrous dysplasia. High-power view shows loosely cellular fibroblastic stroma containing bony trabeculae rimmed with osteoblasts.

  ● Found exclusively in the tibia and fibula, typically on anterior surfaces
  ● Usually presents as a painless area of swelling on the anterior surface of the distal lower extremity; may cause anterior or anterolateral bowing of the area or presents as a pathologic fracture

Radiographic Features

  ● Characteristic features consist of an anterior cortical lucent lesion of the tibial diaphysis that does not involve the medullary canal
  ● Inner cortical margin may exhibit reactive features
  ● Anterior bowing may be seen
  ● May see additional lytic lesions with similar features in the tibia or fibula

Gross Pathology

  ● Resected lesions consist of an anterior intracortical, soft, sometimes gritty fibrous mass

Histopathology

  ● Fibroblastic spindle cells with benign cytologic features; may be loosely arranged or may have a storiform architecture
  ● Bony trabeculae rimmed with osteoblasts exhibit zonal maturation with central immature, thin forms maturing peripherally to thickened mineralized lamellar bone
  ● Rare cytokeratin positive cells may be seen in the stroma, but nests of epithelial cells are not present
  ● May have myxomatous stroma, cystic changes, hemorrhage, and aggregates of multinucleated giant cells

Special Stains and Immunohistochemistry

  ● Cytokeratin: rare positive cells may be present within the stroma; does not warrant the diagnosis of adamantinoma (believed to be a process closely related to osteofibrous dysplasia)

Other Techniques for Diagnosis

- Noncontributory

Differential Diagnosis

▮ Fibrous dysplasia
- Occurs in older patients and does not exhibit osteoblastic rimming of osteoid

▮ Adamantinoma
- Typically occurs in an older age group
- Contains epithelial islands within the stroma that are cytokeratin positive

▮ Well-differentiated intramedullary osteosarcoma
- Intramedullary neoplasm
- Spindle cell stroma of this tumor has pleomorphic cells with atypical nuclei with clumped chromatin

Pearls

- Osteofibrous dysplasia may be a precursor lesion of adamantinoma
- No reported cases of malignant transformation of osteofibrous dysplasia

Selected References

Gleason BC, Liegl-Atzwanger B, Kozakewich HP, et al: Osteofibrous dysplasia and adamantinoma in children and adolescents: a clinicopathologic reappraisal. Am J Surg Pathol 32:363-376, 2008.

Grimer RJ, Carter SR, Tillman RM, Abudu A: Osteofibrous dysplasia of the tibia. J Bone Joint Surg Br 89:141, 2007.

Unni KK, Inwards CY, Bridge J, et al: Tumors of the Bones and Joints, 4th Series, Fascicle 2. Washington, DC, Armed Forces Institute of Pathology, 2005, pp 343-345.

Vigorita VJ: Orthopaedic Pathology. Philadelphia, Lippincott Williams & Wilkins, 1999, pp 307-308.

Nonossifying Fibroma (Fibrous Cortical Defect, Metaphyseal Fibrous Defect)

Clinical Features

- Male-to-female ratio about 1:1
- Peak incidence in second decade
- Distal femur, proximal tibia, and distal tibia are the most common sites
- Usually asymptomatic and found incidentally on radiographs done for other reasons
- Larger lesions may present with pain or pathologic fractures

Radiographic Features

- Eccentric metaphyseal cortical lytic lesions with well-defined sclerotic margins
- Typically no mineralization except when it is resolving (density of calcification increases)

Gross Pathology

- Curettage produces soft and yellow to tan tissue depending on quantity of foamy histiocytes

Figure 16-22. Nonossifying fibroma. Histologic section shows a cellular fibroblastic proliferation with a vague storiform pattern.

- Resected lesions are well-demarcated, eccentric cortical fibrous masses that may be yellow to tan depending on quantity of foamy histiocytes
- Areas of necrosis, hemorrhage, or cystic changes may be present

Histopathology

- Cellular fibroblastic stroma that sometimes exhibits a storiform pattern
- Variable numbers of xanthoma cells, siderophages, and multinucleated giant cells
- Occasional normal mitotic figures
- Hemorrhage with giant cell reaction and cystic changes similar to aneurysmal bone cyst
- Foci of necrosis or reactive bone formation

Special Stains and Immunohistochemistry

- Noncontributory

Other Techniques for Diagnosis

- Noncontributory

Differential Diagnosis

▮ Giant cell tumor
- Occurs in skeletally mature patients
- Located in the epiphysis

▮ Desmoplastic fibroma
- Exhibits dense collagenous stroma

▮ Fibrous dysplasia
- Usually does not exhibit reactive bone with osteoblastic rimming of osteoid and lacks multinucleated giant cells

▮ Benign fibrous histiocytoma
- Histologically, this tumor is identical to nonossifying fibroma
- *Benign fibrous histiocytoma* is the term used when the features of nonossifying fibroma are found in ribs, vertebrae, or flat bones

Pearls

- Most cases of nonossifying fibroma are asymptomatic and are treated only if large enough to become symptomatic
- Multifocal nonossifying fibromas may occur in neurofibromatosis and Jaffe-Campanacci syndrome (multifocal nonossifying fibroma, café-au-lait pigmentation, mental retardation, and nonskeletal anomalies)
- Presence of necrosis and mitotic activity with typical forms are not indicative of an aggressive process

Selected References

Unni KK, Inwards CY, Bridge J, et al: Tumors of the Bones and Joints, 4th Series, Fascicle 2. Washington, DC, Armed Forces Institute of Pathology, 2005, pp 334-336.

Betsy M, Kupersmith LM, Springfield DS: Metaphyseal fibrous defects. J Am Acad Orthop Surg 12:89-95, 2004.

Biermann JS: Common benign lesions of bone in children and adolescents. J Pediatr Orthop 2002; 22:268-273, 2002.

Desmoplastic Fibroma

Clinical Features

- Male-to-female ratio is about equal
- Most cases occur in second decade
- Most common sites are the mandible (mental region), pelvis, and metaphyses of the humerus, femur, and tibia
- Patients present with pain and swelling
- About one fifth of patients present with a pathologic fracture, and some patients present with a deformity of the affected bone

Radiographic Features

- Well-delineated, expansile, lucent mass
- May be multicystic with trabeculations, giving it a soap-bubble appearance

Figure 16-23. Desmoplastic fibroma. Histologic section shows bony trabeculae separated by a proliferation of fibroblastic cells embedded in a collagenous stroma.

- Cortical destruction with extension into the surrounding soft tissue may be seen

Gross Pathology

- Typically has features similar to a soft tissue desmoid and appears as a solid, firm, gray mass sometimes exhibiting a whorled pattern

Histopathology

- Histologic features are similar to those of fibromatosis (desmoid tumor)
- Variably cellular mass composed of spindle-shaped fibroblasts intermixed with collagenous stroma
- Fibroblasts are haphazardly arranged and with slightly enlarged oval to fusiform, mildly hyperchromatic nuclei with inconspicuous nucleoli
- Mitotic figures are usually absent
- May exhibit infiltrative borders, including extension into haversian canals, permeation of bone marrow, and extension into soft tissue

Special Stains and Immunohistochemistry

- Vimentin and MSA positive

Other Techniques for Diagnosis

- Trisomy 8 and trisomy 20 may be found in desmoplastic fibroma of bone

Differential Diagnosis

▌ Low-grade fibrosarcoma
  - Lacks multicystic appearance radiographically
  - Histologically, the fibroblasts are arranged in herringbone pattern rather than haphazardly
  - Cells with variable nuclear pleomorphism, hyperchromasia, nucleoli, and mitotic activity

▌ Fibrous dysplasia
  - In a small biopsy that does not demonstrate osteoid, desmoplastic fibroma may be diagnosed

Pearls

- Extremely rare tumor
- Should be suspected clinically in a young patient with a lytic lesion of the mandible
- Mitotic activity of any significant degree (greater than rare) should raise concern of well-differentiated fibrosarcoma
- Desmoplastic fibromas are rarely associated with Paget disease and fibrous dysplasia

Selected References

Hauben EI, Jundt G, Cleton-Jansen AM, et al: Desmoplastic fibroma of bone: An immunohistochemical study including beta-catenin expression and mutational analysis for beta-catenin. Hum Pathol 36:1025-1030, 2005.

Unni KK, Inwards CY, Bridge J, et al: Tumors of the Bones and Joints, 4th Series, Fascicle 2. Washington, DC, Armed Forces Institute of Pathology, 2005, pp 193-196.

Bridge JA, Swarts SJ, Buresh C, et al: Trisomies 8 and 20 characterize a subgroup of benign fibrous lesions arising in both soft tissue and bone. Am J Pathol 154:729-733, 1999.

West R, Huvos AG, Levine AM, et al: Desmoplastic fibroma of bone arising in fibrous dysplasia. Am J Clin Pathol 79:630-633, 1983.

Dahlin DC, Hoover NW: Desmoplastic fibroma of bone. JAMA 188:685-687, 1964.

Fibrosarcoma

Clinical Features

- Male-to-female ratio is equal
- Cases occur in all age groups; rare in first decade
- Most common sites are distal femur, proximal tibia, pelvis, mandible, and proximal femur and humerus; multicentric forms have been described
- Patients usually present with pain and swelling of several months' duration

Radiographic Features

- Large, eccentric, metaphyseal or diaphyseal lesion that is purely lytic and poorly demarcated
- May see cortical destruction and soft tissue extension
- Tumor may extend to the articular cartilage in skeletally mature patients

Gross Pathology

- Dependent on degree of differentiation
  - Well-differentiated tumors are usually better-delineated, firm, white masses
  - Poorly differentiated tumors are fleshy, gray to brown with ill-defined, infiltrative margins
  - Higher-grade tumors contain areas of necrosis, hemorrhage, and myxoid features

Figure 16-24. Fibrosarcoma. Histologic section shows a proliferation of spindle-shaped cells arranged in interlacing fascicles within a collagenous stroma.

Histopathology

- Well-differentiated tumors are composed of spindle cell fibroblasts arranged in interlacing fascicles within collagenous stroma
  - Tumor cells typically arranged in a herringbone pattern
  - Mild nuclear atypia and occasional mitotic figures
- Higher-grade tumors exhibit less collagenous stroma
  - More significant nuclear atypia
  - Greater mitotic activity
  - Necrosis, hemorrhage, and myxoid areas
- Tumors are graded as follows
  - Grade 1
    - Fibroblasts are of normal size with little nuclear atypia
    - Mitotic activity ranging from 1 to 4 mitotic figures/high-power field
    - Abundant collagenous tissue
  - Grade 2
    - Numerous mitotic figures
    - Increased nuclear atypia
    - Less collagen with greater cellularity
  - Grade 3
    - High cellularity with marked nuclear pleomorphism and prominent nucleoli
    - Abundant mitotic activity with atypical forms
    - Necrosis, hemorrhage, and myxoid change

Special Stains and Immunohistochemistry

- Vimentin strongly positive

Other Techniques for Diagnosis

- Gain of the platelet-derived growth factor-β (*PDGF-β*) gene located at 22q12.3-q13.1

Differential Diagnosis

▌ Desmoplastic fibroma
  - Radiographically has a multicystic appearance not seen in fibrosarcoma
  - Less cellular tumor composed of benign, bland spindle cells arranged haphazardly; lacks herringbone pattern
  - Contains tumor osteoid
  - Lacks mitotic activity and nuclear pleomorphism
▌ Dedifferentiated chondrosarcoma
  - Contain areas of low-grade chondrosarcoma
▌ Malignant fibrous histiocytoma
  - Tumor cells are typically arranged in a storiform pattern and contains neoplastic multinucleated giant cells; lacks herringbone pattern

Pearls

- Fibrosarcoma may be a secondary tumor arising most commonly after irradiation of a previous giant cell tumor and also in Paget disease, enchondroma, osteochondroma, fibrous dysplasia, chronic osteomyelitis, bone infarct, and ameloblastic fibroma

Selected References

Unni KK, Inwards CY, Bridge J, et al: Tumors of the Bones and Joints, 4th Series, Fascicle 2. Washington, DC, Armed Forces Institute of Pathology, 2005, pp 196-199.

Hattinger CM, Tarkkanen M, Benini S, et al: Genetic analysis of fibrosarcoma of bone, a rare tumor entity closely related to osteosarcoma and malignant fibrous histiocytoma of bone. Eur J Cell Biol 83:483-491, 2004.

Papagelopoulos PJ, Galanis EC, Trantafyllidis P, et al: Clinicopathologic features, diagnosis, and treatment of fibrosarcoma of bone. Am J Orthop 31:253-257, 2002.

Vigorita VJ: Orthopaedic Pathology. Philadelphia, Lippincott Williams & Wilkins, 1999, p 309.

Huvos AG, Higinbotham NL: Primary fibrosarcoma of bone: A clinicopathologic study of 130 patients. Cancer 37:939-945, 1976.

Malignant Fibrous Histiocytoma

Clinical Features

- Male-to-female ratio is equal
- Found in all age groups; rare in patients younger than 20 years
- Most common sites are distal femur, proximal femur, proximal tibia, pelvis, and skull
- Patients present with pain of variable duration
- May rarely arise as a secondary tumor in enchondromas, fibrous dysplasia, Paget disease, bones with infarcts, radiated bones, and bones containing metallic prostheses

Radiographic Features

- Radiographic findings are not diagnostic but show a poorly defined, metaphyseal, lytic mass that may exhibit mottled-appearing calcifications
- Cortical expansion causes destruction and extension into soft tissue, resulting in an extraskeletal mass
- Periosteal reaction is minimal or absent

Figure 16-25. Malignant fibrous histiocytoma. High-power view shows atypical multinucleated cells with focally vacuolated eosinophilic cytoplasm.

- Tumor may extend into epiphysis
- Pathologic fracture may be present

Gross Pathology

- Poorly demarcated tumor that may be firm and fibrous or soft and fleshy
- Varies in color from gray to tan to yellow
- Regional necrosis and hemorrhage are common

Histopathology

- Composed of a malignant proliferation of giant cells, histiocytes, fibroblasts, and myofibroblasts arranged in a storiform, swirling, cartwheel, or irregular pattern
- Intermixed are variable numbers of foamy macrophages, siderophages, inflammatory cells, and collagenous matrix
- Spindle fibroblastic cells are usually arranged in storiform pattern and exhibit prominent nuclear pleomorphism, hyperchromasia, and abundant mitotic activity, often with atypical forms
- Mononuclear histiocytic cells also have pleomorphic nuclei and brisk mitotic activity
- Admixed lymphocytic infiltrate; occasional plasma cells and eosinophils may be seen
- May have areas with hemangiopericytoma-like pattern
- Foci of thick eosinophilic fibrillary deposits surrounding individual tumor cells and mimicking tumor osteoid may be seen
- Any of the variants of malignant fibrous histiocytoma in soft tissue may be found in bone tumors
  — Most common types are the storiform-pleomorphic variant and the giant cell–rich variant

Special Stains and Immunohistochemistry

- Vimentin positive
- CD68 typically positive

Other Techniques for Diagnosis

- Increased levels of C-myc protein

Differential Diagnosis

▎ Giant cell tumor
- Giant cell–rich variant of malignant fibrous histiocytoma may be misdiagnosed as a giant cell tumor
- Giant cell tumor does not exhibit significant nuclear pleomorphism and atypical mitoses

▎ Osteosarcoma
- Contains tumor osteoid

▎ Dedifferentiated chondrosarcoma
- Contains areas of low-grade chondrosarcoma

▎ Fibrosarcoma
- Composed of spindle cells arranged in a herringbone pattern
- Does not contain neoplastic multinucleated giant cells

Pearls

- Presence of definitive tumor osteoid within a bone tumor with features of malignant fibrous histiocytoma should be categorized as osteosarcoma
- Diagnosis of malignant fibrous histiocytoma should only be made after exclusion of tumors with myoid, lipomatous, chondroid, and osteoid differentiation; also rule out metastatic spindle cell carcinomas and melanoma

Selected References

Tarkkanen M, Larramendy ML, Böhling T, et al: Malignant fibrous histiocytoma of bone: Analysis of genomic imbalances by comparative genomic hybridisation and C-MYC expression by immunohistochemisty. Eur J Cancer 42:1172-1180, 2006.

Unni KK, Inwards CY, Bridge J, et al: Tumors of the Bones and Joints, 4th Series, Fascicle 2. Washington, DC, Armed Forces Institute of Pathology, 2005, pp 202-207.

Huvos AG, Heilweil M, Bretsky, SS: The pathology of malignant fibrous histiocytoma of bone: A study of 130 patients. Am J Surg Pathol 9:853-871, 1985.

Capanna R, Bertoni F, Bacchini P, et al: Malignant fibrous histiocytoma of bone: The experience at the Rizzoli Institute: report of 90 cases. Cancer 54:177-187, 1984.

Dahlin DC, Unni KK, Matsuno T: Malignant (fibrous) histiocytoma of bone—fact or fancy? Cancer 39:1508-1516, 1977.

Giant Cell Tumor

Clinical Features

- Typically occurs in skeletally mature patients
- Slight female predominance
- Most occur in second, third, and fourth decades
- Most common sites are distal femur, proximal tibia, distal radius, and sacrum
- Most patients present with localized pain
- Muscular atrophy with decreased range of motion of the adjacent joint may be present
- Some patients may present with a pathologic fracture

Radiographic Features

- Lytic epiphyseal mass without sclerosis or periosteal reaction
- May appear to extend into soft tissue but contains an outer rim of thin periosteal bone

Gross Pathology

- Curettage reveals friable, soft tissue of variable color
- Resected specimens reveal an epiphyseal mass that is red, brown, gray, and focally yellow
  — Can extend to the articular cartilage
  — May contain fleshy areas, foci of necrosis, and cystic changes suggestive of aneurysmal bone cyst

Figure 16-26. Giant cell tumor of the ulna. A, Typical circumscribed lytic lesion. **B,** Resected specimen shows a well-defined, fleshy tumor mass. **C,** Histologic section shows a single multinucleated giant cell with multiple nuclei in a background of sheets of mononuclear histiocytic cells and red blood cells.

Histopathology

- Typically consists of large numbers of evenly distributed multinucleated giant cells in a background of sheets of mononuclear histiocytic cells
- Mononuclear histiocytic cells are polygonal or round to oval with cytologically benign nuclei; variable mitotic rate with no atypical forms
- Multinucleated giant cells have features of osteoclasts
  — May contain numerous nuclei, sometimes greater than 100
  — Nuclei have benign cytologic features similar to the mononuclear cells
  — Giant cells are not mitotically active

- Foamy histiocytes, siderophages, reactive bone, and delicate vascular structures containing intravascular tumor may be seen
- Cartilaginous tissue is not found in giant cell tumors unless associated with a fracture

Special Stains and Immunohistochemistry

- Noncontributory

Other Techniques for Diagnosis

- Cytogenetically, giant cell tumors may demonstrate telomeric associations (tas), end-to-end fusion of cytogenetically appearing intact chromosomes; telomeres most commonly involved include 19q, 1p, 15p, 21p, 20q, and 18p
- Overexpression of *c-myc*, hepatocyte growth factor receptor, and vascular endothelial growth factor gene has been associated with more aggressive behavior

Differential Diagnosis

- Giant cell reparative granuloma
  - Lacks uniform distribution of giant cells
  - These giant cells contain much fewer nuclei
  - Tends to be an aggregate of giant cells around foci of hemorrhage
  - Stroma is more fibrotic and contains more abundant hemosiderin and hemorrhage
  - Stromal cells are spindle shaped rather than round to oval
- Nonossifying fibroma
  - Radiographically shows peripheral sclerosis
  - Typically affects younger patients
  - Usually metaphyseal lesions
- Aneurysmal bone cyst
  - Does not typically involve epiphyses
  - Giant cells are arranged around cystic spaces
- Giant cell–rich osteosarcoma
  - Though present only focally, delicate strands of osteoid can be found surrounding aggregates of pleomorphic mononuclear cells exhibiting atypical mitotic activity
- Metastatic carcinoma containing giant cells
  - Positive for epithelial markers: cytokeratin and EMA

Pearls

- Three common epiphyseal tumors, which include giant cell tumor, clear cell chondrosarcoma, and chondroblastoma
- Complete evaluation of clinicopathologic and radiographic features is essential in the diagnosis of giant cell tumor
- Account for about one fifth of all benign bone tumors
- Diagnosis of giant cell tumor in a skeletally immature patient should be questioned
- Paramyxovirus-like nuclear inclusions have been reported in some giant cell tumors

- May be associated with Paget disease of bone (craniofacial bones and pelvis)
- Serum chemistry may be helpful in the differential diagnosis of giant cell tumors
  - Elevated serum calcium and parathyroid hormone suggest hyperparathyroidism (brown tumor)
  - Elevated alkaline phosphatase and normal calcium may indicate a giant cell tumor arising in Paget disease of bone
- Benign pulmonary metastases (e.g., tumor embolization) may occur in patients with giant cell tumors that show intratumoral vascular invasion; however, this is an uncommon event
- Malignant giant cell tumors arise from benign giant cell tumors or in sites of prior benign giant cell tumors
- Tumors with radiographic evidence of aggressive growth should be evaluated carefully histologically

Selected References

Balke M, Schremper L, Gebert C, et al: Giant cell tumor of bone: Treatment and outcome of 214 cases. J Cancer Res Clin Oncol 134:969-973, 2008.

Junming M, Cheng Y, Dong C, et al: Giant cell tumor of the cervical spine: A series of 22 cases and outcomes. Spine 33:380-388, 2008.

Brimo F, Aziz M, Rosen G, et al: Malignancy in giant cell tumor of bone: Is there a reproducible histological threshold? A study of three giant cell tumours with worrisome features. Histopathology 51:864-866, 2007.

Unni KK, Inwards CY, Bridge J, et al: Tumors of the Bones and Joints, 4th Series, Fascicle 2. Washington, DC, Armed Forces Institute of Pathology, 2005, pp 281-298.

Bridge JA, Neff JR, Mouron BJ: Giant cell tumor of bone: Chromosomal analysis of 48 specimens and review of the literature. Cancer Genet Cytogenet 58:2-13, 1992.

Dahlin DC, Cupps RE, Johnson EW: Giant cell tumor: A study of 195 cases. Cancer 25:1061-1070, 1970.

Giant Cell Reparative Granuloma

Clinical Features

- Male-to-female ratio is equal
- 75% of patients are younger than 30 years
- Most common sites are phalanges, metatarsals, metacarpals, mandible, and maxilla
- Patients usually present with pain and swelling of variable duration

Radiographic Features

- Expansile, purely lytic lesion with cortical thinning
- May exhibit trabeculation and periosteal bone formation

Gross Pathology

- Curettage produces fragments of reddish-brown friable tissue

Figure 16-27. Giant cell reparative granuloma. Histologic section shows a single multinucleated giant cell containing few nuclei and surrounded by mononuclear stromal cells and foam cells.

Histopathology

- Consists of spindle cells within collagenous stroma and multinucleated giant cells exhibiting clustering around areas of hemorrhage
- Multinucleated giant cells are fewer in number and contain fewer nuclei than seen in giant cell tumors; mitoses are not seen in this cell population
- Mitotic figures (no atypical forms) may be found but typically are fewer than in giant cell tumors
- Scattered chronic inflammatory cells may be found in the stroma
- Reactive osteoid and bone may be present with and without osteoblastic rimming
- Siderophages, giant cells with phagocytized erythrocytes, and intravascular giant cells may be seen
- Secondary aneurysmal bone cyst formation may be found
- Cartilage is not present unless associated with a fracture

Special Stains and Immunohistochemistry

- Mononuclear stromal cells and multinucleated giant cells express α_1-antitrypsin, α_1-antichymotrypsin, and CD68

Other Techniques for Diagnosis

- Noncontributory

Differential Diagnosis

▍ Aneurysmal bone cyst
- May share histologic features with giant cell reparative granuloma; typically giant cells surround cystic spaces
- In tumors of the hands and feet, the presence of solid foci stromal cells and giant cells is more consistent with a diagnosis of giant cell reparative granuloma over primary aneurysmal bone cyst

▍ Brown tumor in hyperparathyroidism
- Histologically indistinguishable from giant cell reparative granuloma
- Patients have elevated serum calcium and parathyroid hormone levels

▍ Giant cell tumor
- Greater numbers of giant cells, which are generally evenly distributed without clustering
- Giant cells contain greater numbers of nuclei

▍ Nonossifying fibroma
- Aggregate of giant cells is not typical in these tumors
- Rare in bones of hands, feet, mandible, and maxilla

▍ Giant cell–rich osteosarcoma
- Contains delicate strands of osteoid, which can be found focally surrounding aggregates of pleomorphic mononuclear cells exhibiting atypical mitotic activity

▍ Malignant fibrous histiocytoma
- Cytologic features of malignancy can be found even if low grade
- Radiographic features include cortical destruction with soft tissue extension

Pearls

- May enlarge rapidly during pregnancy
- Have been found in association with polyostotic fibrous dysplasia and Paget disease of bone
- Any patient with the clinical diagnosis of giant cell reparative granuloma of bone should have serum calcium, phosphorous, alkaline phosphatase, and parathyroid hormone levels evaluated to rule out hyperparathyroidism

Selected References

De Lange J, van den Akker HP, van den Berg H: Central giant cell granuloma of the jaw: A review of the literature with emphasis on therapy options. Oral Surg Oral Med Oral Pathol Oral Radiol Endod 104:603-615, 2007.

Motamedi MH, Eshghyar N, Jafari SM, et al: Peripheral and central giant cell granulomas of the jaws: A demographic study. Oral Surg Oral Med Oral Pathol Oral Radiol Endod 103:e39-43, 2007.

Unni KK, Inwards CY, Bridge J, et al: Tumors of the Bones and Joints, 4th Series, Fascicle 2. Washington, DC, Armed Forces Institute of Pathology, 2005, pp 357-358.

Vigorita VJ: Orthopaedic Pathology. Philadelphia, Lippincott Williams & Wilkins, 1999, pp 272-273.

Adamantinoma

Clinical Features

- Male-to-female ratio is equal
- Most cases occur in second and third decades
- Most common site is the diaphysis of the tibia (>80%)
- Patients present with pain of variable duration from several weeks to several years

Figure 16-28. Adamantinoma. Histologic section slows strands of epithelial cells with peripheral palisading and stellate reticulum-like stroma.

- May be swelling and pathologic fracture at presentation
- Significant number of patients report a history of trauma, which is most likely coincidental

Radiographic Features

- Eccentric, multicystic (soap-bubble appearance), lobulated, lytic diaphyseal tibial defect
- Usually involves both the cortical and medullary portions of the bone and may be multifocal in the same bone
- Peripheral sclerosis may connect multiple lesions
- Cortical expansion with thinning
- Occasionally cortical penetration with development of a soft tissue mass is seen

Gross Pathology

- Well-circumscribed, lobulated gray mass
- Variable consistency from soft to granular to fibrous
- May contain regional hemorrhage and cystic changes

Histopathology

- Characterized by a hypocellular fibrous stroma containing epithelioid cellular islands
- Epithelioid cellular islands may be composed of various cell types, including basaloid, squamoid, tubular, or spindle cells
  - Nests with basaloid patterns exhibit central loose spindle cells (stellate reticulum-like) with peripheral palisading of cuboidal cells
  - Squamoid cell nests may show keratinization
  - Tubular pattern consists of branching and anastomosing tubular structures lined by a single layer of epithelioid cells, imparting a vascular appearance
  - Spindle cell pattern consists of plump, fibroblast-like spindle cells within a fibrous stroma reminiscent of the sclerosing variant of basal cell carcinoma

- These cells are generally bland without atypia and mitotic activity; rare cases may exhibit mild atypia and occasional mitotic figures

Special Stains and Immunohistochemistry

- Cytokeratin: epithelioid islands are positive

Other Techniques for Diagnosis

- Cytogenetic studies have shown that extra copies of chromosomes 7, 8, 12, 19, and 21 are recurrent in adamantinoma; inversions, translocations, deletions, and marker chromosomes may also be detected

Differential Diagnosis

- Osteofibrous dysplasia
  - Lacks epithelioid cell islands
  - Stroma may contain individual cytokeratin positive cells
  - Cytogenetics may be similar to adamantinoma; osteofibrous dysplasia lacks structural abnormalities such as translocations, inversions, and deletions
- Fibrous dysplasia
  - Lacks cytokeratin-positive epithelial cells
- Metastatic carcinoma
  - Tumor cells typically show significantly more cytologic atypia with nuclear pleomorphism
  - High mitotic rate often with atypical forms

Pearls

- Slow-growing, locally destructive tumors with low metastatic potential
- Typically cured by local resection

Selected References

Jain D, Jain VK, Vasishta RK, et al: Adamantinoma: A clinicopathological review and update. Diagn Pathol 3:8, 2008.

Papagelopoulos PJ, Mavrogenis AF, Galanis EC, et al: Clinicopathological features, diagnosis, and treatment of adamantinoma of the long bones. Orthopedics 30:211-217, 2007.

Unni KK, Inwards CY, Bridge J, et al: Tumors of the Bones and Joints, 4th Series, Fascicle 2. Washington, DC, Armed Forces Institute of Pathology, 2005, pp 299-307.

Vigorita VJ: Orthopaedic Pathology. Philadelphia, Lippincott Williams & Wilkins, 1999, 401-403.

Small Cell Neoplasms

Ewing Sarcoma

Clinical Features

- Male-to-female ratio is about 1.3:1
- Most patients present between ages 5 and 20 years; rare in patients younger than 5 and older than 30 years

Figure 16-29. Ewing sarcoma. A, Radiograph of the radius shows a medullary lesion with expansion and permeation of the cortex, giving a sunburst appearance. **B,** Histologic section shows small, uniform cells with hyperchromatic nuclei and scant, vacuolated cytoplasm.

- Bones in the lower extremities and pelvis are the most common sites; rare in the upper extremities
- Patients present with progressively increasing pain and swelling
- Presence of fever, increased sedimentation rate, leukocytosis, anemia, and malaise may indicate disseminated disease

Radiographic Features

- Poorly marginated lytic or sclerotic diaphyseal mass with periosteal reaction (sunburst or onion-skin pattern)
- Soft tissue mass may be present
- Extensive permeation of bone marrow may be seen on MRI

Gross Pathology

- Intact tumor consists of a gray-white intramedullary mass that is soft, glistening, and moist
- May be watery and have the appearance of pus
- Regional areas of cystic changes and hemorrhage may be present

Histopathology

- Consists of broad sheets of small, uniform cells with hyperchromatic nuclei with inconspicuous nucleoli, scant cytoplasm, and indistinct cell borders; minimal surrounding stroma
- Occasional mitotic activity
- Usually a subgroup of degenerate or apoptotic cells that have hyperchromatic pyknotic nuclei
- Rosettes, lobular architecture, focal spindle cells, and metaplastic bone or cartilage may be present
- Areas of geographic necrosis or small foci of necrosis are usually seen
- Chemotherapy and radiation may cause tumor cells to be more pleomorphic and have larger nuclei with folded forms, multinucleated forms, and prominent nucleoli
- Large cell variant may morphologically resemble lymphoma

Special Stains and Immunohistochemistry

- CD99 (MIC2) positive
- PAS: most tumors exhibit intracytoplasmic glycogen
- Vimentin and cytokeratin: variable expression
- Chromogranin and synaptophysin: negative
- Leukocyte common antigen (LCA), SMA, MSA, and vascular markers negative

Other Techniques for Diagnosis

- Cytogenetic studies demonstrate characteristic chromosomal translocation t(11;22)(q24;q12) in 95% of cases
- Presence of type 1 *EWS/FLI1* fusion gene as opposed to type 2 has prognostic significance, with type 1 exhibiting significant longer survival
- MIC2 overexpression may be demonstrated by in situ hybridization

Differential Diagnosis

▮ Neuroectodermal tumor of bone
- Characteristically shows prominent rosettes
- Positive for chromogranin and synaptophysin
- Worse prognosis

▮ Metastatic neuroblastoma
- Typically occurs in children younger than 5 years
- Urinary catecholamine metabolites may be elevated
- Tends to metastasize to the skull
- Contains Homer-Wright rosettes with fibrillary background
- Expresses neuroendocrine markers; negative for CD99

▮ Lymphoma, leukemia
- Expresses lymphoid markers; negative for CD99

▮ Osteosarcoma, small cell variant
- Foci of tumor osteoid should be present
- Negative for CD99

◼ Mesenchymal chondrosarcoma
  - Foci of chondroid differentiation should be present
  - Tumor expresses S-100 protein
  - Negative for CD99 and MIC2

Pearls

- Rare in blacks, patients younger than 5 years, and patients older than 30 years
- In patients younger than 5 years, metastatic neuroblastoma and leukemia-lymphoma are more common and should be ruled out
- In patients older than 30 years, metastatic small cell carcinoma and large cell lymphoma are more common and should be ruled out
- If greater than 20% of the tumor contains rosettes, primitive neuroectodermal tumor (PNET) should be considered
- Differentiation from PNET is important because the prognosis of Ewing sarcoma appears to be better, even though these tumors are identical by molecular analysis
- Multiple bone involvement at time of diagnosis is not uncommon

Selected References

Riggi N, Suvá ML, Suvá D, et al: EWS-FLI-1 expression triggers a Ewing's sarcoma initiation program in primary human mesenchymal stem cells. Cancer Res 68:2176-2185, 2008.

Peersman B, Vanhoenacker FM, Heyman S, et al: Ewing's sarcoma: Imaging features. JBR-BTR 90:368-376, 2007.

Unni KK, Inwards CY, Bridge J, et al: Tumors of the Bones and Joints, 4th Series, Fascicle 2. Washington, DC, Armed Forces Institute of Pathology, 2005, pp 209-222.

Kissane JM, Askin FB, Foulkes M, et al: Ewing's sarcoma of bone: Clinicopathologic aspects of 303 cases from the Intergroup Ewing's Sarcoma Study. Hum Pathol 14:773-779, 1983.

Lymphoma

Clinical Features

- Male-to-female ratio is 1.5:1
- Most tumors occur in second through eighth decades
- Pelvis and bones of the lower extremities are the most common sites
- Patients present with pain, typically of long duration (>1 year)

Radiographic Features

- Lytic lesion with a moth-eaten appearance
- May be sclerotic, suggesting Paget disease of bone
- Usually no periosteal reaction
- Soft tissue mass may be present; MRI, CT, and isotope scans may be helpful in delineating the extent of disease

Figure 16-30. Lymphoma, large cell type. High-power view shows sheets of large, atypical lymphoid cells.

Gross Pathology

- Typically a soft, white, fleshy mass
- Permeates the medullary cavity
- Cyst formation, necrosis, and hemorrhagic foci may be present

Histopathology

- Diffuse large cell lymphomas are the most common type
- Composed of sheets of large cells that may or may not have cleaved nuclei; most are noncleaved
- Some tumors may contain multilobate nuclei or cells with immunoblastic features
- May exhibit a prominent inflammatory infiltrate consisting of neutrophils and mature lymphocytes, which may suggest a diagnosis of osteomyelitis
- Small cell lymphomas and mixed small cell–large cell lymphomas may also occur
- Spindle cell patterns suggestive of sarcoma or clear cell patterns, signet ring cell variants, and clustering of epithelioid cells suggestive of metastatic carcinoma may occur
- Starry-sky pattern (Burkitt lymphoma) occurs in the maxilla and mandible

Special Stains and Immunohistochemistry

- Tumor cells express lymphoid markers and are usually of B-cell type
  — CD45 and CD20 positive
  — Anaplastic large cell lymphomas may express CD30
  — Large cell lymphomas may express bcl-2
- Hodgkin lymphoma may express CD15 and CD30
- Reticulin stain highlights fine network of reticulin around individual tumor cells

Other Techniques for Diagnosis

- Phenotyping by flow cytometry and gene rearrangement studies may be helpful in ruling out benign processes that may mimic lymphoma

- About 80% of non-Hodgkin lymphomas have clonal chromosome abnormalities

Differential Diagnosis

▋ Neuroectodermal tumor of bone
  - Typically have prominent rosettes
  - Positive for NSE, chromogranin, synaptophysin, CD99
  - Negative for LCA
▋ Metastatic neuroblastoma
  - Usually occurs in children younger than 5 years
  - May have elevated urinary catecholamine metabolites
  - Tends to metastasize to the skull
  - Characterized by Homer-Wright rosettes with fibrillary background
  - Positive for NSE, chromogranin, and synaptophysin
▋ Osteosarcoma, small cell variant
  - Foci of tumor osteoid should be seen
▋ Mesenchymal chondrosarcoma
  - Foci of chondroid differentiation
  - Tumor cells express S-100 protein; negative for LCA
▋ Metastatic small cell carcinoma
  - Positive for cytokeratin and neuroendocrine markers
▋ Langerhans cell histiocytosis
  - Composed of histiocytes with a prominent eosinophilic cellular infiltrate
  - Histiocytes express S-100 protein and CD1a
▋ Sarcoma
  - Occasionally lymphomas will have a spindle cell component, mimicking sarcoma
  - Sarcomas do not express leukocyte and lymphoid markers
▋ Chronic osteomyelitis
  - Typically composed of a polymorphous inflammatory infiltrate with lymphocytes, eosinophils, and neutrophils; lacks large neoplastic lymphocytes
  - Immunophenotypically consists of a mixed population of B and T cells
  - Absence of clonal population by flow cytometry or gene rearrangement

Pearls

- T-cell lymphomas of bone are extremely rare and are most common in Japan
- Primary Hodgkin disease of bone is rare, with the most common types being nodular sclerosing and mixed cellularity; axial skeletal involvement is much more common than appendicular involvement
- Primary lymphoma of bone is diagnosed only if there is no evidence of extraskeletal lymphoma 6 months after original diagnosis of the bone lesion and there is no prior history of extraskeletal lymphoma

- Primary lymphoma of bone is more common in the appendicular skeleton, whereas secondary osseous lymphoma is more common in the axial skeleton
- When metastatic to bone, low-grade secondary osseous lymphomas do not necessarily have a worse prognosis, whereas secondary high-grade osseous lymphomas do have a worse prognosis

Selected References

Lima FP, Bousquet M, Gomez-Brouchet A, et al: Primary diffuse large B-cell lymphoma of bone displays preferential rearrangements of the c-MYC or BCL2 gene. Am J Clin Pathol 129:723-726, 2008.

Unni KK, Inwards CY, Bridge J, et al: Tumors of the Bones and Joints, 4th Series, Fascicle 2. Washington, DC, Armed Forces Institute of Pathology, 2005, pp 231-240.

McCarthy EF: Differential Diagnosis in Pathology: Bone and Joint Disorders. New York, Igaku-Shoin, 1996, pp 126-129.

Multiple Myeloma and Solitary Plasmacytoma

Clinical Features

- Male-to-female ratio is about 2:1
- Most cases occur between ages 50 and 80 years
- Solitary plasmacytoma tends to occur at a slightly younger age
- Vertebrae, ribs, skull, pelvis, and long bones are the most common sites
- Patients with multiple myeloma present with pain, usually of less than 6 months' duration
  — May cause weight loss, peripheral neuropathy, pathologic fracture, fever, anemia, bleeding, hypercalcemia, hypergammaglobulinemia, and renal dysfunction
- Patients with solitary plasmacytoma usually present with pain; about 10% of patients with solitary plasmacytoma are asymptomatic
- Some cases may be associated with POEMS syndrome (*p*olyneuropathy, *o*rganomegaly [hepatosplenomegaly and lymphadenopathy], *e*ndocrinopathy [amenorrhea, diabetes, gynecomastia, hirsutism, or impotence], *M*-protein, and *s*kin changes [hyperpigmentation, hypertrichosis, or clubbing of digits])

Radiographic Features

- In multiple myeloma, there are multiple punched-out lytic lesions, typically without sclerosis or periosteal reaction
- Solitary plasmacytoma may exhibit a lytic lesion in vertebrae with cortical ridging (corduroy cloth) or a bubbly appearance in long bones; cortical expansion may be seen

Gross Pathology

- Soft, gray-red tissue involving the marrow space

Figure 16-31. Multiple myeloma involving the skull. A, Multiple osteolytic, defined round lesions. **B,** Cross section of the scalp shows punched-out lesions. **C,** Histologic section shows sheets of plasma cells.

Histopathology

- Tumor is composed of sheets of small cells with plasmacytic features
  — Eccentric nuclei with stippled chromatin patterns (cartwheel or clock face)
  — Cytoplasm is eosinophilic with perinuclear clearing (perinuclear Golgi zone)

- Intracytoplasmic immunoglobulins may produce grapelike structures (Mott cells or morula)
- Extracytoplasmic immunoglobulins may be found and are represented as Russell bodies (extracellular eosinophilic spherical bodies)
- Plasma cells may be atypical, multinucleated, or immature (plasmablasts have large nuclei and prominent nucleoli)
- Generally, mitotic activity is not prominent unless atypical forms or plasmablasts are present
- Amyloid may be present accompanied by giant cell reaction

Special Stains and Immunohistochemistry

- Predominance of either κ or λ light chains (clonal process)
- CD38, CD10 positive
- Positive for immunoglobulin G (IgG) or IgA, less commonly for either IgM or IgE
- Tumor cells may express EMA but are cytokeratin negative
- Congo red stain with apple-green birefringence is seen if amyloid is present
- Negative for LCA

Other Techniques for Diagnosis

- Serum and urine immunoelectrophoresis is used to demonstrate a monoclonal gammopathy and the presence of light chains
  — Dense band usually in IgG region by serum protein electrophoresis (SPE)
- Flow cytometry will demonstrate light-chain clonality
- Gene rearrangements usually found in IgG chain

Differential Diagnosis

▍ Chronic osteomyelitis
- Typically composed of a polymorphous inflammatory infiltrate with lymphocytes, eosinophils, and neutrophils
- Prominent fibrosis
- κ-to-λ ratio is normal or slightly elevated (about 3:1)

▍ Metastatic carcinoma
- Occasionally the plasma cell infiltrate will mimic an epithelial neoplasm
- Epithelial cells are cytokeratin positive
- EMA is not helpful because myeloma cells can be EMA positive

▍ B-cell immunoblastic lymphoma
- Positive for B-cell markers

Pearls

- Most patients with solitary plasmacytoma progress to multiple myeloma
- About 4% of cases of multiple myeloma are nonsecretory; paraprotein is made, but it is not secreted outside the cell (these patients tend to have a

better prognosis than do those with the secretory form of myeloma)

- Most common sites of solitary plasmacytoma are thoracic and lumbar vertebrae
- κ Light chains are the most common type of light chain produced in multiple myeloma
- IgG and IgA are the most common monoclonal gammopathies produced in multiple myeloma (IgG more common than IgA)
- About 75% of patients with solitary plasmacytoma do not have a serum M-component (paraprotein)
- Presence of immature plasmablastic cells is pathognomonic for myeloma in a subset of the literature
- Multinucleated forms of plasma cells are not diagnostic of myeloma or solitary plasmacytoma; may be found in reactive and inflammatory processes
- Multiple myeloma is the most common primary malignant bone tumor
- Osteosclerotic myeloma is a rare form that presents in younger patients with bone lesions that are sclerotic

Selected References

Edwards CM, Zhuang J, Mundy GR: The pathogenesis of the bone disease of multiple myeloma. Bone 42:1007-1013, 2008.

Bilsky MH, Azeem S: Multiple myeloma: primary bone tumor with systemic manifestations. Neurosurg Clin N Am 19:31-40, 2008.

Unni KK, Inwards CY, Bridge J, et al: Tumors of the Bones and Joints, 4th Series, Fascicle 2. Washington, DC, Armed Forces Institute of Pathology, 2005, pp 222-231.

Vigorita VJ: Orthopaedic Pathology. Philadelphia, Lippincott Williams & Wilkins, 1999, pp 455-463.

Miscellaneous Bone Lesions

Chordoma

Clinical Features

- Male-to-female ratio is 2:1
- Most occur in fourth to seventh decades; occurrence in patients younger than 30 years is rare
- Spheno-occipital tumors tend to occur at a slightly younger age (10 years younger) than sacral tumors
- One half of cases involve the sacrum, and one third occur in the spheno-occipital region; remainder occur in cervical and lumbar regions of the spinal cord
- Symptoms are dependent on site of tumor
  — Sacral tumors present with pain, bladder dysfunction, and constipation
  — Spheno-occipital tumors present with cranial nerve deficits, hypopituitarism, and diplopia

Radiographic Features

- Midline lytic destructive tumor that may contain intralesional calcifications

Figure 16-32. **Chordoma.** Histologic section shows nests and cords of large vacuolated cells within a myxoid mucoid matrix.

- In spheno-occipital tumors, there may be erosion of the sella turcica, clivus, and sphenoid bones

Gross Pathology

- Lobulated gelatinous gray tissue that may appear encapsulated

Histopathology

- Lobulated mass containing vacuolated cells forming nests and cords or strands within a myxoid mucoid matrix
- Cellularity is variable and some tumors may contain solid areas
- Rare mitoses may be present
- Classic *physaliphorous* cells are round to oval and have a central nucleus with a prominent nucleolus; cytoplasm is abundant and eosinophilic with circumferential perinuclear vacuoles imparting a bubbly appearance to the cell cytoplasm; typically found in a myxoid matrix and may form syncytia
- May exhibit foci of chondroid differentiation, especially in spheno-occipital tumors; designated *chondroid chordoma*
- Rare cases exhibit a malignant spindle cell component with features of malignant fibrous histiocytoma; designated *dedifferentiated chordoma*

Special Stains and Immunohistochemistry

- Cytokeratin (CAM-5.2) and EMA positive
- Vimentin and S-100 protein positive

Other Techniques for Diagnosis

- Noncontributory

Differential Diagnosis

▮ Chondrosarcoma
- Tumor cells are negative for cytokeratin and EMA
▮ Metastatic adenocarcinoma
- Does not have a physaliphorous pattern
- Often exhibits glandular differentiation

■ Liposarcoma
  ● Tumor cells are negative for cytokeratin and EMA

Pearls

  ● Chordoma is not an uncommon neoplasm; follows osteosarcoma, chondrosarcoma, and Ewing sarcoma in frequency of primary malignant bone tumors
  ● Classic physaliphorous cells may be rare in some cases
  ● In some studies, chondroid chordoma has a higher survival rate than traditional chordoma
  ● Dedifferentiated chordomas typically occur after several recurrences of a classic chordoma; some of these patients have been irradiated, suggesting that these tumors are radiation induced

Selected References

Cho YH, Kim JH, Khang SK, et al: Chordomas and chondrosarcomas of the skull base: Comparative analysis of clinical results in 30 patients. Neurosurg Rev 31:35-43, 2008.

Sell M, Sampaolo S, Di Lorio G, Theallier A: Chordomas: A histological and immunohistochemical study of cases with and without recurrent tumors. Clin Neuropathol 23:277-285, 2004.

Papagelopoulos PJ, Mavrogenis AF, Galanis EC, et al: Chordoma of the spine: Clinicopathological features, diagnosis, and treatment. Orthopedics 27:1256-1263, 2004.

Aneurysmal Bone Cyst

Clinical Features

  ● Male-to-female ratio is about 1.3:1
  ● More than 75% of cases occur in first two decades
  ● Three fourths occur in vertebrae (posterior aspect and spinous process), distal femur, and proximal tibia
  ● Small bones of the hands and feet and craniofacial bones are also relatively common sites
  ● Pain of variable duration and swelling are presenting symptoms

Radiographic Features

  ● Eccentric metaphyseal or posterior vertebral cystic ballooned lytic lesion initially exhibits a permeative growth pattern with cortical destruction
  ● Periosteal bone formation may be seen
  ● In older lesions, a thin outer bony shell (eggshell) develops, and the cyst becomes trabeculated

Gross Pathology

  ● Hemorrhagic, cystic, honeycomb mass
  ● Fibrous septa separating the cavernous cystic spaces are gritty
  ● Spaces are filled with blood or serosanguineous fluid
  ● Solid, soft-gray to white mass may be present, representing a precursor lesion in secondary aneurysmal bone cysts

Figure 16-33. Aneurysmal bone cyst. A, Cross section shows complex, multiloculated cystic spaces filled with blood. **B,** Histologic section shows cystic spaces filled with red blood cells surrounded by giant cells, fibroblasts, and inflammatory cells.

Histopathology

  ● Composed of numerous cavernous or cystic spaces filled with blood and lacking an endothelial lining
  ● Spaces are separated by fibrous septa lacking smooth muscle and containing fibroblasts, capillaries, inflammatory cells, giant cells, benign osteoid (may resemble osteoblastoma), and benign chondroid tissue
  ● Chondroid areas may have myxoid features, which is characteristic of aneurysmal bone cysts
  ● Mitotic activity may be brisk, but no atypical mitosis or stromal cell nuclear anaplasia is present
  ● Secondary aneurysmal bone cysts have solid areas exhibiting histologic features of the precursor lesion
  ● Secondary aneurysmal bone cyst may occur in many tumors, including the following: osteosarcoma, malignant fibrous histiocytoma, metastatic carcinoma, osteoblastoma, chondroblastoma, chondromyxoid fibroma, giant cell tumor, nonossifying fibroma, fibrous histiocytoma, fibrous dysplasia, eosinophilic granuloma, hemangioma, giant cell reparative granuloma, and unicameral bone cyst

Special Stains and Immunohistochemistry

- Noncontributory

Other Techniques for Diagnosis

- Noncontributory

Differential Diagnosis

▌ Unicameral bone cyst
- Fibrous septa are usually hypocellular, with foci containing occasional giant cells
- Fibrous septa lack inflammatory cells, osteoid, and chondroid tissue

▌ Giant cell tumor
- Located in the epiphyses in skeletally mature patients
- Stromal mononuclear cells and numerous multinucleated giant cells are present

▌ Telangiectatic osteosarcoma
- Uncommon in vertebrae, craniofacial bones, and bones of hands and feet
- Anaplastic tumor with production of tumor osteoid
- May show complex karyotypic abnormalities not found in aneurysmal bone cyst

▌ Secondary aneurysmal bone cyst
- Histologic evidence of a precursor lesion (see "Histopathology") should be identified

Pearls

- Curettings and any solid areas of an excised tumor should be processed completely to evaluate for the presence of a precursor lesion
- Clinicoradiographic correlation is necessary in determining whether the histology represents a secondary aneurysmal bone cyst
- Precursor lesion is found in about half of aneurysmal bone cysts; most common preexisting lesions are giant cell tumor, chondroblastoma, fibrous dysplasia, and chondromyxoid fibroma
- Radiographic features of an aneurysmal bone cyst may mimic a malignant process

Selected References

Saccomanni B: Aneurysmal bone cyst of spine: A review of literature. Arch Orthop Trauma Surg 128:1145-1147, 2007.

Basrir K, Piskin A, Guclü B, et al: Aneurysmal bone cyst recurrence in children: A review of 56 patients. J Pediatr Orthop 27:938-943, 2007.

Mendenhall WM, Zlotecki RA, Gibbs CP, et al: Aneurysmal bone cyst. Am J Clin Oncol 29:311-315, 2006.

Unni KK, Inwards CY, Bridge J, et al: Tumors of the Bones and Joints, 4th Series, Fascicle 2. Washington, DC, Armed Forces Institute of Pathology, 2005, pp 324-330.

Martinez V, Sissons HA: Aneurysmal bone cyst: A review of 123 cases including primary lesions and those secondary to other bone pathology. Cancer 61:2291-2304, 1988.

Unicameral Bone Cyst (Simple Cyst)

Clinical Features

- Male-to-female ratio is about 2:1
- Most cases occur in first two decades
- Most common sites are proximal humerus, mid-humerus, and proximal femur
- Most are asymptomatic, but some patients present with sudden onset of pain due to pathologic fracture

Radiographic Features

- Elongated medullary expanding cystic lesion without cortical disruption
- Bone fragment may be present in the dependent area of the cyst (fallen-fragment sign)
- Cyst may contain fluid that has the density of water

Gross Pathology

- Intramedullary cyst containing clear or straw-colored, nonviscous, serous-like fluid
- May be multiloculated
- Cyst is composed of thin, delicate fibrous tissue

Histopathology

- Cyst wall is composed of thin, hypocellular fibrous tissue
- Occasional giant cells may be seen in the fibrous septa
- Inflammatory changes are absent or minimal
- No osteoid or chondroid tissue

Special Stains and Immunohistochemistry

- Noncontributory

Other Techniques for Diagnosis

- Noncontributory

Differential Diagnosis

▌ Aneurysmal bone cyst
- Contains osteoid and chondroid tissue with fibromyxoid features, and giant cells

▌ Giant cell tumor
- Occurs in the epiphyses of bones in skeletally mature patients
- Composed of mononuclear stromal cells and many more giant cells than are normally seen in unicameral bone cyst

Pearls

- Fracture of unicameral bone cyst may complicate the histology because of the presence of reactive bone; may result in misinterpretation as aneurysmal bone cyst

Selected References

Unni KK, Inwards CY, Bridge J, et al: Tumors of the Bones and Joints, 4th Series, Fascicle 2. Washington, DC, Armed Forces Institute of Pathology, 2005, p 330.

Vigorita VJ: Orthopaedic Pathology. Philadelphia, Lippincott Williams & Wilkins, 1999, pp 256-261.

Dorfman HD, Czerniak B: Bone Tumors. St. Louis, Mosby, 1998, pp 879-891.

McCarthy EF: Differential Diagnosis in Pathology: Bone and Joint Disorders. New York, Igaku-Shoin, 1996, pp 105-107.

Paget Disease of Bone

Clinical Features

- Male-to-female ratio is 2:1
- Most cases occur in fifth and sixth decades; rarely found in patients younger than 40 years
- Most common sites are pelvis, skull, femur, vertebrae, and tibia
- Patients may be asymptomatic or present with pain
- Other symptoms that may occur at presentation or develop later are largely due to hypercalcemia and include deafness and other cranial nerve deficits, high-output heart failure, nephrolithiasis, hyperuricemia, arthritis, fractures, leonine facies, and femoral, tibial, or vertebral bowing

Figure 16-34. Paget disease of bone. A, Gross section of the calvarium shows marked overgrowth of the cortex. **B,** Histologic section shows irregularly thickened bony trabeculae with prominent cement lines.

Radiographic Features

- Bones show increased density with cotton-wool appearance intermixed with lucent areas
- Flame-shaped or V-shaped lytic areas may be seen in long bones; known as a *flame sign* or *blade of grass sign*
- Increased bone density or cortical thickening (window-frame appearance); round occipital and frontal bone radiolucencies (osteitis circumscripta) may be present

Gross Pathology

- Pinkish discoloration of bone due to increased vascularity
- Coarse, irregular, thickened cortex
- Irregular, thickened medullary cancellous bone
- Mosaic pattern of cement lines with rock-hard, dense bone in late stages

Histopathology

- Initially prominent osteoclastic activity with clustering of osteoclasts (large multinucleate forms)
  — Bony trabeculae with Howship lacunae formation
  — Intratrabecular fibrosis with increased vascularization
- Later, prominent osteoblastic activity and production of osteoid with abnormal collagen deposition are seen
- In the final inactive stage, the bony trabeculae are irregularly thickened, and cement lines form a mosaic pattern

Special Stains and Immunohistochemistry

- Noncontributory

Other Techniques for Diagnosis

- Genetic factors may play an important role, with mutations affecting different components of RANK-NF-κB signaling pathway

Differential Diagnosis

▮ Osteoblastic metastatic carcinoma
  - Tumor cells positive for cytokeratin
▮ Chronic osteomyelitis
  - Mixed inflammatory infiltrate consisting of intratrabecular plasma cells, lymphocytes, and occasional neutrophils
▮ Fibrous dysplasia
  - Osteoid islands do not exhibit osteoclastic or osteoblastic activity and do not contain abnormal cement lines
▮ Osteoblastoma
  - Usually occurs in a younger age group
  - May involve the jaw bones but usually does not involve the calvarium
  - Radiographic evidence of calcification may be present within the tumor
  - Histologically, osteoblastoma is sharply demarcated from uninvolved bone

Pearls

- Disease is a manifestation of an imbalance in bone metabolism; dysregulated osteoclastic activity followed by osteoblastic activity
- Symptoms result from hypercalcemia
- Measles virus has been found in osteoclast precursors in Paget disease of bone
- Sarcoma occurs in about 1% of patients with Paget disease of bone; increases to about 20% in patients with polyostotic disease for more than 20 years
- Most common sarcoma arising in Paget disease of bone is osteosarcoma; other tumors that may arise are malignant fibrous histiocytoma, fibrosarcoma, chondrosarcoma, and malignant giant cell tumor
- Survival rate of patients with osteosarcoma arising in Paget disease of bone is much lower than that of classic osteosarcoma
- An increase in the baseline serum alkaline phosphatase level in a patient with Paget disease of bone is suggestive of sarcomatous transformation

Selected References

Layfield R: The molecular pathogenesis of Paget disease of bone. Expert Rev Mol Med 9:1-13, 2007.

Josse RG, Hanley DA, Kendler D, et al: Diagnosis and treatment of Paget's disease of bone. Clin Invest Med 30:E210-223, 2007.

Deyrup AT, Montag AG, Inwards CY, et al: Sarcomas arising in Paget disease of bone: A clinicopathologic analysis of 70 cases. Arch Pathol Lab Med 131:942-946, 2007.

Sharma H, Mehdi SA, MacDuff E, et al: Paget sarcoma of the spine: Scottish Bone Tumor Registry experience. Spine 31:1344-1350, 2006.

Unni KK, Inwards CY, Bridge J, et al: Tumors of the Bones and Joints, 4th Series, Fascicle 2. Washington, DC, Armed Forces Institute of Pathology, 2005, pp 368-370.

Metastatic Tumors

Clinical Features

- Most common sites are axial and proximal appendicular skeleton in adults and include pelvis, ribs, vertebrae, skull, and proximal femur and humerus
- Pain, swelling, and tenderness are the most common symptoms; some patients present with a pathologic fracture
- Most patients (about 80%) present with a history of a primary malignancy

Radiographic Features

- Consist of multiple, irregular, moth-eaten destructive lesions that are usually lytic but can be blastic or mixed lytic-blastic
- Periosteal reaction may be present

Figure 16-35. Metastatic adenocarcinoma. Histologic section shows bone with metastatic adenocarcinoma in a patient with a lung primary.

Gross Pathology

- Usually poorly delineated with infiltrative margins
- Variable in appearance, color, and consistency, depending on their primary tumor type
- Prostatic metastases are osteoblastic and may be dense

Histopathology

- Most metastatic lesions exhibit histologic features suggestive of some line of differentiation (squamous, glandular, mesenchymal, or melanocytic)
- Clear cell patterns, glandular patterns with follicular features, and pigmented spindle cell tumors are indicative of renal cell carcinoma, follicular carcinoma of thyroid, and melanoma, respectively, and generally pose no problems in identifying the primary
- Some tumors are undifferentiated and require immunohistochemistry for determination of the site of origin
- Spindle cell tumors require immunohistochemistry to differentiate true sarcomas from the spindle cell variant of renal cell carcinoma and other spindle cell carcinomas

Special Stains and Immunohistochemistry

- Battery of immunohistochemical stains may be necessary to delineate primary tumor origin, depending on clinical history and morphology

Other Techniques for Diagnosis

- Noncontributory

Differential Diagnosis

▌ Osteosarcoma
- Metastatic carcinoma may produce prominent osteoid, suggesting osteosarcoma
- Negative for cytokeratin

- ■ Primary bone sarcomas
  - Differentiation of primary bone sarcomas (malignant fibrous histiocytoma and fibrosarcoma) can be difficult and requires clinical correlation
- ■ Paget disease
  - May mimic osteoblastic metastases
  - Osteoblasts lining trabecular bone may appear atypical but do not express cytokeratin

Pearls

- Metastatic tumor cells reach bone through arterial embolization or retrograde flow through venous plexuses (e.g., Batson plexus, which lacks valves) or through veins with defective valves
- Metastases to bones distal to the elbows and knees are rare in adults
  - Metastatic acral bone tumors are usually due to metastatic lung carcinoma
  - Metastatic tumors to bone are more common in the appendiceal skeleton in children
- The most common primary malignancies in adults to metastasize to bone are prostate, kidney, thyroid, lung, pancreas, and breast
- In children, the most common are rhabdomyosarcoma, clear cell carcinoma of kidney, and neuroblastoma
- Osteolytic lesions on radiographs are usually thyroid, kidney, lung, or gastrointestinal tract in origin
- Osteoblastic lesions on radiographs are usually metastatic prostate, medulloblastoma, or carcinoid
- Tumor cells in prostatic adenocarcinoma metastasized to bone in patients previously treated may appear histiocytic and require immunohistochemistry (prostate-specific antigen, prostatic acid phosphatase) to identify prostatic origin

Selected References

Ricco AI, Wodajo FM, Malawer M: Metastatic carcinoma of the long bones. Am Fam Physician 76:1489-1494, 2007.

Unni KK, Inwards CY, Bridge J, et al: Tumors of the Bones and Joints, 4th Series, Fascicle 2. Washington, DC, Armed Forces Institute of Pathology, 2005, pp 321-324.

Vigorita VJ: Orthopaedic Pathology. Philadelphia, Lippincott Williams & Wilkins, 1999, pp 472-489.

Joint and Synovial Diseases

Osteoarthritis

Clinical Features

- Male-to-female ratio is equal
- Greater than 80% occur in patients older than 55 years
- Interphalangeal joints of the hands; metacarpophalangeal joint of the thumb, hips, and knees; cervical and lumbar vertebrae; and metatarsophalangeal joint of great toe may be affected
- Other joints may be affected in secondary osteoarthritis
- Patients complain of arthralgia, limitation of motion, joint enlargement, and swelling
- Vertebral involvement may produce paresthesias, muscle weakness, and hyperreflexia
- Secondary osteoarthritis may result from Legg-Calvé-Perthes disease, previous history of gouty arthritis, rheumatoid arthritis, infectious arthritis, pseudogout, Paget disease of bone, osteonecrosis, hemarthrosis, trauma, hemochromatosis, and Wilson disease

Radiographic Features

- Diagnostic features include osteophyte formation, asymmetric joint space narrowing, subchondral osteosclerosis, and subchondral cyst formation

Gross Pathology

- Cartilaginous articular surface is thinned, irregular, or denuded, giving a polished ivory appearance to the outer subchondral bone (bony eburnation)
- Subchondral bone is thickened and sclerotic
- Peripheral osteophyte formation is common

Histopathology

- Articular cartilaginous surface is fibrillated, frayed, and thinned or denuded
- Chondrocytic hyperplasia is represented by aggregates of chondrocytes surrounded by basophilic staining matrix
- Subchondral bone is represented by thickened trabeculae
- Intratrabecular granulation tissue is present and may contain few lymphocytes and plasma cells
- Intratrabecular granulation tissue may undergo myxoid changes, with coalescence producing subchondral cysts
- May be superficial foci of osteonecrosis, subcortical fibrocartilaginous production, and marginal cartilage proliferation, with endochondral ossification producing osteophytes
- Mild synovial cell hyperplasia with subsynovial lymphocytosis
- Fragments of bone and cartilage may become embedded in synovium
- Cartilage may ultimately form loose bodies or "joint mice" by proliferation of chondrocytes, with subsequent fragmentation into the joint space

Special Stains and Immunohistochemistry

- Noncontributory

Other Techniques for Diagnosis

- Noncontributory

Differential Diagnosis

▮ Rheumatoid arthritis
  - Contains a subchondral intratrabecular infiltrate of plasma cells
  - Pannus formation
▮ Osteoarthritis secondary to avascular necrosis
  - Segmental osteonecrosis with bony trabeculae containing empty lacunae
▮ Osteoarthritis secondary to chondrocalcinosis
  - Contains clusters of calcium pyrophosphate crystals within chondroid matrix
  - Crystals are rhomboid and are weakly birefringent

Pearls

- Denervation of joints, most commonly associated with diabetes, may produce osteoarthritic changes and is called *neuropathic joint*
- Spondylosis deformans is a form of osteoarthritis that involves the disks and vertebral bodies of the spine; disk cartilage herniates into the vertebral body (Schmorl node)

Selected References

Benjamin M, McGonagle D: Histopathologic changes at "synovio-entheseal complexes" suggesting a novel mechanism for synovitis in osteoarthritis and spondylarthritis. Arthritis Rheum 56:3601-3609, 2007.

Cushner FD, La Rosa DF, Vigorita VJ, et al: A quantitative histologic comparison: ACL degeneration in the osteoarthritic knee. J Arthroplasty 18:687-692, 2003.

McCarthy EF, Frassica FJ: Pathology of Bone and Joint Disorders with Clinical and Radiographic Correlation. Philadelphia, WB Saunders, 1998, pp 324-337.

Rheumatoid Arthritis

Clinical Features

- Male-to-female ratio is 1:3
- Can occur in all age groups, with most cases occurring in fourth and fifth decades

- Most commonly affects joints of hands, feet, and knees but eventually may involve other joints, including hips, shoulders, ankles, and sternoclavicular joint
- Patients present with arthralgia, stiffness, swelling, erythema, limitation of motion, and joint tenderness

Radiographic Features

- Concentric joint space narrowing, osteopenia, and marginal bony erosions

Gross Pathology

- Synovium is edematous with prominent villous architecture
- Surfaces may have fibrinous deposits
- Articular cartilaginous surface is irregular and fibrillated and may be denuded, resulting in exposure of subchondral bone
- Pannus is present in subchondral bone and extends to the surface of the articular cartilage
- Rice bodies (detached inflamed fibrinous exudate) may be present

Histopathology

- Subsynovial connective tissue contains plasma cell and lymphocytic infiltrate with lymphoid follicle formation
- Perifollicular cuffing of plasma cells and multinucleated giant cells (Grimley-Sokoloff synovial giant cells) may be present
- Pannus is represented by inflamed granulation tissue that undermines and covers the articular cartilaginous surface
- Chondrolysis is represented by cartilage exhibiting decreased staining of chondroid matrix and loss of chondrocytic nuclei
- Subchondral intratrabecular spaces may contain plasma cell infiltrates

Special Stains and Immunohistochemistry

- Noncontributory

Other Techniques for Diagnosis

- Serum autoantibodies: RF (rheumatoid factor)
- Class II major histocompatibility complex alleles DR4, DR1, or both

Differential Diagnosis

▮ Osteoarthritis
  - Osteophytes are more prominent, and articular surface pannus is absent
  - Subchondral granulation tissue may exhibit myxoid changes, and subchondral cysts may be present
  - Chondrolysis is not present
  - Serum RF is negative

Figure 16-36. Rheumatoid arthritis. Histologic section shows a pannus covering the degenerated articular surface.

▌ Chronic osteomyelitis
  ● Presence of intratrabecular plasma cell infiltrates may mimic chronic osteomyelitis
  ● Clinical and radiographic features are different
  ● Serum RF is negative

Pearls

  ● There are no pathognomonic histologic changes of rheumatoid arthritis
  ● About 20% of patients with rheumatoid arthritis develop subcutaneous rheumatoid nodules
  ● Clinical history and laboratory findings provide helpful clinicopathologic correlations

Selected References

Vigorita VJ: Orthopaedic Pathology. Philadelphia, Lippincott Williams & Wilkins, 1999, pp 588-609.

McCarthy EF, Frassica FJ: Pathology of Bone and Joint Disorders with Clinical and Radiographic Correlation. Philadelphia, WB Saunders, 1998, pp 337-345.

Gynther GW, Holmlund AB, Reinholt FP, Lindblad S: Temporomandibular joint involvement in generalized osteoarthritis and rheumatoid arthritis: A clinical, arthroscopic, histologic, and immunohistochemical study. Int J Oral Maxillofac Surg 26:10-16, 1997.

Gout

Clinical Features

  ● Male-to-female ratio is 2:1
  ● Peak incidence in fifth decade
  ● Usually monoarticular and involves large peripheral joints of the lower extremities
  ● Great toe is the most common site
  ● Acute gout presents with joint redness, swelling, and tenderness
  ● Chronic gout consists of painless tophi that may involve the ear helix, feet, hands, fingers, tibia, olecranon bursa, and Achilles tendon

Figure 16-37. Gout. Histologic section shows amorphous material surrounded by histiocytic and multinucleated giant cells.

Radiographic Features

  ● In acute phase, only subcutaneous swelling is seen
  ● In chronic phase, subcutaneous and periarticular masses adjacent to eroded bone are present
  ● Bone erosions are most common in the hands and feet

Gross Pathology

  ● Synovial pasty and chalk-white deposits in the soft tissue

Histopathology

  ● Specimens should be fixed in alcohol rather than formalin so as not to dissolve the crystals
  ● Polarizable needle-shaped uric acid crystals may be found within neutrophils of synovial fluid
  ● In acute gout, the synovium contains neutrophilic and lymphocytic infiltrates
  ● In chronic gout, tophi are represented by pale-staining amorphous material surrounded by histiocytes and multinucleated foreign-body–like giant cells

Special Stains and Immunohistochemistry

  ● Noncontributory

Other Techniques for Diagnosis

  ● Polarized light and compensated polarized light have been used to identify crystals and categorize as uric acid (needle shaped)

Differential Diagnosis

▌ Pseudogout (calcium pyrophosphate deposition disease)
  ● Crystals are rhomboid and birefringent
  ● Crystals appear blue when parallel and yellow when perpendicular to compensated polarized light
  ● Granulomatous inflammation is absent
▌ Infectious granulomatous synovitis
  ● Special stains (acid-fast bacilli, Gomori methenamine silver, PAS) may be positive, but negative stains do not rule out infectious granulomatous synovitis
  ● Cultures and clinicoradiographic correlation are necessary to rule out an infectious etiology

Pearls

  ● If a surgeon is suspicious of gout, recommend submitting surgical tissue specimen in 100% ethanol so that uric acid crystals do not dissolve (uric acid crystals are soluble in formalin and will dissolve)

Selected References

Lam HY, Cheung KY, Law SW, Fung KY: Crystal arthropathy of the lumbar spine: A report of 4 cases. J Orthop Surg (Hong Kong) 15:94-101, 2007.

Vigorita VJ: Orthopaedic Pathology. Philadelphia, Lippincott Williams & Wilkins, 1999, pp 533-537.

McCarthy EF, Frassica FJ: Pathology of Bone and Joint Disorders with Clinical and Radiographic Correlation. Philadelphia, WB Saunders, 1998, pp 346-348.

Pseudogout (Chondrocalcinosis–Calcium Pyrophosphate Deposition Disease)

Clinical Features

- Male-to-female ratio is 1.4:1
- Mean age of 72 years
- Rare before the age of 30 years
- Typically affects the distal radioulnar joint, symphysis pubis, knee, and intervertebral disks
- Many patients are asymptomatic
- Patients may present with symptoms of acute arthritis, including pain, swelling, and redness of the affected joint
- Associated conditions include hyperparathyroidism, hemochromatosis, hypophosphatasia, hypomagnesemia, hypothyroidism, gout, neuropathic joints, amyloidosis, trauma, osteochondritis desiccans, and familial hypocalciuric hypercalcemia

Radiographic Features

- Exhibits linear, punctate intra-articular calcifications within tendons, articular cartilage, and menisci

Gross Pathology

- Articular cartilage contains linear white deposits
- Synovium exhibits white deposits of crystalline material

Histopathology

- Aggregates of crystals are present within cartilage and synovium
- Crystals are rhomboid and birefringent; the crystals appear blue when parallel and yellow when perpendicular to compensated polarized light
- Inflammation is absent
- If crystals are absent, the chondroid matrix may exhibit reduced basophilia and mucoid changes, which are considered diagnostic of pseudogout

Special Stains and Immunohistochemistry

- Noncontributory

Other Techniques for Diagnosis

- Polarized light and compensated polarized light have been used to identify crystals and categorize as calcium pyrophosphate, which appears yellow when parallel and blue when perpendicular to compensated polarized light

Differential Diagnosis

▌ Gout
- Crystals are needle shaped and not birefringent; they are yellow when parallel and blue when perpendicular to compensated polarized light
- Granulomatous inflammation is present

▌ Tumoral calcinosis
- Radiographically, this process is represented by fused, round to oval soft tissue radiodensities
- Composed of nodular calcifications surrounded by macrophages and giant cells
- Intracytoplasmic giant cell calcifications, metaplastic bone, and psammoma bodies may be present
- No polarizable crystals are present
- May be associated with a history of chronic renal dialysis

Pearls

- By the age of 80 years, 20% of patients have joint deposits of calcium pyrophosphate
- About 25% of patients who undergo knee replacement surgery have deposits of calcium pyrophosphate in the native joints

Selected References

Fenoy AJ, Menezes AH, Donovan KA, Kralik SF: Calcium pyrophosphate dihydrate crystal deposition in the craniovertebral junction. J Neurosurg Spine 8:22-29, 2008.

Saffer P: Chondrocalcinosis of the wrist. J Hand Surg [Br] 29:486-493, 2004.

McCarthy EF, Frassica FJ: Pathology of Bone and Joint Disorders with Clinical and Radiographic Correlation. Philadelphia, WB Saunders, 1998, pp 348-350.

Ryan LM, McCarty DJ: Arthritis associated with calcium containing crystals. In Stein JH (ed): Internal Medicine. St. Louis, Mosby, 1998, pp 1276-1279.

Synovial Chondromatosis

Clinical Features

- Male-to-female ratio is 2:1
- Most cases occur in fourth and fifth decades
- Most commonly affected joints are knees (70%), hips, and elbows
- Patients present with pain, swelling, and limitation of motion of variable duration (averaging 5 years)

Figure 16-38. Synovial chondromatosis. Histologic section shows discrete nodules of mature hyaline cartilage.

Radiographic Features

- Well-marginated ring-shaped and stippled radiodensities in the joint or bursa
- May be fusion of these densities, forming a mass
- Bone erosion may be seen

Gross Pathology

- Synovium contains single or multiple well-circumscribed nodules of cartilaginous tissue
- Detached free cartilaginous nodules may be in the joint space
- Bosselated, larger nodules with outer granular surfaces representing fused smaller nodules may be identified
- Tendons and bursa may be involved

Histopathology

- Synovium contains multiple discrete nodules of hyaline cartilage, which may exhibit myxoid changes, calcification, or peripheral ossification
- Clusters of atypical chondrocytes showing nuclei with open chromatin; small multinucleated forms, and mitotic figures can also be seen
- Cartilaginous nodules may exhibit endochondral ossification
- Chondrocytes with clear cell features and prominent eosinophilic cytoplasm may be seen

Special Stains and Immunohistochemistry

- Noncontributory

Other Techniques for Diagnosis

- Noncontributory

Differential Diagnosis

▌ Secondary synovial chondrometaplasia
- Evidence of preexisting joint disease (history or radiographic features of chondral fracture, osteonecrosis, or osteoarthritis)
- Histologically, the cartilaginous nodule has a central nidus of detached hypocellular articular cartilage or detached, necrotic subchondral bone that is surrounded by concentric rings of metaplastic cartilage composed of benign-appearing chondrocytes

▌ Synovial chondrosarcoma
- May mimic synovial chondrometaplasia radiographically, but the radiodensities are poorly circumscribed or demarcated
- Histologically, the cellularity is increased without clusters or cloning
- Solid sheets of crowded chondrocytes exhibit more significant atypia and mitotic activity
- Spindle-shaped forms are located around the periphery of nodules, and necrosis may be present
- Myxoid features may be more prominent

▌ Secondary joint involved chondrosarcoma
- Clinical and radiographic features suggest that the tumor is not arising in synovium but rather in bone with extension into the joint space

Pearls

- Chondrocytic atypia present in synovial chondrometaplasia to the degree that, in a different location (proximal or axial skeleton, not synovium), the diagnosis of chondrosarcoma might be made
- Clinicoradiographic correlation is important in evaluating these lesions so that they are not overdiagnosed as chondrosarcomas
- Malignant transformation has been reported

Selected References

Galat DD, Ackerman DB, Spoon D, et al: Synovial chondromatosis of the foot and ankle. Foot Ankle Int 29:312-317, 2008.

Murphey MD, Vidal JA, Fanburg-Smith JC, Gajewski DA: Imaging of synovial chondromatosis with radiologic pathologic correlation. Radiographics 27:1465-1488, 2007.

Unni KK, Inwards CY, Bridge J, et al: Tumors of the Bones and Joints, 4th Series, Fascicle 2. Washington, DC, Armed Forces Institute of Pathology, 2005, pp 386-389.

McCarthy EF, Frassica FJ: Pathology of Bone and Joint Disorders with Clinical and Radiographic Correlation. Philadelphia, WB Saunders, 1998, pp 307-310.

Pigmented Villonodular Synovitis

Clinical Features

- Male-to-female ratio is 1:2
- Majority occur in third and fourth decades
- Knee is the most common joint involved (80%)
- Hip, shoulder, and ankle are also commonly involved

Figure 16-39. Pigmented villonodular synovitis. Histologic section shows subsynovial cellular infiltrate of mononuclear cells, multinucleated giant cells, foam cells, and scattered hemosiderin-laden macrophages.

- Usually presents with a long history of pain, swelling, limitation of motion, and joint stiffness
- Some patients present with hemarthroses

Radiographic Features

- Routine radiographs usually reveal soft tissue swelling
- May exhibit evidence of degenerative joint disease, represented by subchondral cysts and erosions on both sides of the joint
- Lucent bone lesions may be present
- CT or MRI reveals pedunculated lesions in the joint

Gross Pathology

- Synovium is brown and thickened; contains papillary villous projections and nodular structures
- Cut surface shows variable coloring, including yellow and red areas, depending on lipid and hemosiderin content
- Pedunculated or polypoid masses may be seen

Histopathology

- Cellular infiltrates of mononuclear cells within the subsynovial connective tissue
  — Mononuclear cells have oval nuclei with vesicular or clumped chromatin and prominent cytoplasm
  — Mitotic activity may be brisk
- Hemosiderin-laden mononuclear cells, multinucleated giant cells, and foam cells are present
- In older lesions areas of fibrosis are common

Special Stains and Immunohistochemistry

- Mononuclear cells and multinucleated giant cells express CD68 and HAM-56

Other Techniques for Diagnosis

- Cytogenetic studies: trisomy 7, trisomy 5, and aneuploid mononuclear cell lines may be seen
- Structural rearrangements of 1p11-13 may be seen

Differential Diagnosis

▌Hemosiderotic synovitis
- Usually occurs in patients with hemophilia, on anticoagulant therapy, or having a past history of post-traumatic hemarthroses, or in the presence of synovial vascular tumors (hemangioma)
- Villous synovial projections are delicate and do not form nodules
- Mononuclear cells in pigmented villonodular synovitis are not present, and foam cells and multinucleated giant cells are not typical

▌Giant cell tumor of bone
- Does not exhibit radiolucent lesions on both sides of the joint
- Giant cells are larger, have many more nuclei, and do not stain with histiocytic markers

▌Rheumatoid synovitis
- Synovial plasma cell and lymphocytic infiltrates with follicle formation
- Hemosiderin is not prominent

▌Traumatic synovitis
- Foam cells and multinucleated giant cells are not present

▌Detritic synovitis
- Foreign material is found associated with an inflammatory response

Pearls

- Extra-articular nodular form of pigmented villonodular synovitis is called *giant cell tumor of tendon sheath*; occurs most often in older males and more commonly involves the fingers
- Secondary bone invasion occurs in about one fourth to one half of patients
- Most cases are monoarticular
- Polyarticular involvement may occur, but it is seen in younger patients, tends to be familial, and may be associated with multiple lentigines syndrome, pectus excavatum, or fibrous dysplasia
- Malignant pigmented villonodular synovitis has been reported
  — Histologic features suggesting malignancy include cells with large, atypical nuclei containing large nucleoli and prominent eosinophilic cytoplasm; areas of necrosis and infiltrative borders are seen

Selected References

Carpintero P, Gascon E, Mesa M, et al: Clinical and radiologic features of pigmented villonodular synovitis of the foot: Report of eight cases. J Am Podiatr Med Assoc 97:415-419, 2007.

Unni KK, Inwards CY, Bridge J, et al: Tumors of the Bones and Joints, 4th Series, Fascicle 2. Washington, DC, Armed Forces Institute of Pathology, 2005, pp 383-384.

Somerhausen NS, Flecher CD: Diffuse-type giant cell tumor: Clinicopathologic and immunohistochemical analysis of 50 cases with extraarticular disease. Am J Surg Pathol 24:479-492, 2000.

McCarthy EF, Frassica FJ: Pathology of Bone and Joint Disorders with Clinical and Radiographic Correlation. Philadelphia, WB Saunders, 1998, pp 310-312.

Robin D. LeGallo and Mark R. Wick

17

Soft Tissue

Nodular Fasciitis

Clinical Features

- Most common pseudoneoplastic proliferation in soft tissue
- Primarily affects young adults aged 20 to 40 years; occasionally seen in children
- Presents as a rapidly growing solitary mass; may be painful
- Inconsistently associated with recognized previous trauma (10% to 15%)
- Can involve any site; flexor aspect of forearm, chest, and back are common sites

Gross Pathology

- Located in the deep dermis or subcutis; occasionally occurs intramuscularly
- Round to oval, nodular, well-circumscribed mass; usually smaller than 3 cm
- Cut surface may be fibrous, myxoid, or cystic

Histopathology

- "Tissue culture" appearance with long fascicles of spindled cells with a whorled growth pattern
- Loose, feathery collagenous stroma with myxoid or microcystic appearance

Figure 17-1. Nodular fasciitis. Bland, plump spindle cells show a "cell culture" growth pattern. Rare extravasated red cells are present.

- Zonal pattern with cellular periphery and loose, feathery center that may be cystic
- Scattered inflammatory cells, typically lymphocytes and macrophages, and extravasated red blood cells
- Giant cells that may have a ganglion-like appearance
- Frequent mitotic figures; no abnormal mitotic figures
- Variants
  — Intravascular fasciitis
    ◆ Affects primarily children and adolescents
    ◆ Involves arteries and veins
  — Cranial fasciitis
    ◆ Affects infants younger than 1 year
    ◆ Involves the scalp and skull
  — Ossifying fasciitis
    ◆ Periosteal location
    ◆ Similar to myositis ossificans but lacks triphasic zonal pattern

Special Stains and Immunohistochemistry

- Vimentin and smooth muscle actin (SMA) positive
- Immunohistochemistry is not helpful in excluding other myofibroblastic or smooth muscle proliferations

Other Techniques for Diagnosis

- Noncontributory

Differential Diagnosis

▮ Kaposi sarcoma
- Ill-defined margins
- Prominent vasculature, extravasated red blood cells
- Found in immunocompromised individuals; typically patients with acquired immunodefiency syndrome (AIDS)
- Immunoreactive for human herpesvirus type 8 (HHV-8) and latent nuclear antigen 1 (LNA-1)

▮ Myxoma
- Characterized by a paucity of cells, myxoid matrix, and sparse vascularity

▮ Fibrous histiocytoma (dermatofibroma)
- Spindle cell proliferation admixed with epithelioid and foamy histiocytes
- Typically arranged in a storiform pattern
- Lacks prominent vasculature and extravasated red blood cells

▮ Fibromatosis (desmoid tumor)
- Typically involves the abdomen or trunk
- Usually shows infiltrative margins

- Dense collagenous stroma usually lacking inflammatory component or myxoid areas
- Lacks thin-walled vessels and extravasated red blood cells
- Nuclear immunoreactivity for β-catenin

Pearls

- Nodular fasciitis is commonly misdiagnosed as a sarcoma
- Believed to be a reactive rather than a neoplastic condition
- Benign lesion with an excellent prognosis
- May progress through myxoid, cellular, and fibrous phases
- Conservative surgical resection is the treatment of choice

Selected References

Hornick JL, Fletcher CD: Intraarticular nodular fasciitis—a rare lesion: Clinicopathologic analysis of a series. Am J Surg Pathol 30:237-241, 2006.

Sarangarajan R, Dehner LP: Cranial and extracranial fasciitis of childhood: A clinicopathologic and immunohistochemical study. Hum Pathol 30:87-92, 1999.

Montgomery EA, Meis JM: Nodular fasciitis: Its morphologic spectrum and immunohistochemical profile. Am J Surg Pathol 15:942-948, 1991.

Patchefsky AS, Enzinger FM: Intravascular fasciitis: A report of 17 cases. Am J Surg Pathol 5:29-36, 1981.

Price EB Jr, Sillaphant WM, Shuman R: Nodular fasciitis: A clinicopathologic analysis of 65 cases. Am J Clin Pathol 35:122-136, 1961.

Proliferative Fasciitis and Myositis

Clinical Features

- Typically occurs in adults (usually about 50 years of age)

Figure 17-2. Proliferative fasciitis. Numerous ganglion-like cells are seen in a collagenous stroma.

- Firm, palpable, rapidly growing subcutaneous or intramuscular nodule; may be painful
  — Proliferative fasciitis
    ◆ Most common site is forearm, followed by leg and trunk
    ◆ Often associated with a history of trauma
  — Proliferative myositis
    ◆ Commonly located in the flat muscles of the trunk and shoulder girdle

Gross Pathology

- Poorly circumscribed, gray-white soft tissue mass
- Typically measures 1 to 3 cm in diameter
- Proliferative myositis is commonly a pale, gray, scarlike induration involving muscle and overlying fascia

Histopathology

- Ill-defined lesions characterized by large myofibroblasts that have large vesicular nuclei, prominent nucleoli, and abundant eosinophilic cytoplasm (ganglion-like cells) admixed with immature spindle cells in a matrix composed of varying proportions of mucoid material and collagen
- Often numerous mitotic figures in spindled and ganglion-like cells; they are not atypical
  — Proliferative fasciitis
    ◆ Histologic features similar to those of proliferative myositis except for a lack of intramuscular location
    ◆ Typically grows along fibrous septa with an interlobular distribution
  — Proliferative myositis
    ◆ Endomysial and epimysial growth separates bundles of atrophic skeletal muscle, creating a checkerboard pattern

Special Stains and Immunohistochemistry

- Noncontributory

Other Techniques for Diagnosis

- Noncontributory

Differential Diagnosis

▮ Rhabdomyosarcoma
- Tumor of children, rarely seen in adults
- Presence of rhabdomyoblasts rarely with cytoplasmic cross-striations
- Immunoreactivity for desmin, muscle-specific actin (MSA), myogenin, and MyoD1

▮ Ganglioneuroblastoma
- Intermixed neuroblasts and ganglion cells in a background of schwannian spindle cell stroma
- S-100 protein is present in the schwannian stroma
- Tumor of young children; extremities an unusual location

▌ Nodular fasciitis
- Typically has well-defined margins
- Spindle cell proliferation with scattered inflammatory cells and extravasated red blood cells
- Lacks prominent ganglion-like cells

Pearls

- Pathogenesis of proliferative fasciitis and myositis remains unexplained; fascial or muscular injury is thought to be a likely contributor
- Benign, self-limited, reactive process treated with conservative surgical excision
- Proliferative fasciitis and proliferative myositis are similar reactive proliferations that are best distinguished by their locations

Selected References

Wong NL: Fine needle aspiration cytology of pseudosarcomatous reactive proliferative lesions of soft tissue. Acta Cytol 46:1049-1055, 2002.

Meis JM, Enzinger FM: Proliferative fasciitis and myositis of childhood. Am J Surg Pathol 16:364-372, 1992.

El-Jabbour JN, Bennett MH, Burke MM, et al: Proliferative myositis: An immunohistochemical and ultrastructural study. Am J Surg Pathol 15:654-659, 1991.

Chung EB, Enzinger FM: Proliferative fasciitis. Cancer 36:1450-1458, 1975.

Myositis Ossificans

Clinical Features

- Commonly affects young, athletic adults; usually involves the extremities
- Uncommon in children
- Presents as a solitary, tender mass; often associated with a history of trauma (>50% of cases)
- Radiographic findings show characteristic zonal ossification

Gross Pathology

- Well-circumscribed, gray-yellow lesions with gritty areas

Histopathology

- Typically shows a triphasic pattern with distinct zonation
  — Central cellular region
    ◆ Resembles nodular fasciitis
    ◆ Cells have bland nuclear features and a variable mitotic rate
    ◆ Occasional multinucleated giant cells
  — Intermediate region is composed of immature osteoid
  — Peripheral zone is composed of mature, "purposeful" lamellar bone

Special Stains and Immunohistochemistry

- Noncontributory

Other Techniques for Diagnosis

- Noncontributory

Differential Diagnosis

▌ Extraskeletal osteosarcoma
- Characterized by disorderly growth of hyperchromatic, pleomorphic cells with delicate lacelike osteoid formation, often with faint bluish calcification
- Absence of zonation

Pearls

- Myositis ossificans is a benign, self-limited process with an excellent prognosis
- Spontaneous regression can occur

Selected References

Wilson JD, Montague CJ, Salcuni P, et al: Heterotopic mesenteric ossification ("intraabdominal myositis ossificans"): Report of five cases. Am J Surg Pathol 23:1464-1470, 1999.

Clapton WK, James CL, Morris LL, et al: Myositis ossificans in childhood. Pathology 24:311-314, 1992.

Nuovo MA, Norman A, Chumas J, Ackerman LV: Myositis ossificans with atypical clinical, radiographic, or pathologic findings: a review of 23 cases. Skeletal Radiol 21:87-101, 1992.

Ackerman LV: Extra-osseous localized non-neoplastic bone and cartilage formation (so-called myositis ossificans): Clinical and pathological confusion with malignant neoplasms. J Bone Joint Surg Am 40:279-298, 1958.

Ischemic Fasciitis

Clinical Features

- Also referred to as *atypical decubital fibroplasia*
- Occurs over bony prominences or other pressure points in debilitated patients

Figure 17-3. Ischemic fasciitis. A transition is seen between fibrin-rich necrosis and stellate myofibroblastic cells.

- Shoulders, chest wall, hip, and buttock are the most common locations
- Usually presents as a painless subcutaneous or deep mass

Gross Pathology

- Poorly circumscribed, multinodular mass up to 10 cm in diameter
- May have overlying ulceration

Histopathology

- Typical zonation pattern
  — Central necrotic region
    ◆ Liquefactive or coagulative necrosis with fibrin deposition
  — Peripheral fibroblastic and vascular proliferation
    ◆ Granulation tissue–like with plump endothelial cells
    ◆ Atypical fibroblasts with abundant eosinophilic cytoplasm and ganglion-like features
    ◆ Vascular thrombosis and fibrinoid necrosis

Special Stains and Immunohistochemistry

- Noncontributory

Other Techniques for Diagnosis

- Noncontributory

Differential Diagnosis

▌ Epithelioid sarcoma
- Typically seen on the extremities of younger patients
- Atypical cells are immunoreactive for keratin and epithelial membrane antigen (EMA)
▌ Myxoid liposarcoma
- Lacks the zonation of ischemic fasciitis
- Delicate plexiform vasculature and presence of lipoblasts

Pearls

- Ischemic fasciitis is a benign, reactive process likely related to intermittent ischemia
- Surgical excision is the treatment of choice; can recur owing to persistence of underlying cause

Selected References

Ilaslan H, Joyce M, Bauer T, Sundaram M: Decubital ischemic fasciitis: Clinical, pathologic, and MRI features of pseudosarcoma. AJR Am J Roentgenol 187:1338-1341, 2006.

Perosio PM, Weiss SW: Ischemic fasciitis: A juxta-skeletal fibroblastic proliferation with a predilection for elderly patients. Mod Pathol 6:69-72, 1993.

Elastofibroma

Clinical Features

- Usually presents as a deeply seated mass located in the lower subscapular area

Figure 17-4. Elastofibroma. A, Thick and fragmented elastic fibers are seen in a collagenous background. **B,** Verhoeff–van Gieson elastic stain highlights the abnormal elastic fibers.

- Almost exclusively seen in late adulthood and rarely in younger patients
- More commonly found in females

Gross Pathology

- Firm, rubbery, soft tissue mass with ill-defined margins
- Cut surface is gray-white and glistening with entrapped foci of fat
- Focal cystic degeneration is often seen

Histopathology

- Poorly defined lesion composed of thickened, coarse, slightly basophilic elastic fibers and scant fibroblastic cells embedded in a heavily collagenized stroma
- Entrapped mature adipose tissue is typically seen

Special Stains and Immunohistochemistry

- Verhoeff-van Gieson elastic stain highlights elastic fibers

Other Techniques for Diagnosis

- Noncontributory

Differential Diagnosis

❚ Fibrolipoma
- Characterized by predominance of mature adipocytes with intervening fibrous connective tissue
- Lacks elastic fibers

Pearls

- Histology of elastofibroma is described as "spaghetti and meatballs" owing to long and globular elastic fibers
- Increased incidence in manual laborers; related to repetitive motion injury
- Can usually be diagnosed by radiology or by fine-needle aspiration

Selected References

Yamazaki K: An ultrastructural and immunohistochemical study of elastofibroma: CD 34, MEF-2, prominin 2 (CD133), and factor XIIIa-positive proliferating fibroblastic stromal cells connected by Cx43-type gap junctions. Ultrastruct Pathol 31:209-219, 2007.

Hisaoka M, Hashimoto H: Elastofibroma: Clonal fibrous proliferation with predominant CD34-positive cells. Virchows Arch 448:195-199, 2006.

Superficial Fibromatoses

Clinical Features

- Presents as a small, slow-growing, subcutaneous nodule or thickening
  - Palmar fibromatosis (Dupuytren contracture)
    - Palmar surface of the hand; may result in contractures
    - Almost exclusively in adults, males affected more than females
    - Often bilateral, especially in alcoholics
  - Plantar fibromatosis (Ledderhose disease)
    - Plantar, non-weight-bearing area of the foot
    - Occurs in both children and adults
    - Often multinodular
  - Penile fibromatosis (Peyronie disease)
    - Dorsal aspect of the shaft of the penis
    - Exclusively seen in adults

Gross Pathology

- Single or multiple, gray-white, firm nodules or scarlike tissue in the subcutis

Histopathology

- Proliferative and involutional phases
- Proliferative phase shows variably cellular fascicles of bland, spindled cells often arranged in a nodular pattern
- Occasionally prominent giant cells in plantar lesions
- Mitotic figures may be seen
- Involutional or residual phase shows paucicellular, densely collagenized tissue

Special Stains and Immunohistochemistry

- SMA positive
- Immunohistochemistry not helpful in excluding other myofibroblastic or smooth muscle proliferations

Other Techniques for Diagnosis

- Gains of chromosomes 7 or 8 are common, but in general, cytogenetic study is not required

Differential Diagnosis

❚ Calcifying aponeurotic fibroma
- Primarily affects children and adolescents
- Characterized by an infiltrative growth pattern
- Hyalinized nodules with stippled calcification, often with chondroid features
❚ Fibroma of tendon sheath
- Well-circumscribed, sometimes multinodular mass firmly attached to tendon sheath
- Hypocellular with bland spindle cells widely separated by hyalinized collagenous stroma
❚ Fibrosarcoma (infantile and adult types)
- Infantile fibrosarcoma usually affects children younger than 1 year
- Adult fibrosarcoma is only rarely found in distal extremities
- Highly cellular, infiltrative tumor composed of uniform fibroblasts with hyperchromatic nuclei and scant cytoplasm, arranged in a distinctive herringbone pattern
- High mitotic rate is common; atypical mitotic figures may be seen
- Areas of necrosis or hemorrhage may be seen

Figure 17-5. Inclusion body fibromatosis. Plump spindle cells contain cytoplasmic round, eosinophilic inclusions.

Pearls

- Superficial fibromatosis may be multifocal
- Plantar or palmar fibromatosis may be highly cellular and mistaken for sarcoma
- Associated conditions may include diabetes, cirrhosis, and epilepsy; some fibromatoses may have a hereditary component
- Surgical excision is the treatment of choice

Selected References

Evans HL: Multinucleated giant cells in plantar fibromatosis. Am J Surg Pathol 26:244-248, 2002.

Montgomery E, Lee JH, Abraham SC, Wu TT: Superficial fibromatoses are genetically distinct from deep fibromatoses. Mod Pathol 14:695-701, 2001.

Allen PW: The fibromatoses: A clinicopathologic classification based on 140 cases. Am J Surg Pathol 1:255-270, 1977.

Fibrous Hamartoma of Infancy

Clinical Features

- Rapidly growing, painless subcutaneous mass in young children, sometimes congenital
- Common sites include trunk, shoulder, axilla, and groin
- Most cases occur within the first 2 years of life

Gross Pathology

- Poorly defined deep dermal or subcutaneous mass
- Gray, firm cut surface with yellow flecks
- Usually 2 to 5 cm but may be larger

Histopathology

- Triphasic appearance comprising an admixture of fibrous tissue, adipose tissue, and bundles of immature mesenchymal cells
- Often has a stellate configuration and infiltrates surrounding fat

Figure 17-6. Fibrous hamartoma of infancy. The triphasic population of collagen fascicles, primitive myoid bundles, and fat forms a stellate lesion.

Special Stains and Immunohistochemistry

- SMA positive
- Immunohistochemistry is not helpful in excluding other myofibroblastic or smooth muscle proliferations

Other Techniques for Diagnosis

- Noncontributory

Differential Diagnosis

- Lipofibromatosis
  - Lacks a primitive mesenchymal component
- Lipoblastoma
  - Lobulated mass with fat lobules separated by fibrous bands
  - Lacks a primitive mesenchymal component
  - Myxoid stroma and lipoblasts are present
- Embryonal rhabdomyosarcoma
  - Lacks fibrous and adipose tissue
  - Positive for desmin, myogenin, and MyoD1

Pearls

- Fibrous hamartoma of infancy is a benign lesion usually cured with local excision

Selected References

Dickey GE, Sotelo-Avila C: Fibrous hamartoma of infancy: Current review. Pediatr Dev Pathol 2:236-243, 1999.

Coffin CM, Dehner LP: Fibroblastic-myofibroblastic tumors in children and adolescents: A clinicopathologic study of 108 examples in 103 patients. Pediatr Pathol 11:569-588, 1991.

Groisman G, Lichtig C: Fibrous hamartoma of infancy: An immunohistochemical and ultrastructural study. Human Pathol 22:914-918, 1991.

Lipofibromatosis

Clinical Features

- Previously referred to as *infantile fibromatosis, nondesmoid type*
- Occurs in childhood, between birth and second decade; males affected more than females
- Slowly growing, painless mass most commonly presenting in an extremity or on the trunk; rare cases in the head and neck
- May cause isolated macrodactyly

Gross Pathology

- Poorly defined subcutaneous mass with admixed adipose tissue
- Usually 1 to 3 cm

Histopathology

- Bands of bland spindled cells and collagen traversing through mature adipose tissue
- Infiltrative borders

Figure 17-7. Lipofibromatosis. Fascicles of bland spindle cells and collagen are admixed with mature adipose tissue.

Special Stains and Immunohistochemistry

- SMA positive
- Immunohistochemistry is not helpful in excluding other myofibroblastic or smooth muscle proliferations

Other Techniques for Diagnosis

- Noncontributory

Differential Diagnosis

▍ Fibrous hamartoma of infancy
- Contains a primitive mesenchymal component

▍ Lipoblastoma
- Lobulated mass with fat lobules separated by fibrous bands
- Myxoid stroma and presence of lipoblasts

▍ Desmoid-type fibromatosis
- Contains moderately cellular areas of fibrous growth, which infiltrates into fat; adipose tissue is not a primary component

Pearls

- Lipofibromatosis has a high rate of local recurrence but no metastatic potential
- Wide local excision is standard treatment

Selected References

Deepti AN, Madhuri V, Walter NM, Cherian RA: Lipofibromatosis: Report of a rare paediatric soft tissue tumour. Skeletal Radiol 37:555-558, 2008.

Kenney B, Richkind KE, Friedlaender G, Zambrano E: Chromosomal rearrangements in lipofibromatosis. Cancer Genet Cytogenet 179:136-139, 2007.

Fetsch JF, Miettinen M, Laskin WB, et al: A clinicopathologic study of 45 pediatric soft tissue tumors with an admixture of adipose tissue and fibroblastic elements, and a proposal for classification as lipofibromatosis. Am J Surg Pathol 24:1491-1500, 2000.

Calcifying Aponeurotic Fibroma

Clinical Features

- Also known as *juvenile aponeurotic fibroma* or *Keasby tumor*
- Most commonly affects children but may also occur in adults
- Presents as a slow-growing, painless mass, usually on the palmar or plantar surfaces of the hands or feet, rarely in other locations

Gross Pathology

- Poorly circumscribed, firm, gray-white, rubbery nodule usually smaller than 3 cm
- Gritty cut surface

Histopathology

- Bland oval plump fibroblasts in a heavily collagenized stroma
- Foci of stippled to confluent amorphous calcifications surrounded by rounded chondrocyte-like cells
- Infiltrative margins with extension into adipose tissue
- Osteoclast-like giant cells may be associated with calcification

Special Stains and Immunohistochemistry

- Noncontributory

Other Techniques for Diagnosis

- Noncontributory

Differential Diagnosis

▍ Fibromatosis (palmar, plantar)
- Characterized by fascicles of spindled uniform-appearing fibroblasts with varying amount of collagen

Figure 17-8. Calcifying aponeurotic fibroma. Nodular calcifications are surrounded by chondrocyte-like cells with intervening spindle cells in a hyalinized stroma.

- Growth along fascial planes and tendons
- Absence of calcification or chondroid differentiation
- Usually found in adults, but plantar fibromatosis occasionally seen in children
▌ Chondroma
- Typically occur in adults
- Characteristically a lobulated lesion composed of mature hyaline cartilage
- Undergoes calcification in a diffuse rather than in a focal manner
▌ Giant cell tumor of tendon sheath
- Numerous giant cells, plump mononuclear cells, and variable amounts of xanthoma cells
- Not calcified and no chondroid differentiation

Pearls

- Calcifying aponeurotic fibroma is a locally aggressive lesion characterized by local recurrence (>50% recur)
- Younger lesions are less heavily calcified, and older lesions show more extensive calcification and chondroid differentiation
- Surgical excision is the preferred treatment

Selected References

Fetsch JF, Miettinen M: Calcifying aponeurotic fibroma: A clinicopathologic study of 22 cases arising in uncommon sites. Hum Pathol 29:1504-1510, 1998.

Coffin CM, Dehner LP: Fibroblastic-myofibroblastic tumors in children and adolescents: A clinicopathologic study of 108 examples in 103 patients. Pediatr Pathol 11:569-588, 1991.

Allen PW, Enzinger FM: Juvenile aponeurotic fibroma. Cancer 26:857-867, 1970.

Myofibroma and Myofibromatosis

Clinical Features

- Also known as *infantile congenital myofibromatosis* or *congenital myofibromatosis* in children

Figure 17-9. Myofibroma. Plump, bland ovoid cells are arranged in a hemangiopericytomatous growth pattern.

- Most common fibrous tumor of infancy
- About 90% occur within the first 2 years of life; however, adults may be affected
- *Myofibroma* refers to a solitary lesion (common), whereas *myofibromatosis* denotes multiple skin and soft tissue lesions with variable visceral involvement
  — Solitary subcutaneous nodules typically involve the head and neck but can occur anywhere
  — Multicentric form may involve the lungs, heart, bones, and gastrointestinal tract

Gross Pathology

- Cut surface is rubbery gray-white with a lobulated or whorled appearance
- May have central necrosis or cyst formation
- Margins may be well defined or focally infiltrative
- Size from 0.5 cm up to 8 cm

Histopathology

- Typically shows a biphasic pattern or zonal phenomenon
  — *Peripheral areas* show fascicular or whorled growth of plump, spindled cells with eosinophilic cytoplasm (myofibroblasts)
  — *Central areas* of the lesion are more cellular with oval cells and a staghorn-appearing, hemangiopericytoma-like vasculature
- Variable mitotic activity but no atypical division figures
- Scattered lymphoplasmacytic infiltrate typically present
- Polypoid protrusion into vascular spaces is typical at the edge of the lesion
- Focal areas of hemorrhage, calcification, and necrosis may be seen centrally
- May be well circumscribed or infiltrative

Special Stains and Immunohistochemistry

- SMA and MSA positive
- Desmin variable
- Immunohistochemistry is not helpful in excluding other myofibroblastic or smooth muscle proliferations

Other Techniques for Diagnosis

- Noncontributory aside from ruling out other selected lesions such as infantile fibrosarcoma

Differential Diagnosis

▌ Nodular fasciitis
- Usually seen in older children
- Solitary, well-circumscribed nodule
- Zonation tends to be reversed, with a more cellular periphery and collagenized center
- Tends to be more myxoid, with more inflammatory cells and extravasated red blood cells
▌ Infantile fibrosarcoma
- Most commonly involves the extremities or trunk

- Highly cellular, infiltrative tumor with herringbone pattern of growth
- Numerous mitotic figures
- Translocation t(12;15)(p13;q26), producing an *ETV6-NTRK* fusion demonstrable by molecular or cytogenetic studies

Pearls

- Patients with solitary and multiple lesions of myofibroma or myofibromatosis confined to soft tissues have an excellent prognosis; visceral involvement imparts a worse prognosis depending on the particular locations and extent of growth
- Lesions may spontaneously regress
- Surgical resection is the standard treatment

Selected References

Zand DJ, Huff D, Everman D, et al: Autosomal dominant inheritance of infantile myofibromatosis. Am J Med Genet 126:261-266, 2004.

Coffin CM, Dehner LP: Fibroblastic-myofibroblastic tumors in children and adolescents: A clinicopathologic study of 108 examples in 103 patients. Pediatr Pathol 11:569-588, 1991.

Daimaru Y, Hashimoto H, Enjoji M: Myofibromatosis in adults (adult counterpart of infantile myofibromatosis). Am J Surg Pathol 13:859-865, 1989.

Chung EB, Enzinger FM: Infantile myofibromatosis. Cancer 48:1807-1818, 1981.

Gardner Fibroma

Clinical Features

- Benign lesion of childhood and early adulthood that has a strong association with desmoid-type fibromatosis and familial adenomatous polyposis (Gardner syndrome)
- Poorly defined, plaquelike soft tissue mass in superficial and deep tissues of back and paraspinal region, head and neck, extremities, and chest

Gross Pathology

- Ill-defined firm mass with a white-gray, rubbery cut surface
- Ranges in size from 1 to 12 cm

Histopathology

- Sheets of densely hyalinized bundles of collagen containing scant, small spindle cells
- Collagen fibers are separated by cracks or clefts
- Infiltrative borders are seen with entrapped connective tissue

Special Stains and Immunohistochemistry

- CD34 positive
- β-Catenin: most are positive with nuclear labeling

Other Techniques for Diagnosis

- Noncontributory

Differential Diagnosis

- Desmoid-type fibromatosis
  - More cellular spindle cell proliferation with fascicular growth pattern
- Nuchal fibroma
  - Bundles of hyalinized collagen with entrapped adnexal structures and connective tissues
  - Frequently has proliferation of small nerves similar to traumatic neuroma
  - Distinct clinical presentation, occurs in the posterior neck of middle-aged adult (males affected more than females); associated with diabetes mellitus in about half of cases
  - CD34 and β-catenin stains typically negative
- Elastofibroma
  - Densely eosinophilic elastic fibers intermixed with collagen as highlighted with the Verhoeff-van Gieson elastic stain
  - Occurs in older patients, frequently in subscapular location
  - Not associated with familial adenomatous polyposis

Pearls

- Gardner fibroma may be the first presentation of familial adenomatous polyposis (Gardner syndrome)
- About half of patients will develop desmoid-type fibromatosis
- Surgical resection is the standard treatment

Selected References

Coffin CM, Hornick JL, Zhou H, Fletcher CD: Gardner fibroma: A clinicopathologic and immunohistochemical analysis of 45 patients with 57 fibromas. Am J Surg Pathol 31:410-416, 2007.

Allen PW: Nuchal-type fibroma appearance in a desmoid fibromatosis. Am J Surg Pathol 25:828-829, 2001.

Wehrli BM, Weiss SW, Yandow S, Coffin CM: Gardner-associated fibromas (GAF) in young patients: A distinct fibrous lesion that identifies unsuspected Gardner syndrome and risk for fibromatosis. Am J Surg Pathol 25:645-651, 2001.

Desmoid-Type Fibromatosis

Clinical Features

- Also referred to as aggressive or deep fibromatosis
- Typically occurs in adolescents and young adults, but age range is wide
- Comprises a group of proliferative tumors that present as deep-seated masses
- Shoulder region, chest wall, thigh, and mesentery are favored sites
  — Musculoaponeurotic fibromatosis
    ◆ Lesions are associated intimately with muscular aponeuroses

Figure 17-10. Desmoid-type fibromatosis. Moderately cellular fascicles of bland spindle cells in a collagenized stroma diffusely infiltrate surrounding fat.

— Abdominal fibromatosis
  ◆ Rectus muscle is the favored location
  ◆ Occurs almost exclusively in women who are pregnant or postpartum
— Mesenteric fibromatosis
  ◆ Found in mesentery of the bowel or retroperitoneum
  ◆ Often associated with previous history of abdominal surgery
  ◆ May be associated with Gardner syndrome (familial adenomatous polyposis, mesenteric fibromatosis, osteomas, and multiple epidermal inclusion cysts)

Gross Pathology

- May appear well defined but actually has infiltrative margins
- Often grows along fascial planes
- Firm tumor that often has a gritty cut surface
- Sectioning reveals a glistening, white, trabeculated surface

Histopathology

- Composed of uniform-appearing, spindle-shaped fibroblasts and abundant collagen
- Infiltrative margins
- Extremely rare mitotic figures
- Delicate, thin-walled vessels with open lumens
- Myxoid matrix may be seen, primarily in abdominal fibromatosis

Special Stains and Immunohistochemistry

- β-Catenin: positive nuclear immunoreactivity
- SMA positive

Other Techniques for Diagnosis

- Recurrent chromosomal abnormalities include trisomies 8 and 20 and loss of 5q, not usually needed for diagnosis

Differential Diagnosis

▌ Nodular fasciitis
  - Usually smaller than 3 cm
  - Loose, feathery collagenous stroma with myxoid or microcystic appearance
  - Scattered chronic inflammatory cells
  - Frequent mitotic figures may be seen
  - Extravasated red blood cells
▌ Low-grade fibromyxoid sarcoma
  - Alternating collagenized and myxoid zones with prominent curvilinear vessels
  - May contain hyaline collagen rosettes
  - Negative for nuclear β-catenin
  - Presence of t(7;16)(q33;p11), producing an *FUS-CREB3L2* fusion in molecular or cytogenetic analysis
▌ Fibrosarcoma (infantile and adult types)
  - Most commonly affects children younger than 1 year; occasionally seen in adults
  - Highly cellular, infiltrative tumor composed of fibroblasts with hyperchromatic nuclei and scant cytoplasm arranged in a herringbone pattern
  - Mitoses are obvious, and atypical mitotic figures may be seen
  - Areas of necrosis or hemorrhage may be present
  - Infantile fibrosarcoma harbors t(12;15)(p13;q26), producing an *ETV6-NTRK* fusion demonstrable by molecular or cytogenetic studies

Pearls

- Desmoid-type fibromatosis has a high recurrence rate and may be locally aggressive but typically has no metastatic potential
- Surgical removal with a wide margin of resection is preferred treatment
- Recurrence rate ranges between 25% and 80%
- There are no pathologic features that can predict recurrence

Selected References

Carlson JW, Fletcher CD: Immunohistochemistry for beta-catenin in the differential diagnosis of spindle cell lesions: analysis of a series and review of the literature. Histopathology 51:509-514, 2007.

Bhattacharya B, Dilworth HP, Iacobuzio-Donahue C, et al: Nuclear beta-catenin expression distinguishes deep fibromatosis from other benign and malignant fibroblastic and myofibroblastic lesions. Am J Surg Pathol 29:653-659, 2005.

De Wever I, Dal Cin P, Fletcher CD, et al: Cytogenetic, clinical, and morphologic correlations in 78 cases of fibromatosis: A report from the CHAMP Study Group. Chromosomes and Morphology. Mod Pathol 13:1080-1085, 2000.

Coffin CM, Dehner LP: Fibroblastic-myofibroblastic tumors in children and adolescents: A clinicopathologic study of 108 examples in 103 patients. Pediatr Pathol 11:569-588, 1991.

Calcifying Fibrous (Pseudo) Tumor

Clinical Features

- Benign fibrous tumor that occurs predominantly in adolescents and young adults
- Most common in subcutaneous and deep soft tissues of extremities, trunk, groin, and neck but has been described in many locations, including viscera
- Originally thought to be pseudoneoplastic, but not currently

Gross Pathology

- Typically a circumscribed solid mass, 3 to 5 cm, but may be larger
- Cut surface is solid, firm, and gray-white

Histopathology

- Hypocellular, sclerotic tissue with a sparse lymphoplasmacytic infiltrate and discrete calcifications
- Calcification may be psammomatous or dystrophic
- Germinal center formation may be seen at lesion periphery

Special Stains and Immunohistochemistry

- Noncontributory

Other Techniques for Diagnosis

- Noncontributory

Figure 17-11. Calcifying fibrous tumor. Paucicellular, sclerotic lesion contains lymphoplasmacytic infiltrate and psammomatous calcifications.

Differential Diagnosis

- Inflammatory myofibroblastic tumor
  - Typically more cellular and less densely collagenized
  - Calcifications are extremely uncommon
  - Frequently positive for anaplastic lymphoma kinase-1 (ALK-1) in 40% of cases by immunohistochemistry
- Nodular fasciitis
  - Typically more cellular with a myxedematous stroma
  - Lacks calcifications
  - Loosely apposed lesional cells
- Desmoid-type fibromatosis
  - Characterized by fascicles of spindle-shaped fibroblasts with varying amounts of collagen and infiltrative borders
  - Calcifications are uncommon
  - Positive for β-catenin nuclear reactivity
- Calcifying aponeurotic fibroma
  - Stippled calcification with surrounding chondroid differentiation
  - Infiltrative margins
  - Inflammation not typical
  - Typically seen on hands and feet of young children

Pearls

- Calcifying (pseudo) tumor is a benign lesion with rare reports of recurrence
- Treatment is complete surgical resection

Selected References

Lau SK, Weiss LM: Calcifying fibrous tumor of the adrenal gland. Hum Pathol 38:656-659, 2007.

Kirby PA, Sato Y, Tannous R, Dehner LP: Calcifying fibrous pseudotumor of the myocardium. Pediatr Dev Pathol 9:384-387, 2006.

Nascimento AF, Ruiz R, Hornick JL, Fletcher CD: Calcifying fibrous "pseudotumor": Clinicopathologic study of 15 cases and analysis of its relationship to inflammatory myofibroblastic tumor. Int J Surg Pathol 10:189-196, 2002.

Hill KA, Gonzalez-Crussi F, Chou PM: Calcifying fibrous pseudotumor versus inflammatory myofibroblastic tumor: A histological and immunohistochemical comparison. Mod Pathol 14:784-790, 2001.

Fetsch JF, Montgomery EA, Meis JM: Calcifying fibrous pseudotumor. Am J Surg Pathol 17:502-508, 1993.

Inflammatory Myofibroblastic Tumor

Clinical Features

- Previously known as *inflammatory pseudotumor* and *plasma cell granuloma*
- Most often occurs in children and young adults but has a wide age range
- Commonly seen in the lung; the most frequent extrapulmonary sites are mesentery and omentum, but it can involve any location

Figure 17-12. Inflammatory myofibroblastic tumor. Loose fascicles of spindled cells with large vesicular nuclei are admixed with an inflammatory infiltrate.

- Systemic symptoms and signs may be present, including fever, weight loss, anemia, increased erythrocyte sedimentation rate, and elevated C-reactive protein levels

Gross Pathology

- Typically circumscribed, but nonencapsulated; often multinodular
- Cut surface is solid, firm, and gray-white

Histopathology

- Variably cellular tumor comprising spindle cells and mixed inflammatory cells in a myxoid or collagenized background
- Some lesions contain large histiocytoid ganglion-like cells
- May be hypocellular and resemble scars
- Mitotic figures may be numerous but are not atypical

Special Stains and Immunohistochemistry

- SMA positive
- ALK-1 protein present in about 40% of cases, more frequently in childhood tumors

Other Techniques for Diagnosis

- Rearrangement of *ALK* locus at 2p23 by molecular or cytogenetic analysis

Differential Diagnosis

▌ Leiomyoma
- Characterized by fascicles of uniform, spindle-shaped smooth muscle cells in short interlacing fascicles with negligible mitotic activity
- Well circumscribed
- Extremely rare in the deep soft tissues

- Lacks a mixed inflammatory infiltrate
- Immunohistochemistry not useful for differential diagnosis unless ALK-1 is positive (favoring a diagnosis of inflammatory myofibroblastic tumor)

▌ Leiomyosarcoma
- Characterized by fascicles of cytologically atypical spindle cells with hyperchromatic nuclei and variable but present mitotic activity
- Lacks a mixed inflammatory infiltrate
- Typically, middle-aged and elderly adults are affected

▌ Desmoid-type fibromatosis
- Fascicles of spindle-shaped fibroblasts with variable amounts of collagen and infiltrative borders
- Positive for β-catenin with nuclear labeling

▌ Embryonal rhabdomyosarcoma
- Primitive spindle cells, usually in a myxoid background; focal strap cells may be present
- Usually lacks inflammation
- Positive for myogenin and MyoD1

▌ Inflammatory malignant fibrous histiocytoma
- Usually occurs in older adults; retroperitoneum is the most common location
- Atypical hyperchromatic cells with prominent mixed inflammation rich in xanthomatous cells
- Negative for SMA and ALK-1

▌ Metastatic sarcomatoid carcinoma
- May have areas of squamous differentiation
- At least focally positive for keratin, EMA, MOC31, or p63

▌ Spindle cell melanoma
- Variably cellular spindle cell lesion with variable cellular pleomorphism, prominent nucleoli, and nuclear pseudoinclusions
- May show perineural invasion extending beyond the tumoral component
- Positive for S-100 protein; rarely for tyrosinase, melan-A, or HMB-45

Pearls

- Inflammatory myofibroblastic tumor is currently considered a neoplastic process
- Treatment is based on surgical resection
- May recur after excision

Selected References

Coffin CM, Hornick JL, Fletcher CD: Inflammatory myofibroblastic tumor: Comparison of clinicopathologic, histologic, and immunohistochemical features including ALK expression in atypical and aggressive cases. Am J Surg Pathol 31:509-520, 2007.

Cook JR, Dehner LP, Collins MH, et al: Anaplastic lymphoma kinase (ALK) expression in the inflammatory myofibroblastic tumor: a comparative immunohistochemical study. Am J Surg Pathol 25:1364-1371, 2001.

Coffin CM, Dehner LP, Meis-Kindblom JM: Inflammatory myofibroblastic tumor, inflammatory fibrosarcoma, and related lesions: An historical review with differential diagnostic considerations. Semin Diagn Pathol 15:102-110, 1998.

Coffin CM, Watterson J, Priest JR, Dehner LP: Extrapulmonary inflammatory myofibroblastic tumor (inflammatory pseudotumor): A clinicopathologic and immunohistochemical study of 84 cases. Am J Surg Pathol 19:859-872, 1995.

Solitary Fibrous Tumor

Clinical Features

- Typically occurs in middle-aged adults but has a wide age range
- Presents as a localized, slow-growing, painless mass
- Most commonly involves the pleura; extrapleural sites include subcutaneous and deep soft tissues, orbit, retroperitoneum, mediastinum, pericardium, and other locations

Gross Pathology

- Ranges in size from 1 to 27 cm
- Typically well circumscribed with a firm, tan-white cut surface; sometimes multinodular
- Focal necrosis, hemorrhage, and cystic degeneration may be seen

Histopathology

- Characterized by uniform spindle cells with attenuated nuclei, haphazardly arranged in a collagenized background; collagen focally surrounds individual cells
- Alternating hypercellular and hypocellular areas

Figure 17-13. Solitary fibrous tumor. Monotonous ovoid and spindle tumor cells arranged in a "patternless pattern" around a hyalinized vasculature.

- Hemangiopericytoma-like vasculature
- Epithelioid areas may be present
- Low mitotic activity (<3 mitotic figures/10 high-power fields [hpf])
- Criteria for malignancy include dense cellularity, numerous mitotic figures, obvious cytologic atypia, necrosis, and infiltrative growth

Special Stains and Immunohistochemistry

- CD34 positive in about 85% of cases
- CD99 and bcl-2 positive in about 75% of cases

Other Techniques for Diagnosis

- Not contributory

Differential Diagnosis

- Hemangiopericytoma
  - Characterized by staghorn vascular spaces of varying sizes lined by flattened endothelium
  - Perivascular and intervascular proliferation of uniform spindle-shaped tumor cells
  - May show faint positivity for CD34; CD57 also positive in 50% to 60% cases
  - Negative for keratin, EMA, and CD99
- Synovial sarcoma
  - Monophasic spindle cell or biphasic spindle cell and epithelioid tumors with high nuclear-to-cytoplasmic ratios
  - Herringbone growth pattern is common
  - May show myxoid, squamoid, or collagenized images focally
  - Mitotic activity is usually easily seen
  - Intratumoral calcifications are sometimes present
  - Immunoreactive for keratin or EMA, CD99, and bcl-2; CD34 negative
- Fibrosarcoma (infantile and adult types)
  - Usually found in children younger than 1 year; occasionally seen in adults
  - Infantile form most commonly involves the extremities
  - Highly cellular, infiltrative tumor composed of spindle cells with hyperchromatic nuclei and scant cytoplasm
  - Mitotic figures are usually seen
  - Tumor cells are arranged in a herringbone pattern, at least focally
  - May show areas of hemorrhage and necrosis
  - Negative for CD34, CD99, and bcl-2

Pearls

- Solitary fibrous tumor can occur at any location
- Has "patternless pattern" of spindle cells with hemangiopericytoma-like vasculature

- Usually behaves in an indolent manner but may recur or metastasize even if histologically banal; borderline tumor
- Surgical resection is the preferred treatment

Selected References

Alawi F, Stratton D, Freedman PD: Solitary fibrous tumor of the oral soft tissues: A clinicopathologic and immunohistochemical study of 16 cases. Am J Surg Pathol 25:900-910, 2001.

Brunnemann RB, Ro JY, Ordonez NG, et al: Extrapleural solitary fibrous tumor: A clinicopathologic study of 24 cases. Mod Pathol 12:1034-1042, 1999.

Hasegawa T, Matsuno Y, Shimoda T, et al: Extrathoracic solitary fibrous tumors: Their histological variability and potentially aggressive behavior. Hum Pathol 30:1464-1473, 1999.

Vallat-Decouvelaere AV, Dry SM, Fletcher CD: Atypical and malignant solitary fibrous tumors in extrathoracic locations: Evidence of their comparability to intra-thoracic tumors. Am J Surg Pathol 22:1501-1511, 1998.

Low-Grade Fibromyxoid Sarcoma

Clinical Features

- Related to "hyalinizing spindle cell tumor with giant rosettes"
- Typically seen in young adults but can occur in children and elderly
- Deep soft tissue mass most often in proximal extremities or trunk
- May be present for several years before diagnosis

Gross Pathology

- Usually a large and nonencapsulated but well-circumscribed mass
- Cut surface is firm, white, or tan, sometimes with a myxoid appearance

Figure 17-14. Low-grade fibromyxoid sarcoma. Well-circumscribed tumor with alternating hyalinized and myxoid tumor fascicles.

Histopathology

- Biphasic low-grade spindle cell proliferation
- Myxoid nodules of bland fusiform cells with a prominent arcade of hyalinized vessels, around which tumor cells aggregate
- Collagenized areas are arranged in short haphazard fascicles with a whorling growth pattern
- Rosettes may be present, characterized by hyalinized nodules cuffed by tumor cells
- Mitotic figures are absent or sparse
- Higher-grade foci may be present; this does not appear to affect prognosis adversely

Special Stains and Immunohistochemistry

- Negative for muscle-related and neural markers, CD34, bcl-2, and CD99

Other Techniques for Diagnosis

- Presence of t(7;16)(q34;p11), producing an *FUS-CREBL2* fusion, can be demonstrated by cytogenetic or molecular analysis in most cases

Differential Diagnosis

▌ Low-grade myxofibrosarcoma
- Almost exclusively myxoid with long, curvilinear vessels
- Mild cytologic atypia and pseudolipoblasts
- Older patients; more superficial location

▌ Synovial sarcoma
- Monophasic spindle cell or biphasic spindle cell and epithelioid tumors with high nuclear-to-cytoplasmic ratios
- Herringbone growth pattern is common
- May show myxoid, squamoid, or collagenized images focally
- Mitotic activity usually easily seen
- Intratumoral calcifications sometimes present
- Immunoreactive for keratin or EMA

▌ Desmoid-type fibromatosis
- Lacks alternating myxoid and collagenized zonation
- Highly infiltrative borders
- Positive for β-catenin by nuclear labeling

▌ Myxoid neurofibroma
- Lacks zonation
- Slender, wavy nuclei with tapered ends
- Positive for S-100 protein, CD56, and CD57

Pearls

- Low-grade fibromyxoid sarcoma can be deceptively circumscribed; margins are usually positive if shelled out
- Has a propensity to recur
- Metastases do rarely occur years after resection; long-term follow-up is necessary
- Surgical excision is standard therapy

Selected References

Guillou L, Benhattar J, Gengler C, et al: Translocation-positive low-grade fibromyxoid sarcoma: Clinicopathologic and molecular analysis of a series expanding the morphologic spectrum and suggesting potential relationship to sclerosing epithelioid fibrosarcoma: A study from the French Sarcoma Group. Am J Surg Pathol 31:1387-1402, 2007.

Vernon SE, Bejarano PA: Low-grade fibromyxoid sarcoma: A brief review. Arch Pathol Lab Med 130:1358-1360, 2006.

Billings SD, Giblen G, Fanburg-Smith JC: Superficial low-grade fibromyxoid sarcoma (Evans tumor): A clinicopathologic analysis of 19 cases with a unique observation in the pediatric population. Am J Surg Pathol 29:204-210, 2005.

Panagopoulos I, Storlazzi CT, Fletcher CD, et al: The chimeric FUS/CREB3l2 gene is specific for low-grade fibromyxoid sarcoma. Genes Chromosomes Cancer 40:218-228, 2004.

Folpe AL, Lane KL, Paull G, Weiss SW: Low-grade fibromyxoid sarcoma and hyalinizing spindle cell tumor with giant rosettes: A clinicopathologic study of 73 cases supporting their identity and assessing the impact of high-grade areas. Am J Surg Pathol 24:1353-1360, 2000.

Evans HL: Low-grade fibromyxoid sarcoma: A report of 12 cases. Am J Surg Pathol 17:595-600, 1993.

Low-Grade Myofibroblastic Sarcoma

Clinical Features

- Also known as *myofibrosarcoma*
- Distinctive low-grade tumor with myofibroblastic differentiation
- Tumor of middle-aged adults, rarely reported in children
- Most commonly involves head and neck

Gross Pathology

- Firm mass with white cut surface and poorly defined margins

Histopathology

- Moderately cellular spindle cell lesion arranged in fascicles and whorls
- Modest nuclear hyperchromasia and mild cellular pleomorphism
- Infiltrates adjacent tissues
- Mitotic figures are variable in number

Special Stains and Immunohistochemistry

- Desmin, MSA, SMA: at least one is positive

Other Techniques for Diagnosis

- Electron microscopy shows intercellular fibronexuses, cytoplasmic thin filaments, dense bodies, and intermediate-type gap junctions

Differential Diagnosis

- Deep fibromatosis
  - Lacks cellular pleomorphism
  - Positive for β-catenin with nuclear labeling

- Low-grade fibromyxoid sarcoma
  - Alternating hypocellular myxoid areas and collagenized foci
  - Possible presence of hyalinizing rosettes
  - Margins usually less infiltrative
  - Presence of t(7;16)(q34;p11), producing an *FUS-CREBL2* fusion, is characteristic
- Infantile fibrosarcoma
  - Almost exclusively seen in young children
  - Lacks myogenic differentiation by immunohistochemistry and electron microscopy
  - Presence of t(12;15)(p13;q26), producing an *ETV6-NTRK3* fusion, is typical
- Myofibroma and myofibromatosis
  - Almost exclusively seen in young children
  - Less cellular and lacks significant pleomorphism
  - Hemangiopericytoma-like growth pattern
  - Biphasic growth, in terms of cellularity

Pearls

- Wide surgical resection is necessary for low-grade myofibroblastic sarcoma
- Local recurrence is common; metastases are rare but may be seen after many years
- High-grade myofibroblastic sarcomas are likely a different clinicopathologic entity, synonymous with *malignant fibrous histiocytoma* or *high-grade pleomorphic sarcoma*

Selected References

Fisher C: Myofibrosarcoma. Virchows Arch 445:215-223, 2004.

Gonzalez-Campora R, Escudero AG, Rios Martin JJ, et al: Myofibrosarcoma (low-grade myofibroblastic sarcoma) with intracytoplasmic hyaline (fibroma-like) inclusion bodies. Ultrastruct Pathol 27:7-11, 2003.

Mentzel T, Dry S, Katenkamp D, Fletcher CD: Low-grade myofibroblastic sarcoma: Analysis of 18 cases in the spectrum of myofibroblastic tumors. Am J Surg Pathol 22:1228-1238, 1998.

Smith DM, Mahmoud HH, Jenkins JJ 3rd, et al: Myofibrosarcoma of the head and neck in children. Pediatr Pathol Lab Med 15:403-418, 1995.

Infantile Fibrosarcoma

Clinical Features

- Occurs primarily in children younger than 2 years; about 25% are congenital
- Most common on extremities, followed by trunk and head and neck
- May mimic a vascular lesion both clinically and radiographically; large "hemangiomas" in young children should undergo biopsy if they enlarge

Gross Pathology

- Infiltrative borders
- Firm, fleshy, lobulated mass, often large
- Cut surface is gray-white to tan-yellow

Figure 17-15. Infantile fibrosarcoma. Cellular fascicles of spindle cells are arranged in herringbone growth pattern.

Histopathology

- Cellular tumor is characterized by apposed, spindle-shaped fibroblasts arranged in interlacing fascicles or a herringbone pattern
- Frequent mitotic activity is seen, sometimes with atypical forms
- Necrosis and hemorrhage are common
- Myxoid or collagenous stroma may be seen
- May have focal hemangiopericytoma-like vasculature
- Scattered chronic inflammatory cells and focal extramedullary hematopoiesis are seen

Special Stains and Immunohistochemistry

- Negative for epithelial, myogenous, and neural markers, CD34, bcl-2, and CD99

Other Techniques for Diagnosis

- Up to 90% of cases have t(12;15)(p13;q26) that creates a fusion gene, *ETV6-NTRK3 (TEL-TRCKC)*; this may be cryptic on conventional karyotyping and requires reverse transcription polymerase chain reaction or fluorescent in situ hybridization studies
- Trisomy 11 is the most common additional chromosomal abnormality, followed by trisomies 8, 17, and 20

Differential Diagnosis

- Fibromatosis
  - Lacks dense cellularity, mitotic figures, and herringbone pattern of growth
  - No hemorrhage or necrosis

- Myofibroma and myofibromatosis
  - Infantile fibrosarcoma may contain foci indistinguishable from those of myofibroma, shows more cellular and atypical areas as well
  - Biphasic areas of cellular density
  - Possible intravascular polypoid projections
- Spindle cell rhabdomyosarcoma
  - Intersecting short cellular fascicles with variable stromal collagen
  - Possible presence of strap cells
  - Positive for desmin, myogenin, and MyoD1
- Synovial sarcoma (monophasic)
  - May have herringbone or hemangiopericytoma-like growth patterns
  - Immunoreactivity for cytokeratin, EMA, CD99, and bcl-2
  - Presence of t(X;18) is characteristic
  - Extremely rare in infancy
- Malignant peripheral nerve sheath tumor
  - Composed of elongated cells with variably pleomorphic, serpentine nuclei
  - Cellular growth in fascicles and whorls, with possible neural "tactoid" formation
  - Nuclear palisading potentially present
  - May be positive for S-100 protein, CD56, CD57, or collagen type IV
  - Extremely rare in infancy

Pearls

- Wide surgical excision is the preferred treatment for infantile fibrosarcoma
- Chemotherapy is reserved for unresectable tumors
- About 15% to 30% of cases recur, but metastases are rare
- Presence of t(12;15) is also seen in cellular mesoblastic nephroma of the kidney

Selected References

Sandberg AA, Bridge JA: Updates on the cytogenetics and molecular genetics of bone and soft tissue tumors: Congenital (infantile) fibrosarcoma and mesoblastic nephroma. Cancer Genet Cytogenet 132:1-13, 2002.

Bourgeois JM, Knezevich SR, Mathers JA, Sorensen PH: Molecular detection of the ETV6-NTRK3 gene fusion differentiates congenital fibrosarcoma from other childhood spindle cell tumors. Am J Surg Pathol 24:937-946, 2000.

Coffin CM, Jaszcz W, O'Shea PA, Dehner LP: So-called congenital-infantile fibrosarcoma: Does it exist and what is it? Pediatr Pathol 14:133-150, 1994.

Adult Fibrosarcoma

Clinical Features

- Rare malignant spindle cell tumor with possible herringbone growth pattern
- Tumor of middle-aged to elderly adults

- Located in deep tissue of extremities, trunk, or head and neck; rarely other locations
- In rare cases seen as a second pattern in dermatofibrosarcoma protuberans or other low-grade sarcomas
- May be seen as a postirradiation neoplasm

Gross Pathology

- Firm, lobulated mass usually 3 to 10 cm in diameter
- Small tumors may be well circumscribed
- Cut surface is gray-white to tan-yellow with hemorrhage or necrosis

Histopathology

- Variably hyperchromatic spindle cells with eosinophilic or amphophilic cytoplasm, may show a herringbone growth pattern; some lesions resemble desmoid fibromatosis but have mitotic figures
- Variable mitotic activity
- Lacks significant pleomorphism
  — Well-differentiated fibrosarcoma: shows an orderly arrangement of spindle cells with minimal pleomorphism and variable amounts of collagen; mitotic figures are infrequent
  — Poorly differentiated fibrosarcoma: a cellular lesion with nuclear hyperchromasia, mild pleomorphism, and numerous mitotic figures; hemorrhage and necrosis are common

Special Stains and Immunohistochemistry

- Negative for epithelial, myogenous, and neural markers as well as CD34, CD99, bcl-2, and nuclear β-catenin

Other Techniques for Diagnosis

- Noncontributory except to rule out other tumors, especially monophasic synovial sarcoma (t[X;18])

Differential Diagnosis

▌ Desmoid-type fibromatosis
  - Lacks dense cellularity, nuclear hyperchromasia, and herringbone growth
  - No hemorrhage or necrosis
  - Positive for nuclear β-catenin
▌ Synovial sarcoma (monophasic)
  - May have herringbone or hemangiopericytoid growth patterns
  - Commonly shows areas of hypercellularity and hypocellularity
  - Immunoreactivity for cytokeratin, EMA, CD99, bcl-2, and CD57
  - Presence of t(X;18)
▌ Malignant peripheral nerve sheath tumor
  - Composed of elongated cells with variably pleomorphic, serpentine nuclei

- Cells arranged in fascicles or whorls; possible formation of neural tactoids
- Nuclear palisading sometimes seen
- May be positive for S-100 protein, CD56, CD57, and collagen type IV

▌ Dedifferentiated and spindle cell liposarcoma
  - May be seen de novo through the clonal evolution of well-differentiated liposarcoma
  - Dedifferentiated areas may mimic fibrosarcoma, but extensive sampling reveals low-grade adipocytic component
  - Most commonly occurs in the retroperitoneum
▌ Low-grade fibromyxoid sarcoma
  - Alternating hypocellular myxoid areas and collagenized spindle cell foci
  - Lacks herringbone and desmoid-like patterns of growth
  - Presence of t(7;16) is diagnostic

Pearls

- Wide resection, with or without adjuvant radiotherapy, for adult fibrosarcoma is standard therapy; chemotherapy may be indicated for high-grade tumors
- Local recurrence in 10% to 50% of cases, and high-grade tumors may produce hematogenous metastases
- Fibrosarcoma is a pathologic diagnosis of exclusion

Selected References

Hansen T, Katenkamp K, Brodhun M, Katenkamp D: Low-grade fibrosarcoma: Report on 39 not otherwise specified cases and comparison with defined low-grade fibrosarcoma types. Histopathology 49:152-160, 2006.

Scott SM, Reiman HM, Pritchard DJ, Ilstrup DM: Soft tissue fibrosarcoma: A clinicopathologic study of 132 cases. Cancer 64:925-931, 1989.

Pritchard DJ, Soule EH, Taylor WF, Ivins JC: Fibrosarcoma: A clinicopathologic and statistical study of 199 tumors of the soft tissues of the extremities and trunk. Cancer 33:888-897, 1974.

Sclerosing Epithelioid Fibrosarcoma

Clinical Features

- Distinctive variant of fibrosarcoma
- Tumor of middle-aged adults, but has been reported in children
- Common locations include deep soft tissue of extremities, trunk, chest wall, or head and neck; may be painful

Gross Pathology

- Firm, oval, or lobulated soft tissue mass ranging in size from 2 to 20 cm
- Cut surface is gray-white; may have myxoid or cystic areas

Figure 17-16. **Sclerosing epithelioid fibrosarcoma.** Small epithelioid cells with nuclear atypia are set in a sclerotic matrix.

Histopathology

- Nests or cords of uniform, round to oval tumor cells with eosinophilic to clear cytoplasm embedded in a densely hyalinized stroma
- May have fascicular, myxoid, or cystic areas and hemangiopericytoma-like vasculature
- Mitotic figures are infrequent

Special Stains and Immunohistochemistry

- Vimentin positive
- EMA variable

Other Techniques for Diagnosis

- Electron microscopy confirms fibroblastic/myofibroblastic differentiation with abundant rough endoplasmic reticulum and skeins of thin filaments that are helpful in distinguishing this tumor from mimics of other cell lineages
- Few chromosomal and molecular abnormalities have been reported, two of which showed rearrangements of 10p11

Differential Diagnosis

- Metastatic carcinoma
  - Histology may suggest lobular breast carcinoma or signet ring cell adenocarcinoma
  - Positive for keratin, p63, MOC31, or CA72.4
- Sclerosing lymphoma
  - Positive for leukocyte common antigen (CD45) and B-cell markers (CD20, CD79a, and PAX5)
- Deep fibromatosis
  - Cells tend to be more fusiform, and margins are infiltrative
  - Positive for β-catenin (nuclear)
- Sclerosing rhabdomyosarcoma
  - Eosinophilic, hyperchromatic, and pleomorphic cells
  - Positive for desmin, myogenin, and MyoD1

- Sclerosing, well-differentiated liposarcoma
  - Usually contains lipomatous areas if well sampled
  - Nuclear pleomorphism and lipoblasts are present
- Low-grade fibromyxoid sarcoma
  - Shows clinical and histologic overlap with sclerosing epithelioid fibrosarcoma, and distinction may be difficult
  - Alternating bundles of hypocellular myxoid areas with collagenized spindle cells
  - Presence of t(7;16)

Pearls

- Wide surgical resection is mainstay of therapy for sclerosing epithelioid fibrosarcoma
- Local recurrence in about 50% of cases; distant metastases are common

Selected References

Guillou L, Benhattar J, Gengler C, et al: Translocation-positive low-grade fibromyxoid sarcoma: Clinicopathologic and molecular analysis of a series expanding the morphologic spectrum and suggesting potential relationship to sclerosing epithelioid fibrosarcoma. A study from the French Sarcoma Group. Am J Surg Pathol 31:1387-1402, 2007.

Ogose A, Kawashima H, Umezu H, et al: Sclerosing epithelioid fibrosarcoma with der(10)t(10;17)(p11;q11). Cancer Genet Cytogenet 152:136-140, 2004.

Antonescu CR, Rosenblum MK, Pereira P, et al: Sclerosing epithelioid fibrosarcoma: A study of 16 cases and confirmation of a clinicopathologically distinct tumor. Am J Surg Pathol 25:699-709, 2001.

Meis-Kindblom JM, Kindblom LG, Enzinger FM: Sclerosing epithelioid fibrosarcoma: A variant of fibrosarcoma simulating carcinoma. Am J Surg Pathol 19:979-993, 1995.

Myxofibrosarcoma

Clinical Features

- Also known as *myxoid malignant fibrous histiocytoma*
- Almost exclusively occurs in older adults and elderly people
- Usually presents as a slow-growing, painless mass in subcutaneous or deep tissues of the proximal extremities, rarely on trunk or head and neck

Gross Pathology

- Mulitlobulated or single ill-defined mass with gelatinous, myxoid cut surface

Histopathology

- Multilobulated lesion demarcated with incomplete fibrous septa containing a myxoid stroma and pleomorphic cells
  — Low-grade myxofibrosarcoma
    ◆ Abundant myxoid matrix with scattered spindled or stellate hyperchromatic tumor cells with irregular borders and eosinophilic cytoplasm

Figure 17-17. Low-grade myxofibrosarcoma. Demarcated, paucicellular tumor with small spindle cells in abundant myxoid matrix.

◆ Pseudolipoblasts show eccentric, pleomorphic nuclei and abundant vacuolated cytoplasm
◆ Long curvilinear blood vessels with perivascular condensation of tumor cells is characteristic
— High-grade myxofibrosarcoma
  ◆ Cellular tumor composed of fascicles or sheets of highly pleomorphic fusiform or stellate cells, many of which are multinucleated
  ◆ Myxoid stroma that is less apparent but variable throughout the lesion
  ◆ Numerous mitotic figures and atypical mitoses
  ◆ Hemorrhage and necrosis common
  ◆ Rarely, has an epithelioid phenotype

Special Stains and Immunohistochemistry

● Vimentin positive

Other Techniques for Diagnosis

● Karyotypes tend to be complex but with no specific recurrent abnormalities

Differential Diagnosis

▌ Low-grade fibromyxoid sarcoma
  ● Alternating bundles of hypocellular myxoid areas with collagenized spindle cells
  ● Delicate, plexiform vasculature
  ● Presence of hyalinizing rosettes
  ● Tends to be in younger patients
  ● Presence of t(7;16)(q33;p11), producing an *FUS-CREB3L2* fusion
▌ Myxoid liposarcoma
  ● Bland spindled or fusiform cells with presence of true lipoblasts
  ● Tumor cells are less pleomorphic

● Vasculature is delicate and arborizing and lacks condensed perivascular tumor cells
● Deeply seated tumor that most commonly occurs in the thighs of adults
● Presence of t(12;16)(q13;p11), producing an *FUS-DDIT3* fusion
▌ Myxoma
  ● Paucicellular lesion with small, bland nuclei that lack pleomorphism
  ● Usually intramuscular

Pearls

● Wide surgical resection with radiation, chemotherapy, or both for high-grade lesions is standard therapy for myxofibrosarcoma
● Low-grade tumors show local recurrence in up to 50% of cases but rarely metastasize
● High-grade tumors have a high rate of local recurrence and metastasize in about one third of cases

Selected References

Nascimento AF, Bertoni F, Fletcher CD: Epithelioid variant of myxofibrosarcoma: Expanding the clinicomorphologic spectrum of myxofibrosarcoma in a series of 17 cases. Am J Surg Pathol 31:99-105, 2007.

Willems SM, Debiec-Rychter M, Szuhai K, et al: Local recurrence of myxofibrosarcoma is associated with increase in tumour grade and cytogenetic aberrations, suggesting a multistep tumour progression model. Mod Pathol 19:407-416, 2006.

Antonescu CR, Baren A: Spectrum of low-grade fibrosarcomas: A comparative ultrastructural analysis of low-grade myxofibrosarcoma and fibromyxoid sarcoma. Ultrastruct Pathol 28:321-332, 2004.

Mentzel T, Calonje E, Wadden C, et al: Myxofibrosarcoma: Clinicopathologic analysis of 75 cases with emphasis on the low-grade variant. Am J Surg Pathol 20:391-405, 1996.

Giant Cell Tumor of Tendon Sheath

Clinical Features

● Also referred to as *nodular tenosynovitis*; diffuse form is termed *pigmented villonodular synovitis*
● Typically found in adults but may affect any age; more commonly occurs in women
● Present as a slow-growing, small mass usually in the hands, but may affect feet, wrists, knees, and rarely other joints

Gross Pathology

● Well-circumscribed, lobulated, gray-white mass

Histopathology

● Cellular tumors with a nodular architecture composed of varying amounts of mononuclear stromal cells admixed with osteoclast-like giant cells, xanthoma cells, and inflammation

Figure 17-18. Giant cell tumor of tendon sheath. High-power view shows osteoclast-like giant cells and mononuclear cells with eccentric nuclei and eosinophilic cytoplasm.

- Stroma may be hyalinized, and hemosiderin is invariably present
- Mitotic figures are usually present
- Malignant giant cell tumor of tendon sheath
  — Rare tumors
  — Typical giant cell tumor of tendon sheath containing or recurring as frank sarcomatous elements
  — Destructive localized growth, increased mitotic activity (more than 10 mitotic figures/20 hpf), and extensive necrosis are typically seen in clinically malignant cases

Special Stains and Immunohistochemistry

- CD68 positive
- MSA and desmin variably positive

Other Techniques for Diagnosis

- Structural abnormalities of chromosome 1p are common

Differential Diagnosis

▌ Giant cell malignant fibrous histiocytoma
- Characterized by bizarre, pleomorphic tumor cells arranged in a storiform pattern
- High mitotic rate and necrosis
▌ Fibroma of tendon sheath
- Typically hypocellular lesion composed of spindled fibroblasts in a collagenized stroma
- Lacks osteoclast-like giant cells and inflammatory cells

Pearls

- Giant cell tumor of tendon sheath is a benign lesion but may recur in 5% to 30% of cases, usually in a nondestructive fashion amenable to repeat excision

- Rare malignant forms that tend to have multiple local recurrences have been reported and may metastasize to the same extremity, lymph nodes, and lung
- Complete surgical resection is the preferred treatment

Selected References

Li CF, Wang JW, Huang WW, et al: Malignant diffuse-type tenosynovial giant cell tumors: A series of 7 cases comparing with 24 benign lesions with review of the literature. Am J Surg Pathol 32:587-599, 2008.

Somerhausen NS, Fletcher CD: Diffuse-type giant cell tumor: Clinicopathologic and immunohistochemical analysis of 50 cases with extraarticular disease. Am J Surg Pathol 24:479-492, 2000.

Sciot R, Rosai J, Dal Cin P, et al: Analysis of 35 cases of localized and diffuse tenosynovial giant cell tumor: A report from the Chromosomes and Morphology (CHAMP) study group. Mod Pathol 12:576-579, 1999.

O'Connell JX, Fanburg JC, Rosenberg AE: Giant cell tumor of tendon sheath and pigmented villonodular synovitis: immunophenotype suggests a synovial cell origin. Hum Pathol 26:771-775, 1995.

Ushijima M, Hashimoto H, Tsuneyoshi M, Enjoji M: Giant cell tumor of the tendon sheath (nodular tenosynovitis): A study of 207 cases to compare the large joint group with the common digit group. Cancer 57:875-884, 1986.

Deep Benign Fibrous Histiocytoma

Clinical Features

- Rare benign fibrohistiocytic tumor usually presenting in early adulthood
- Slow-growing, painless nodule, predominantly on head and neck and lower extremities
- Most often involves subcutaneous tissue; deep lesions rare

Gross Pathology

- Well-defined lesion with a tan-white cut surface
- Focal areas of hemorrhage may be seen

Histopathology

- Well-defined or focally infiltrative margins
- Bland spindle cells arranged in short fascicles or storiform pattern; hemangiopericytoma growth pattern may be seen
- Scattered chronic inflammatory cells are common; foam cells and giant cells may be seen
- Typically has few mitotic figures; no atypical mitoses

Special Stains and Immunohistochemistry

- Noncontributory

Other Techniques for Diagnosis

- Noncontributory

Differential Diagnosis

▌ Nodular fasciitis
  ● Loose, feathery collagenous stroma with myxoid or microcystic appearance
  ● Scattered mixed chronic inflammatory cells and extravasated red blood cells are common
  ● Prominent thin-walled blood vessels
▌ Leiomyoma
  ● Characterized by interlacing fascicles of well-differentiated smooth muscle
  ● Immunoreactivity for SMA and desmin
▌ Solitary fibrous tumor
  ● Spindle cells arranged in a "patternless pattern;" hemangiopericytoma growth pattern common
  ● Background tends to be collagenized; hyalinized blood vessels common
  ● Immunoreactivity for CD34 and CD99
▌ Malignant fibrous histiocytoma
  ● Large, deep tumor with infiltrative borders
  ● Pleomorphic spindle cells with a less organized pattern of growth
  ● High mitotic activity with atypical mitotic figures
  ● Hemorrhage and necrosis

Pearls

  ● Tumors are benign but may recur if not completely excised
  ● Surgical resection is the treatment of choice

Selected References

Gleason BC, Fletcher CD: Deep "benign" fibrous histiocytoma: Clinicopathologic analysis of 69 cases of a rare tumor indicating occasional metastatic potential. Am J Surg Pathol 32:354-362, 2008.

Fletcher CD: Benign fibrous histiocytoma of subcutaneous and deep soft tissue: A clinicopathologic analysis of 21 cases. Am J Surg Pathol 14:801-809, 1990.

Smith NM, Davies JB, Shrimankar JS, Malcolm AJ: Deep fibrous histiocytoma with giant cells and bone metaplasia. Histopathology 17:365-367, 1990.

Malignant Fibrous Histiocytoma

Clinical Features

  ● *Malignant fibrous histiocytoma* (MFH) often used synonymously with *high-grade pleomorphic sarcoma*
  ● Most common malignant soft tissue tumor in adults, usually occurring in the sixth and seventh decades
  ● Common sites include proximal extremities and retroperitoneum; inflammatory MFH usually found in the retroperitoneum
  ● Presents as an enlarging, painless mass

Gross Pathology

  ● Solitary, multilobulated, fleshy, tan-white to gray mass; often large

Figure 17-19. Pleomorphic malignant fibrous histiocytoma. Markedly pleomorphic tumor cells with atypical mitotic figures show no discernible line of differentiation.

  ● Most are located in the deep soft tissue, usually within skeletal muscle
  ● Areas of hemorrhage and necrosis are common

Histopathology

  ● Cellular tumor characterized by large pleomorphic cells with large, hyperchromatic nuclei and prominent nucleoli
  ● May show a storiform architecture
  ● Abundant mitotic activity; often, atypical mitoses are present
  ● Areas of hyalinization and necrosis may be seen; xanthoma cells are also common
  ● Various subtypes are described
    — Myxoid MFH
      ◆ Greater than 50% of tumor composed of myxoid areas
      ◆ Combination of myxoid areas and conventional MFH
      ◆ Prominent vascularity
      ◆ Numerous xanthoma cells may be present
    — Inflammatory MFH
      ◆ Presence of an intense, acute and chronic inflammatory infiltrate
    — Pleomorphic MFH
      ◆ Displays bizarre tumor giant cells
      ◆ Numerous mitotic figures, including atypical mitoses
    — Giant cell MFH
      ◆ Presence of osteoclast-like giant cells admixed with conventional MFH areas
      ◆ Must differentiate from giant cell tumor of bone with extraosseous extension; giant cell component is similar; however, background cells appear malignant in giant cell MFH

Special Stains and Immunohistochemistry

- Vimentin positive
- CD68 often positive

Other Techniques for Diagnosis

- Electron microscopy reveals histiocyte-like cells with prominent lysosomes, Golgi, and surface ruffles
- Cytogenetic studies: MFH may be associated with deletion of chromosome 1

Differential Diagnosis

▐ Myxoid liposarcoma
- Composed of vacuolated lipoblasts in a myxoid matrix
- Delicate plexiform capillary pattern is common
- Typically immunoreactivity for S-100 protein

▐ Pleomorphic liposarcoma
- Characterized by bizarre giant lipoblasts
- May be immunoreactive for S-100 protein

▐ Pleomorphic rhabdomyosarcoma
- Large, pleomorphic rhabdomyoblasts, which may show cytoplasmic cross-striations
- Rhabdomyoblasts are immunoreactive for desmin, myogenin, and MyoD1

▐ Leiomyosarcoma
- Prominent fascicular growth pattern
- Immunoreactive for SMA and desmin

Pearls

- MFH is an aggressive tumor with a tendency to recur (myxoid and inflammatory types have lower rates of metastatic spread)
- Distant metastases occur most commonly in the lung, followed by bone and liver
- Depth and location are important prognostic factors
- Surgical resection with wide margins is the treatment of choice
- MFH may be associated with previous radiation exposure

Selected References

Nakayama R, Nemoto T, Takahashi H, et al: Gene expression analysis of soft tissue sarcomas: Characterization and reclassification of malignant fibrous histiocytoma. Mod Pathol 20:749-759, 2007.

Fletcher CD: The evolving classification of soft tissue tumours: An update based on the new WHO classification. Histopathology 48:3-12, 2006.

Coindre JM, Mariani O, Chibon F, et al: Most malignant fibrous histiocytomas developed in the retroperitoneum are dedifferentiated liposarcomas: A review of 25 cases initially diagnosed as malignant fibrous histiocytoma. Mod Pathol 16:256-262, 2003.

Daw NC, Billups CA, Pappo AS, et al: Malignant fibrous histiocytoma and other fibrohistiocytic tumors in pediatric patients: The St. Jude Children's Research Hospital experience. Cancer 97:2839-2847, 2003.

Montgomery E, Fisher C: Myofibroblastic differentiation in malignant fibrous histiocytoma (pleomorphic myofibrosarcoma): A clinicopathological study. Histopathology 38:499-509, 2001.

Brooks JJ: Fact or fiction: Malignant fibrous histiocytoma. Am J Surg Pathol 16:1023-1024, 1992.

Lipoma

Clinical Features

- Most common mesenchymal tumor, usually presents in adulthood; uncommon in children
- Slow-growing, mobile, soft mass in the subcutaneous tissue; occasionally found in deeper tissue
- Most common locations include back, shoulder, neck, and abdomen

Gross Pathology

▐ Subcutaneous lipoma
- Soft, well-circumscribed, lobulated tumors that are thinly encapsulated
- Cut surface shows soft, pale, yellow, homogeneous, mature-appearing adipose tissue
- Typically no areas of hemorrhage or necrosis

▐ Deep lipoma
- Usually larger and less well defined
- May infiltrate surrounding skeletal muscle or soft tissue

Histopathology

- Composed of mature adipose tissue with cells that vary only slightly in size with small, eccentric, compressed nuclei
- Lobular architecture with thin, internal fibrous septa
- Thin, fibrous capsule is typically seen in superficial tumors; deep lipomas may show infiltrative margins with extension into adjacent muscle
- Areas of myxoid change are common

Figure 17-20. Intramuscular lipoma. Uniform mature fat cells entrap skeletal muscle fibers.

- No mitotic activity
- Histologic variants are characterized as follows
  — Intramuscular lipoma
    ◆ Adipose tissue infiltrating mature skeletal muscle, which may show degenerative changes
  — Lumbosacral lipoma
    ◆ Primarily affects children younger than 10 years and is occasionally associated with spina bifida or tethered spinal cord
  — Chondroid lipoma
    ◆ Usually deeply seated lesion in the extremities of adults; females affected more than males
    ◆ Multilobular tumor composed of lipoblasts and mature fat in a myxoid to cartilaginous matrix
  — Hibernoma
    ◆ Slow-growing, painless mass typically found in the scapular region of young adults
    ◆ Composed of lobules of mature lipocytes showing granular, vacuolated cytoplasm and golden-brown lipofuscin pigment (brown fat)
  — Lipoma arborescens
    ◆ Poorly circumscribed fatty infiltration of synovial tissues
    ◆ Causes swelling of affected joints; most commonly seen in adult males

Special Stains and Immunohistochemistry

- S-100 protein positive

Other Techniques for Diagnosis

- Recurrent chromosomal abnormalities include aberrations of 12q13-15 (*HMGIC* gene) and 6p21-23 and loss of 13q

Differential Diagnosis

▌ Myxoma
- Hypovascular, paucicellular tumor characterized by an abundant myxoid stroma
- Typically intramuscular
- Uniform-appearing fibroblast-like cells

▌ Well-differentiated liposarcoma
- Commonly located in the retroperitoneum or deep soft tissue
- Characterized by atypical, often multinucleated adipocytes and lipoblasts admixed with mature, uniform adipocytes
- Thick fibrous septa are common

▌ Myxoid liposarcoma
- Composed of lipoblasts in various stages of maturation, including primitive mesenchymal cells and differentiated lipoblasts
- Prominent myxoid matrix; large pools of myxoid material may be seen
- Delicate arborizing, plexiform capillary network
- Presence of t(12;16)(q13;p11), producing an *FUS-CHOP* fusion

Pearls

- Lipoma and its variants are benign tumors cured by local excision; occasionally recur if incompletely excised (especially true of the intramuscular lipoma)
- Lipoma-like tumors in the retroperitoneal soft tissue should be classified as well-differentiated liposarcomas because of the natural history of these lesions

Selected References

Bassett MD, Schuetze SM, Disteche C, et al: Deep-seated, well differentiated lipomatous tumors of the chest wall and extremities: The role of cytogenetics in classification and prognostication. Cancer 103:409-416, 2005.

Sandberg AA: Updates on the cytogenetics and molecular genetics of bone and soft tissue tumors: Lipoma. Cancer Genet Cytogenet 150:93-115, 2004.

Furlong MA, Fanburg-Smith JC, Miettinen M: The morphologic spectrum of hibernoma: A clinicopathologic study of 170 cases. Am J Surg Pathol 25:809-814, 2001.

Meis JM, Enzinger FM: Chondroid lipoma: A unique tumor simulating liposarcoma and myxoid chondrosarcoma. Am J Surg Pathol 17:1103-1112, 1993.

Kindblom LG, Angervall L, Stener B, Wickbom I: Intermuscular and intramuscular lipomas and hibernomas: A clinical, roentgenologic, histologic, and prognostic study of 46 cases. Cancer 33:754-762, 1974.

Angiolipoma

Clinical Features

- Most commonly affects young adults; rare in young children and elderly people
- Potentially painful superficial mass most commonly seen on the forearm or trunk; often multifocal

Figure 17-21. Angiolipoma. Mature adipose tissue with a branching network of small vascular channels, many of which contain fibrin thrombi.

Gross Pathology

- Well-circumscribed encapsulated nodule with yellow or red cut surface; usually smaller than 3 cm

Histopathology

- Mature adipose tissue with numerous grouped delicate vessels, some of which may contain fibrin thrombi
- Vascularity is variable and tends to be densest at the periphery of the lesional lobules

Special Stains and Immunohistochemistry

- Noncontributory

Other Techniques for Diagnosis

- Cytogenetic studies to date have shown a normal karyotype

Differential Diagnosis

▌ Involuting juvenile hemangioma
- Regressive change in preexisting juvenile hemangioma; usually seen in children
- Lobular lesion with ectatic vessels infiltrated by mature adipose tissue; microthrombi are not a component

▌ Intramuscular hemangioma and hemangiomatosis
- Also called *infiltrating angiolipoma* in older literature
- Deep vascular lesion infiltrating muscle, which has largely been replaced by fat
- Poorly circumscribed lesion lacking microthrombi

▌ Kaposi sarcoma
- Ill-defined tumors with infiltrative margins
- Slitlike vascular spaces with lymphoplasmacytic inflammation and extravasated red blood cells; adipose tissue is not a major component
- Intralesional hyaline globules may be seen
- Seen in HIV patients or on the legs of elderly patients
- HHV-8 and LNA-1 immunoreactivity in 85% of cases

Pearls

- Angiolipoma is one of the painful lesions associated with the ANGEL mnemonic (*a*ngiolipoma, *n*euroma, *g*lomus tumor, *e*ccrine spiradenoma, *l*eiomyoma)
- Angiolipomas are benign and cured by surgical excision

Selected References

Sciot R, Akerman M, Dal Cin P, et al: Cytogenetic analysis of subcutaneous angiolipoma: Further evidence supporting its difference from ordinary pure lipomas. A report of the CHAMP Study Group. Am J Surg Pathol 21:441-444, 1997.

Hunt SJ, Santa Cruz DJ, Barr RJ: Cellular angiolipoma. Am J Surg Pathol 14:75-81, 1990.

Dixon AY, McGregor DH, Lee SH: Angiolipomas: An ultrastructural and clinicopathological study. Hum Pathol 12:739-747, 1981.

Spindle Cell Lipoma and Pleomorphic Lipoma

Clinical Features

- Tumor of older individuals; seen on the posterior neck or shoulders
- Mobile, subcutaneous mass

Gross Pathology

- Well-circumscribed mass with yellow to tan cut surface

Histopathology

- Spindle cell lipoma
  - Mature fat admixed with haphazardly arranged fascicles of bland spindle cells; ropy collagen is characteristic; myxoid change is common
  - No mitotic figures
- Pleomorphic lipoma
  - Variably numerous multinucleated hyperchromatic floret-like cells admixed with mature fat
  - Ropy collagen characteristic
  - No mitotic figures

Special Stains and Immunohistochemistry

- S-100 protein positive in adipocytes
- CD34 positive in spindle and pleomorphic cells

Other Techniques for Diagnosis

- Karyotype is often diploid, but partial loss of chromosomes 13 and 16 is common

Differential Diagnosis

▌ Well-differentiated liposarcoma or atypical lipomatous tumor
- Deeply seated lesion in the extremities or retroperitoneum

Figure 17-22. Pleomorphic lipoma. Mature fat, floret-like giant cells, and ropy collagen are characteristic.

- Atypical stromal cells are variably prominent
- Rare mitotic figures and no ropy collagen as seen in spindle cell or pleomorphic lipoma
- Amplification of 12q14-15 as a supernumerary ring chromosome
▮ Pleomorphic liposarcoma
- Extremities are the most common location
- Pleomorphic lipoblasts in an otherwise high-grade sarcoma
- Mitotically active
- Negative for CD34
▮ Lipofibromatosis
- Poorly circumscribed lesion, usually on extremities of children
- Organized fascicles of bland spindle cells with abundant collagen admixed with mature adipose tissue
- Infiltrative borders

Pearls

- Spindle cell or pleomorphic lipoma represents a morphologic spectrum of clinically and genetically similar tumors, and features of both can be seen in the same lesion
- Benign lesion cured by surgical excision

Selected References

Domanski HA, Carlen B, Jonsson K, et al: Distinct cytologic features of spindle cell lipoma: A cytologic-histologic study with clinical, radiologic, electron microscopic, and cytogenetic correlations. Cancer 93:381-389, 2001.

Fanburg-Smith JC, Devaney KO, Miettinen M, Weiss SW: Multiple spindle cell lipomas: A report of 7 familial and 11 nonfamilial cases. Am J Surg Pathol 22:40-48, 1998.

Yue XH, Liu YQ: Pleomorphic lipoma. Am J Surg Pathol 20:898-899, 1996.

Lipoblastoma and Lipoblastomatosis

Clinical Features

- Typically occurs in infancy or early childhood; most patients are younger than 5 years; more common in boys
- Usually presents as a painless, superficial mass on the extremities but may occur in any location
- Lipoblastomatosis
  — Diffuse form of lipoblastoma
  — Tends to infiltrate muscle

Gross Pathology

- Well-circumscribed, lobular tumors averaging 5 cm (1 to 20 cm); lipoblastomatosis has infiltrative borders
- Cut surface often shows myxoid to gelatinous tissue with fibrous strands

Histopathology

- Typically has a lobular architecture separated by fibrous septa of variable cellularity

Figure 17-23. Lipoblastoma. Nodular growth of mature adipose tissue admixed with lipoblasts in a highly myxoid stroma.

- Adipose tissue in various stages of maturation; usually with identifiable lipoblasts
- Variably myxoid stroma

Special Stains and Immunohistochemistry

- Noncontributory

Other Techniques for Diagnosis

- Cytogenetic and molecular studies: associated with rearrangements of chromosome 8q11-13 involving the *PLAG1* gene

Differential Diagnosis

▮ Myxoid liposarcoma
- Found primarily in adults
- Prominent myxoid matrix with a characteristic delicate plexiform capillary network
- Presence of lipoblasts and mild nuclear atypia
- Lacks the lobular configuration of lipoblastoma
- Presence of t(12;16)(q13;p11), producing an *FUS-CHOP* fusion
▮ Lipofibromatosis
- Ill-defined tumors with infiltrative margins
- Composed of mature adipocytes with cellular fascicles of spindled cells
- Lacks lobular architecture, myxoid stroma, and lipoblasts

Pearls

- Lipoblastoma and lipoblastomatosis are benign lesions that may recur if not completely excised
- Recurrences are often less myxoid and more lipoma-like

Selected References

Hicks J, Dilley A, Patel D, et al: Lipoblastoma and lipoblastomatosis in infancy and childhood: Histopathologic, ultrastructural, and cytogenetic features. Ultrastruct Pathol 25:321-333, 2001.

Chen Z, Coffin CM, Scott S, et al: Evidence by spectral karyotyping that 8q11.2 is nonrandomly involved in lipoblastoma. J Mol Diagn 2:73-77, 2000.

Collins MH, Chatten J: Lipoblastoma/lipoblastomatosis: A clinicopathologic study of 25 tumors. Am J Surg Pathol 21:1131-1137, 1997.

Chung EB, Enzinger FM: Benign lipoblastomatosis: An analysis of 35 cases. Cancer 32:482-492, 1973.

Well-Differentiated Liposarcoma and Atypical Lipomatous Tumor

Clinical Features

- Most common form of liposarcoma
- Primarily occurs in adult life; peak incidence between 50 and 70 years
- Common sites include thigh, retroperitoneum, spermatic cord, and posterior mediastinum
- Usual presentation is that of an insidiously growing, ill-defined mass that has attained a large size by the time it is identified

Gross Pathology

- Well-circumscribed to irregular mass that may exceed 30 cm
- Cut surface is usually fatty with fibrous bands but may be predominantly fibrous or myxoid
- Areas of fat necrosis are common

Histopathology

- Composed of variably sized adipocytes with variable nuclear atypia and hyperchromasia
- Varying numbers of vacuolated or signet ring cell lipoblasts
- Fibrous septa containing occasional hyperchromatic stromal cells with nuclear atypia; floret-like cells may be seen
  — Lipoma-like liposarcoma
    ◆ Predominantly mature fat, atypical cells are hard to find; most common in retroperitoneum
  — Sclerosing liposarcoma
    ◆ Collagenous stroma admixed with variable amounts of adipose-tissue containing pleomorphic, hyperchromatic stromal cells and rare lipoblasts
  — Inflammatory liposarcoma
    ◆ Dense chronic inflammatory infiltrate superimposed on lipoma-like or sclerosing forms of liposarcoma
    ◆ Hyperchromatic, atypical stromal cells are scattered throughout

Special Stains and Immunohistochemistry

- S-100 protein positive
- MDM2 variably positive

Other Techniques for Diagnosis

- Giant supernumerary marker ring chromosome composed of the 12q14-15 region represents *MDM2* amplification

Differential Diagnosis

▌ Panniculitis
  - Mature adipose tissue showing fat necrosis, acute inflammation, and lipid-laden macrophages
▌ Spindle cell or pleomorphic lipoma
  - Typically seen on upper trunk superficially
  - Uniform spindle cells admixed with mature adipose tissue
  - Pleomorphic lipoma pattern is characterized by hyperchromatic, multinucleated, floret-like giant cells
  - Both often contain ropy collagen fibers
  - CD34 positive in spindled and pleomorphic cells
  - Lacks *MDM2* amplification
▌ Angiomyolipoma
  - Typically seen in the kidney but may occur in the soft tissues
  - Composed of mature fat, smooth muscle, and thick-walled vessels
  - Positive for HMB-45, MART-1, or PNL2

Pearls

- The nomenclature for well-differentiated liposarcoma (WDL) and atypical lipomatous tumor (ALT) is not always consistent, but WDL is often used for deep masses, whereas ALT is reserved for more superficial lesions that are amenable to complete surgical resection
- The identification of lipoblasts is neither necessary nor sufficient to warrant a diagnosis of WDL or ALT
- Lipoma-like, sclerosing, and inflammatory patterns often coexist in liposarcomas of the retroperitoneum
- WDL and ALT rarely metastasize but show frequent recurrences and have the potential to dedifferentiate
- Surgical excision with wide margins of resection is the treatment of choice

Selected References

Evans HL: Atypical lipomatous tumor, its variants, and its combined forms: A study of 61 cases, with a minimum follow-up of 10 years. Am J Surg Pathol 31:1-14, 2007.

Sirvent N, Coindre JM, Maire G, et al: Detection of MDM2-CDK4 amplification by fluorescence in situ hybridization in 200 paraffin-embedded tumor samples: Utility in diagnosing adipocytic lesions and comparison with immunohistochemistry and real-time PCR. Am J Surg Pathol 31:1476-1489, 2007.

Binh MB, Sastre-Garau X, Guillou L, et al: MDM2 and CDK4 immunostainings are useful adjuncts in diagnosing well-differentiated and dedifferentiated liposarcoma subtypes: A comparative analysis of 559 soft tissue neoplasms with genetic data. Am J Surg Pathol 29:1340-1347, 2005.

Rosai J, Akerman M, Dal Cin P, et al: Combined morphologic and karyotypic study of 59 atypical lipomatous tumors:

Evaluation of their relationship and differential diagnosis with other adipose tissue tumors (a report of the CHAMP Study Group). Am J Surg Pathol 20:1182-1189, 1996.

Lucas DR, Nascimento AG, Sanjay BK, Rock MG: Well-differentiated liposarcoma. The Mayo Clinic experience with 58 cases. Am J Clin Pathol 102:677-683, 1994.

Myxoid and Round Cell Liposarcoma

Clinical Features

- Represents 30% to 50% of liposarcomas
- Primarily occurs in young to middle-aged adults; rare in children
- Most common site is deep tissue of thigh; rare in retroperitoneum or superficial locations

Figure 17-24. Myxoid liposarcoma. Numerous vacuolated lipoblasts are seen in a loose myxoid stroma with a characteristic chicken-wire vasculature.

Figure 17-25. Round cell myxoid liposarcoma. The tumor cells have hyperchromatic round nuclei, and there is little myxoid stroma.

Gross Pathology

- Poorly circumscribed mass with fatty to myxoid cut surface
- Areas of hemorrhage or necrosis are common and may represent more poorly differentiated areas (round cell component)

Histopathology

- Composed of lipoblasts in various stages of maturation, ranging from primitive mesenchymal cells to well-differentiated lipoblasts
- Prominent myxoid matrix; large pools of myxoid material may be seen
- Arborizing, plexiform capillary network
- Rare mitotic activity
- Mast cells are common

Special Stains and Immunohistochemistry

- S-100 protein positive
- MDM2 variably positive

Other Techniques for Diagnosis

- Presence of t(12;16)(q13;p11), producing an *FUS-DDIT3* fusion (also called *TLS-CHOP*) in 90% of cases, identified by cytogenetic or molecular genetic techniques
- Less commonly, t(12;22)(q13;p11), producing an *EWS-DDIT3* fusion

Differential Diagnosis

▌ Lipoblastoma
  - Lobulated mass with fibrous septa
  - Lacks delicate vascular network
  - Lesion of young children; extremely rare in adults
  - Alterations at 8q11-13 involving *PLAG1*
▌ Spindle cell or pleomorphic lipoma
  - Typically presents on superficial upper trunk in adults
  - Uniform spindle-shaped cells admixed with mature adipose tissue
  - Pleomorphic lipoma pattern is characterized by hyperchromatic, multinucleated floret-like giant cells
  - Both often contain ropy collagen fibers
  - CD34 positive in spindled and pleomorphic cells
  - Lacks *MDM2* amplification

Pearls

- Round cell liposarcoma is considered a higher-grade variant of myxoid liposarcoma, and a transition between the histologic features of both is often present; more than 5% round cell sarcoma represents an adverse prognostic factor
- Surgical excision with wide margins of resection is the treatment of choice

Selected References

Downs-Kelly E, Goldblum JR, Patel RM, et al: The utility of fluorescence in situ hybridization (FISH) in the diagnosis of myxoid soft tissue neoplasms. Am J Surg Pathol 32:8-13, 2008.

Fiore M, Grosso F, Lo Vullo S, et al: Myxoid/round cell and pleomorphic liposarcomas: Prognostic factors and survival in a series of patients treated at a single institution. Cancer 109:2522-2531, 2007.

Antonescu CR, Elahi A, Humphrey M, et al: Specificity of TLS-CHOP rearrangement for classic myxoid/round cell liposarcoma: Absence in predominantly myxoid well-differentiated liposarcomas. J Mol Diagn 2:132-138, 2000.

Tallini G, Akerman M, Dal Cin P, et al: Combined morphologic and karyotypic study of 28 myxoid liposarcomas: Implications for a revised morphologic typing (a report from the CHAMP Group). Am J Surg Pathol 20:1047-1055, 1996.

Pleomorphic Liposarcoma

Clinical Features

- High-grade sarcoma representing about 10% of liposarcomas
- Most common site is extremities; occasionally occurs in the abdomen or retroperitoneum
- Tumor occurs in elderly people

Gross Pathology

- Large, multinodular mass with yellow to tan cut surface
- Areas of hemorrhage or necrosis common

Histopathology

- Pleomorphic, multivacuolated lipoblasts with scalloped hyperchromatic nuclei
- Background lesion is a high-grade spindle cell and pleomorphic sarcoma
- Mitotic figures are easily identified, and necrosis is common
- Eosinophilic hyaline globules may be present
- Epithelioid variant shows pleomorphic lipoblasts in a background of cohesive hyperchromatic polygonal cells with variable amounts of eosinophilic cytoplasm

Figure 17-26. Pleomorphic liposarcoma. Haphazard growth of markedly pleomorphic cells without discernible lipoblasts.

Special Stains and Immunohistochemistry

- S-100 protein and MDM2 variably positive

Other Techniques for Diagnosis

- Complex karyotype, often with large ring-marker chromosomes or double minutes

Differential Diagnosis

❚ Pleomorphic lipoma
- Posterior neck and shoulder most common location; superficial
- Basic histologic image is that of lipoma
- Presence of ropy collagen
- Mitotic figures extremely rare or absent

❚ Dedifferentiated liposarcoma
- Pleomorphic lipoblasts
- Has a coexisting or preexisting lower-grade liposarcoma component

❚ High-grade pleomorphic sarcoma or malignant fibrous histiocytoma
- No lipoblasts
- Lacks S-100 protein immunoreactivity

❚ Pleomorphic rhabdomyosarcoma
- Pleomorphic rhabdomyoblasts may mimic lipoblasts
- Immunoreactivity for desmin, myogenin, MyoD1, or myoglobin

Pearls

- Pleomorphic liposarcoma is a high-grade sarcoma with a high propensity for local recurrence and metastasis, usually to the lungs
- Surgical excision with wide margins of resection is the treatment of choice, often with adjuvant radiotherapy

Selected References

Fiore M, Grosso F, Lo Vullo S, et al: Myxoid/round cell and pleomorphic liposarcomas: Prognostic factors and survival in a series of patients treated at a single institution. Cancer 109:2522-2531, 2007.

Downes KA, Goldblum JR, Montgomery EA, Fisher C: Pleomorphic liposarcoma: A clinicopathologic analysis of 19 cases. Mod Pathol 14:179-184, 2001.

Gebhard S, Coindre JM, Michels JJ, et al: Pleomorphic liposarcoma: Clinicopathologic, immunohistochemical, and follow-up analysis of 63 cases: A study from the French Federation of Cancer Centers Sarcoma Group. Am J Surg Pathol 26:601-616, 2002.

Dedifferentiated Liposarcoma

Clinical Features

- Nonlipomatous component arising from low-grade liposarcoma
- Occurs in about 10% of well-differentiated liposarcomas, most commonly in retroperitoneum

Figure 17-27. Dedifferentiated liposarcoma. An abrupt transition is seen between the well-differentiated sclerosing liposarcoma and a high-grade nonlipogenic component.

- Majority arise de novo in a primary liposarcoma; less frequently, they are seen in recurrences
- Most dedifferentiated liposarcomas show high-grade dedifferentiation, but low-grade dedifferentiation (actually divergent differentiation) can occur

Gross Pathology

- Large, multinodular mass, often with a distinct solid component in an overtly fatty background

Histopathology

- The dedifferentiated component is a nonlipogenic tumor that often has the appearance of a high-grade pleomorphic sarcoma, malignant fibrous histiocytoma, or fibrosarcoma
- An abrupt transition with the well-differentiated liposarcoma is common, but the transition may be gradual
- Heterologous differentiation along myogenic, osseous, or neurogenic lines can be seen
- Low-grade dedifferentiation is represented by a low-grade myogenous or fibroblastic or myofibroblastic component

Special Stains and Immunohistochemistry

- The dedifferentiated component is often only positive for vimentin but may show immunoreactivity for heterologous lineage markers

Other Techniques for Diagnosis

- Usually shows the same ring-marker chromosomes composed of 12q14-15, as seen in well-differentiated liposarcoma

Differential Diagnosis

▌ High-grade pleomorphic sarcoma or malignant fibrous histiocytoma

- May be indistinguishable from high-grade dedifferentiated liposarcoma if low-grade areas have not been sampled
- Lacks adjacent low-grade liposarcoma

Pearls

- Dedifferentiated liposarcoma is usually a high-grade sarcoma but has a less aggressive course than other pleomorphic sarcomas
- Sampling should be thorough to recognize the low-grade liposarcoma component
- Presence of heterologous elements does not affect prognosis
- Surgical excision with wide margin is preferred treatment, with or without adjuvant therapy

Selected References

Binh MB, Guillou L, Hostein I, et al: Dedifferentiated liposarcomas with divergent myosarcomatous differentiation developed in the internal trunk: A study of 27 cases and comparison to conventional dedifferentiated liposarcomas and leiomyosarcomas. Am J Surg Pathol 31:1557-1566, 2007.

Fabre-Guillevin E, Coindre JM, Somerhausen Nde S, et al: Retroperitoneal liposarcomas: Follow-up analysis of dedifferentiation after clinicopathologic reexamination of 86 liposarcomas and malignant fibrous histiocytomas. Cancer 106:2725-2733, 2006.

Elgar F, Goldblum JR: Well-differentiated liposarcoma of the retroperitoneum: A clinicopathologic analysis of 20 cases, with particular attention to the extent of low-grade dedifferentiation. Mod Pathol 10:113-120, 1997.

Henricks WH, Chu YC, Goldblum JR, Weiss SW: Dedifferentiated liposarcoma: A clinicopathological analysis of 155 cases with a proposal for an expanded definition of dedifferentiation. Am J Surg Pathol 21:271-281, 1997.

Rhabdomyoma

Clinical Features

- Rare benign extracardiac tumor with skeletal muscle differentiation; less than 2% of all skeletal muscle tumors
- Three distinct clinical and morphologic subtypes exist
  — Fetal rhabdomyoma
    ♦ Typically occurs in children younger than 3 years; may be congenital
    ♦ Mass in the subcutaneous or mucosal tissue of the head and neck
  — Adult rhabdomyoma
    ♦ Average age is 60 years; more common in males
    ♦ Polypoid mass in the head and neck region; may present with upper airway obstruction
    ♦ May be multinodular and rarely multifocal
  — Genital rhabdomyoma
    ♦ Presents as a polypoid mass in the vagina or vulva of young to middle-aged women
    ♦ May cause vaginal bleeding

Gross Pathology

- Circumscribed, lobulated tumor with a finely granular, red-brown cut surface
- Typically ranges in size from 2 to 10 cm

Histopathology

▌ Fetal rhabdomyoma
- Classic or myxoid form shows primitive spindle cells in a loose myxoid stroma
- Intermediate or cellular form has a fascicular growth pattern with strap cells or plump rhabdomyoblasts
- Both forms contain cells with cross-striations, negligible mitotic figures, and a lack of necrosis

▌ Adult rhabdomyoma
- Large, round to polygonal rhabdomyocytes with eosinophilic, granular, or vacuolated cytoplasm and small peripheral nuclei
- Tumor cells show variable cross-striation and focal vacuolization owing to glycogen content; "spider" cells are common

▌ Genital rhabdomyoma
- Plump polygonal or fusiform cells in various stages of myogenic differentiation in a fibrous stroma with dilated vessels

Special Stains and Immunohistochemistry

- MSA, desmin, and myoglobin positive
- Myogenin and MyoD1 may be positive in scattered cells

Other Techniques for Diagnosis

- Electron microscopy: cells with large nuclei and prominent nucleoli; thick and thin myofilaments with Z lines and A and I bands

Differential Diagnosis

Adult Rhabdomyoma

▌ Granular cell tumor
- Sheet of polygonal cells with coarsely granular eosinophilic cytoplasm and small central nuclei; no strap cells
- Positive for S-100 protein in 85% of cases; no myogenic markers

▌ Hibernoma
- Characterized by round to oval cells with central nuclei and granular or vacuolated cytoplasm containing lipofuscin pigment (brown fat)

▌ Paraganglioma
- Organoid arrangement of round to oval cells with central nuclei, eosinophilic granular cytoplasm, a delicate capillary network
- Positive for chromogranin, synaptophysin, and CD56; lacks myogenic markers

▌ Rhabdomyosarcoma
- In adults, usually pleomorphic; poorly circumscribed lesion with marked nuclear pleomorphism, mitotic activity, and necrosis
- A higher percentage of cells are positive for myogenin and MyoD1; infrequent staining for myoglobin

Fetal and Genital Rhabdomyoma

▌ Embryonal rhabdomyosarcoma (ERMS)
- A distinction between fetal rhabdomyoma and ERMS may be difficult
- ERMS lacks circumscription, shows less differentiation, and manifests mitotic figures or necrosis
- Myogenin and MyoD1 stain less than 50% of the tumor cells; rare cell positivity for myoglobin

▌ Botryoid rhabdomyosarcoma
- Spindled to rounded rhabdomyoblasts in an abundant myxoid matrix with a condensed cambium layer under an epithelial surface

Pearls

- Rhabdomyomas are adequately treated with complete excision
- Local recurrence possible if incompletely removed; some fetal rhabdomyomas have recurred as rhabdomyosarcomas

Selected References

Walsh SN, Hurt MA: Cutaneous fetal rhabdomyoma: A case report and historical review of the literature. Am J Surg Pathol 32:485-491, 2008.

Braaten K, Young RH: Ovarian serous cystadenoma with associated genital rhabdomyoma. Hum Pathol 36:1240-1241, 2005.

Cronin CT, Keel SB, Grabbe J, Schuler JG: Adult rhabdomyoma of the extremity: A case report and review of the literature. Hum Pathol 31:1074-1080, 2000.

Kodet R, Fajstavr J, Kabelka Z, et al: Is fetal cellular rhabdomyoma an entity or a differentiated rhabdomyosarcoma? A study of patients with rhabdomyoma of the tongue and sarcoma of the tongue enrolled in the intergroup rhabdomyosarcoma studies I, II, and III. Cancer 67:2907-2913, 1991.

Rhabdomyosarcoma

Clinical Features

- Tumors with almost exclusive skeletal muscle differentiation
- Most common sarcomas of childhood
  — Embryonal rhabdomyosarcoma
    - Common sites include the head and neck, genitourinary tract, abdomen, retroperitoneum, and paratesticular region
    - Primarily affects young children

Figure 17-28. Embryonal rhabdomyosarcoma. Pleomorphic, primitive spindle cells with tapered eosinophilic cytoplasm are seen in myxoid stroma.

Figure 17-29. Alveolar rhabdomyosarcoma. Monomorphic, hyperchromatic round cells cling to fibrovascular septa. Tumor giant cells are abundant.

◆ Botryoid rhabdomyosarcoma is a favorable variant that occurs beneath the mucosal surfaces of the genitourinary tract or head and neck in young children
◆ Spindle cell rhabdomyosarcoma is a favorable subtype when seen in the paratesticular soft tissue of adolescents
— Alveolar rhabdomyosarcoma
◆ Most commonly presents as a deep mass in the extremities or buttocks
◆ Typically affects adolescents
— Pleomorphic rhabdomyosarcoma
◆ Presents as a deep mass in the extremities
◆ Typically affects adults

Gross Pathology

- Soft, poorly circumscribed lobulated mass with a gray-tan cut surface
- Focal areas of necrosis are common
- Botryoid rhabdomyosarcomas are polypoid, grape-like masses with a gray-white cut surface

Histopathology

❚ Embryonal rhabdomyosarcoma
- Hyperchromatic, primitive spindled cells, often with a myxoid stroma
- Alternating hypocellular and hypercellular areas with cells condensed around blood vessels
- Rare strap cells with eosinophilic cytoplasm, tapered ends, and cross-striations
- Anaplasia is defined by large hyperchromatic tumor cells at least 3 times the size of neighboring nuclei, with atypical mitotic figures
  — Botryoid rhabdomyosarcoma
    ◆ Polypoid architecture
    ◆ Cambium layer (condensation of tumor cells) under intact epithelium in at least one microscopic field
  — Spindle cell rhabdomyosarcoma
    ◆ Fascicular growth pattern within a variably collagenized background
❚ Alveolar rhabdomyosarcoma
- Classic alveolar pattern shows round hyperchromatic tumor cells clinging to fibrovascular cores with central dyshesion
- Solid alveolar pattern represented by sheets or nests of monomorphic tumor cells with round nuclei and a fine chromatin pattern
- Scattered tumor giant cells
- Differentiating rhabdomyoblasts are oval cells with eccentric eosinophilic cytoplasm
❚ Pleomorphic rhabdomyosarcoma
- Large, pleomorphic cells with abundant eosinophilic cytoplasm
- Admixture of small, primitive, undifferentiated cells and spindle cells

Special Stains and Immunohistochemistry

- Desmin and MSA positive
- Myogenin and MyoD1: nuclear reactivity
- Myoglobin positive only in cells with overt skeletal muscle differentiation

Other Techniques for Diagnosis

- Electron microscopy: rhabdomyoblasts show cytoplasmic thick and thin filaments and dilated endoplasmic reticulum
- Cytogenetic and molecular studies
  — Alveolar rhabdomyosarcoma: 75% have either t(2;13)(q35;q14) or t(1;13)(p36;q14), producing a *PAX3* or *PAX7-FKHR* fusion

— Embryonal rhabdomyosarcoma: commonly show loss of heterozygosity at 11q15 or hyperdiploidy with gains of chromosome 2, 7, 8, 12, and 13

Differential Diagnosis

▌ Neuroblastoma
- Usually in patients younger than 5 years, occurring in the adrenal or along the sympathetic chain
- Small round cells with variable neuropil and ganglion cell differentiation; rosettes may be seen
- Nests of tumor cells separated by delicate curvilinear vascular network
- Immunoreactivity for neuron-specific enolase (NSE), synaptophysin, and NB84; lacks myogenic markers

▌ Ewing sarcoma (EWS) and primitive neuroectodermal tumor (PNET)
- Sheets of monomorphic round cells with a rim of eosinophilic to clear cytoplasm
- Rosettes may be seen
- Lacks tumor giant cells and rhabdomyoblasts
- Immunoreactivity for CD99 with strong membranous pattern and nuclear Fli-1; lacks myogenic markers
- Presence of t(11;22)(q24;q12), producing an *EWS-FLI-1* fusion by cytogenetic or molecular techniques is characteristic

▌ Desmoplastic small round cell tumor (DSRCT)
- Characteristically involves abdomen of adolescents
- Undifferentiated small cells in nested pattern separated by desmoplastic stroma
- Polyphenotypic immunophenotype with reactivity for keratin and EMA, neural markers (synaptophysin, CD56), and desmin; negative for myogenin and MyoD1
- Presence of t(11;22)(p13;q12), producing an *EWS-WT1* fusion by cytogenetic or molecular techniques is characteristic

▌ Inflammatory myofibroblastic tumor
- Can mimic the spindle cell or embryonal rhabdomyosarcoma
- Ganglion cell–like myofibroblasts and mixed inflammatory background
- Immunoreactivity for SMA and ALK-1 (40%); negative for myogenin and MyoD1

▌ Monophasic synovial sarcoma
- In the differential diagnosis of spindle cell rhabdomyosarcoma
- Cellular lesion with herringbone or hemangiopericytoma-like pattern of growth
- Immunoreactive for cytokeratin, EMA, bcl-2, or CD99; negative for myogenin and MyoD1
- The presence of t(X,18)(p11.2;q11.2), producing an *SYT-SSX1/2* fusion by cytogenetic or molecular techniques is characteristic

▌ Malignant lymphoma
- Diffuse population of atypical lymphoid cells
- Tumor cells are immunoreactive for CD45

Pearls

- Surgical excision with adjuvant chemotherapy and radiotherapy is standard therapy for rhabdomyosarcoma
- Risk stratification for rhabdomyosarcoma is based on histology, patient age, tumor stage, and site of origin
- Alveolar rhabdomyosarcoma has a worse prognosis than other subtypes; may involve bone marrow
- Anaplasia is considered a poor prognosis in intermediate-risk embryonal rhabdomyosarcomas
- Metastases usually involve the lungs and regional lymph nodes

Selected References

Parham DM, Qualman SJ, Teot L, et al: Correlation between histology and PAX/FKHR fusion status in alveolar rhabdomyosarcoma: A report from the Children's Oncology Group. Am J Surg Pathol 31:895-901, 2007.

Morotti RA, Nicol KK, Parham DM, et al: An immunohistochemical algorithm to facilitate diagnosis and subtyping of rhabdomyosarcoma: The Children's Oncology Group experience. Am J Surg Pathol 30:962-968, 2006.

Nishio J, Althof PA, Bailey JM, et al: Use of a novel FISH assay on paraffin-embedded tissues as an adjunct to diagnosis of alveolar rhabdomyosarcoma. Lab Invest 86:547-556, 2006.

Parham DM, Ellison DA: Rhabdomyosarcomas in adults and children: An update. Arch Pathol Lab Med 130:1454-1465, 2006.

Ferrari A, Dileo P, Casanova M, et al: Rhabdomyosarcoma in adults: A retrospective analysis of 171 patients treated at a single institution. Cancer 98:571-580, 2003.

Folpe AL, McKenney JK, Bridge JA, Weiss SW: Sclerosing rhabdomyosarcoma in adults: Report of four cases of a hyalinizing, matrix-rich variant of rhabdomyosarcoma that may be confused with osteosarcoma, chondrosarcoma, or angiosarcoma. Am J Surg Pathol 26:1175-1183, 2002.

Furlong MA, Mentzel T, Fanburg-Smith JC: Pleomorphic rhabdomyosarcoma in adults: A clinicopathologic study of 38 cases with emphasis on morphologic variants and recent skeletal muscle-specific markers. Mod Pathol 14:595-603, 2001.

Leiomyoma (Cutaneous and Deep Soft Tissue)

Clinical Features

- Clinical presentation depends on location and can range from painful cutaneous swellings to deep masses in the extremities, abdomen, or retroperitoneum
- Based on their location, leiomyomas are categorized as follows
  - Cutaneous leiomyoma
    - Most commonly involves extensor surfaces of extremities or genital skin
    - Extremity lesions differentiate toward the pilar arrector muscle; they are often multiple and usually painful
    - Typically seen in adolescents and young adults but may occur in childhood

Figure 17-30. Leiomyoma. Interlacing fascicles of well-differentiated smooth muscle without nuclear atypia or mitotic figures.

— Angioleiomyoma
  ◆ Differentiates toward vascular smooth muscle
  ◆ Typically found in women
  ◆ Solitary, often painful mass, usually on the extremities
— Deep leiomyoma
  ◆ Arises in the deep tissues of the extremities, abdomen, or retroperitoneum
  ◆ Rare tumor found almost exclusively in adults
  ◆ Radiograph often shows intralesional calcification
  ◆ A diagnosis to be made with caution; most deep smooth muscle tumors of soft tissue are malignant

Gross Pathology

- Typically measures less than 2 cm; deep tumors may be larger
- Sectioning shows a firm, trabeculated, gray-white, bulging surface
- Focal areas of calcification or hyalinization may be present

Histopathology

▋ Cutaneous leiomyoma
  ● Typically has ill-defined margins
  ● Well-differentiated smooth muscle cells arranged in interlacing fascicles
  ● Eosinophilic cytoplasm and oval, blunt-ended nuclei with perinuclear vacuoles
  ● Focal calcification, hyalinization, ossification, and myxoid degeneration may be seen
  ● No mitotic activity
  ● Atrophic epidermis
▋ Angioleiomyoma
  ● Well-defined margins

- Prominent, irregular, interconnecting vascular spaces surrounded by well-differentiated smooth muscle; may be solid or contain large vascular spaces
▋ Deep leiomyoma
  ● Interlacing fascicles of well-differentiated smooth muscle spindle cells with blunt ends and perinuclear vacuoles
  ● Variable degenerative atypia, calcification, and ossification apparent, but true pleomorphism should be absent
  ● Mitotic figures should be absent

Special Stains and Immunohistochemistry

● SMA and desmin positive

Other Techniques for Diagnosis

● Noncontributory

Differential Diagnosis

▋ Cutaneous fibrous histiocytoma (dermatofibroma)
  ● Characterized by spindle cells arranged in a storiform pattern with entrapment of collagen
  ● Immunoreactive for factor XIIIa
▋ Leiomyosarcoma
  ● Characterized by spindle-shaped cells with cigar-shaped nuclei, atypical nuclear features, and mitotic activity
  ● Cells are arranged in interlacing fascicles
  ● Focal necrosis, hyalinization, and myxoid change may be seen

Pearls

● Cutaneous leiomyomas are benign tumors that are treated by surgical excision
● Cutaneous leiomyomas may show an autosomal dominant pattern of inheritance
● Retroperitoneal smooth muscle tumors in women are often estrogen dependent
● Diagnosis of retroperitoneal leiomyoma is controversial, and some observers regard all smooth muscle tumors in that location as sarcomas de facto

Selected References

Sandberg AA: Updates on the cytogenetics and molecular genetics of bone and soft tissue tumors: Leiomyoma. Cancer Genet Cytogenet 158:1-26, 2005.

Billings SD, Folpe AL, Weiss SW: Do leiomyomas of deep soft tissue exist? An analysis of highly differentiated smooth muscle tumors of deep soft tissue supporting two distinct subtypes. Am J Surg Pathol 25:1134-1142, 2001.

Fletcher CD, Kilpatrick SE, Mentzel T: The difficulty in predicting behavior of smooth-muscle tumors in deep soft tissue. Am J Surg Pathol 19:116-117, 1995.

Kilpatrick SE, Mentzel T, Fletcher CD: Leiomyoma of deep soft tissue: Clinicopathologic analysis of a series. Am J Surg Pathol 18:576-582, 1994.

Leiomyosarcoma

Clinical Features

- Usually seen in patients between 40 and 70 years of age, but can occur at any age
- Retroperitoneum or pelvis is the most common location, but leiomyosarcoma may also arise from large veins and in deep tissues of extremities
- Retroperitoneal and intra-abdominal tumors are more common in women
- Usual presentation is that of an enlarging mass with symptoms related to displacement of adjacent organs

Gross Pathology

- Relatively well-circumscribed, fleshy mass with a gray-white, whorled, cut surface
- Focal hemorrhage, necrosis, or cystic change may be seen

Histopathology

- Variably cellular tumor composed of fascicles of spindle cells with eosinophilic cytoplasm and cigar-shaped nuclei with perinuclear vacuoles
- Cellular pleomorphism may be minimal to marked; tumor giant cells and osteoclast-like giant cells possible
- Mitotic rate usually 5 mitotic figures/10 hpf, but any mitotic activity should raise suspicion of malignancy
- Areas of hyalinization and coagulative tumor necrosis often seen
- Epithelioid differentiation, myxoid change, nuclear palisading, or prominent lymphoid inflammation may occasionally be present

Special Stains and Immunohistochemistry

- SMA, h-caldesmon positive
- Desmin typically positive

Figure 17-31. Leiomyosarcoma. Cellular tumor with short intersecting fascicles composed of hyperchromatic spindle cells with bluntly tapered ends.

Other Techniques for Diagnosis

- Electron microscopy: thin filaments (actin and myosin) with dense bodies, pinocytosis, and external basal lamina
- Cytogenetic studies: most leiomyosarcomas have complex karyotypes but no diagnostic abnormality
- Alterations in the Rb1–cyclin D pathway are common

Differential Diagnosis

- ❚ Leiomyoma
  - Low-power appearance similar to that of well-differentiated leiomyosarcoma
  - Absent mitotic activity and minimal cytologic atypia
  - No coagulative necrosis
- ❚ Cellular schwannoma or malignant peripheral nerve sheath tumor
  - Elongated cells with wavy, serpentine nuclei
  - Nuclear palisading is common, but this can also be seen in leiomyosarcoma
  - At least focal positivity for S-100 protein, CD56, or CD56, with a lack of smooth muscle markers
- ❚ Malignant fibrous histiocytoma
  - Pleomorphic and spindle cells arranged in a storiform pattern, often in a collagenized or myxoid stroma
  - High-grade leiomyosarcomas may have a similar appearance
  - Negative for SMA, MSA, desmin, and h-caldesmon
- ❚ Monophasic synovial sarcoma
  - Fascicles of spindle cells with variable nuclear pleomorphism and a herringbone or hemangiopericytoma-like growth pattern
  - Variable mitotic rate
  - Immunoreactivity for cytokeratin, EMA, bcl-2, or CD99; lacks smooth muscle markers
  - The presence of t(X;18)(p11.2;q11.2), producing an *SYT-SSX1/2* fusion by cytogenetic or molecular techniques, is characteristic
- ❚ Spindle cell rhabdomyosarcoma
  - Often occur in the paratesticular region in adolescent males
  - Focal strap cell differentiation may be seen
  - Nuclear immunoreactivity for myogenin and MyoD1
- ❚ Extragastrointestinal stromal tumor
  - May have an epithelioid, spindle cell, or mixed phenotype; myxoid change may be present
  - Fascicular growth is not prominent
  - Immunoreactive for C-kit (CD117) and CD34
- ❚ Inflammatory myofibroblastic tumor
  - Spindle cell lesion with ganglion cell–like myofibroblasts and prominent inflammation
  - Usually lacks the fascicular growth pattern of leiomyosarcoma
  - Immunoreactive for SMA, but lacks desmin and h-caldesmon; positive for ALK-1 (40%)
- ❚ Fibrosarcoma (infant and adult type)
  - Most often affects children younger than 1 year; occasionally seen in adults

- Usually found in the extremities
- Highly cellular, infiltrative tumor with hyperchromatic nuclei and scant cytoplasm; herringbone growth pattern
- High mitotic rate; atypical mitotic figures may be seen
- Negative for SMA, desmin, and h-caldesmon

Pearls

- Leiomyosarcoma is often a large tumor; local recurrence and metastases to lungs and liver are common
- Tumor location, depth, and size are more important prognostic factors than histologic features
- Surgical excision with wide resection margins is the treatment of choice
- Deep smooth muscle tumors with discernible mitotic activity should be considered malignant

Selected References

Sandberg AA: Updates on the cytogenetics and molecular genetics of bone and soft tissue tumors: leiomyosarcoma. Cancer Genet Cytogenet 161:1-19, 2005.

Farshid G, Pradhan M, Goldblum J, Weiss SW: Leiomyosarcoma of somatic soft tissues: A tumor of vascular origin with multivariate analysis of outcome in 42 cases. Am J Surg Pathol 26:14-24, 2002.

Oda Y, Miyajima K, Kawaguchi K, et al: Pleomorphic leiomyosarcoma: clinicopathologic and immunohistochemical study with special emphasis on its distinction from ordinary leiomyosarcoma and malignant fibrous histiocytoma. Am J Surg Pathol 25:1030-1038, 2001.

Rubin BP, Fletcher CD: Myxoid leiomyosarcoma of soft tissue, an underrecognized variant. Am J Surg Pathol 24:927-936, 2000.

de Saint Aubain Somerhausen N, Fletcher CD: Leiomyosarcoma of soft tissue in children: Clinicopathologic analysis of 20 cases. Am J Surg Pathol 23:755-763, 1999.

Granular Cell Tumor

Clinical Features

- Typically occurs in adults (fourth through sixth decades); females are affected more than males
- Presents as a dermal, subcutaneous, or submucosal mass, infrequently multiple
- Tongue is a common site of involvement

Gross Pathology

- Poorly circumscribed nodule
- Typically small (<3 cm) and firm with a yellow-white cut surface

Histopathology

- Composed of sheets of large, polygonal cells with abundant coarse, eosinophilic, granular cytoplasm
- May grow in sheets, nests, or trabeculae; occasionally exhibit pronounced desmoplasia

Figure 17-32. Granular cell tumor. Large polygonal cells with small vesicular nuclei have abundant eosinophilic, granular cytoplasm.

- May have small nuclei or larger vesicular nuclei with nucleoli
- Minimal nuclear pleomorphism and rare mitotic activity
- Pseudoepitheliomatous hyperplasia often seen in overlying squamous epithelium
- Histologic features worrisome for malignancy include necrosis, more than 2 mitotic figures/10 hpf, tumor cell spindling, vesicular chromatin with large nucleoli, and cellular pleomorphism

Special Stains and Immunohistochemistry

- S-100 protein, CD68 positive
- Periodic acid–Schiff (PAS): cells typically show cytoplasmic positivity

Other Techniques for Diagnosis

- Electron microscopy shows cytoplasmic membrane-bound granules consistent with phagolysosomes

Differential Diagnosis

▌ Adult rhabdomyoma
  - Characterized by round to polygonal cells with cytoplasmic cross-striations
  - Immunoreactivity for desmin, myogenin, and myoglobin
▌ Hibernoma
  - Cells have vacuolated to granular cytoplasm with distinct cell borders
  - Lipid droplets can be detected by oil red O stain

Pearls

- Granular cell tumor is a benign neural tumor typically treated by local excision
- Most granular cell tumors behave in a benign manner; however, malignant granular cell tumors do exist (about 1%); histologic criteria to differentiate

between benign and malignant tumors are not well established

- Metastasis is the only definitive feature defining malignant tumors
- Pseudoepitheliomatosis may be mistaken for squamous cell carcinoma

Selected References

Fanburg-Smith JC, Meis-Kindblom JM, Fante R, Kindblom LG: Malignant granular cell tumor of soft tissue: Diagnostic criteria and clinicopathologic correlation. Am J Surg Pathol 22:779-794, 1998.

Filie AC, Lage JM, Azumi N: Immunoreactivity of S100 protein, alpha-1-antitrypsin, and CD68 in adult and congenital granular cell tumors. Mod Pathol 9:888-892, 1996.

Nakazato Y, Ishizeki J, Takahashi K, Yamaguchi H: Immunohistochemical localization of S-100 protein in granular cell myoblastoma. Cancer 49:1624-1628, 1982.

Schwannoma

Clinical Features

- Also called *neurilemmoma*
- Can occur at any age; typically in adulthood
- Common sites of involvement are intracranial sites (cerebellopontine angle), posterior mediastinum, retroperitoneum, flexor surface of extremities, and head and neck
- Slow-growing, usually painless tumors
- Most often sporadic; less than 5% occur in patients with neurofibromatosis type 2 (NF2)

Gross Pathology

- Ovoid or fusiform mass, usually smaller than 5 cm
- Well-defined and typically encapsulated with pink to tan, firm cut surface
- Focal areas of cystic degeneration may be seen

Figure 17-33. Schwannoma. Loose Antoni B areas alternate with cellular Antoni A foci with nuclear palisading and Verocay bodies.

Histopathology

- Well-defined capsule consisting of epineurium
- Presence of compact hypercellular areas (Antoni A areas) and hypocellular, myxoid areas (Antoni B areas)
- Nuclear palisading around fibrillary processes (Verocay bodies)
- Cells are spindled and contain elongated, wavy nuclei with tapered ends
- Hyalinized vessels are characteristic
- Focal areas of hemorrhage, hemosiderin deposition, and xanthomatous change
- Rarely have glandular structures or pure epithelioid morphology
- Ancient schwannoma
  — Prominent degenerative changes, including cyst formation, calcification, hyalinized vessels, hemorrhage, and cytologic atypia
- Cellular schwannoma
  — Composed almost entirely of Antoni A areas (must be distinguished from malignant peripheral nerve sheath tumor)
  — Mitotically active but cellularity exceeds mitotic figures

Special Stains and Immunohistochemistry

- S-100 protein strongly positive
- Leu-7 (CD57), CD56, and GFAP positive
- Collagen IV: surround individual tumor cells

Other Techniques for Diagnosis

- Electron microscopy: tumor cells contain electron-dense basement membrane material and characteristic Luse bodies (long-spaced collagen)

Differential Diagnosis

▌ Neurofibroma
- Characterized by fascicles and whorls of elongated cells with wavy, serpentine nuclei with wavy collagen fibers; often has a myxoid stroma
- Lacks Antoni A and Antoni B areas

▌ Leiomyoma
- Characterized by interlacing bundles of spindle cells with oval, blunt-ended nuclei
- Lacks Antoni A and Antoni B areas
- Positive for SMA

▌ Malignant peripheral nerve sheath tumor
- Infiltrative, highly cellular tumors characterized by elongated cells with pleomorphic nuclei
- Prominent mitotic activity
- Necrosis is common
- Less intense positivity for S-100 protein

Pearls

- Schwannoma is a benign tumor showing almost exclusively Schwann cell differentiation; malignant transformation is exceedingly rare

- Surgical removal with nerve preservation is the recommended treatment
- Cellular schwannoma may be misclassified as a malignant peripheral nerve sheath tumor; strong S-100 protein reactivity favors cellular schwannoma

Selected References

Begnami MD, Palau M, Rushing EJ, et al: Evaluation of NF2 gene deletion in sporadic schwannomas, meningiomas, and ependymomas by chromogenic in situ hybridization. Hum Pathol 38:1345-1350, 2007.

Nascimento AF, Fletcher CD: The controversial nosology of benign nerve sheath tumors: Neurofilament protein staining demonstrates intratumoral axons in many sporadic schwannomas. Am J Surg Pathol 31:1363-1370, 2007.

Agaram NP, Prakash S, Antonescu CR: Deep-seated plexiform schwannoma: A pathologic study of 16 cases and comparative analysis with the superficial variety. Am J Surg Pathol 29:1042-1048, 2005.

McMenamin ME, Fletcher CD: Expanding the spectrum of malignant change in schwannomas: Epithelioid malignant change, epithelioid malignant peripheral nerve sheath tumor, and epithelioid angiosarcoma. A study of 17 cases. Am J Surg Pathol 25:13-25, 2001.

Fletcher CD, Davies SE, McKee PH: Cellular schwannoma: A distinct pseudosarcomatous entity. Histopathology 11:21-35, 1987.

Neurofibroma

Clinical Features

- Usually occur in the dermal or subcutaneous tissues throughout the body
- People of any age can be affected, but seen most commonly in young adults
- Lesions may be localized, diffuse, or plexiform, the latter two having a strong association with NF1

Figure 17-34. Neurofibroma. Small wavy spindle cells are admixed with dense collagen bundles.

- — NF1, von Recklinghausen disease
  - ◆ Autosomal dominant, chromosome 17
  - ◆ Positive family history in most cases
  - ◆ Multiple neurofibromas at different areas of the body
  - ◆ Café-au-lait spots (hyperpigmented skin lesions)
  - ◆ Lisch nodules (pigmented iris hamartomas)

Gross Pathology

- Well-defined fusiform lesion often in association with a nerve trunk
- Firm, gray-white cut surface
- Diffuse lesions show ill-defined, plaquelike thickening of the subcutaneous tissues
- Plexiform lesions are a multinodular conglomerate of lesions likened to a "bag of worms"

Histopathology

- Low to moderately cellular lesion composed of cells with wavy nuclei and eosinophilic cytoplasm interspersed with wisps of collagen
- Stroma may show small amounts of mucoid material or be myxoid and is occasionally hyalinized
- Tumor is well circumscribed but usually not encapsulated
- Mild nuclear atypia is common and does not mean malignant transformation
- May contain melanin pigment (pigmented neurofibroma) or show epithelioid morphology (epithelioid neurofibroma)
- Plexiform neurofibroma
  - — Almost exclusively associated with NF1
  - — Irregularly expanded nerve bundles giving a multinodular appearance
  - — Tend to be hypocellular with a prominent myxoid matrix
  - — Variable degrees of nuclear pleomorphism may be seen
  - — Infrequent mitotic activity
- Diffuse neurofibroma
  - — Neoplastic cells expand the dermal and subcutaneous tissues and envelop subcutaneous and adnexal structures

Special Stains and Immunohistochemistry

- S-100 protein positive

Other Techniques for Diagnosis

- Biallelic loss of *NF1* tumor suppressor gene on chromosome 17q11.2 may be demonstrated by molecular techniques

Differential Diagnosis

▌ Schwannoma
- Encapsulated by epineurium and composed almost exclusively of fascicles of Schwann cells

- Lacks the myxoid background, and hyalinized vessels are common
- Presence of both Antoni A and Antoni B areas
▮ Myxoma
  - May be intramuscular, cutaneous, or juxta-articular
  - Composed of spindled to stellate cells in a prominent myxoid background
  - Negative for S-100 protein
▮ Malignant peripheral nerve sheath tumor
  - Cellular tumor characterized by pleomorphic cells with wavy nuclei
  - Prominent mitotic activity
  - Areas of tumor necrosis
  - Less strongly positive for S-100 protein

Pearls

- Localized, sporadic neurofibroma is a benign lesion treated by conservative excision; malignant transformation is exceedingly rare
- Malignant transformation occurs in about 3% of neurofibromas associated with NF1, most commonly in deep-seated and plexiform lesions, and is characterized by increased cellularity, mitotic activity, and diffuse nuclear atypia

Selected References

De Luca A, Bernardini L, Ceccarini C, et al: Fluorescence in situ hybridization analysis of allelic losses involving the long arm of chromosome 17 in NF1-associated neurofibromas. Cancer Genet Cytogenet 150:168-172, 2004.

Fetsch JF, Michal M, Miettinen M: Pigmented (melanotic) neurofibroma: A clinicopathologic and immunohistochemical analysis of 19 lesions from 17 patients. Am J Surg Pathol 24:331-343, 2000.

Liapis H, Dehner LP, Gutmann DH: Neurofibroma and cellular neurofibroma with atypia: A report of 14 tumors. Am J Surg Pathol 23:1156-1158, 1999.

McCarron KF, Goldblum JR: Plexiform neurofibroma with and without associated malignant peripheral nerve sheath tumor: A clinicopathologic and immunohistochemical analysis of 54 cases. Mod Pathol 11:612-617, 1998.

Paraganglioma

Clinical Features

- Occurs in patients between 40 and 60 years of age
- Presents with different symptoms depending on location
  - Carotid body tumor
    ◆ Painless, slowly enlarging mass in the neck
  - Jugulotympanic paraganglioma
    ◆ Dizziness, tinnitus, cranial nerve palsy, and conductive hearing loss
  - Vagal paraganglioma
    ◆ Horner syndrome and vocal cord paralysis
  - Retroperitoneal paraganglioma
    ◆ Back pain and a palpable mass

Figure 17-35. Paraganglioma. Nests of polygonal tumor cells with nuclear atypia and eosinophilic cytoplasm create a Zellballen pattern.

Gross Pathology

- Lobular, red-brown, well-circumscribed masses
- May measure from a few centimeters up to 20 cm in diameter

Histopathology

- Trabecular or organoid arrangement of round to polygonal cells (Zellballen) with central nuclei and eosinophilic, faintly granular cytoplasm
- Variable nuclear hyperchromasia and pleomorphism
- Extensive delicate vascular network
- Infrequent mitotic activity
- Malignant paraganglioma
  - No reliable histologic criteria can predict malignancy
  - Aggressive behavior has been associated with tumor necrosis, vascular invasion, and increased mitotic activity
  - Metastatic spread is the only reliable criterion for malignancy

Special Stains and Immunohistochemistry

- NSE, chromogranin positive
- S-100 protein highlights sustentacular network surround tumor nests
- Cytokeratin typically negative

Other Techniques for Diagnosis

- Electron microscopy: cytoplasmic dense-core neurosecretory granules

Differential Diagnosis

▮ Carcinoid tumor
  - Sheets of small, uniform cells with central nuclei, stippled chromatin, and abundant finely granular cytoplasm
  - Immunoreactivity for cytokeratin

- Alveolar soft part sarcoma
  - Occurs in the deep soft tissue; usually thigh
  - Characterized by uniform, polygonal cells with eosinophilic, granular, cytoplasm, and central nuclei
  - Organoid growth pattern
  - Vascular invasion commonly seen

Pearls

- Paraganglioma usually follows a benign clinical course
- Overall incidence of malignant transformation is about 10%; no reliable histologic criteria can predict malignancy
- Definite familial incidence has been observed
- May be associated with von Hippel-Lindau disease and multiple endocrine neoplasia syndromes
- May be associated with Carney triad: paraganglioma, pulmonary chondroma, and gastric leiomyosarcoma

Selected References

Cascon A, Landa I, Lopez-Jimenez E, et al: Molecular characterization of a common SDHB deletion in paraganglioma patients. J Med Genet 45:233-238, 2008.

Plaza JA, Wakely PE Jr, Moran C, et al: Sclerosing paraganglioma: Report of 19 cases of an unusual variant of neuroendocrine tumor that may be mistaken for an aggressive malignant neoplasm. Am J Surg Pathol 30:7-12, 2006.

Elder EE, Xu D, Hoog A, et al: Ki-67 and hTERT expression can aid in the distinction between malignant and benign pheochromocytoma and paraganglioma. Mod Pathol 16:246-255, 2003.

Carney JA: Gastric stromal sarcoma, pulmonary chondroma, and extra-adrenal paraganglioma (Carney Triad): Natural history, adrenocortical component, and possible familial occurrence. Mayo Clin Proc 74:543-552, 1999.

Linnoila RI, Keiser HR, Steinberg SM, Lack EE: Histopathology of benign versus malignant sympathoadrenal paragangliomas: Clinicopathologic study of 120 cases including unusual histologic features. Hum Pathol 21:1168-1180, 1990.

Malignant Peripheral Nerve Sheath Tumor

Clinical Features

- Typically presents as an enlarging mass arising in association with a major nerve trunk, frequently on the proximal extremities
- About 3% to 10% of patients with NF1 develop a malignant peripheral nerve sheath tumor (MPNST)
- About 50% of cases are found in patients with NF1; often develops after 10 to 20 years
- Sporadic cases typically develop in adults, with a male-to-female ratio of 1:1
- Cases associated with neurofibromatosis occur at a younger age and show a 4:1 male-to-female ratio

Gross Pathology

- Arises as a fusiform, deep-seated mass, often within a major nerve

Figure 17-36. Malignant peripheral nerve sheath tumor. Fascicles of pleomorphic spindle cells with dense cellularity alternate with less cellular areas. Focal necrosis is present.

- Tumors are typically poorly defined and frequently infiltrate along adjacent nerve or into adjacent soft tissue
- Tan-white, fleshy cut surface with focal areas of hemorrhage and necrosis

Histopathology

- Cellular spindle cell tumor with fascicular growth pattern
- Alternating hypercellular and hypocellular zones often with areas of myxoid stroma
- Nuclear palisading and whorled nodules of spindle cells may be seen
- Perivascular tumor cell condensation and growth along nerve twigs is common
- Spindle cells show hyperchromatic wavy or buckled nuclei and show minimal to marked pleomorphism
- High mitotic activity and necrosis are common
- Benign or malignant heterologous elements such as bone, cartilage, and skeletal muscle may be seen
- Malignant triton tumor
  - Presence of rhabdomyoblastic differentiation
- MPNST
  - Tumor showing areas of conventional MPNST admixed with nests of round to polygonal epithelioid cells with round nuclei, prominent nucleoli, and clear to eosinophilic cytoplasm

Special Stains and Immunohistochemistry

- S-100 protein focally and weakly positive in most cases
- CD56 and CD57 variably positive
- Collagen IV positive around individual tumor cells

Other Techniques for Diagnosis

- Electron microscopy reveals interdigitating cell processes, complete or partial external lamina, cell junctions, and pinocytotic vesicles
- Cytogenetic studies show numerous structural and numeral abnormalities, none of which are diagnostic

Differential Diagnosis

- Cellular schwannoma
  - Hypercellular tumor composed almost entirely of Antoni A areas
  - Typically well circumscribed rather than infiltrative
  - Tumor cells are more uniform with less nuclear pleomorphism
  - Mitotic activity and necrosis are infrequent
  - Strong positivity for S-100 protein
- Leiomyosarcoma
  - Characterized by spindle cells with eosinophilic cytoplasm and atypical cigar-shaped nuclei arranged in short interlacing fascicles
  - Cellular pleomorphism is often pronounced, and mitotic figures are numerous
  - Immunoreactivity for SMA and desmin
- Fibrosarcoma
  - Highly cellular, infiltrative tumor composed of fibroblasts with hyperchromatic nuclei and scant cytoplasm arranged in an almost exclusive herringbone pattern
  - High mitotic rate; atypical mitotic figures may be seen
  - Negative for markers of neural differentiation
- Synovial sarcoma (monophasic)
  - Characterized by fascicles and whorls of spindle-shaped cells with a high nuclear-to-cytoplasmic ratio
  - Immunoreactivity for cytokeratin, EMA, CD99, and bcl-2
  - Presence of t(X;18)(p11;q11)
- Clear cell sarcoma (melanoma of soft parts)
  - Characterized by uniform cells with central round to oval nuclei, prominent basophilic nucleoli, and clear to eosinophilic cytoplasm with glycogen
  - Intracellular melanin (frequently inconspicuous)
  - Groups of cells separated by delicate fibrous septa; collagen IV stain surrounds groups rather than individual tumor cells
  - Immunoreactivity for S-100 protein, HMB-45, and melan-A
  - Presence of t(12;22)(q13;q12), producing an *EWS-ATF1* fusion

Pearls

- MPNSTs have a high likelihood of local recurrence and distant metastasis
- Metastases usually involve the lungs, liver, and bone; lymph node involvement is rare
- These tumors have a propensity to spread for considerable distances along the nerve sheath

Selected References

Anghileri M, Miceli R, Fiore M, et al: Malignant peripheral nerve sheath tumors: Prognostic factors and survival in a series of patients treated at a single institution. Cancer 107:1065-1074, 2006.

Stasik CJ, Tawfik O: Malignant peripheral nerve sheath tumor with rhabdomyosarcomatous differentiation (malignant triton tumor). Arch Pathol Lab Med 130:1878-1881, 2006.

Allison KH, Patel RM, Goldblum JR, Rubin BP: Superficial malignant peripheral nerve sheath tumor: a rare and challenging diagnosis. Am J Clin Pathol 124:685-692, 2005.

Zhou H, Coffin CM, Perkins SL, et al: Malignant peripheral nerve sheath tumor: A comparison of grade, immunophenotype, and cell cycle/growth activation marker expression in sporadic and neurofibromatosis 1-related lesions. Am J Surg Pathol 27:1337-1345, 2003.

Watanabe T, Oda Y, Tamiya S, et al: Malignant peripheral nerve sheath tumours: High Ki67 labelling index is the significant prognostic indicator. Histopathology 39:187-197, 2001.

Hemangioma

Clinical Features

- Capillary hemangioma (infantile and juvenile hemangioma)
  - Most common vascular tumor of infancy, usually presenting in the first few weeks of life
  - Commonly occurs in the head and neck; may involve the subcutaneous tissue or occasionally the viscera; diffuse soft tissue growth is termed *hemangiomatosis*
  - Typically presents as a crimson skin lesion that becomes raised over time (strawberry hemangioma)
  - Usually grows through first year of life and regresses over time
- Cavernous hemangioma
  - Commonly seen in children, with a predilection for skin of the head and neck (port-wine nevus)

Figure 17-37. Hemangioma. Tightly packed small vascular channels are lined by a flattened endothelium.

- Typically involves deeper tissue than capillary hemangiomas do
- May occur in abdominal viscera, notably liver and spleen
- Less likely to regress over time
- Occasionally associated with Maffucci syndrome (multiple enchondromas and vascular proliferations)

■ Epithelioid hemangioma
  - Also termed *angiolymphoid hyperplasia with eosinophilia*
  - Presents in head and neck as a pruritic red lesion; may be multifocal
  - Most common in third to fifth decades; slightly more common in men
  - May recur after excision

■ Pyogenic granuloma (lobular capillary hemangioma [LCH])
  - Essentially the same as a capillary hemangioma, although LCH does not usually present in infancy
  - Typically a polypoid growth in the skin or oral mucosa
  - Commonly associated with pregnancy or oral contraceptive use

■ Spindle cell hemangioma
  - Typically presents as a subcutaneous nodule on a distal extremity; may be multifocal
  - Most common in the second to third decades but can occur at any age

■ Intramuscular hemangioma
  - Presents as a slowly growing deep mass that may be painful
  - Lower extremities are most commonly affected, followed by head and neck, upper extremities, and trunk
  - Most common in adolescents and young adults
  - Has a tendency to recur if incompletely excised

Gross Pathology

- Hemangiomas may be dermal or deeply seated and well circumscribed or infiltrative
- Most have a spongy, dark-red cut surface

Histopathology

■ Capillary hemangioma
  - Lobular architecture with arborizing, small vascular channels lined by plump to flattened endothelial cells, separated by scant connective tissue stroma
  - Cellular lesions show inconspicuous capillary lumina; solid growth pattern and variable mitotic activity (*cellular hemangioma*)
  - Involutional changes include vascular ectasia and replacement by fat or fibrous tissue

■ Cavernous hemangioma
  - Typically found in subcutaneous tissue
  - Characterized by dilated, blood-filled, medium- to large-caliber vascular spaces, lined by flat endothelial cells

■ Epithelioid hemangioma
  - Well-circumscribed dermal lesion comprising small to medium-sized blood vessels
  - Vascular channels lined by plump endothelial cells with abundant eosinophilic cytoplasm and vesicular oval nuclei
  - Background typically shows a lymphocytic infiltrate, sometimes with germinal centers; variable numbers of interspersed mast cells, eosinophils, and plasma cells

■ Pyogenic granuloma
  - Well circumscribed with a lobular architecture
  - Characterized by small, arborizing vascular channels and bland endothelium

■ Spindle cell hemangioma
  - Poorly circumscribed lesion
  - Biphasic population of solid masses of spindle cells combined with cavernous vascular channels; may contain thrombi
  - Cells lining ectatic channels are attenuated, whereas spindle cells tend to be plump, often with cytoplasmic vacuoles

■ Intramuscular angioma
  - Capillary or cavernous channels admixed with mature skeletal muscle and a variable amount of fat

Special Stains and Immunohistochemistry

- Thrombomodulin, CD34, CD31, and Fli-1 highlight endothelial cells
- GLUT1 positive in capillary hemangioma of juvenile type only

Other Techniques for Diagnosis

- Noncontributory

Differential Diagnosis

■ Hemangiopericytoma
  - Almost always seen in adult population
  - Typically occurs in deep soft tissue of legs, pelvis, or retroperitoneum
  - Cellular blunt spindle cell tumor characterized by staghorn blood vessels
  - Perivascular and intervascular proliferation of uniform pericytic cells

■ Angiosarcoma
  - Angiosarcomas are extraordinarily rare in children
  - Typically found in skin or viscera; rare in deep soft tissue
  - Characterized by irregular anastomosing vascular channels lined by atypical endothelial cells
  - Mitotic activity are usually present
  - Hemorrhage and necrosis are common

■ Kaposi sarcoma
  - Fascicles of uniform spindle cells forming slitlike vascular spaces
  - Extravasated red blood cells common

- PAS-positive hyaline globules (intracellular and extracellular)
- Most common in AIDS patients and elderly patients of Mediterranean descent
- Immunoreactive for HHV-8 and LNA-1 in 80% to 85% of cases

Pearls

- Von Hippel-Lindau disease is characterized by cerebellar hemangioblastomas, widespread visceral angiomatous lesions, and renal cell carcinoma
- Sturge-Weber syndrome is characterized by venous angiomatous lesions in the leptomeninges and ipsilateral port-wine nevi of the face
- Strawberry hemangiomas tend to resolve spontaneously without treatment
- Epithelioid hemangiomas and intramuscular angiomas are more likely to recur following excision

Selected References

Goh SG, Calonje E: Cutaneous vascular tumours: An update. Histopathology 52:661-673, 2008.

Dadras SS, North PE, Bertoncini J, et al: Infantile hemangiomas are arrested in an early developmental vascular differentiation state. Mod Pathol 17:1068-1079, 2004.

Brenn T, Fletcher CD: Cutaneous epithelioid angiomatous nodule: A distinct lesion in the morphologic spectrum of epithelioid vascular tumors. Am J Dermatopathol 26:14-21, 2004.

North PE, Waner M, Mizeracki A, Mihm MC Jr: GLUT1: A newly discovered immunohistochemical marker for juvenile hemangiomas. Hum Pathol 31:11-22, 2000.

Calonje E, Fletcher CD: Sinusoidal hemangioma: A distinctive benign vascular neoplasm within the group of cavernous hemangiomas. Am J Surg Pathol 15:1130-1135, 1991.

Glomus Tumor

Clinical Features

- Tumor differentiates toward modified smooth muscle of the glomus body
- Typically seen in young adults
- Usually involves distal extremities, especially fingers and toes; deep or visceral tumors are rare
- Red and blue subcutaneous nodule that is painful; may be multifocal

Gross Pathology

- Typically smaller than 1 cm; well-circumscribed dermal or subcutaneous nodule

Histopathology

- Sheets or nests of uniform, round cells with oval nuclei and pale eosinophilic cytoplasm
- Groups of glomus cells may surround dilated vessels (*glomangioma*)
- Minimal mitotic activity
- May show focal degenerative nuclear atypia

Figure 17-38. Glomus tumor. Nodular proliferation of uniform round cells with central nuclei and pale cytoplasm.

Special Stains and Immunohistochemistry

- SMA and h-caldesmon positive
- CD34 variably positive
- CD31 and thrombomodulin negative in tumor cells

Other Techniques for Diagnosis

- Noncontributory

Differential Diagnosis

- ▋ Cellular or cavernous hemangioma
  - Cellular hemangioma is characterized by small, arborizing vascular channels lined by flat endothelial cells
  - No glomus cells
  - Focal cavernous hemangioma-like areas may be present in glomangioma
  - Positive for thrombomodulin, CD31, and CD34; negative for SMA
- ▋ Paraganglioma
  - Trabecular or organoid arrangement of round to polygonal cells with oval nuclei and eosinophilic, granular cytoplasm
  - Extensive and delicate capillary network, dividing tumor into compartments (Zellballen)
  - Positive for neuroendocrine markers (synaptophysin, chromogranin, and NSE); negative for keratin and SMA

Pearls

- Glomus tumor is benign and typically treated by excision; about 5% to 10% recur
- Malignant glomus tumors (glomangiosarcoma) are exceedingly rare; they are typically large, in deep or visceral locations, with infiltrative growth, nuclear atypia, and brisk mitotic activity

Selected References

Mentzel T, Dei Tos AP, Sapi Z, Kutzner H: Myopericytoma of skin and soft tissues: Clinicopathologic and immunohistochemical study of 54 cases. Am J Surg Pathol 30:104-113, 2006.

Miettinen M, Paal E, Lasota J, Sobin LH: Gastrointestinal glomus tumors: A clinicopathologic, immunohistochemical, and molecular genetic study of 32 cases. Am J Surg Pathol 26:301-311, 2002.

Folpe AL, Fanburg-Smith JC, Miettinen M, Weiss SW: Atypical and malignant glomus tumors: Analysis of 52 cases, with a proposal for the reclassification of glomus tumors. Am J Surg Pathol 25:1-12, 2001.

Tsuneyoshi M, Enjoji M: Glomus tumor: A clinicopathologic and electron microscopic study. Cancer 50:1601-1607, 1982.

Hemangiopericytoma and Myopericytoma

Clinical Features

▌ Hemangiopericytoma
- Has at least borderline malignant potential; shows differentiation toward modified pericytes
- Occurs in adults; usually deep, most frequently in legs, pelvis, or retroperitoneum
- Often large on clinical detection
- Hypoglycemia may be associated with tumors of the pelvis or retroperitoneum (Doege-Potter syndrome)

▌ Myopericytoma
- Same as hemangiopericytoma, except that lesion is subcutaneous, usually on distal extremities

Gross Pathology

- Solitary, well-circumscribed, often lobulated mass with gray-white to red-brown cut surface
- Focal hemorrhage or cystic degeneration may be seen

Figure 17-39. Hemangiopericytoma. Bland ovoid tumor cells with indistinct cytoplasmic borders are arranged around a ramifying vascular network.

Histopathology

▌ Hemangiopericytoma
- Thin-walled staghorn vascular channels lined by a single layer of flat endothelium, surrounded by perivascular and intervascular proliferation of uniform-appearing oval to spindle-shaped pericytes showing ill-defined cytoplasmic borders
- Reticulin-rich network surrounding individual pericytes
- Focal hyalinization and myxoid change may be present
- Mitotic rate typically less than 4 mitotic figures/10 hpf
- May have variable admixed adipose tissue "lipomatous hemangiopericytoma"
- Criteria characterizing "malignant" hemangiopericytomas are not clearly defined, but aggressive behavior associated with brisk mitotic activity, nuclear atypia, necrosis, and hemorrhage; *all* hemangiopericytomas have at least borderline malignant potential

▌ Myopericytoma
- Same as hemangiopericytoma, except with plump, spindled to round myoid cells that surround vessels with a hemangiopericytoid pattern

Special Stains and Immunohistochemistry

- CD34: equivocal positivity
- SMA positive in myopericytoma but negative in conventional hemangiopericytoma

Other Techniques for Diagnosis

- Electron microscopy: pericytes contain rough endoplasmic reticulum, mitochondria, free polyribosomes, and thin filaments
- Cytogenetic studies: hemangiopericytoma may be associated with structural aberrations involving the long arm of chromosome 12

Differential Diagnosis

▌ Solitary fibrous tumor
- Semantic difference; the World Health Organization has combined hemangiopericytoma and solitary fibrous tumor into one entity
- Patternless architecture of spindle cells in a variably hyalinized stroma; hemangiopericytoid vasculature is common
- Often pleural but can occur in any location
- Positive for CD34, CD99, and bcl-2

▌ Fibrous histiocytoma with hemangiopericytoma-like areas
- Spindle cells and histiocytoid cells arranged in a storiform pattern
- Often shows admixed inflammatory cells
- "Dissection" of collagen by tumor cells at lesion periphery

▍Glomangioma
  ● Dilated vessels surrounded by sheets of round cells with central nuclei and pale eosinophilic cytoplasm
  ● Positive for SMA
▍Synovial sarcoma (monophasic)
  ● Composed of hyperchromatic blunt spindle cells with a hemangiopericytoma-like growth pattern
  ● Immunoreactivity for cytokeratin or EMA; positivity for CD99 and bcl-2, but not CD34
  ● Presence of t(X;18)(p11;q11)

Pearls

  ● Hemangiopericytoma is a diagnosis of exclusion because the hemangiopericytoma-like pattern may be seen in a variety of other tumors
  ● Long-term survival following surgical resection is typical; metastases may appear 10 to 20 years later and usually involve lung or bone
  ● Natural history is difficult to predict; occasional tumors with aggressive morphologic characteristics may have more rapid evolution
  ● Tumor recurrence often precedes the appearance of distant metastases

Selected References

Gengler C, Guillou L: Solitary fibrous tumour and haemangiopericytoma: Evolution of a concept. Histopathology 48:63-74, 2006.

Thompson LD, Miettinen M, Wenig BM: Sinonasal-type hemangiopericytoma: A clinicopathologic and immunophenotypic analysis of 104 cases showing perivascular myoid differentiation. Am J Surg Pathol 27:737-749, 2003.

Espat NJ, Lewis JJ, Leung D, et al: Conventional hemangiopericytoma: Modern analysis of outcome. Cancer 95:1746-1751, 2002.

Ferrari A, Casanova M, Bisogno G, et al: Hemangiopericytoma in pediatric ages: A report from the Italian and German Soft Tissue Sarcoma Cooperative Group. Cancer 92:2692-2698, 2001.

Guillou L, Gebhard S, Coindre JM: Lipomatous hemangiopericytoma: A fat-containing variant of solitary fibrous tumor? Clinicopathologic, immunohistochemical, and ultrastructural analysis of a series in favor of a unifying concept. Hum Pathol 31:1108-1115, 2000.

Hemangioendothelioma

Clinical Features

  ● Considered to be a low-grade variant of endothelial malignancy; may be seen in several anatomic locations
▍Epithelioid hemangioendothelioma
  ● Occurs in any age group but is rare in children
  ● Usually involves dermal or subcutaneous tissues of extremities; rarely multicentric; bone or visceral involvement is possible

Figure 17-40. Epithelioid hemangioendothelioma. Nests of epithelioid cells with cytoplasmic vacuoles are embedded in a fibromyxoid stroma.

  ● Often surrounds a preexisting blood vessel, most commonly a vein, and may be associated with edema or thrombophlebitis
▍Kaposiform hemangioendothelioma
  ● Occurs principally in children, often in first year of life
  ● Most common locations are superficial and deep soft tissues of extremities or retroperitoneum
  ● Often associated with consumptive coagulopathy and thrombocytopenia (Kasabach-Merritt syndrome), especially with deep lesions
▍Retiform hemangioendothelioma and papillary intralymphatic angioendothelioma (Dabska tumor)
  ● Seen at all ages; retiform hemangioendothelioma is more common in adults, and Dabska tumor is more common in children
  ● The limbs are the most commonly affected

Gross Pathology

  ● Violaceous plaques or subcutaneous nodules; often multinodular
  ● Infiltrative borders and gray to white variegated cut surfaces
  ● Epithelioid hemangioendotheliomas associated with large vessels may resemble organizing thrombi

Histopathology

▍Epithelioid hemangioendothelioma
  ● Cords and nests of polygonal endothelial cells with eosinophilic cytoplasm and oval nuclei
  ● Intracellular cytoplasmic lumens with intraluminal red blood cells
  ● Intramural growth into preexisting vessels with perivascular extension of tumor
  ● Tumor cells typically have bland, round to oval nuclei but may show some pleomorphism

- Background stroma is myxoid or hyalinized
- Typically low mitotic rate

▮ Kaposiform hemangioendothelioma
  - Tumor nodules separated by fibrous septa; nodules may resemble capillary hemangioma or have the spindle cell morphology of Kaposi sarcoma
  - Glomeruloid structures, consisting of small nodules of tumor cells, are characteristic
  - Extravasated red blood cells, intratumoral hemorrhage, and hemosiderin are common

▮ Retiform hemangioendothelioma and papillary intralymphatic angioendothelioma (Dabska tumor)
  - Both tumors are characterized by plump cells lining lymphatic-like vascular channels, with or without intraluminal papillary projections
  - Retiform hemangioendothelioma shows narrow, arborizing vascular spaces lined by the plump endothelium and separated by sclerotic stroma, often containing a lymphocytic infiltrate
  - Dabska tumor contains intraluminal tufts of plump endothelium and resembles deep lymphangioma; characteristic deposits of basement membrane are seen in cellular tufts

Special Stains and Immunohistochemistry

- Factor VIIIa, CD31, CD34, thrombomodulin, podoplanin, and Fli-1 positive
- GLUT1 negative
- Keratin may be focally positive in epithelioid hemangioendothelioma
- Reticulin highlights constituent vessels

Other Techniques for Diagnosis

- Recurrent t(1;3)(p36;q25) has been reported in epithelioid hemangioendothelioma

Differential Diagnosis

▮ Epithelioid sarcoma
  - Usually occurs in the distal extremities of adolescents and young adults
  - Coalescing nodules of polygonal cells with central areas of necrosis
  - Positive for cytokeratin and EMA; negative for endothelial markers except for CD34

▮ Epithelioid angiosarcoma
  - Solid growth with sievelike vascular channels rather than the architectural patterns of hemangioendothelioma
  - Greater nuclear atypia, mitotic activity, and necrosis than are seen in epithelioid hemangioendothelioma

▮ Kaposiform hemangioendothelioma and Kaposi sarcoma
  - Kaposi sarcoma
    — Extraordinarily rare in children; typically associated with immunosuppression
    — Lacks areas reminiscent of cellular hemangioma
    — Positive for HHV-8 and LNA-1, unlike hemangioendotheliomas

Pearls

- Hemangioendotheliomas have borderline biologic behavior with the ability to recur but rare metastasis; epithelioid hemangioendotheliomas are the most aggressive of the group, metastasizing in up to 33% of cases
- Surgical excision is standard treatment; medical therapy may be indicated for unresectable lesions or to treat consumptive coagulopathy

Selected References

Fukunaga M, Suzuki K, Saegusa N, Folpe AL: Composite hemangioendothelioma: Report of 5 cases including one with associated Maffucci syndrome. Am J Surg Pathol 31:1567-1572, 2007.

Debelenko LV, Perez-Atayde AR, Mulliken JB, et al: D2-40 immunohistochemical analysis of pediatric vascular tumors reveals positivity in kaposiform hemangioendothelioma. Mod Pathol 18:1454-1460, 2005.

Lyons LL, North PE, Mac-Moune Lai F, et al: Kaposiform hemangioendothelioma: A study of 33 cases emphasizing its pathologic, immunophenotypic, and biologic uniqueness from juvenile hemangioma. Am J Surg Pathol 28:559-568, 2004.

Fanburg-Smith JC, Michal M, Partanen TA, et al: Papillary intralymphatic angioendothelioma (PILA): A report of twelve cases of a distinctive vascular tumor with phenotypic features of lymphatic vessels. Am J Surg Pathol 23:1004-1010, 1999.

Calonje E, Fletcher CD, Wilson-Jones E, Rosai J: Retiform hemangioendothelioma: A distinctive form of low-grade angiosarcoma delineated in a series of 15 cases. Am J Surg Pathol 18:115-125, 1994.

Zukerberg LR, Nickoloff BJ, Weiss SW: Kaposiform hemangioendothelioma of infancy and childhood: An aggressive neoplasm associated with Kasabach-Merritt syndrome and lymphangiomatosis. Am J Surg Pathol 17:321-328, 1993.

Dabska M: Malignant endovascular papillary angioendothelioma of the skin in childhood: Clinicopathologic study of 6 cases. Cancer 24:503-510, 1969.

Angiosarcoma

Clinical Features

- Rare tumor comprising less than 1% of sarcomas; usually seen in adults
- Predilection for skin and superficial soft tissue, breast, bone, liver, and spleen; rare in deep soft tissue
- May be associated with chronic lymphedema (typically postmastectomy), previous therapeutic radiation, or arteriovenous fistulas in renal transplant recipients
- Angiosarcomas of liver are associated with prior exposure to polyvinyl chloride and thorium dioxide (Thorotrast)

Gross Pathology

- Cutaneous angiosarcomas present as an ill-defined, bruiselike lesion or ulcerated hemorrhagic nodules, or plaques simulating erysipelas

Figure 17-41. Angiosarcoma. Hyperchromatic, pleomorphic tumor cells form primitive vascular channels containing red blood cells.

- Commonly large hemorrhagic, ill-defined masses with spongy quality and blood-filled spaces

Histopathology

- Primarily constituted by epithelioid or fusiform cells with rudimentary vascular differentiation; pleomorphism, mitoses, and widespread tissue infiltration are common
- Tumor cells in vascular spaces may be attenuated or plump with hyperchromatic nuclei
- Spindle cell areas may resemble fibrosarcoma or other spindle cell tumors

Special Stains and Immunohistochemistry

- Thrombomodulin, CD31, CD34, and Fli-1 positive
- Cytokeratin may be positive in epithelioid variant of angiosarcoma

Other Techniques for Diagnosis

- Electron microscopy may demonstrate cytoplasmic Weibel-Palade bodies in roughly 25% of cases

Differential Diagnosis

▌ Hemangioma
- Complete tubular vascular channels lined by uniform, flattened endothelial cells
- Lacks pleomorphism, mitotic activity, necrosis, and irregular tissue infiltration

▌ Papillary endothelial hyperplasia (intravascular hemangioendothelioma of Masson)
- An unusual variant of organizing thrombus characterized by numerous intravascular anastomosing pseudopapillae lined by endothelial cells
- Lacks nuclear pleomorphism and mitotic activity; no extravascular component

▌ Epithelioid hemangioendothelioma
- Polygonal epithelioid endothelial cells in cords and clusters, eosinophilic cytoplasm and oval, bland nuclei
- Little if any nuclear pleomorphism and limited mitotic activity; cytoplasmic vacuoles

Pearls

- Angiosarcomas are treated with radical surgery and radiation therapy
- Clinical course is characterized by frequent recurrence and distant metastasis, most commonly to lungs, lymph nodes, and bone
- Prognosis is related to size, multifocality, and ability to achieve a complete excision

Selected References

Deyrup AT, McKenney JK, Tighiouart M, et al: Sporadic cutaneous angiosarcomas: A proposal for risk stratification based on 69 cases. Am J Surg Pathol 32:72-77, 2008.

Al-Abbadi MA, Almasri NM, Al-Quran S, Wilkinson EJ: Cytokeratin and epithelial membrane antigen expression in angiosarcomas: An immunohistochemical study of 33 cases. Arch Pathol Lab Med 131:288-292, 2007.

Sher T, Hennessy BT, Valero V, et al: Primary angiosarcomas of the breast. Cancer 110:173-178, 2007.

Bocklage T, Leslie K, Yousem S, Colby T: Extracutaneous angiosarcomas metastatic to the lungs: Clinical and pathologic features of twenty-one cases. Mod Pathol 14:1216-1225, 2001.

Meis-Kindblom JM, Kindblom LG: Angiosarcoma of soft tissue: A study of 80 cases. Am J Surg Pathol 22:683-697, 1998.

Wehrli BM, Janzen DL, Shokeir O, et al: Epithelioid angiosarcoma arising in a surgically constructed arteriovenous fistula: a rare complication of chronic immunosuppression in the setting of renal transplantation. Am J Surg Pathol 22:1154-1159, 1998.

Lymphangioma

Clinical Features

- Rare tumors typically occurring as congenital tumors; most present before the age of 2 years
- Typically present as a poorly defined soft tissue or cutaneous mass in the head and neck or axillary region
- Abdominal or visceral involvement may be found
- Subcategorized into the following types
  — Cystic lymphangioma (cystic hygromas)
     ◆ Superficially located
     ◆ Commonly involves the neck region
  — Cavernous lymphangioma
     ◆ Commonly involves skeletal muscle or deeper soft tissue

Gross Pathology

- Commonly appears as a soft, cystic, gray-white tumor

Figure 17-42. Lymphangioma. Dilated lymphatic channels are separated by inflamed fibrous stroma.

- Cystic lymphangiomas are typically well circumscribed, whereas cavernous lymphangiomas have infiltrative margins

Histopathology
- Characterized by anastomosing, thin-walled, irregular lymphatic channels lined by flat endothelial cells
- Proteinaceous intraluminal fluid containing lymphocytes and red blood cells
- Stromal fibrosis and chronic inflammatory infiltrate are common; lymphoid aggregates are often seen
- Cavernous lymphangiomas have infiltrative margins and often extend into adjacent adipose tissue

Special Stains and Immunohistochemistry
- Noncontributory

Other Techniques for Diagnosis
- Noncontributory

Differential Diagnosis
▊ Hemangioma
- Arborizing, small vascular channels lined by flattened endothelial cells

Pearls
- Lymphangiomas are treated by surgical excision
- Overall excellent prognosis; may rarely recur

Selected References

Fukunaga M: Expression of D2-40 in lymphatic endothelium of normal tissues and in vascular tumours. Histopathology 46:396-402, 2005.

Galambos C, Nodit L: Identification of lymphatic endothelium in pediatric vascular tumors and malformations. Pediatr Dev Pathol 8:181-189, 2005.

Hornick JL, Fletcher CD: Intraabdominal cystic lymphangiomas obscured by marked superimposed reactive changes: Clinicopathological analysis of a series. Hum Pathol 36:426-432, 2005.

Guillou L, Fletcher CD: Benign lymphangioendothelioma (acquired progressive lymphangioma): A lesion not to be confused with well-differentiated angiosarcoma and patch stage Kaposi's sarcoma. Clinicopathologic analysis of a series. Am J Surg Pathol 24:1047-1057, 2000.

Gomez CS, Calonje E, Ferrar DW, et al: Lymphangiomatosis of the limbs: Clinicopathologic analysis of a series with a good prognosis. Am J Surg Pathol 19:125-133, 1995.

Myxoma

Clinical Features
- Usually well-defined, deep mass; may be intramuscular, cutaneous, or juxta-articular
- Intramuscular tumors are common in older patients and are found within the large muscles of the body
- Juxta-articular tumors typically occur around the knee or other large joints
- May be associated with Carney complex
  — Autosomal dominant
  — Characterized by myxomas, skin pigmentation, and endocrine hyperactivity

Gross Pathology
- Round to ovoid tumors with a gray-white, gelatinous cut surface

Histopathology
- Hypocellular tumor with well-circumscribed margins; often with a pseudocapsule at the interface of tumor and surrounding soft tissue

Figure 17-43. Myxoma. Paucicellular lesion shows bland spindle cells in abundant myxoid stroma.

- Few stellate or bipolar cells with oval nuclei (spider cells)
- Abundant loose, paucicellular, myxoid stroma

Special Stains and Immunohistochemistry

- Vimentin positive

Other Techniques for Diagnosis

- Noncontributory

Differential Diagnosis

▌ Nerve sheath myxoma
- Characterized by parallel layers of spindle cells with wavy nuclei at the periphery

▌ Myxoid neurofibroma
- Wavy, spindle nuclei; often areas show a collagenized stroma
- Positive for S-100 protein

▌ Aggressive angiomyxoma
- Most common in the vulvar region in women of reproductive age but may be seen in the perineum of males; intramuscular location is unusual
- Prominent thick- and thin-walled vessels
- Matrix is often collagenized
- Usually positive for SMA and desmin

Pearls

- Myxomas are benign tumors with rare local recurrence; surgical excision is the preferred treatment and is usually curative

Selected References

Okamoto S, Hisaoka M, Meis-Kindblom JM, et al: Juxta-articular myxoma and intramuscular myxoma are two distinct entities: Activating Gs alpha mutation at Arg 201 codon does not occur in juxta-articular myxoma. Virchows Arch 440:12-15, 2002.

van Roggen JF, McMenamin ME, Fletcher CD: Cellular myxoma of soft tissue: A clinicopathological study of 38 cases confirming indolent clinical behaviour. Histopathology 39:287-297, 2001.

Nielsen GP, O'Connell JX, Rosenberg AE: Intramuscular myxoma: A clinicopathologic study of 51 cases with emphasis on hypercellular and hypervascular variants. Am J Surg Pathol 22:1222-1227, 1998.

Ossifying Fibromyxoid Tumor

Clinical Features

- Occurs primarily in adults; slight male predominance
- Painless, well-defined mass in the upper and lower extremities; may also occur in the head and neck
- Typically affects the deep subcutis

Gross Pathology

- Well-circumscribed, lobulated, subcutaneous mass
- May be partially surrounded by a shell of bony tissue

Figure 17-44. Ossifying fibromyxoid tumor. Bland ovoid cells are randomly arranged in a fibromyxoid stroma. Focal calcification is present.

Histopathology

- Variably cellular tumor with uniform, round to polygonal cells arranged in nests or cords
- Cells have uniform, bland, round to oval nuclei with eosinophilic to clear cytoplasm and ill-defined cytoplasmic borders
- Abundant myxoid to hyaline matrix
- Metaplastic bone formation is common and is typically seen at the periphery

Special Stains and Immunohistochemistry

- Vimentin and S-100 protein positive

Other Techniques for Diagnosis

- Noncontributory

Differential Diagnosis

▌ Myxoid chondrosarcoma (extraskeletal)
- Anastomosing cords of round to oval, atypical chondrocytes
- Abundant myxoid matrix
- Intervening fibrous septa

Pearls

- Surgical excision is the preferred treatment for ossifying fibromyxoid tumor
- Local recurrence is seen in about 25% of patients; metastases are exceedingly rare

Selected References

Folpe AL, Weiss SW: Ossifying fibromyxoid tumor of soft parts: A clinicopathologic study of 70 cases with emphasis on atypical and malignant variants. Am J Surg Pathol 27:421-431, 2003.

Holck S, Pedersen JG, Ackermann T, Daugaard S: Ossifying fibromyxoid tumour of soft parts, with focus on unusual clinicopathological features. Histopathology 42:599-604, 2003.

Miettinen M: Ossifying fibromyxoid tumor of soft parts: Additional observations of a distinctive soft tissue tumor. Am J Clin Pathol 95:142-149, 1991.

Guarner J, Dominguez-Malagon HR, Meneses-Garcia A: Ossifying fibromyxoid tumor. Am J Surg Pathol 14:1167-1170, 1990.

Enzinger FM, Weiss SW, Liang CY: Ossifying fibromyxoid tumor of soft parts: A clinicopathological analysis of 59 cases. Am J Surg Pathol 13:817-827, 1989.

Angiomatoid Fibrous Histiocytoma

Clinical Features

- Typically seen in children and young adults but can occur at any age
- The extremities, head and neck, and trunk are common locations; often occur in locations of normal lymph nodes

Gross Pathology

- Well-circumscribed, lobulated, multicystic mass; usually about 5 cm in size
- Cystic spaces are often filled with hemorrhagic fluid

Histopathology

- Low-power appearance shows multinodular proliferation, often with central cystic spaces with a prominent lymphoid cuff
- Cells are spindle or ovoid and often surround pseudoangiomatoid spaces
- Cells are usually cytologically bland, but nuclear atypia and mitotic activity may be seen
- A prominent fibrous pseudocapsule contains a prominent lymphoplasmacytic infiltrate

Figure 17-45. Angiomatoid fibrous histiocytoma. Nodule of bland spindle cells with myxoid change surrounded by a fibrous pseudocapsule with a dense lymphocytic infiltrate.

Special Stains and Immunohistochemistry

- Desmin and CD68 are usually positive
- EMA and CD99 may be positive

Other Techniques for Diagnosis

- Presence of t(2;22)(q34;q12), producing an *EWSR1-CREB1* fusion; t(12;22)(q13;q12), producing an *EWSR1-ATF1* fusion, or t(12;16)(q13;p11), producing an *FUS-ATF1* fusion, can be demonstrated in most cases by cytogenetic or molecular techniques

Differential Diagnosis

- Benign fibrous histiocytoma
  - Lacks the inflammatory fibrous pseudocapsule and pseudoangiomatoid spaces
  - Well-circumscribed nodular lesion with storiform architecture

Pearls

- Angiomatoid fibrous histiocytoma is a low-grade lesion that occasionally recurs; metastases are exceedingly rare
- Surgical excision is standard therapy

Selected References

Thway K: Angiomatoid fibrous histiocytoma: A review with recent genetic findings. Arch Pathol Lab Med 132:273-277, 2008.

Rossi S, Szuhai K, Ijszenga M, et al: EWSR1-CREB1 and EWSR1-ATF1 fusion genes in angiomatoid fibrous histiocytoma. Clin Cancer Res 13:7322-7328, 2007.

Hasegawa T, Seki K, Ono K, Hirohashi S: Angiomatoid (malignant) fibrous histiocytoma: A peculiar low-grade tumor showing immunophenotypic heterogeneity and ultrastructural variations. Pathol Int 50:731-738, 2000.

Fanburg-Smith JC, Miettinen M: Angiomatoid "malignant" fibrous histiocytoma: A clinicopathologic study of 158 cases and further exploration of the myoid phenotype. Hum Pathol 30:1336-1343, 1999.

Fletcher CD: Angiomatoid "malignant fibrous histiocytoma": An immunohistochemical study indicative of myoid differentiation. Hum Pathol 22:563-568, 1991.

Costa MJ, Weiss SW: Angiomatoid malignant fibrous histiocytoma: A follow-up study of 108 cases with evaluation of possible histologic predictors of outcome. Am J Surg Pathol 14:1126-1132, 1990.

Synovial Sarcoma

Clinical Features

- Typically found in adolescents or young adults but can occur at any age
- Presents as a deep-seated, often painful mass; has often been present for years
- Usually arises near the joint in close relation to tendons and bursa but not in the joint space itself; lower extremities are commonly affected

Figure 17-46. Biphasic synovial sarcoma. Glandular structures are seen interspersed with spindle cells.

Figure 17-47. Monophasic synovial sarcoma. Fascicles of uniform spindle cells exhibit a herringbone growth pattern.

- Synovial sarcoma has been described in virtually every location, including viscera

Gross Pathology

- Typically a well-circumscribed mass with a gray-white or variegated cut surface; rapidly growing tumors tend to be more infiltrative
- Variably sized cyst formation may be seen
- Attachment to surrounding tendons or walls of joint capsules may be present

Histopathology

▌ Biphasic synovial sarcoma
- Characterized by fascicles of spindle cells admixed with groups of epithelial cells that form clefts, cysts, cords, nests, tubules, or papillae

- Epithelial cells are cuboidal to columnar with ovoid nuclei and a moderate amount of cytoplasm
- Eosinophilic or mucinous secretions are common in overtly epithelial cell groups; squamous metaplasia can occur
- Spindle cell component shows herringbone-like or hemangiopericytoma-like growth
- Calcification is seen in about 25% of cases; myxoid, chondroid, or osseous foci are less common
- Mast cells are common

▌ Monophasic synovial sarcoma
- Spindle cell form predominates over purely epithelial synovial sarcoma
- Fascicles of spindle cells, often with herringbone or hemangiopericytoid growth pattern; epithelial component is inconspicuous
- At low power, a biphasic pattern of alternating loose and dense areas is seen
- Calcification, myxoid change, hyalinization, and mast cell infiltration may be present
- Mitotic figures can be identified but usually are not numerous

▌ Poorly differentiated synovial sarcoma
- Small cell tumor composed of hyperchromatic round to spindled cells with high nuclear-to-cytoplasmic ratios; hemangiopericytoma-like growth is common
- Mitotic figures are readily identified and necrosis is common
- Rhabdoid differentiation may be present

Special Stains and Immunohistochemistry

- Cytokeratin, EMA, E-cadherin: epithelial component is positive, and mesenchymal-like component often shows focal positivity for at least one of these markers
- CD99: membranous staining in either or both components
- CD56, CD57, and bcl-2: cytoplasmic staining in either or both components
- SYT: nuclear staining
- S-100 protein: focal nuclear staining in 33% of cases
- CD34, Fli-1, and CD117 negative

Other Techniques for Diagnosis

- Presence of t(X;18)(p11;q11) can be demonstrated in greater than 90% of synovial sarcomas by cytogenetic or molecular techniques; fusion genes are *SYT-SSX1/SSX2* or *SSX4*

Differential Diagnosis

▌ Hemangiopericytoma
- Characterized by numerous thin-walled and branching staghorn vessels of variable caliber lined by a single layer of flattened endothelium; this vascular pattern is present throughout the entire tumor

- Reticulin network surrounding individual tumor cells
- Lacks epithelial differentiation by immunohistochemistry and is positive for CD34 in 70% to 80% of cases
- Absence of t(X:18)
- Rare lesion; diagnosis is one of ultimate exclusion

▌ EWS and PNET
- May be difficult to distinguish from poorly differentiated synovial sarcoma, especially in a small biopsy
- Monomorphic round cell tumor with high nuclear-to-cytoplasmic ratios and fine chromatin; cellular rosettes may be present
- Spindle cell change may occur but is usually focal
- Like synovial sarcoma, PNET is positive for CD99 and may express epithelial antigens, especially low-molecular-weight keratins
- Usually negative for CD56 and bcl-2; positive for Fli-1
- Presence of t(11;22)(q24;q12) can be demonstrated by cytogenetic or molecular techniques and is diagnostic

▌ Fibrosarcoma
- Most often affects children younger than 1 year; occasionally seen in adults
- Typically found in the extremities
- Variably cellular, infiltrative tumor composed of fusiform cells with hyperchromatic nuclei and eosinophilic or amphophilic cytoplasm, arranged in a herringbone pattern
- Variable mitotic rate; atypical mitotic figures may be seen
- Lacks a biphasic growth pattern
- Negative for epithelial antigens, CD99, and t(X;18)

▌ MPNST
- Characterized by fascicles of elongated cells with serpiginous nuclei; nuclear palisading or cellular tactoids may be present
- Typically shows at least some nuclear pleomorphism and high mitotic activity
- Often associated with a major nerve or neurofibromatosis
- Immunophenotype may overlap with that of synovial sarcoma; both may show focal S-100 protein positivity; MPNST may show focal epithelial differentiation but lacks CD99 and SYT

▌ Solitary fibrous tumor
- Frequently pleural but has been reported in soft tissue sites as well
- Well-circumscribed, often exophytic mass with gray-white firm cut surface
- Short fascicles or "patternless pattern" of spindle cells in variably collagenized stroma, often with hemangiopericytoma-like vasculature
- Positive for CD34, bcl-2, and CD99 in 85% to 90% of cases; lacks epithelial immunoreactivity

Pearls
- Synovial sarcoma is an aggressive tumor that is frequently complicated by distant metastasis to the lungs and lymph nodes; this may become manifest late in the course of disease
- Favorable prognostic characteristics include age younger than 25 years, tumor size less than 5 cm, low mitotic rate, and heavy calcification

Selected References

Hartel PH, Fanburg-Smith JC, Frazier AA, et al: Primary pulmonary and mediastinal synovial sarcoma: A clinicopathologic study of 60 cases and comparison with five prior series. Mod Pathol 20:760-769, 2007.

He R, Patel RM, Alkan S, et al: Immunostaining for SYT protein discriminates synovial sarcoma from other soft tissue tumors: Analysis of 146 cases. Mod Pathol 20:522-528, 2007.

Kanemitsu S, Hisaoka M, Shimajiri S, et al: Molecular detection of SS18-SSX fusion gene transcripts by cRNA in situ hybridization in synovial sarcoma using formalin-fixed, paraffin-embedded tumor tissue specimens. Diagn Mol Pathol 16:9-17, 2007.

Ferrari A, Gronchi A, Casanova M, et al: Synovial sarcoma: A retrospective analysis of 271 patients of all ages treated at a single institution. Cancer 101:627-634, 2004.

Chan JA, McMenamin ME, Fletcher CD: Synovial sarcoma in older patients: Clinicopathological analysis of 32 cases with emphasis on unusual histological features. Histopathology 43:72-83, 2003.

de Silva MV, McMahon AD, Paterson L, Reid R: Identification of poorly differentiated synovial sarcoma: A comparison of clinicopathological and cytogenetic features with those of typical synovial sarcoma. Histopathology 43:220-230, 2003.

Bergh P, Meis-Kindblom JM, Gherlinzoni F, et al: Synovial sarcoma: Identification of low and high risk groups. Cancer 85:2596-2607, 1999.

Epithelioid Sarcoma

Clinical Features

- Typically seen in adolescents and young adults (usually in second and third decades), males affected more than females
- Presents as a slowly growing, painless nodule or plaque, usually occurring on the flexor surfaces of the extremities; epithelioid sarcoma is the most common sarcoma of distal extremities
- Central, deeply seated lesions in pelvis and genital tract have been termed *proximal epithelioid sarcomas*

Gross Pathology

- Poorly defined multinodular mass with infiltrating margins, ranging in size from 0.5 to 5 cm
- Gray-white cut surface; focal areas of necrosis and hemorrhage are common
- Overlying skin may be ulcerated

Figure 17-48. Epithelioid sarcoma. Cytologic features of epithelioid sarcoma include round, eccentric vesicular nuclei with prominent nucleoli and eosinophilic cytoplasm.

Histopathology

- Multinodular proliferation of epithelioid and spindle cells commonly with central necrosis
- Epithelioid cells have round vesicular nuclei, prominent nucleoli, and ample eosinophilic cytoplasm; proximal epithelioid sarcoma may exhibit a rhabdoid phenotype
- Spindle cells have similar cytologic features in a collagenized stroma
- Central zones of degeneration and necrosis resemble infectious or palisading granuloma
- Extensive hyalinization and scattered chronic inflammatory infiltrate may be present

Special Stains and Immunohistochemistry

- Cytokeratin or EMA positive in more than 90% of cases
- Vimentin positive
- CD34 positive in about 50% of cases
- S-100 protein may be focally positive
- INI1/SMARCB1: loss of immunoreactivity in proximal type of epithelioid sarcoma

Other Techniques for Diagnosis

- Electron microscopy: tumor cells show prominent masses of filaments, cell processes, and intercellular junctions

Differential Diagnosis

▌ Granuloma annulare
- Palisading histiocytes around central zones of necrobiotic collagen and stromal mucin
- May be dermal or subcutaneous
- Cells are negative for epithelial markers (cytokeratin and EMA) and positive for CD68 or factor XIIIa

▌ Synovial sarcoma
- Deeper and usually more proximal than epithelioid sarcoma
- Characterized by fascicles of spindle cells admixed with obvious nests of epithelial cells (biphasic pattern), but purely epithelioid synovial sarcoma may resemble epithelioid sarcoma
- Lacks nodular growth with central necrosis; cells usually have less abundant cytoplasm than those of epithelioid sarcoma
- Shows vimentin and epithelial marker immunoreactivity; negative for CD34
- Presence of t(X;18)(p11;q11) is diagnostic of synovial sarcoma as demonstrated by cytogenetic or molecular techniques

▌ Epithelioid angiosarcoma
- Most often affects the scalp of elderly patients but can occur at other sites, especially in the setting of lymphedema
- Hemorrhagic, multinodular, and infiltrative tumor with solid growth or with rudimentary vascular channels
- Tumor cells are plump and hyperchromatic with distinct nucleoli and eosinophilic cytoplasm
- Immunoreactive for CD34, CD31, thrombomodulin, and Fli-1; may "aberrantly" express keratin but not EMA

▌ Epithelioid malignant peripheral nerve sheath tumor
- Usually a deep tumor associated with a major nerve but may be cutaneous; superficial lesions are usually well circumscribed and not multinodular
- Tumor cells are round to polygonal with large vesicular nuclei and prominent central or eccentric nucleoli
- Positive for S-100 protein, CD56, CD57, and nestin and may show focal positivity for epithelial markers; negative for CD34

▌ Malignant melanoma
- Frequently has an in situ component at the dermoepidermal junction
- Positive for S-100 protein, HMB-45, melan-A, tyrosinase, and PNL2; negative for epithelial markers and CD34

Pearls

- Epithelioid sarcoma is an aggressive neoplasm with a propensity for multiple recurrences before metastasizing
- Most common metastatic site is lung, but it may involve regional lymph nodes as well
- Overall prognosis is poor; survival is related to tumor size, depth, mitotic rate, and necrosis and presence of vascular invasion

Selected References

Casanova M, Ferrari A, Collini P, et al: Epithelioid sarcoma in children and adolescents: A report from the Italian Soft Tissue Sarcoma Committee. Cancer 106:708-717, 2006.

Laskin WB, Miettinen M: Epithelioid sarcoma: New insights based on an extended immunohistochemical analysis. Arch Pathol Lab Med 127:1161-1168, 2003.

Hasegawa T, Matsuno Y, Shimoda T, et al: Proximal-type epithelioid sarcoma: A clinicopathologic study of 20 cases. Mod Pathol 14:655-663, 2001.

Debiec-Rychter M, Sciot R, Hagemeijer A: Common chromosome aberrations in the proximal type of epithelioid sarcoma. Cancer Genet Cytogenet 123:133-136, 2000.

Miettinen M, Fanburg-Smith JC, Virolainen M, et al: Epithelioid sarcoma: An immunohistochemical analysis of 112 classical and variant cases and a discussion of the differential diagnosis. Hum Pathol 30:934-942, 1999.

Guillou L, Wadden C, Coindre JM, et al: "Proximal-type" epithelioid sarcoma, a distinctive aggressive neoplasm showing rhabdoid features: Clinicopathologic, immunohistochemical, and ultrastructural study of a series. Am J Surg Pathol 21:130-146, 1997.

Chase DR, Enzinger FM: Epithelioid sarcoma: Diagnosis, prognostic indicators, and treatment. Am J Surg Pathol 9:241-263, 1985.

Extraskeletal Ewing Sarcoma and Peripheral Neuroectodermal Tumor

Clinical Features

- Primarily affects adolescents and young adults but has a wide age range; makes up 15% of pediatric sarcomas
- Often presents as a rapidly growing deep mass; occasionally painful
- Common sites include chest, paravertebral region, abdomen and pelvis, and extremities

Figure 17-49. Ewing sarcoma. Sheets of overlapping uniform undifferentiated round cells is only one pattern of this tumor.

Gross Pathology

- Typically a lobulated, soft, tan-gray tumor with focal hemorrhage and necrosis
- Usually measures 5 to 10 cm in maximum diameter

Histopathology

- Cellular tumor comprising monomorphic round cells with finely dispersed chromatin, small nucleoli, and scant clear or amphophilic cytoplasm
- Growth is in sheets, nests, or islands, but EWS and PNET may have an alveolar pattern or show focal spindle cell change; cellular discohesion is common
- Tumor cells often contain intracytoplasmic glycogen with PAS staining
- Variable mitotic rate and apoptosis are often present
- Cellular rosettes may be seen

Special Stains and Immunohistochemistry

- CD99 strongly positive with a membrane pattern
- FLi-1: nuclear positivity
- Neural markers, including NSE, synaptophysin, CD57, and PGP 9.5 variably positive
- Keratin: 20% of cases positive for low-molecular-weight keratins
- PAS: intracytoplasmic positivity with abrogation of staining after pretreatment with diastase

Other Techniques for Diagnosis

- Electron microscopy: tumor cells have intracytoplasmic glycogen pools, primitive organelles, and macular junctions
- Presence of t(11;22)(q24;q12), producing an *EWS-FLI1* fusion (80-85%) or t(21;22)(q12;q12), producing an *EWS-ERG* fusion (5-10%) can be demonstrated by cytogenetic or molecular techniques; other variant translocations involving EWS or FUS have been reported

Differential Diagnosis

▮ Neuroblastoma
- Typically seen in young children arising from adrenal gland or sympathetic nerve trunk
- Characterized by the presence of cellular neuropil or ganglion cell differentiation
- Absence of intracellular glycogen
- Positive for CD56 and NB84; negative for keratin, CD99, and Fli-1
- Frequent chromosomal aberrations involve 17q, 1p, and 11q; *MYCN* amplification is present in 15% of cases but is not seen in EWS or PNET

▮ Alveolar rhabdomyosarcoma
- May have solid or alveolar architecture; monomorphic round tumor cells adhere to fibrovascular septa
- Focal overt rhabdomyoblastic differentiation may be seen with abundant eccentric pink cytoplasm; tumor giant cells are common

- Immunoreactivity for desmin, myogenin, and MyoD1; may be positive for CD99 but with a cytoplasmic pattern
- Presence of t(2;13)(q35;q14) or t(1;13)(p36;q14) can be demonstrated by cytogenetic or molecular techniques in 75% of cases
▌ Lymphoma
  - Characterized by diffuse growth of atypical round cell with irregular nuclear membranes
  - Most lymphomas show immunoreactivity for leukocyte common antigen (LCA; CD45), and lymphoblastic lymphoma expresses CD34, CD99, CD117, and TdT; either B-cell or T-cell antigens are also present
  - Lymphoblastic lymphoma is frequently positive for CD99 and Fli-1, and additional markers must be used (e.g., TdT) to distinguish it from EWS and PNET
▌ Desmoplastic small round cell tumor
  - Most common in the abdomen of adolescent and young-adult males
  - Diffuse peritoneal spread
  - Nests of small round cells with uniform, hyperchromatic nuclei, indistinct nucleoli, and scant cytoplasm, separated by a desmoplastic stroma
  - Polyphenotypic immunoprofile with coexpression of vimentin, keratin, neural markers, and desmin, the latter with a dotlike pattern
  - Presence of t(11;22)(p13;q12), producing an *EWS-WT1* fusion, can be demonstrated by cytogenetic or molecular techniques
▌ Poorly differentiated synovial sarcoma
  - Difficult to distinguish from EWS and PNET, especially in a small biopsy
  - Hyperchromatic tumor cells, often with a hemangiopericytoma-like growth pattern
  - Positive for CD99, bcl-2, CD57, and EMA and keratin; negative for Fli-1
  - Presence of t(X;18)(p11;q11) demonstrable by cytogenetic or molecular techniques

Pearls

- EWS and PNET are high-grade sarcomas, but current therapy has significantly improved the prognosis
- Common sites of distant metastasis include lung and bone
- Large tumor size and necrosis are factors that adversely affect prognosis

Selected References

Lewis TB, Coffin CM, Bernard PS: Differentiating Ewing's sarcoma from other round blue cell tumors using a RT-PCR translocation panel on formalin-fixed paraffin-embedded tissues. Mod Pathol 20:397-404, 2007.

Sanati S, Lu DW, Schmidt E, et al: Cytologic diagnosis of Ewing sarcoma/peripheral neuroectodermal tumor with paired prospective molecular genetic analysis. Cancer 111:192-199, 2007.

Folpe AL, Goldblum JR, Rubin BP, et al: Morphologic and immunophenotypic diversity in Ewing family tumors: A study of 66 genetically confirmed cases. Am J Surg Pathol 29:1025-1033, 2005.

Collini P, Sampietro G, Bertulli R, et al: Cytokeratin immunoreactivity in 41 cases of ES/PNET confirmed by molecular diagnostic studies. Am J Surg Pathol 25:273-274, 2001.

Folpe AL, Hill CE, Parham DM, et al: Immunohistochemical detection of FLI-1 protein expression: A study of 132 round cell tumors with emphasis on CD99-positive mimics of Ewing's sarcoma/primitive neuroectodermal tumor. Am J Surg Pathol 24:1657-1662, 2000.

Dehner LP: Primitive neuroectodermal tumor and Ewing's sarcoma. Am J Surg Pathol 17:1-13, 1993.

Desmoplastic Small Round Cell Tumor

Clinical Features

- Primarily affects young adults
- More commonly occurs in males (4:1 ratio)
- Usually found in the abdomen with extensive peritoneal spread, but also has been reported in other locations
- Presents with abdominal pain, distention, and ascites

Gross Pathology

- Large lobulated tumors with a gray-white cut surface
- Myxoid and necrotic areas typically seen

Histopathology

- Well-demarcated nests of small round cells with uniform, hyperchromatic nuclei, indistinct nucleoli, and scant cytoplasm, separated by desmoplastic stroma
- Nests vary in size, and cords or individual tumor cells also may infiltrate fibrous stroma

Figure 17-50. Desmoplastic small round cell tumor. Variably sized islands of hyperchromatic tumor cells separated by abundant desmoplastic stroma. This case shows overt epithelial differentiation.

- High mitotic rate and necrosis
- Occasional rhabdoid features or overt epithelial differentiation may be seen

Special Stains and Immunohistochemistry

- Cytokeratin and EMA positive in most cases
- NSE typically positive
- Vimentin positive
- Desmin positive (perinuclear dotlike pattern)
- WT-1 (C-terminus) positive

Other Techniques for Diagnosis

- Electron microscopy: tumor cells show minimal differentiation with scant organelles; perinuclear whorls of microfilaments are common, and dense core neurosecretory granules may be seen
- Presence of t(11;22)(p13;q12), producing an *EWS-WT1* fusion, can be demonstrated by cytogenetic or molecular techniques

Differential Diagnosis

- Extraskeletal EWS and PNET
  - Usually seen in chest wall, extremities, paravertebral region, or retroperitoneum
  - Cellular tumor characterized by sheets or nests of uniform round cells with finely dispersed chromatin, small nucleoli, and scant cytoplasm
  - Tumor cells may contain intracytoplasmic glycogen
  - Rich, delicate vasculature surrounding groups of tumor cells
  - Lacks desmoplastic stroma
  - Positive for CD99 and Fli-1
  - Presence of t(11;22)(q24;q12), producing an *EWS-FLI1* fusion or variants, can be demonstrated by cytogenetic or molecular techniques
- Alveolar rhabdomyosarcoma
  - May have solid or alveolar architecture; monomorphic round tumor cells adhere to fibrovascular septa
  - Focal overt rhabdomyoblastic differentiation with abundant plump eosinophilic cytoplasm; tumor giant cells are common
  - Diffuse cytoplasmic staining for desmin and nuclear labeling for myogenin and MyoD1
  - Presence of t(2;13)(q35;q14) or t(1;13)(p36;q14) can be demonstrated by cytogenetic or molecular techniques in 75% of cases
- Small cell carcinoma
  - Large intra-abdominal tumor is an atypical presentation of carcinoma
  - Positive for cytokeratin, EMA, NSE, chromogranin, CD56, or synaptophysin; negative for vimentin and desmin

Pearls

- The line of differentiation of DSRCT is uncertain
- DSRCT is an aggressive tumor and often unresectable at the time of presentation; most patients die within 5 years

- Variant chromosomal translocations have been described and are often associated with an atypical histology

Selected References

Chang F: Desmoplastic small round cell tumors: Cytologic, histologic, and immunohistochemical features. Arch Pathol Lab Med 130:728-732, 2006.

Hassan I, Shyyan R, Donohue JH, et al: Intraabdominal desmoplastic small round cell tumors: A diagnostic and therapeutic challenge. Cancer 104:1264-1270, 2005.

Zhang PJ, Goldblum JR, Pawel BR, et al: Immunophenotype of desmoplastic small round cell tumors as detected in cases with EWS-WT1 gene fusion product. Mod Pathol 16:229-235, 2003.

Lae ME, Roche PC, Jin L, et al: Desmoplastic small round cell tumor: A clinicopathologic, immunohistochemical, and molecular study of 32 tumors. Am J Surg Pathol 26:823-835, 2002.

Sandberg AA, Bridge JA: Updates on the cytogenetics and molecular genetics of bone and soft tissue tumors: Desmoplastic small round-cell tumors. Cancer Genet Cytogenet 138:1-10, 2002.

Gerald WL, Miller HK, Battifora H, et al: Intra-abdominal desmoplastic small round-cell tumor: Report of 19 cases of a distinctive type of high-grade polyphenotypic malignancy affecting young individuals. Am J Surg Pathol 15:499-513, 1991.

Alveolar Soft Part Sarcoma

Clinical Features

- Rare malignant soft tissue tumor presenting in late adolescence and young adulthood; rarely affects young children and elderly people
- Arises predominantly in the upper extremity and less often in the retroperitoneum, mesentery, and omentum; tumors in younger patients often involve the head and neck region

Figure 17-51. Alveolar soft part sarcoma. Organoid growth pattern of polygonal cells with cellular dyshesion.

- Typically presents as a slow-growing, painless mass but may present with symptoms related to distant metastases usually involving lung and brain

Gross Pathology

- Poorly defined soft tissue mass
- Yellow-gray cut surface, often with focal areas of hemorrhage and necrosis

Histopathology

- Organoid or nested growth pattern with islands of cells separated by delicate sinusoidal spaces
- Central cellular discohesion may impart an alveolar appearance
- Epithelioid cells with abundant eosinophilic, granular, or clear cytoplasm and regular, uniform nuclei, often with central nucleoli
- Intracytoplasmic crystals and intracytoplasmic glycogen often present; best seen with PAS stain
- Typically low mitotic rate
- Vascular invasion is typically present

Special Stains and Immunohistochemistry

- Desmin variably positive
- MyoD1 often positive in cytoplasm only
- TFE3: positive nuclear staining
- PAS highlights intracytoplasmic glycogen and crystals

Other Techniques for Diagnosis

- Electron microscopy: may show characteristic membrane-bound or free rhomboid crystals
- Presence of t(X;17)(p11;q25), producing an *ASPL-TFE3* fusion, can be demonstrated by cytogenetic or molecular techniques

Differential Diagnosis

- ∎ Alveolar rhabdomyosarcoma
  - Organoid architecture is not as prominent
  - Cells have higher nuclear-to-cytoplasmic C ratios and nuclear hyperchromasia; rhabdomyoblasts and giant cells may be seen
  - Nuclear immunoreactivity toward myogenin and MyoD1
  - Alveolar rhabdomyosarcoma shows t(2:13) or t(1:13) in 75% of cases
- ∎ Paraganglioma
  - Characterized by trabecular or organoid arrangement of round to polygonal cells with central nuclei and eosinophilic granular cytoplasm
  - Uncommon in extremity, usually seen along sympathetic chain
  - Positive for neuroendocrine markers (synaptophysin, chromogranin, and NSE)
- ∎ Granular cell tumor
  - Composed of sheets of large, polygonal cells with abundant coarse, eosinophilic, granular cytoplasm; lacks organoid pattern seen in alveolar soft part sarcoma

- Cells have small vesicular nuclei with prominent nucleoli
- Positive for S-100 protein
- ∎ Metastatic renal cell carcinoma (clear cell)
  - Tumor cells typically show more prominent cytoplasmic clearing
  - Lacks PAS positive crystals
  - Positive for EMA, CD10, and RCC

Pearls

- Alveolar soft part sarcoma is a high-grade sarcoma with a poor prognosis, although it may have a prolonged course
- Distant metastases to lung and brain are present at diagnosis in up to one third of cases but may occur late in the course
- Large tumor size, older age, and metastases at diagnosis portend a worse prognosis

Selected References

Zarrin-Khameh N, Kaye KS: Alveolar soft part sarcoma. Arch Pathol Lab Med 131:488-491, 2007.

Bu X, Bernstein L: A proposed explanation for female predominance in alveolar soft part sarcoma: Noninactivation of X; autosome translocation fusion gene? Cancer 103:1245-1253, 2005.

Argani P, Lal P, Hutchinson B, et al: Aberrant nuclear immunoreactivity for TFE3 in neoplasms with TFE3 gene fusions: A sensitive and specific immunohistochemical assay. Am J Surg Pathol 27:750-761, 2003.

Weiss SW: Alveolar soft part sarcoma: Are we at the end or just the beginning of our quest? Am J Pathol 160:1197-1199, 2002.

Portera CA Jr, Ho V, Patel SR, et al: Alveolar soft part sarcoma: Clinical course and patterns of metastasis in 70 patients treated at a single institution. Cancer 91:585-591, 2001.

Cullinane C, Thorner PS, Greenberg ML, et al: Molecular genetic, cytogenetic, and immunohistochemical characterization of alveolar soft-part sarcoma: Implications for cell of origin. Cancer 70:2444-2450, 1992.

Lieberman PH, Brennan MF, Kimmel M, et al: Alveolar soft-part sarcoma: A clinico-pathologic study of half a century. Cancer 63:1-13, 1989.

Clear Cell Sarcoma

Clinical Features

- Also referred to as *malignant melanoma of soft parts*
- Typically occurs in adults aged 20 to 40 years
- Extremities are most common location (lower affected more than upper), often distal; frequently associated with tendons or aponeuroses
- Usually presents as a slowly enlarging mass; may be painful

Gross Pathology

- Lobulated mass with a gray-white cut surface
- Focal areas of hemorrhage, necrosis, and dark-brown pigmentation may be seen

Figure 17-52. Clear cell sarcoma. Nests of polygonal cells with abundant clear cytoplasm are separated by a delicate fibrovascular network.

Histopathology

- Nests and fascicles of round or fusiform cells with vesicular nuclei showing a single, prominent, basophilic nucleolus and clear to eosinophilic cytoplasm
- Thin fibrous septa typically surround nests, but background may be hyalinized
- Multinucleated giant cells are common; rhabdoid cells may be present
- Variable mitotic rate, typically fewer than 2 mitotic figures/10 hpf
- Intracellular melanin pigment occasionally seen

Special Stains and Immunohistochemistry

- S-100 protein, HMB-45 positive
- HMB-45, melan-A, tyrosinase, and Mart-1 variably positive

Other Techniques for Diagnosis

- Electron microscopy: schwannian cell features including interdigitating cell processes and melanosomes
- Presence of t(12;22)(q13;q12), producing an *EWS-ATF1* fusion, can be demonstrated by cytogenetic or molecular techniques

Differential Diagnosis

- Spindle cell malignant melanoma
  - Typically located within the dermis
  - Associated with junctional activity in the overlying skin
  - Characterized by cells with elongated, hyperchromatic nuclei

- Fibrosarcoma
  - Most often affects children younger than 1 year; occasionally seen in adults
  - Typically found in the extremities
  - Highly cellular, infiltrative tumor composed of fibroblasts with hyperchromatic nuclei and scant cytoplasm arranged in a distinctive herringbone pattern
  - High mitotic rate; atypical mitotic figures may be seen
- Epithelioid malignant peripheral nerve sheath tumor
  - Characterized by cords and nests of polygonal cells with round nuclei, prominent nucleoli, and clear to eosinophilic cytoplasm
  - Often positive for S-100 protein and NSE; occasionally positive for EMA

Pearls

- Clear cell sarcoma is a highly aggressive tumor with a poor prognosis
- Local recurrence and metastases are common; metastases often occur within 3 years
- Common sites of metastasis include lungs, lymph nodes, and bone
- Adverse prognostic factors include large tumor size, vascular invasion, and tumor necrosis

Selected References

Kawai A, Hosono A, Nakayama R, et al: Clear cell sarcoma of tendons and aponeuroses: A study of 75 patients. Cancer 109:109-116, 2007.

Coindre JM, Hostein I, Terrier P, et al: Diagnosis of clear cell sarcoma by real-time reverse transcriptase-polymerase chain reaction analysis of paraffin embedded tissues: Clinicopathologic and molecular analysis of 44 patients from the French sarcoma group. Cancer 107:1055-1064, 2006.

Ferrari A, Casanova M, Bisogno G, et al: Clear cell sarcoma of tendons and aponeuroses in pediatric patients: A report from the Italian and German Soft Tissue Sarcoma Cooperative Group. Cancer 94:3269-3276, 2002.

Sandberg AA, Bridge JA: Updates on the cytogenetics and molecular genetics of bone and soft tissue tumors: Clear cell sarcoma (malignant melanoma of soft parts). Cancer Genet Cytogenet 130:1-7, 2001.

Deenik W, Mooi WJ, Rutgers EJ, et al: Clear cell sarcoma (malignant melanoma) of soft parts: A clinicopathologic study of 30 cases. Cancer 86:969-975, 1999.

Lucas DR, Nascimento AG, Sim FH: Clear cell sarcoma of soft tissues: Mayo Clinic experience with 35 cases. Am J Surg Pathol 16:1197-1204, 1992.

Enzinger FM: Clear-cell sarcoma of tendons and aponeuroses: An analysis of 21 cases. Cancer 18:1163-1174, 1965.

Perivascular Epithelioid Cell Tumor

Clinical Features

- Tumor with putative perivascular cell differentiation composed of clear epithelioid cells with coexpression of smooth muscle and melanocytic markers ("myomelanocytes")

Figure 17-53. Perivascular epithelioid cell tumor (PEComa). Haphazard arrangement of spindle and epithelioid cells has cleared out cytoplasm.

- Most common locations are uterus and falciform ligament; other soft tissue and visceral sites are rare; marked female predominance
- The perivascular epithelioid cell tumor (PEComa) family includes angiomyolipoma, lymphangioleiomyoma and lymphangioleiomyomatosis, and clear-cell "sugar" tumor of lung, all of which may be associated with tuberous sclerosis
  — PEComa of internal female genitalia
    ◆ Tumor of middle-aged women
    ◆ May present with pelvic pain or vaginal bleeding
  — Clear cell myomelanocytic tumor of the falciform ligament or ligamentum teres
    ◆ Occurs in young women during first or second decade
    ◆ Presents as painful abdominal mass

Gross Pathology

- Firm, gray-white mass; may show cystic change, hemorrhage, or necrosis
- Maximum size ranges from 1 to 20 cm; intra-abdominal and retroperitoneal tumors tend to be largest

Histopathology

- Highly vascular tumor with thin-walled vessels, the walls of which blend with ovoid or fusiform neoplastic cells
- Epithelioid tumor cells often contain clear cytoplasm; spindle cells have more granular eosinophilic cytoplasm
- Falciform ligament tumors tend to have an exclusively spindle cell morphology

- Small centrally placed nuclei and small nucleoli are typical, although pleomorphism and high nuclear grade may be seen
- Mitotic activity tends to be low; numerous mitotic figures or atypical forms may be an indicator of more aggressive behavior

Special Stains and Immunohistochemistry

- HMB-45 positive in more than 95% of cases
- Melan-A, MiTF, S-100 protein, tyrosinase, and PNL2 variably positive
- SMA positive
- Desmin variably positive
- Cytokeratin, CD117, and CD34 typically negative

Other Techniques for Diagnosis

- Electron microscopy: smooth muscle and melanocytic differentiation with premelanosomes
- Cytogenetics: numeric and structural abnormalities including loss of 1p, 16p, 17p, 18p, and 19 and gains of 2q, 3q, 5, 12q, and X

Differential Diagnosis

▌ Clear cell sarcoma (malignant melanoma of soft parts)
- Most commonly seen in the extremities; rare in abdomen or visceral organs
- Tends to be strongly positive for S-100 protein but lacks evidence of smooth muscle differentiation
- Presence of t(12;22)(q13;q12), producing an *EWS-ATF1* fusion, can be demonstrated in most cases
▌ Gastrointestinal stromal tumor
- Positive for CD117 and CD34 and lacks melanocytic differentiation
▌ Leiomyoma and leiomyosarcoma
- Epithelioid and clear cells usually make up only part of the tumor
- Lacks melanocytic differentiation
▌ Clear cell carcinomas
- Positive for keratin; lack melanocytic and smooth muscle differentiation

Pearls

- PEComas are rare tumors, and criteria for malignancy are not well established; about 10% to 20% behave in a malignant fashion
- Large size, infiltrative borders, high nuclear grade, greater than 1 mitotic figure/50 hpf, necrosis, and vascular invasion may be indicative of aggressive behavior
- Falciform ligament tumors are usually indolent
- Common sites of metastases include liver, lung, and bone

Selected References

Fadare O: Perivascular epithelioid cell tumors (PEComas) and smooth muscle tumors of the uterus. Am J Surg Pathol 31:1454-1455; author reply, 1455-1456, 2007.

Pan CC, Jong YJ, Chai CY, et al: Comparative genomic hybridization study of perivascular epithelioid cell tumor: Molecular genetic evidence of perivascular epithelioid cell tumor as a distinctive neoplasm. Hum Pathol 37:606-612, 2006.

Folpe AL, Mentzel T, Lehr HA, et al: Perivascular epithelioid cell neoplasms of soft tissue and gynecologic origin: A clinicopathologic study of 26 cases and review of the literature. Am J Surg Pathol 29:1558-1575, 2005.

Vang R, Kempson RL: Perivascular epithelioid cell tumor ('PEComa') of the uterus: A subset of HMB-45-positive epithelioid mesenchymal neoplasms with an uncertain relationship to pure smooth muscle tumors. Am J Surg Pathol 26:1-13, 2002.

Folpe AL, Goodman ZD, Ishak KG, et al: Clear cell myomelanocytic tumor of the falciform ligament/ligamentum teres: A novel member of the perivascular epithelioid clear cell family of tumors with a predilection for children and young adults. Am J Sur Pathol 24:1239-1246, 2000.

Hornick JL, Fletcher CD: PEComa: What do we know so far? Histopathology 48:75-82, 2006.

Pea M, Martignoni G, Zamboni G, Bonetti F: Perivascular epithelioid cell. Am J Surg Pathol 20:1149-1153, 1996.

Carmela D. Tan and E Rene Rodriguez

18

Heart, Pericardium, and Blood Vessels

Heart

Cardiomyopathy

Clinical Features

▌ Hypertrophic cardiomyopathy
- Myocardial disease characterized by left ventricular hypertrophy in the absence of systemic hypertension, aortic valve stenosis, or infiltrative diseases
- Associated with normal systolic function and diastolic dysfunction; systolic dynamic obstruction of the left ventricular outflow tract occurs in 25%
- Estimated prevalence of unexplained left ventricular hypertrophy on echocardiography compatible with a diagnosis of hypertrophic cardiomyopathy is 1 in 500

- Clinical presentation varies from asymptomatic to congestive heart failure, syncope, dyspnea, chest pain, and sudden death
- Associated with sudden death in athletes during exercise

▌ Dilated cardiomyopathy
- Most common cause of congestive heart failure in young patients and one of the leading indications for heart transplantation
- Patient presentation related to systolic dysfunction and progressive cardiac chamber enlargement with secondary mitral or tricuspid regurgitation
- Usually idiopathic, but can be caused by toxins, drugs, and metabolic derangements, and can be associated with myocarditis, alcohol abuse,

Figure 18-1. Hypertrophic cardiomyopathy. A, Movat-stained histologic section shows disorganization in the arrangement of myocyte bundles with interstitial fibrosis. **B,** Disarray can also be observed in the myofibrils of individual myocytes. **C,** Dysplastic small intramural coronary arteries are often observed with a narrowed lumen, irregularly thickened wall, and adventitial fibrosis.

pregnancy, familial incidence, nutritional deficiencies, neuromuscular disorders, and endocrine abnormalities
- Idiopathic dilated cardiomyopathy is a diagnosis of exclusion; heart failure is out of proportion to the presence of any concomitant coronary artery disease, systemic hypertension, or valvular heart disease
▌ Restrictive cardiomyopathy
- Patients present with symptoms associated with diastolic dysfunction, reduced diastolic volume, and normal systolic function
- Caused by endomyocardial scarring (idiopathic restrictive cardiomyopathy, endomyocardial fibrosis, Löffler syndrome, and endocardial fibroelastosis), storage disease (hemochromatosis, glycogen storage disease, Fabry disease), or myocardial infiltrate (amyloidosis, sarcoidosis, and radiation fibrosis)

- Idiopathic restrictive cardiomyopathy
  — Rare entity with autosomal dominant transmission and associated with skeletal myopathy
- Endomyocardial fibrosis
  — Recognized as a tropical disease, occurring most often in sub-Saharan Africa, affecting children and young adults
- Löffler syndrome (Löffler endomyocarditis and endocarditis parietalis fibroplastica)
  — Occurs in older patients and in men (more often than women) who live in the temperate zone
  — Often associated with reactive or neoplastic eosinophilia
- Endocardial fibroelastosis
  — Classified as primary or secondary; secondary form much more common

Figure 18-2. Arrhythmogenic right ventricular cardiomyopathy. A, Histologic section of right ventricular wall shows a markedly thinned myocardium with fatty infiltration of the wall. **B,** Movat stain shows fibrous replacement of the myocytes.

— Primary form may be related to intrauterine myocarditis with left ventricular dilation

— Secondary form is associated with congenital heart disease involving the left ventricle such as aortic stenosis, hypoplastic left heart syndrome, and coarctation of the aorta

● Hemochromatosis

— Primary hemochromatosis is an autosomal recessive disorder in which excessive iron absorption leads to iron overload

— Secondary hemochromatosis is associated with ineffective erythropoiesis, chronic liver disease, or multiple blood transfusions

▌ Arrhythmogenic right ventricular dysplasia and cardiomyopathy

● Inherited heart muscle disease that may present with arrhythmias, heart failure, or sudden death

● Arrhythmias are usually of right ventricular origin associated with global or regional dysfunction of the right ventricle

● Increasingly recognized as an important cause of sudden cardiac death

● Clinical diagnosis is based on major and minor diagnostic criteria proposed in 1994 by the European Society of Cardiology and Scientific Council on Cardiomyopathies of the International Society and Federation of Cardiology

Gross Pathology

▌ Hypertrophic cardiomyopathy

● Left ventricular hypertrophy, which may be symmetrical or asymmetrical

● Asymmetrical forms include thickening of subaortic ventricular septum (which is at least 1.5 times that of the left ventricular free wall), mid-ventricular segment, or apical region

● Systolic anterior motion of the anterior mitral leaflet leads to a contact lesion in the septum seen as an area of endocardial fibrosis

● Mechanical trauma to the anterior mitral leaflet and chordae result in thickening and fibrosis

● Foci of small scars often observed in the septum do not correspond to areas supplied by the major epicardial coronary arteries

▌ Dilated cardiomyopathy

● Increased cardiac weight with four-chamber dilation

● Normal or decreased left ventricular wall thickness due to chamber dilation

● Mural thrombi may be present

● Endocardial fibrosis is focal and may be related to organized thrombus or jet lesions from valvular regurgitation

● Valves are normal or may exhibit secondary changes associated with insufficiency such as dilated annulus or thickening of free edges

- Coronary arteries are normal or may exhibit mild atherosclerotic change within limits expected for the patient's age
∎ Restrictive cardiomyopathy
  - Idiopathic restrictive cardiomyopathy
    — Firm myocardium with normal left ventricular wall thickness
    — Normal left ventricular cavity size
    — Often biatrial dilation
    — Endocardium is not grossly thickened
  - Endomyocardial fibrosis
    — Thick, white scarring of the left ventricular endocardium at the inflow tract and apex with encasement of papillary muscles and subvalvular apparatus resulting in valvular regurgitation
    — Fibrosis of right ventricular apex seen in half of the cases
  - Löffler syndrome
    — Fibrosis of endocardium characteristically with large mural thrombi at the inflow tract and apex of both ventricles
  - Endocardial fibroelastosis
    — Left ventricle is usually contracted but may be dilated
    — Diffuse endocardial thickening that may obscure trabeculae carneae
  - Hemochromatosis
    — Left ventricular hypertrophy with rusty-brown discoloration of myocardium
∎ Arrhythmogenic right ventricular dysplasia and cardiomyopathy
  - Replacement of right ventricular myocardium by adipose and fibrous tissue
  - In early disease, these changes are segmental and present in the apex, right ventricular inflow tract, and right ventricular outflow tract
  - Progressive loss of myocardium leads to diffuse involvement with right ventricular dilation and localized ventricular aneurysms
  - Left ventricular involvement is seen in advanced stages with preferential involvement of posterolateral wall

Histopathology

∎ Hypertrophic cardiomyopathy
  - Hypertrophy and disarray of myocytes with interstitial fibrosis
  - Disarray is maximal in the middle or deeper region of the interventricular septum
  - Intramural small coronary arteries are dysplastic with narrowed lumens due to medial hyperplasia with or without intimal thickening
  - Replacement fibrosis and myocardial scars
  - Should not be diagnosed on the basis of right ventricular endomyocardial biopsy
∎ Dilated cardiomyopathy
  - Histopathologic findings are nonspecific
  - Myocyte hypertrophy with enlarged hyperchromatic nuclei, mixed with myocyte atrophy and degeneration

- Interstitial fibrosis sometimes associated with sparse inflammatory cell infiltrates
∎ Restrictive cardiomyopathy
  - Idiopathic restrictive cardiomyopathy
    — Diffuse interstitial fibrosis that surrounds individual myocytes
  - Endomyocardial fibrosis
    — Hyalinized collagen scarring of the endocardium with few mesenchymal cells
    — Fibrosis extends into the inner myocardium
  - Löffler syndrome
    — Three stages have been described
      ◆ Acute necrotic stage: shows intense eosinophilic infiltrate in myocardium with arteritis
      ◆ Thrombotic stage: characterized by superimposed thrombosis on thickened endocardium and thrombi in intramyocardial vessels
      ◆ Fibrotic stage: shows thick endocardium with loosely arranged vascularized fibrous tissue in the deepest layer; vessels show intimal thickening and perivascular fibrosis
    — Once the fibrotic stage is reached, the distinction between endomyocardial fibrosis and Löffler syndrome based on pathologic features may not be possible
  - Endocardial fibroelastosis
    — Diffuse fibrosis of endocardium with prominent elastic fibers
  - Hemochromatosis
    — Hemosiderin deposition within myocytes
∎ Arrhythmogenic right ventricular dysplasia and cardiomyopathy
  - Transmural extensive fatty replacement of the myocardium with fibrosis and myocyte atrophy
  - Lymphocytic infiltrates associated with myocyte damage may be present

Special Stains and Immunohistochemistry

- Masson trichrome highlights interstitial fibrosis and myofibrillar loss
- Movat pentachrome highlights fibrosis and elastosis
- Prussian blue highlights iron deposition in myocytes and macrophages
- Periodic acid–Schiff (PAS) with and without diastase highlights glycogen accumulation in myocytes, including basophilic degeneration

Other Techniques for Diagnosis

∎ Dilated cardiomyopathy
  - Electron microscopy: myocyte degeneration with myofibrillar loss in some myocytes and myocyte hypertrophy in others; dilation of T tubules, increased number of mitochondria, and increased glycogen, lipid vacuoles, myelin figures, and phagolysosomes

- Toxic cardiomyopathy (specifically doxorubicin)
  - Grading of doxorubicin endomyocardial biopsies requires at least three pieces of myocardium and examination of 10 plastic-embedded semithin sections stained with toluidine blue
    - Grade 0: normal myocardium by light and electron microscopy
    - Grade 1: occasional isolated myocytes with myofibrillar loss or vacuolar degeneration (distended sarcoplasmic reticulum and T-tubular system) involving less than 5% of cells
    - Grade 1.5: scattered, single myocytes with myofibrillar loss or vacuolar degeneration affecting 5% to 15% of myocytes
    - Grade 2: clusters of affected myocytes affecting 16% to 25% of cells
    - Grade 2.5: 26% to 35% of myocytes affected
    - Grade 3: diffuse myocyte damage affecting more than 35% of cells; myocyte cell necrosis (total loss of contractile elements, loss of organelles, and mitochondrial and nuclear degeneration)
- Metabolic cardiomyopathy
  - Fabry disease
    - Electron microscopy: electron-dense intracellular lamellar bodies or myelin figures corresponding to the accumulation of glycolipids
  - Mitochondrial cardiomyopathy
    - Electron microscopy: proliferation of mitochondria, which are pleomorphic in size and shape and have abnormal cristae and paracrystalline inclusions
  - Glycogen storage disease
    - Electron microscopy: markedly increased sarcoplasmic free glycogen; glycogen in lysosomes; vacuoles containing autophagic material

Differential Diagnosis

- Hypertrophic cardiomyopathy versus metabolic cardiomyopathy
  - Myocyte sarcoplasmic vacuolization or granularity should raise suspicion for storage disease and mitochondrial abnormalities; electron microscopy is necessary for complete evaluation
  - Fabry disease due to mutations in lysosomal α-galactosidase A
  - Adult-onset glycogen storage disease with left ventricular hypertrophy and Wolff-Parkinson-White syndrome due to mutations in the $\gamma2$ regulatory subunit of the adenosine monophosphate-activated protein kinase (PRKAG2)
  - X-linked hypertrophic cardiomyopathy (Danon disease) with skeletal myopathy and mental retardation due to mutations in lysosome-associated membrane protein (LAMP2)
  - Mitochondrial cardiomyopathy due to mutations in mitochondrial DNA

- Symmetrical hypertrophic cardiomyopathy versus physiologic hypertrophy in response to exercise ("athlete's heart")
- Hypertrophic cardiomyopathy versus age-related subaortic bulging of the interventricular septum (sigmoid or catenoid septum)
  - Anatomic variant commonly seen in elderly patients, which may be accentuated by concomitant systemic hypertension, simulating asymmetrical hypertrophic cardiomyopathy
- Hypertrophic cardiomyopathy versus diseases associated with left ventricular hypertrophy in infants and young children
  - Infiltrative cardiomyopathies including type II Pompe disease, Hunter disease, and Hurler disease
  - Noonan syndrome resulting from *PTPN11* (protein-tyrosine phosphatase, nonreceptor type 11) gene mutation presenting with cardiofacial abnormalities, including pulmonic valve stenosis and atrial septal defect
  - Infants of insulin-dependent diabetic mothers
- Restrictive cardiomyopathy versus constrictive pericarditis
  - Diastolic filling is restricted in constrictive pericarditis by rigid, thickened pericardium with fibrous pericardial adhesions
  - Endomyocardial biopsy has proved useful in establishing diagnosis of infiltrative cardiomyopathies
  - A normal endomyocardial biopsy would direct the clinical workup to re-evaluate the pericardium

Pearls

- Traditional functional classification of cardiomyopathies has been challenged in recent years as the genetic basis of a number of cardiomyopathies has become evident; moreover, hypertrophic cardiomyopathy and some infiltrative diseases may progress to a dilated form late in the course of the disease.
  - Hypertrophic cardiomyopathy
    - Familial in at least 50% of cases with autosomal dominant mode of inheritance but variable clinical expression as to age of onset and severity
    - Sometimes referred to as disease of the sarcomere because mutations have been identified in 13 sarcomeric protein genes
    - Most common gene mutations involve the β-myosin heavy chain (*MYH7*, chromosome locus 14q12) and myosin-binding protein C (*MYBPC3*, chromosome locus 11p11.2)
    - Endomyocardial biopsy is almost never diagnostic but can be helpful to rule out other diagnoses
    - Disarray may be absent in small myectomy specimens, but presence of coronary artery dysplasia and interstitial and endocardial fibrosis is suggestive of hypertrophic cardiomyopathy

- Dilated cardiomyopathy
  — Recent studies indicate that at least 30% of dilated cardiomyopathy cases may be familial
  — Pattern of inheritance is variable and includes autosomal dominant, autosomal recessive, and X-linked
  — Mutations are more varied and are found in genes encoding sarcomeric proteins, intermediate filaments, dystrophin-associated protein complex components, nuclear membrane proteins, and phospholamban
- Arrhythmogenic right ventricular dysplasia and cardiomyopathy
  — Familial occurrence in about 30% to 50% of cases with predominantly autosomal dominant pattern of inheritance and incomplete penetrance
  — Most common mutations are in genes encoding desmosomal proteins (desmoplakin, plakophilin, and plakoglobin)
- There is a considerable overlap and variation in the phenotypic expression of genetic mutations associated with cardiomyopathy
- Endomyocardial biopsy is able to establish the diagnosis in patients with unexplained cardiomyopathy with a high degree of sensitivity and specificity

Selected References

Maron BJ, Towbin JA, Thiene G, et al: Contemporary definitions and classification of the cardiomyopathies: An American Heart Association scientific statement from the Council on Clinical Cardiology, Heart Failure and Transplantation Committee; Quality of Care and Outcomes Research and Functional Genomics and Translational Biology Interdisciplinary Working Groups; and Council on Epidemiology and Prevention. Circulation 113:1807-1816, 2006.

Arad M, Maron BJ, Gorham JM, et al: Glycogen storage diseases presenting as hypertrophic cardiomyopathy. N Engl J Med 352:362-372, 2005.

Chimenti C, Pieroni M, Maseri A, Frustaci A: Histologic findings in patients with clinical and instrumental diagnosis of sporadic arrhythmogenic right ventricular dysplasia. J Am Coll Cardiol 43:2305-2313, 2004.

Ardehali H, Qasim A, Cappola T, et al: Endomyocardial biopsy plays a role in diagnosing patients with unexplained cardiomyopathy. Am Heart J 147:919-923, 2004.

Gilbert-Barness E, Barness LA: Nonmalformative cardiovascular pathology in infants and children. Pediatr Dev Pathol 2:499-530, 1999.

Felker GM, Hu W, Hare JM, et al: The spectrum of dilated cardiomyopathy: The Johns Hopkins experience with 1,278 patients. Medicine (Baltimore) 78:270-283, 1999.

Olsen EG, Spry CJ: Relation between eosinophilia and endomyocardial disease. Prog Cardiovasc Dis 27:241-254, 1995.

Katritsis D, Wilmshurst PT, Wendon JA, et al: Primary restrictive cardiomyopathy: Clinical and pathologic characteristics. J Am Coll Cardiol 18:1230-1235, 1991.

Myocarditis

Clinical Features

- Lymphocytic myocarditis
  - Frequently asymptomatic or has a subclinical course that later progresses to dilated cardiomyopathy
  - May present as unexplained acute onset of congestive heart failure, arrhythmias, or sudden death
  - Viruses are the most common cause of myocarditis, particularly in children
- Giant cell myocarditis
  - Typically affects young and middle-aged adults
  - Most patients present with rapidly progressive heart failure, often with refractory ventricular arrhythmia, rarely with heart block or chest pain mimicking myocardial infarction
  - Poor prognosis and often fatal if untreated

Figure 18-3. Lymphocytic myocarditis. Histologic section shows interstitial infiltrate of lymphocytes with rare eosinophils. Note the thinning of the myocytes in areas of myocyte necrosis.

Figure 18-4. Giant cell myocarditis. Histologic section shows extensive areas of myocyte dropout with a mixed inflammatory infiltrate consisting of multinucleated giant cells, lymphocytes, eosinophils, and hemosiderin-laden macrophages.

▌Eosinophilic myocarditis
- Hypersensitivity myocarditis
  — Believed to be an allergic delayed hypersensitivity reaction to diverse pharmacologic drugs and nutritional supplements
  — Reported complication of smallpox vaccination in young individuals
  — Associated with prolonged continuous administration of vasopressors, particularly dobutamine
  — Signs and symptoms are nonspecific and include typical allergic reaction (fever, rash, and blood eosinophilia), arrhythmias, sudden death, and congestive heart failure
- Acute necrotizing eosinophilic myocarditis
  — Thought to represent the most severe form of hypersensitivity myocarditis but can also be associated with viral infections, cancer, connective tissue diseases, and Churg-Strauss syndrome
  — Presents with fulminant heart failure and can be rapidly fatal
- Hypereosinophilic syndrome
  — Characterized by eosinophilia in the blood and bone marrow and tissue infiltration with eosinophils in multiple organs
  — Predominantly affects males between 20 and 50 years old
  — Cardiac involvement is most common and can present with restrictive physiology
  — Mural thrombi are frequently formed and can lead to systemic embolization

Gross Pathology

- Variable degrees of cardiac hypertrophy and possible chamber dilation may be seen
- Affected myocardium appears as pale foci, sometimes with minute hemorrhages
- Irregular and geographic fibrous scars without predilection to particular sites and affecting both ventricles and interventricular septum develop in giant cell myocarditis if patient survives
- In hypereosinophilic syndrome, endocardial damage leads to mural thrombosis
- Associated fibrinous pericarditis and pericardial effusion

Histopathology

▌Lymphocytic myocarditis
- Focal to diffuse interstitial mononuclear cell infiltrate, predominantly lymphocytes, with associated myocyte necrosis
- In endomyocardial biopsies, sparse lymphocytic infiltrate not associated with myocyte damage is diagnosed as borderline myocarditis based on the Dallas criteria
- Repeat biopsies showing persistent lymphocytic infiltrate is called *persistent myocarditis*, a less intense infiltrate is *resolving myocarditis*, and absence of inflammatory infiltrate is *resolved myocarditis*

▌Giant cell myocarditis
- Multifocal to diffuse infiltrate consisting of lymphocytes and macrophages with multinucleated giant cells
- Eosinophils are often present
- Occasional poorly formed granulomas may be seen
- Geographic areas of myocyte damage or necrosis with varying degrees of fibrosis are evident on low magnification

▌Eosinophilic myocarditis
- Patchy interstitial and perivascular infiltrates consisting of many eosinophils mixed with histiocytes, lymphocytes, and plasma cells
- May involve the endocardium and epicardium
- Lesions are all of the same age
- Usually only minimal myocyte necrosis and interstitial fibrosis
- Acute necrotizing eosinophilic myocarditis shows intense and diffuse infiltrates with extensive myocyte necrosis
- Hypereosinophilic syndrome also shows eosinophilic infiltrates with myocyte necrosis
- Charcot-Leyden crystals can be seen

Special Stains and Immunohistochemistry

- Gram, Gomori methenamine silver (GMS), PAS, and Ziehl-Neelsen stains to demonstrate causative organisms in infectious myocarditis

Other Techniques for Diagnosis

- In situ hybridization and polymerase chain reaction for viral detection; most commonly detected viruses are enteroviruses (Coxsackie B), parvovirus B19, adenovirus, human herpesvirus type 6, cytomegalovirus, influenza virus A and B, Epstein-Barr virus, and hepatitis C virus (HCV)

Differential Diagnosis

▌Lymphocytic myocarditis
- Myocarditis associated with Lyme disease, leptospirosis, typhoid fever, syphilis, chlamydia and rickettsial infections, and AIDS
- Myocarditis associated with collagen vascular disease and autoimmune disorders
- Toxic myocarditis
  — Includes toxin-induced myocardial injury (e.g., diphtheria exotoxin) and dose-related, direct toxic effects of drugs to myocardium
  — Seen in patients who were on vasopressor agents, have elevated endogenous catecholamine, or are cocaine abusers
  — Small foci of myocardial necrosis with contraction bands
  — Inflammatory infiltrates are predominantly macrophages
  — Lesions are of varying ages
- Microbiologic, serologic, and clinical correlation help make the diagnosis

■ Giant cell myocarditis
- Sarcoidosis
  - Dense fibrous scars toward the base of the heart involving the septum more heavily than the free wall of the left or right ventricle can be seen in sarcoidosis
  - Characterized by well-formed granulomas and fibrosis with few or no eosinophils
  - Generally lacks myocyte necrosis
  - Rarely present as isolated cardiac involvement; lymph node or lung involvement almost always present
- Rheumatic myocarditis
  - Endocardial and interstitial Aschoff granulomas with giant cells
- Infectious granulomatous diseases
  - Giant cells may be seen in tuberculosis, cryptococcosis, syphilitic myocarditis, or measles myocarditis
  - Myocardial involvement is rarely isolated
  - Special stains for microorganisms should be performed
- Foreign-body reaction
  - Birefringent material under polarized light
  - Myocardial reaction to pacemaker leads, assist devices
■ Eosinophilic myocarditis
- Parasitic infestation with peripheral eosinophilia (e.g., *Trichinella* species)
■ Neutrophilic infiltrates
- Usually seen in systemic bacterial and fungal infections in the immunocompromised host or spread by direct extension
  - Focal neutrophilic infiltrates with myocyte necrosis and microabscesses
- Myocardial infarction
  - A zone of necrosis with neutrophilic infiltration at the periphery corresponding to a territory supplied by an epicardial coronary artery

Pearls

■ Lymphocytic myocarditis
- Detection of viral genome, specifically enteroviruses, is an independent predictor of poor clinical outcome in patients with dilated cardiomyopathy
■ Giant cell myocarditis
- Up to 20% of patients have other inflammatory diseases, especially inflammatory bowel disease or autoimmune disorders
- Most commonly associated tumor is thymoma
- Giant cell myocarditis is known to recur in transplanted hearts
■ Hypersensitivity myocarditis
- Diagnosis requires high clinical index of suspicion
- Endomyocardial biopsy necessary to establish the diagnosis

- No correlation between the duration and dose of the drug and the severity of myocarditis
- Treatment requires removal of the offending substance; immunosuppressive therapy may be indicated in severe cases

Selected References

Ginsberg F, Parrillo JE: Eosinophilic myocarditis. Heart Fail Clin 1:419-429, 2005.

Kuhl U, Pauschinger M, Seeberg B, et al: Viral persistence in the myocardium is associated with progressive cardiac dysfunction. Circulation 112:1965-1970, 2005.

Calabrese F, Thiene G: Myocarditis and inflammatory cardiomyopathy: Microbiological and molecular biological aspects. Cardiovasc Res 60:11-25, 2003.

Cooper LT Jr, Berry GJ, Shabetai R: Idiopathic giant-cell myocarditis: Natural history and treatment. Multicenter Giant Cell Myocarditis Study Group Investigators. N Engl J Med 336:1860-1866, 1997.

Amyloidosis

Clinical Features

- Symptoms are nonspecific and can present with restrictive cardiomyopathy, congestive heart failure, atypical chest pain, and arrhythmias
- Preponderance of male patients
- Amyloid deposition in the heart may be associated with systemic amyloidosis, hereditary amyloidosis, or senile cardiac amyloidosis

Gross Pathology

- Cardiac amyloidosis usually leads to cardiomegaly with ventricular hypertrophy
- Cut surface may show a variable appearance ranging from normal to firm and rubbery myocardium
- Tiny, semitranslucent, waxy nodules may be seen on the endocardium, more prominent in the left atrium; in severe cases, they are visible in all chambers and on the valvular endocardium

Histopathology

- Characteristic interstitial deposition of extracellular amorphous material surrounding individual myocytes results in atrophy and loss of myocytes
- Other patterns of infiltration are nodular, subendocardial, vascular, and mixed
- Amyloid involvement of valves, conduction system, and aorta may be seen
- Mononuclear inflammatory cell infiltrates can be found and correlate with poor prognosis

Special Stains and Immunohistochemistry

- Congo red: apple-green birefringence under polarized light
- Thioflavin T or thioflavin S: ultraviolet fluorescence of the amyloid deposits

Figure 18-5. Amyloidosis. Abundant eosinophilic material is deposited around myocytes, which show marked variation in size on cross section, indicating hypertrophy and degeneration (**A**). Individual myocytes are outlined by amyloid deposits that fluoresce with thioflavin stain (**B**). Immunohistochemical staining with λ light chain is positive in this case (**C**).

- Sulfated alcian blue: highlights green-staining amyloid surrounding individual myocytes and red-staining interstitial fibrosis
- Immunohistochemical staining with the following is useful in cardiac amyloidosis: transthyretin, κ and λ light chains, heavy chains, amyloid A, and atrial natriuretic peptide

Other Techniques for Diagnosis

- Electron microscopy: interstitial expansion by extracellular, nonbranching, randomly oriented fibrils measuring 8 to 10 nanometers in diameter

Differential Diagnosis

▌ Hyalinized collagen
  - May appear similar to amyloid on hematoxylin and eosin–stained sections
  - Congo red may have false-positive birefringence in collagen if staining method is not optimal

Pearls

- Cardiac amyloidosis can be divided into primary (light and heavy chains), secondary (amyloid A), hereditary (mutant transthyretin), senile systemic (wild-type transthyretin), isolated atrial (atrial natriuretic peptide), and hemodialysis-related (β_2-microglobulin)
- Deposits in the heart are most common in primary and age-related forms of amyloidosis
- Endomyocardial biopsy is a safe method to establish the diagnosis
- In early disease, amyloid deposits may be visible only with electron microscopy
- Immunohistochemistry should be done to identify the type of protein, as it has prognostic and therapeutic implications
- Congo red staining varies with the type of amyloid
- Thioflavin T is more sensitive than Congo red and easy to perform but requires fluorescence microscopy

Selected References

Westermark P, Benson MD, Buxbaum JN, et al: Amyloid: Toward terminology clarification. Report from the Nomenclature Committee of the International Society of Amyloidosis. Amyloid 12:1-4, 2005.

Kholova I, Niessen HW: Amyloid in the cardiovascular system: A review. J Clin Pathol 58:125-133, 2005.

Rahman JE, Helou EF, Gelzer-Bell R, et al: Noninvasive diagnosis of biopsy-proven cardiac amyloidosis. J Am Coll Cardiol 43:410-415, 2004.

Strege RJ, Saeger W, Linke RP: Diagnosis and immunohisto-chemical classification of systemic amyloidoses: Report of 43 cases in an unselected autopsy series. Virchows Arch 433:19-27, 1998.

Sarcoidosis

Clinical Features

- Involves young or middle-aged adults of either sex
- Lung, lymph nodes, skin, and eyes commonly involved; rarely, isolated cardiac involvement has been reported
- Cardiac involvement present in about 25% of sarcoidosis patients in autopsy series, with less than 5% having associated symptoms
- Patients present with arrhythmias, heart block and heart failure, or sudden death

Gross Pathology

- Granulomatous infiltration may be visible as patchy, irregular white firm areas
- Transmural myocardial scars not associated with coronary atherosclerosis represent healed granulomas
- Preferential sites of involvement, in decreasing order of frequency, are left ventricular free wall at the base

Figure 18-6. Cardiac sarcoidosis. Epithelioid granulomas with multinucleated giant cells are seen in areas of replacement fibrosis. Unlike giant cell myocarditis, the granulomas are discrete in a background of dense fibrous tissue with an infiltrative border.

of and including papillary muscles, basal and cephalic portion of interventricular septum, and right ventricular free wall

Histopathology

- Noncaseating, well-formed granulomas composed of epithelioid histiocytes and multinucleated giant cells with or without lymphocytic infiltrates and no stainable microorganisms
- Granulomas may involve the endocardium, myocardium, epicardium, and pericardium
- Typically minimal myocyte necrosis
- Collagenous stroma around granulomas
- Myocardial scars with few or no residual granulomas in burnt-out or treated cases

Special Stains and Immunohistochemistry

- Noncontributory

Other Techniques for Diagnosis

- Noncontributory

Differential Diagnosis

▌ Giant cell myocarditis
- Poorly formed granulomas with greater extent of myocyte necrosis and increased eosinophils compared with sarcoidosis
- Appears clinically distinct with a more fulminant course and shorter time from symptom onset to death or transplantation

▌ Infectious myocarditis
- Infectious etiology should be excluded by performing stains for fungi and mycobacteria

▌ Myocardial infarction
- Scarring and thinning of the ventricle may be mistaken for healed myocardial infarcts, but normal coronary arteries should rule out ischemic heart disease

Pearls

- Endomyocardial biopsy has poor sensitivity in detecting cardiac sarcoidosis; therefore, a negative endomyocardial biopsy does not exclude the diagnosis of sarcoidosis
- Extensive myocardial scarring and ventricular aneurysm may be related to natural history of the disease or previous corticosteroid therapy

Selected References

Ardehali H, Howard DL, Hariri A, et al: A positive endomyocardial biopsy result for sarcoid is associated with poor prognosis in patients with initially unexplained cardiomyopathy. Am Heart J 150:459-463, 2005.

Okura Y, Dec GW, Hare JM, et al: A clinical and histopathologic comparison of cardiac sarcoidosis and idiopathic giant cell myocarditis. J Am Coll Cardiol 41:322-329, 2003.

Silverman KJ, Hutchins GM, Bulkley BH: Cardiac sarcoid: A clinicopathologic study of 84 unselected patients with systemic sarcoidosis. Circulation 58:1204-1211, 1978.

Roberts WC, McAllister HA Jr, Ferrans VJ: Sarcoidosis of the heart: A clinicopathologic study of 35 necropsy patients (group 1) and review of 78 previously described necropsy patients (group 11). Am J Med 63:86-108, 1977.

Valvular Diseases

Morphologic and Functional Correlations

▌ Stenotic valves with or without regurgitation
  - Diffuse fibrous thickening with a variable amount of calcification
  - No valvular tissue loss, perforations, or vegetations
  - No valvular tissue excess
  - Fusion of valve commissures
  - Chordae tendineae are fibrotic, fused, and shortened
  - Attached papillary muscle is normal

▌ Purely regurgitant valves
  - Usually mild and focal fibrous thickening and absent calcification
  - Perforations or vegetations may be present
  - Excess valvular tissue may be present
  - No commissural fusion
  - Chordae tendineae are elongated or ruptured
  - Attached papillary muscle may be ruptured

Figure 18-8. Aortic valve. Only one commissure is identified in this surgically excised congenitally malformed unicommissural aortic valve with eccentrically located orifice (*upper left*). A bicuspid aortic valve has two cusps with a slitlike opening of the valve. The larger of the cusps shows a calcified median raphe. A fenestration is present in the smaller cusp (*upper right*). Calcific aortic stenosis due to severe nodular calcification of all three cusps is shown (*lower left*). Rheumatic aortic stenosis shows fusion of all the commissures with thick retracted cusps resulting in a fixed triangular orifice (*lower right*).

Etiology of Valvular Dysfunction

▌ Mitral valve
  - Mitral stenosis
    — Congenital
    — Acquired
    — Postinflammatory and rheumatic
    — Mitral annular calcification
  - Mitral regurgitation
    — Congenital
    — Acquired
      ◆ Mitral valve prolapse
      ◆ Postinflammatory and rheumatic
      ◆ Mitral annular calcification
      ◆ Infective endocarditis
      ◆ Ruptured papillary muscle
      ◆ Papillary muscle dysfunction secondary to ischemia and infarct
      ◆ Distortion of left ventricular geometry

▌ Aortic valve
  - Aortic stenosis
    — Congenital
      ◆ Unicuspid aortic valve
      ◆ Calcification of bicuspid aortic valve
    — Acquired
      ◆ Senile calcific aortic stenosis
      ◆ Postinflammatory and rheumatic
  - Aortic regurgitation
    — Congenital
      ◆ Bicuspid aortic valve

Figure 18-7. Mitral valve. In the upper specimen, postinflammatory scarring of the mitral valve results in commissural fusion and stenosis of the orifice. The chordae are fused, thickened, and shortened. Shown at the same magnification, the lower specimen, a segmental resection of a mitral valve, shows a diffusely thickened, expanded leaflet with mild billowing typical of mitral valve prolapse. The chordae are elongated and irregularly thickened, as seen on the ventricular aspect of the right lower specimen.

— Acquired
  - Postinflammatory and rheumatic
  - Infective endocarditis
  - Aortic dilation and aneurysm
  - Aortic dissection

Clinical Features

- Rheumatic heart disease
  - Findings of acute rheumatic fever include pericardial friction rubs, weak heart sounds, tachycardia, and arrhythmias; usually occur 10 days to 6 weeks after the pharyngitis episode
  - Findings in chronic rheumatic heart disease include evidence of valvular stenosis or regurgitation, congestive heart failure, arrhythmias, thromboembolic complications, and infective endocarditis; usually occur 20 to 25 years after the acute disease
- Mitral valve prolapse
  - Prevalence is estimated at 2% to 3% of the population, with equal distribution among men and women
  - Most patients do not develop symptoms
  - Prolapse occurs most commonly in the middle scallop of the posterior mitral valve leaflet as identified on echocardiography
  - Commonly idiopathic
  - Known association with connective tissue disorders including Marfan syndrome, Ehlers-Danlos syndrome, osteogenesis imperfecta, and pseudoxanthoma elasticum
  - Men appear to have a higher incidence of complications, which include severe mitral regurgitation, infective endocarditis, thromboembolic events, and sudden death
- Calcific aortic valve disease
  - Senile calcific aortic stenosis is more common in males, with a peak incidence in the seventh and eighth decades of life
  - Calcification of a congenital bicuspid aortic valve peaks in the fifth and sixth decades of life
  - Calcific disease of the aortic valve results in left ventricular hypertrophy, with symptoms including angina, syncope, and congestive heart failure
- Mitral annular calcification
  - More common and more severe in women, primarily those older than 60 years
  - Associated with aging, hypertension, aortic stenosis, chronic renal disease, and atherosclerosis
  - Often asymptomatic, but potential complications include acquired mitral stenosis or regurgitation, conduction system disturbances, endocarditis, and systemic embolism
- Pure aortic regurgitation
  - Pure aortic insufficiency can be due to lesions of the valve or the aorta
  - Aortic root dilation is currently the most common cause of aortic insufficiency, followed by congenital bicuspid valve associated with ascending aortic aneurysm
- Carcinoid heart disease
  - Carcinoid syndrome is characterized by episodic bronchospasm, flushing of the skin, telangiectasia, and diarrhea, usually associated with gastrointestinal carcinoid tumors that have metastasized to the liver
  - Cardiac involvement manifests as right-sided valvular disease that progresses to right-sided heart failure
  - Valvular dysfunction results in pure regurgitation of the tricuspid valve and predominantly regurgitation of the pulmonic valve
  - Left-sided involvement is rare and associated with the presence of right-to-left shunt, pulmonary metastases, or bronchial carcinoids

Gross Pathology

- Rheumatic heart disease
  - Involves, in descending order of frequency, mitral, aortic, tricuspid, and pulmonic valves
  - Acute rheumatic fever may show small verrucous vegetations along the lines of closure
  - Chronic rheumatic heart disease shows diffuse thickening and fibrous retraction of valve leaflets with or without calcification, fusion of the commissures, and shortened, fused, and thickened chordae
  - Narrowed valvular orifice due to commissural fusion
  - Calcific deposits are found at the free edge and commissures, which may become ulcerated
- Mitral valve prolapse
  - Myxomatous degeneration may involve any valve but most frequently involves the mitral valve
  - Diffuse leaflet thickening and redundancy with increased surface area
  - Interchordal hooding or billowing (parachute) deformity may be seen
  - Cut surface reveals abundant gray translucent myxoid material affecting the base, midportion, and free edge of the leaflet
  - Elongated chordae with irregular thickening are commonly seen, and sometimes rupture occurs
  - Often with annular dilation
- Calcific aortic valve disease
  - Senile calcific aortic stenosis shows fibrosis and calcification of the base and body of the cusps filling up the sinuses of Valsalva and rarely involving the free edge
  - Calcification of a congenital bicuspid aortic valve typically begins in the median raphe or false commissure and extends to the body of the cusps
  - Absent or minimal commissural fusion is seen in degenerative aortic valve stenosis

- Mitral annular calcification
  - Calcification develops in the ring of the mitral valve, usually at the base of the posterior leaflet, forming a solid bar causing distortion and elevation of the posterior leaflet
  - Lesion may also extend into the myocardium and medially into the septum, where it may cause disruption of the bundle of His
  - Calcium mass may erode through the valve leaflet, ulcerate, and predispose to thrombosis and infection
  - Central softening and liquefaction of the calcification may occur and should not be mistaken for abscess
- Pure aortic regurgitation
  - Floppy valves are large, redundant, mildly thickened, and gelatinous in consistency
  - In aortic regurgitation secondary to dilation of the aortic root, the aortic cusps can be normal, with only focal and minimal fibrosis in the body; free edges are thickened; commissures are not fused
- Carcinoid heart disease
  - White fibrotic plaques on the tricuspid and pulmonic valve, mural endocardium, and occasionally intima of great vessels
  - Fibrous plaques located predominantly on the ventricular aspect of tricuspid valve and almost exclusively on the arterial aspect of pulmonic valve
  - Plaques cause thickening and retraction of the leaflets
  - Plaques may also cause adherence of the valve to the mural endocardium of the right ventricle or intima of the pulmonary artery

Histopathology

- Rheumatic heart disease
  - Acute rheumatic fever may show inflammation and Aschoff bodies in all layers of the heart, including valves and papillary muscles
  - Aschoff bodies consist of foci of fibrinoid degeneration surrounded by lymphocytes, occasional plasma cells, and Anitschkow or Aschoff cells
  - Anitschkow cells are macrophages with abundant cytoplasm and central round to oval vesicular nuclei with a central bar of condensed chromatin (caterpillar-like); may become multinucleated to form Aschoff giant cells
  - Chronic rheumatic heart disease shows diffuse fibrosis, neovascularization, or calcification of the valve
  - Focal chronic inflammatory cell infiltrate (mainly lymphocytic) may be seen
- Mitral valve prolapse
  - Accumulation of mucopolysaccharides in the spongiosa with disruption of the collagenous bundles in the fibrosa and fragmentation of elastic fibers
  - Absence of neovascularization or inflammation
  - Surface thrombus formation may be seen
  - Mucopolysaccharide infiltration of the chordae tendineae

- Calcific aortic valve disease
  - Calcification begins in the fibrosa layer
  - Lipid deposits and chronic inflammatory cell infiltrates are commonly found
  - Osseous metaplasia may develop in the calcium deposits
- Mitral annular calcification
  - Calcification may be associated with mild inflammation and foreign-body giant cells
- Pure aortic regurgitation
  - Fibrous thickening of the free edges
  - Myxomatous degeneration with accumulation of mucopolysaccharides in the spongiosa
- Carcinoid heart disease
  - Plaque is cellular and contains fibroblasts, myofibroblasts, smooth muscle cells, and collagen embedded in a myxoid matrix
  - Plaques have a stuck-on appearance on the underlying valve and endocardium, which are intact
  - Usually there are no elastic lamellae (i.e., no fibroelastosis) within the carcinoid plaque

Special Stains and Immunohistochemistry

- Movat delineates the different layers of the valve and highlights mucopolysaccharide accumulation, fibrosis, and disruption and fragmentation of elastic fibers

Other Techniques for Diagnosis

- Noncontributory

Differential Diagnosis

- Stenosis versus regurgitant: see "Morphologic and Functional Correlations" under "Valvular Diseases"

Pearls

- An etiologic diagnosis can be formulated in most instances with careful gross evaluation of operatively excised valves
- Histologic evaluation is necessary to establish diagnosis in infective endocarditis and metabolic diseases involving cardiac valves (e.g., Fabry disease, mucopolysaccharidoses, carcinoid syndrome)

Selected References

Hayek E, Gring CN, Griffin BP: Mitral valve prolapse. Lancet 365:507-518, 2005.

Roberts WC, Ko JM: Frequency by decades of unicuspid, bicuspid, and tricuspid aortic valves in adults having isolated aortic valve replacement for aortic stenosis, with or without associated aortic regurgitation. Circulation 111:920-925, 2005.

Simula DV, Edwards WD, Tazelaar HD, et al: Surgical pathology of carcinoid heart disease: A study of 139 valves from 75 patients spanning 20 years. Mayo Clin Proc 77:139-147, 2002.

Feldman T: Rheumatic heart disease. Curr Opin Cardiol 11:126-130, 1996.

Waller B, Howard J, Fess S: General concepts in the morphologic assessment of operatively excised cardiac valves. Part I. Clin Cardiol 17:41-46, 1994.

Waller B, Howard J, Fess S: General concepts in the morphologic assessment of operatively excised cardiac valves. Part II. Clin Cardiol 17:208-214, 1994.

King BD, Clark MA, Baba N, et al: "Myxomatous" mitral valves: Collagen dissolution as the primary defect. Circulation 66:288-296, 1982.

Pomerance A: Pathological and clinical study of calcification of the mitral valve ring. J Clin Pathol 23:354-361, 1970.

Infective Endocarditis

Clinical Features

- Risk factors for infective endocarditis are structural valvular abnormalities, congenital heart diseases, prosthetic heart valves, and injection drug use
- *Staphylococcus aureus* has become the most common cause of infective endocarditis owing to nosocomial infections and medical and surgical interventions including indwelling catheters and devices
- Most subacute cases of native valve endocarditis are due to *Streptococcus viridans*
- Prosthetic valve endocarditis is usually caused by *Staphylococcus epidermidis* and *S. aureus*
- Endocarditis caused by fastidious gram-negative bacilli of the HACEK group (*Haemophilus parainfluenzae*, *H. aphrophilus*, *H. paraphrophilus*, *H. influenzae*, *Actinobacillus actinomycetemcomitans*, *Cardiobacterium hominis*, *Eikenella corrodens*, *Kingella kingae*, and *K. denitrificans*) accounts for about 5% to 10% of native valve community-acquired endocarditis in patients who are not injection drug users
- Symptoms are nonspecific and include fever, chills, fatigue, and weight loss
- Special attention to potential sources of bacteremia, new regurgitant murmurs, and embolic phenomena including septic lung emboli is emphasized
- Infection of a mechanical prosthetic valve may lead to valve dehiscence or paravalvular leak

Figure 18-9. Infective endocarditis. An aortic cusp shows perforation with large yellow-red vegetations on the ventricular aspect.

Gross Pathology

- Aortic and mitral valves are most commonly affected
- Valvular insufficiency is caused by destruction or perforation of the valve and bulky vegetations that prevent proper coaptation of the leaflets
- Cusp or leaflet may have an irregular, ulcerated free border or perforation of the body and ruptured chordae
- Healed endocarditis may result in aneurysms and perforation with smooth borders
- Tissue prosthetic valve usually shows vegetations on both inflow and outflow surfaces
- Mechanical prosthetic valve infection starts at the sewing ring and results in a periprosthetic or ring abscess

Histopathology

- Acute vegetations consist of fibrin, platelets, neutrophils, and bacteria
- Subacute vegetations have granulation tissue at the base with both acute and chronic inflammatory cells as well as histiocytes and multinucleated giant cells

Special Stains and Immunohistochemistry

- Gram, PAS, GMS, Warthin-Starry, Fite, and Ziehl-Neelsen stains are useful in detecting microorganisms in tissues
- Antibodies to *Tropheryma*, *Chlamydia*, *Bartonella*, and *Coxiella* species are available only in specialized laboratories

Other Techniques for Diagnosis

- Serologic tests are useful for the diagnosis of *Bartonella*, *Coxiella*, and *Legionella* endocarditis
- Polymerase chain reaction followed by direct sequencing of 16S recombinant RNA genes from valve tissue are also used to detect *Tropheryma*, *Bartonella*, and *Coxiella* species

Differential Diagnosis

■ Nonbacterial thrombotic endocarditis
- Usually occurs in association with chronic inflammatory disease, hypercoagulable state, and underlying malignancy, especially adenocarcinomas
- Aseptic vegetation may embolize or serve as a substrate for infection
- Aortic and mitral valves are most commonly affected
- Right-sided lesions are usually associated with intravenous catheters
- Vegetations are present on the atrial surfaces of atrioventricular valves and ventricular surfaces of semilunar valves
- Small (1- to 5-mm), multiple, nondestructive vegetations are loosely attached to the underlying valve leaflets, usually on previously normal valves
- Composed of platelets mixed with fibrin and a few red blood cells

- Inflammatory reaction is absent
- Organization may be seen at the base of the lesion with fibroblastic proliferation
▋ Libman-Sacks endocarditis
  - Occurs in patients with systemic lupus erythematosus (SLE)
  - Only 6% to 20% are symptomatic
  - Rare source of emboli
  - Most often develop on mitral and tricuspid valves
  - Relatively adherent, sessile, small (3- to 4-mm), pink to yellow-tan vegetations occurring singly or in clusters on the atrial and ventricular surfaces of the valve, anywhere from the free edge to the base, with extension onto the endocardium, chordae tendineae, and papillary muscles
  - Sterile vegetations consist of fibrin and mononuclear cells with fibroblastic proliferation and neovascularization
  - Necrosis with hematoxylin bodies rarely seen
  - Healed endocarditis results in fibrous plaque

Pearls

- Up to 20% of patients with infective endocarditis have negative blood cultures, which may result from previous antibiotic administration or infection with highly fastidious bacteria and unusual organisms such as *Bartonella* species, *Coxiella burnetii*, *Brucella* species, *Tropheryma whippelii*, and *Chlamydia* and *Legionella* species

Selected References

Lalani T, Kanafani ZA, Chu VH, et al: Prosthetic valve endocarditis due to coagulase-negative staphylococci: Findings from the International Collaboration on Endocarditis Merged Database. Eur J Clin Microbiol Infect Dis 25:365-368, 2006.

Baddour LM, Wilson WR, Bayer AS, et al: Infective endocarditis: Diagnosis, antimicrobial therapy, and management of complications: A statement for healthcare professionals from the Committee on Rheumatic Fever, Endocarditis, and Kawasaki Disease, Council on Cardiovascular Disease in the Young, and the Councils on Clinical Cardiology, Stroke, and Cardiovascular Surgery and Anesthesia, American Heart Association, endorsed by the Infectious Diseases Society of America. Circulation 111:e394-e434, 2005.

Fowler VG Jr, Miro JM, Hoen B, et al: Staphylococcus aureus endocarditis: A consequence of medical progress. JAMA 293:3012-3021, 2005.

Houpikian P, Raoult D: Blood culture-negative endocarditis in a reference center: Etiologic diagnosis of 348 cases. Medicine (Baltimore) 84:162-173, 2005.

Prosthetic Valves

Most Commonly Implanted Prosthetic Heart Valves

▋ Bioprosthetic valves
  - Stented bioprosthetic valves
    — Leaflets made from bovine pericardium or porcine aortic valve treated with a chemical preservative
    — Mounted on flexible plastic or titanium metal frame (stent) covered with synthetic fabric (sewing cuff); three stent posts (struts) further support the cusps
  - Stentless bioprosthetic valve
    — Chemically treated porcine aortic valve and a portion of the aortic root reinforced with a pliable exterior cuff
▋ Mechanical valves
  - Hinged bileaflet D-shaped tilting disks made of pyrolytic carbon
  - Housing made of a short hollow tube with a sewing cuff
▋ Homografts
  - Cryopreserved human aortic roots

Common Complications and Modes of Failure of Prosthetic Heart Valves

▋ Thrombus formation
  - May become a source of thromboemboli or become infected
  - May hinder or entrap leaflets at hinge points in mechanical valves
  - Thrombi usually form in the outflow side of bioprosthetic valves, filling up the concave aspect of the cusps
▋ Infection
  - May progress to ring abscess, leading to valve dehiscence or paravalvular leak
▋ Pannus overgrowth
  - Fibrous tissue overgrowth from the sewing ring extends to valvular cusps, resulting in stiff thickened cusps, commissural fusion, and stenosis
  - Retraction of cusps results in insufficiency
▋ Paravalvular leak
  - Early leaks are complications arising from suturing technique or separation from an annulus with calcification or infection
  - Late paravalvular leak results from tissue retraction during healing
▋ Structural deterioration
  - Most frequent cause of failure in bioprosthetic valves
    — Mineralization of tissue valves causes stiffening and often tearing of cusps
    — Connective tissue matrix degradation leads to cuspal tears and perforations or cuspal stretching
    — Tears also occur at flexure sites and at attachment sites to the stent and stent posts
  - Fractures of metallic components of mechanical valves rarely occurs

Pearls

- Most patients with bioprosthetic valves do not require lifetime anticoagulation, but valves wear out or become stenotic with mineralization and pannus overgrowth

- Mechanical valves are more durable but require anticoagulation
- Homografts are efficient in terms of hemodynamics and usually do not require prolonged anticoagulation but are of limited availability and require more demanding surgical technique; no valves are available for mitral position
- Ross procedure is advantageous in children with congenital heart disease; this technique uses the patient's pulmonic valve and pulmonary trunk to replace the aortic valve and aortic root with a homograft implanted in the pulmonary position

Selected References

Schoen FJ: Pathology of bioprostheses and other tissue heart valve replacements. In Silver MD (ed): Cardiovascular Pathology, 2nd ed. New York, Churchill Livingstone, 1991, pp 1547-1606.

Silver MD, Wilson GJ: Pathology of mechanical heart valve prostheses and vascular grafts made of artificial materials. In Silver MD (ed): Cardiovascular Pathology, 2nd ed. New York, Churchill Livingstone, 1991, pp 1487-1546.

Myxoma

Clinical Features

- Most common primary cardiac tumor in adults
- Clinical manifestations include constitutional symptoms, an embolic phenomenon, and valvular stenosis
- Sporadic tumors more prevalent in women; peak incidence in fifth decade
- Familial tumors often present earlier, with equal sex distribution and more frequent right atrial or multiple site involvement

Gross Pathology

- Most frequently found in the left atrium attached to the fossa ovalis but may be found in any cardiac chamber and sometimes attached to valves
- Usually pedunculated with short stalk; rarely sessile
- Varies from a soft, gelatinous, papillary mass to a firm, smooth mass
- Cut surface shows a variegated appearance, frequently with areas of hemorrhage and cyst formation
- Calcification may be focal or extensive

Histopathology

- Tumor is composed of polygonal, bipolar, or stellate myxoma or lepidic cells that have round to oval nuclei with inconspicuous nucleoli, eosinophilic cytoplasm, and indistinct borders
- Cells may be scattered singly, aggregate in small nests or cords, or form rings surrounding vascular channels
- Minimal pleomorphism and mitoses
- Background typically consists of myxoid and loose fibrous tissue with scattered lymphocytic and histiocytic infiltrate, especially hemosiderin-laden macrophages
- Surface thrombus may be identified
- Rarely, ossification and mucinous glands may be seen

Figure 18-10. Cardiac myxoma. A, Gross photograph of a myxoma with a smooth outer surface and a short pedicle. Cut surface is myxoid with areas of hemorrhage. **B,** The histologic section shows concentrically arranged layers of elongated neoplastic (lepidic) cells around blood vessels and cords of tumor cells in abundant eosinophilic stroma.

Special Stains and Immunohistochemistry

- Reactive with vimentin, CD34, and α_1-antichymotrypsin

Other Techniques for Diagnosis

- Noncontributory

Differential Diagnosis

▌ Organized thrombus
- Hypocellular fibrous endocardial tumors or organized intravascular thrombi
- Spindle mesenchymal cells are not arranged in cords, nests, or ring structures
- Base of endocardial lesions does not contain the lymphocytic infiltrates or prominent thick-walled vessels that are often present in myxoma
- Differentiation between thromboembolus and myxoma embolus may not be possible at times

▌ Myxoid sarcomas
- Most cardiac sarcomas are also found in the left atrium and often have myxoid stroma
- Foci of atypical spindle cells with nuclear pleomorphism, hypercellularity, and increased mitotic activity
- Tumor cells do not form cords or ring structures around blood vessels
- Tumor cells often exhibit storiform growth pattern with arborizing vessels

▌ Papillary fibroelastoma
- Typically located on valves
- Soft and papillary tumors can be grossly misdiagnosed as myxoma but are readily distinguished from myxoma on histology

Pearls

- Neoplastic nature is supported by demonstration of chromosomal abnormalities and aneuploidy
- Villous or papillary surface is associated with embolic events
- Tumor production of interleukin-6 is correlated with constitutional symptoms, including fever, weight loss, and fatigue
- Surgical excision is curative; recurrence is more frequent in familial tumors
- Some familial myxomas are manifestations of Carney complex (myxomas at various sites, endocrine tumors, and spotty pigmentation of the skin)

Selected References

Acebo E, Val-Bernal JF, Gomez-Roman JJ, Revuelta JM: Clinicopathologic study and DNA analysis of 37 cardiac myxomas: A 28-year experience. Chest 123:1379-1385, 2003.

Burke AP, Virmani R: Cardiac myxoma: A clinicopathologic study. Am J Clin Pathol 100:671-680, 1993.

Dewald GW, Dahl RJ, Spurbeck JL, et al: Chromosomally abnormal clones and non-random telomeric translocations in cardiac myxomas. Mayo Clin Proc 62:558-567, 1987.

McCarthy PM, Piehler JM, Schaff HV, et al: The significance of multiple, recurrent, and "complex" cardiac myxomas. J Thorac Cardiovasc Surg 91:389-396, 1986.

Rhabdomyoma

Clinical Features

- Benign congenital cardiac tumor believed to be a hamartoma
- Most common cardiac tumor in infancy and childhood; most are found in infants 1 year or younger
- Usually occurs in patients with tuberous sclerosis but may be sporadic or arise in patients with structural congenital heart disease
- Symptoms related to tuberous sclerosis, fetal hydrops, congestive heart failure, arrhythmias, and intracardiac obstruction in the perinatal period

Gross Pathology

- White, solid, well-circumscribed nodules
- Multiple tumors can measure less than 0.1 cm
- Most often found in the ventricular septum or the left ventricle

Histopathology

- Well-circumscribed tumors composed of large, vacuolated, atypical myocytes with central nuclei and a thin peripheral rim of cytoplasm
- Radial cytoplasmic strands extending from the nucleus to the cell wall are responsible for the term *spider cells*
- Intervening clear cytoplasm contains abundant glycogen

Special Stains and Immunohistochemistry

- PAS highlights abundant glycogen content in cells
- Reactive with muscle markers desmin, smooth muscle actin, and myoglobin; also reactive with hamartin, tuberin, and ubiquitin

Other Techniques for Diagnosis

- Electron microscopy: intercalated disklike structures around the cell periphery with abundant glycogen and a decreased number of small mitochondria

Differential Diagnosis

▌ Glycogen storage disease (e.g., Pompe disease)
- Myocytes show vacuolization owing to abundant cytoplasmic glycogen
- Involves the myocardium in a more diffuse manner; distinct tumor nodules not seen

■ Histiocytoid cardiomyopathy
- Cardiac hamartoma often manifesting as ventricular tachyarrhythmias or sudden death in infants and children
- Clusters of large round to oval cells with pale granular cytoplasm resembling histiocytes
- Ultrastructural studies show proliferation of mitochondria, absence of T tubules, and few myofibrils

Pearls

- Tumors increase in size until 32 weeks of gestation and then regress progressively
- Multiple rhabdomyomas are associated with tuberous sclerosis in 50% to 80% of cases
- Cardiac rhabdomyomas may be the earliest marker of disease in tuberous sclerosis caused by mutations in TSC1, encoding the protein hamartin, and TSC2, encoding the protein tuberin
- Surgical excision is recommended only in patients with severe hemodynamic compromise or persistent arrhythmias

Selected References

Bader RS, Chitayat D, Kelly E, et al: Fetal rhabdomyoma: Prenatal diagnosis, clinical outcome, and incidence of associated tuberous sclerosis complex. J Pediatr 143:620-624, 2003.

Becker AE: Primary heart tumors in the pediatric age group: A review of salient pathologic features relevant for clinicians. Pediatr Cardiol 21:317-323, 2000.

Burke AP, Virmani R: Cardiac rhabdomyoma: A clinicopathologic study. Mod Pathol 4:70-74, 1991.

Fibroma

Clinical Features

- Rare, benign congenital cardiac tumor, probably a fibrous hamartoma
- Usually seen in infancy and childhood
- Clinical presentation is related to left ventricular outflow obstruction, ventricular dysfunction, and conduction disturbances, depending on the location and extent of tumor
- Cardiomegaly is the most common radiologic finding

Gross Pathology

- Usually a single large mural lesion in the ventricular septum or left ventricular free wall
- Round, homogeneous mass of whorled, rubbery, white fibrous tissue
- May show circumscribed or infiltrative borders

Histopathology

- Cellular tumor consisting of spindle-shaped fibroblasts and mild to extensive stromal collagen deposition, commonly with elastic fibers

- Minimal pleomorphism and rare mitotic figures
- Often shows irregular, infiltrating margin
- Calcification is common
- Lymphocytic infiltrate around small vessels may be seen
- Tumor cellularity decreases with age, and collagen content increases with age

Special Stains and Immunohistochemistry

- Reactive with vimentin; may be focally reactive with smooth muscle actin

Other Techniques for Diagnosis

- Noncontributory

Differential Diagnosis

■ Fibrosarcoma
- Frequent site of involvement is the left atrium
- May resemble a cellular fibroma in newborns and infants but contains more frequent mitoses

■ Inflammatory pseudotumor
- Rare cardiac tumor
- Less cellular mass showing a prominent mixed inflammatory cell infiltrate

Pearls

- Residual tumor after incomplete resection usually remains stable for years
- Spontaneous regression has been reported
- Occasional association with nevoid basal cell carcinoma syndrome (Gorlin-Goltz syndrome) manifesting with enlarged occipital circumference, odontogenic keratocysts of the jaws, epidermal cysts, rib anomalies, ovarian fibromas, and multiple basal cell carcinomas of the skin

Selected References

Thomas-de-Montpreville V, Nottin R, Dulmet E, Serraf A: Heart tumors in children and adults: Clinicopathological study of 59 patients from a surgical center. Cardiovasc Pathol 16:22-28, 2007.

Cho JM, Danielson GK, Puga FJ, et al: Surgical resection of ventricular cardiac fibromas: Early and late results. Ann Thorac Surg 76:1929-1934, 2003.

Burke AP, Rosado-de-Christenson M, Templeton PA, Virmani R: Cardiac fibroma: Clinicopathologic correlates and surgical treatment. J Thorac Cardiovasc Surg 108:862-870, 1994.

Papillary Fibroelastoma

Clinical Features

- Benign endocardial tumor that seldom causes symptoms and usually is an incidental finding on echocardiography or at autopsy
- Most commonly located on the aortic valve but can be found anywhere on any valve, endocardial surfaces, or chordae tendineae

Figure 18-11. Papillary fibroelastoma. A, Gross photograph of papillary fibroelastomas shows delicate branching papillary structures best appreciated when examined underwater. **B** and **C,** Movat-stained section shows a dense central core of collagen at the base. The papillary fronds consist of central fibrous cores surrounded by concentric layers of elastic fibers. A thin myxoid layer rich in acid mucopolysaccharides and an overlying layer of endothelial cells surround the fibroelastic core.

- Right-sided papillary fibroelastomas are usually asymptomatic; left-sided tumors may present with symptoms of embolization or prolapse into coronary ostia
- Most commonly diagnosed in the fifth and sixth decades of life

Gross Pathology

- Typically small, frondlike, soft to fibrotic outgrowths that may be sessile or attached by a short stalk
- Soft polypoid lesions are best examined underwater to appreciate the papillary villous configuration of the tumor, which has been likened to a sea anemone
- May occasionally be multiple

Histopathology

- Branching papillary fronds composed of an avascular dense central core surrounded by a myxoid loose connective tissue stroma
- Papillae are covered by an endothelial cell lining
- Central core contains collagen and elastin

Special Stains and Immunohistochemistry

- Movat highlights elastic fibers and collagenous core

Other Techniques for Diagnosis

- Noncontributory

Differential Diagnosis

▌ Papillary myxoma
- Contains typical polygonal or stellate myxoma cells arranged in ringlike structures around vascular channels
- Usually attached to the atrial septum; rarely seen on valve surfaces
- Most do not contain elastic tissue

▌ Lambl excrescences
- Probably related to age, typically found in elderly patients
- Often multiple, usually smaller than 0.5 cm, and found on cardiac valves along the line of closure and nodule of Arantius
- Not seen on the arterial side of semilunar valves or on mural endocardium
- Characterized by broad-based filiform processes without a central stalk

Pearls

- Tumor resembles large Lambl excrescences both grossly and microscopically

- Pathogenesis is unknown; suggested mechanisms are a reaction to prior endocardial damage, hamartomatous origin, and organizing thrombi
- Mobile tumors as detected on echocardiography are independent predictors of risk for embolic events and sudden cardiac death
- Surgical excision is curative

Selected References

Gowda RM, Khan IA, Nair CK, et al: Cardiac papillary fibroelastoma: A comprehensive analysis of 725 cases. Am Heart J 146:404-410, 2003.

Sun JP, Asher CR, Yang XS, et al: Clinical and echocardiographic characteristics of papillary fibroelastomas: A retrospective and prospective study in 162 patients. Circulation 103:2687-2693, 2001.

Rubin MA, Snell JA, Tazelaar HD, et al: Cardiac papillary fibroelastoma: An immunohistochemical investigation and unusual clinical manifestations. Mod Pathol 8:402-407, 1995.

Cardiac Sarcomas

Clinical Features

- Most common primary malignant tumors of the heart are sarcomas, representing about 95% of cases; the other 5% are hematologic malignancies (primarily non-Hodgkin lymphomas)
- Cardiac sarcomas include angiosarcoma, myxosarcoma, liposarcoma, fibrosarcoma, leiomyosarcoma, rhabdomyosarcoma, osteosarcoma, synovial sarcoma, neurofibrosarcoma, malignant fibrous histiocytoma, malignant mesenchymoma, and undifferentiated sarcoma
- Tumors are often asymptomatic until advanced stage
- Symptoms are related to intracavitary obstruction, embolic phenomena, local invasion causing arrhythmia, congestive heart failure, or pericardial effusion; constitutional symptoms are frequent
- Left atrium is commonly involved in most sarcomas
- Angiosarcoma
  - Most common primary malignant tumor of the heart
  - Characteristically located in the right-sided chambers, commonly originating from the right atrium
  - More common in males, with a peak incidence in the fourth decade
  - Patients often present with signs and symptoms of cardiac tamponade, pericardial constriction, right ventricular outflow obstruction, or pulmonary metastases
- Rhabdomyosarcoma
  - Occurs in infants, children, and young adults, with mean age at presentation in the second to third decade

  - Slightly more common in males
  - Can involve any chamber, with no predilection for left atrium

Gross Pathology

- Bulky, invasive masses that can have both intramural and intracavitary extension and epicardial infiltration
- Some tumors can have polypoid growth
- Tend to be multicentric
- Involvement of valvular structures by direct extension
- Firm cut surface with hemorrhages, cysts, or calcifications
- Angiosarcoma
  - Large, dark, multilobular hemorrhagic mass
  - May diffusely infiltrate local structures and pericardium
- Rhabdomyosarcoma
  - Can be found either in atrium or in ventricle
  - Soft, gray, bulky, invasive tumor that may appear myxoid or gelatinous

Histopathology

- Classified similar to soft tissue sarcomas (see Chapter 17)
- About 24% of primary cardiac sarcomas are unclassifiable and designated as undifferentiated sarcomas
- Undifferentiated sarcomas may be composed of pleomorphic, epithelioid, spindle, or small cells
- Sarcomas with more than 10 mitoses per high-power field and tumors with necrosis are considered high grade

Special Stains and Immunohistochemistry

- Vimentin positive in undifferentiated sarcomas
- Smooth muscle actin and muscle-specific actin focally positive in undifferentiated sarcomas, not specific for leiomyosarcoma
- CD34 and CD31 highlight endothelial cells
- Desmin highlights rhabdomyoblasts; also positive in some leiomyosarcomas
- Cytokeratin positive in epithelial cell component of synovial sarcoma
- S-100 focally positive in malignant peripheral nerve sheath tumors (neurofibrosarcoma)

Other Techniques for Diagnosis

- Synovial sarcoma: cytogenetic analysis for t(X;18)(p11.2;q11.2) chromosomal translocation

Differential Diagnosis

▌ Myxoma
- Lacks cellular pleomorphism and hypercellularity
- Absence of mitoses

- Absence of necrosis (groups of cells with neutrophilic infiltrate)
- Presence of capillary vessels surrounded by myxoma cells
- Chondroid differentiation not seen

Pearls

- Extensive sampling of tumor is important because some sarcomas can have hypocellular myxoid areas
- Prognosis is poor owing to advanced stage at presentation
- Reported survival rates at 1 and 3 years are 47% and 24%, respectively
- Histologic type and presence of differentiation do not correlate with prognosis
- Surgical approach ranges from open biopsy to complete resection to tumor debulking

Selected References

Bakaeen FG, Reardon MJ, Coselli JS, et al: Surgical outcome in 85 patients with primary cardiac tumors. Am J Surg 186:641-647, 2003.

Burke AP, Virmani R: Tumors of the Heart and Great Vessels. Atlas of Tumor Pathology, 3rd Series, Fascicle 16. Washington, DC, Armed Forces Institute of Pathology, 1996, pp 127-170.

Tazelaar HD, Locke TJ, McGregor CG: Pathology of surgically excised primary cardiac tumors. Mayo Clin Proc 67:957-965, 1992.

Burke AP, Cowan D, Virmani R: Primary sarcomas of the heart. Cancer 69:387-395, 1992.

Pericardium

Acute Pericarditis

Clinical Features

- Patients present with chest pain, pericardial friction rub, electrocardiographic changes, and constitutional symptoms

Gross Pathology

- Fibrinous and serofibrinous pericarditis are most common and cause a dry, dull, roughened pericardial surface with fibrinous adhesions
- Variable type and amount of effusion in pericardial sac, including serous, fibrinous, purulent, bloody, and caseous accumulations, depending on cause

Histopathology

- Histology generally not helpful in determining underlying cause
- Inflammatory cell infiltrates with neutrophils and lymphocytes, proliferation of capillaries, edema, and fibrin deposition

Special Stains and Immunohistochemistry

- Special stains for microorganisms (GMS, PAS, Ziehl-Neelsen) may identify causative organisms in infectious cases

Other Techniques for Diagnosis

- Noncontributory

Differential Diagnosis

- Idiopathic, viral infection, acute myocardial infarction, Dressler syndrome, uremia, bacterial infection (tuberculous and nontuberculous), chest irradiation, rheumatic fever, connective tissue diseases (rheumatoid arthritis, SLE, scleroderma), trauma, drugs, and neoplasms

Pearls

- Normal pericardium is a fibroelastic tissue lined by mesothelium
- Normal pericardial sac contains 15 to 50 mL of clear, straw-colored fluid
- Acute pericarditis that subsides in a few days is most often idiopathic
- Hemorrhagic effusions are often caused by malignancy and infection

Selected References

Ariyarajah V, Spodick DH: Acute pericarditis: Diagnostic cues and common electrocardiographic manifestations. Cardiol Rev 15:24-30, 2007.

Zayas R, Anguita M, Torres F, et al: Incidence of specific etiology and role of methods for specific etiologic diagnosis of primary acute pericarditis. Am J Cardiol 75:378-382, 1995.

Waller BF, Taliercio CP, Howard J, et al: Morphologic aspects of pericardial heart disease: Part I. Clin Cardiol 15:203-209, 1992.

Waller BF, Taliercio CP, Howard J, et al: Morphologic aspects of pericardial heart disease: Part II. Clin Cardiol 15:291-298, 1992.

Constrictive Pericarditis

Clinical Features

- Idiopathic in about half of cases
- A restrictive or constrictive clinical picture, with biventricular equalization of pressures, elevated jugular venous pressure, and significantly decreased cardiac output
- Effect on ventricular contraction may be mild to marked, depending on degree of constriction
- Enlarged congested liver or hypoperfused lungs may be seen

Gross Pathology

- Significant fibrous thickening of pericardium, with or without calcification

- Dense pericardial adhesions with obliteration of pericardial space

Histopathology

- Marked fibrosis, associated calcifications, neovascularization, and mild chronic lymphoplasmacytic cell infiltrate
- Hemosiderin-laden macrophages may be seen
- Occasional granulomas in constrictive tuberculous pericarditis

Special Stains and Immunohistochemistry

- Noncontributory

Other Techniques for Diagnosis

- Noncontributory

Differential Diagnosis

- Chest irradiation and previous cardiac surgery; classically caused by tuberculosis

Pearls

- Histology is generally not helpful in determining underlying cause
- Occasional patients with clinically constrictive physiology will have pericardial biopsy showing no fibrosis or calcification

Selected References

Oh KY, Shimizu M, Edwards WD, et al: Surgical pathology of the parietal pericardium: A study of 344 cases (1993-1999). Cardiovasc Pathol 10(4):157-168, 2001.

Ling LH, Oh JK, Schaff HV, et al: Constrictive pericarditis in the modern era: Evolving clinical spectrum and impact on outcome after pericardiectomy. Circulation 100:1380-1386, 1996.

Myers RB, Spodick DH: Constrictive pericarditis: Clinical and pathophysiologic characteristics. Am Heart J 138:219-232, 1999.

Pericardial Cysts

Clinical Features

- Asymptomatic except when large; chest pain is the most common symptom
- Often found incidentally on chest radiographs
- Most commonly located in the cardiophrenic angle but may also be seen in the any of the mediastinal compartments

Gross Pathology

- Thin-walled, uniloculated cysts with smooth lining and filled with clear fluid
- Typically small but may vary in size and weigh up to 300 g
- May occasionally communicate with the pericardial sac

Histopathology

- Cyst wall composed of fibrous connective tissue and lined by a layer of flattened mesothelial cells

Special Stains and Immunohistochemistry

- Noncontributory

Other Techniques for Diagnosis

- Noncontributory

Differential Diagnosis

■ Loculated effusion
- Does not have a cyst wall with lining

■ Bronchogenic cyst
- Most commonly found in the anterior or middle mediastinum, may be intracardiac or intrapericardial
- Contains mucoid material
- Lined by pseudostratified ciliated columnar cells with smooth muscle and cartilage in the wall

Pearls

- Pericardial cysts are considered congenital lesions but are diagnosed in adulthood

Selected References

Wick MR: Cystic lesions of the mediastinum. Semin Diagn Pathol 22:241-253, 2005.

Patel J, Park C, Michaels J, et al: Pericardial cyst: Case reports and a literature review. Echocardiography 21:269-272, 2004.

Stoller JK, Shaw C, Matthay RA: Enlarging, atypically located pericardial cyst: Recent experience and literature review. Chest 89:402-406, 1986.

Localized Fibrous Tumor of the Pericardium

Clinical Features

- Extremely rare benign pericardial tumor
- Often are incidental findings; some patients present with dyspnea and pericardial effusion

Gross Pathology

- May be broad based or attached to the pericardium by a stalk; rarely, arise from the epicardium and encase the heart
- Round to ovoid, white, well-circumscribed mass with a firm, whorled cut surface
- Cystic change may be seen
- No invasion into the myocardium

Histopathology

- Consists of patternless proliferation or short fascicles of spindled fibroblasts with thick collagen bundles
- Alternating hypocellular and hypercellular areas
- Hemangiopericytoma-like vascular pattern

- Minimal pleomorphism, mitotic activity, and necrosis
- May have focal calcification

Special Stains and Immunohistochemistry

- Vimentin and CD34 positive
- Cytokeratin, actin, and S-100 negative

Other Techniques for Diagnosis

- Noncontributory

Differential Diagnosis

▌ Sarcomatoid mesothelioma
- Invasion of underlying tissue
- Presence of marked nuclear pleomorphism and hyperchromasia
- Negative for CD34

Pearls

- Surgical excision is usually curative

Selected References

Andreani SM, Tavecchio L, Giardini R, Bedini AV: Extrapericardial solitary fibrous tumour of the pericardium. Eur J Cardiothorac Surg 14:98-100, 1998.

el-Naggar AK, Ro JY, Ayala AG, et al: Localized fibrous tumor of the serosal cavities: Immunohistochemical, electron-microscopic, and flow-cytometric DNA study. Am J Clin Pathol 92:561-565, 1989.

Primary Malignant Tumors of the Pericardium

Clinical Features

- Clinical findings of dyspnea, constrictive pericarditis, pericardial effusion, and cardiac tamponade are frequent
- Male predominance
- Pericardial mesothelioma
  — Represents less than 2% of malignant mesotheliomas of serosal membranes
  — May be localized or diffuse
  — Male predominance
- Pericardial angiosarcoma
  — Less common than primary angiosarcoma of the heart

Gross Pathology

- Tumors are found in the parietal and visceral pericardium (epicardium) as coalescent nodules that obliterate the pericardial space and may diffusely encase the heart and great vessels
- Pericardial mesothelioma
  — Solitary or localized mesothelioma is rare
  — Usually invades the heart only superficially
- Pericardial angiosarcoma
  — Invades the myocardium, and in one fourth of cases, intracavitary extension is seen

Histopathology

▌ Pericardial mesothelioma
- Epithelioid, sarcomatoid, and mixed types have all been reported
- Histology similar to mesothelioma of pleura and peritoneum

▌ Pericardial angiosarcoma
- Anastomosing vascular channels lined by atypical endothelial cells with abundant mitotic activity and areas of necrosis
- Solid areas of epithelioid anaplastic cells or spindle cells are often present

Special Stains and Immunohistochemistry

- Reticulin stain highlights a vascular pattern in angiosarcoma
- CK5/6, calretinin, WT-1, HBME-1, thrombomodulin, mesothelin, podoplanin, D2-40, and h-caldesmon are considered positive markers in mesothelioma
- CD31, CD34, and von Willebrand factor are positive in angiosarcoma

Other Techniques for Diagnosis

- Pericardial mesothelioma
  — Electron microscopy: numerous long, slender, smooth microvilli on cellular surface and intracellular and intercellular lumens with length-to-diameter ratio greater than 10 in epithelioid mesothelioma; epithelial differentiation of sarcomatoid mesotheliomas includes presence of intercellular junctions, surface microvilli, tonofilaments, and basal lamina formation
- Pericardial angiosarcoma
  — Electron microscopy: vasoformative structures and Weibel-Palade bodies

Differential Diagnosis

▌ Metastatic adenocarcinoma
- A panel of positive markers for adenocarcinomas arising from different sites (thyroid transcription factor-1, carcinoembryonic antigen, Leu-M1, MOC-31, BG-8, B72.3, Ber-EP4, and CA19-9) can be used in the evaluation of malignant pericardial tumors

▌ Epithelioid angiosarcoma versus mesothelioma
- Epithelioid angiosarcoma shows strong and diffuse reactivity for vimentin and absent to weak staining with cytokeratin
- Mesotheliomas will have more intense staining with cytokeratin and less intense vimentin staining
- Additional immunohistochemical stains (see "Special Stains and Immunohistochemistry") can establish the diagnosis in most instances

Pearls

- No definite association has been found between asbestos exposure and pericardial mesothelioma

- Pericardial mesothelioma may spread to adjacent pleura, mediastinum, diaphragm, and lymph nodes but rarely presents with distant metastases
- In advanced disease, differentiation between primary cardiac and pericardial angiosarcoma may not be possible

Selected References

Suster S, Moran CA: Applications and limitations of immunohistochemistry in the diagnosis of malignant mesothelioma. Adv Anat Pathol 13:316-329, 2006.

Val-Bernal JF, Figols J, Gomez-Roman JJ: Incidental localized (solitary) epithelial mesothelioma of the pericardium: Case report and literature review. Cardiovasc Pathol 11:181-185, 2002.

Lin BT, Colby T, Gown AM, et al: Malignant vascular tumors of the serous membranes mimicking mesothelioma: A report of 14 cases. Am J Surg Pathol 20:1431-1439, 1996.

Thomason R, Schlegel W, Lucca M, et al: Primary malignant mesothelioma of the pericardium: Case report and literature review. Tex Heart Inst J 21:170-174, 1994.

Metastatic Tumors of the Heart and Pericardium

Clinical Features

- Twenty to 40 times more common than primary tumors
- Signs and symptoms vary but include dyspnea on exertion, cough, chest pain, pericardial effusion, and conduction abnormalities
- Most commonly develop through lymphatic spread from primary epithelial tumors (lung and breast) in the thoracic cavity and usually metastasize to the pericardium
- Hematogenous spread occurs from melanoma, leukemia, sarcoma, and renal cell carcinoma and shows small myocardial metastases
- Intracavitary extension from the inferior vena cava into the right atrium most commonly occurs with renal cell carcinoma and hepatocellular carcinoma

Gross Pathology

- Metastatic tumors most commonly involve the pericardium
- In the heart, lesions are commonly found as epicardial and myocardial nodules or bulky intracavitary masses
- Valves and endocardium are relatively spared

Histopathology

- Carcinomas, lymphomas, and leukemias, in descending order of frequency, are the most common histologic types of malignancy seen
- Melanoma also often metastasizes to the heart

Special Stains and Immunohistochemistry

- Identical to primary tumor

Other Techniques for Diagnosis

- Identical to primary tumor

Differential Diagnosis

- See "Primary Malignant Tumors of the Pericardium"

Pearls

- In children, common metastatic tumors include non-Hodgkin lymphoma, neuroblastoma, sarcomas, Wilms tumor, and hepatoma
- Clinical evidence of cardiac involvement by metastatic neoplasms is found in only about 10% of patients; most of the cardiac symptoms result from pericardial effusions and pericardial constriction

Selected References

Butany J, Leong SW, Carmichael K, Komeda M: A 30-year analysis of cardiac neoplasms at autopsy. Can J Cardiol 21:675-680, 2005.

Roberts WC: Primary and secondary neoplasms of the heart. Am J Cardiol 80:671-682, 1997.

Abraham KP, Reddy V, Gattuso P: Neoplasms metastatic to the heart: Review of 3314 consecutive autopsies. Am J Cardiovasc Pathol 3:195-198, 1990.

Chan HS, Sonley MJ, Moes CA, et al: Primary and secondary tumors of childhood involving the heart, pericardium, and great vessels: A report of 75 cases and review of the literature. Cancer 56:825-836, 1985.

The Vasculitides

- Widely used criteria for classification of vasculitis are those of the American College of Rheumatology and the Chapel Hill Consensus Conference on the Nomenclature of Systemic Vasculitis
- Classification criteria were developed for use in clinical trials and epidemiologic studies; they were not intended for use as diagnostic criteria
- Useful information for the classification of vasculitis includes
  — Size of predominant vessels involved
    - Large vessels include the aorta and its major branches
    - Medium vessels include muscular arteries and small arteries that can be observed with the naked eye or visualized by arteriography
    - Small vessels include small arteries, arterioles, capillaries, and postcapillary venules, vessels that are typically 500 μm or less
    - Overlap in the size of involved vessels is often observed, but predominant vessels involved usually produce the typical clinical manifestations
  — Demographic profile, particularly age group and ethnicity
  — Organ tropism
  — Immune complex deposition

— Presence of antineutrophil cytoplasmic and anti–glomerular basement membrane antibodies in serum

● Pathologic evaluation alone is usually insufficient and may not always be required to make a clinical diagnosis

Large-Vessel Vasculitis

Clinical Features

▌ Giant cell arteritis

● Frequently involves the aorta and its major branches

● More commonly found in older females; rare in blacks and Asians

● Patients present with a variety of symptoms, including fatigue, headaches, jaw claudication, diplopia, and vision loss; common cause of fever of unknown origin in elderly patients

● Often associated with polymyalgia rheumatica

● Aortic involvement results in aneurysms, less often leads to stenosis, and is clinically manifest in only a minority of patients

● End-organ ischemia may result from luminal stenosis or occlusion of extracranial branches of the external and internal carotid arteries, most commonly involving the temporal artery; may involve vertebral or ophthalmic arteries

▌ Takayasu arteritis

● Typically occurs in patients younger than 40 years with female predominance; worldwide distribution, but higher frequency in Japan, Southeast Asia, and India

● Involvement of the aorta and its major branches, with frequent involvement of the subclavian and carotid arteries; may also involve coronary, pulmonary, mesenteric, and renal arteries

● Patients often present with fever, malaise, arthralgia, myalgia, and weight loss

● Causes ischemic symptoms (pulselessness, claudication, and blindness), loss or asymmetry of pulses and blood pressure, bruits, renovascular hypertension, and sometimes aortic aneurysms

Gross Pathology

● Aortic aneurysms will show wrinkled intima with a tree-bark appearance, indistinct medial layer, and variably thickened adventitia

● Stenotic lesions show fibrous thickening of the vessel wall with reduction in the lumen caliber of the aorta and major arteries; thrombosis may occur

Histopathology

▌ Giant cell arteritis

● Characterized by focal granulomatous inflammation of large and medium-sized arteries

● In the aorta, areas of laminar medial necrosis surrounded by granulomatous inflammation is common

Figure 18-12. Giant cell aortitis. A, Aorta shows a central area of inflammation disrupting the media, which in turn is acellular. The areas of absent smooth muscle cells correspond to laminar necrosis. In addition, there is fibrointimal hyperplasia, adventitial fibrosis, and mononuclear inflammation. **B,** Numerous multinucleated giant cells are admixed with the lymphohistiocytic infiltrates. **C,** Movat stain shows elastic lamellae within the eosinophilic areas of laminar medial necrosis.

Figure 18-13. Giant cell arteritis. A, A temporal artery biopsy shows transmural granulomatous inflammation with giant cells in the media and adventitia of this muscular artery. **B,** Movat stain shows disruption of the internal elastic lamina in the areas with inflammation and marked intimal hyperplasia. Fibrinoid necrosis is occasionally observed.

- In temporal arteries, infiltrates are centered along the internal elastic lamina
- Mixed inflammatory cell infiltrate consisting mainly of lymphocytes, plasma cells, and histiocytes with occasional neutrophils and eosinophils
- Giant cells are variably present, ranging from 44% to 100% of cases
- Healing or healed lesions show irregular fibrointimal proliferation, focal fibrosis, and scarring of the media and diminished inflammatory cell infiltrate

▌ Takayasu arteritis
- Variable inflammatory response, including a necrotizing acute inflammatory cell infiltrate, granulomatous inflammation with giant cells, or a chronic lymphocytic infiltrate
- Acute phase shows inflammation and neovascularization in the outer two thirds of media, adventitia, and adventitial fat
- Healing lesions may show minimal inflammatory component; often shows only medial scarring with focal loss of elastic lamellae and marked intimal and adventitial thickening and fibrosis

Special Stains and Immunohistochemistry
- Movat highlights the disrupted internal elastic lamina, aortic elastic lamellae, and fibrosis
- Trichrome demonstrates scarring in the vessel wall

Other Techniques for Diagnosis
- Noncontributory

Differential Diagnosis
▌ Giant cell arteritis and Takayasu disease
- Major discriminating clinical feature is the age of the patient; giant cell arteritis is common after 50 years, and Takayasu disease rarely occurs after 50 years

▌ Chronic sclerotic phase of aortitis
- Healed phase of Takayasu or giant cell arteritis may not be diagnosed with certainty
- Other causes of inflammatory aortitis, including infectious (syphilitic) disease and rheumatologic diseases (rheumatoid arthritis, ankylosing spondylitis, relapsing polychondritis, SLE, Behçet disease, and sarcoidosis), need to be considered in the differential diagnosis with correlative clinical information necessary to arrive at a diagnosis

▌ Age-related changes (arteriosclerosis)
- Concentric intimal thickening, fragmentation, and reduplication of the internal elastic lamina and foci of calcification may be seen
- Lacks inflammatory cell component

Pearls
▌ Giant cell arteritis and Takayasu arteritis cannot be confidently differentiated based on histopathologic features only

▌ Giant cell arteritis
- Because of the frequent involvement of temporal arteries in giant cell arteritis, "temporal arteritis" has often been used interchangeably with "giant cell arteritis" in the literature; however, *giant cell arteritis* is the preferred term because not all patients with giant cell arteritis have temporal arteritis, and not all cases of temporal arteritis are caused by giant cell arteritis
- Rate of positive temporal artery biopsies ranges between 10% and 20% of specimens; negative predictive value of temporal artery biopsy is about 90%
- Lesions of giant cell arteritis are typically segmental
  — At least three hematoxylin and eosin stain levels and one elastic stain of the temporal artery must be evaluated
  — Multiple sections of the aorta should be submitted

▌Takayasu arteritis
- Frequently diagnosed by clinical criteria and vascular imaging
- Stenotic lesions are found in up to 98% of patients and aneurysms in 27%
- Abdominal aorta is affected in about 40% of patients
- Most common sites requiring surgical intervention are aortic arch and branch vessels

▌Isolated aortitis
- Most often discovered after surgical resection of ascending aortic aneurysms
- Histopathologic features similar to those of giant cell aortitis, but patients lack evidence of systemic disease
- Favorable outcome even without medical therapy

Selected References

Maksimowicz-McKinnon K, Clark TM, Hoffman GS: Limitations of therapy and a guarded prognosis in an American cohort of Takayasu arteritis patients. Arthritis Rheum 56:1000-1009, 2007.

Miller DV, Isotalo PA, Weyand CM, et al: Surgical pathology of noninfectious ascending aortitis: A study of 45 cases with emphasis on an isolated variant. Am J Surg Pathol 30:1150-1158, 2006.

Bongartz T, Matteson EL: Large-vessel involvement in giant cell arteritis. Curr Opin Rheumatol 18:10-17, 2006.

Rojo-Leyva F, Ratliff NB, Cosgrove DM 3rd, Hoffman GS: Study of 52 patients with idiopathic aortitis from a cohort of 1,204 surgical cases. Arthritis Rheum 43:901-907, 2000.

Genereau T, Lortholary O, Pottier MA, et al: Temporal artery biopsy: A diagnostic tool for systemic necrotizing vasculitis. French Vasculitis Study Group. Arthritis Rheum 42:2674-2681, 1999.

Jennette JC, Falk RJ, Andrassy K, et al: Nomenclature of systemic vasculitides: Proposal of an international consensus conference. Arthritis Rheum 37:187-192, 1994.

Medium-Vessel Vasculitis

Clinical Features

▌Polyarteritis nodosa (PAN)
- Idiopathic systemic disease characterized by vasculitis involving medium-sized and small muscular arteries
- Most patients are in the fourth to sixth decades; male-to-female ratio is 2:1
- Patients usually have nonspecific systemic symptoms of weight loss and fever with focal symptoms in the specific organ involved (peripheral neuropathy, testicular pain, livedo reticularis, myalgias, and gastrointestinal infarction)
- Associated with deposition of circulating immune complexes in hepatitis B infection
- May become manifest in the course of hairy cell leukemia, rheumatoid arthritis, and Sjögren syndrome

- Arteriography detects aneurysms or occlusions of visceral arteries; commonly involved vessels are renal, coronary, hepatic, and mesenteric arteries; lung involvement (bronchial arteries) in up to 30% of patients

▌Kawasaki disease (mucocutaneous lymph node syndrome, infantile PAN)
- Acute self-limited disease typically affects infants and children (range, 6 months to 15 years; peaks at 13 to 24 months)
- Increased incidence in Japan and Korea
- In the United States, children of American Asian and Pacific Island origin have higher incidence compared with African American and white children
- Clinical criteria include fever for at least 5 days and at least four of the following clinical features: conjunctival injection, cervical lymphadenopathy, oral mucosal changes, polymorphous rash, and swelling or redness of the extremities
- Typically affects coronary arteries, but any muscular artery may be involved; subclavian, axillary, iliac, femoral, renal, and superior mesenteric artery involvement has been observed

Gross Pathology

▌PAN
- Tendency to occur at arterial branching sites
- Aneurysms or stenosis of the arteries may be seen
- Thrombosis is common

▌Kawasaki disease
- Coronary ectasia or aneurysm can be seen in the acute stage
- Regression of aneurysms is seen in half of the cases within 1 to 2 years
- Progression of aneurysms to stenotic lesions occurs in about 10%

Histopathology

▌PAN
- Lesions are usually in various stages of development
- Acute injury is characterized by transmural inflammation with focal segmental destruction of the wall and deposition of amorphous eosinophilic material (fibrinoid necrosis)
- Inflammation is initially neutrophilic but later is composed predominantly of lymphocytes and macrophages
- Healing lesions consist of granulation tissue within the vessel wall and may show luminal narrowing owing to thrombosis or fibrointimal proliferation
- Aneurysms and pseudoaneurysms may develop owing to weakening of the vessel wall

▌Kawasaki disease
- Inflammation consisting of lymphocytes and macrophages is first seen in the intima and adventitia, then progresses into the media

- Panarteritis is associated with neutrophilic infiltration, disruption of the internal elastic lamina, smooth muscle degeneration, and edema in the media
- Healed lesions show fibrointimal proliferation, recanalization, thinning of the media, destruction of the internal elastic lamina, and fibrosis in the adventitia

Special Stains and Immunohistochemistry

- Elastic highlights destruction of the elastic lamina
- Trichrome stains fibrin red
- Movat highlights both elastin and collagen

Other Techniques for Diagnosis

- Noncontributory

Differential Diagnosis

▌ PAN
- Isolated or single-organ vasculitis
  — Often an unexpected finding in surgical specimens resected for inflammatory processes or mass lesions
  — Isolated vasculitis has been reported from the gastrointestinal tract, gallbladder, appendix, breast, uterus, ovary, and testis
  — Although the histologic features are similar to those of PAN, use of PAN in the diagnosis is discouraged because it can be misleading
  — Necrotizing or granulomatous inflammation of the vessels can be present
  — Cured with resection and does not require systemic therapy
  — May be the first manifestation of a systemic vasculitis; clues to systemic disease include presence of systemic symptoms, acute-phase reactants, and serologic autoimmune markers
  — Long-term follow-up is necessary to confirm absence of systemic involvement
- Kawasaki disease
  — Fibrinoid necrosis is absent, and inflamed media is edematous
  — Predominance of mononuclear cells (T lymphocytes and macrophages) rather than neutrophils in the acute phase
- Small-vessel vasculitis
  — If involvement of only small arteries is seen in a biopsy, differentiation between medium-vessel and small-vessel vasculitis cannot be made accurately because small arteries can be affected in both conditions
- Vasculitis associated with connective tissue disorders
  — Most commonly arises in the setting of rheumatoid arthritis, SLE, or Sjögren syndrome and is correlated with disease activity
  — May involve vessels of any size; small-vessel involvement predominates
  — Clinically manifest with cutaneous or visceral organ involvement (usually renal or gastrointestinal)

- Cholesterol atheroembolism
  — Can present with multiorgan involvement including renal failure, tissue necrosis, or visceral organ infarction
  — Cholesterol emboli derived from ulcerated plaques in the aorta often affect the kidneys, intestines, and extremities
  — Embolization can occur spontaneously but is often triggered by invasive procedures, cardiovascular surgery, anticoagulation, and thrombolytic therapy
  — Occlusion of small arteries and arterioles by cholesterol emboli; cholesterol crystals induce foreign-body giant cell reaction and variable infiltrates of neutrophils, eosinophils, and mononuclear cells
- Segmental mediolytic arteriopathy
  — Presence of visceral ischemia, intra-abdominal hemorrhage, and multiple arterial aneurysms is usually mistaken for PAN
  — Abrupt gaps in the arterial wall due to loss of medial smooth muscle; gaps are bridged by fibrin deposits and hemorrhage
  — Vacuolar degeneration of smooth muscle cells results in intramural hemorrhage and dissection
  — Inflammation if present is minimal and limited to the adventitial fibrinous deposits

Pearls

▌ PAN
- Involvement of arterioles, venules, or capillaries (including pulmonary capillaritis and glomerulonephritis) is not consistent with a diagnosis of PAN as proposed in the Chapel Hill Consensus Conference
- Classic PAN has little association with antineutrophil cytoplasmic antibody (ANCA)
- Fibrinoid necrosis should not be equated with PAN
- Most patients have a chronic relapsing course; high-dose corticosteroids and often cyclophosphamide are typically beneficial
- Factors associated with a poor prognosis include age greater than 50 years and gastrointestinal, renal, or cardiac involvement
- Five-year survival rate approaches 80% in treated patients; often fatal if untreated

▌ Kawasaki disease
- Diagnosis is usually based on clinical criteria rather than tissue biopsy or angiography
- Coronary artery aneurysm develops in 15% to 25% of untreated cases; male patients, infants younger than 6 months of age, children older than 8 years, patients who did not receive intravenous immunoglobulin treatment or who have persistent fever despite treatment are at highest risk for this complication
- Giant aneurysms (diameter of coronary lumen ≥ 8 mm) are at risk for rupture in the acute phase and become stenotic with progressive intimal hyperplasia and thrombosis in the chronic phase

Selected References

Colmegna I, Maldonado-Cocco JA: Polyarteritis nodosa revisited. Curr Rheumatol Rep 7:288-296, 2005.

Takahashi K, Oharaseki T, Naoe S, et al: Neutrophilic involvement in the damage to coronary arteries in acute stage of Kawasaki disease. Pediatr Int 47:305-310, 2005.

Newburger JW, Takahashi M, Gerber MA, et al: Diagnosis, treatment, and long-term management of Kawasaki disease: A statement for health professionals from the Committee on Rheumatic Fever, Endocarditis and Kawasaki Disease, Council on Cardiovascular Disease in the Young, American Heart Association. Circulation 110:2747-2771, 2004.

Kato H, Sugimura T, Akagi T, et al: Long-term consequences of Kawasaki disease: A 10- to 21-year follow-up study of 594 patients. Circulation 94:1379-1385, 1996.

Lightfoot RW Jr, Michel BA, Bloch DA, et al: The American College of Rheumatology 1990 criteria for the classification of polyarteritis nodosa. Arthritis Rheum 33:1088-1093, 1990.

Pauci-immune Small-Vessel Vasculitis

Clinical Features

▌ Wegener granulomatosis
- Syndrome characterized by a necrotizing granulomatous vasculitis involving the upper and lower respiratory tract and glomerulonephritis
  — Head and neck involvement includes the nose, middle ear, eyes, sinuses, and subglottis, with symptoms of sinusitis, rhinitis, proptosis, septal perforation, or airway stenosis
  — Pulmonary manifestations include cough, hemoptysis, cavitary nodular densities, and lung infiltrates
  — Renal disease characterized by hematuria and proteinuria; occasionally renal failure
- Typically affects individuals in their fifth and sixth decades, with equal male-to-female distribution

Figure 18-14. Necrotizing arteritis. A testicular muscular-type artery shows fibrinoid necrosis with focal transmural acute inflammation.

- Strong association with ANCA
  — Autoantibodies directed against components of neutrophil granules and monocytes lysosomes
  — c-ANCA (cytoplasmic): antiproteinase-3 antibodies; present in up to 90% of cases
  — p-ANCA (perinuclear): antimyeloperoxidase antibodies; nonspecific; found in 5% to 10% of cases
  — Up to 20% of patients are negative for ANCA, especially those with the limited form of the disease

▌ Churg-Strauss syndrome (allergic granulomatosis and angiitis)
- Systemic necrotizing vasculitis associated with severe asthma, peripheral blood and tissue eosinophilia, extravascular granulomas, and multiple organ involvement
- Typically diagnosed in middle age, with slight male predominance
- Symptoms of allergic disease, eosinophilia, and systemic vasculitis usually do not occur simultaneously, and time interval between asthma and vasculitis is variable
- Affects multiple organ systems
  — Pulmonary infiltrates often noted on radiography; granulomatous pulmonary mass lesions and capillaritis causing alveolar hemorrhage more unusual in Churg-Strauss syndrome than in Wegener granulomatosis or microscopic polyangiitis
  — Mononeuritis multiplex, polyneuropathy, and central nervous system vasculitis
  — Nodules on extensor surfaces of joints; rash and palpable purpura on the lower extremities
  — Cardiac involvement is a significant cause of mortality; may be complicated by small coronary artery vasculitis and myocardial ischemia, mural thrombosis, endomyocardial fibrosis, cardiomyopathy, and acute or constrictive pericarditis
  — Gastrointestinal symptoms are related to eosinophilic gastroenteritis and mesenteric artery vasculitis
  — Kidneys are affected in one fourth of patients
  — Associated with p-ANCA in 40% to 60% of cases and less commonly with c-ANCA (10%)
  — ANCA-positive patients tend to have glomerulonephritis, pulmonary hemorrhage, and peripheral neuropathy; ANCA-negative patients manifest with cardiac involvement

▌ Microscopic polyangiitis
- Syndrome characterized by necrotizing small-vessel vasculitis with few or no immune deposits affecting arterioles, venules, and capillaries in the skin, kidneys, and lungs (glomeruli and pulmonary capillaries)

- Mean age of onset is 50 years, with slight male predominance
- Symptoms are nonspecific and include hemoptysis, hematuria, proteinuria, palpable purpura, neuropathy, myalgias, and arthralgias
- Serum-positive p-ANCA is characteristic (70% of cases)

Gross Pathology

- Noncontributory

Histopathology

■ Wegener granulomatosis
- Geographic areas of parenchymal necrosis (coagulative or suppurative), often surrounded by epithelioid histiocytes, are frequently seen in nasal and oral cavities, paranasal sinuses, trachea, or lung parenchyma
- Neutrophilic microabscesses with necrotic centers and nuclear debris
- Granulomas are small and poorly formed with palisading histiocytes around microabscesses or necrotic foci
- Hyperchromatic multinucleated giant cells are randomly dispersed
- Lymphocytes and plasma cells are typically present; eosinophils may be seen but are not abundant
- Necrotizing vasculitis affects small to medium-sized arteries and veins and may be minimal or absent in biopsy tissue
- Necrotizing vasculitis with partial or complete destruction of the vessel wall by granulomatous or nongranulomatous inflammation
- Other variants of pulmonary involvement include bronchocentric injury, intense stromal eosinophilia, bronchiolitis obliterans–organizing pneumonia-like, and pulmonary hemorrhage with capillaritis
- Head and neck lesions show similar changes of tissue necrosis, granulomatous inflammation, and vasculitis, but these changes often are not found concurrently in biopsies, probably because of sampling limitations
- Kidney lesions include focal segmental necrotizing glomerulonephritis, crescentic glomerulonephritis, glomerular thrombosis, interstitial granulomatous inflammation, and papillary necrosis

■ Churg-Strauss syndrome
- Typically affects small and medium-sized arteries and veins
- Vasculitis is characterized by fibrinoid necrosis with eosinophil-rich infiltrate; can be granulomatous or nongranulomatous
- Inflammatory cells are an admixture of eosinophils, neutrophils, lymphocytes, plasma cells, histiocytes, and multinucleated giant cells

- Pulmonary lesions consist of eosinophilic pneumonia, extravascular eosinophilic granuloma, and necrotizing vasculitis
- Skin biopsies reveal eosinophil-rich leukocytoclastic vasculitis, dermal eosinophilia, and extravascular necrotizing granuloma
- Cardiac involvement is that of eosinophilic myocarditis
- Glomerulonephritis can be focal, segmental, or crescentic glomerulonephritis

■ Microscopic polyangiitis
- Destruction of the vessel wall by polymorphonuclear and mononuclear infiltrates, often with leukocytoclasia and segmental fibrinoid necrosis
- Associated hemorrhage is common
- Cutaneous lesions often involve upper and middle dermal venules with a histologic pattern of leukocytoclastic vasculitis
- Pulmonary lesions show inflammation and necrosis of interalveolar septa and capillaries with neutrophils, nuclear dusts, and intra-alveolar hemorrhage
- Renal lesions are those of necrotizing and crescentic glomerulonephritis
- Lesions are typically of the same age
- May affect small and medium-sized arteries, but arterial involvement is not necessary for diagnosis
- Occasional thrombosis present in arteritis results in tissue infarction and ulceration
- Granulomatous inflammation is not seen

Special Stains and Immunohistochemistry

- Trichrome stains fibrin red
- Movat highlights both elastin and collagen

Other Techniques for Diagnosis

- Immunofluorescence microscopy: little or no staining with immunoglobulins (immunoglobulin G [IgG]) in the affected vessels (including glomeruli) for Wegener granulomatosis, Churg-Strauss syndrome, and microscopic polyangiitis; hence, these vasculitides are often referred to as *pauci-immune (ANCA-associated) small-vessel vasculitis*
- Electron microscopy: no immune complex–type deposits are detected

Differential Diagnosis

- There are no histologic features that are specific for the different types of small-vessel vasculitis; further classification is based on clinical criteria and serology in conjunction with biopsy of the relevant organ

■ PAN
- Proposed distinguishing feature of PAN is the absence of involvement of small vessels (i.e., arterioles, venules, or capillaries)
- Vasculitis is characterized by lesions of varying ages, including focal and segmental fibrinoid necrosis and occasional multinucleated giant cells, but granulomatous inflammation is not seen

- Does not cause pulmonary capillaritis or glomerulonephritis
- When small and medium-sized arteries are involved, necrotizing arteritis as a component of microscopic polyangiitis is histologically indistinguishable from that of PAN
- Positive ANCA is rare in PAN

▌ Goodpasture syndrome
- Clinical presentation of pulmonary-renal syndrome of alveolar hemorrhage and rapidly progressive glomerulonephritis similar to microscopic polyangiitis
- Associated with glomerular and alveolar capillary basement membrane antibodies; antigen target is an α_3 chain of type IV collagen
- Linear immunoglobulin deposition of IgG, often with C3, in glomerular and alveolar capillary basement membrane on immunofluorescence microscopy

▌ Drug-induced vasculitis
- Associated with recent medication use, most commonly antibiotics and diuretics
- Often isolated skin involvement; time interval from drug exposure to onset of rashes is highly variable
- Neutrophilic or lymphocytic vasculitis in superficial small vessels; if present, tissue eosinophilia is a clue to possible drug etiology
- Usually no ANCA association
- Drug-related vasculitis with positive ANCA: hydralazine, pantoprazole, propylthiouracil, carbimazole, minocycline, and cimetidine

▌ Infection-induced vasculitis
- Commonly implicated infectious agents are hepatitis B, mycoplasma, meningococci, streptococci, *Staphylococcus aureus*, *Pseudomonas* species, *Yersinia* species, *Legionella* species, *Helicobacter pylori*, herpesvirus, adenovirus, cytomegalovirus, parvovirus B19, *Mycobacterium tuberculosis*, *Rickettsia* species, and fungi
- Histology shows superficial neutrophilic small-vessel vasculitis
- Septic vasculitis will show luminal thrombosis with neutrophils, hemorrhage, microabscesses, and necrosis
- Eccentric or segmental vessel wall necrosis is more characteristic of systemic vasculitides

▌ Vasculitis associated with circulating immune complexes
- Immune complex deposition can occur in solid organ and hematologic malignancies, connective tissue disorders, chronic active hepatitis, and inflammatory bowel diseases

▌ Sarcoidosis
- Characterized by tight, compact granulomas usually without necrosis
- Granulomas typically distributed along interlobular septa and bronchovascular pathways
- Non-necrotizing granulomas within the media of vessels are frequently seen

- Necrosis is not a prominent feature
- Commonly lung involvement; rarely kidney involvement
- No association with c-ANCA or p-ANCA

▌ Eosinophilic pulmonary infiltrates
- Churg-Strauss syndrome needs to be differentiated from eosinophilic pneumonia, idiopathic hypereosinophilic syndrome, allergic bronchopulmonary aspergillosis, parasitic infections, and Hodgkin disease

▌ Epstein-Barr virus–associated lymphoproliferative disorders with propensity for angioinvasion
- Extranodal natural killer and T-cell lymphoma, nasal type (angiocentric lymphoma)
  — Most commonly involves the nasal and nasopharyngeal areas
  — Atypical lymphoid cells are small to medium in size
  — Tumor necrosis often present; neutrophilic infiltration rare
- Lymphomatoid granulomatosis
  — T-cell–rich, B-cell–proliferative disorder
  — Predilection for lung, but skin and central nervous system can also be affected
  — Destructive nodular infiltrates with central necrosis and prominent vascular and perivascular infiltration
  — Infiltrates consist of small lymphocytes, histiocytes, plasma cells, and atypical intermediate to large B cells
  — Absence of granulomatous inflammation

Pearls

- Vasculitis involving arterioles, capillaries, and venules allows for the diagnosis of small-vessel vasculitis
- ANCA testing by indirect immunofluorescence microscopy confirmed by enzyme-linked immuno-sorbent assay has about 99% sensitivity and 70% specificity; negative ANCA test does not rule out a diagnosis of pauci-immune small-vessel vasculitis
- Induction and remission therapy in pauci-immune ANCA-positive small-vessel vasculitis is similar for all subtypes and consists of systemic glucocorticoids and cyclophosphamide

▌ Wegener granulomatosis
- Etiology is unknown; evidence suggests an immune-mediated mechanism with a synergistic effect of ANCA and proinflammatory stimuli most likely of infectious origin
- Chronic carriage of *S. aureus* in the upper airways is associated with increased risk for relapses
- Evolution of inflammatory vascular lesions and symptoms over time may cause a change in the diagnosis of patients from microscopic polyangiitis to Wegener granulomatosis if patients subsequently develop granulomatous lesions

- Limited forms of Wegener granulomatosis spare the kidney
- c-ANCA levels are often used to monitor disease activity
▮ Churg-Strauss syndrome
  - Clinical manifestations may evolve over time or be suppressed by oral glucocorticoid therapy for asthma; sometimes, vasculitis precedes development of asthma
  - More frequent involvement of peripheral nerves, skin, and heart; less frequent involvement of kidneys; less frequently positive for ANCA than are Wegener granulomatosis and microscopic polyangiitis
  - Eosinophils may not be found or become less abundant in biopsies from patients treated with corticosteroids
  - Increased mortality rate is seen when two or more of the following are present at the time of diagnosis: elevated serum creatinine, proteinuria, and gastrointestinal, cardiac, and central nervous system involvement
▮ Microscopic polyangiitis
  - Previously referred to as *microscopic polyarteritis and microscopic periarteritis*; however, arterial involvement is not a constant feature
  - Known clinical and histologic overlap with Wegener granulomatosis

Selected References

Sable-Fourtassou R, Cohen P, Mahr A, et al: Antineutrophil cytoplasmic antibodies and the Churg-Strauss syndrome. Ann Intern Med 143:632-638, 2005.

Travis WD: Pathology of pulmonary vasculitis. Semin Respir Crit Care Med 25:475-482, 2004.

Guillevin L, Pagnoux C, Mouthon L: Churg-Strauss syndrome. Semin Respir Crit Care Med 25:535-545, 2004.

Jennette JC, Thomas DB, Falk RJ: Microscopic polyangiitis (microscopic polyarteritis). Semin Diagn Pathol 18:3-13, 2001.

Lie JT: Wegener's granulomatosis: Histological documentation of common and uncommon manifestations in 216 patients. Vasa 26:261-270, 1997.

Travis WD, Hoffman GS, Leavitt RY, et al: Surgical pathology of the lung in Wegener's granulomatosis. Review of 87 open lung biopsies from 67 patients. Am J Surg Pathol 15:315-333, 1991.

Leavitt RY, Fauci AS, Bloch DA, et al: The American College of Rheumatology 1990 criteria for the classification of Wegener's granulomatosis. Arthritis Rheum 33:1101-1107, 1990.

Masi AT, Hunder GG, Lie JT, et al: The American College of Rheumatology 1990 criteria for the classification of Churg-Strauss syndrome (allergic granulomatosis and angiitis). Arthritis Rheum 33:1094-1100, 1990.

Devaney KO, Travis WD, Hoffman G, et al: Interpretation of head and neck biopsies in Wegener's granulomatosis: A pathologic study of 126 biopsies in 70 patients. Am J Surg Pathol 14:555-564, 1990.

Immune Complex Small-Vessel Vasculitis

Clinical Features

▮ Henoch-Schönlein purpura
  - Most common form of small-vessel vasculitis in children (typically ages 3 to 15 years); males affected twice as commonly as females; rarely affects adults
  - Commonly preceded by an upper respiratory tract infection
  - Manifestations include nonthrombocytopenic palpable purpura, arthralgias, arthritis, colicky abdominal pain, and bloody diarrhea
  - Renal involvement with hematuria or mild proteinuria in up to 50% of cases; rarely a progressive renal disease
  - Serum IgA levels are increased in more than 50% of patients
▮ Cryoglobulinemic vasculitis
  - Mixed cryoglobulins are composed of monoclonal IgM and polyclonal IgG in type II and polyclonal IgM and IgG in type III
  - Can be essential or secondary to connective tissue diseases, hematologic malignancies, and infections
  - Mixed cryoglobulins are found in 55% to 90% of patients with chronic HCV infection, but cryoglobulinemic vasculitis is present in fewer than 5% of these patients
  - Syndrome is characterized by purpura, arthralgias, and weakness, usually with peripheral nervous system and renal involvement
  - Serologic tests show HCV viremia, anti-HCV antibodies, mixed cryoglobulins, high titers of rheumatoid factor, and low complement levels
  - Clonal B-lymphocyte expansion is responsible for autoantibody production with increased incidence of developing non-Hodgkin lymphoma

Gross Pathology

- Noncontributory

Histopathology

▮ Henoch-Schönlein purpura
  - Small-vessel vasculitis involving postcapillary venules, arterioles, and capillaries
  - Characterized by neutrophilic infiltrate with fibrin deposits and nuclear debris in small, predominantly superficial dermal vessels
  - Renal lesions vary from focal to diffuse mesangial proliferation to crescentic glomerulonephritis
▮ Cryoglobulinemic vasculitis
  - Skin biopsy shows leukocytoclastic vasculitis in superficial and deep dermal plexus
  - Some patients have lymphocytic vasculitis and involvement of medium-sized arteries
  - Membranoproliferative glomerulonephritis type I is the most common renal lesion; fibrinoid necrosis and crescents are absent to rare

Special Stains and Immunohistochemistry

- Noncontributory

Other Techniques for Diagnosis

▍Immunofluorescence microscopy
  - Henoch-Schönlein purpura: glomerular (mesangial, capillary wall, arteriolar) and dermal vascular staining with IgA and C3
  - Cryoglobulinemic vasculitis: vascular staining with IgM, IgG, or C3

▍Electron microscopy
  - Henoch-Schönlein purpura: with renal involvement, prominent electron-dense mesangial deposits are seen
  - Cryoglobulinemic vasculitis: mesangial and subendothelial deposits and intraluminal monocytes

Differential Diagnosis

▍Cutaneous leukocytoclastic vasculitis (hypersensitivity vasculitis)
  - Localized, self-limited cutaneous vasculitis often triggered by drugs or preceding infection
  - Similar histologic features of leukocytoclastic vasculitis in superficial vessels
  - Ulcers or subcutaneous nodules uncommon and suggest involvement of arteries in the dermal-subcutis interface in other systemic vasculitis
  - Diagnosis of exclusion; no systemic vasculitis or glomerulonephritis

▍Hypocomplementemic urticarial vasculitis
  - Chronic or recurrent urticaria with leukocytoclastic vasculitis and deposition of immunoglobulins and complement around vessels
  - Hypocomplementemia observed in patients with systemic manifestations including arthralgia or arthritis, uveitis or episcleritis, glomerulonephritis, recurrent abdominal pain, chronic obstructive pulmonary disease, and positive lupus band test on skin biopsy
  - Low serum C1q levels with anti-C1q autoantibodies
  - Associated with SLE and Sjögren syndrome

▍Drug-induced vasculitis
  - See "Differential Diagnosis" under "Pauci-immune Small-Vessel Vasculitis"

▍Infection-induced vasculitis
  - See "Differential Diagnosis" under "Pauci-immune Small-Vessel Vasculitis"

▍Malignancy-associated (paraneoplastic) vasculitis
  - Most common underlying malignancies are lymphomas and leukemias
  - Histopathology shows leukocytoclastic vasculitis, rarely lymphocytic vasculitis

▍Connective tissue disease–associated vasculitis
  - Frequently associated with SLE, rheumatoid arthritis, and Sjögren syndrome, and less commonly with dermatomyositis, scleroderma, and relapsing polychondritis

  - Affects small and medium-sized vessels
  - Can have neutrophilic, lymphocytic, or granulomatous infiltrates
  - Can be complicated by the presence of antiphospholipid antibodies that lead to vascular thrombosis
  - Can be positive for p-ANCA and, less commonly, c-ANCA

▍Pauci-immune small-vessel vasculitis
  - Skin lesions can be part of the initial presentation in Wegener granulomatosis, Churg-Strauss syndrome, and microscopic polyangiitis
  - Absence or paucity of immunoglobulin or complement deposits in vascular lesions

▍IgA nephropathy (Berger disease)
  - Renal lesions are histologically indistinguishable from Henoch-Schönlein purpura
  - Disease localized to the kidney; no systemic manifestations

Pearls

▍Henoch-Schönlein purpura
  - Etiologic agent is currently unknown
  - Typically self-limited; most cases spontaneously regress in 2 to 3 weeks without sequelae
  - Renal failure is the most common cause of morbidity and mortality; poor prognostic features include development of nephrotic syndrome and renal biopsy showing more than 50% of glomeruli with crescents
  - Treatment involves supportive therapy; corticosteroids only for severe systemic symptoms

▍Cryoglobulinemic vasculitis
  - There is no established classification or diagnostic criteria for cryoglobulinemic vasculitis
  - Diagnosis is established with serologic and histopathologic examination
  - Overlap of symptoms with Sjögren syndrome, autoimmune hepatitis, and B-cell lymphoproliferative disorders is recognized

Selected References

Carlson JA, Chen KR: Cutaneous vasculitis update: Small vessel neutrophilic vasculitis syndromes. Am J Dermatopathol 28:486-506, 2006.

Monti G, Pioltelli P, Saccardo F, et al: Incidence and characteristics of non-Hodgkin lymphomas in a multicenter case file of patients with hepatitis C virus-related symptomatic mixed cryoglobulinemias. Arch Intern Med 165:101-115, 2005.

Ferri C, Sebastiani M, Giuggioli D, et al: Mixed cryoglobulinemia: Demographic, clinical, and serologic features and survival in 231 patients. Semin Arthritis Rheum 33:355-374, 2004.

Saulsbury FT: Henoch-Schönlein purpura in children: Report of 100 patients and review of the literature. Medicine (Baltimore) 78:395-409, 1999.

Mills JA, Michel BA, Bloch DA, et al: The American College of Rheumatology 1990 criteria for the classification of Henoch-Schonlein purpura. Arthritis Rheum 33:1114-1121, 1990.

Buerger Disease (Thromboangiitis Obliterans)

Clinical Features

- Inflammatory and occlusive vascular disorder affecting small and medium-sized arteries and veins
- Typically involves the vessels of the distal upper and lower extremities; rare involvement of mesenteric arteries and veins
- Found almost exclusively in young men who are heavy smokers; occasionally reported in women smokers
- Onset before age of 40 years
- Patients with advanced disease may present with claudication, ischemic ulcers, or gangrene

Gross Pathology

- Segmental involvement of arteries or veins with acute or organized thrombosis and luminal narrowing

Histopathology

- Involves both small and medium-sized arteries and veins
- Acute lesions are diagnostic and consist of cellular inflammatory thrombus and mild acute transmural inflammation without fibrinoid necrosis
- Microabscesses are noted within the thrombus, often with multinucleated giant cells
- Older lesions show organizing thrombosis with chronic inflammation resulting in luminal occlusion; recanalization is often seen
- Internal elastic lamina remains intact in acute and chronic lesions
- Superficial migratory thrombophlebitis with or without inflammatory thrombus is seen in fewer than half of the patients

Special Stains and Immunohistochemistry

- Elastic highlights the intact elastic lamina

Other Techniques for Diagnosis

- Noncontributory

Differential Diagnosis

▐ Organizing thromboemboli
- Giant cells and prominent inflammatory infiltrate within the organizing thrombus are not seen
- Acute inflammation within the vessel wall is not seen
▐ Necrotizing arteritis
- Characterized by granulomatous or nongranulomatous inflammation with fibrinoid necrosis and destruction of the internal elastic lamina

Pearls

- Tobacco use appears to be a universal factor associated with this condition

- No laboratory or serologic tests are useful in establishing diagnosis
- Cessation of smoking with or without steroid therapy usually renders a good prognosis

Selected References

Olin JW, Shih A: Thromboangiitis obliterans (Buerger's disease). Curr Opin Rheumatol 18:18-24, 2006.

Ohta T, Ishioashi H, Hosaka M, Sugimoto I: Clinical and social consequences of Buerger disease. J Vasc Surg 39:176-180, 2004.

Fibromuscular Dysplasia

Clinical Features

- Noninflammatory, nonatherosclerotic vascular diseases that affect medium and small muscular arteries
- Can affect any artery, but the most commonly involved are the renal arteries (60% to 75%, bilateral in 35%) and carotid or vertebral arteries (25% to 30%)
- About 28% of cases have multiple arteries involved
- Most patients are asymptomatic; most common presentations are renovascular hypertension, cervical or epigastric systolic, and diastolic bruit
- Multisystem involvement mimics systemic necrotizing vasculitis with mesenteric ischemia, renal failure, syncope, stroke, end-organ ischemia, or extremity ischemia
- Typically affects young adults, more commonly women in the third and fourth decades
- Angiography shows the classic string-of-beads appearance

Gross Pathology

- Artery may show stenosis or segmental narrowing with or without dilations

Histopathology

▐ Medial fibromuscular dysplasia is divided into three subtypes
- Medial fibroplasia is the most common histologic type and characterized by thick fibromuscular ridges alternating with areas of medial thinning
  — Smooth muscle cells are disorganized and separated by moderate accumulation of collagen and ground substance
  — External elastic lamina is frequently fragmented
  — Intima is normal
  — Internal elastic lamina is disrupted in advanced lesions with microaneurysm formation
- Medial hyperplasia causes concentric luminal stenosis by proliferation of smooth muscle exhibiting minimal disorganization

- Perimedial fibroplasia shows excessive accumulation of elastic tissue between the outer media and adventitia with effacement of the external elastic lamina
▮ Intimal fibroplasia
  - Segmental concentric or eccentric accumulation of loose fibrous tissue without lipids or inflammatory cells
  - Internal elastic lamina is frequently fragmented or reduplicated
  - Media and adventitia are normal
▮ Adventitial (periarterial) fibroplasia
  - Dense collagen replaces the adventitia and extends into the periadventitial soft tissue
  - Intima and media including external elastic lamina are intact

Special Stains and Immunohistochemistry

- Elastic stain highlights destruction of the elastic lamina

Other Techniques for Diagnosis

- Noncontributory

Differential Diagnosis

▮ Atherosclerosis
  - Occurs in older population with high atherosclerotic risk factors
  - Atherosclerotic disease tends to affect the renal artery ostia and proximal portion; in contrast, fibromuscular dysplasia affects the distal two thirds and branches of the artery
  - Fibroatheromatous plaques with focal disruption of the elastic lamina and medial atrophy
▮ Healed arteritis
  - Medial destruction and focal loss of the elastic lamina may lead to aneurysm
  - Often granulation tissue or fibrosis is seen in the media
  - Residual inflammatory cell infiltrate may be seen
▮ Neurofibromatosis
  - Aneurysms and stenotic arterial lesions often involve the renal arteries, aorta, carotid, vertebral, and mesenteric vessels
  - Nodular intimal proliferation of spindle cells in a mucoid matrix, with disruption of the internal elastic lamina and attenuation of the media
  - Characteristic skin and skeletal abnormalities and tumorous growths in neurofibromatosis allows for clinical differentiation

Pearls

- Dissections, aneurysms, and arteriovenous fistulas are complications of fibromuscular dysplasia
- Classic angiographic findings are suggestive of this condition

- Percutaneous balloon angioplasty is performed for arterial stenosis; surgery is used to treat microaneurysms

Selected References

Slovut DP, Olin JW: Fibromuscular dysplasia. N Engl J Med 350:1862-1871, 2004.

Luscher TF, Lie JT, Stanson AW, et al: Arterial fibromuscular dysplasia. Mayo Clin Proc 62:931-952, 1987.

Heritable Disorders of Blood Vessels

Clinical Features

▮ Marfan syndrome
  - Autosomal dominant trait with variable clinical manifestations, including bilateral ectopia lentis, tall stature, long slender limbs, arachnodactyly, pectus excavatum or carinatum, and scoliosis
  - Aortic dissection follows a period of progressive aortic dilation
  - Patients with a second type of Marfan syndrome exhibit some of the cardiovascular and skeletal manifestations of Marfan syndrome but lack ocular abnormalities
▮ Loeys-Dietz syndrome
  - Autosomal dominant disorder characterized by a triad of arterial tortuosity and aneurysm, hypertelorism, and bifid uvula or cleft palate
  - Aneurysms in thoracic arterial branches are common, in addition to thoracic aortic aneurysm
  - High incidence of pregnancy-related complications and aortic dissection or rupture in young patients
▮ Ehlers-Danlos syndrome type IV (vascular Ehlers-Danlos syndrome)
  - Autosomal dominant group of heritable connective tissue disorders characterized by skin hyperextensibility, joint hypermobility, and tissue fragility
  - Only form of Ehlers-Danlos syndrome associated with increased risk for premature death owing to arterial, intestinal, or uterine ruptures
  - A major event is the presenting feature in about 70% of patients

Gross Pathology

- Aneurysmal aortic wall may be thin with a bluish tinge of the intima
- Dissection may be evident with a hematoma between the split media
- Chronic dissection shows a false lumen lined by white opalescent neointima
- Occasional intimal lacerations are not associated with intramural dissection and heal with neointima lining an ellipsoid intimal depression

Figure 18-15. Cystic medial degeneration. A, The hematoxylin and eosin stain shows areas of blue discoloration in the media. **B,** Movat stain shows corresponding mucopolysaccharide deposits with fragmentation and loss of elastic lamellae.

Figure 18-16. Aortic dissection. A, An acute dissection shows a false lumen filled with recent thrombus in the media. **B,** The intimomedial flap of a chronic dissection is shown with a thick neointima lining the plane of dissection.

Histopathology

- Cystic medial degeneration shows fragmentation and loss of elastic lamellae with or without significant proteoglycan deposition
- Laminar medial necrosis is characterized by loss of smooth muscle cells in the media with collapse of the elastic lamellae and fibrosis

- Aortic dissection
  — Dissection typically occurs between the inner two thirds and outer one third of the media
  — False lumen may be lined by blood, fibrin and thrombus, granulation tissue, or neointima, depending on the age of the lesion
  — Inner media usually shows medial necrosis

— Acute inflammation is usually limited to fibrinous deposits, extending minimally into the media
— Healed dissection is recognized by a linear vascularized collagenous scar tissue in the media

Special Stains and Immunohistochemistry

- Movat demonstrates loss of the elastic lamellae, loss of smooth muscle cells with fibrosis, and proteoglycan deposition

Other Techniques for Diagnosis

▌ Marfan syndrome
- Classic Marfan syndrome patients have mutations in the *fibrillin 1* gene
- Marfan syndrome type 2 is linked to mutations in the gene encoding transforming growth factor-β receptor 2 (*TGFBR2*)

▌ Loeys-Dietz syndrome
- Associated with mutations in *TGFBR1* and *TGFBR2*

▌ Ehlers-Danlos syndrome
- Caused by mutations in type III procollagen gene, *COL3A1*

Differential Diagnosis

▌ Medial changes are nonspecific, but quantitative differences are found between normal aging aorta and diseased or dilated aorta
- Conditions associated with cystic medial degeneration include normal aging process, systemic hypertension, bicuspid aortic valve, and Marfan syndrome

▌ Infectious aortitis
- Etiologic agents include *Staphylococcus aureus*, streptococci, *Salmonella* species, *Escherichia coli*, and *Mycobacteria* and *Clostridium* species
- Results from hematogenous seeding, septic embolization from infective endocarditis, or direct extension of infection from a contiguous site

- Abdominal aorta and femoral arteries more commonly affected than thoracic aorta
- Causes aortic rupture or produces saccular (mycotic) aneurysms
- Medial necrosis with marked acute inflammatory infiltrates in the media
- Inflammatory reaction in the adventitia common and includes neutrophilic infiltrates, microabscesses, edema, and granulation tissue

Pearls

- Ascending aortic aneurysms are clinically distinct from descending thoracic and abdominal aortic aneurysms
- Pathologic changes in the media vary considerably from one area to the next, necessitating multiple and extensive histologic sampling of the specimen

Selected References

Robinson PN, Arteaga-Solis E, Baldock C, et al: The molecular genetics of Marfan syndrome and related disorders. J Med Genet 43:769-787, 2006.

Homme JL, Aubry MC, Edwards WD, et al: Surgical pathology of the ascending aorta: A clinicopathologic study of 513 cases. Am J Surg Pathol 30:1159-1168, 2006.

Loeys BL, Schwarze U, Holm T, et al: Aneurysm syndromes caused by mutations in the TGF-beta receptor. N Engl J Med 355:788-798, 2006.

Pepin M, Schwarze U, Superti-Furga A, Byers PH: Clinical and genetic features of Ehlers-Danlos syndrome type IV, the vascular type. N Engl J Med 342:673-680, 2000.

Hahn RT, Roman MJ, Mogtader AH, Devereux RB: Association of aortic dilation with regurgitant, stenotic and functionally normal bicuspid aortic valves. J Am Coll Cardiol 19:283-288, 1992.

Elizabeth J. Cochran

19 Central Nervous System

Astrocytic Tumors

Diffuse Astrocytoma, Anaplastic Astrocytoma, Gliomatosis Cerebri, Glioneuronal Tumor with Neuropil-like Islands, Gliosarcoma, and Glioblastoma Multiforme (WHO Grades II, III, IV)

Clinical Features

- Account for 33% of all primary brain tumors and about 75% of diffuse gliomas
- Produce neurologic findings, including seizures; symptoms are related to mass effect, or focal neurologic deficits are related to the location of the tumor
- Computed tomography (CT) scans show an ill-defined area of low density
- Low-grade astrocytomas do not show contrast enhancement; higher-grade tumors, including anaplastic astrocytomas, gliosarcoma, and glioblastoma multiforme (GBM), typically enhance and frequently show ring enhancement
- Gliomatosis cerebri shows diffuse enlargement of involved areas without a focal mass identifiable (T1 hypointensity, T2 hyperintensity); no enhancement

Figure 19-1. A, Low-grade astrocytoma. Cellular infiltrate of neoplastic astrocytes showing nuclear enlargement, nuclear membrane irregularity, and slight hyperchromasia. **B, Anaplastic astrocytoma.** Highly cellular tumor composed of neoplastic astrocytes with moderate nuclear pleomorphism, hyperchromatism, nuclear membrane irregularity, and mitoses. **C, Glioblastoma multiforme (GBM).** Notice the prominent area of necrosis with pseudopalisading. **D, GBM.** Neoplastic astrocytes surrounding endothelial proliferation (glial fibrillary acidic protein stain).

- Astrocytoma occurs commonly in cerebral hemispheres in adults (mean age, 30 to 40 years) and in the brain stem in children; occasionally occur in cerebellum or spinal cord
- Anaplastic astrocytoma is typically found in adults (mean age, 45 years); pontine lesions are more common in children
- Gliomatosis cerebri
  — Glioma, usually astrocytic, which involves at least three cerebral lobes of the brain; usually bilateral involvement and without defined focal mass identifiable
  — Peak occurrence between ages 40 and 50 years
  — Wide-ranging signs and symptoms; generalized cognitive impairment, often without focal neurologic deficits
- GBM
  — Most frequently occurring brain tumor; up to 15% of all intracranial neoplasms and up to 75% of all astrocytic neoplasms
  — Overall, usually occurs in individuals between ages 45 and 75 years (80% occur in those older than 50 years); most commonly involves the cerebral hemispheres
  — Usually affects the brain stem in children

  — Primary glioblastoma occurs de novo as a grade IV neoplasm
    ◆ Most GBMs are primary and have a short (<3 months) clinical history
    ◆ Usually occur at older ages (mean age, 62 years)
  — Secondary glioblastomas occur in the setting of a previously diagnosed grade II or III astrocytoma
    ◆ Mean age of occurrence is 45 years

Gross Pathology

- Low-grade tumors have a variable gross appearance ranging from subtle, barely visible lesions to large, soft, gelatinous, gray-white ill-defined masses that blur the gray-white border and expand the cortex and white matter
- GBMs are typically large and often involve more than one lobe
  — Extension across the corpus callosum results in involvement of both hemispheres (*butterfly glioma*)
  — Hemorrhage and large areas of necrosis are characteristic
- Gliomatosis cerebri: diffuse enlargement of affected brain regions; usually, no distinct mass is seen

- Giant cell GBMs and gliosarcoma may each be sharply circumscribed and firm owing to presence of connective tissue components

Histopathology

- ▌ Astrocytoma (WHO grade II)
  - Hypercellular (relative to normal brain), infiltrative, ill-defined lesions typically centered in the white matter or less commonly the cerebral cortex
  - Presence of a single mitosis should not prompt designation as an anaplastic astrocytoma
  - Sample size is important in this determination; a small sample with a mitosis should suggest an anaplastic designation, but a single mitosis in a large resection should not prompt a higher-grade diagnosis
- ▌ Fibrillary astrocytomas: most common type
  - Neoplastic astrocytes are slightly pleomorphic and enlarged, with hyperchromatic angular cigar-shaped nuclei
  - Cytoplasm is often not visible, or scant asymmetrical cell processes are evident
  - Loose fibrillary glial matrix is present in more cellular areas
- ▌ Protoplasmic astrocytomas: rare variant of low-grade astrocytoma
  - Nuclei are round to oval, and fibrillary processes are not evident
  - Cells reside in loose mucoid matrix with prominent microcysts
- ▌ Gemistocytic astrocytoma
  - Neoplastic astrocytes have large cell bodies with abundant eosinophilic cytoplasm and short fibrillary processes and eccentric nuclei
  - Presence of at least 20% of gemistocytes is necessary for this designation
  - This subtype has a high tendency to progress to anaplastic astrocytoma
  - Mitotic figures are typically scant or absent
- ▌ Anaplastic astrocytoma (WHO grade III)
  - Tumor shows higher cellularity, increased nuclear pleomorphism, and hyperchromasia
  - Mitotic figures are present (see previous discussion of mitoses in astrocytoma)
- ▌ Gliomatosis cerebri (WHO grade III)
  - Growth pattern of diffuse glioma, most often astrocytoma, but may be mixed or oligodendroglioma
  - Astrocytic cells often contain elongated nuclei (may be confused with microglia)
  - Mitoses are usually sparse; endothelial proliferation and necrosis are absent
  - With longer survival, autopsy may show focal areas of higher grade (glioblastoma)
- ▌ Glioneuronal tumor with neuropil-like islands (WHO grade II or III)
  - Fibrillary or gemistocytic astrocytic components alternate with islands of neuropil-like tissue

containing neurocytic cells, frequently peripherally ringing the neuropil islands
  - Ganglion cells may also be present
  - Usually behaves in an aggressive and malignant fashion
- ▌ GBM (WHO grade IV)
  - Infiltrative, highly cellular tumor with a wide range of abnormal cytology
  - Most often present, at least focally, are cells with hyperchromatic, pleomorphic nuclei and ill-defined fibrillary cytoplasm
  - The following may also be seen: small cells (primitive appearing), multinucleated cells, giant cells, lipidized cells, granular cells, and epithelioid change
  - Numerous mitotic figures are always present
  - Rarely, metaplastic elements are present, including squamous or adenoid differentiation, bone, or cartilage
  - Required for diagnosis of GBM
    - Abundant vascular endothelial cell proliferation or areas of necrosis with or without pseudopalisading
- ▌ Variants of glioblastoma
  - Giant cell glioblastoma (WHO grade IV)
    - Large, bizarre cells with markedly pleomorphic nuclei and multinucleation
    - May have increased reticulin network and appear more circumscribed
  - Gliosarcoma (WHO grade IV)
    - Defined by the presence of a sarcomatous component in addition to a malignant astrocytic component of the neoplasm
    - Astrocytic component is high grade and may occasionally display adenoid or squamous metaplasia
    - Sarcomatous component shows histology suggesting fibrosarcoma or malignant fibrous histiocytoma most frequently
  - Small cell astrocytoma (WHO grade III or IV)
    - Monomorphous oval nuclei, mild nuclear hyperchromasia, occasional small nucleoli, scant cytoplasm, many mitoses
    - Endothelial proliferation or pseudopalisading necrosis may be present (if present, grade IV; if absent, grade III)
    - May exhibit architectural features causing confusion with oligodendroglioma, such as chicken-wire vasculature, clear halos, perineuronal satellitosis, and calcifications

Special Stains and Immunohistochemistry

- Glial fibrillary acidic protein (GFAP) positive in grade II; higher-grade tumors are highly variable in expression
- Mib-1 (Ki-67): labeling index is low in low-grade astrocytomas (<5%) and high in anaplastic

astrocytomas (5% to 10%) and glioblastomas (15% to 20%)

- Cytokeratin: may see cross-reactivity with AE1/AE3 cytokeratin antibody
- Epithelial membrane antigen (EMA) typically negative
- Positive for TP53; may help to identify a low-grade astrocytoma from reactive astrocytosis and from a pilocytic astrocytoma
- Reticulin highlights mesenchymal and sarcomatous components in gliosarcoma and desmoplastic component in giant cell GBM
- Periodic acid–Schiff (PAS) positive in granular cell change

Other Techniques for Diagnosis

- Electron microscopy
  — Astrocytes show cytoplasmic intermediate filaments and cell processes; poorly formed cell junctions may be seen
- Cytogenetics
  — *TP53* mutation: 59% of astrocytomas, 53% of anaplastic astrocytomas, 65% of secondary glioblastomas, 84% of giant cell GBMs, and 28% of primary glioblastomas
  — Loss of heterozygosity of chromosome 10q: 35% to 60% of anaplastic astrocytomas, and about equal frequencies in primary and secondary glioblastomas (60% to 70%)
  — *PTEN* mutation: 4% of secondary GBMs, 32% of primary GBMs, and 33% of giant cell GBMs
  — *EGFR* gene amplification, 8% of secondary glioblastomas, 5% of giant cell GBMs, and 36% of primary glioblastomas
  — Small-cell subtype: high frequency of *EGFR* amplification

Differential Diagnosis

▌ Metastasis (metastatic carcinoma or metastatic melanoma)
- Metastatic carcinoma: cytokeratin and EMA positive
- Metastatic melanoma: S-100 and HMB-45 typically positive
- GFAP negative

▌ Lymphoma
- May show radiologic findings similar to those in GBM
- Typically located in periventricular regions
- Angiocentric distribution
- Leukocyte common antigen (LCA) positive; most are of B-cell lineage (CD20 positive)

▌ Reactive astrocytosis
- Small cystlike spaces are not typically seen in reactive processes
- Cellularity is not as high as in astrocytomas
- Reactive astrocytes lack hyperchromatic and pleomorphic nuclei
- More regular arrangement of cells

▌ Oligodendroglioma
- Cells show cytologic features of oligodendrocytes, including perinuclear halos
- Composed of uniform round cells with minimal cytologic atypia
- Negative for GFAP
- Characteristic genetic profile: deletions of chromosomes 1p and 19q

▌ Demyelinating diseases
- Characteristically have numerous foamy macrophages and inflammatory cells
- Areas of demyelination may be identified with myelin stains

Pearls

- Patients with well-differentiated diffuse astrocytomas may be treated with surgery, radiation, or both; most patients die of the disease within 10 years; progression to a high-grade tumor commonly occurs (secondary GBM)
- Anaplastic astrocytoma may be treated with surgery and radiation; patients typically die in 2 to 3 years
- GBM is a highly aggressive tumor with a poor outcome; death usually results within 1 year; younger patients may have a slightly better outcome
- Astrocytomas of the brain stem occur most commonly in the first decade in the ventral pons, encasing the basilar artery and associated with a poor prognosis

Selected References

Edgar M, Rosenblum MK: Mixed glioneuronal tumors, recently described entities. Arch Pathol Lab Med 131:228-233, 2007.

Takei H, Bhattacharjee MB, Rivera A, et al: New immunohistochemical markers in the evaluation of central nervous system tumors: A review of seven selected adult and pediatric brain tumors. Arch Pathol Lab Med 131:234-241, 2007.

von Deimling A, Burger PC, Nakazato Y, et al: Diffuse astrocytoma. In Louis DN, Ohgaki H, Wiestler OD, Cavenee W (eds): World Health Organization: Classification of Tumours of the Central Nervous System. Lyon, IARC, 2007, pp 25-29.

Kleihues P, Burger PC, Rosenblum MK, et al: Anaplastic astrocytoma. In Louis DN, Ohgaki H, Wiestler OD, Cavenee W (eds): World Health Organization: Classification of Tumours of the Central Nervous System. Lyon, IARC, 2007, pp 30-32.

Kleihues P, Burger PC, Aldape KD, et al: Glioblastoma. In Louis DN, Ohgaki H, Wiestler OD, Cavenee W (eds): World Health Organization: Classification of Tumours of the Central Nervous System. Lyon, IARC, 2007, pp 33-49.

Fuller GN, Kros JM: Gliomatosis cerebri. In Louis DN, Ohgaki H, Wiestler OD, Cavenee W (eds): World Health Organization: Classification of Tumours of the Central Nervous System. Lyon, IARC, 2007, pp 50-52.

Perry A, Aldape KD, George DH, Burger PC. Small cell astrocytoma: An aggressive variant that is clinicopathologically and genetically distinct from anaplastic oligodendroglioma. Cancer 101:2318-2326, 2004.

Pilocytic Astrocytoma (WHO Grade I)

Clinical Features

- Occurs predominantly in children and young adults; usually presents in the first two decades
- Most common glioma in children
- Most frequently occurs in the cerebellum; may be seen in the optic nerve, third ventricle, hypothalamus, brain stem, cerebral hemispheres, or thalamus
- When arising in the brain stem, it is usually exophytic dorsally or extends into the cerebellopontine angle
- Patients can present with either focal or nonlocalized neurologic deficits or symptoms of increased intracranial pressure; may present with seizures

Gross Pathology

- Typically well-circumscribed, soft, gray, discrete tumors
- Cyst formation in about 50% of cases

Histopathology

- Most commonly demonstrates a biphasic pattern consisting of pilocytic areas and microcystic components
  — Loose, microcystic areas typically contain eosinophilic granular bodies or protein droplets
  — Pilocytic component shows elongated cells with densely packed fibrillary cytoplasm and Rosenthal fibers (tapered, eosinophilic, corkscrew-shaped hyaline structures); Rosenthal fibers are not always seen or necessary for diagnosis
- A diffuse variant of pilocytic astrocytomas having a dense fibrillary component and lacking microcystic areas has been described and has a good prognosis

- Neoplastic astrocytes are usually piloid and have uniform nuclei with minimal pleomorphism
- Multinucleated giant cells are commonly seen
- Mitotic activity is rare; more frequently seen in tumors of infants
- Vascular proliferation and areas of hyalinization are common features
- Focal areas of calcification may be seen, but necrosis is uncommon
- Although grossly circumscribed, the tumor may have microscopic infiltration into adjacent brain tissue
- Occasionally hypercellular tumors with increased pleomorphism and multinucleation (features associated with long-standing lesions) are seen

Special Stains and Immunohistochemistry

- GFAP positive
- Negative for TP53
- Mib-1 labeling index ranges from 0% to 4% (mean, 1%)

Other Techniques for Diagnosis

- Electron microscopy: pilocytic astrocytes show abundant intermediate filaments; eosinophilic granular bodies contain intermediate filaments, osmiophilic granules, and myelin figures
- Cytogenetics: gains are seen most often in chromosomes 5 and 7

Differential Diagnosis

▌ Diffuse astrocytoma
- Typically lack circumscription and contrast enhancement
- Tissue infiltration and malignant behavior are much more common
- Usually lacks biphasic pattern, Rosenthal fibers, and eosinophilic granular bodies

Figure 19-2. Pilocytic astrocytoma. A, Classic architecture of densely fibrillated areas alternating with microcystic areas. **B,** Diffuse pilocytic astrocytoma consisting only of densely packed elongated cells. Rosenthal fibers are also present.

- Pleomorphic xanthoastrocytoma
  - Lacks biphasic pattern
  - Typically more cellular and has increased nuclear pleomorphism
  - Xanthomatous cells are not seen in pilocytic astrocytoma
- Ganglion cell tumors
  - Show clustered atypical neurons, which are immunohistochemically positive with neuronal markers
- Hemangioblastoma
  - Also associated with cyst formation
  - Highly vascular with abundant reticulin formation
  - Contains foamy cells filled with lipid

Pearls

- Important to distinguish pilocytic astrocytomas from fibrillary or diffuse astrocytomas because treatment and prognosis are different
- Typically cured by complete resection; overall prognosis is excellent
- Rare tumors have an aggressive clinical course, and transformation to glioblastoma has been reported

Selected References

Scheithauer BW, Hawkins C, Tihan T, et al: Pilocytic astrocytoma. In Louis DN, Ohgaki H, Wiestler OD, Cavenee W (eds): World Health Organization: Classification of Tumours of the Central Nervous System. Lyon, IARC, 2007, pp 14-20.

Tihan T, Davis R, Elowitz E, et al: Practical value of Ki-67 and p53 labeling indexes in stereotactic biopsies of diffuse and pilocytic astrocytomas. Arch Pathol Lab Med 124:108-113, 2000.

Tomlinson FH, Scheithauer BW, Hayostek CJ, et al: The significance of atypia and histologic malignancy in pilocytic astrocytomas of the cerebellum: A clinicopathologic and flow cytometric study. J Child Neurol 9:301-310, 1994.

Pilomyxoid Astrocytoma (WHO Grade II)

Clinical Features

- Considered a variant of pilocytic astrocytoma
- Occurs in infants and young children (mean age, 18 months) and involves the chiasm and hypothalamus most often
- Has been reported in temporal lobe, thalamus, posterior fossa, and spinal cord
- Presenting symptoms may be nonlocalizing: failure to thrive, developmental delay, vomiting and feeding difficulties, generalized weakness, and altered levels of consciousness
- Focal neurologic symptoms also occur: visual disturbances and endocrine dysfunction
- Tendency to disseminate through cerebrospinal fluid and to recur

Gross Pathology

- Myxoid ill-defined mass

Histopathology

- Monomorphous, hypercellular, compact small bipolar cells set in a myxoid and fibrillary background
- An angiocentric pattern of arrangement of cells suggestive of perivascular pseudorosettes is often evident
- Limited peripheral parenchymal involvement
- Rare nuclear pleomorphism
- Usually lacks Rosenthal fibers and eosinophilic granular bodies
- Mitotic figures may be present
- Vascular proliferation and necrosis reported in some cases

Special Stains and Immunohistochemistry

- GFAP: diffuse positivity
- Vimentin positive
- Neuronal markers: negative
- Mib-1 labeling index ranges from 2% to 20%

Other Techniques for Diagnosis

- Cytogenetics: only rare case reports

Differential Diagnosis

- Pilocytic astrocytoma
  - Occurs also in the chiasm and hypothalamus
  - Rosenthal fibers and eosinophilic granular bodies present
  - Biphasic architecture

Pearls

- Report of transition of a pilomyxoid astrocytoma to a pilocytic astrocytoma supports a close relationship between these two entities
- Pilomyxoid astrocytoma is locally aggressive with a tendency to recur (76%) and disseminate through the cerebrospinal fluid (14%); overall survival is 63 months
- Focal areas of pilomyxoid features in an otherwise typical pilocytic astrocytoma do not indicate a diagnosis of pilomyxoid astrocytoma

Selected References

Brat DJ, Scheithauer BW, Fuller GN, Tihan T. Newly codified glial neoplasms of the 2007 WHO Classification of Tumours of the Central Nervous System: Angiocentric glioma, pilomyxoid astrocytoma and pituicytoma. Brain Pathol 17:319-324, 2007.

Ceppa EP, Bouffet E, Griebel R, Robinson C: The pilomyxoid astrocytoma and its relationship to pilocytic astrocytoma: Report of a case and a critical review of the entity. J Neurooncol 81:191-196, 2007.

Komotar RJ, Mocco J, Jones JE, et al: Pilomyxoid astrocytoma: diagnosis, prognosis, and management. Neurosurg Focus 18:E7, 2005.

Tihan T, Fisher PG, Kepner JL, et al: Pediatric astrocytomas with monomorphous pilomyxoid features and a less favorable outcome. J Neuropath Exp Neurol 58:1061-1068, 1999.

Pleomorphic Xanthoastrocytoma (WHO Grade II)

Clinical Features

- Rare astrocytic neoplasm usually found in children and young adults (66% are younger than 18 years)
- Superficial location in the cerebral hemisphere (most frequently temporal lobe) often involving the meninges; rare involvement of the deep gray matter, cerebellum, spinal cord, sella, suprasellar region, and retina
- Patients present typically with long history of seizures and occasional headaches; seldom with focal neurologic signs
- CT and magnetic resonance imaging (MRI) show a well-defined enhancing mass, adjacent to the meninges, that is solid or cystic with a mural nodule

Gross Pathology

- Well-defined, cystic mass with a mural nodule or a solid mass
- Often attached to the meninges; may spread along brain surface

Histopathology

- Varied histologic pattern ranging from single or multinucleated giant cells to irregular spindle cells showing intracellular lipid accumulation (xanthomatous change)
- Reticulin network surrounding individual tumor cells; desmoplasia often present

Figure 19-3. Pleomorphic xanthoastrocytoma. Infiltrate of neoplastic astrocytic cells with marked nuclear pleomorphism and xanthomatous changes. Eosinophilic granular bodies are present.

- Patchy lymphocytic infiltrates often seen
- Variable degrees of vascular sclerosis
- Eosinophilic granular bodies or protein droplets prominent
- Usually absent or inconspicuous mitotic activity and necrosis
- When numerous mitoses ($\geq$5 mitoses/10 high-power fields [hpf]) and necrosis are present, high rates of recurrence are seen (pleomorphic xanthoastrocytoma with anaplastic features)
- Neuronal differentiation may be present

Special Stains and Immunohistochemistry

- GFAP, S-100 protein, and CD34 positive
- Reticulin highlights fibrous network surrounding tumor cells
- Synaptophysin and neurofilament variably positive
- Mib-1 labeling index: less than 1%

Other Techniques for Diagnosis

- Electron microscopy: cells typically show abundant intermediate filaments, lysosomes, lipid droplets, basal lamina, and secondary lysosomes
- About 20% show ultrastructural features indicating neuronal differentiation: microtubules, dense core granules, and clear vesicles
- Cytogenetic analyses: gains of chromosomes 3 and 7 and alterations of chromosome 1

Differential Diagnosis

▌ Glioblastoma
- Important distinction from pleomorphic xanthoastrocytoma because of poor prognosis associated with glioblastoma
- Most lack reticulin investment and eosinophilic granular bodies
- Usually not cystic with mural nodules; always a high mitotic index and endothelial proliferation or necrosis

▌ Pilocytic astrocytoma
- Biphasic pattern is characteristic
- Rosenthal fibers are commonly found
- Usually less cellular and without xanthomatous changes

▌ Ganglion cell tumors
- Atypical neurons that are positive for neuronal markers (synaptophysin and neurofilament) are a defining feature
- Usually lack xanthomatous changes

Pearls

- Surgical resection is usually sufficient to control tumor
- Subtotally resected and recurrent tumors have been treated with radiation, with unclear results
- These tumors are hypothesized to arise from subpial astrocytes and often display neuronal differentiation

Selected References

Giannini C, Paulus W, Louis DN, Liberski P: Pleomorphic xanthoastrocytoma. In Louis DN, Ohgaki H, Wiestler OD, Cavenee W (eds): World Health Organization: Classification of Tumours of the Central Nervous System. Lyon, IARC, 2007, pp 22-24.

McClendon RE, Gray L, Shah LM, Friedman AH: Pleomorphic xanthoastrocytoma. In McClendon RE, Rosenblum MK, Bigner DD (eds): Russell and Rubenstein's Pathology of Tumors of the Nervous System. New York, Oxford, 2006.

Giannini C, Scheithauer BW, Lopes MBS, et al: Immunophenotype of pleomorphic xanthoastrocytoma. Am J Surg Pathol 26:479-485, 2002.

Kepes JJ: Pleomorphic xanthoastrocytoma: The birth of a diagnosis and a concept. Brain Pathol 3:269-274, 1993.

Subependymal Giant Cell Astrocytoma (WHO Grade I)

Clinical Features

- Most common neoplastic process involving the brain in patients with tuberous sclerosis
  - Tuberous sclerosis is an autosomal dominant disorder with markedly variable penetrance and an incidence between 1 per 9000 and 1 per 10,000 births
  - Central nervous system (CNS) abnormalities include cortical hamartomas (tubers), subcortical glioneuronal hamartomas, subependymal glial nodules, subependymal giant cell astrocytoma (SEGA); other organs affected are skin, eyes, kidney, and heart
  - Neurologic symptoms in tuberous sclerosis usually occur shortly after birth and include seizures and infantile spasms; cognitive disability and autism may become evident at older ages

Figure 19-4. Subependymal giant cell astrocytoma. Infiltrate of astrocytic-appearing cells with abundant, frequently spindled eosinophilic cytoplasm. Prominent nucleoli are frequent.

- Caused by mutation in two genes: *TSC1* (encoding hamartin) on chromosome 9 and *TSC2* (encoding tuberin) on chromosome 16
- SEGA rarely occurs without association with tuberous sclerosis
  - Occurs in 10% of persons with tuberous sclerosis
  - Usually develops during childhood or adolescence
  - Clinical symptoms are usually secondary to obstructive hydrocephalus and occur when large SEGAs block cerebrospinal fluid (CSF) flow

Gross Pathology

- Typically an exophytic, solid, fleshy, well-defined, tan mass arising in the wall of the lateral ventricle

Histopathology

- Variable cellular morphology, including
  - Polygonal cells with abundant eosinophilic cytoplasm suggestive of gemistocytic astrocytes
  - Spindle-shaped cells with fibrillary cytoplasm forming streams and bundles
  - Large pleomorphic cells with nuclei exhibiting prominent nucleoli, suggestive of neuronal differentiation (sometimes multinucleated)
  - Focal microcalcifications and scattered mast cells are common features
  - Ill-defined pseudorosette formation may be seen
  - Variable mitotic activity
  - Vascular proliferation and necrosis are uncommon
  - High-grade cytologic features do not appear to impose an adverse clinical course

Special Stains and Immunohistochemistry

- GFAP, S-100 protein, synaptophysin, and neurofilament positive
- Class III β-tubulin and neuropeptides (somatostatin and met-enkephalin) positive
- Mib-1 (Ki-67): few positive cells (low proliferative index)

Other Techniques for Diagnosis

- Cytogenetics: associated with abnormalities involving long arm of chromosome 9 (*TSC1*) and short arm of chromosome 16 (*TSC2*)

Differential Diagnosis

▌ Gemistocytic astrocytoma
  - May be confused because both lesions contain astrocytic cells with abundant pink glassy cytoplasm
  - Intraparenchymal tumor rather than an exophytic intraventricular mass
  - Typically shows an infiltrative architecture
  - No mast cell infiltrate and microcalcifications

▐ Subependymal glial nodule
  - Considered to be a precursor to SEGA
  - More frequently calcified than SEGA
  - Usually asymptomatic; shows no growth on serial brain scans
  - Histologically identical to SEGA

Pearls

  - Debate still exists as to whether SEGAs can occur outside the setting of tuberous sclerosis
  - Believed to be an astrocytic neoplasm; however, studies have shown that many tumors show a more glioneuronal phenotype
  - Tumors occasionally recur, but unlike gemistocytic astrocytoma, no malignant transformation has been shown, although local invasion has been reported
  - Only about 50% of tuberous sclerosis patients have a positive family history, suggesting a high rate of spontaneous mutation

Selected References

Lopes MBS, Wiestler OD, Stemmer-Rachamimov AO, Sharma MC: Tuberous sclerosis complex and subependymal giant cell astrocytoma. In Louis DN, Ohgaki H, Wiestler OD, Cavenee W (eds): World Health Organization: Classification of Tumours of the Central Nervous System. Lyon, IARC, 2007, pp 218-221.

Goh S, Butler W, Thiele EA: Subependymal giant cell tumors in tuberous sclerosis complex. Neurology 63:1457-1461, 2004.

Burger PC, Scheithauer BW, Vogel FS: The brain: Tumors. In Surgical Pathology of the Nervous System and Its Coverings, 4th ed. New York, Churchill Livingston, 2002, pp 220-223.

Oligodendroglial Tumors

Oligodendroglioma (WHO Grade II) and Anaplastic Oligodendroglioma (WHO Grade III)

Clinical Features

  - Reported to represent between 12% and 20% of all infiltrating gliomas
  - Typically occurs in adults (peak, fifth and sixth decades)
  - Patients present with a long history of progressively worsening neurologic symptoms
  - Commonly cause severe headache and epileptic seizures
  - CT and MRI show a well-defined mass, often with calcifications

Gross Pathology

  - Typically white-matter tumors; infiltration into the cortex is common, and infiltration into leptomeninges may be seen
  - Soft, ill-defined, gray-pink tumors

Figure 19-5. A, Low-grade oligodendroglioma. Moderately cellular tumor composed of cells with round hyperchromatic nuclei and clear cytoplasm, giving the characteristic fried-egg appearance. **B, Anaplastic oligodendroglioma.** Notice the mitoses, high cellularity, nuclear enlargement, and hyperchromatism.

  - Mucoid degeneration with a gelatinous appearance may be seen
  - Cyst formation and focal intratumoral hemorrhage are common

Histopathology

▐ Oligodendroglioma
  - Low to moderately cellular tumor composed of cells with round nuclei that are larger than normal oligodendrocytes and show atypia; nuclei are hyperchromatic and may appear lobate (cytologic features are well demonstrated with smear preparations)
  - Formalin-fixed, paraffin-embedded tissue often causes the tumor cells to swell, resulting in an enlarged cell with well-defined cell membranes and clear cytoplasm; fried-egg appearance (not seen on smear preparations, frozen sections, or quickly fixed tissue)
  - Few glial fibrillary processes are seen

- Two morphologic variants of oligodendroglial cells may also be present
  — Minigemistocytes or microgemistocytes, exhibiting small pools of eosinophilic cytoplasm
  — Gliofibrillary oligodendrocytes, exhibiting paranuclear eosinophilic fibrils
- A dense network of branching capillaries (chicken-wire appearance) is seen throughout tumor
- Mitotic activity is usually low
- Microcalcifications and mucoid and microcystic degeneration are helpful diagnostic features
- Focal hemorrhage is commonly seen
- Cortex is often involved; perinuclear satellitosis is often present

▌ Anaplastic oligodendroglioma
- Same cytologic features described previously but with increased nuclear atypia and cellular pleomorphism while retaining round nuclear outlines
- Increased cellularity is evident
- Mitotic activity is marked (minimum of 6 mitoses/10 hpf)
- Endothelial vascular proliferation has been shown in several studies to correlate with aggressive behavior and poor prognosis
- Presence of geographic necrosis (with or without pseudopalisading) has also been found to correlate with aggressive behavior and poor prognosis but is not an independent prognostic factor in all studies

▌ Oligodendroglioma with neurocytic differentiation
- Foci of Homer-Wright rosettes and perivascular pseudorosettes associated with small round dark nuclei (reminiscent of internal granular cell layer neurons) have been reported in otherwise typical oligodendrogliomas

Special Stains and Immunohistochemistry

- GFAP positive in reactive astrocytes; GFAP also positive in gliofibrillary oligodendrocytes and minigemistocytes
- Synaptophysin, Neu-N, and neurofilament negative except in rare specimen with foci of neurocytic differentiation
- Cytokeratin negative
- Mib-1: disease-free survival is significantly shorter in patients with a labeling index of more than 5% compared with patients with a labeling index of less than 5%

Other Techniques for Diagnosis

- Electron microscopy: presence of microtubules
- Cytogenetics: losses of 1p and 19q are almost always found together in oligodendrogliomas (50% to 80%)

Differential Diagnosis

▌ Diffuse astrocytoma
- Tumor cells have greater nuclear irregularity and pleomorphism, no perinuclear halos, and fibrillary cytoplasm

- GFAP positive
- *TP53* mutations; no losses of chromosomes 1p and 19q

▌ Small cell variant of anaplastic astrocytoma and glioblastoma
- Cytologically monotonous, but oval, not round, nuclei
- Numerous mitoses, pseudopalisading necrosis, vascular proliferation
- GFAP positive cytoplasmic processes
- No loss of chromosomes 1p and 19q
- Amplification of *EGFR* and *EGFRvIII*, loss of chromosome 10q

▌ Central neurocytoma
- Usually within the ventricle attached to the septum pellucidum
- Well circumscribed without infiltrative borders, neurocytic rosettes
- Positive for synaptophysin

▌ Dysembryoplastic neuroepithelial tumor (DNET)
- Usually found in younger individuals with a long history of seizures
- Most are located in the temporal lobe
- Histologically consists of a glioneuronal element, glial nodules, and cortical dysplasia

▌ Clear cell ependymoma
- Usually affects younger individuals
- Forms perivascular pseudorosettes consisting of cells with elongated, tapering processes and ependymal rosettes and canals
- GFAP positive

▌ Pilocytic astrocytoma
- Affects children usually
- Cerebellar location, but also in hypothalamus, optic nerve, and brain stem
- Elongated cells with prominent fibrillary cytoplasm
- GFAP positive

Pearls

- Loss of 1p and 19q is a strong predictor of response to chemotherapy (procarbazine, lomustine, vincristine [PCV] and temozolomide), possibly radiation therapy, and long survival in low- and high-grade oligodendrogliomas
- Combined loss of 1p and 19q is rare in other gliomas
- Testing for deletions of 1p and 19q may be indicated to help in diagnostic classification when a glioma does not clearly show morphologic features allowing definitive designation as oligodendroglioma
- Overall, patients have a survival time of 3 to 5 years for all oligodendrogliomas
- Other factors associated with increased survival: younger age, frontal location, complete surgical removal, and radiation
- Most patients with anaplastic oligodendroglioma die of local recurrence; CSF dissemination or systemic metastases occur rarely

Selected References

Aldape K, Burger PC, Perry A: Clinicopathologic aspects of 1p/19q loss and the diagnosis of oligodendroglioma. Arch Pathol Lab Med 131:242-251, 2007.

Perry A, Scheithauer BW, Macaulay RJB, et al: Oligodendrogliomas with neurocytic differentiation: A report of four cases with diagnostic and histogenetic implications. J Neuropathol Exp Neurol 61:947-955, 2002.

Giannini C, Scheithauer BW, Weaver AL, et al: Oligodendrogliomas: Reproducibility and prognostic value of histologic diagnosis and grading. J Neuropathol Exp Neurol 60:248-262, 2001.

Cairncross JG, Ueki K, Zlatescu MC, et al: Specific genetic predictors of chemotherapeutic response and survival in patients with anaplastic oligodendrogliomas. J Natl Cancer Inst 90:1473-1479, 1998.

Mixed Gliomas

Oligodendroglioma and Astrocytoma (WHO Grade II), Anaplastic Oligodendroglioma and Astrocytoma (WHO Grade III), and Glioblastoma Multiforme with Oligodendroglial Features (WHO Grade IV)

Clinical Features

- Account for 5% to 10% of gliomas
- Clinical signs and symptoms at presentation are similar to those seen in pure gliomas

Gross Pathology

- Gross features similar to those seen with pure gliomas

Histopathology

- May exhibit distinct areas of astrocytic and oligodendroglial differentiation or have intermingled astrocytic and oligodendroglial cells
- Percentages of each glial component necessary to qualify the glioma as mixed are not universally agreed on
▌ Oligodendroglioma and astrocytoma (WHO grade II)
  - Low to moderate cellularity and cytologic atypia
  - Rare mitotic figures
▌ Anaplastic oligodendroglioma and astrocytoma (WHO grade III)
  - Higher cellularity and increased cytologic atypia
  - Abundant mitotic activity
  - Endothelial proliferation
  - Anaplastic features may be present in either glial component
▌ Glioblastoma multiforme with oligodendroglial features (WHO grade IV)
  - Recent study has found that the presence of necrosis with or without pseudopalisading is associated with a worse prognosis than an anaplastic oligoastrocytoma without necrosis, and suggested use of designation *GBM with oligodendroglial features*

Special Stains and Immunohistochemistry

- See "Special Stains and Immunohistochemistry" for astrocytomas and oligodendrogliomas

Other Techniques for Diagnosis

- Cytogenetics
  — Mixed tumors usually exhibit homogeneous genetic profiles
  — Analysis of oligoastrocytomas suggests two distinct genetic subsets
    ◆ Mutation in *TP53* gene or loss of heterozygosity of 17p indicates relationship to astrocytomas
    ◆ Loss of heterozygosity of 1p and 19q indicates genetic resemblance to oligodendrogliomas (reported in 20% to 30% of oligoastrocytomas)

Differential Diagnosis

▌ Pure astrocytoma
  - Consists of only a neoplastic astrocytic component
  - Lacks unequivocal neoplasia in other glial cell line
▌ Pure oligodendroglioma
  - Consists of only a neoplastic oligodendroglial component
  - Lacks unequivocal neoplasia in other glial cell line

Pearls

- The prognosis in this neoplasm is still better than that of a GBM without an oligodendroglioma component, independent of 1p and 19q deletion status
- Some studies show that oligoastrocytomas and pure oligodendrogliomas respond similarly to chemotherapy and show no significant differences in survival; in addition, it has been reported that patients with pure oligodendrogliomas or oligoastrocytomas do better than those with pure astrocytomas
- Combined loss of 1p and 19q is associated with improved survival in oligoastrocytomas compared with oligoastrocytomas without deletions of 1p and 19q

Selected References

Von Deimling A, Reifenberger G, Kros JM, et al: Oligoastrocytoma. In Louis DN, Ohgaki H, Wiestler OD, Cavenee W (eds): World Health Organization: Classification of Tumours of the Central Nervous System. Lyon, IARC, 2007, pp 63-65.

Von Deimling A, Reifenberger G, Kros JM, et al: Anaplastic oligoastrocytoma. In Louis DN, Ohgaki H, Wiestler OD, Cavenee W (eds): World Health Organization: Classification of Tumours of the Central Nervous System. Lyon, IARC, 2007, pp 66-67.

Miller CR, Dunham CP, Scheithauer BW, Perry A: Significance of necrosis in grading of oligodendroglial neoplasms: A clinicopathologic and genetic study of newly diagnosed high-grade gliomas. J Clin Oncol 24:5419-5426, 2006.

Perl A, Fuller CE, Banerjee R, et al: Ancillary FISH analysis for 1p and 19q status: Preliminary observations in 287 gliomas and oligodendroglioma mimics. Front Biosci 8:a1-a9, 2003.

Ependymal Tumors

Ependymoma (WHO Grade II) and Anaplastic Ependymoma (WHO Grade III)

Clinical Features

- Typically occur in children and young adults
- Account for about 3% to 9% of all neuroepithelial tumors; most frequent neuroepithelial tumors of the spinal cord (50% to 60% of spinal gliomas)
- Occur at any site along the ventricular system; most commonly in the fourth ventricle and spinal cord, followed by the lateral ventricles
- Tumors in children are more commonly in the infratentorial region at a mean age of 6.4 years
- In adults, spinal tumors present between the ages of 30 and 40 years
- Patients often present with symptoms of hydrocephalus, including nausea, vomiting, and headache; patients occasionally develop seizures
- Posterior fossa tumors may cause visual disturbances or cerebellar ataxia

Gross Pathology

- Soft gray-pink tumors that may be solid or cystic
- Areas of hemorrhage or necrosis may be present
- Typically protrude from the ventricular lining and fill the ventricular lumen; well demarcated, but may invade the adjacent brain parenchyma

Histopathology

▍ Ependymoma
- Cellular tumors composed of monomorphic cells with round to oval hyperchromatic nuclei and long fibrillary cell processes
- Characteristically form perivascular pseudorosettes and true rosettes
- Perivascular pseudorosettes consist of tumor cells radially arranged around blood vessels
- True ependymal rosettes consist of columnar cells radially arranged around a central lumen; not present in most ependymomas
- Calcification, as well as metaplastic cartilage or bone, may be seen
- Necrosis without pseudopalisading may be present in ependymoma, grade II

▍ Ependymoma variants
- Cellular ependymoma (WHO grade II)
  — Increased cellularity without appreciable increase in mitotic rate or other features associated with anaplasia
  — Increased occurrence in extraventricular sites
- Papillary ependymoma (WHO grade II)
  — Extensive papillary formations
- Clear cell ependymoma
  — Cells exhibit round nuclei and perinuclear halos
  — Anaplastic histologic features are often present

Figure 19-6. Ependymoma. A, Low-power view shows a moderately cellular glial tumor with classic perivascular pseudorosettes. **B,** High-power view shows classic ependymal rosettes. Notice glial cells radially arranged to form a canal (phosphotungstic acid–hematoxylin stain). **C,** Myxopapillary ependymoma. Glial cells exhibiting perivascular arrangement with abundant interposed mucin deposition.

  — Occur more frequently in supratentorial compartment than in infratentorial compartment
- Tanycytic ependymoma (WHO grade II)
  — Occur more commonly in spinal cord
  — Composed of elongated spindled glial cells forming fascicles
  — Ependymal rosettes often not present; perivascular pseudorosettes may be ill-defined

▌ Anaplastic ependymoma
- Morphologic criteria that consistently correlate with prognosis are not well established
- Increased cellularity and increased mitotic activity
- Often endothelial proliferation and necrosis with pseudopalisading
- Perivascular pseudorosettes persist

Special Stains and Immunohistochemistry

- GFAP: marked cytoplasmic immunoreactivity, especially prominent in the perivascular pseudorosettes
- Cytokeratin: AE1/AE3 immunoreactivity present in most ependymomas; focal and variably strong positivity with other keratin antibodies
- EMA: dotlike cytoplasmic immunoreactivity present in most neoplastic cells
- CD99: diffuse and dotlike cytoplasmic immunoreactivity with accentuation at membrane surface
- Mib-1 labeling index in more than 5% associated with decreased survival

Other Techniques for Diagnosis

- Electron microscopy: cells show polarity with well-formed terminal bars; typically have surface microvilli, cilia, intercellular junctions (zonula adherens), and blepharoplasts
- Cytogenetics: chromosome 22 deletions involving *NF2* tumor suppressor gene (member of protein 4.1 family) are most common; clear cell ependymomas have been reported to exhibit losses on chromosome 18

Differential Diagnosis

▌ Metastatic adenocarcinoma
- Morphology more consistently epithelial
- Cytokeratin positivity specific for site of origin; less likely positive in ependymoma

▌ Fibrillary or diffuse astrocytoma
- Poorly defined infiltrative tumor
- Lacks rosette formation
- EMA typically negative

▌ Astroblastoma
- Rare tumor
- Located away from the ventricle
- Shows marked and diffuse vascular sclerosis
- Tumor cells have short, broad processes
- Lacks true rosette formation

▌ Choroid plexus papilloma or carcinoma
- Papillary architecture and no rosette formation
- Negative or only focally positive for GFAP
- Carcinomas have a loose papillary architecture and consist of sheets of pleomorphic cells with a high mitotic rate; extensive necrosis is common

Figure 19-7. Choroid plexus papilloma. Columnar epithelium overlying classic papillary architecture with central fibrovascular core.

Pearls

- Complete surgical resection may offer long survival time; many eventually recur, and death often results
- Patients with spinal ependymomas do much better because complete surgical resection is more feasible
- May occasionally occur in the deep white matter away from the ventricle

Selected References

Kurt E, Zheng POP, Hop WCJ, et al: Identification of relevant prognostic histopathologic features in 69 intracranial ependymomas, excluding myxopapillary ependymomas and subependymomas. Cancer 106:388-395, 2006.

Rajaram V, Gutmann DH, Prasad SK, et al: Alterations of protein 4.1 family members in ependymomas: A study of 84 cases. Mod Pathol 18:991-997, 2005.

Kawano N, Yasui Y, Utsuki S, et al: Light microscopic demonstration of the microlumen of ependymoma: A study of the usefulness of antigen retrieval for epithelial membrane antigen (EMA) immunostaining. Brain Tumor Pathol 21:17-21, 2004.

Foulade M, Helton K, Dalton J, et al: Clear cell ependymoma: A clinicopathologic and radiographic analysis of 10 patients. Cancer 98:2232-2244, 2003.

Myxopapillary Ependymoma (WHO Grade I)

Clinical Features

- Represents about 10% to 13% of all ependymomas
- Typically presents in young adults at an average age of 36 years
- Occurs more frequently in males (2.5:1)
- Occurs almost exclusively in the conus-cauda-filum terminale region
- Also reported in subcutaneous tissue overlying the sacrococcyx, and in the presacral and postsacral regions
- Rarely occurs outside of this region (fourth or lateral ventricles, brain parenchyma)

- Signs and symptoms include low back pain, sciatica, and focal neurologic deficits referable to the tumor location

Gross Pathology

- Lobulated, circumscribed, soft gray tumors in the filum terminale or attached to nerve roots

Histopathology

- Composed of papillae lined by monotonous elongated or columnar cells surrounding a central vascular core
- Occasionally fascicular architecture is present
- Abundant perivascular mucin pools and a fibrillary background

Special Stains and Immunohistochemistry

- GFAP, vimentin, and S-100 protein positive
- PAS and Alcian blue highlight perivascular mucin
- Cytokeratin negative
- Mib-1: low

Other Techniques for Diagnosis

- Ultrastructural examination shows collagen-rich stroma, cells with basal lamina, and cellular interdigitation

Differential Diagnosis

▌ Metastatic adenocarcinoma (mucin secreting)
- Rarely involves the filum terminale
- Consists of pleomorphic tumor cells with high mitotic rate
- Hemorrhage and necrosis are typical
- Strong cytokeratin positivity
▌ Chordoma
- Characterized by a lobular architecture with cords of epithelial and physaliphorous cells
- Lacks papillary architecture and fibrillary background
- GFAP negative
▌ Schwannoma
- Abundant reticulin
- GFAP negative
▌ Paraganglioma
- Morphologic features of neuroendocrine differentiation
- Immunoreactive for neuroendocrine markers

Pearls

- Typically slow-growing tumors with a favorable prognosis
- Treatment includes surgical resection and radiation therapy for incompletely excised tumors
- Survival is excellent following complete resection; slightly lower survival rate for incompletely excised lesions
- Tumors occurring in soft tissues have been associated with aggressive behavior and metastases

Selected References

McLendon RE, Rosenblum MK, Schiffer D, Wiestler OD: Myxopapillary ependymoma. In Louis DN, Ohgaki H, Wiestler OD, Cavenee W (eds): World Health Organization: Classification of Tumours of the Central Nervous System. Lyon, IARC, 2007, pp. 72-73.

Ng, HK: Ependymoma, subependymoma, and myxopapillary ependymoma. In McLendon RE, Rosenblum MK, Bigner DD (eds): Russell & Rubinstein's Pathology of Tumors of the Nervous System, 7th ed. New York, Oxford University Press, 2006, pp 201-221.

Prayson RA: Myxopapillary ependymomas: A clinicopathologic study of 14 cases including MIB-1 and p53 immunoreactivity. Mod Pathol 10:304-310, 1997.

Subependymoma (WHO Grade I)

Clinical Features

- Most frequently found in adult males (male-to-female ratio, 4:1)
- Most occur in the fourth (50% to 60%) or lateral (40% to 50%) ventricles; less commonly in the spinal cord
- Many are found incidentally at autopsy, but some cause symptoms, usually related to increased intracranial pressure due to obstruction of the ventricular system
- Symptoms related to mass effect may also be seen (focal neurologic signs, seizures)

Gross Pathology

- Firm, tan-white, polypoid nodules of varying size
- Arise from the lining of the ventricle or from the septum pellucidum and protrude in the ventricular lumen; usually well circumscribed
- Focal hemorrhage, calcifications, and cystic changes may be present

Histopathology

- Characterized by clusters of monomorphic tumor cells (resembling normal ependymal cells) in a dense fibrillary matrix of glial cell processes
- Microcystic architecture is a common feature
- Small blood vessel proliferation or focal hemorrhage may be seen within the tumor
- Mitotic activity is rare to absent
- Ependymal pseudorosettes may be seen but are not a typical finding; true rosettes are rare
- Microcalcifications are common
- Microcysts filled with basophilic amorphous material are common

Special Stains and Immunohistochemistry

- GFAP positive, but may be variable in extent
- S-100 protein diffusely positive
- Mib-1: usually less than 1%

Other Techniques for Diagnosis

- Typically have a normal karyotype
- Ultrastructural examination shows features typical of ependymal cells (surface microvilli, intercellular junctions, and cilia)

Differential Diagnosis

▌Ependymoma
- Generally found in younger individuals
- Usually symptomatic, producing hydrocephalus, visual disturbances, or cerebellar ataxia
- More cellular and characterized by rosette and prominent pseudorosette formation

Pearls

- For symptomatic lesions, surgical resection is the treatment of choice and is often curative
- Tumors showing both ependymal and subependymal features are generally classified as ependymomas
- Believed to arise from subependymal glial cells (tanycytes) or astrocytes of the subependymal plate; may be a hamartomatous proliferation

Selected References

McLendon RE, Schiffer D, Rosenblum MK, Wiestler OD: Subependymoma. In Louis DN, Ohgaki H, Wiestler OD, Cavenee W (eds): World Health Organization: Classification of Tumours of the Central Nervous System. Lyon, IARC, 2007, pp 70-71.

Ragel BT, Osborn AG, Whang K, et al: Subependymomas: An analysis of clinical and imaging features. Neurosurgery 58:881-890, 2006.

Brown DF, Rushing EJ: Subependymomas: Clinicopathological study of 14 tumors. Arch Pathol Lab Med 123:873, 1999.

Other Neuroepithelial Tumors

Astroblastoma (No WHO Grade at Present)

Clinical Features

- Rare neoplasm occurring most frequently in children and young adults; uncommon in older adults; one study has noted a female predominance
- Patients typically present with symptoms of mass effect; may have focal neurologic deficits, headache, or seizures
- Most often located near or at the surface of the cerebral hemispheres; may arise in the corpus callosum, cerebellum, optic nerves, brain stem, or cauda equina
- MRI shows a well-defined, contrast-enhancing mass with solid or cystic components; the solid component has a characteristic bubbly appearance and little associated T2 hyperintensity

Gross Pathology

- Small cyst formation and focal necrosis may be seen, especially in larger tumors

Histopathology

- Key feature is the astroblastic pseudorosette composed of broad, nontapering, nonfibrillar processes that radiate toward a central blood vessel
- Depending on the tumor grade, cells may be monomorphic with inconspicuous nucleoli or show pleomorphic, hyperchromatic nuclei with obvious nucleoli
- Marked perivascular hyalinization is characteristic and may coalesce to occupy extensive areas
- Typically noninfiltrative interface with surrounding brain tissue
- Low grade
  — Uniform distribution of perivascular pseudo-rosettes
  — Low mitotic activity (mean, 1 mitosis/10 hpf)
  — Minimal cellular pleomorphism
  — No vascular proliferation or necrosis with pseudopalisading
- High grade
  — Increased cellularity (focal or multifocal)
  — High mitotic rate (>5 mitoses/10 hpf)
  — Nuclear anaplasia
  — Vascular proliferation and necrosis with pseudopalisading

Special Stains and Immunohistochemistry

- GFAP, S-100, and vimentin: strong immunoreactivity
- EMA: focal membranous immunoreactivity
- Cytokeratin (low molecular weight): variable
- Mib-1 index: low grade, 3%; high grade, 15%

Other Techniques for Diagnosis

- Electron microscopy: tumor cells contain abundant intermediate filaments and exhibit microvilli, poorly developed intercellular junctions, and rare cilia
- In comparative genomic hybridization studies, most frequently found was gain of chromosome arm 20q, and slightly less frequent was gain of chromosome 19

Differential Diagnosis

▌Ependymoma
- Most are infratentorial and within or close to a ventricle
- Lacks vascular hyalinization
- Shows formation of true rosettes
- Cells have elongated fibrillary processes and fibrillary background

▌Angiocentric glioma
- In contrast to astroblastoma, angiocentric gliomas are infiltrating lesions composed of piloid cells that exhibit circumferential arrangements of neoplastic cells around vessels in addition to radial arrangements (as seen in astroblastomas)

▮ Papillary meningioma
- Contain distinct areas of meningothelial differentiation
- Characteristically EMA positive
- GFAP negative

Pearls

- Cell of origin is debated because astroblastomas exhibit features of both astrocytes and ependymal cells; they are suggested to be of tanycytic derivation
- Complete resection typically results in long-term survival
- Focal astroblastic features may be seen in low-grade and high-grade astrocytomas

Selected References

Port JD, Brat DJ, Burger PC, Pomper MG: Astroblastoma: Radiologic-pathologic correlation and distinction from ependymoma. Am J Neuroradiol 23:243-247, 2002.

Brat DJ, Hirose Y, Cohen KJ, et al: Astroblastoma: Clinicopathologic features and chromosomal abnormalities defined by comparative genomic hybridization. Brain Pathol 10:342-352, 2000.

Chordoid Glioma (WHO Grade II)

Clinical Features

- Uncommon glioma arising in region of third ventricle
- Mean age, 46 years; range, 12 to 70 years
- Females affected more than males
- Signs and symptoms usually secondary to obstructive hydrocephalus; reported symptoms include headache, weight loss, endocrine disturbances, autonomic disturbances, psychosis, and focal neurologic deficits

Gross Pathology

- Well-circumscribed, fusiform, ovoid shape containing cysts; may be attached to the hypothalamus

Histopathology

- Cords and clusters of epithelioid cells, myxoid and mucinous background
- Neoplastic cells have abundant eosinophilic cytoplasm, round to oval nuclei, and inconspicuous nucleoli
- Sparse to abundant lymphoplasmacytic infiltrates with Russell bodies
- Rare mitotic figures, no necrosis, and endothelial proliferation
- Does not infiltrate into surrounding brain, but Rosenthal fibers are present in adjacent brain

Special Stains and Immunohistochemistry

- PAS and Alcian blue positive background
- GFAP and vimentin: strong diffuse immunoreactivity
- CD34, EMA, and cytokeratin: focal positivity

- E-cadherin, neuron-specific enolase (NSE), neurofilament, and S-100: variable positivity
- Synaptophysin and desmin negative
- Mib-1 labeling index: generally less than 2%

Other Techniques for Diagnosis

- Electron microscopy: abundant intermediate filaments in cytoplasm, microvilli, focal basal lamina, and hemidesmosomes

Differential Diagnosis

▮ Chordoma
- Limited cytokeratin immunoreactivity in chordoid glioma, compared with diffuse and strong reactivity in chordoma
- Physaliferous cells characteristic

▮ Chordoid meningioma
- Presence of whorls and psammoma bodies, nuclear pseudoinclusions
- No immunoreactivity for GFAP; usually positive for EMA
- Both may have inflammatory infiltrates

Pearls

- Gross total resection is optimal treatment, but adherence to hypothalamus may prevent complete resection and lead to significant morbidity and poor outcome
- Cell of origin is hypothesized to originate from tanycytes (glial progenitor cells with astrocytic and ependymal features) found in circumventricular organs (lamina terminalis in anterior third ventricular wall)
- Metaplastic elements have been reported (chondroid)

Selected References

Buccoliero AM, Caldarella A, Gallina P, et al: Chordoid glioma: Clinicopathologic profile and differential diagnosis of an uncommon tumor. Arch Pathol Lab Med 128:e141-145, 2004.

Cenacchi G, Roncaroli F, Cerasoli S, et al: Chordoid glioma of the third ventricle: An ultrastructural study of three cases with a histogenetic hypothesis. Am J Surg Pathol 25:401-405, 2001.

Brat DJ, Scheithauer BW, Stugaitis SM, et al: Third ventricular chordoid glioma: A distinct clinicopathologic entity. J Neuropathol Exper Neurol 57:283-290, 1998.

Angiocentric Glioma (WHO Grade I)

Clinical Features

- Slow-growing glioma
- Reported in patients ranging in age from 2 to 70 years, but occurs most commonly in childhood and adolescence
- Long-standing history of seizures is common

- Occurs in cerebrum, most often frontoparietal lobe; also temporal lobe

Gross Pathology

- Not yet described

Histopathology

- Superficial cortical location with subpial accumulation
- Infiltration of surrounding parenchyma
- Monomorphous slender bipolar cells with angiocentricity
- Circumferential (more common) or radial arrangements around vessels of all sizes
- Occasional fascicular architecture
- Rare mitoses

Special Stains and Immunohistochemistry

- GFAP: variable degrees of positivity, often around vessels
- S-100 and vimentin positive
- EMA surface and paranuclear dotlike positivity
- Neu-N, chromogranin, and synaptophysin negative
- Mib-1 index: 1% to 5%

Other Techniques for Diagnosis

- Ultrastructure: perivascular cells contain cytoplasmic intermediate filaments and exhibit basement membrane; cell junctions and microvilli are described
- Cytogenetics: not yet fully studied; gains of chromosome 11 described

Differential Diagnosis

▌ Astrocytoma
- Lacks monomorphic nuclear appearance of angiocentric glioma
- No angiocentricity

▌ Pilocytic astrocytoma
- Not infiltrative
- EMA negative

▌ Pilomyxoid astrocytoma
- Mucinous and myxoid background
- Usual location in hypothalamus
- Contrast enhancing
- Occurs in very young

▌ Ependymoma
- Usually in or adjacent to a ventricle
- Exhibits only radially arranged perivascular pseudorosettes and ependymal rosettes

▌ Astroblastoma
- Radially arranged perivascular pseudorosettes with marked vessel sclerosis

Pearls

- Newly described entity
- Surgical excision is usually curative

Selected References

Brat DJ, Scheithauer BW, Fuller GN, Tihan T: Newly codified glial neoplasms of the 2007 WHO classification of tumors of the central nervous system: Angiocentric glioma, pilomyxoid astrocytoma, and pituicytoma. Brain Pathol 17:319-324, 2007.

Wang M, Tihan T, Fojiani AM, et al: Monomorphous angiocentric glioma: A distinctive epileptogenic neoplasm with features of infiltrating astrocytoma and ependymoma. J Neuropath Exp Neurol 64:875-881, 2005.

Neuronal and Glioneuronal Neoplasms

Gangliocytoma (WHO Grade I) and Ganglioglioma (WHO Grades II and III)

Clinical Features

- Gangliocytomas are WHO grade I
- Most gangliogliomas are WHO grade I; criteria for grade II gangliogliomas are not yet established
- Anaplastic gangliogliomas are uncommon (WHO grade III)
- Low incidence (1.3% of all brain tumors), but is the most common neoplasm in patients with chronic intractable focal epilepsy
- Typically supratentorial and usually involves the temporal lobe (70%)
- Most present in the first three decades; may be found in all ages
- CT and MRI usually show a complex solid or cystic mass; often with calcification

Gross Pathology

- Well-circumscribed gray granular mass that is variably solid and cystic; mural nodule within the cystic component often seen
- May extend into the leptomeninges and subarachnoid space
- Extensive calcification, hemorrhage, or necrosis may be seen

Figure 19-8. Ganglioglioma. Mixed glial-neuronal neoplasm composed of neoplastic astrocytes intermixed with atypical clustered ganglion cells.

Histopathology

▌ Gangliocytoma
  - Composed entirely of neurons forming ill-defined groups
  - Often exhibits cytologic atypia

▌ Ganglioglioma
  - Tumor composed of atypical ganglion cells as well as a neoplastic glial component
  - Neoplastic neurons are characterized by haphazard clustering, lack of orderly distribution, and, often, an abnormal location (in white matter)
  - Abnormal neurons may be small or large; often they are binucleated and have large nuclei and prominent nucleoli
  - Variably cellular glial component most commonly consisting of a neoplastic astrocytic population; oligodendroglial foci are rarely seen
  - Astrocytic component may be pilocytic with Rosenthal fibers and eosinophilic granular bodies
  - Atypical glial cells with large, bizarre, hyperchromatic nuclei with intranuclear cytoplasmic inclusions may be seen
  - Tumor cells may be located in a reticulin-rich stroma
  - Foci of perivascular chronic inflammation is common histologic feature
  - Microcalcifications are often present
  - Microcystic cavities may be present
  - Mitotic figures are rare
  - Atypical ganglioglioma (WHO grade II): increased cellularity and mitoses in the astrocytic component
  - Anaplastic ganglioglioma (WHO grade III): further increased mitotic activity in the astrocytic component

Special Stains and Immunohistochemistry

  - Synaptophysin, S-100 protein, NSE, and Neu-N: neurons are positive
  - Neurofilament: neurons may be positive
  - Silver stain (Bielschowsky) highlights cell processes of ganglion cells
  - CD 34: neuronal component is positive
  - GFAP: astrocytic component is positive
  - Mib-1: low index (<3%) in typical ganglioglioma (grade I); elevated in atypical (grade II) and anaplastic (grade III) gangliogliomas

Other Techniques for Diagnosis

  - Electron microscopy: neurons contain dense-core neurosecretory granules and occasionally exhibit synapses
  - Cytogenetic analyses: gangliogliomas; gains of chromosome 7 are most often found, and *TSC2* gene mutation is reported in glial component

Differential Diagnosis

▌ Variants of ganglioglioma
  - Desmoplastic infantile ganglioglioma and astrocytoma, WHO grade I
    — Most occur before 2 years of age
    — Large cystic masses, superficially located, most often occurring in frontal and parietal lobes, may involve more than one lobe
    — Dense fibrotic masses
    — Fibrous stroma with intermixed clusters or scattered astrocytes
    — Eosinophilic granular bodies and Rosenthal fibers
    — Ganglion cells and small neurocytic cells present in desmoplastic infantile ganglioglioma but may be sparse
  - Dysplastic gangliocytoma of the cerebellum (Lhermitte-Duclos)
    — Benign cellular proliferation of dysplastic ganglion cells
    — Diffusely enlarged cerebellar folia secondary to ganglion cells that enlarge and distort the molecular and internal granular cell layers
    — Pathognomic of Cowden disease

▌ Pilocytic astrocytoma
  - Similar radiographic findings
  - Biphasic tumor consisting of pilocytic areas and a microcystic background
  - Lacks clusters of atypical neurons

▌ DNET
  - Both tumors show similar clinical picture
  - Composed of a multinodular architecture with a mucoid collagenous background
  - Neurons in DNET are typically normal; lacks clustering of pleomorphic neurons

▌ Fibrillary or diffuse astrocytoma
  - Entrapped non-neoplastic neurons may suggest ganglioglioma
  - Tumor cells are negative for neuronal markers; positive for GFAP
  - Mib-1 index: higher in astrocytomas than gangliogliomas

▌ Pleomorphic xanthoastrocytoma
  - Pleomorphic, xanthomatous cells characterize the neoplasm
  - Exhibits both CD34 and GFAP positivity
  - Usually lacks a neuronal component

Pearls

  - Surgical resection for gangliocytoma and ganglioglioma is usually curative; no radiation or chemotherapy is needed
  - Eosinophilic granular bodies are evidence of chronicity and slow growth; they are not diagnostic of gangliogliomas and may be seen in pilocytic astrocytoma, pleomorphic xanthoastrocytoma, and other low-grade astrocytomas
  - Malignant transformation of the glial cells is extremely rare (anaplastic ganglioglioma)

- Ganglion cells may be difficult to appreciate on frozen section; patient age, radiographic findings, and clinical history are helpful

Selected References

Becker AJ, Wiestler OD, Figarella-Branger D, Blumcke I: Ganglioglioma and gangliocytoma. In Louis DN, Ohgaki H, Wiestler OD, Cavenee W (eds): World Health Organization: Classification of Tumours of the Central Nervous System. Lyon, IARC, 2007, pp 103-105.

Blumcke I, Wiestler OD: Gangliogliomas: An intriguing tumor entity associated with focal epilepsies. J Neuropathol Exper Neurol 61:575-584, 2002.

McLendon RE, Provenzale J: Glioneuronal tumors of the central nervous system. Brain Tumor Pathol 19:51-58, 2002.

Prayson RA, Khajavi K, Comair YG: Cortical architecture abnormalities and MIB-1 immunoreactivity in gangliogliomas: A study of 60 patients with intracranial tumors. J Neuropathol Exper Neurol 54:513-520, 1995.

Dysembryoplastic Neuroepithelial Tumor (WHO Grade I)

Clinical Features

- Typically found in the first decade in the setting of drug-resistant epilepsy
- Occurs most often in the temporal lobe cortex; also reported in frontal, parietal, and occipital cortexes and selected infratentorial areas

Gross Pathology

- May be well defined or poorly demarcated
- Variable size; most measure a few centimeters
- Gyral expansion with vague multinodular formation and mucoid viscous appearance

Figure 19-9. Dysembryoplastic neuroepithelial tumor. Neurons floating in a mucoid matrix with oligodendroglial-like cells.

- Small cyst formation often seen
- Distortion of the overlying skull may be present

Histopathology

- Cortical, multinodular, microcystic, mucoid tumor
- Three classic histologic features
  — Glioneuronal element ("specific component")
    ◆ Oligodendroglial-like cells and normal-appearing neurons floating in mucin-rich spaces
    ◆ Up to 50% of DNETs lack this element
  — Glial nodules
    ◆ Aggregates of oligodendroglial-like cells mixed with astrocytes resembling an oligoastrocytoma
  — Cortical dysplasia
    ◆ Architectural disarray with loss of normal laminations
- Presence of the nodular architecture in association with the glioneuronal element is sufficient to make a diagnosis of DNET
- Eosinophilic granular bodies may be present
- Endothelial proliferation may be present

Special Stains and Immunohistochemistry

- Synaptophysin, NSE, and Neu-N highlight neuronal component
- GFAP stains astrocytic component
- S-100 protein stains oligodendroglial-like cells
- Alcian blue highlights mucoid background (acid mucopolysaccharide)
- Mib-1: usually low labeling index, but up to 8% reported

Other Techniques for Diagnosis

- Ultrastructure
  — Oligodendroglial-like cells in the glial nodules or specific glial neuronal component have round or oval nuclei and scant cytoplasm with short processes
  — Cytoplasm contains mitochondria, free ribosomes, rough endoplasmic reticulum, and lysosomes
  — Occasional astrocytic (intermediate filaments) and neuronal differentiation (dense core granules) are seen
- Cytogenetics: do not exhibit loss of chromosome arms 1p and 19q (three cases studied)

Differential Diagnosis

▍ Ganglioglioma
- Dominant feature is bizarre, pleomorphic, or binucleate neurons
- Shows a neoplastic glial component in addition to the abnormal neurons
- Lacks multinodular architecture
- Typically shows perivascular lymphoid infiltrate and may have abundant collagenous stroma

- Oligodendroglioma
  - Lacks distinct multinodular architecture
  - No glioneuronal element
  - Difficult to distinguish from DNET in small biopsies
- Oligoastrocytoma
  - Lacks distinct multinodular architecture
  - No glioneuronal element
- Pilocytic astrocytoma
  - Composed of biphasic dense and loose piloid astrocytes without floating neurons or associated cortical dysplasia

Pearls

- Histogenesis is currently unknown; may be hamartomatous rather than neoplastic
- Surgical resection is reserved for patients with intractable seizures
- Most patients remain seizure free and without tumor recurrence after resection
- Recurrence is rare, and there are only two case reports of malignant transformation

Selected References

Daumas-Duport C, Pietsch T, Hawkins C, Shankar SK: Dysembryoplastic neuroepithelial tumor. In Louis DN, Ohgaki H, Wiestler OD, Cavenee W (eds): World Health Organization: Classification of Tumours of the Central Nervous System. Lyon, IARC, 2007, pp 99-102.

Daumas-Duport C, Scheithauer BW, Chodkiewicz JP, et al: Dysembryoplastic neuroepithelial tumor: A surgically curable tumor of young patients with intractable partial seizures. Report of 39 cases. Exp Clin Studies 23:545-556, 1988.

Central and Extraventricular Neurocytoma (WHO Grade II)

Clinical Features

- Incidence is 0.25% to 0.50% of all brain tumors
- Typically occurs in young adults (ages 20 to 40 years)
- Central neurocytoma: intraventricular tumors are usually found in the lateral or third ventricles, adjacent to the foramen of Monro
  - Extraventricular neurocytomas occur in parenchyma, away from the ventricular system; reported in cerebrum, cerebellum, midbrain, and spinal cord
  - Central neurocytomas present with signs of increased intracranial pressure including headache, nausea, vomiting, seizures, visual disturbance, and papilledema
  - CT and MRI characteristically show a heterogeneously contrast-enhancing, partially calcified intraventricular (or in extraventricular lesions, parenchymal) mass; cysts and calcification are common

Figure 19-10. **Central neurocytoma.** The neoplasm is composed of a monotonous population of small round cells with a fine chromatin pattern and occasional nuclei-free islands suggesting neuropil.

- Cerebellar liponeurocytoma
  - Rare low-grade (WHO grade II) neoplasm composed of neurocytes with focal lipomatous differentiation
  - Mean age of occurrence, 50 years

Gross Pathology

- Well-circumscribed, lobulated tumor
- Typically, infiltration into the surrounding brain parenchyma is not seen
- Often hemorrhagic, focally calcified, and cystic
- Cerebellar liponeurocytoma: usually in cerebellar hemispheres

Histopathology

- Central neurocytomas
  - Hypercellular tumor composed of diffuse sheets of monotonous uniform cells punctuated by anuclear areas composed of a fibrillar matrix, reminiscent of neuropil
  - Perivascular clearing composed of cell processes resembling ependymal pseudorosettes may be seen
  - A delicate vascular stroma and microcalcifications are often present
  - Nuclei have regular outlines with delicate chromatin and small inconspicuous nucleoli
  - Mitotic activity, endothelial proliferation, and necrosis are rare
  - Rare cases exhibit ganglion cells
- Atypical neurocytomas
  - Defined by elevation of Mib-1 index (>2%) with or without the presence of endothelial proliferation, necrosis, and increased atypia
- Extraventricular neurocytomas
  - Cytologically very similar to central neurocytomas
  - Architectural pattern is more varied, such as clusters, ribbons, or rosettes, in addition to sheets

- Higher degree of ganglionic differentiation and possibly glial differentiation
- Cerebellar liponeurocytoma
  - Composed of neurocytes, some showing lipidization

Special Stains and Immunohistochemistry

- Synaptophysin: diffusely positive
- NSE and Neu-N positive
- Chromogranin and neurofilament usually negative
- GFAP negative in central neurocytomas; variable in extraventricular neurocytomas
- Mib-1 index: less than 2% in typical neurocytomas; more than 2% shortens recurrence-free survival
- Cerebellar liponeurocytoma: in addition to neuronal markers, focal GFAP positivity is often present

Other Techniques for Diagnosis

- Cytogenetic analyses: gains at 2p, 10q, and 18q; frequent deletions of both arms of 17 and small deletions in 1p

Differential Diagnosis

- Oligodendroglioma
  - Poorly circumscribed with an infiltrative border
  - Typically not located in the ventricle
  - Lacks salt-and-pepper nuclei, neuropil islands, and ganglion cell differentiation
  - Synaptophysin negative
- Ependymoma (especially clear cell variant)
  - Cells have long fibrillary processes
  - Characteristically shows true rosettes
  - Typically protrudes from ventricular lining
  - GFAP positive and synaptophysin negative
- Neuroblastoma (primitive neuroectodermal tumor)
  - Hyperchromatic atypical cells with frequent mitoses
  - Lack of fine chromatin and neuropil islands
  - Intraparenchymal with tendency to seed neuraxis
  - Immunohistochemical profiles are the same

Pearls

- Most are slow-growing tumors that are essentially cured by surgical resection; associated with an excellent prognosis
- Recurrence is associated with subtotal resection, atypical histology, and elevated Mib-1 proliferation index

Selected References

Figarella-Branger D, Soylemezoglu F, Burger PC: Central neurocytoma and extraventricular neurocytoma. In Louis DN, Ohgaki H, Wiestler OD, Cavenee W (eds): World Health Organization: Classification of Tumours of the Central Nervous System. Lyon, IARC, 2007, pp 106-109.

Kleihues P, Chimelli L, Giangaspero F, Ohgaki H: Cerebellar liponeurocytoma. In Louis DN, Ohgaki H, Wiestler OD, Cavenee W (eds): World Health Organization: Classification of Tumours of the Central Nervous System. Lyon, IARC, 2007, pp 110-112.

Giangaspero F, Cenacchi G, Losi L, et al: Extraventricular neoplasms with neurocytoma features. Am J Surg Pathol 21:206-212, 1997.

Papillary Glioneuronal Tumor (No WHO Grade at Present)

Clinical Features

- Generally behave as grade I
- Rare neoplasm; wide age range, from 4 to 75 years (mean age, 23 years)
- Seizures, headaches, visual disturbances, language or gait disturbances, and mood changes have been reported as presenting symptoms
- Occurs in cerebral parenchyma, most commonly in frontal and temporal lobes
- MRI shows well-circumscribed solid and cystic masses with contrast enhancement; may have a cyst with a mural nodule

Gross Pathology

- Well-circumscribed solid and cystic mass, may have a mural nodule in a cyst

Histopathology

- Architecturally composed of pseudopapillae and solid areas
- Pseudopapillae exhibit pseudostratified, small cuboidal cells without atypia around hyalinized vessels
- Solid areas contain mixtures of neurocytes and ganglion cells and cells intermediate between the two within a fibrillar or basophilic mucoid matrix
- Rosenthal fibers, calcification, and old hemorrhage are seen
- Mitoses are rare or absent
- No endothelial proliferation or necrosis

Special Stains and Immunohistochemistry

- GFAP: cells of pseudopapillae positive
- Synaptophysin: cells from solid areas (neurocytes and ganglion cells) positive
- Neu-N: cells from solid areas (neurocytes and ganglion cells) positive
- Neurofilament: cells from solid areas and ganglion cells positive
- Chromogranin: cells from solid areas (neurocytes and ganglion cells) negative
- Mib-1 index: range, 1% to 3%

Other Techniques for Diagnosis

- Ultrastructural examination: pseudopapillae lining cells show astrocytic features with intermediate filaments; solid area cells show neuronal features such as microtubules, dense core, and clear vesicles and occasionally synaptic junctions
- Cytogenetic analyses: no definitive studies at present

Differential Diagnosis

▌ Papillary ependymoma
  - Lacks solid component exhibiting neuronal elements
▌ Papillary meningioma
  - EMA positive
  - GFAP negative
  - Synaptophysin and Neu-N negative
▌ Choroid plexus papillomas
  - Papillary formations not consistently GFAP positive
  - Lacks solid areas composed of neuronal elements
▌ Metastatic papillary adenocarcinoma
  - Cytokeratin positive
  - GFAP, synaptophysin, and Neu-N negative
▌ Astroblastoma
  - Lacks neuronal elements

Pearls

  - Good prognosis
  - No reports of recurrence after gross total resection

Selected References

Atri S, Sharma MC, Sarkar C, et al: Papillary glioneuronal tumor: A report of a rare case and review of the literature. Child Nerv Syst 23:349-353, 2007.

Edgar M, Rosenblum MK: Mixed glioneuronal tumors, recently described entities. Arch Pathol Lab Med 131:228-233, 2007.

Komori T, Scheithauer BW, Anthony DC, et al: Papillary glioneuronal tumor: A new variant of mixed neuronal-glial neoplasm. Am J Surg Pathol 22:1171-1183, 1998.

Rosette-Forming Glioneuronal Tumor of the Fourth Ventricle (WHO Grade I)

Clinical Features

  - Rare neoplasm occurring at mean age of 32 years (range, 12 to 59 years)
  - Women affected more than men
  - Signs and symptoms secondary to obstructive hydrocephalus, ataxia, visual disturbances, and vertigo

Gross Pathology

  - Soft, gelatinous, well demarcated

Histopathology

  - Composed of neurocytic and glial cells
  - Neurocytic component exhibits small round nuclei and scant cytoplasm and forms perivascular pseudorosettes and Homer-Wright rosettes, often accompanied by a microcystic, myxoid background; rarely, ganglion cells may be seen
  - Glial component exhibits piloid and spindle-shaped cells, may be more extensive than the neuronal component
  - Rosenthal fibers and eosinophilic granular bodies may be seen
  - Degenerative changes are often seen consisting of sclerotic vessels, collagen, calcifications, and hemosiderin-laden macrophages
  - Endothelial proliferation may be seen
  - Mitoses are rare
  - Well-defined tumor-parenchyma interface

Special Stains and Immunohistochemistry

  - Synaptophysin: positive granular staining of neurocytic component
  - NSE positive in neurocytic component
  - GFAP and S-100 positive in glial component
  - Mib-1 index: less than 3%

Other Techniques for Diagnosis

  - Ultrastructure: glial component has bundles of intermediate filaments; neurocytic component exhibits cells with small round nuclei, ribosomes, and rough endoplasmic reticulum; Golgi apparatus, sparse dense core granules, and microtubules in the rosette formations
  - Occasional presynaptic specializations

Differential Diagnosis

▌ Pilocytic astrocytoma
  - Usually occurs in younger individuals
  - Lacks neurocytic component and Homer-Wright rosettes
▌ Central neurocytoma
  - Does not have a biphasic appearance with the piloid astrocytic component alternating with the neurocytic component
▌ Papillary glioneuronal neoplasm
  - More often occurs in cerebrum rather than fourth ventricle
  - Does not display Homer-Wright rosettes
  - Exhibits papillary architecture formed by astrocytic cells

Pearls

  - Indolent growth
  - Multifocal tumor nodules have been reported

Selected References

Edgar M, Rosenblum MK: Mixed glioneuronal tumors, recently described entities. Arch Pathol Lab Med 31:228-233, 2007.

Komori T, Scheithauer BW, Hirose T: A rosette-forming glioneuronal tumor of the fourth ventricle: Infratentorial form of dysembryoplastic neuroepithelial tumor? Am J Surg Pathol 26:582-591, 2002.

Paraganglioma of the Spinal Cord (WHO Grade I)

Clinical Features

  - Benign, encapsulated neoplasm arising from neural crest cells, occurring in cauda equina and filum terminale

- Constitutes 3.5% of all neoplasms in this location
- Mean age of occurrence is 48 years
- Patients most commonly present with back pain or sciatica and urinary or fecal incontinence; sensory or motor deficits are less common; symptoms secondary to hormonal manifestations are uncommon

Gross Pathology

- Most are intradural and encapsulated (80%)
- Red-brown soft tissue; may contain cysts
- Usually attached to filum terminale

Histopathology

- Nests (Zellballen) of small uniform cells surrounded by sustentacular cells
- Delicate vascular network (organoid pattern)
- Cells are polygonal or columnar with round nuclei and fine chromatin and granular eosinophilic cytoplasm
- Perivascular pseudorosette formation may occur
- Mitoses and necrosis are infrequent
- Ganglion cell differentiation present in up to 45%
- Divergent differentiation is reported (homologous or heterologous components)
- Melanotic and oncocytic variants have been described

Special Stains and Immunohistochemistry

- Chromogranin, synaptophysin, and NSE positive
- Neurofilament: variable staining
- GFAP and cytokeratin negative
- Sustentacular cells: S-100 and GFAP positive
- Mib-1 index: low

Other Techniques for Diagnosis

- Ultrastructure: cytoplasmic dense core secretory granules and intermediate filaments
- Cytogenetics
  - Mutations in succinic dehydrogenase genes (part of mitochondrial complex II)
  - Associated with the following autosomal dominant syndromes: von Hippel-Lindau disease (VHL), multiple endocrine neoplasia type II (MEN II), and neurofibromatosis type 1 (NF1)

Differential Diagnosis

▌ Ependymoma
- GFAP positive
- Fibrillary pattern with perivascular pseudorosettes and ependymal rosettes

▌ Metastatic carcinoma
- Cytologically anaplastic, lacking organoid pattern of uniform cells
- Not encapsulated

Pearls

- Most are slow growing and curable with complete resection

- Recurrence may occur with subtotal resection
- Subarachnoid space dissemination reported
- Morphologic criteria to distinguish between benign and aggressive tumors not described

Selected References

Pytel P, Krausz T, Wollmann R, Utset MF: Ganglioneuromatous paraganglioma of the cauda equina: A pathological case study. Hum Pathol 36:444-446, 2005.

Miliaras GC, Kyritsis AP, Polyzoidis KS: Cauda equina paraganglioma: A review. J Neurooncol 65:177-190, 2003.

Embryonal Tumors

Medulloblastoma (WHO Grade IV)

Clinical Features

- Malignant neoplasm of cerebellum composed of primitive cells usually with neuronal differentiation
- Most occur before 16 years of age (peak, 17 years)
- May occur in adulthood; most often between 21 and 40 years
- Symptoms include signs of cerebellar dysfunction (gait abnormalities, ataxia) or increased intracranial pressure

Gross Pathology

- Most occur in vermis and may bulge into or fill the fourth ventricle
- Involvement of the hemispheres is more common in older individuals
- Hemispheric lesions are more likely desmoplastic
- Solid, variably demarcated (from well to poorly defined), homogeneous mass

Figure 19-11. Medulloblastoma. Highly cellular tumor, spreading in the subarachnoid space, composed of small cells with carrot-shaped nuclei and indistinct cytoplasm forming Homer-Wright rosettes.

Histopathology

- Highly cellular tumor composed of undifferentiated cells with variable growth patterns
- Classically consists of small, round to carrot-shaped uniform cells with hyperchromatic nuclei and wispy cytoplasm, often with distinct fibrillary background composed of cell processes
- Homer-Wright rosettes may be seen (40%) but are often absent
- High mitotic rate is common
- Individual cell and small areas of necrosis are frequently present
- Distinct streaming (single-filing) or palisading of tumor cells is often seen
- Morphologic subtypes
  - Nodular and desmoplastic medulloblastoma (previously called *cerebellar neuroblastoma*)
    - Pale nodular areas lacking reticulin are surrounded by hypercellular sheets containing abundant reticulin
    - Nodules contain cells with neuronal maturation, and often a fibrillary matrix is present
    - Surrounding cells are more primitive and have high mitotic rates
  - Medulloblastoma with extensive nodularity
    - Large pale areas composed of neurocytic cells and neuropil with scant internodular component
  - Large cell and anaplastic medulloblastoma
    - Anaplastic changes are the presence of marked nuclear pleomorphism, cell wrapping and molding, high mitotic and Mib-1 indexes, and abundant apoptosis
    - Large cell changes are defined by cells with large round nuclei with prominent nucleoli, abundant mitoses, and apoptosis
    - Often, both large cells and anaplastic changes are found in the same neoplasm
  - Medullomyoblastoma
    - Rhabdomyoblastic differentiation is present
    - Spindle cells or globular cells that are positive for desmin, actin, or myoglobin
  - Melanotic medulloblastoma
    - Contains cells with melanin pigment
    - May also see ill-defined tubules or papillary formations

Special Stains and Immunohistochemistry

- Synaptophysin, microtubule-associated protein 2, neurofilament (low- and intermediate-molecular-weight), vimentin, NSE positive
- Cytokeratin negative
- GFAP may show focal positivity in tumors with astrocytic differentiation or may represent entrapped astrocytes
- Mib-1 index: more than 20%

Other Techniques for Diagnosis

- Electron microscopy: undifferentiated neuroepithelial cells with scant cytoplasm and few organelles; may show prominent cytoplasmic processes
- More differentiated neoplasms have microtubules, dense core vesicles, and synapses
- Cytogenetics: isochromosome 17q (30% to 40%)

Differential Diagnosis

- Atypical teratoid/rhabdoid tumor
  - Usually in children younger than 2 years
  - Presence of rhabdoid cells
  - Unique immunohistochemical profile positive for EMA, vimentin, SMA, cytokeratin, and synaptophysin; negative Ini protein antibody
  - *hSNF4/INI1* deletion or mutation (found in 85%)
- Peripheral primitive neuroectodermal tumor (PNET) and extraosseous Ewing sarcoma of the craniospinal vault
  - Morphologically indistinguishable from medulloblastoma and supratentorial PNET
  - CD99: membranous staining
  - *EWS-FLI1* fusion gene detectable by fluorescent in situ hybridization (FISH)
- Ependymoma
  - Generally less cellular, and cells have more cytoplasm; infrequent mitotic activity
  - Form perivascular pseudorosettes and ependymal rosettes
  - GFAP positive
  - Synaptophysin and chromogranin negative
- Pilocytic astrocytoma
  - Similar location and age range
  - Less cellular tumor consisting of biphasic pattern with elongated astrocytic areas (piloid) and a microcystic architecture
  - GFAP diffusely positive
  - Synaptophysin and chromogranin negative
- Lymphoma and leukemia
  - History of lymphoma and leukemia is often known
  - Lack nodular architecture and rosette formation
  - Lymphomatous infiltrate is positive for LCA (CD45) and, if B-cell type, CD20
- Metastatic neuroendocrine carcinoma
  - Typically found in older individuals
  - Lacks rosette formation
  - Positive for cytokeratin

Pearls

- Propensity for leptomeningeal dissemination
- Surgical resection with craniospinal radiation is the typical treatment
- Negative prognostic factors: incomplete surgical resection, large cell and anaplastic subtype, isochromosome 17q, loss of 17p, or amplification of *MYCC* or *MYCN*
- Good prognostic factor: presence of extensive nodularity

Selected References

Kazmi SA, Perry A, Pressey JG, et al: Primary Ewing sarcoma of the brain: A case report and literature review. Diagn Mol Pathol 16:108-111, 2007.

Giangaspero F, Wellek S, Masuoka J, et al: Stratification of medulloblastoma on the basis of histopathological grading. Acta Neuropathol 112:5-12, 2006.

McManamy CS, Lamont JM, Taylor RE, et al: Morphophenotypic variation predicts clinical behavior in childhood non-desmoplastic medulloblastomas. J Neuropath Exp Neurol 62:627-632, 2003.

Eberhart CG, Kepner JL, Goldthwaithe PT, et al: Histopathologic grading of medulloblastomas. Cancer 94:552-560, 2002.

Supratentorial Primitive Neuroectodermal Neoplasms (Neuroblastoma, Ganglioneuroblastoma, Ependymoblastoma, Medulloepithelioma) (WHO Grade IV)

Clinical Features

- Neoplasms of primitive neuroepithelial cells occurring in hemispheres, brain stem, or spinal cord
- May display differentiation along neuronal (neuroblastoma, ganglioneuroblastoma), astrocytic, ependymal (ependymoblastoma), or mesenchymal lines (medulloepithelioma)
- Mean age of presentation is 5.5 years (range, 4 to 20 years)
- Signs and symptoms are referable to the site of the mass lesion

Gross Pathology

- Appear as a well-circumscribed, tan-gray, homogeneous mass
- Small cyst formation and calcification are common
- Hemorrhage and necrosis may be present
- Ependymoblastoma and medulloepithelioma usually arise close to the ventricles
- Medulloepitheliomas are often massive lesions with abundant necrosis and hemorrhage

Histopathology

- Hypercellular tumors that appear well circumscribed but are infiltrative
- Homer-Wright rosettes are often present, but poorly formed pseudorosettes consisting of perivascular anuclear zones showing loose fibrillary processes are more common
- Presence of fibrous connective tissue stroma will produce a lobular pattern; this is most prominent when leptomeninges are invaded (desmoplastic form)
- The tumor cells are usually small (round to carrot shaped) and have monomorphic but hyperchromatic nuclei and inconspicuous nucleoli; a moderate degree of nuclear pleomorphism occasionally seen
- Neuronal differentiation is seen in 25% to 50% of cases involving the brain

- Ganglioneuroblastoma
  - Cells will have larger nuclei, vesicular chromatin, nucleoli, and more abundant fibrillar cytoplasm
  - Mitotic activity is variable (usually numerous)
- Medulloepithelioma
  - Papillary or trabecular pattern
  - May display differentiation along neural, glial, and mesenchymal lines
- Ependymoblastoma
  - Distinguished by multilayered rosettes in a background of primitive cells (true rosettes consisting of stratified, small, mitotically active cells with basally oriented nuclei radially arranged around a central lumen)

Special Stains and Immunohistochemistry

- Ganglioneuroblastoma and neuroblastoma
  - Synaptophysin and S-100 positive
  - NSE and neurofilament positive
  - Cytokeratin negative
  - Mib-1 index: markedly variable, 0% to 85%
- Ependymoblastoma
  - GFAP positive
  - Cytokeratin positive
- Medulloepithelioma
  - Nestin and vimentin positive
  - EMA, cytokeratin, and NF variably positive
  - GFAP and S-100 negative

Other Techniques for Diagnosis

- Electron microscopy: tumor cells have microtubules within bipolar processes; typically few neurosecretory granules and sparse cytoplasmic organelles
- Cytogenetics: variable chromosomal losses and gains

Differential Diagnosis

- Central neurocytoma
  - Located within the lateral or third ventricle
  - Lacks distinct rosette formation
  - Cells are uniform and have low mitotic activity
- Peripheral PNET and extra-osseus Ewing sarcoma of the craniospinal vault
  - Morphologically indistinguishable from medulloblastoma and supratentorial PNET
  - CD99: membranous staining
  - *EWS-FLI1* fusion gene detectable by FISH
- Metastatic neuroendocrine carcinoma
  - Typically found in older individuals
  - Lacks rosette formation
  - Positive for cytokeratin
- Desmoplastic infantile ganglioglioma
  - Large cystic masses in infancy (usually younger than 18 months)
  - Typically involves frontal and parietal lobes

- Usually involves leptomeninges, prominent collagenous stroma
- Divergent differentiation along astrocytic and neuronal lines
- Composed of GFAP-positive spindle cells and often inconspicuous ganglion cells

Pearls

- Children younger than 2 years have a poorer prognosis than those older than 2 years
- Cerebrospinal pathway seeding does occur, and metastases outside the CNS have been reported
- Ependymoblastoma: particularly poor prognosis; death occurs in less than 6 months

Selected References

McLendon RE, Judkins AR, Egerhart CG, et al: Central nervous system primitive neuroectodermal tumors. In Louis DN, Ohgaki H, Wiestler OD, Cavenee W (eds): World Health Organization: Classification of Tumours of the Central Nervous System. Lyon, IARC, 2007, pp 141-146.

McLendon RE, Provenzale J: Glioneuronal tumors of the central nervous system. Brain Tumor Pathol 19:51-58, 2002.

Molloy PT, Yachnis AT, Rorke LB, et al. Central nervous system medulloepithelioma: A series of eight cases including two arising in the pons. J Neurosurg 84:430-436, 1996.

Dorsay TA, Rovira MJ, Ho VB, Kelly J: Ependymoblastoma: MR presentation. A case report and review of the literature. Pediatr Radiol 25:433-435, 1995.

Atypical Teratoid/Rhabdoid Tumor (WHO Grade IV)

Clinical Features

- Rare malignant neoplasm occurring most commonly in children younger than 3 years
- About 50% of cases occur in the posterior fossa, with a predilection for the cerebellopontine angle; other reported sites include suprasellar region, pineal region, cerebrum, and spinal cord
- May be intra-axial or extra-axial, with predilection for leptomeningeal dissemination
- Symptoms may be nonlocalizing, consisting of lethargy, vomiting, and failure to thrive; in posterior fossa tumors, focal signs are usually cranial nerve palsies

Gross Pathology

- Gray-white tissue with necrosis and hemorrhage

Histopathology

- Sheets or nests of large cells, each with a round nucleus, prominent nucleolus, plump cell body with homogeneous cytoplasm, or a dense round distinct cytoplasmic inclusion (rhabdoid cells)

- Frequently co-occurrence of foci or sheets of primitive neuroectodermal neoplastic cells, most often a minority component
- An epithelial (adenomatous or papillary pattern) or mesenchymal (loosely packed spindle cells) neoplastic component may also be present (about 33%)
- Epithelial component is least common
- Abundant mitoses and necrosis
- Leptomeningeal spread may be evident on the surface of the cerebellum

Special Stains and Immunohistochemistry

- EMA, vimentin, and smooth muscle actin positive
- GFAP, synaptophysin, and cytokeratin (high- and low-molecular-weight cocktail) frequently positive
- Neurofilament, chromogranin, S-100, desmin, and HMB-45 may be positive
- Ini negative
- Mib-1 index: more than 50%

Other Techniques for Diagnosis

- Ultrastructure: rhabdoid cell cytoplasm contains bundles of intermediate filaments
- Cytogenetics: *hSNF4/INI1* deletion or mutation (found in 85%)

Differential Diagnosis

▌ Medulloblastoma
  - Rhabdoid cells not seen, EMA negative, Ini positive
▌ Choroid plexus carcinoma
  - Not usually in posterior fossa; cytokeratin positive, EMA negative

Pearls

- Resistant to standard therapy for primitive neuroectodermal neoplasms; mean survival time is 10 to 15 months
- Presence of rhabdoid cells is not diagnostic of atypical teratoid/rhabdoid tumor
- Immunohistochemistry and evaluation for the presence of a mutation of the *hSNF5/INI1* gene should be performed
- Seeding of the subarachnoid space is common

Selected References

Bambakidis NC, Robinson S, Cohen M, Cohen AR: Atypical teratoid/rhabdoid tumors of the central nervous system: Clinical, radiographic and pathologic features. Pediatr Neurosurg 37:64-70, 2002.

Packer RJ, Biegel JA, Blaney S, et al: Atypical teratoid/rhabdoid tumor of the central nervous system: report on workshop. J Pediatr Hematol Oncol 24:337-342, 2002.

Rorke LB, Packer RJ, Biegel JA: Central nervous system atypical teratoid/rhabdoid tumors of infancy and childhood: definition of an entity. J Neurosurg 85:56-65, 1996.

Choroid Plexus Tumors

Choroid Plexus Papilloma (WHO Grade I), Atypical Choroid Plexus Papilloma (WHO Grade II), and Choroid Plexus Carcinoma (WHO Grade III)

Clinical Features

- Choroid plexus papillomas (WHO grade I)
  - Slow-growing benign tumors accounting for less than 1% of brain tumors
  - Characteristically found in the fourth ventricle (40%), lateral ventricle (50%), or third ventricle (5%) or at the cerebellopontine angle
  - Commonly found in the first and second decades (50% found before age 20); more often occur in the lateral ventricles when in young individuals and in the fourth ventricle in adults
- Choroid plexus carcinomas (WHO grade III)
  - Typically occur in patients younger than 10 years; rare in adults
  - Most carcinomas affecting the choroid plexus in adults represent metastatic carcinomas
- Patients often present with signs and symptoms secondary to hydrocephalus owing to the overproduction of cerebrospinal fluid or obstruction

Gross Pathology

- Well-demarcated, pedunculated, or cauliflower-like masses
- Papillomas do not invade into the adjacent tissue
- Carcinomas characteristically invade the surrounding tissue and are often necrotic and hemorrhagic

Histopathology

- Choroid plexus papilloma
  - Papillary architecture is composed of a single orderly layer of columnar cells surrounding a distinct fibrovascular core
  - A mild degree of nuclear stratification, crowding of the nuclei, focal necrosis, and nuclear atypia may be seen
  - Stromal calcifications; may see metaplastic bone or cartilage
  - Mitotic activity is typically minimal
  - Small foci of ependymal differentiation may be seen
- Atypical choroid plexus papilloma
  - Defined by increase in mitoses (≥2 mitoses/10 randomly selected hpf)
  - Hypercellularity, nuclear pleomorphism, solid growth pattern, and necrosis may also be present
- Choroid plexus carcinoma
  - Typically show a loose papillary architecture consisting of sheets of pleomorphic cells
  - Extensive necrosis and high mitotic activity (>5 mitoses/hpf)
  - Brain invasion

Special Stains and Immunohistochemistry

- S-100 protein positive (more uniform in papillomas than in carcinomas)
- Cytokeratin 8 and 18, vimentin positive
- Transthyretin (prealbumin): approximately 70% are positive
- GFAP: papillomas may be focally positive; carcinomas typically negative
- EMA variable to negative
- Carcinoembryonic antigen (CEA) usually negative
- Ini protein positive
- Synaptophysin variable positivity
- Mib-1 index: range in papillomas is 2% to 5%; range in carcinomas is 14% to 18%

Other Techniques for Diagnosis

- Electron microscopy: cells of both papillomas and carcinomas typically show cilia, microvilli, basement membrane, and desmosomes
- Cytogenetics
  - Inactivating mutation of the *hSNF5/INI1* gene has been reported in several series of choroid plexus carcinomas and in one series of papillomas
  - A variety of other cytogenetic abnormalities have been described in choroid plexus papillomas and carcinomas

Differential Diagnosis

- Normal choroid plexus
  - Apical hobnail cuboidal cells instead of crowded, more columnar cells with some atypia are present in normal choroid plexus
- Metastatic carcinoma
  - Usually found in older adults
  - Not usually associated with the ventricle
  - Typically positive for EMA and often also for CEA
  - Usually negative for S-100 protein and GFAP
- Ependymoma (especially papillary subtype)
  - Intraventricular location is common for both tumors
  - Solid nonpapillary areas may be evident with both perivascular pseudorosette and true rosette formation
  - GFAP positive; usually more diffuse than in choroid plexus neoplasms
- Atypical teratoid and rhabdoid tumors
  - Important part of differential diagnosis in children with posterior fossa tumors
  - Epithelial areas form part, not all, of the neoplasm
  - Rhabdoid cells and primitive neuroectodermal cell components are also present
  - Ini protein negative

Pearls

- GFAP positivity demonstrates that choroid plexus tumors may show ependymal differentiation
- In choroid plexus papilloma, overall prognosis is good with surgical resection, but incompletely resected tumors may occasionally recur

- Leptomeningeal spread may occur in both papillomas and carcinomas but is rare in papillomas
- Choroid plexus carcinoma has an overall poor prognosis
  — Brain invasion and cerebrospinal fluid spread is typically seen
  — Systemic metastases are rarely seen

Selected References

Paulus W, Brandner S: Choroid plexus tumors. In Louis DN, Ohgaki H, Wiestler OD, Cavenee W (eds): World Health Organization: Classification of Tumours of the Central Nervous System. Lyon, IARC, 2007, pp 82-85.

Krishnan S, Brown PD, Scheithauer BW, et al: Choroid plexus papillomas: A single institutional experience. J Neurooncol 68:49-55, 2004.

Gessi M, Giangaspero F, Pietsch T: Atypical teratoid/rhabdoid tumors and choroid plexus tumors: When genetics "surprise" pathology. Brain Pathol 13:409-414, 2003.

Pineal Parenchymal Tumors

Pineocytoma (WHO Grade I) and Pineal Parenchymal Tumor of Intermediate Differentiation (WHO Grades II and III)

Clinical Features

- Rare tumors accounting for less than 1% of all intracranial neoplasms
- Typically occur in adults
- Localized to the region of the pineal gland and surrounding structures, may extend into the third ventricle and compress the colliculi and cerebral aqueduct
- Variable clinical presentation: ophthalmologic dysfunction, mental status changes, and symptoms related to increased intracranial pressure or endocrine abnormalities
- Computed tomography shows a round, homogeneous, contrast-enhancing mass

Gross Pathology

- Well-circumscribed tumor typically less than 3 cm in diameter
- Gray-tan homogeneous tumor often with small cyst formation
- Small areas of hemorrhage may be present
- Necrosis is not a typical finding

Histopathology

▍ Pineocytoma
- Sheets of tumor cells without a distinct pattern or an irregular lobular arrangement with large aggregates of tumor cells separated by fibrous septa
- Small and uniform cells with hyperchromatic nuclei, finely granular chromatin, inconspicuous nucleoli, and eosinophilic cytoplasmic processes

- Forms large (pineocytomatous) rosettes with abundant fibrillary cell processes in the center, sometimes with cytoplasmic club-shaped terminal expansion; may or may not be centered around blood vessels
- Calcification may be present
- Ganglion cells and multinucleated giant cells are occasionally seen
- Mitotic activity is minimal, and necrosis is not seen

▍ Pineal parenchymal tumor of intermediate differentiation
- Diffuse or lobulated tumors of moderate cellularity
- Mild to moderate nuclear atypia and sparse to moderately frequent mitoses

Special Stains and Immunohistochemistry

- Synaptophysin, chromogranin, NSE, and S-100 protein positive
- Retinal S antigen and rhodopsin positive
- GFAP highlights background residual reactive astrocytes
- Mib-1 labeling index
  — Pineocytoma: low
  — Pineal parenchymal tumor of intermediate differentiation: 3% to 10%

Other Techniques for Diagnosis

- Electron microscopy: cells have oval nuclei and cytoplasm containing numerous organelles, including smooth and rough endoplasmic reticulum, Golgi complexes, mitochondria, lysosomes, intermediate filaments, microtubules, synapse-like junctions, and membrane-bound electron-dense granules; cell processes are typically prominent
- Cytogenetic analyses
  — Pineocytomas: show loss of all or part of chromosomes 22, 11, and 12
  — Pineal parenchymal tumor of intermediate differentiation: abnormalities on chromosomes 4, 12, and 22

Differential Diagnosis

▍ Normal pineal gland
- Normal lobular architecture is a helpful distinguishing feature
- May show irregular calcifications

▍ Pineal cyst
- Radiographically shows a distinct cystic structure
- Rarely symptomatic; mean age of symptomatic occurrence is 30 years
- Women are affected more than men
- Lacks large rosettes typically seen in pineocytoma
- Consists of a glial-lined cavity surrounded by reactive glial tissue

▍ Pineoblastoma
- Occurs typically in young individuals
- Shows well-formed, small perivascular rosettes
- Consists of undifferentiated, monomorphic, small round blue cells

■ Astrocytoma
- Lacks lobular architecture and rosettes
- GFAP positive
- Synaptophysin negative

Pearls

- Pineocytoma
  — Slow-growing neoplasm with excellent prognosis; metastases are not reported with these tumors
  — Treatment consists of conservative surgery after the development of symptoms
- Five-year survival rate for pineal parenchymal tumor of intermediate differentiation ranges from 39% to 74%
- Factors associated with improved survival are presence of neurofilament immunoreactivity, low mitoses, and absence of necrosis

Selected References

Hirato J, Nakazato Y: Pathology of pineal region tumors. J Neurooncol 54:239-249, 2001.

Jouvet A, Sainte-Pierre G, Fauchon F, et al: Pineal parenchymal tumors: A correlation of histological features with prognosis in 66 cases. Brain Pathol 10:49-60, 2000.

Taylor MD, Mainprize TG, Squire JA, Rutka JT: Molecular genetics of pineal region neoplasms. J Neurooncol 54:219-238, 2001.

Pineoblastoma (WHO Grade IV)

Clinical Features

- Constitute 45% of all pineal tumors
- Typically found in children within the first two decades
- Variable clinical presentation: ophthalmologic dysfunction; mental status changes, symptoms related to increased intracranial pressure, or endocrine abnormalities
- CT and MRI show a large, lobulated, poorly defined, contrast-enhancing mass

Gross Pathology

- Poorly defined soft, friable mass with hemorrhage and necrosis
- Infiltration into adjacent brain parenchyma and meninges is common

Histopathology

- Highly cellular neoplasm composed of primitive poorly differentiated tumor cells
- Diffuse sheets of neoplastic cells with focal rosette formation
- Round or oval hyperchromatic nuclei, typically with single nucleoli, scant cytoplasm, and indistinct cell borders
- Homer-Wright rosettes or, less commonly, Flexner-Wintersteiner true rosettes

- Mitotic activity is often prominent; hemorrhage and necrosis are common

Special Stains and Immunohistochemistry

- Synaptophysin positive, diffuse, or dotlike
- Chromogranin and NSE positive
- Retinal S antigen positive
- GFAP typically negative

Other Techniques for Diagnosis

- Cytogenetic analyses: patients with germline mutations in *Rb* gene (chromosome 13q14) are predisposed to tumor occurrence as part of trilateral retinoblastoma disease
- This mutation has not been reported in sporadic pineoblastomas

Differential Diagnosis

■ Pineocytoma and pineal parenchymal tumor of intermediate differentiation
- Pineocytomas have better-differentiated cells with more abundant cytoplasm and pineocytomatous rosettes
- Pineal parenchymal tumors of intermediate differentiation have moderate cellularity, less atypia, and fewer mitosis

Pearls

- Aggressive tumor typically with craniospinal seeding; rare extracranial metastases

Selected References

Nakazato Y, Jouvet A, Scheithauer BW: Pineoblastoma. In Louis DN, Ohgaki H, Wiestler OD, Cavenee W (eds): World Health Organization: Classification of Tumours of the Central Nervous System. Lyon, IARC, 2007, pp 126-127.

Hirato J, Nakazato Y: Pathology of pineal region tumors. J Neurooncol 54:239-249, 2001.

Taylor MD, Mainprize TG, Squire JA, Rutka JT: Molecular genetics of pineal region neoplasms. J Neurooncol 54:219-238, 2001.

Papillary Tumor of the Pineal Region (WHO Grades II and III)

Clinical Features

- Wide age range (5 to 66 years); mean, 32 years
- Presentation is usually with headache due to obstructive hydrocephalus, without focal neurologic signs
- MRI shows a well-circumscribed T1-hypointense, T2-hyperintense enhancing mass in the pineal region, ranging in size from 1.7 to 5 cm

Gross Pathology

- Well-circumscribed, usually solid

Histopathology

- Papillary architecture with perivascular pseudorosettes; ependymal rosettes have been reported
- Cells are cuboidal to columnar and have well-defined cytoplasm
- Necrosis is usually present; mitoses are sparse, and vascular proliferation is not usually present

Special Stains and Immunohistochemistry

- Cytokeratin (AE1/AE3, CAM5.2, CK18) and S-100 positive
- GFAP: focal positivity
- Synaptophysin, chromogranin, and NSE weakly and focally positive
- EMA variably positive
- Mib-1 labeling index: 4% to 5%

Other Techniques for Diagnosis

- Ultrastructure: microvilli, zipper-like junctions, abundant rough endoplasmic reticulum, dilated cisternae, annulatae lamellae, dense core vesicles, and microtubules
- Cytogenetics: most commonly found are losses of chromosomes 10 and 22q and gain of chromosome 4

Differential Diagnosis

▌ Choroid plexus papilloma
- Distinctly epithelial morphology and well-defined papillary formations
- No ependymal rosettes
- Usually no necrosis

▌ Ependymoma
- Fibrillary cytoplasm
- GFAP: prominent perivascular pseudorosette positivity
- EMA: consistent dotlike positivity
- Cytokeratin: focally positive

Pearls

- Newly defined entity
- Tumor recurrence and progression is frequent (72%) and is associated with incomplete resection and increased mitoses

Selected References

Boco T, Aalaei S, Musacchio M, et al: Papillary tumor of the pineal region. Neuropathology 28:87-92, 2008.

Fèvre-Montange M, Hasselblatt M, Figarella-Branger D, et al: Prognosis and histopathologic features in papillary tumors of the pineal region: A retrospective multicenter study of 31 cases. J Neuropathol Exp Neurol 65:1004-1011, 2006.

Jouvet A, Fauchon F, Liberski P, et al: Papillary tumor of the pineal region. Am J Surg Pathol 27:505-512, 2003.

Other Neoplasms and Related Entities

Peripheral Nerve Sheath Tumors

Clinical Features

▌ Schwannoma (WHO grade I)
- Benign tumor composed of Schwann cells; also called *neurilemmoma*
- Found in all ages, most commonly in the fourth through sixth decades
- Most commonly involves peripheral nerves in skin and subcutaneous tissues of the head and neck region and flexor surfaces of extremities
- Accounts for about 10% of intracranial tumors (usually arises from sensory cranial nerves, most often eighth cranial nerve) and about 30% of spinal tumors
- Associated with neurofibromatosis type 2 (NF2) (bilateral vestibular schwannomas)

Figure 19-12. A, Schwannoma. Compact spindle cells (Antoni A tissue) and Verocay bodies. **B, Neurofibroma.** Sparsely cellular proliferation of spindle cells with wavy nuclei and cytoplasmic processes.

- Peripheral tumors typically present as asymptomatic masses; spinal tumors often present with radicular pain or signs of spinal cord compression; tumors of cranial nerve VIII cause hearing difficulties, tinnitus, or facial paresthesias
■ Neurofibroma (WHO grade I)
  - Common benign tumor composed of Schwann cells, fibroblasts, and perineural cells
  - Occur sporadically most frequently but also associated with NF1
  - Multiple subtypes
    — Localized cutaneous neurofibroma: most common subtype, usually solitary and not associated with NF; cases associated with NF1 are often multiple
    — Diffuse cutaneous neurofibroma: uncommon, occurs primarily in children and young adults, forms large, ill-defined plaques
    — Localized intracranial neurofibroma: causes segmental, fusiform enlargement of the nerve; multiple lesions occur primarily in a background of NF1
    — Plexiform neurofibroma: transformation of multiple fascicles of nerve into neurofibroma with preservation of normal anatomic configuration, affecting larger nerves or a nerve plexus and occurring almost exclusively in patients with NF1
    — Massive soft tissue neurofibroma: the least common variant found in patients with NF1, typically massive tumors resulting in marked enlargement of the affected extremity or regional soft tissue
■ Malignant peripheral nerve sheath tumor (MPNST) (WHO grade II, III, or IV)
  - May arise from Schwann cells, fibroblasts, or perineural cells
  - Most present as mass lesions in association with medium to large peripheral nerves of the extremities
  - Intracranial lesions usually involve the vagus or vestibular nerves
  - About 50% are associated with NF1
  - Tumors occur most commonly in third to sixth decades, but earlier in association with NF1
■ Perineurioma (WHO grade I, II, or III)
  - Present in teens or young adulthood with muscle weakness in distribution of a peripheral nerve or as mass lesion in deep soft tissue
  - Several types described with varying presentations
    — Extraneural soft tissue perineurioma: subcutaneous tissues of trunk and limbs; painless mass, in children or adults
    — Sclerosing perineurioma: hands of young adult men
    — Reticular perineurioma: in upper limbs of women (31 to 61 years)
    — Intraneural perineurioma: in children and young adults, in extremities

Gross Pathology
■ Schwannoma
  - Typically solitary, encapsulated, round to oval mass measuring up to 10 cm (multiple lesions are seen in NF)
  - Cut surface shows firm, tan-white to bright-yellow, glistening tissue
  - Small cyst formation and focal hemorrhage may be seen (cysts are typically absent in cellular schwannomas)
  - Nerve is often identified
■ Neurofibroma
  - Solid, tan-white, soft to mucoid tumors surrounded by a thin capsule
  - Tumor incorporates the nerve, so no nerve is typically identified
■ Plexiform neurofibroma
  - Typically forms a complex tangle of enlarged nerves resembling a bag of worms
■ Malignant peripheral nerve sheath tumor
  - Large infiltrative, nonencapsulated mass with a fleshy, tan cut surface
  - Hemorrhage and necrosis are common
■ Perineurioma
  - Circumscribed and firm; intraneural subtype is associated with peripheral nerve

Histopathology
■ Schwannoma
  - Shows biphasic pattern alternating between highly cellular, compact areas and loose, spongy areas of low cellularity
  - Compact, cellular areas are termed *Antoni A* and consist of interlacing fascicles of elongated, regular spindle cells with long, pencil-shaped nuclei
  - Sparsely cellular areas consisting of loose, spongy tissue with small, uniform cells termed *Antoni B*
  - Tumors showing marked nuclear pleomorphism, hyperchromasia (degenerative atypia), and thick, hyalinized blood vessels are called *ancient schwannomas*
  - Areas of nuclear palisading with nuclei arranged in linear stacks are called *Verocay bodies*; more commonly seen in spinal schwannomas
  - Axons may be seen at the periphery of the tumor
  - Mitotic activity is minimal
  - Perivascular whorls resembling meningioma may occasionally be seen
  - Vessels are often hyalinized, and foci of lipid-laden macrophages may be present
  - Two subtypes
    — Cellular schwannoma
      ◆ Increased likelihood of recurrence, but lacks ability to metastasize
      ◆ Highly cellular, consisting predominantly of Antoni A areas

◆ Variable mitotic activity; typically show 1 to 4 mitoses/10 hpf

◆ Frequent capsular, subcapsular, and perivascular lymphocytic infiltrates

◆ Small foci of necrosis may be seen

— Melanotic schwannoma

◆ Usually grossly pigmented and contains Schwann cells with melanosomes

◆ About 10% behave more aggressively than the nonmelanotic schwannomas

▮ Neurofibroma

● Typically hypocellular tumor consisting of interlacing fascicles of elongated spindle cells with wavy nuclei; minimal nuclear pleomorphism is typical

● Background shows variable degrees of mucopolysaccharide matrix, collagen, and reticulin

● Minimal mitotic activity

● Plexiform neurofibroma: consists of multiple hypocellular, pale fascicles of spindle cells

● Mucinous or myxoid background

▮ Malignant peripheral nerve sheath tumor

● Highly cellular tumors with moderate to marked nuclear pleomorphism (sarcomatous appearance)

● High mitotic rate (more than 5/10 hpf)

● Areas of geographic necrosis may be seen

● Greatly variable morphology, but often spindle cells forming a herringbone or fascicular pattern are seen

● Up to 20% of cases show unusual histologic features, including epithelioid cells and divergent mesenchymal or glandular differentiation

▮ Perineurioma

● Extraneural and sclerosing subtypes: vary from spindle-shaped elongated cells to epithelioid; variable architectural patterns, including whorling, lamellar, and storiform

● Reticular subtype: prominent myxoid stroma, netlike growth pattern

● Intraneural subtype: spindle cells arranged in pseudo onion-bulb arrangement around axons and Schwann cells

Special Stains and Immunohistochemistry

▮ Schwannomas

● S-100 positive

● GFAP: variable focal positivity

● Collagen IV and laminin positive

▮ Neurofibroma

● S-100 positive

● Collagen IV, laminin variable

● EMA: few positive cells

▮ Perineurioma

● EMA positive

● Collagen IV, laminin positive

● Claudin-1, GLUT1 positive

● S-100 negative

● Mib-1 index: ranges from 5% to 15%

▮ MPNST

● S-100 positive in up to 70%, but higher-grade lesions show less positivity

● Mib-1 index: ranges from 5% to 65%

Other Techniques for Diagnosis

▮ Conventional and cellular schwannoma

● Electron microscopy: well-differentiated, elongated cells with long cytoplasmic processes surrounded by a complete basal lamina; characteristically shows intercellular long-spacing collagen (Luse bodies)

● Cytogenetics: loss of the *NF2* gene product on chromosome 22 (also called *Merlin*) in 60%

▮ Neurofibroma

● Electron microscopy: mixture of cells including Schwann cells and perineurial cells

● Cytogenetics: plexiform subtype associated with NF1; sporadic neurofibromas commonly also have mutations in the *NF1* gene

▮ MPNST

● Electron microscopy: poorly differentiated cells showing nuclear pleomorphism and an incomplete basement membrane; usually no Luse bodies

● Cytogenetics: 50% associated with NF1

▮ Perineurioma

● Electron microscopy: elongated cells and nuclei, delicate chromatin, pinocytotic vesicles, basal lamina, and tight junctions

● Cytogenetics: loss of chromosome 22 or 22q

Differential Diagnosis

▮ Meningioma

● Often shows prominent whorled pattern and psammoma bodies

● Rare in lumbosacral region (common site for schwannomas)

● Negative or faint staining for S-100 protein

● Positive staining for EMA (70%)

Pearls

● Large neurofibromas associated with NF and plexiform neurofibromas have an increased potential for malignant transformation (MPNST)

● Multiple schwannomas may be seen in various syndromes (schwannomatosis, NF); isolated bilateral schwannomas of cranial nerve VIII are pathognomonic of NF2

● MPNSTs are high-grade, aggressive tumors with tendency to recur and metastasize (often metastasize to lung)

● EMA positivity in perineuriomas may be faint and difficult to see because of thin processes

● Perineuriomas are usually cured with complete resection, but rare malignant cases are reported

Selected References

Macarenco RS, Ellinger F, Oliveira AM: Perineurioma: A distinctive and underrecognized peripheral nerve sheath neoplasm. Arch Pathol Lab Med 31:625-636, 2007.

Scheithauer BW, Louis DN, Hunter S, et al: Tumors of the cranial and paraspinal nerves. In Louis DN, Ohgaki H, Wiestler OD, Cavenee W (eds): World Health Organization: Classification of Tumours of the Central Nervous System. Lyon, IARC, 2007, pp 151-162.

Scheithauer BW, Woodruff JM, Erlandson RA: Tumors of the peripheral nervous system. Atlas of Tumor Pathology, 3rd Series, Fascicle 24. Bethesda, MD, Armed Forces Institute of Pathology, 1999.

Meningioma (WHO Grade I), Atypical Meningioma (WHO Grade II), and Anaplastic Meningioma (WHO Grade III)

Clinical Features

- Common tumor accounting for 24% to 30% of all primary intracranial neoplasms
- Typically found in middle-aged adults; occasionally seen in children
- More commonly occurs in females (3:2); intraspinal tumors show a 10:1 female-to-male ratio
- About 90% of tumors are intracranial
- Patients usually present with symptoms related to an enlarging intracranial mass or increased intracranial pressure; may have focal neurologic deficits or rarely seizures
- CT and MRI show dura-based, richly vascular, contrast-enhancing, well-defined masses; clusters of calcifications may be seen
- Rarely arises from the optic nerve, causing visual symptoms, or within the spinal cord, causing radicular pain; may also rarely involve the ventricular system

Figure 19-13. Meningioma. Syncytial pattern of neoplastic cells displaying a classic meningothelial appearance with round to oval nuclei. Several whorls are present.

Gross Pathology

- Firm, well-defined, tan-white tumor often showing attachment to a segment of dura; may show a yellow or gelatinous cut surface owing to lipid or mucin accumulation
- Frequent infiltration of bone and scalp
- Frequently causes hyperostosis of skull
- Calcification is commonly seen
- Atypical or anaplastic meningioma
  - Typically causes considerable cerebral edema
  - Brain invasion is frequently present

Histopathology

- Extremely diverse tumor with numerous histologic variants
- Classic meningioma (WHO grade I)
  - Syncytial, fibrous, and transitional variants (transitional variant is most common): *syncytial pattern* is created by sheets of tumor cells that have indistinct cell borders; *fibrous meningiomas* show elongated cells in a collagenous background; *transitional meningiomas* show a pattern that is intermediate between the syncytial and fibrous types or composed of a mixture of syncytial and fibrous patterns
    - Neoplastic cells are arranged in a whorled or lobulated architecture
    - Tumor cells have a meningothelial appearance with round to oval nuclei, dispersed chromatin, inconspicuous nucleoli, and eosinophilic cytoplasm
    - Prominent round intranuclear inclusions are typical
    - Psammoma bodies are often noted throughout the tumor; less commonly seen in pure fibrous types
    - Focal nuclear pleomorphism is often present
    - Scattered mitotic figures may be seen
  - Other variants
    - Psammomatous meningioma (WHO grade I)
      - Shows abundant psammoma bodies throughout the tumor
    - Secretory meningioma (WHO grade I)
      - Cytoplasm contains round, eosinophilic, hyaline structures resembling psammoma bodies (pseudopsammoma bodies)
      - Structures are PAS positive and diastase resistant
    - Microcystic meningioma (WHO grade I)
      - Consists of a delicate, microcystic architecture with cystic spaces filled with clear fluid
      - Often shows greater degree of cytologic atypia or areas of xanthomatous cells with vacuolated cytoplasm
    - Lymphoplasmacytic meningioma (WHO grade I)
      - Shows a pronounced lymphoplasmacytic response

— Metaplastic meningioma (WHO grade I)
  ◆ Metaplastic areas may consist of myxoid, chordoid, osteoblastic, lipoblastic, or xanthomatous differentiation
— Angiomatous meningioma (WHO grade I)
  ◆ Abundant vessels with sparse meningothelial cells
  ◆ Vessels are usually hyalinized, and degenerative nuclear atypia is common
- Prognostically important variants
  — Chordoid meningioma (WHO grade II)
    ◆ Rare variant
    ◆ Consists of small groups or cords of epithelioid cells in a mucin-rich background (resembles a chordoma)
  — Clear cell meningioma (WHO grade II)
    ◆ Composed of cells with clear cytoplasm
    ◆ Cytoplasm contains glycogen (PAS positive)
    ◆ Suggestion of aggressive growth and high recurrence rates
  — Papillary meningioma (WHO grade III)
    ◆ Typically occurs in younger individuals
    ◆ Tumor cells arranged around blood vessels resembling ependymoma-like pseudorosettes
    ◆ Aggressive clinical course (55% recurrence rate; 20% metastasis rate)
  — Rhabdoid meningioma (WHO grade III)
    ◆ Tumor may exhibit exclusively rhabdoid cellular morphology, but more commonly presents mixed with rhabdoid cells and typical meningioma cells
    ◆ Rhabdoid cells have eccentric nuclei and hyaline paranuclear inclusions
    ◆ Reported cases have high Mib-1 index and many mitoses, which have been associated with a high rate of recurrence and aggressive growth

▌ Atypical meningioma (WHO grade II)
- Exhibits increased mitoses (≥4 mitoses/10 hpf), brain invasion, or the presence of at least three of following four microscopic features: tumor showing sheetlike growth pattern, nuclei with macronucleoli, hypercellularity, and small cell formation or spontaneous necrosis

▌ Anaplastic meningioma (WHO grade III)
- Exhibits focal or diffuse loss of meningothelial differentiation at the light microscopic level (areas showing sarcomatous, carcinomatous, or melanoma-like appearance) *or* marked elevation in mitotic rate (≥20 mitoses/10 hpf)

Special Stains and Immunohistochemistry

- EMA, claudin-1: most are positive
- S-100 protein: occasionally positive; fibrous meningiomas: 80% are positive
- Cytokeratin: usually negative; secretory meningiomas usually positive
- GFAP negative
- Mib-1: labeling index correlates with grade and recurrence rate; in general, an index greater than 4% is associated with increased recurrence; mean values of Mib-1 index: benign, 3.8%; atypical, 7.2%; anaplastic, 14.7%
- CD34: 60% of fibrous meningiomas are positive
- Progesterone receptor: variably positive; less likely to be positive in atypical or anaplastic meningiomas

Other Techniques for Diagnosis

- Electron microscopy: cells have nuclei with interdigitating, irregular membranes, desmosomes, and intranuclear cytoplasmic inclusions
- Cytogenetics
  — Monosomy 22 is most commonly found
  — With increasing grade, cytogenetic abnormalities increase; most often found are abnormalities of chromosomes 1, 6, 10, 14, and 18
  — Meningiomas are found in NF2 (*NF2* locus on chromosome 22q), and mutations in the *NF2* gene are found in 60% of sporadic meningiomas

Differential Diagnosis

▌ Schwannoma
- Biphasic tumor consisting of highly cellular areas (Antoni A) admixed with loose spongy areas of lower cellularity (Antoni B)
- Usually lacks distinct whorled architecture and psammoma bodies
- Typically found in posterior fossa or spinal cord
- S-100 protein and EMA usually positive

▌ Ependymoma
- Located within the ventricle; not usually associated with the meninges
- Typically occurs in children or young adults
- Cells have long fibrillary processes
- Rosettes are commonly seen
- GFAP positive

▌ Meningeal hyperplasia
- Single or multiple foci of meningothelial cells (more than 10 cell layers thick)
- Usually associated with a predisposing factor (hemorrhage, chronic renal failure, trauma)
- Discontinuous growth pattern and no invasion or adjacent tissue

▌ Hemangiopericytoma
- Contains numerous variably sized, slitlike and staghorn vessels
- No psammoma bodies
- Negative for EMA, and patchy, weak positivity for CD34

▌ Solitary fibrous tumor
- Shows hemangiopericytoma-like vascular pattern
- CD34 positive

Pearls

- Treatment is complete surgical resection; typically offers an excellent prognosis with classic meningiomas
- Radiation therapy has been shown to be beneficial in recurrent or unresectable tumors
- Benign meningiomas have a recurrence rate of up to 25%; atypical meningiomas are associated with a 29% to 52% recurrence rate; anaplastic meningiomas have recurrence rate range of 50% to 94%

Selected References

Nakasu S, Li DH, Okabe H, et al: Significance of MIB-1 staining indices in meningiomas. Am J Surg Pathol 25:472-478, 2001.

Perry A, Scheithauer BW, Stafford SL, et al: "Malignancy" in meningiomas: A clinicopathologic study of 116 patients with grading implications. Cancer 85:2046-2056, 1999.

Perry A, Stafford SL, Scheithauer BW, et al: Meningioma grading: An analysis of histologic parameters. Am J Surg Pathol 21:1455-1465, 1997.

Perry A, Scheithauer BW, Nascimento AG: The immunophenotypic spectrum of meningeal hemangiopericytoma: A comparison with fibrous meningioma and solitary fibrous tumor of meninges. Am J Surg Pathol 21:1354-1360, 1997.

Hemangiopericytoma (WHO Grade II) and Anaplastic Hemangiopericytoma (WHO Grade III)

Clinical Features

- Dura-based sarcoma accounts for less than 1% of all CNS tumors
- Typically associated with meninges and located within the cranial rather than the spinal compartment
- Most originate in the meninges and often mimic meningiomas

Figure 19-14. Hemangiopericytoma. Classic staghorn vascular pattern is evident in this neoplasm composed of polygonal to spindle-shaped cells.

- Usually found in adults; no sex predilection
- Most patients present with headache and focal neurologic deficits
- CT and MRI show a diffusely enhancing, sharply defined lesion with dural attachment suggestive of meningioma; bone destruction may be seen

Gross Pathology

- Typically forms a discrete, lobulated, tan-gray, fleshy mass
- May show invasive architecture with destruction of adjacent bone; usually no calcifications
- Markedly vascular tumor that bleeds profusely at surgery
- Cut surface is solid, focally hemorrhagic, and often with large vascular spaces

Histopathology

- Variably cellular tumor with numerous small slitlike and large staghorn vascular channels
- Some tumors show predominantly spindle cells with collagenous background
- Tumor cells typically have plump oval or elongated nuclei with inconspicuous nucleoli and scant cytoplasm
- Typically lacks areas of necrosis
- Lacks tight whorls, psammoma bodies, or nuclear pseudoinclusions as seen in meningiomas
- Anaplastic hemangiopericytoma
  - Presence of necrosis or more than 5 mitoses/10 hpf; and at least two of the following microscopic features
    - Hemorrhage
    - Moderate to high nuclear atypia
    - Moderate to high cellularity

Special Stains and Immunohistochemistry

- Reticulin: surrounds individual cells
- CD34: patchy positivity
- CD99, factor XIIIa, bcl-2, and vimentin: strong diffuse positivity
- EMA: weak, focal positivity
- Factor VIII: endothelial cells are positive; tumor cells are negative
- Mib-1 labeling index: 5% to 10%

Other Techniques for Diagnosis

- Electron microscopy: cells with basal lamina, primitive intercellular junctions, and whorled masses of intermediate filaments
- Molecular analysis: abnormalities of chromosomes 12 and 3

Differential Diagnosis

▌ Meningioma
- Presence of psammoma bodies, whorls, calcification, and pseudoinclusions

- Typically lack large staghorn blood vessels and abundant reticulin
- EMA positive; CD34 negative; CD99 negative; bcl-2 negative

▌ Solitary fibrous tumor

- Areas of hyalinization and collagen deposition are frequent
- Typically lacks highly cellular areas seen in hemangiopericytoma
- Sparse reticulin deposition, around clusters of cells
- Strong and diffuse positivity for CD34, vimentin, and bcl-2

Pearls

- High rate of local recurrence with frequent late distant metastases typically involving the bone, liver, or lung
- Surgical resection followed by radiotherapy is the usual treatment
- Postoperative radiation, chemotherapy, or both decreases tumor recurrence and may increase survival
- Anaplastic hemangiopericytomas are associated with increased rates of recurrence and decreased survivals
- Mib-1 labeling index unrelated to grade

Selected References

Rajaram V, Brat DJ, Perry A: Anaplastic meningioma versus meningeal hemangiopericyoma: Immunohistochemical and genetic markers. Hum Pathol 35:1413-1418, 2004.

Ecker RD, Marsh WR, Pollock BE, et al: Hemangiopericytoma in the central nervous system: Treatment, pathological features, and long-term follow up in 38 patients. J Neurosurg 98:1182-1187, 2003.

Tihan T, Viglione M, Rosenblum MK, et al: Solitary fibrous tumors in the central nervous system: A clinicopathologic review of 18 cases and comparison to meningeal hemangiopericytomas. Arch Pathol Lab Med 127:432-439, 2003.

Perry A, Scheithauer BW, Nascemento AG: The immuno-phenotypic spectrum of meningeal hemangiopericytoma: A comparison with fibrous meningioma and solitary fibrous tumor of meninges. Am J Surg Pathol 21:1354-1360, 1997.

Hemangioblastoma (WHO Grade I)

Clinical Features

- Low-grade neoplasm, associated with VHL: autosomal dominant disorder characterized by hemangioblastomas of the CNS and retina, renal cell carcinoma, pheochromocytoma, pancreatic islet cell tumor, endolymphatic sac tumor, and visceral cysts
- About 25% of cerebellar hemangioblastomas occur in patients with VHL
- Of patients with VHL, 70% develop hemangioblastomas

Figure 19-15. Hemangioblastoma. Abundant vascular channels and numerous lipid-laden stromal cells.

- Sporadic cases are typically found in adults (fourth and fifth decades) and are usually single; multiple tumors are commonly seen in patients with VHL and occur at younger ages (third and fourth decades)
- Typically occurs in the cerebellum (80%); less commonly found in the spinal cord, brain stem, or cerebrum
- Symptoms are usually related to increased intracranial pressure when the tumor is in the posterior fossa; back pain and weakness or pain in extremities are seen in spinal cord tumors
- Tumor production of erythropoietin may cause secondary polycythemia

Gross Pathology

- Well-circumscribed, highly vascular mass, usually largely cystic with a solid mural nodule
- Cyst fluid is clear, often yellow, and may be hemorrhagic
- Neoplasm may be yellow owing to high lipid content and commonly has areas of hemorrhage

Histopathology

- Characteristically shows a prominent dense network of capillaries lined by hyperplastic endothelial cells and pericytes; interspersed large thin-walled vessels are also present
- Interstitial stromal cells are large and have abundant vacuolated lipid-rich pale cytoplasm; nuclei are large, usually without nucleoli, and occasionally show slight to moderate pleomorphism
- Cyst wall is composed of reactive astrocytes and Rosenthal fibers that may resemble a pilocytic astrocytoma
- Mitotic activity is rare to absent

Special Stains and Immunohistochemistry

- GFAP: entrapped astrocytes positive; stromal cells negative
- Vimentin: stromal cells positive
- Inhibin A and oil red O (on fresh tissue): stromal cells positive
- S-100 and NSE: stromal cells variably positive
- EMA, cytokeratin, CD34, and factor VIII: stromal cells negative
- Reticulin highlights vessels and is present around tumor cells
- Mib-1 index: sparse positive nuclei (<2%)

Other Techniques for Diagnosis

- Ultrastructure: three cell types are identified: endothelial cells, pericytes, and stromal cells; the stromal cells contain lipid droplets, microfilaments, and electron-dense granules (associated with erythropoietin-like substance)
- Cytogenetics: VHL is caused by deletions or mutations in a tumor suppressor gene (chromosome 3p25-26)
- Germline mutations in this gene are found in some individuals presenting with hemangioblastoma
- Loss or inactivation of *VHL* gene is found in up to 50% of patients with sporadic neoplasms

Differential Diagnosis

▌ Pilocytic astrocytoma
- Classically cells have elongated nuclei and fibrillary cytoplasm
- GFAP diffusely positive

▌ Metastatic clear cell renal cell carcinoma
- May occur in association with hemangioblastoma in VHL
- Usually not cystic
- Mitotic figures usually abundant
- Typically positive for EMA, cytokeratin (CAM5.2), and CD10; negative for inhibin A and NSE

▌ Paraganglioma
- Typically synaptophysin and chromogranin positive

▌ Meningioma (angiomatous)
- EMA positive and inhibin A negative

Pearls

- The stromal cell is considered the neoplastic component of the tumor, but its histogenesis has not been clarified
- Complete surgical resection offers excellent results; rare reports of tumor recurrence after incomplete resection
- Recent study suggests symptom progression is secondary to the increasing size of the cyst rather than growth of the neoplasm

Selected References

Aldape KD, Plate KH, Vortmeyer AO, et al: Hemangioblastoma. In Louis DN, Ohgaki H, Wiestler OD, Cavenee W (eds): World Health Organization: Classification of Tumours of the Central Nervous System. Lyon, France, IARC, 2007, pp 184-186.

Takei H, Bhattacharjee MB, Rivera A, et al: New immunohistochemical markers in the evaluation of central nervous system tumors: A review of seven selected adult and pediatric brain tumors. Arch Pathol Lab Med 131:234-241, 2007.

Hoang MP, Amirkhan MH: Inhibin alpha distinguishes hemangioblastoma from clear cell renal cell carcinoma. Am J Surg Pathol 27:1152-1156, 2003.

Malignant Lymphoma (Non-Hodgkin and Hodgkin)

Clinical Features

- Primary CNS lymphomas (PCNSLs) make up 6.6% of all primary brain tumors and occur in both immunocompetent and immunocompromised hosts
- PCNSL is non-Hodgkin type, and about 5% of primary cases are associated with acquired immunodeficiency syndrome (AIDS)
- Incidence of PCNSL has increased over the past 25 years, only partially attributable to occurrence in those with human immunodefiency virus (HIV) infection
- The peak ages of occurrence in the immunocompetent individual are in the sixth and seventh decades, with a slightly higher occurrence in men than women
- Immunocompromised host mean age is 37 years in transplant recipients and 39 years in AIDS patients
- Most common location is in the parenchyma of the cerebral hemispheres, forming discrete or diffuse lesions
  — Occurs, with decreasing frequency, in the thalamus and basal ganglia, corpus callosum, ventricles, and cerebellum
  — Less common sites of occurrence are the leptomeninges, eye, and spinal cord

Figure 19-16. Malignant lymphoma. Classic angiocentric pattern for a malignant lymphoma involving the brain.

- Overall, up to 50% are multiple, but multifocality is more common in the immunocompromised patient (85%)
- Meningeal involvement is more common in secondary lesions
- The typical clinical presentation of PCNSL is with focal neurologic signs or symptoms (70%), followed by neuropsychiatric symptoms (43%) and increased intracranial pressure (33%)
- Primary Hodgkin disease in the CNS is extremely rare; more common is to have CNS involvement with known systemic disease

Gross Pathology

- An ill-defined mass involving the deep periventricular tissue or occurring superficially in the brain, causing thickening of the cortex, is most common
- Tumor may be yellow or gray-white, show areas of hemorrhage or necrosis, and be solid or cystic
- Hodgkin disease typically involves the dura, meninges, and skull-base structures

Histopathology

- ▌ Non-Hodgkin lymphoma
  - In both the immunocompetent and immunocompromised hosts, most are diffuse large B-cell type (>95%)
  - Less commonly, low-grade B-cell type, marginal zone B-cell lymphoma, Burkitt lymphoma, or T-cell types
  - Patchy clusters of cells with a predilection for perivascular spaces (evokes a deposition of reticulin fibers); diffuse sheets may also be seen
  - Individual cells are usually large and round with scant circumscribed cytoplasm and pleomorphic nuclei with nucleoli
  - Mitoses, apoptosis, and geographic necrosis are common
- ▌ Hodgkin disease
  - Most common subtypes involving the brain are nodular sclerosing and mixed cellularity
  - Characterized by neoplastic Reed-Sternberg cells (large, binucleated cells with each nucleus containing a single prominent nucleolus; abundant eosinophilic cytoplasm) in a background of mixed inflammatory cells, including lymphocytes, plasma cells, neutrophils, eosinophils, and macrophages

Special Stains and Immunohistochemistry

- LCA (CD45) positive
- B- and T-cell markers: CD20/CD3 positive depending on lineage
- Epstein-Barr virus (EBV) in situ hybridization positive in lymphomas in AIDS patients and other immunocompromised hosts

Other Techniques for Diagnosis

- Cytogenetics: gains of *MALT1* and *bcl-2* in 18q21 are the most common abnormality

Differential Diagnosis

- ▌ Metastatic neuroendocrine carcinoma
  - Well-defined tumors typically lacking an infiltrative margin
  - Cell cohesion and nuclear molding typically present
  - Cytokeratin, synaptophysin, and chromogranin positive
  - LCA and CD20 negative
- ▌ Oligodendroglioma
  - Monomorphic oligodendroglial cells with perinuclear halos and less well-defined cytoplasm compared with lymphoma cells
  - Cells typically do not infiltrate through the vessel walls as in lymphoma
  - Microcalcifications are characteristic
  - LCA and CD20 negative
  - Deletions of chromosomes 1p and 19q frequent
- ▌ Reactive lymphocytosis (as in viral encephalitis and demyelinating diseases)
  - Lymphocytes do not show significant cytologic atypia
  - Lacks monoclonality (usually predominantly T lymphocytes, less B lymphocytes)
  - Cluster in perivascular regions, but do not form solid sheets of cells in the parenchyma
  - Consider progressive multifocal leukoencephalopathy (PML) and toxoplasmosis in the immunocompromised host
- ▌ Medulloblastoma and PNET
  - Rosette formation may be seen
  - Positive for synaptophysin, NSE, and neurofilament
  - Negative for LCA

Pearls

- Treatment with steroids before biopsy is to be avoided if possible because the treatment may disrupt cellular morphology so completely that pathologic diagnosis is not possible
- Surgical resection and radiation treatment have not been of long-term therapeutic benefit; radiation therapy is associated with marked neurotoxic effects, especially in older patients
- Methotrexate chemotherapy alone or in combination with other agents has resulted in durable responses, but most patients eventually relapse
- Prognostic markers: the following have been associated with a poor prognosis
  - Age greater than 60 years
  - Poor performance status
  - Increased lactate dehydrogenase level
  - Increased CSF protein
  - Deep location of tumor mass in the brain

Selected References

Commins DL: Pathology of primary central nervous system lymphoma. Neurosurg Focus 21:E2, 2006.

Batchelor T, Loeffler JS: Primary CNS lymphoma. J Clin Oncol 24:1281-1288, 2006.

Plotkin SR: Update on primary central nervous system lymphoma. Curr Opin Neurol 18:645-653, 2005.

Ferreri AJM, Reni M: Prognostic factors in primary central nervous lymphomas. Hematol Oncol Clin N Am 19:629-649, 2005.

Germ Cell Tumors

Clinical Features

- Intracranial counterpart of germ cell tumors found in gonads and other extracranial sites
- About 90% of patients present before age 20; more common in males
- Symptoms include signs of increased intracranial pressure, hydrocephalus, visual abnormalities, or various endocrinopathies, including diabetes insipidus or precocious puberty
- Typically located in the midline; most often involving the pineal or pituitary region (two thirds in pineal region, one third in pituitary region)

Gross Pathology

- See Chapters 11 and 12

Histopathology

- See Chapters 11 and 12

Special Stains and Immunohistochemistry

- See Chapters 11 and 12

Other Techniques for Diagnosis

- Cytogenetic analysis: most frequent chromosomal abnormalities in germinomas of the pineal region are loss of 13q and 18q

Figure 19-17. Germinoma. Large polygonal and well-defined cells with abundant clear cytoplasm and nuclei with prominent nucleoli, intermixed with lymphocytes.

Differential Diagnosis

- Pineocytoma and pineoblastoma
  - Presence of pineocytomatous rosettes or small blue cells
  - Human chorionic gonadotropin, human placental lactogen, placental alkaline phosphatase, and cytokeratin negative
- See Chapters 11 and 12 for other differential diagnoses

Pearls

- Overall, intracranial germ cell tumors are rare; represent 3% to 11% of all brain tumors in children and 1% in adults
- Sacrococcygeal teratomas are often identified in the neonatal period; more common in females and usually benign

Selected References

Hirato J, Nakazato Y: Pathology of pineal region tumors. J Neurooncol 54:239-249, 2001.

Rickert CH, Simon R, Bergmann M, et al: Comparative genomic hybridization in pineal region germ cell tumors. J Neuropathol Exp Neurol 59:815-821, 2000.

Balmaceda C, Modak S, Finlay J: Central nervous system germ cell tumors. Semin Oncol 25:243-250, 1998.

Neuraxial Cysts: Rathke Cleft Cyst, Colloid Cyst, and Enterogenous Cyst

Clinical Features

- Rathke cleft cyst (RCC)
  - Usually located in the sella or suprasellar region
  - Often asymptomatic and found at autopsy, but may produce compressive symptoms (headache, hypopituitarism, hyperprolactinemia, and visual disturbance) owing to accumulated colloid secretions
- Colloid cyst (CC)
  - Usually within third ventricle near the foramen of Monro
  - May cause obstructive hydrocephalus
  - Rarely associated with sudden death
  - Mean age of occurrence is 40 years
- Enterogenous cyst (EntC)
  - Located within the spinal canal, usually in the cervical and upper thoracic levels
  - Rarely located intracranially
  - Usually intradural, extramedullary, and anterior to the cord
  - May be associated with vertebral abnormalities
  - Usually occurs in children and young adults

Gross Pathology

- Each cyst is thin walled with a smooth lining and filled with gray-white mucoid material
- CC often contains particularly dense cyst contents

Figure 19-18. Rathke cleft cyst. A, The cyst wall is lined by ciliated columnar epithelium overlying anterior pituitary tissue. **B,** Mucin stain showing positive goblet cells.

Figure 19-19. A, Colloid cyst. The cyst wall is lined by cuboidal to columnar epithelium, overlying a fibrous stroma. **B, Enterogenous cyst.** The cyst wall is lined by ciliated or mucin-secreting columnar epithelium reminiscent of respiratory or intestinal linings, respectively.

Histopathology

- Cysts are lined by epithelium ranging from simple columnar or cuboidal cells to a pseudostratified layer of cells; cilia and mucin production are typically seen
- In RCC, cyst often overlies anterior pituitary gland cells
- Squamous metaplasia may be seen in RCC

Special Stains and Immunohistochemistry

- Cytokeratin and EMA: RCC, CC, and EntC lining cells positive
- Vimentin: RCC is positive; CC and EntC variably positive
- GFAP: RCC, CC, and EntC negative

Other Techniques for Diagnosis

- Ultrastructure: ciliated and nonciliated epithelial cells with junctional complexes and microvilli, resting on a continuous basal lamina

Differential Diagnosis

- Craniopharyngioma versus RCC
  - Presence of squamous metaplasia in RCC may make distinction difficult, but RCC usually lacks keratin formation
  - Craniopharyngiomas contain solid epithelial islands, distinctive stellate reticulum, and basally palisaded epithelium
- Distinction between RCC, CC, and EntC
  - Difficult to distinguish histologically
  - Location is likely to be helpful
- Ependymal cyst
  - Most are in the deep white matter
  - Epithelial lining of low cuboidal to columnar cells that are frequently ciliated
  - Cyst lining is positive for GFAP and S-100 protein
- Arachnoid cyst
  - No epithelial lining; lined by meningothelial cells
  - Lining cells positive for EMA; negative for GFAP and S-100 protein

▌ Cysticercosis of ventricular system or subarachnoid space
  ● Presence of fragments of parasite on biopsy indicates correct diagnosis

  Pearls
  ● Each cyst is benign and usually cured by complete excision

Selected References

Osborn AG, Preece MT: Intracranial cysts: Radiologic-pathologic correlation and imaging approach. Radiology 239:650-664, 2006.

Takei H, Fuller GN, Powell SZ: Intracranial cysts of endodermal or respiratory epithelial origin. In McLendon RE, Rosenblum MK, Bigner DD (eds): Russell and Rubinstein's Pathology of Tumors of the Nervous System, 7th ed. New York, Hodder Arnold, 2006, pp 591-598.

Kleinschmidt-DeMasters BK, Lillehei KO, Stears JC: The pathologic, surgical, and MR spectrum of Rathke cleft cysts. Surg Neurol 44:19-27, 1995.

Pituitary Adenoma (Including Typical and Atypical Adenomas), Pituitary Carcinoma, and Pituitary Hyperplasia

Clinical Features

▌ Pituitary adenomas
  ● Most frequently found in women in their third through sixth decades; rarely seen in children
  ● Represent about 15% of all intracranial neoplasms
  ● May occasionally be found incidentally at autopsy
  ● Patients present with endocrinopathy in two thirds of the cases (hormone secretion by tumor or pressure on stalk or hypothalamus) or with visual complaints (a nonsecretory tumor is more likely to grow large enough to compress optic tracts)

Figure 19-20. Pituitary adenoma. Sinusoidal pattern of uniform cells with distinct cytoplasm and round nuclei containing salt-and-pepper chromatin.

  ● Functional tumors have variable presentation depending on what hormone they secrete
    — Growth hormone (GH)–secreting adenomas produce acromegaly
    — Prolactin (PRL)–secreting adenomas produce galactorrhea
    — Adrenocorticotropic hormone (ACTH)–secreting adenomas produce Cushing disease or Nelson syndrome
    — Gonadotrophic adenomas (follicle-stimulating hormone [FSH] or luteinizing hormone [LH] producing) are not usually biochemically active and present as nonfunctioning tumors
    — Thyroid-stimulating hormone (TSH)–producing adenomas produce hyperthyroidism
  ● May be associated with MEN I
  ● Atypical pituitary adenoma
    — Accounts for about 5% of adenomas
    — Defined histopathologically (see under "Histopathology")
▌ Pituitary carcinoma: defined only by the presence of metastasis
▌ Pituitary hyperplasia
  ● Clinical presentation is the same as for adenomas
  ● Radiologic studies may show diffuse enlargement of pituitary gland without a discernible rim of normal tissue

Gross Pathology

  ● Range in size from microadenomas to several centimeters, with enlargement of the sella and occasionally extrasellar extension
  ● Soft masses with occasional cystic degeneration or necrosis in larger lesions
  ● Invasive pituitary adenoma
    — Shows extensive dural, vascular, osseous, neural, or sinus invasion; this designation is best made radiographically or intraoperatively
    — Invasion is present in about 50% of all adenomas

Histopathology

  ● Tumor has a nested architecture with large groups of cells surrounded by incomplete reticulin network; may show focal papillary architecture
  ● Compression of adjacent normal pituitary gland may be seen
  ● Tumor is generally composed of monomorphic cells with round nuclei and inconspicuous nucleoli; a moderate degree of nuclear pleomorphism may occasionally be seen (see characteristics specific to hormone production)
  ● Oncocytic differentiation may occasionally be present
  ● Mitotic figures are rare
  ● Microcalcifications may be present
  ● Large adenomas may show focal necrosis, infarction, or hemorrhage (pituitary apoplexy)
  ● Complete tumor infarction may rarely occur

- Characteristics specific to hormone production
  — PRL-containing adenomas
    - Sparsely granulated adenomas
      ◇ Usually are responsive to dopamine agonists and show changes secondary to treatment
      ◇ Small cells in fibrous stroma and focal staining for PRL
      ◇ Untreated tumors are chromophobic with abundant cytoplasm and strong PRL positivity
    - Densely granulated adenomas: acidophilic to chromophobic cells with strong diffuse positivity to PRL
    - Acidophil stem cell adenoma: oncocytic change and variably positive to PRL and GH with CAM5.2 fibrous bodies
  — GH-containing adenomas
    - Sparsely granulated adenomas: weak positivity for GH, and CAM5.2 identifies fibrous bodies
    - Densely granulated adenomas: eosinophilic cytoplasm and perinuclear dotlike reactivity with CAM5.2
    - Mammosomatotroph adenoma: may also produce and secrete prolactin in addition to GH or PRL and TSH (plurihormonal adenoma)
  — ACTH-containing adenomas
    - May be sparsely or densely granulated
    - Most microadenomas are densely granulated
    - Composed of basophilic cells with strong PAS positivity and CAM5.2 positivity
    - Adjacent nonadenomatous gland shows Crooke hyaline change (concentric whorls of hyaline material in cytoplasm)
  — TSH-secreting adenomas
    - Usually large infiltrative masses with fibrosis and atypia
    - Composed of chromophobic cells
- Nonfunctioning adenomas
  — Most are gonadotrophic adenomas without clinical evidence of hormonal secretion
  — Solid sheets, nests, or sinusoidal pattern of acidophilic cells; pseudopapillae and rosettes may also be seen
  — Oncocytic change may be present
  — Positive for FSH and LH
- Plurihormonal adenomas
  — Most frequent combinations include GH, PRL, and one or more of the following: TSH, FSH, or LH
- Silent subtype 3 adenoma
  — Often positive for PRL, GH, and TSH
  — Intense stromal fibrosis and high vascularity
  — Characteristic ultrastructure
  — Aggressive behavior and poor prognosis
- Atypical adenomas
  — Usually show invasive growth
  — Increased mitoses, and Mib-1 labeling index greater than 3%
  — Extensive nuclear positivity for TP53

- Invasive pituitary adenoma
  — Defined by invasion into bone, sphenoid or cavernous sinus, and diaphragm sellae; same histologic features as typical pituitary adenomas; no reliable light or electron microscopic findings help distinguish this subtype
  — May show elevation of Mib-1 and TP53 positivity
- Pituitary hyperplasia
  — Pituitary acini expanded by cells of one hormonal type with intermixed cells staining for all hormones
  — Reticulum network remains intact but expanded
  — Often difficult to distinguish from normal gland
- Pituitary carcinoma
  — Rare pituitary tumor
  — Morphologically cannot be separated from typical pituitary adenoma
  — Two thirds are functional and produce PRL or ACTH
  — Definitive diagnosis is based on the presence of distant metastases

Special Stains and Immunohistochemistry

- Variably positive or negative staining for pituitary gland hormones (see detailed description under "Histopathology")
- Mib-1: correlation between invasiveness and high Mib-1 index has been reported; labeling index of greater than 3% for atypical adenomas
- Extensive positivity for TP53 in atypical adenomas

Other Techniques for Diagnosis

- Electron microscopy: distribution and morphology of secretory granules help to classify adenomas
- Several genomic alterations have been associated with invasiveness (overexpression of *EGFR* in recurrent GH adenomas)

Differential Diagnosis

▌ Normal pituitary gland
  - Small clusters of monomorphic cells with uniform nuclei completely surrounded by reticulin network
▌ Craniopharyngioma
  - Distinctive morphology: cords and solid areas of squamous epithelium with palisaded basal cells, keratin formation, and calcification
▌ Hypophysitis
  - May occur as a primary process confined to the gland or secondary to systemic disease
▌ Lymphocytic hypophysitis (primary)
  - More common in women, especially peripartum
  - Partial or total pituitary hypofunction
  - Lymphoplasmacytic infiltrate of gland; lymphoid follicles may be seen

- Granulomatous hypophysitis (primary)
  - Well-formed granulomas composed of epithelioid histiocytes, giant cells, and lymphocytes
  - Infectious etiology should be considered
  - May be the primary manifestation of sarcoidosis
  - Idiopathic form exists; hypothesized to be of autoimmune origin
- RCC
  - Single layer of ciliated cuboidal to columnar cells forming a cyst wall, often overlying pituitary gland
  - Squamous metaplasia may occur
- Spindle cell oncocytoma of the adenohypophysis (WHO grade I)
  - Suspected to derive from folliculostellate cells of anterior pituitary gland
  - Interlacing spindle and epithelioid cells with eosinophilic oncocytic cytoplasm
  - May see nuclear atypia
  - EMA and S-100 positive
  - GFAP, cytokeratin, and synaptophysin negative
- Granular cell tumor of the neurohypophysis
  - Polygonal cells with granular cytoplasm
  - GFAP and cytokeratin negative

Pearls

- Hemorrhagic necrosis of a pituitary adenoma (pituitary apoplexy) constitutes a surgical emergency (occurs in less than 1% of cases)

Selected References

Fuller GN, Scheithauer BW, Roncaroli F, Wesseling P: Spindle cell oncocytoma of the adenohypophysis. In Louis DN, Ohgaki H, Wiestler OD, Cavenee W (eds): World Health Organization: Classification of Tumours of the Central Nervous System. Lyon, IARC, 2007, pp 245-246.

Al-Brahim NYY, Asa SL: My approach to pathology of the pituitary gland. J Clin Pathol 59:1245-1253, 2006.

Al-Shraim M, Asa SL: The 2004 World Health Organization classification of pituitary tumors: What is new? Acta Neuropathol 111:1-7, 2006.

Kontogeorgos G: Classification and pathology of pituitary tumors. Endocrine 28:27-35, 2005.

Pituicytoma (WHO Grade I)

Clinical Features

- Low-grade glial neoplasm arising in the neurohypophysis or infundibulum
- Extremely rare; occurs in adults; men are affected more than women
- Signs and symptoms are secondary to mass effect: visual disturbance, headache, and hypopituitarism; may also see compression of infundibulum and secondary hyperprolactinemia

Gross Pathology

- Circumscribed solid mass

Histopathology

- Spindle cells forming fascicles or storiform pattern
- Cells range from elongated to rounded and contain nuclei with little atypia
- No mitoses
- No intermixed axons or axonal swellings

Special Stains and Immunohistochemistry

- GFAP positive, but may vary in intensity and extent
- Vimentin and S-100 positive
- Neurofilament, synaptophysin, and chromogranin negative
- Cytokeratin and pituitary hormones negative
- Mib-1 labeling: 0.5% to 2.0%

Other Techniques for Diagnosis

- Noncontributory

Differential Diagnosis

- Pituitary adenoma
  - Morphologically composed of epithelial cells forming sheets, trabeculae, or ribbons
  - Cytokeratin positive
  - GFAP negative
- Granular cell tumor of the neurohypophysis (WHO grade I)
  - Polygonal cells with abundant granular cytoplasm forming nodules or sheets
  - S-100, CD68, α_1-antitrypsin, and α_1-antichymotrypsin positive
  - GFAP, synaptophysin, and cytokeratin negative
- Spindle cell oncocytoma of the adenohypophysis
  - Spindle and epithelioid cells
  - GFAP negative
  - EMA positive
- Pilocytic astrocytoma
  - Characteristically has dense and loose architecture
  - Presence of Rosenthal fibers and eosinophilic granular bodies

Pearls

- Pituicytes are specialized cells of posterior pituitary with glial characteristics
- Indolent growth and no reports of malignant transformation

Selected References

Fuller GN, Wesseling P: Granular cell tumor of the neurohypophysis. In Louis DN, Ohgaki H, Wiestler OD, Cavenee W (eds): World Health Organization: Classification of Tumours of the Central Nervous System. Lyon, IARC, 2007, pp 241-242.

Figarella-Branger D, Dufour H, Fernandez C, et al: Pituicytomas, a mis-diagnosed benign tumor of the neurohypophysis: Report of three cases. Acta Neuropathol (Berlin) 104:313-319, 2002.

Brat DJ, Scheithauer BW, Staugaitis SM, et al: Pituicytoma: A distinctive low-grade glioma of the neurohypophysis. Am J Surg Pathol 24:362-368, 2000.

Craniopharyngioma (WHO Grade I)

Clinical Features

- Represents about 3% of all intracranial tumors
- Usually suprasellar; may be found within the sella, both suprasellar and infrasellar (dumbbell shape) or in the third ventricle, or rarely in the pineal region
- Has two peaks of incidence: children and older adults (fifth and sixth decades)
- Two histologic subtypes
  — Adamantinomatous variant usually presents in the first or second decade
  — Papillary variant typically occurs in adults (mean age, 45 years)
- Presenting symptoms are of three types
  — Visual abnormalities
  — Symptoms secondary to pituitary or hypothalamic dysfunction (typically short stature, diabetes insipidus, delayed sexual development, obesity, psychomotor retardation)
  — Symptoms secondary to increased intracranial pressure
- On MRI, adamantinomatous subtypes show cystic lesions frequently with calcifications; the solid areas are isointense and enhancing; papillary subtypes do not calcify

Gross Pathology

- Classically forms a variably sized, lobulated suprasellar mass that may distort the roof of the third ventricle and infiltrate adjacent brain; usually interdigitates with surrounding brain tissue

Figure 19-21. Craniopharyngioma. Section shows adamantinomatous squamous epithelium exhibiting keratinization and typical peripherally palisading nuclei.

- Adamantinomatous type shows cysts filled with thick, dark-brown fluid (resembling motor oil) and small glistening cholesterol crystals, and calcification; poorly circumscribed and frequently infiltrates surrounding brain tissue
- Papillary type is entirely solid or has a small cystic component; more circumscribed than the adamantinomatous variant

Histopathology

- Two subtypes; mixture of both subtypes may be seen
  — Adamantinomatous variant
    - Lobules of basally palisading squamous epithelium underlying a stellate reticulum of loose cells topped by keratin formation
    - Keratin pearls or wet keratin (nodules of plump eosinophilic, keratinized cells with ghost nuclei) are characteristic histologic features; often associated with calcification
    - Degeneration results in cystic cavities filled with fluid or acellular debris
    - Typically these tumors show local invasion of the surrounding brain tissue
    - Adjacent brain tissue usually shows marked chronic inflammation, cholesterol clefts, foreign-body giant cells, and Rosenthal fiber–rich astrocytosis
  — Papillary variant
    - Papillary architecture composed of well-differentiated epithelial cells with distinct fibrovascular cores
    - No microcyst formation, nuclear palisading, keratin pearls, wet keratin, calcification, or significant inflammatory component

Special Stains and Immunohistochemistry

- Cytokeratin highlights epithelial component
- Mib-1 labeling index: no association between index and recurrence

Other Techniques for Diagnosis

- Electron microscopy: epithelial component shows well-formed desmosomes and bundles of tonofilaments
- Cytogenetics: mutations of the *β-catenin* gene in more than 70% (adamantinomatous type)

Differential Diagnosis

▌ RCC
- Well-defined, thin-walled, fluid-filled cyst lined by a single layer of columnar and mucus-secreting cells
- Lacks papillary or solid architecture, keratin formation, and calcification

▌ Pilocytic astrocytoma
- Confusion with pilocytic astrocytoma may arise because of reactive astrocytosis and Rosenthal fibers surrounding the neoplasm

- Consists of pilocytic areas (elongated astrocytic cells with Rosenthal fibers) and a microcystic background
- Lacks cholesterol crystals and chronic inflammatory infiltrate
- Negative for cytokeratin, positive for GFAP
▌ Epidermoid cyst
  - Squamous epithelium lacks basal palisading, keratohyaline granules, and wet keratin
▌ Xanthogranuloma
  - Composed of chronic inflammation, macrophages, and cholesterol clefts
  - No significant component of epithelium

Pearls

- Histogenesis is debated; one hypothesis is that craniopharyngiomas occur from a developmental remnant of the Rathke cleft pouch; the other is that they arise from metaplastic squamous cells of the anterior pituitary gland
- Incomplete resection leads to recurrence even though most lesions are slow growing; postoperative radiotherapy may be given to tumors that are incompletely resected or recurrent, with improved patient survival
- Malignant change is extremely rare, with only a few cases reported in the literature, two occurring in the setting of prior radiation therapy

Selected References

Rodriguez FJ, Scheithauer BW, Tsunoda S, et al: The spectrum of malignancy in craniopharyngioma. Am J Surg Pathol 31:1020-1028, 2007.

Rushing EJ, Giangaspero F, Paulus W, Burger PC: Craniopharyngioma. In Louis DN, Ohgaki H, Wiestler OD, Cavenee W (eds): World Health Organization: Classification of Tumours of the Central Nervous System. Lyon, IARC, 2007, pp 238-240.

Crotty TB, Scheithauer BW, Young WF Jr, et al: Papillary craniopharyngioma: A clinicopathological study of 48 cases. J Neurosurg 83:206-214, 1995.

Chordoma

Clinical Features

- Rare tumors (1% of all intracranial tumors; 4% of primary bone tumors)
- Arise from notochord remnants, usually in or near the midline, anywhere from the sella turcica to the sacrum
- About one third occur in the sacrum, one third in the spheno-occipital region or clivus, and one third in the vertebrae
- Typically found in adults (peak in fourth decade); rare in children
- Patients with sacral chordomas present with pain, anal sphincter dysfunction, or neurologic symptoms secondary to pressure on the adjacent nerve roots

Figure 19-22. Chordoma. Classic trabecular pattern of the physaliferous cells in a mucoid background.

- Intracranial tumors generally produce headache and cranial nerve palsies
- Radiographically, tumors are expansile, are destructive of bone, and extend into soft tissue; MRI scans show hypointense signal on T1-weighted images and high signal intensity on T2-weighted images and enhancement after contrast administration

Gross Pathology

- Locally invasive and destructive lesions that commonly destroy adjacent bone and entrap regional nerves
- Typically lobulated gelatinous or mucoid gray masses

Histopathology

- May be divided into conventional, chondroid, or dedifferentiated subtypes
  - Conventional chordoma
    - Well-defined, lobular architecture separated by bands of fibrous tissue that may exhibit chronic inflammation
    - Lobules are composed of cords of epithelial-appearing cells and a mucoid background
    - Cells have variably sized central nuclei and abundant, pale-pink to clear, vacuolated cytoplasm (physaliphorous cells)
    - Necrosis and recent or old hemorrhage may be present
    - Mitoses are infrequent
  - Chondroid chordoma
    - Variant of chordoma that contains cartilaginous areas resembling chondrosarcoma
    - Distinction is important because it usually has a better prognosis than either typical chordoma or high-grade chondrosarcoma

— Dedifferentiated chordoma
  ◆ Rarely, chordomas show transformation into a malignant tumor with features of malignant fibrous histiocytoma, chondrosarcoma, or malignant undifferentiated spindle cell tumor or dedifferentiated chordoma

Special Stains and Immunohistochemistry

- PAS and PAS with diastase stains identify glycogen in cytoplasm (PAS positive; PAS with diastase sensitive)
- Mucin stain: stroma stains lightly
- Alcian blue: stroma strongly positive
- Mixed mesenchymal and epithelial immunophenotype of neoplastic cells
  — Vimentin positive
  — Cytokeratin (CK8, CK15, CK18, and CK19) positive
  — S-100 protein: most are positive
  — Brachyury (newly described protein found in notochord and notochord-derived tumors) positive

Other Techniques for Diagnosis

- Electron microscopy: distinct features of epithelial cells, including well-formed desmosomes and intracytoplasmic lumens; extracellular mucin is typically abundant
- Cytogenetic analyses have shown losses in chromosomes 1 and 3 and gains in chromosome 7

Differential Diagnosis

▌ Chondrosarcoma
- Vacuolated (physaliphorous) cells are not characteristic
- Negative for cytokeratin and EMA, positive for S-100
▌ Myxopapillary ependymoma
- Almost exclusively found in the filum terminale
- Pseudopapillary architecture with elongated monomorphic cells
- Positive for GFAP
▌ Metastatic mucinous adenocarcinoma
- Cytologically more anaplastic appearing with pleomorphism, hyperchromatism
- Necrosis and mitoses
- Likely S-100 negative
▌ Chordoid meningioma
- Foci of whorls, intranuclear pseudoinclusions, and psammoma bodies
- Cytokeratin negative
▌ Chordoid glioma
- Typically arise in third ventricular and suprasellar regions
- GFAP positive; most cells are negative for EMA and cytokeratin

Pearls

- Treatment typically involves an attempt at complete resection and postoperative radiotherapy

- Chordomas often recur and occasionally show distant metastases to lymph nodes, lung, or skin
- Chondroid chordomas occur more frequently in skull base than sacrum
- Dedifferentiated chordomas occur more frequently in sacrum
- Factors associated with a worse prognosis include
  — Female sex
  — Age more than 40 years at time of diagnosis
  — Presence of mitotic activity or necrosis
  — Large tumor volume
  — Incomplete resection

Selected References

Rosenberg AE: Chordoma and related lesions, chondrosarcoma and osteosarcoma of the cranium. In McClendon RE, Rosenblum MK, Bigner DD (eds): Russell and Rubenstein's Pathology of Tumors of the Nervous System. New York, Oxford, 2006, pp. 765-786.

Vujovic S, Handerson S, Presneau N, et al: Brachyury, a crucial regulator of notochordal development, is a novel biomarker for chordomas. J Pathol 209:157-165, 2006.

Radner H, Katenkamp D, Reifenberger G, et al: New developments in the pathology of skull base tumors. Virchows Arch 438:321-335, 2001.

Secondary Tumors

Clinical Features

- Metastases typically occur through hematogenous route or by direct extension from skull or spinal column lesions
- Direct extension
  — Carcinomas metastatic to bone (commonly breast, prostate, or lung) may expand and compress brain or spinal cord
  — May also metastasize directly to dura
  — Head and neck neoplasms may extend along nerves in a patchy way, appearing metastatic

Figure 19-23. Metastatic ductal carcinoma from the breast. Solid proliferation of malignant epithelial cells with focal necrosis.

- Hematogenous route
  - Up to 10% of carcinomas metastatic to CNS are not recognized before presentation of CNS metastasis
  - Metastatic tumors are the most common neoplasms of the CNS
  - About 30% of intracranial brain tumors in adults are due to metastatic carcinoma
  - Common primary sites of malignancy that may metastasize to the brain in adults include, in decreasing order of frequency, lung carcinoma (especially small cell and adenocarcinoma), breast carcinoma, melanoma, renal cell carcinoma, and colon carcinoma
  - Metastases are usually multiple and radio-graphically show distinct, contrast-enhancing masses with a surrounding zone of cerebral edema
  - Patients often present with headaches, focal neurologic deficits, or altered mental status
- Carcinomatous meningitis
  - Metastases involving the meninges, predominantly the subarachnoid space, without an intraparenchymal mass lesion
  - More commonly occurs with adenocarcinoma of lung, breast, or stomach
  - Headache, stroke, encephalopathy, and cranial nerve deficit are typical presenting symptoms
  - Cytologic examination of the CSF is positive in about 60% of cases

Gross Pathology

- Typically gray-white to tan and well-circumscribed masses with a pushing rather than an infiltrative margin
- Hemorrhage and necrosis are common, especially in melanoma, choriocarcinoma, and renal cell carcinoma
- Brown-black pigmentation is common in metastatic melanoma

Histopathology

- Histologic features similar to those of the primary tumors
- Discrete lesions usually displacing rather than infiltrating the adjacent brain tissue; small cell carcinoma often shows limited infiltrative borders
- Neoplastic cells often have prominent perivascular distribution with more viable tumor located around blood vessels
- Necrosis is typically extensive
- Vascular proliferation is not a characteristic feature
- Meningeal carcinomatosis shows tumor cells freely floating within the subarachnoid space with extension along Virchow-Robin spaces and into superficial brain parenchyma

Special Stains and Immunohistochemistry

- Cytokeratin, EMA: carcinomas
- S-100 protein, HMB-45: malignant melanoma
- LCA: lymphoma
- GFAP negative in most metastatic neoplasms

Other Techniques for Diagnosis

- Electron microscopy: features similar to those of the primary neoplasm
- Cytogenetics: same genetic abnormalities as found in primary neoplasm

Differential Diagnosis

- Glial neoplasms with epithelioid, sarcomatous, or small-cell differentiation
  - Infiltrative tumors with areas morphologically typical for glioma
  - Positive for GFAP
  - May be positive for cytokeratin AE1/3, but usually not other cytokeratins
  - EMA positivity reported in some gliomas
- Primitive neuroectodermal neoplasms including medulloblastomas
  - Cytokeratin negative
  - CD99 and EWS/FLI-1 negative
  - Uncommon in adults
- Anaplastic meningioma
  - Cytokeratin usually negative
  - EMA positive
  - Usually focal areas morphologically suggestive of meningioma
- Choroid plexus carcinoma (versus metastatic papillary adenocarcinoma)
  - Choroid plexus carcinomas are rare in adults
  - S-100 variably positive
  - GFAP positive in 20%

Pearls

- Most patients with brain metastasis have multiple lesions
- Features reliably used to distinguish metastatic carcinomas from primary CNS tumors on frozen section include cell cohesion, tumor circumscription, and prominent fibrous septa around groups of tumor cells; smear preparations are usually better for evaluation of cytologic characteristics

Selected References

Wesseling P, von Deimling A, Aldape KD: Metastatic tumors of the CNS. In Louis DN, Ohgaki H, Wiestler OD, Cavenee W (eds): World Health Organization: Classification of Tumours of the Central Nervous System. Lyon, IARC, 2007, pp 248-249.

Srodon M, Westra WH: Immunohistochemical staining for thyroid transcription factor-1: A helpful aid in discerning primary site of tumor origin in patients with brain metastases. Hum Pathol 33:642-645, 2002.

Giordana MT, Cordera S, Boghi A: Cerebral metastases as first symptom of cancer: A clinico-pathologic study. J Neurooncol 50: 265-273, 2000.

Non-neoplastic Conditions

Vascular Malformations

Clinical Features

❚ Arteriovenous malformation (AVM)
  ● Commonly found in adults; occasionally seen in children
  ● Presentation is usually before 40 years of age
  ● Two thirds are discovered when the patient presents with signs or symptoms of intracerebral hemorrhage; most of the remaining are discovered during evaluation for headache, seizures, or focal neurologic deficits; few are discovered incidentally
  ● Multiple AVMs are associated with hereditary hemorrhagic telangiectasia (Osler-Weber-Rendu disease)
❚ Cavernous hemangioma
  ● Patients may present with seizures or focal neurologic deficits
  ● Average age of onset is 30 years
  ● Hemorrhages are common but are usually small and do not cause significant mass effect
  ● About 20% are incidental findings at autopsy
  ● Most are found in the cerebrum; other common locations include brain stem, cerebellum, spinal cord, and leptomeninges
  ● Familial forms (autosomal dominant) exist
    — About 50% of familial cases occur in Hispanic-American individuals
    — Multiple angiomas are found
❚ Capillary telangiectasia
  ● Usually found in the brain stem (basis pontis) or spinal cord
  ● Typically an incidental postmortem finding and of little clinical significance
❚ Venous hemangioma
  ● Typically found in the subarachnoid space of the spinal cord (usually lower thoracic); may be seen within the brain
  ● Rarely symptomatic; typically an incidental postmortem finding
  ● Angiography shows veins with a caput medusa appearance

Gross Pathology

❚ AVM
  ● Variable size with large lesions causing displacement of the adjacent brain tissue
  ● Typically arises in the vicinity of the middle cerebral artery

Figure 19-24. A, Arteriovenous malformation. Numerous intraparenchymal arteries and veins. **B, Cavernous hemangioma.** Numerous dilated thin-walled blood vessels without intervening brain parenchyma. **C, Capillary telangiectasia.** Numerous capillaries are scattered in the basis pontis.

  ● Consists of a mass of tangled and tortuous vessels with intervening and surrounding brain parenchyma
  ● Often has thrombosed or dilated vessels
  ● Necrosis of the brain parenchyma and old and recent hemorrhage is common
❚ Cavernous hemangioma
  ● Most commonly found in the subcortical white matter or brain stem

- Well-defined mass composed of compact tangles of vessels
- Typically measure less than 3 cm in diameter
- Thrombosis is commonly found
- Evidence of prior bleeding in the form of a peripheral rim of hemosiderin is present in virtually all lesions
▪ Capillary telangiectasia
  - Usually small with a diameter of less than 2 cm
  - Poorly defined lesions typically causing an ill-defined stippling or discoloration of the brain parenchyma
▪ Venous hemangioma
  - Composed of network of thin-walled, dilated, blood-filled veins

Histopathology

▪ AVM
  - Composed of variably sized arteries and veins without intervening capillaries
  - Vessel walls show varying degrees of fibrosis, thinning, and dilation
  - Necrosis and hemosiderin-laden macrophages are often seen in brain tissue if thrombosed vessels are present
▪ Cavernous hemangioma
  - Compact network of vessels without smooth muscle or elastic lamella
  - Vessels are tightly packed with no brain parenchyma between the vascular network
  - Hemosiderin and reactive gliosis seen in the surrounding brain parenchyma
  - Calcification is common
▪ Capillary telangiectasia
  - Composed of thin-walled, delicate, dilated vessels without smooth muscle
  - Hemorrhage is rare
  - Intervening and adjacent brain parenchyma is unremarkable without gliosis or hemosiderin
▪ Venous hemangioma
  - Consists of a small collection of delicate veins formed of endothelium and collagen without smooth muscle
  - Veins lie within brain parenchyma that only rarely shows gliosis or hemorrhage

Special Stains and Immunohistochemistry

- Elastic highlights elastic lamella of the arteries seen in AVMs
- Trichrome highlights collagen and smooth muscle of vessel walls

Other Techniques for Diagnosis

- Cytogenetic analysis: in familial cavernous angiomas, mutations in three genes have been identified in association with disease, on chromosomes 7p, 7q, and 3q

Differential Diagnosis

- Discussed earlier under "Histopathology"
- Difficult to distinguish venous angioma from capillary telangiectasia

Pearls

- AVMs are the most dangerous because of their size and likelihood to rupture
- First hemorrhage from AVMs carries 10% to 15% mortality rate
- Surgical removal, stereotactic radiotherapy, and embolization are common methods of treatment for AVMs
- Increased occurrence of aneurysms in patients with AVMs

Selected References

Labauge P, Denier C, Bergametti F, Tournier-Lasserve E: Genetics of cavernous angiomas. Lancet Neurol 6:237-244, 2007.

Zabramski JM, Henn JS, Coons S: Pathology of cerebral vascular malformations. Neurosurg Clin N Am 10:395-410, 1999.

The Arteriovenous Malformation Study Group: Arteriovenous malformations of the brain in adults. N Engl J Med 340:1812-1818, 1999.

Challa VR, Moody DM, Brown WR: Vascular malformations of the central nervous system. J Neuropathol Exper Neurol 54:609-621, 1995.

Cerebral Infarction and Intracerebral Hematomas

Clinical Features

▪ Ischemic cerebral infarctions
  - Patients typically present with sudden onset of neurologic impairment
  - Neurologic deficits vary depending on location and size of infarction
  - Atherosclerosis and cardiac emboli (mural thrombi or valvular heart disease) are the most common causes; multiple infarcts are often related to emboli
  - May radiographically mimic malignant glioma
  - Multiple ischemic infarcts may cause dementia (multi-infarct dementia; see "Dementia" for further discussion)
▪ Venous cerebral infarcts
  - Result from thrombosis of the dural sinuses and cerebral veins; are classified as primary or secondary; are most often hemorrhagic
  - Primary (aseptic) infarcts are associated with hypercoagulable states, including dehydration, pregnancy, oral contraceptive use, and hemolytic anemias
  - Secondary (septic) infarcts are associated with bacterial infections of the face or sinuses, subdural abscesses, and meningitis

Figure 19-25. Acute cerebral infarct. A, Several acutely hypoxic neurons are present. Note the brightly eosinophilic cytoplasm and the pyknotic nucleus. **B,** Acutely infarcted brain tissue showing red neurons, necrosis, and acute inflammation.

Figure 19-26. Amyloid angiopathy. A, Intraparenchymal arteriole containing amorphous eosinophilic material in the media. **B,** Thioflavin S–stained arterioles viewed under ultraviolet light are positive for amyloid deposition.

▐ Intracerebral hematomas
- Associated with hypertension, aneurysms (hematomas occur secondary to blood under high pressure from ruptured or leaking aneurysm), vascular malformations, amyloid angiopathy, and neoplasms (most commonly metastatic, occasionally primary)
- Bleeding typically causes significant mass effect with compression of adjacent structures
- Hypertension-associated hemorrhages most commonly develop in deep gray matter, cerebellum, or pons
- Amyloid-associated hemorrhages are typically lobar (frontal, temporal, parietal, or occipital), occur in elderly individuals, and occur secondary to weakening of the arterial walls owing to deposition of Aβ amyloid

Gross Pathology
▐ Ischemic infarcts
- Grossly recognizable 2 to 4 days after stroke
- Acute lesions are discolored, soft, and swollen; confined to the distribution of a single blood vessel
- Subacute infarcts contain soft, friable necrotic brain tissue
- Old infarcts show cavitation
▐ Venous infarcts
- More commonly involve white matter and are often hemorrhagic
- Bilateral parasagittal hemorrhagic infarcts are associated with superior sagittal sinus occlusion
▐ Intracerebral hematomas
- Well-defined lesion consisting of fresh or organizing hemorrhage

- With organization, a fibrous capsule is formed around the hematoma
- In older lesions, adjacent brain tissue is yellow-brown (accumulation of hemosiderin-laden macrophages)

Histopathology

▌ Ischemic infarcts due to arterial compromise
  - Show varying features, depending on the age of the infarct
    — *Six to 24 hours:* eosinophilic neurons become visible
    — *Twelve to 24 hours:* polymorphonuclear leukocyte infiltrate (peaks at about 24 hours and gone by 7 days) and cerebral edema (peaks at 3 to 4 days)
    — *Days 2 to 3:* infiltration of lipid-laden macrophages and vascular proliferation
    — *Day 7:* beginning of cavitation is evident; proliferation of surrounding astrocytes
    — *Days 14 to 30:* sheets of lipid-laden macrophages; clustering of macrophages around blood vessels is common
    — *More than 3 months:* cystic space surrounded by numerous fibrillary astrocytes
  - General rule is that a 1-cm infarct takes 3 months to become cystic
  - Exact timing of microscopic changes varies from brain to brain and is dependent on infarct size
▌ Venous infarcts
  - Similar histologic features as described previously
  - Typically more hemorrhagic
▌ Intracerebral hematomas
  - Consist of organizing hemorrhage with numerous hemosiderin-laden macrophages
  - Proliferation of fibroblasts at periphery forms capsule
  - Reactive astrocytosis is evident in surrounding brain
  - Underlying cause of hematoma should be looked for: vascular malformation, neoplasm, hyaline arteriolosclerosis in hypertension, and acellular thickening of the small and medium-sized arteries in amyloid angiopathy

Special Stains and Immunohistochemistry

- CD68, HAM-56 highlight macrophages
- PAS: myelin debris within macrophages is positive
- GFAP: reactive astrocytes are positive
- Congo red identifies vascular amyloid deposition; shows apple-green birefringence in polarized light
- Thioflavin-S identifies vascular amyloid, is fluorescent under ultraviolet light
- Aβ amyloid immunohistochemistry: positive in vessels in amyloid angiopathy

Other Techniques for Diagnosis

- Electron microscopy: vessels containing Aβ amyloid show bundles of 10-nm filaments in the adventitia at the media-adventitia interface

Differential Diagnosis

▌ Glioma (oligodendroglioma or astrocytoma)
  - Distinction from reactive process is difficult in small biopsies
  - Typically lacks macrophages (macrophage markers are negative)
▌ GBM
  - Foamy macrophages and necrosis may be seen
  - Shows marked cytologic atypia, which is absent in areas of infarction
  - Mitoses present; elevated Mib-1 staining
▌ Demyelinating diseases
  - Usually occur in younger individuals
  - Multiple sclerosis (MS) is typically a multifocal disease with numerous small plaques without respect for vascular territory
  - Axons are relatively preserved (neurofilament positive) in areas of demyelination and are destroyed in areas of infarction
  - Presence of T lymphocytes in perivascular distribution
▌ Encephalitis
  - Areas of necrosis typically seen
  - Abundant acute and chronic inflammatory cells
  - Organisms (bacteria, viral inclusions, parasites) may be seen

Pearls

- Uncommonly, cerebral infarctions may radiographically mimic a neoplasm, prompting biopsy to rule out a neoplasm
- Lymphocytes are typically scant or absent in infarcts; if present within lesion or around blood vessels, consider vasculitis (primary or secondary)

Selected References

Vinters HV: Cerebrovascular disease—practical issues in surgical and autopsy pathology. Curr Top Pathol 95:51-99, 2001.
Garcia JH, Menan H: Vascular diseases. In Neuropathology: The Diagnostic Approach. St. Louis, Mosby, 1997, pp 263-320.

Vasculitis

Clinical Features

- Involvement of the CNS by vasculitis may be divided into primary or secondary; secondary vasculitis may occur in systemic vasculitis, often in association with collagen vascular diseases, or in infectious processes
▌ Infectious vasculitis
  - Occasionally seen with chronic infections, such as tertiary syphilis and tuberculosis
  - Associated with cerebritis due to aspergillosis and mucormycosis infections
  - Viral infections of the brain causing vasculitis include varicella-zoster virus (VZV), cytomegalovirus (CMV), herpes simplex virus, and HIV

Figure 19-27. Vasculitis. Section of a medium-sized blood vessel showing fibrinoid necrosis of the wall, multinucleated giant cells, and chronic inflammation.

▌Vasculitis in association with collagen vascular diseases and other noninfectious causes
  ● Brain involvement is uncommon in patients with systemic vasculitides
  ● Occurs in polyarteritis nodosa and Wegener granulomatosis and less commonly in Takayasu arteritis, Behçet disease, Kawasaki disease, and Sjögren syndrome
  ● Systemic lupus erythematosus (SLE) is more likely to cause vasculopathy and is rarely associated with cerebral vasculitis; similar morphologic findings to malignant hypertension
  ● CNS vasculitis may be associated with radiation damage and illicit drugs (e.g., amphetamines, cocaine)
  ● Vasculitis also uncommonly occurs in association with deposition of Aβ protein (amyloid angiopathy) in the cerebral cortical and leptomeningeal vessels
▌Primary (or isolated) vasculitis of the CNS, also known as *granulomatous vasculitis*, occurs without systemic involvement
  ● Occurs in fourth to sixth decades
  ● Affects leptomeningeal, cortical, and subcortical small and medium-sized arteries and less frequently veins and venules
  ● Radiologic evaluation includes cerebral angiogram; may be negative with small-vessel involvement
  ● MRI shows lesions indicative of ischemia and inflammation involving the meninges, cortex, and white matter, usually bilaterally
  ● Severe headaches, focal or multifocal neurologic deficits, altered cognition or consciousness, and uncommonly stroke

Gross Pathology

  ● Uncomplicated vasculitis may not be recognized grossly
  ● Complications include brain infarction and hemorrhage

Histopathology

▌Primary vasculitis
  ● Segmental acute and/or chronic inflammation of small arteries and arterioles with intimal proliferation and fibrosis in association with fibrinoid necrosis of the vessel wall
  ● Granulomatosis response (multinucleated giant cells) may be present (<50%)
  ● Thrombosis of the affected vessels may be evident
  ● Brain adjacent to affected vessels may show ischemia, infarction, or hemorrhage
▌Secondary vasculitis
  ● In infection-associated processes, viral inclusions or fungal organisms occasionally seen in the parenchyma or vessel walls, respectively
  ● Special stains (see later) may help identify microorganisms
  ● Occasionally, affected vessels show aneurysmal dilation due to septic emboli (mycotic aneurysms); usually due to fungal and bacterial infections

Special Stains and Immunohistochemistry

  ● Special stains for organisms: PAS, Gomori methenamine silver (GMS), and acid-fact bacilli (AFB)
  ● Elastic highlights elastic lamina

Other Techniques for Diagnosis

  ● In situ hybridization: DNA or RNA radioactive probes may be useful in identifying viral agents

Differential Diagnosis

▌Primary CNS lymphoma
  ● Perivascular lymphoid cells have atypical morphology and are mostly of B-cell origin
▌MS and acute demyelinating encephalomyelitis (ADEM)
  ● Inflammatory infiltrate is typically perivascular and is not associated with wall destruction
  ● Both MS and ADEM are characterized by areas of demyelinated (not usually necrotic) brain parenchyma
▌Viral encephalitis
  ● Perivascular and parenchymal lymphocytic inflammation without vessel wall destruction
  ● Microglial nodules are characteristic
▌Sarcoidosis
  ● Characterized by perivascular and parenchymal granulomas without necrosis; no destruction of the vessel walls
  ● Predilection for hypothalamic and suprasellar regions
▌Nonvasculitic autoimmune inflammatory meningoencephalitis (NAIM)
  ● Newly codified entity associated with autoimmune thyroiditis (Hashimoto encephalopathy) and other autoimmune disorders (Sjögren syndrome, SLE)
  ● Clinical manifestations are variable but usually include cognitive impairment and behavioral changes

- Typically steroid responsive
- Pathologic studies are few; perivascular lymphocytic infiltrate without vasculitis and variable parenchymal involvement has been described

Pearls

- Primary CNS vasculitis is typically focal and segmental; a negative biopsy does not exclude the diagnosis

Selected References

Volcy M, Toro ME, Uribe CS, Toro G: Primary angiitis of the central nervous system: Report of five biopsy-confirmed cases from Colombia. J Neurol Sci 227:85-89, 2004.

Josephs KA, Rubino FA, Diskson DW: Nonvasculitic autoimmune inflammatory meningoencephalitis. Neuropathology 24:149-152, 2004.

Chu CT, Gray L, Goldstein LB, Hulette CM: Diagnosis of intracranial vasculitis: A multidisciplinary approach. J Neuropathol Exp Neurol 57:30-38, 1998.

Parisi JE, Moore PM: The role of biopsy in vasculitis of the central nervous system. Semin Neurol 14:341-349, 1994.

Brain Abscess

Clinical Features

- Most occur during the third and fourth decades; males are affected more than females
- May be due to local extension from an extracerebral infection, including ear, sinus, or dental infections; hematogenous spread from a systemic infection is less common; penetrating head trauma may also cause brain abscess
- Immunosuppressed individuals (AIDS patients, transplant recipients, cancer patients) at greater risk
- Occasionally brain abscess may be a complication of neurosurgery

Figure 19-28. Brain abscess. Section shows a central area of purulent material, surrounded by vascular and fibroblast proliferation and numerous chronic inflammatory cells (periodic acid–Schiff stain).

- Features of local or systemic infections are often absent
- Presenting signs and symptoms are often nonspecific but may include headache, fever, and altered level of consciousness
- Various organisms, including bacteria, fungi, mycobacteria, and parasites (cysticercosis and toxoplasmosis), are the causative agents; bacteria are the most frequently isolated organisms (*Streptococci*, *Staphylococci*, *Fusobacterium*, and *Bacteroides* species are most common) in patients with intact immune systems
- Gram-negative rods, *Aspergillus*, *Candida*, and *Mucor* species occur in the neutropenic patient; T-cell dysfunction is associated with *Toxoplasma*, *Listeria*, *Nocardia*, *Cryptococcus*, and *Mycobacteria* species
- Typically found in the white matter or at the gray-white junction; usually seen in the frontal, temporal, or parietal lobe
- CT shows a cystic mass with ring enhancement and surrounding edema; MRI gives better resolution

Gross Pathology

- Well-defined area of central necrosis surrounded by hyperemic and edematous brain tissue
- Older lesions show a distinct organized fibrous capsule surrounding the necrotic tissue
- *Aspergillus* infection especially associated with hemorrhagic necrosis

Histopathology

- Characteristically shows three distinct zones
  — Central area of necrosis with abundant acute inflammatory cells
  — Zone of acute or chronically inflamed granulation tissue, consisting of fibroblastic and vascular proliferation
  — Peripheral area of edematous brain tissue with a reactive gliosis and a fibrous capsule in later stages
- Organisms may be identified within or adjacent to the necrotic tissue
- Caseating granulomas are characteristic of tuberculosis
- Multinucleated giant cells are usually seen in fungal or tuberculous infection
- May identify parasite (most commonly cysticercosis and toxoplasmosis)
- Gummas in syphilis are rare tumor-like, nonsuppurative lesions

Special Stains and Immunohistochemistry

- Special stains: Gram, PAS, GMS, AFB, Fite, and Warthin-Starry may identify microorganisms

Other Techniques for Diagnosis

- Culture of the necrotic tissue may yield positive results
- Polymerase chain reaction (PCR) may identify mycobacteria (tuberculosis) and selected other bacteria
- Immunohistochemistry: available for identification of toxoplasmosis

Differential Diagnosis

▌ GBM
- On imaging studies, high-grade astrocytoma, brain metastasis, and brain abscess may have similar characteristics
- Histologic examination shows high cellularity, neoplastic astrocytes and associated mitoses, necrosis, and endothelial proliferation

Pearls

- Mortality rates are variable depending on the etiologic agent; overall mortality rates have dropped dramatically owing to better diagnostic and treatment modalities
- Tissue for culture should be taken in operating room rather than in pathology laboratory

- *Aspergillus* species brain infection has been reported in patients with asthma and chronic steroid use as their only risk factor

Selected References

Kleinschmidt-DeMasters BK: Central nervous system aspergillosis: A 20-year retrospective series. Hum Pathol 33:116-124, 2002.

Calfee DP, Wispelwey B: Brain abscess. Semin Neurol 20:353-360, 2000.

Pendlebury WW, Perl DP, Munoz DG: Multiple microabscesses in the central nervous system: A clinicopathologic study. J Neuropathol Exper Neurol 48:290-300, 1989.

Encephalitis and Meningoencephalitis

Clinical Features

- Infection of the cerebral parenchyma characterized by altered level of consciousness, seizures, and focal neurologic deficits
- Infection of both the meninges and parenchyma often occurs (meningoencephalitis)

▌ Common causative agents: viral
- Viral encephalitis: togaviruses (Eastern equine encephalitis), flaviviruses (St. Louis encephalitis),

Figure 19-29. A, Acute meningitis. Low-power view shows dense acute inflammatory infiltrate of the leptomeninges. **B, HIV encephalitis.** A microglial nodule containing a multinucleated giant cell. **C, Viral encephalitis.** Low-power view shows classic perivascular lymphocytic infiltrate of the brain parenchyma. **D, Rabies encephalitis.** Classic intracytoplasmic inclusions in cytoplasm of the Purkinje cell of the cerebellum.

Continued

Figure 19-29, cont'd. E, Toxoplasmosis. An area of encephalitis showing acute inflammation and two cysts containing *Toxoplasma bradyzoites*. **F, Cysticercosis.** Shown is the wall of a cyst of cysticercus. **G, Cysticercosis, gross photograph.** A cluster of cysts (racemose form) of cysticercosis occurs in the ventricles and cisterns of the brain. **H, *Cryptococcus* meningitis.** Mucin stain shows numerous round microorganisms. Notice the lack of staining of the capsule and the absent inflammatory response (periodic acid–Schiff stain).

enteroviruses, and herpesvirus are the most common causative agents
- Herpesvirus infections of the nervous system include herpes simplex virus types 1 and 2 (HSV-1, HSV-2), EBV, CMV, VZV, and human herpesvirus type 6 (HHV-6)
  — HSV-1
    ◆ Causes frontotemporal lobe encephalitis (usually asymmetrical) occurring in immunocompetent older children and adults
    ◆ Most common sporadic encephalitis without seasonal occurrence
  — HSV-2
    ◆ Usually causes aseptic meningitis in adults (women are affected more than men) and neonates; less commonly a cause of encephalomyelitis in adult immunocompetent or immunocompromised hosts

  — CMV
    ◆ Encephalitis occurs most often in AIDS patients; congenital CMV infection also occurs (meningitis and encephalitis)
  — EBV
    ◆ Variable CNS involvement: meningitis, encephalitis, cranial nerve involvement, cerebellitis, and neuromuscular involvement; usually severe neurologic impairment does not occur
  — HHV-6
    ◆ Meningoencephalitis occurs in immunosuppressed patients
- West Nile virus encephalitis
  — Currently the most common cause of epidemic viral encephalitis in the United States
- HIV infection
  — Brain impairment secondary to HIV virus usually occurs in late-stage AIDS patients

- Common causative agents: bacterial
  - Tuberculous meningitis
  - Spirochete infections include both syphilis (*Treponema pallidum*) and Lyme disease (*Borrelia burgdorferi*)
  - Whipple disease caused by *Tropheryma whippelii*
    — Systemic disease; often intestinal dysfunction with weight loss, lymphadenopathy, and arthralgias
- Common causative agents: parasitic
  - Parasite infections are numerous and include trichinosis, strongyloidiasis, cysticercosis, echinococcosis, toxoplasmosis, schistosomiasis, and amebiasis (*Entamoeba histolytica* and *Naegleria*, *Acanthamoeba* species)
    — Cysticercosis is most common parasite worldwide
      ◆ Patients present with seizures
      ◆ Parasite may localize in the subarachnoid space, parenchyma, or ventricles
    — Toxoplasmosis and most fungal infections are seen in immunocompromised hosts (e.g., patients with AIDS)
- Common causative agents: fungal
  - Common fungal infections include candidiasis, histoplasmosis, blastomycosis, cryptococcosis, aspergillosis, mucormycosis, and coccidioidomycosis

Gross Pathology

- Encephalitis
  - Brain may appear normal or be edematous
  - Herpes simplex type 1 infection most commonly affects the temporal lobes, orbital and insular cortexes, and cingulate gyri causing hemorrhagic necrosis
  - AIDS dementia complex: generalized cortical atrophy; gray discoloration of white matter
- Meningoencephalitis
  - If meninges are involved, exudate may be present in subarachnoid space

Histopathology

- Viral encephalitis
  - Predominantly lymphocytic infiltrate involving the leptomeninges with extension into the underlying brain parenchyma
  - Infiltrate is primarily located in a perivascular distribution
  - Microglial nodules are characteristic histologic findings
- Herpesvirus encephalitis
  - Extensive hemorrhage and tissue destruction
  - Cowdry type A inclusions (nuclear inclusions consisting of an eosinophilic body surrounded by a clear halo)
  - Inclusions may be found in neurons, astrocytes, or oligodendrocytes
- Cytomegalovirus
  - Cowdry type A inclusions (may be nuclear or cytoplasmic) most commonly involving ependymal cells, neurons, or glial cells

- Rabies encephalitis
  - Negri bodies (large intracytoplasmic eosinophilic inclusions typically involving neurons of the Purkinje cells, and pyramidal cells of the hippocampus)
- HIV encephalitis and leukoencephalopathy
  - Diffuse microglial activation and microglial nodules containing multinucleated giant cells
  - Diffuse astrocytosis and perivascular chronic inflammation
  - Diffuse pallor of white matter
- Tuberculous meningitis and tuberculoma
  - Caseating granulomas with a lymphoplasmacytic inflammation
  - Parenchymal involvement consists of granulomatous inflammation with central necrosis
  - Endarteritis obliterans may cause ischemic infarction
  - Meningeal involvement is particularly severe on base of brain
- Neurosyphilis: meningovascular and parenchymal forms
  - Meningovascular
    — Meninges show a lymphoplasmacytic infiltrate predominantly around blood vessels; may progress to a vasculitis with intimal proliferation and luminal narrowing, resulting in ischemic changes
    — Spirochetes may be present in the meninges
  - Parenchymal form (general paresis)
    — Invasion of the brain leads to neuronal loss and a reactive gliosis
    — Many rod-shaped microglia in brain parenchyma; perivascular lymphocytes and plasma cells
    — Spirochetes may be present
- Other causes of meningitis and encephalitis
  - In fungal and parasitic infections, a predominantly chronic inflammatory infiltrate is in subarachnoid space or parenchyma
  - Parenchymal infection with fungi or parasites consists of cerebritis, which may progress to abscess (dependent on host immune response)
  - *Aspergillus* species cause hemorrhagic necrosis owing to vessel infiltration by hyphae
  - In Whipple disease, aggregates of PAS-positive macrophages

Special Stains and Immunohistochemistry

- Special stains for microorganisms such as Gram, PAS, GMS, AFB, and Fite
- Immunohistochemistry for selected agents such as herpesvirus, *Toxoplasma* species

Other Techniques for Diagnosis

- Culture of the CSF or the necrotic brain tissue
- In situ hybridization using DNA or RNA probes or PCR on CSF or tissue for viruses (e.g., mycobacteria, treponemes [Lyme disease], *Tropheryma whippelii*)

Differential Diagnosis

■ Sarcoidosis
  - Only rarely involves the CNS and is usually limited to the meninges
  - Characterized by noncaseating granulomas
  - Special stains for organisms are negative
■ Noninfectious vasculitis
  - No organisms identified
  - Inflammation likely to be primarily in vessel wall
■ Nonspecific autoimmune encephalomyelitis
  - Associated with autoimmune disorders
  - Characteristically steroid responsive
■ Paraneoplastic encephalitis
  - Clinical signs and symptoms may precede diagnosis of underlying neoplasm
  - Characterized by perivascular lymphocytes and microglial modules
  - Analysis of cerebrospinal fluid for related antibodies is indicated (e.g., anti-Hu, anti-Jo)

Pearls

  - Patients with viral or bacterial meningitis typically do not undergo brain biopsy; with clinical features of encephalitis, biopsy may be performed to isolate the causative organism and to rule out a vasculitis or demyelinating disease
  - Cowdry type A inclusions are usually only found during the first few days of herpes infection; later, only nonspecific features of encephalitis are found

Selected References

Scaravilli F, Bazille C, Gray F: Neuropathologic contributions to understanding AIDS and the central nervous system. Brain Pathol 17:197-208, 2007.

Davis LE, DeBiasi R, Goade DE, et al: West Nile virus neuroinvasive disease. Ann Neurol 60:286-300, 2006.

Gyure KA: Infections. In Prayson RA, Goldblum JR (eds): Neuropathology. Philadelphia, Elsevier, 2005, pp 287-338.

Kleinschmidt-DeMasters BK, Gilden DH: The expanding spectrum of herpesvirus infections of the nervous system. Brain Pathol 11:440-451, 2001.

Progressive Multifocal Leukoencephalopathy

Clinical Features

  - Demyelinating disease typically seen in immunocompromised patients, typically those with AIDS, hematologic cancer, or organ transplantation
  - Caused by infection of oligodendrocytes with a papovavirus that produces focal areas of demyelination
  - Patients present with visual deficits, personality changes (dementia), and motor deficits
  - Typically multifocal; when single, may mimic a neoplasm on CT or MRI

Figure 19-30. Progressive multifocal leukoencephalopathy. A, Low-power view shows multiple irregular areas of demyelination (myelin stain). **B,** Classic intranuclear viral inclusion in oligodendroglial cell is evident in the center of the photomicrograph.

  - CT and MRI show white matter lesions without mass effect; most often involve occipital lobe; typically nonenhancing

Gross Pathology

  - Variably sized, patchy areas of softening or discoloration of the white matter

Histopathology

  - Sparse perivascular lymphocytes and moderate to numerous macrophages are seen
  - Within the areas of demyelination, reactive gliosis, with both oligodendrocytes and astrocytes showing considerable nuclear atypia (may mimic glial neoplasm)
  - Infected glial cells (mostly oligodendrocytes and astrocytes) are diagnostic and consist of cells with enlarged, glassy, dark, round nuclei; best appreciated at the edge of the lesion

Special Stains and Immunohistochemistry

  - JC virus immunohistochemistry positive in infected cells
  - Klüver stain shows areas of demyelination

- Neurofilament shows relative preservation of axons; there may be axonal loss in the center of a lesion

Other Techniques for Diagnosis

- Electron microscopy: characteristic intranuclear inclusions consisting of stick-and-ball–shaped virion particles
- In situ hybridization for JC virus DNA on CSF or tissue sample confirms the diagnosis

Differential Diagnosis

▌ Malignant glioma (astrocytoma or oligodendroglioma)
- Lacks macrophage component, areas of demyelination, inflammation, and inclusions

▌ MS
- May create a difficult diagnostic problem
- Do not see oligodendrocytes with characteristic inclusions
- Immunohistochemistry and in situ hybridization for JC virus are negative

Pearls

- PML is associated with reactivation of JC virus in an immunocompromised patient
- JC virus is a polyomavirus believed to be acquired in most individuals at a young age, persisting in a latent form in the kidney
- PML has an aggressive clinical course, with death usually resulting in a few months
- There have been several recent reports of PML developing after treatment with natalizumab (a monoclonal antibody to α_4-integrins) in patients with MS and Crohn disease

Figure 19-31. A, Multiple sclerosis. Edge of an active plaque of multiple sclerosis showing abrupt loss of myelin, macrophages, reactive astrocytes, and perivascular lymphocytes (myelin stain). **B, Acute hemorrhagic leukoencephalitis.** An area of acute parenchymal hemorrhage is evident surrounding a necrotic vessel.

Selected References

Kleinschmidt-DeMasters BK, Tyler KL: Progressive multifocal leukoencephalopathy complicating treatment with Natalizumab and Interferon Beta-1a for multiple sclerosis. N Engl J Med 353:369-374, 2005.

Koralnik IJ, Schellingerhout D, Frosch MP: Case 14-2004: A 66-year-old man with progressive neurologic deficits. N Engl J Med 350:1882-1893, 2004.

Weber T, Major EO: Progressive multifocal leukoencephalopathy: Molecular biology, pathogenesis and clinical impact. Intervirology 40:98-111, 1997.

Aksamit AJ Jr: Progressive multifocal leukoencephalopathy: A review of the pathology and pathogenesis. Microsc Res Tech 32:302-311, 1995.

Demyelinating Diseases

Clinical Features

▌ MS
- Signs and symptoms are markedly variable: visual symptoms, paralysis, ataxia, motor and sensory disturbances, optic neuritis, bladder and bowel dysfunction
- Classically disseminated in space and time
- Wide range of onset: 15 to 55 years
- Women are more commonly affected
- Plaques are commonly located adjacent to the lateral ventricles: optic pathway, cerebellum, and spinal cord are also often affected
- Large plaques causing significant mass effect may radiographically mimic brain tumors

▌ Marburg type of MS (*acute MS*)
- Rare variant set apart because of its aggressive course
- Death occurs usually 1 to 6 months after onset
- Usually involves cerebral hemispheres; large confluent lesions

▌ Concentric sclerosis of Baló
- Distinguished by separate concentric rings of demyelinated and myelinated white matter visible, in some instances, on MRI and seen microscopically
- Clinically similar to Marburg variant

▌ Devic disease (neuromyelitis optica): involvement of optic nerve and spinal cord predominates

- Likely distinct from MS pathogenetically
- Associated with serum autoantibody NMO-IgG
■ ADEM
  - Found in both children and adults
  - Acute demyelinating disease, usually monophasic, may be associated with or follow infection or vaccination; may also occur without identified predisposing factors
  - Acute presentation with neurologic symptoms: ataxia, headache, and weakness
■ Acute hemorrhagic leukoencephalitis (Hurst disease)
  - Believed to be a hyperacute form of ADEM
  - Clinical presentation: fever, nausea, vomiting, focal neurologic deficits, and seizures
  - Progression to coma and death or recovery with severe disability

Gross Pathology

■ MS
  - Plaques appear as well-defined, pink to gray gelatinous lesions
  - Plaques are often periventricular
■ Acute demyelinating encephalomyelitis
  - Lesions are usually in cerebral white matter bilaterally and brain stem
■ Acute hemorrhagic leukoencephalitis
  - Brain swelling
  - White matter exhibits scattered petechial hemorrhages and necrotic foci

Histopathology

■ MS
  - Active plaques are discrete, hypercellular lesions composed primarily of macrophages and reactive astrocytes
  - Macrophages have round uniform nuclei, vacuolated or granular cytoplasm (containing myelin debris), and distinct cell borders
  - Occasional mitotic figures may be seen (in astrocytes called *Creutzfeldt cells*)
  - Perivascular cuffs of lymphocytes (predominantly T cells) are prominent in active lesions
  - Inactive plaques are hypocellular and exhibit fibrillary astrocytosis and few macrophages
  - Marburg variant shows abundant Luxol fast blue (LFB)-containing macrophages in the demyelinated plaques
  - Baló concentric sclerosis variant shows alternating bands of myelinated and unmyelinated white matter with myelin stain
  - Devic disease: lesions are particularly destructive and may cavitate, contain abundant macrophages and inflammatory cells, and axonal loss in addition to myelin loss
■ ADEM
  - Characterized by foci of demyelination, which are usually perivenous or perivenular

- Numerous lipid-laden macrophages and a perivascular, mononuclear cell infiltrate
- All lesions show similar levels of activity or age
■ Acute hemorrhagic leukoencephalitis
  - Fibrinoid necrosis of white matter blood vessels with surrounding hemorrhage and demyelination or necrosis
  - Neutrophils and lymphocytes surround vessels

Special Stains and Immunohistochemistry

- LFB with PAS shows discrete areas of demyelination and highlights macrophages containing myelin debris (LFB-positive debris implies acute process, PAS-positive debris implies subacute process)
- Neurofilament: shows relative preservation of axons in demyelinated areas

Other Techniques for Diagnosis

- Electron microscopy: breakdown of myelin and ingestion by macrophages, demyelinated axons, sparse oligodendrocytes, and inflammatory cells

Differential Diagnosis

■ Cerebral infarction
  - Symptoms are typically acute
  - Variable histologic features depending on the age of the infarct
  - Neurofilament immunostain shows axonal loss equal to myelin loss
■ Progressive multifocal leukoencephalopathy
  - Typically found in an immunocompromised host
  - Glial cells have characteristic nuclear inclusions
  - Immunohistochemistry and in situ hybridization for JC virus confirms diagnosis
■ Astrocytoma
  - Do not see macrophage component that characterizes demyelinating diseases
  - Lacks areas of demyelination
  - No perivascular lymphocytes
■ Leukodystrophies
  - Adrenoleukodystrophy or adrenomyeloneuropathy
    — Presence of inflammatory cells may lead to confusion with MS
    — Clinical features are distinct from MS
    — Diffuse nature of lesion rather than focal plaques
    — Elevated levels of long-chain fatty acids in plasma
  - Other leukodystrophies
    — Often inherited and with distinctive clinical presentations
    — Diffuse nature of lesion rather than focal plaques
    — Morphologic findings may also be distinctive (metachromatic deposits or globoid cells)

Pearls

- In MS, solitary plaques may radiographically resemble a neoplasm (tumefactive MS), prompting biopsy of the lesion

- In ADEM, most patients eventually recover with resolution of symptoms and eventual remyelination
- In acute hemorrhagic leukoencephalitis, much higher fatality rate

Selected References

Love S: Demyelinating diseases. J Clin Pathol 59:1151-1159, 2006.

Kleinschmidt-DeMasters BK, Simon JH: Dysmyelinating and demyelinating disorders. In Prayson RA, Goldblum JR (eds): Neuropathology. Philadelphia, Elsevier, 2005, pp 181-222.

Lucchinetti CF, Brueck W, Rodriguez M, Lassmann H: Multiple sclerosis: Lessons from neuropathology. Semin Neurol 18:337-349, 1998.

Zagzag D, Miller DC, Kleinman GM, et al: Demyelinating disease versus tumor in surgical neuropathology: Clues to a correct pathologic diagnosis. Am J Surg Pathol 17:537-545, 1993.

Dementia

Clinical Features

▌ Alzheimer disease
- Most common cause of dementia
- Affects adults of all ages; older age is an important risk factor
- Patients present with memory loss and cognitive impairment; progresses over several years

▌ Lewy body dementia
- Presents with cognitive impairment with prominent behavioral abnormalities, hallucinations, and fluctuating clinical course followed by parkinsonian signs and symptoms

▌ Vascular dementia
- Pathologic substrate of vascular dementia is variable
- Presence of infarcts in brain regions is strategically critical for cognition; multiple lacunar infarcts in deep gray matter (less frequently cortex) or white matter, and multiple large infarcts have each been shown to cause dementia
- Presence of multiple white matter infarcts often in association with hypertension has been called *subcortical arteriosclerotic leukoencephalopathy (Binswanger disease)*
- Clinical course is more variable than in Alzheimer disease: usually relatively sudden onset of impairment and tendency for stepwise progression and fluctuation
- Cerebral autosomal dominant arteriopathy with subcortical infarcts and leukoencephalopathy (CADASIL)
  — Most common form of hereditary (autosomal dominant) stroke leading to dementia
  — Characteristic white matter hyperintensities on MRI
  — Wide range of onset of first stroke: 28 to 60 years of age

▌ Creutzfeldt-Jakob disease
- Believed to be caused by a proteinaceous, infectious particle called a *prion*

Figure 19-32. A, Alzheimer disease. A neuritic plaque, diffuse plaque, and neurofibrillary tangle in the cerebral cortex (modified Bielschowsky stain). **B, Parkinson disease.** A pigmented substantia nigra neuron containing a classic Lewy body in the cytoplasm. Note the brightly eosinophilic body surrounded by a halo.

- Classic nonfamilial patients develop a rapidly progressive dementia with myoclonus and ataxia
- Characteristic electroencephalogram findings of periodic sharp wave complexes

▌ Frontotemporal lobar degeneration (FTLD)
- *FTLD is a general term that encompasses several neurodegenerative diseases in which the most severe pathology involves the frontal and temporal lobes*
- Included in this category are the following entities: frontotemporal dementia and parkinsonism linked to chromosome 17 (FTDP-17), Pick disease (PiD), frontotemporal lobar degeneration with ubiquitin-positive deposits with or without motor neuron disease (FTLD-U, FTLD-MND), dementia lacking distinctive histology (DLDH), progressive supranuclear palsy (PSP), and corticobasal degeneration (CBD); a detailed discussion of these entities is beyond the scope of this chapter
- Clinical presentation is usually with language or behavioral changes; motor weakness, eye movement abnormalities, and extrapyramidal signs may also be present

Gross Pathology

▊ Alzheimer disease
- Brain weight is decreased
- Gyral atrophy affecting primarily frontal, temporal, and parietal lobes
- Increased size of lateral ventricles is typical, especially temporal horns

▊ Lewy body dementia
- Marked depigmentation of the substantia nigra and locus ceruleus
- Usually diffuse cortical atrophy and ventricular enlargement

▊ Vascular dementia
- Caused by multiple cerebral infarcts in various combinations of size and location (cortical, subcortical)
- Multiple white matter infarcts suggest subcortical arteriosclerotic leukoencephalopathy or CADASIL

▊ Creutzfeldt-Jakob disease
- Mild cerebral cortical or cerebellar atrophy

▊ Frontotemporal lobar degeneration
- In FTDP-17, PiD, FTLD-U, and FTLD-MND: atrophy of frontotemporal cortexes, often in association with anterior basal ganglia atrophy
- Perirolandic cortical atrophy and substantia nigra pallor is seen in CBD
- Substantia nigra pallor and atrophy of midbrain, subthalamic nucleus, and cerebellar peduncles are seen in PSP

Histopathology

▊ Alzheimer disease
- Characteristically, two major histologic lesions are seen
  — Neurofibrillary tangles: intraneuronal cytoplasmic fibrillary accumulations especially prominent within the association cortexes and mesial temporal lobe (entorhinal cortex and hippocampus)
    ◆ Flame-shaped or globose, depending on whether location is cortical or subcortical
  — Senile plaques: found throughout the cerebral cortex; less dense in subcortical gray matter and cerebellum
    ◆ Multiple subtypes
    ◆ Diffuse plaque contains Aβ protein
    ◆ Neuritic plaque composed of Aβ protein and tau protein

▊ Lewy body dementia
- Cortical Lewy bodies
  — Eosinophilic, cytoplasmic round inclusions with no halo
  — Found in lower layers of cortex, especially prominent in the anterior cingulate gyrus and parahippocampal gyrus
- Lewy bodies are also in pigmented nuclei (most commonly in the substantia nigra) and consist of intracytoplasmic eosinophilic inclusions surround by a clear halo that are found within the affected neurons

▊ Vascular dementia
- Ischemic necrosis of varying ages; acute (eosinophilic neurons and edema) to old (cystic cavity with glial scar)
- Arteriolosclerosis is typically severe when multiple lacunes are present
- CADASIL: thickening of the walls of arteries due to the deposition of granular eosinophilic material (PAS positive) associated with infarcts in the white matter

▊ Creutzfeldt-Jakob disease
- Spongiform degeneration with neuronal loss and astrocytosis seen in the affected gray matter; white matter is typically not involved; no inflammatory cells
- About 10% of cases have prion amyloid plaques in cerebellum
- Familial form of prion disease (Gerstmann-Sträussler-Scheinker disease) exhibits plaques and neurofibrillary tangles in the neocortex

▊ Frontotemporal lobar degeneration
- FTDP-17, FTLD-U, FTLD-MND: varying degrees of neuronal loss and astrocytosis in the frontal and temporal lobes; basal ganglia and substantia nigra may show neuronal loss
- PiD: severe neuronal loss and astrocytosis in frontotemporal lobes with Pick bodies and Pick cells
- PSP: neuronal loss in substantia nigra, subthalamic nucleus, dentate nucleus, and additional deep gray matter and brain stem nuclei
- CBD: neuronal loss in substantia nigra, basal ganglia, and motor and sensory cortexes

Special Stains and Immunohistochemistry

▊ Alzheimer disease
- Bielschowsky silver stain identifies neurofibrillary tangles and neuritic plaques
- Aβ antibodies identify amyloid component of plaque; tau antibodies identify neuritic plaques and neurofibrillary tangles

▊ Lewy body dementia
- α-Synuclein antibodies identify cortical and subcortical Lewy bodies

▊ Vascular dementia
- Klüver and neurofilament immunostain in white matter to evaluate white matter
- CADASIL: granular eosinophilic deposits may be visualized immunohistochemically

▊ Creutzfeldt-Jakob disease
- Prion protein immunohistochemistry positive

▊ Frontotemporal lobar degeneration
- FTDP-17: tau-positive deposits
- PiD: Pick bodies (cytoplasmic neuronal inclusions): silver and tau positive; Pick cells (ballooned neurons) are neurofilament positive

- FTLD-U and FTLD-MND: TDP-53 and ubiquitin positive neuronal nuclear and cytoplasmic deposits, dystrophic neurites, and glial cytoplasmic inclusions
- DLDH: no positive inclusions
- PSP: a variety of tau-positive structures are present; most prominent are the neurofibrillary tangles and tufted astrocytes
- CBD: a variety of tau-positive structures are present; most prominent are the astrocytic plaques and threadlike processes

Other Techniques for Diagnosis

- Alzheimer disease
  - Several gene mutations identified in early onset familial Alzheimer disease
    — Amyloid precursor protein (chromosome 21)
    — Presenilin 1 (chromosome 14)
    — Presenilin 2 (chromosome 1)
- Vascular dementia
  - CADASIL
    — Ultrastructural examination of the brain or vessels from skin biopsy shows deposition of specific granular osmiophilic material (GOM) evident in basal lamina adjacent to degenerating smooth muscle cells of arteries
    — Cytogenetics: mutation in *Notch3* gene on chromosome 19
- Creutzfeldt-Jakob disease
  - Western blot for protease-resistant prion protein
  - Genetic analysis for mutation in prion protein gene
- Frontotemporal lobar degeneration
  - FTDP-17: mutation in *tau* gene on chromosome 17
  - FTLD-U: *progranulin* gene mutation, valosin-containing protein mutation, linkage to chromosome 9q

Differential Diagnosis

- Kufs disease (adult form of neuronal ceroid lipofuscinosis)
  - Rare storage disease involving the central nervous system of adults
  - Age of onset is about 30 years

- Slowly progressive disease with dementia; some patients have myoclonic epilepsy and ataxia, whereas others have behavioral and motor disturbances
- Excessive deposition of lipofuscin-like substance in neurons and gastrointestinal tract
- Status spongiosus
  - May be mistaken for spongiform degeneration of Creutzfeldt-Jakob disease
  - Found in acute infarcts and end-stage neurodegenerative diseases
  - Vacuoles are predominantly pericellular rather than in the neuropil or intraneuronal

Pearls

- Premortem diagnosis of Alzheimer disease is usually based primarily on clinical symptoms; definitive diagnosis can only be made on tissue examination
- Dementia with atypical clinical presentation is more likely to warrant biopsy
- In prion disease, infectious agent is resistant to formalin fixation; treatment of fixed tissue with formic acid before processing, embedding, and cutting is suggested to decrease infectivity of tissue
- Important to snap-freeze portion of brain biopsy for possible genetic or biochemical studies when clinical history is dementia

Selected References

Cairns NJ, Bigio EH, Mackenzie IRA, et al: Neuropathologic diagnostic and nosologic criteria for frontotemporal lobar degeneration: Consensus of the consortium for frontotemporal lobar degeneration. Acta Neuropathol 144:5-22, 2007.

Cochran EJ: Neurodegenerative diseases. In Prayson RA, Goldblum JR (eds): Neuropathology. Philadelphia, Elsevier, 2005, pp 223-286.

Kalimo H, Ruchous M-M, Viitanen M, Kalaria RN: CADASIL: A common form of hereditary arteriopathy causing brain infarcts and dementia. Brain Pathol 12:371-384, 2002.

McKeith IG, Galaski D, Kosaka K, et al: Consensus guidelines for the clinical and pathologic diagnosis of dementia with Lewy bodies (DBL): Report of the consortium on DBL international workshop. Neurology 47:1113-1124, 1996.

Michael J. Davis and Richard J. Grostern

20

Eye and Orbit

Adult Ocular Lesions

External Lesions

Malignant Melanoma of the Conjunctiva

Clinical Features

- Usually pigmented (may be amelanotic), elevated lesion, anywhere on conjunctiva
- Usually movable, but may be fixed to sclera
- Indistinct edges
- Rare in dark-skinned people
- Incidence increasing in the United States

Gross Pathology

- Noncontributory

Histopathology

- Mixtures of cell types, including small polyhedral cells, spindle cells, epithelioid cells, and balloon cells
- Normal polarity is lost
- Invasion of overlying epithelium by tumor cells
- May have epithelial cysts if arising from nevus
- Often inflammation is found at the base of the lesion
- Analogous to superficial spreading melanomas of skin

Special Stains and Immunohistochemistry

- S-100 protein (low specificity) has been found
- HMB-45 antigen is less sensitive but more specific for melanomas; can be used to distinguish between benign and malignant lesions
- S-100 protein and NK1/C3 markers can be used to determine extent of lesion

Other Techniques for Diagnosis

- Noncontributory

Figure 20-1. Conjunctival melanoma. Numerous polyhedral and spindle cells are present in this conjunctival melanoma.

Differential Diagnosis

- ▌ Primary acquired melanosis (PAM)
  - Unique to conjunctiva; equivalent to melanoma in situ of skin
  - PAM usually lacks mitoses but has varying degrees of atypia
- ▌ Nevus
  - Congenital lesion, without growth
  - May become pigmented only in adulthood
  - Cysts present on histopathology about 50% of time
- ▌ Secondary melanoma
  - Metastatic from skin or uvea
  - Direct extension of intraocular uveal melanoma
- ▌ Racial (congenital) ocular melanosis
  - In heavily pigmented individuals
  - Histopathologically completely benign

Pearls

- Two thirds arise from preexisting PAM; one third arise de novo or from preexisting nevi
- Thickness can predict prognosis: less than 15 mm, excellent prognosis; more than 15 mm, high mortality from metastases
- Sentinel node biopsy (preauricular and deep cervical nodes) should be considered in melanomas more than 2 mm thick
- Breslow and Clark staging probably does not apply

Selected References

Kurli M, Finger PT: Melanocytic conjunctival tumors. Ophthalmol Clin N Am 1815-1824, 2005.
Seregard S: Conjunctival melanoma. Surv Ophthalmol 42:321-350, 1998.
Liesegang TJ: Pigmented conjunctival and scleral lesions. Mayo Clin Proc 69:151-161, 1994.

Primary Acquired Melanosis of the Conjunctiva

Clinical Features

- Acquired unilateral diffuse or patchy pigmentation
- More common in whites
- Can arise anywhere on conjunctiva
- Freely mobile
- Indistinct edges with dusty pigmentation
- Average age of onset, 40 to 50 years
- Potential for malignant degeneration into melanoma

Gross Pathology

- Noncontributory

Histopathology

- Usually divided into PAM without atypia and PAM with atypia
- Ranges from mild hyperpigmentation of the epithelium (epithelial cells) with no atypical melanocytes to clusters of deep atypical melanocytes

Figure 20-2. Primary acquired melanosis of the conjunctiva. Atypical melanocytes replace many of the deeper layers of the conjunctival epithelium.

(crossover with malignant melanoma), usually arranged in pagetoid configuration
- Prominent nucleoli (in atypical lesions)
- Lacks epithelial cysts of nevi and some melanomas
- May be arranged in nests, which may indicate poorer prognosis
- Similar to melanoma in situ of skin

Special Stains and Immunohistochemistry
- HMB-45 immunostaining may help distinguish benign from malignant lesions

Other Techniques for Diagnosis
- Noncontributory

Differential Diagnosis
▌ Conjunctival melanoma (see "Malignant Melanoma of the Conjunctiva")
  - More atypia than PAM
  - Loss of normal polarity with mitotic figures
  - Melanocytes invade overlying epithelium or underlying stroma
▌ Conjunctival nevus
  - Cells always arranged in nests
  - Benign appearance
  - Congenital
  - Adjacent epithelial cells lack pigmentation
▌ Racial melanosis
  - Bilateral
  - Occurs in dark-skinned people
▌ Pigmented papilloma
  - Benign papillomatous lesion with pigmented monolayer of basal cells
  - Lacks malignant features
▌ Drug deposits (adrenochrome granules from epinephrine use)
▌ Mascara deposits (inadvertent and intentional tattooing)

Pearls
- About 46% chance of malignant transformation (into melanoma) if atypical melanocytes are in the basal epithelial layer; much greater chance if melanocytes invade the epithelium in a pagetoid manner or are arranged in deep nests (75% to 90%)
- Some sources advocate biopsy of all PAM lesions; others advocate biopsy only with proven growth or if obviously thick

Selected References

Kurli M, Finger PT: Melanocytic conjunctival tumors. Ophthalmol Clin N Am 1815-1824, 2005.

Liesegang TJ: Pigmented conjunctival and scleral lesions. Mayo Clin Proc 69:151-161, 1994.

Jakobiec FA, Folberg R, Iwamoto T: Clinicopathologic characteristics of premalignant and malignant melanocytic lesions of the conjunctiva. Ophthalmology 96:147-166, 1989.

Pterygium and Pinguecula

Clinical Features
- Fleshy hypertrophic lesions of ocular surface overlying sclera (pinguecula) or sclera and cornea (pterygium)
- Usually over nasal globe, occasionally temporal, usually bilateral

Gross Pathology
- Noncontributory

Histopathology
- Basophilic (elastotic or actinic) degeneration of substantia propria
- Overlying epithelium may have acanthosis, dyskeratosis, or orthokeratosis
- Histopathologically similar to each other; however, pterygium invades superficial cornea, but pinguecula does not

Figure 20-3. Pterygium and pinguecula. Conjunctival epithelium with underlying actinic (elastotic) degeneration.

Special Stains and Immunohistochemistry

- Noncontributory

Modern Techniques for Diagnosis

- Noncontributory

Differential Diagnosis

▌ Squamous cell carcinoma of conjunctiva and cornea (invasive or in situ)
  - Easily differentiated by lack of dysplasia in pterygium and pinguecula
▌ Pseudopterygium as a result of previous penetrating injury with superficial scar formation

Pearls

- Commonly removed, commonly recur
- Less chance of recurrence if excision is combined with conjunctival autograft

Selected Reference

Robin JB, Schanzlin DJ, Verity SM, et al: Peripheral corneal disorders (review). Surv Ophthalmol 31:1-36, 1986.

Squamous Cell Carcinoma of the Conjunctiva and Cornea

Clinical Features

- Gelatinous, with superficial vessels
- Papilliform or leukoplakic lesion
- Usually in the interpalpebral fissure at the corneal limbus, extending into the corneal center
- Thickened, well-demarcated area

Gross Pathology

- Noncontributory

Figure 20-4. Squamous cell carcinoma. Nonkeratinized epithelium of conjunctiva with conjunctival intraepithelial neoplasia. *Upper arrow* indicates a dysplastic region with a sharp line of demarcation to normal-appearing conjunctiva (*lower arrow*).

Histopathology

- Replacement of epithelium by atypical pleomorphic epithelial cells
- Mitoses are common
- Usually will stay within the epithelium (in situ, also known as conjunctival or corneal intraepithelial neoplasia [CIN]), occasionally invades deeper structures, including globe
- Three types of invasive conjunctival squamous cell carcinoma have been reported
  - Spindle cell: spindle-shaped cells difficult to distinguish from fibroblasts
  - Mucoepidermoid carcinoma: also has mucus-secreting cells
  - Adenoid squamous carcinoma: extracellular hyaluronic acid but no intracellular mucin; aggressive form and may invade globe or orbit
- Rarely metastasizes

Special Stains and Immunohistochemistry

- Noncontributory

Other Techniques for Diagnosis

- Noncontributory

Differential Diagnosis

▌ Sebaceous gland carcinoma
  - More common in conjunctiva and eyelid than is squamous cell carcinoma
  - Similar dysplasia, but tends to have a more malignant appearance with a high proportion of cells that display intracytoplasmic vacuolization (sebaceous differentiation)
  - May be a more malignant variant of squamous cell carcinoma
▌ Pterygium and pinguecula
  - No dysplasia in pterygium and pinguecula
▌ Squamous papilloma
  - Typical finger-like projections with fibrovascular cores
  - Goblet cells common
  - Often associated with human papillomavirus (HPV)
▌ Oncocytoma
  - Rare tumor of the caruncle
  - Cystic cavities lined by proliferating epithelium
▌ Lipodermoid
  - Congenital lesion with typical clinical appearance
  - Histopathologically similar to dermoid cyst

Pearls

- Exposure to solar ultraviolet radiation is a major etiologic factor
- HPV and human immunodeficiency virus (HIV) are also etiologic factors
- Diagnosis is usually known before excision
- May recur, but usually stays in situ if the primary tumor was in situ

Selected References

Pe'er J: Ocular surface squamous neoplasia. Ophthalmol Clin N Am 18:1-13, 2005.

Robin JB, Schanzlin DJ, Verity SM, et al: Peripheral corneal disorders (review). Surv Ophthalmol 31:1-36, 1986.

Waring GO III, Roth AM, Ekins MB: Clinical and pathological descriptions of 17 cases of corneal intraepithelial neoplasia. Am J Ophthalmol 97:547-549, 1984.

Sebaceous Gland Carcinoma

Clinical Features

- More common in women
- Most common in patients 60 to 80 years of age
- Represents 5% of all malignant eyelid tumors
- Second most common eyelid tumor after basal cell carcinoma (more common than squamous cell carcinoma of the eyelid)
- Wide range of presentations, from a small firm nodule resembling chalazion to diffuse plaquelike thickening of the tarsus, to unilateral chronic diffuse blepharitis or conjunctivitis
- Overall mortality of about 20%
- May spread through direct extension into adjacent structures (orbit, nasal cavity, sinuses, intracranial cavity) or by the intraepithelial route (pagetoid invasion), lending an impression of multiple primary tumors
- Originates from sebaceous glands of the eyelid and conjunctiva, usually meibomian glands of the tarsus, and from the glands of Zeis (accessory lacrimal glands in conjunctival fornix)
- More common in upper eyelid

Gross Pathology

- Noncontributory

Figure 20-5. Sebaceous gland carcinoma with typical comedo pattern. Notice numerous cells with vacuolated cytoplasms and many mitotic figures.

Histopathology

- Irregular lobular masses of cells with sebaceous differentiation indicated by prominent cytoplasmic vacuolizations
- Frequent mitoses
- Nuclear atypia, pleomorphism
- Varies from highly differentiated to poorly differentiated (which may resemble anaplastic carcinoma)
- Four histologic patterns have been identified
  - Lobular: neoplastic cells form well-demarcated lobules
  - Comedocarcinoma: large lobules with central necrotic foci
  - Papillary: fronds of neoplastic cells, sometimes mistaken for squamous carcinoma or squamous papilloma, although careful examination reveals sebaceous differentiation
  - Mixed: mixture of previous three
- Small biopsies may identify strictly intraepithelial tumors, which may be manifestations of pagetoid spread; more extensive biopsy is usually advised

Special Stains and Immunohistochemistry

- Fat stains of frozen tissue show that many cells contain lipid
- Experienced ophthalmic pathologists can most often make the diagnosis without frozen sections
- *BRST1* marker is positive in sebaceous carcinoma, negative in basal cell carcinoma and squamous carcinoma

Other Techniques for Diagnosis

- Noncontributory

Differential Diagnosis

▮ Chalazion (stye)
  - Lipogranulomatous inflammation on biopsy
▮ Basal cell carcinoma
  - Spreads only through direct extension (unifocal)
  - Lack sebaceous differentiation
▮ Squamous carcinoma
  - Can be difficult to differentiate histopathologically
  - Lacks sebaceous differentiation
  - Hyperkeratosis, parakeratosis, keratin inclusions, and dyskeratosis
▮ Sebaceous adenoma
  - Sometimes associated with visceral malignancy (Muir-Torre syndrome)
  - Solitary benign nodule
  - Predilection for the eyebrow and eyelid

Pearls

- Poor prognosis is indicated by location in the upper lid, size of 10 mm or more, duration greater than 6 months, infiltrative growth pattern, and moderate to poor sebaceous differentiation

- Early diagnosis and treatment with wide local excision may improve prognosis
- Sometimes referred to as "the great masquerader" because it can mimic many other conditions
- Can be found in younger patients who have undergone orbital irradiation (e.g., for retinoblastoma)

Selected References

Shields JA, Demirci H, Marr BP, et al: Sebaceous carcinoma of the ocular region: A review. Surv Ophthalmol 50:103-122, 2005.

Burnier MN Jr, Burnier SV, Correia CP, et al: The immunohistochemical profile of sebaceous cell carcinomas of the eyelid. Presented at the Association for Research in Vision and Ophthalmology (ARVO), May 2000.

Kass LG, Hornblass A: Sebaceous carcinoma of the ocular adnexa. Surv Ophthalmol 33:477-490, 1989.

Rao NA, Hidayat AA, McLean IW, Zimmerman LE: Sebaceous gland carcinoma of the ocular adnexa: A clinicopathologic study of 104 cases with five-year follow-up data. Hum Pathol 13:113-122, 1982.

Internal Lesions

Malignant Melanoma

Clinical Features

- Most common primary malignant intraocular tumor
- Incidence of 5 to 7 per 1 million general population per year
- Incidence of 20 per million per year in whites older than 50 years
- Lifetime risk of 1 in 2,500 for whites
- Median age at presentation is in the sixth decade
- About 1% occur in patients younger than 20 years
- Slightly more prevalent in men and in blue-eyed patients
- No known hereditary component, although a few familial occurrences have been reported
- Patient may be asymptomatic
- Patient may complain of blurred vision because of direct tumor involvement of macula, detachment of retina from subretinal fluid produced by tumor, vitreous hemorrhage, or massive size of tumor obscuring vision

Figure 20-6. A, Typical spindle B choroidal melanoma. *White arrow* indicates a spindle A cell, whereas most of the cells are of the spindle B variety. **B, Epithelioid melanoma.** Large flat cells with prominent nucleoli and marked pleomorphism. This histopathologic appearance is an ominous prognosticator. **C, Cross section of whole globe with choroidal melanoma.** *Arrow* indicates a dome-shaped mass under the retina (*arrowhead*). **D, Choroidal melanoma with extraocular extension.** Choroidal tumor is indicated by *white arrow*, extraocular tumor by *black arrow*.

- Elevated lesion noted in fundus, sometimes with orange pigment on its surface
- Slow growing
- Anterior (ciliary body) position may be associated with segmental cataract
- Anterior (ciliary body) tumors more difficult to visualize
- Anterior (ciliary body) tumors may present with dilated external blood vessel (sentinel vessel)
- Anterior (ciliary body) tumors in rare cases take on a diffuse growth pattern 180 to 360 degrees around the ciliary body, commonly known as a *ring melanoma*
- Choroidal melanomas can be flat and diffuse, making clinical diagnosis more difficult
- Ultrasonography demonstrates solid tumor with low to medium internal reflectivity

Gross Pathology

- Mushroom-shaped or dome-shaped pigmented mass in choroid or ciliary body
- When these tumors arise in the choroid (as opposed to the ciliary body) they may rupture through the overlying Bruch membrane and extend into the subretinal space (giving a mushroom or collar-button shape)
- Size and location are important prognostic factors (size greater than 1 cm^3 and location at the ciliary body or over the optic nerve are poor prognosticators)
- Extrascleral extension can be seen, usually through scleral canals with vortex veins; this too is an important poor prognosticator
- Occasionally may extend into the subconjunctival space and be mistaken for a primary conjunctival lesion

Histopathology

- Most tumors probably arise from preexisting nevi in the choroid (not retinal pigment epithelium); others arise de novo
- Cell types (Callender histologic classification is most commonly used)
  - Spindle A
    - About 5% of melanomas (second least common)
    - Highly cohesive cells with spindle-shaped nuclei having a central stripe of chromatin (caused by nuclear fold)
    - Cell boundaries not easily identified
    - Rare mitoses
    - High survival rate (>90%)
    - Pure spindle A tumors behave more like nevi than malignant melanomas
  - Spindle B
    - Common type (about 35% to 40% of all melanomas)
    - Plump spindle cells with prominent nucleoli but without chromatin bar

- Indistinct cell boundaries
- Mitotic figures are rare, although more common than in spindle A
- Often arranged in fascicular (herringbone) pattern
- Moderate survival rate (about 75%)
  - Epithelioid
    - Rarest type (about 3%)
    - Noncohesive, large cells with large nuclei and abundant cytoplasm
    - High degree of pleomorphism
    - Mitoses are common
    - Poor prognosis; survival of about 28%
  - Mixed
    - Most common type (about 45%)
    - By definition contains a mixture of epithelioid and spindle cell types
    - Usually spindles predominate, but the occasional epithelioid cell classifies the tumor as mixed and negatively affects prognosis
    - Survival rate about 40%
  - Necrotic
    - Rare
    - Tumor is so necrotic as to be unidentifiable in cell type
    - Survival approximates that of mixed cell type
    - Most tumors have some necrosis
    - Balloon cells commonly found and may represent aging apoptotic cells
    - Inflammatory infiltrates commonly seen within tumor, composed mostly of T-cell lymphocytes
    - Macrophages (melanophages) are commonly seen scattered throughout melanomas
    - Degree of pigmentation varies between tumors and even within an individual tumor (varies from amelanotic to deeply pigmented)

Special Stains and Immunohistochemistry

- Frequently HMB-45 positive (about 50%)
- Very commonly S-100 positive (>90%)

Other Techniques for Diagnosis

- Noncontributory

Differential Diagnosis

▌ Choroidal nevus
- Smaller than melanoma
- Exclusively spindle cell type (usually spindle A)
- Uncommonly have serous subretinal fluid associated
- Never extend out of globe
- Mitoses not present

▌ Cavernous hemangioma of the choroid
- Hamartoma that may occur in isolation or in association with Sturge-Weber syndrome (encephalotrigeminal angiomatosis)
- Round or oval, slightly elevated orange-red lesion, usually 3 to 15 mm in diameter

- Occasional leakage of fluid, similar to melanoma
- Ultrasound helpful in differentiating from melanoma (high versus medium internal reflectivity)
- Histopathologically shows many large cavernous blood-filled spaces

▮ Metastatic carcinoma
- Most common intraocular tumor
- Usually in posterior pole, near vascular arcades
- Fast growing
- May be multifocal
- Ultrasonography may help to differentiate from melanoma
- Breast and lung are the two most common metastatic tumors to the eye
- Up to 12% of all carcinomas may metastasize to choroid (based on autopsy studies)
- In 20% to 45% of cases, ocular findings precede the diagnosis of the primary tumor
- Histopathology varies depending on site of primary tumor

▮ Choroidal melanocytoma (magnocellular nevus)
- Deeply pigmented (jet-black) benign tumor of choroidal melanocytes
- Usually occurs adjacent to optic nerve
- Tends to be flat or minimally elevated
- More common in heavily pigmented people
- Probably has the same low malignant potential as nevus
- Histologically composed of deeply pigmented plump polyhedral nevus cells containing large melanosomes

▮ Subretinal hemorrhage
- Deep red, may appear brown or black
- Ultrasonography useful in differentiating from melanoma

▮ Schwannoma
- Rare tumor of Schwann cells surrounding ciliary nerves
- Clinically and ultrasonographically similar to choroidal melanoma
- Histologically difficult to differentiate from spindle cell melanoma, although characteristically lacks the prominent nucleoli of melanoma
- Electron microscopy may be helpful in making diagnosis (Antoni patterns)

▮ Choroidal osteoma
- An unusual benign osseous, creamy-white lesion of posterior pole
- Usually relatively flat
- Ultrasonography shows calcification

Pearls

- About 4% of eyes enucleated from white patients with blind, painful eyes and opaque media harbor unsuspected choroidal melanoma (which may provoke pain, leading to enucleation more commonly than in nonpainful blind eyes)

- Metastases are usually a late occurrence and may happen years after enucleation
- Liver is by far the most common site of metastasis
- Mistaken clinical diagnosis rate by experienced ophthalmologists of approximately 1%
- Overall 15-year mortality rate is about 40% to 50%, significantly worse for large tumors and better for small tumors
- Treatment options include external-beam irradiation, plaque brachytherapy with iodine-125, transpupillary thermal therapy, local excision, and enucleation
- Choroidal melanomas are not known to be chemoresponsive, nor are the metastases

Selected References

The Collaborative Ocular Melanoma Study Group: The COMS randomized trial of iodine 125 brachytherapy for choroidal melanoma. V. Twelve-year mortality rates and prognostic factors: COMS report no 28. Arch Ophthalmol 124:1683-1693, 2006.

The Collaborative Ocular Melanoma Study Group: Histopathologic characteristics of uveal melanomas in eyes enucleated from the Collaborative Ocular Melanoma Study. COMS report no. 6. Am J Ophthalmol 125:745-766, 1998.

Albert DM: The ocular melanoma story. LIII Edward Jackson memorial lecture: Part II. Am J Ophthalmol 123:729-741, 1997.

Albert DM, Rubenstein RA, Scheie HG: Tumor metastasis to the eye. I. Incidence in 213 adult patients with generalized malignancy. Am J Ophthalmol 63:723-726, 1967.

Ciliary Body Adenoma

Clinical Features

- Also known as *Fuchs adenoma, Fuchs reactive hyperplasia, coronal adenoma, Fuchs epithelioma,* and *benign ciliary epithelioma*
- Present in more than 25% of older people
- Little clinical significance

Figure 20-7. Ciliary body (Fuchs) adenoma. Chords of ciliary epithelium interspersed with abundant eosinophilic material.

Gross Pathology

- Small mass in ciliary body sometimes noted on dissection of an eye in the histopathology lab

Histopathology

- Benign proliferation of cords of nonpigmented ciliary epithelium
- Abundant eosinophilic basement membrane material is present among the cords

Special Stains and Immunohistochemistry

- Noncontributory

Other Techniques for Diagnosis

- Noncontributory

Differential Diagnosis

▌ Amelanotic melanoma
  - Spindle or epithelioid cell types
  - Usually has some pigment
▌ Medulloepithelioma
  - Congenital lesion
  - Slowly enlarging
  - Made up of poorly differentiated neuroectodermal tissue
▌ Metastatic carcinoma
  - Usually rapidly growing
  - Most commonly breast and lung carcinomas

Pearls

- Proliferative rather than neoplastic
- May rarely cause occlusion of the anterior chamber angle
- Rarely misdiagnosed as a ciliary body melanoma

Selected References

Bateman JB, Foos RY: Coronal Adenomas. Arch Ophthalmol 97:2379-2384, 1979.

Shields JA, Eagle RC, Shields CL, DePotter PD: Acquired neoplasms of the nonpigmented ciliary epithelium (adenoma and adenocarcinoma). Ophthalmology 103:2007-2016, 1996.

Iris Nevus and Melanoma

Clinical Features

- Included as a separate entity because of distinct behavior compared with ciliary body and choroidal melanoma
- Nevi and melanoma are the most common tumors of the iris
- No sex predilection
- Average age of involvement is between 40 and 50 years
- Nonaggressive tumor (overall chance of metastasis about 2% to 4%)

Figure 20-8. Iris melanoma. *Black arrow* indicates posterior pigment epithelium of iris. Note the overall hypercellularity of the stroma with a population of spindle-shaped melanocytes displaying moderate pleomorphism.

- May have prominent vascularity
- Predisposition for inferior iris
- May present as a discrete mass, a diffuse mass (cottage cheese–like), iris heterochromia, hyphema, glaucoma, or chronic uveitis
- Varies in pigmentation from amelanotic to deeply pigmented

Gross Pathology

- Noncontributory

Histopathology

- Vary from more benign to purely malignant
  — More benign tumors usually have an abundance of slender spindle cells with few prominent nucleoli (may be considered a nevus)
  — More malignant tumors have plump spindle cells with prominent nucleoli or epithelioid cells (worst prognosis)
- Arise from iris stroma, not from posterior pigment epithelium

Special Stains and Immunohistochemistry

- Most tumors show positive staining for HMB-45, but this does not predict prognosis

Other Techniques for Diagnosis

- Noncontributory

Differential Diagnosis

▌ Iris nevus
  - Benign-appearing spindle cells
  - May slowly enlarge, but usually does not lead to glaucoma or hyphema

- Increased incidence in people who have neurofibromatosis type 1 (called a *Lisch nodule*, histopathologically identical to nevus)
- ▌ Ciliary body melanoma with anterior extension
  - Much more malignant in histopathologic appearance with poor prognosis
- ▌ Iridocorneal endothelial syndrome (ICE) variant
  - Iris nevus syndrome—diffuse hyperpigmentation with inflammation
  - Usually associated with glaucoma or corneal decompensation
- ▌ Cyst of posterior iris epithelium
  - May follow surgery or trauma
  - Ultrasound will detect fluid-filled cavity
- ▌ Metastatic tumors to the iris
  - Most commonly lung and breast carcinoma
- ▌ Iris freckle (ephelis)
  - Small, without discrete mass
  - Increase in pigmentation without an increase in the number of melanocytes
- ▌ Inflammatory mass
  - Collection of lymphocytes and plasma cells
- ▌ Penetrating ocular trauma
  - Foreign body with inflammatory reaction
  - Iris prolapse simulating iris mass
- ▌ Iris leiomyoma
  - Rare
  - May be difficult to differentiate from nevus and melanoma (all spindle cell tumors)

Pearls

- Most arise from preexisting nevi
- Constitute 5% to 10% of all uveal melanomas
- Can often be successfully excised

Selected References

Yap-Veloso MI, Simmons RB, Simmons RJ: Iris melanomas: Diagnosis and management. Int Ophthalmol Clin 37:87-100, 1997.

Kersten RC, Tse DT, Anderson R: Iris melanoma: Nevus or malignancy? Surv Ophthalmol 29:423, 1985.

Arentsen JJ, Green WR: Melanoma of the iris: Report of 72 cases treated surgically. Ophthalmic Surg 6:23-27, 1975.

Childhood Ocular Lesions

Retinoblastoma

Clinical Features

- A common childhood malignancy, occurring in 1 in 16,000 to 23,000 live births
- Third most common intraocular malignancy after metastasis and uveal melanoma
- No racial or sex predilection
- Bilateral in 20% to 30% of cases

- Average age of diagnosis is between 12 and 18 months, with 89% diagnosed before age 3 years
- Average age at diagnosis is lower in bilateral cases
- Rare after age 10 years; has rarely been reported in adults
- Usually presents as leukocoria (literally, "white pupil") but may present as strabismus, intraocular inflammation, hemorrhage, or trauma
- Highly malignant with great metastatic potential
- Most common method of spread is by direct invasion of optic nerve with extension into central nervous system
- May spread by invasion of leptomeninges and dissemination into cerebrospinal fluid
- Hematogenous spread can lead to distant metastases throughout the entire body
- May spread through lymphatics
- Retinoblastoma has one of the highest rates of spontaneous regression of any malignant tumor (regressed retinoblastoma, also called *retinocytoma* or *retinoma*)
- Heredity
  - The retinoblastoma (*RB*) gene is a tumor suppressor gene on the q14 band of chromosome 13, and retinoblastoma arises as a result of mutations in both copies of the gene
  - May arise in a sporadic or inherited fashion
  - Somatic mutation results in unilateral tumor
  - Germline mutation is likely to result in bilateral or multifocal tumors
  - Can be inherited as a genotypically recessive gene but phenotypically behaves like a dominant gene; if one faulty copy of the gene is transmitted, there is greater than a 90% chance of acquiring the second mutation
  - *Trilateral retinoblastoma* refers to retinoblastoma tumor arising in the pineal gland in addition to bilateral retinoblastoma; this occurs with germline mutations
  - About one third of tumors are germline, and two thirds are somatic
  - About 10% of all retinoblastoma cases are familial
  - The risk for a bilateral (germline) retinoblastoma survivor's having an affected offspring is about 45%
  - The risk for a unilateral (somatic) retinoblastoma survivor's having an affected offspring is about 7% to 15%

Gross Pathology

- Chalky-white tumor arising from the retina
- May grow in an endophytic pattern (into vitreous) or an exophytic pattern (into subretinal space), or more commonly in some combination of both

Histopathology

- Basic cell type has a large basophilic nucleus of variable size and shape and scanty cytoplasm

Figure 20-9. Large retinoblastoma. A, Low-power view. Notice the overall architecture of the tumor with basophilic tumor cells clustered around blood vessels within a background of necrosis (*black arrows*). *White arrows* indicate areas of calcification within the tumor. **B,** Tumor cells clustered around blood vessel in a pseudorosette pattern with adjacent necrosis. **C,** High-power view demonstrating many mitotic figures, a fleurette (*yellow arrow*), and a Flexner-Wintersteiner rosette (*black arrow*). **D,** Invasion of the tumor into the choroid. Retinal pigment epithelium (*black arrows*) separates the retina from the choroid, and there is tumor on both sides.

- Mitoses are frequent
- Tumor cells are clustered around blood vessels with intervening areas of necrosis and scattered calcification ("Islands of blue tumor in a sea of pink necrosis with purple flecks of calcium"— M. E. Smith)
- The Flexner-Wintersteiner rosette is pathognomonic of retinoblastoma and consists of a single row of tumor cells surrounding a central lumen; these are found exclusively in retinoblastoma
- The Homer-Wright rosette is also commonly found and consists of a single row of tumor cells surrounding a jumbled eosinophilic center; these are found in retinoblastoma, neuroblastoma, and medulloblastoma
- Groups of partially differentiated retinoblasts elongate and resemble photoreceptors; they then form a flower-like configuration known as a *fleurette*

- Blood vessels commonly have a cuff of basophilia, which most likely represents accumulation of DNA from necrotic and apoptotic retinoblastoma cells
- Calcification is usually present
- Histopathologic factors that help determine the chance of metastases include extension of the tumor into the optic nerve beyond the lamina cribrosa, extension of tumor to the surgical margin of optic nerve, massive invasion of the choroid by the tumor, and extraocular tumor
- Fully differentiated forms of retinoblastoma are referred to as *retinocytomas* and lack malignant characteristics

Special Stains and Immunohistochemistry

- The typical histopathologic appearance of these tumors makes special stains clinically unimportant

Other Techniques for Diagnosis

- Noncontributory

Differential Diagnosis

- The differential diagnosis of leukocoria (white pupil) in a young child is broad
- General categories include cataract, developmental ocular abnormalities, ocular inflammation and infection, other tumors, vascular abnormalities, trauma, and retinal detachment
- The diagnosis of retinoblastoma is usually an easy histopathologic diagnosis

Pearls

- Treatment of unilateral cases is usually by enucleation, with adjuvant chemotherapy and radiation therapy reserved for cases with evidence of extraocular spread or cases with histopathologic risk factors for metastasis
- Treatment of bilateral cases usually involves enucleation of the more severely affected eye (if there is no potential for useful vision) with subsequent chemotherapy (chemoreduction) combined with radiation, cryotherapy, and/or laser photocoagulation; bilateral enucleation is also a consideration
- The risk for subsequent neoplasms in germline retinoblastoma survivors is high, and the overall mortality rate from second tumors is as high as 30%
- The most common second neoplasm is osteosarcoma, especially in irradiated fields (orbit); however, soft tissue sarcomas, malignant melanoma, carcinomas, malignancies of the hematopoietic system, and brain tumors occur at a higher rate in individuals with germline mutations
- Overall long-term survival rate is about 85%, although a mortality rate as high as 60% after 35 years has been reported in patients with bilateral retinoblastoma

Selected References

Abramson DH: Second nonocular cancers in retinoblastoma: unified hypothesis. The Franceschetti Lecture. Ophthalmic Genet 20:193-204, 1999.

Usalito M, Wheeler S, O'Briend J: New approaches in the clinical management of retinoblastoma. Ophthalmol Clin North Am 12:255-264, 1999.

Albert DM: Historic review of retinoblastoma. Ophthalmology 94:654-662, 1987.

Abramson DH, Ellsworth RM, Kitchin D, et al: Second nonocular tumors in retinoblastoma survivors: Are they radiation induced? Ophthalmology 91:1351-1355, 1984.

Sang DN, Albert DM: Retinoblastoma: Clinical and histopathologic features. Hum Pathol 13:133-147, 1982.

Adult Orbital Lesions

Orbital Lymphoma, Including Lymphoid Hyperplasia and Malignant Lymphoma of the Orbit

Clinical Features

- Average age of onset is 50 to 70 years; rare before age 20 years
- Females slightly more affected than males
- Insidious presentation
- No inflammatory signs; little (if any) pain
- May present with gradually progressive proptosis or as a visible "salmon patch" of the conjunctiva
- Lacrimal gland involved in 30% of cases
- Imaging reveals an infiltrative lesion, which molds to surrounding structures (globe, orbital bones)
- Most common in superior anterior orbit

Gross Pathology

- Noncontributory

Figure 20-10. A, Lymphoid infiltrate with marked pleomorphism. Orbital biopsy from the patient in Figure 20-2. **B, Lymphoma of the anterior orbit.** Clinical photograph of a patient showing a typical "salmon patch" in the inferior conjunctival fornix.

Histopathology

- Range of features depends on degree of malignancy of lesion
- More benign lesions (lymphoid hyperplasia)
  — Dense lymphoid infiltrate consisting of mature-appearing lymphocytes
  — Cell population has benign features (no pleomorphism, low mitotic activity, moderate amount of polyclonality and polymorphism)
  — Well-defined germinal centers
- True lymphomas
  — Usually non-Hodgkin B-cell lymphomas
  — Cells can be small or large, cleaved or noncleaved
  — Mucosa-associated lymphoid tissue (MALT) lymphomas account for up to 50% of all orbital lymphomas
  — May be classified according to the Modified Rappaport Classification or the Revised European-American Lymphoma Classification
- Differentiation between lymphoid hyperplasia and true lymphoma is often difficult; occasionally the term *atypical lymphoid hyperplasia* is evoked by pathologists

Special Stains and Immunohistochemistry

- Because most are B-cell tumors, they express CD20
- κ and λ light chains may indicate monoclonality
- Polymorphism among the populations of more benign lesions may show positive T-cell, plasma cell, or macrophage markers

Other Techniques for Diagnosis

- Noncontributory

Differential Diagnosis

- ▌ Orbital pseudotumor
  - More inflammatory onset
  - Varies according to stage and type, but usually a polymorphic infiltrate of benign-appearing lymphocytes with or without fibrosis
  - May include germinal centers
  - Occasionally, granulomatous inflammation
- ▌ Orbital cellulitis
  - Imaging usually reveals a periosteal abscess or adjacent sinusitis
  - More likely to occur in younger individuals
  - In most cases does not come to biopsy, although true abscesses of orbit are often drained
  - Acute inflammatory signs
- ▌ Solid tumors of orbit
  - Including lacrimal gland tumors, primary and metastatic orbital tumors
- ▌ Graves orbitopathy
  - Extraocular muscles are always the site of primary involvement
  - Interstitial edema and lymphocytic inflammatory infiltrate within the endomysial connective tissue are early findings
  - May lead to edema and inflammatory infiltration around muscles and eventually fibrosis
  - Lacks germinal centers
- ▌ Vascular lesions
  - Includes hemangioma, lymphangioma, varix, and arteriovenous fistula

Pearls

- Strictly conjunctival and epibulbar tumors are less likely to be associated with systemic disease
- About 13% to 19% of patients have known systemic lymphoma at the time of diagnosis
- Up to 25% of all patients with orbital lymphoma can be expected to have evidence of systemic lymphoma within 5 years
- Bilaterality is not uncommon and does not necessarily predict a higher likelihood of systemic disease
- Treatment is usually with orbital external-beam irradiation; alternative treatments include local cryotherapy, chemotherapy, interferon treatment, and surgical excision
- Systemic evaluation should be performed and may include hematologic evaluation with bone marrow biopsy, bone scan, and head, chest, and abdomen radioimaging

Selected References

Bardenstain DS: Ocular adnexal lymphoma: Classification, clinical disease, and molecular biology. Ophthalmol Clin N Am 18:187-197, 2005.

Harris NL, Jaffe ES, Stein H, et al: A revised European-American classification of lymphoid neoplasm: A proposal from the International Lymphoma Study Group. Blood 84:1361-1392, 1994.

Knowles DM, Jakobiec FA, McNally L, et al: Lymphoid hyperplasia and malignant lymphoma occurring in the ocular adnexa (orbit, conjunctiva, and eyelids): A prospective multiparametric analysis of 108 cases during 1977 to 1987. Hum Pathol 21:959-973, 1990.

Mederios LJ, Harris NL: Lymphoid infiltrates of the orbit and conjunctiva: A morphologic and immunophenotypic study of 99 cases. Am J Surg Pathol 13:459-471, 1989.

Rosenberg S: National Cancer Institute-sponsored study of classifications of Non-Hodgkins lymphomas: Summary and description of a working formulation for clinical usage. Cancer 49:2112-2135, 1982.

Orbital Pseudotumor (Idiopathic Orbital Inflammation)

Clinical Features

- Lymphoid tumors are not included as part of this topic
- Non-neoplastic, nonspecific inflammatory space-occupying orbital lesion
- Presents as proptosis, chemosis, lid swelling, and erythema, usually accompanied by pain

Figure 20-11. Sclerosing orbital pseudotumor. Dense fibrosis and inflammatory infiltrate with germinal centers are present.

- Usually unilateral, but may be bilateral (especially in children)
- Equal sex incidence
- Most common in fourth to sixth decades
- May present acutely, subacutely, or chronically
- May be recurrent
- May present as myositis, dacryoadenitis, nonspecific connective tissue inflammation, or deep orbital inflammation with accompanying cranial nerve dysfunction
- Can also involve the eye and produce optic nerve edema, scleritis, and intraocular inflammation
- First-line treatment is usually oral prednisone in high doses (60 to 80 mg)

Gross Pathology
- Noncontributory

Histopathology
- Histopathologic findings vary depending on which tissue is primary involved
- Early disease
  — Edema
  — Paucicellular polymorphic inflammatory infiltrate consisting of mature lymphocytes, plasma cells, eosinophils (especially in children), and neutrophils
  — Frequent perivascular lymphocytic cuffing
- Late disease
  — Increasing fibrosis
  — Less inflammatory infiltrate
  — Germinal centers occasionally found
- Lymphoid elements are usually widely separated by fibrosis (in contrast to sheets of lymphoid elements found in lymphoid tumors)
- Granulomatous foci are occasionally found

Special Stains and Immunohistochemistry
- Markers for monoclonality will usually not be positive

Other Techniques for Diagnosis
- Noncontributory

Differential Diagnosis
- Orbital cellulitis
  - Imaging will usually reveal a periosteal abscess or adjacent sinusitis
  - More likely to occur in younger individuals
  - In most cases does not come to biopsy, although true abscesses of orbit are often drained
- Thyroid orbitopathy
  - Extraocular muscles are almost always the site of primary involvement
  - Usually lacks eosinophils and germinal centers
- Orbital lymphoma
  - More insidious onset
  - Monoclonal tumor
- Posterior scleritis
  - May present with acute pain, proptosis, and ocular and periocular inflammation
  - Imaging reveals no orbital mass or infiltration
- Solid tumors of orbit
  - Including lacrimal gland tumors and primary and metastatic orbital tumors
- Granulomatous disease
  - Sinus involvement expected
- Ruptured dermoid cyst
  - May present in an adult with no prior knowledge of the dermoid
  - See "Dermoid and Epidermoid Cysts"
- Vascular lesions
  - Includes hemangioma, lymphangioma, varix, and arteriovenous fistula

Pearls
- About 6% to 15% of orbital pseudotumors occur during the first two decades of life
- More likely to be bilateral in children
- Acute pseudotumor is extremely radiosensitive

Selected References

Kennerdell JS, Dresner SC: The nonspecific orbital inflammatory syndromes. Surv Ophthalmol 29:93-103, 1984.
Chavis RM, Garner A, Wright JE: Inflammatory orbital pseudotumor: A clinicopathologic study. Arch Ophthalmol 96:1817-1822, 1978.

Thyroid Orbitopathy (Thyroid Ophthalmopathy, Dysthyroid Orbitopathy, and Graves Orbitopathy)

Clinical Features
- Graves disease: autoimmune process that includes any combination of hyperthyroidism, ophthalmopathy, and infiltrative dermatopathy
- Usually associated with hyperthyroidism, although patient may be hypothyroid or euthyroid

Figure 20-12. Thyroid orbitopathy. Interstitial inflammatory infiltrate within striated extraocular muscle.

- Ophthalmopathy is clinically apparent in 50% of patients with Graves disease but requires intervention in only 3 % to 5%
- Women are affected 3 to 4 times more often than men
- Usually begins as mild irritation of the eyes, followed by upper eyelid retraction, proptosis, and diplopia
- Acute anterior orbital inflammatory signs and symptoms may develop
- Advanced disease can lead to glaucoma, compressive optic neuropathy, and corneal blindness from exposure
- A detailed classification of ocular changes in thyroid orbitopathy is included in the NOSPECS classification
- Imaging will reveal enlargement of extraocular muscle bellies without involvement of the tendons
- Diagnosis is usually clinical, although biopsy of extraocular muscles or orbital fat is occasionally performed

Gross Pathology

- Thin strips of extraocular muscle or small pieces of orbital fat and connective tissue

Histopathology

- Inflammation and enlargement of extraocular tissues, most commonly the extraocular muscles
- Histologic findings vary with the stage and extent of disease
- Interstitial edema and lymphocytic inflammatory infiltrate within the endomysial connective tissue are early findings
- Inflammatory infiltrate consists mostly of lymphocytes and plasma cells with scattered mast cells

- Eosinophils and germinal centers are not a prominent feature
- Later the inflammation spreads to perimysium and epimysium
- Eventual fibrosis and fatty infiltration of the muscle occurs

Special Stains and Immunohistochemistry

- Noncontributory

Other Techniques for Diagnosis

- Noncontributory

Differential Diagnosis

▮ Orbital pseudotumor
  - Involvement usually not restricted to muscles
  - When muscles are involved, the tendon is not spared as it is in thyroid orbitopathy
  - Eosinophils and germinal centers are more common than in thyroid orbitopathy
▮ Orbital cellulitis
  - Imaging usually reveals a periosteal abscess or adjacent sinusitis
  - More likely to occur in younger individuals
  - In most cases does not come to biopsy, although true abscesses of the orbit are often drained
▮ Metastatic tumors to extraocular muscles
  - Most commonly carcinoma of breast and lung
▮ Other orbital inflammatory, infiltrative, and neoplastic conditions
  - Usually do not present with muscular involvement, and the diagnosis is made clinically

Pearls

- Most common cause of unilateral and bilateral proptosis in adults
- Smoking is a known risk factor for the development and progression of thyroid orbitopathy
- Treatment is aimed at the predominant sign or symptom
  — Eyelid procedures for corneal exposure
  — Radiotherapy and a systemic steroid for acute cases of massive swelling of the extraocular muscles can improve diplopia and resolve optic nerve compression
  — Strabismus surgery for stable symptomatic diplopia unresponsive to other treatment
  — Orbital decompression surgery for acute optic nerve compression unresponsive to radiotherapy and steroids

Selected References

Jakobiec FA, Bilyk JR, Font RL: Orbit: Noninfectious orbital inflammations—thyroid-related orbitopathy. In Spencer W (ed): Ophthalmic Pathology: An Atlas and Textbook, 4th ed, vol 4. Philadelphia, WB Saunders, 1996, pp 2811-2828.

Trokel SL, Jakobiec FA: Correlation of CT scanning and pathologic features of ophthalmic Graves' disease. Ophthalmology 88:553-564, 1981.

Werner SC: Modification of the classification of the eye changes of Graves' disease. Am J Ophthalmol 83:725-727, 1977.

Childhood Orbital Lesions

Cystic

Dermoid and Epidermoid Cysts

Clinical Features

- Most common cystic orbital tumors
- Most common orbital tumors in pediatric age group
- Choristomatous tumors
- Result from primitive epithelial or dermal elements that are sequestered in fetal suture lines
- Propensity for superotemporal and superonasal anterior quadrants of the orbit
- Always present from birth, but may become apparent only during adulthood

Gross Pathology

- Large single or multiloculated cystic cavity
- Keratin center has cheesy yellow appearance

Histopathology

- Single or multilobulated cyst lined by stratified squamous epithelium
- Dermoid has accompanying pilosebaceous apparatus; epidermoid contains only epidermal elements
- May have extensive foreign-body giant cell reaction within wall of cyst if the cyst has previously ruptured
- Center is filled with keratin, hair shafts, and lipid material

Special Stains and Immunohistochemistry

- Noncontributory

Other Techniques for Diagnosis

- Noncontributory

Figure 20-13. Dermoid cyst. The wall of the cyst with a lumen appears toward the top of the photograph. A pilosebaceous apparatus is seen in the wall of this cyst, which had previously ruptured and provoked an intense granulomatous giant cell reaction (*arrow*).

Differential Diagnosis

- ▌ Rhabdomyosarcoma
  - Solid mass
  - Rapidly progressive
  - Rhabdomyoblasts with malignant features
- ▌ Hemangioma
  - Densely packed capillaries with plump endothelial lining
  - May have a lobular pattern
- ▌ Meningocele and encephalocele
- ▌ Microphthalmos with cyst
  - See "Microphthalmos with Cyst"
- ▌ Orbital cellulitis
  - Inflamed dermoid may mimic cellulitis
  - Imaging will usually help with diagnosis

Pearls

- Ultrasound and radiography useful in detecting cystic nature of lesion
- Dumbbell-shaped dermoid may project anteriorly from lateral orbit, erode lateral wall of orbit, and straddle the temporal fossa and orbit

Selected References

Yanoff M, Fine BS: Ocular Pathology, 4th ed. Chicago, Mosby-Wolfe, 1996, pp 505-507.

Sherman RP, Rootman J, LaPoint JS: Dermoids: Clinical presentation and management. Br J Ophthalmol 68:642-652, 1984.

Capillary Hemangioma of the Orbit

Clinical Features

- Also known as *hemangioma of infancy, strawberry hemangioma,* and *benign hemangioendothelioma*
- Most common periocular vascular tumor in infancy and childhood
- More common in females (2:1)
- About 30% are evident at birth and 95% by 6 months of age, often with explosive growth for 3 to 6 months
- Most spontaneously involute by 4 to 8 years of age
- Usually present with proptosis
- Mass may increase in size with crying, owing to increased venous congestion
- Half may develop amblyopia, either from deprivation caused by occlusion or from astigmatism
- When located near the surface, diagnosis is easy, and the tumor is commonly referred to as *strawberry nevus*
- Generally occur in otherwise healthy children; at 1% to 2% overall incidence

Gross Pathology

- Circumscribed soft, red lobular mass
- Feeding vessels may be apparent

Figure 20-14. Capillary hemangioma of the orbit. Numerous densely packed capillaries lined by plump endothelial cells. Periodic acid–Schiff staining helps delineate individual vessels.

Histopathology

- Densely packed capillaries lined by plump endothelial cells
- May have lobular pattern
- Lumens often difficult to identify
- Mitotic figures may be seen during active phase
- With time, fibrosis develops within each lobule, effacing the endothelial cells

Special Stains and Immunohistochemistry

- Reticulin stain sometimes necessary to help delineate the lumens

Other Techniques for Diagnosis

- Noncontributory

Differential Diagnosis

▌ Rhabdomyosarcoma
- See "Orbital Rhabdomyosarcoma"
▌ Lymphangioma
- See "Lymphangioma"
▌ Congenital hydrops
▌ Epidermoid and dermoid cysts
- See "Epidermoid and Dermoid Cysts"

Pearls

- Deep tumors can be difficult to differentiate from rhabdomyosarcoma, necessitating biopsy
- Superficial tumors can be treated with intralesional steroid injections or systemic steroid
- Small superficial tumors may also be surgically excised
- Deep orbital injection of steroid has been associated with central retinal artery occlusion and is thus contraindicated
- Because of a high rate of spontaneous involution, treatment is instituted only under vision-threatening circumstances

- *Kasabach-Merritt syndrome* refers to a large sequestration of platelets (usually) in gastrointestinal hemangiomas leading to thrombocytopenia and hemorrhage

Selected References

Kushner BJ: Hemangiomas. Arch Ophthalmol 118:835-836, 2000.

Mulliken JB, Young AE: Vascular birthmarks: Hemangiomas and malformations. Philadelphia, JB Lippincott, 1988.

Kushner BJ: Intralesional corticosteroid injection for infantile adnexal hemangioma. Am J Ophthalmol 93:496-506, 1982.

Haik BG, Jakobiec FA, Ellsworth RM, Jones IS: Capillary hemangioma of the lids and orbit: An analysis of the clinical features and therapeutic results in 101 cases. Ophthalmology 86:760-792, 1979.

Lymphangioma

Clinical Features

- Defined as a choristoma of the orbit because lymphatics are not normally found there
- Frequently presents in a child younger than 10 to 15 years (although may present in adulthood) with acute onset of fulminant proptosis, presumably secondary to spontaneous hemorrhage
- Fluctuating clinical course with multiple recurrences is typical
- During severe exacerbations may lead to compressive optic neuropathy, glaucoma, or large refractive shift
- Mass may enlarge during or after an upper respiratory infection

Gross Pathology

- Diffusely infiltrating mass, usually not removed in toto because of inaccessible location

Figure 20-15. Lymphangioma. Within a background of connective tissue, many thin-walled structures are identified (*arrows*), some of which are filled with faint eosinophilic material.

Histopathology

- Unencapsulated lesion affecting any orbital structure
- Blood- and lymph-filled, thin-walled vascular channels of varying caliber
- Channels lined by an attenuated endothelial layer with interrupted basement membrane, anchoring fibrils, and general absence of pericytes

Special Stains and Immunohistochemistry

- Noncontributory

Other Techniques for Diagnosis

- Noncontributory

Differential Diagnosis

▮ Hemangioma
- Capillary hemangiomas found in children usually present in the first year of life
- Histopathologically distinct—see "Capillary Hemangioma of the Orbit"
▮ Primary and metastatic malignancies of the orbit
- Include primary rhabdomyosarcoma, metastatic neuroblastoma, other metastatic tumors of childhood, and solid tumor of leukemia (chloroma)
▮ Cephalocele
- Continuous with central nervous system
- Contains cerebrospinal fluid
- Imaging helps to differentiate
- Microphthalmos usually not present
- Neural tissue with overlying meninges present on histopathology
▮ Orbital pseudotumor
- See "Orbital Pseudotumor (Idiopathic Orbital Inflammation)"

Pearls

▮ Clinical management is difficult
- Systemic steroids have little effect
- Surgery is usually reserved for cases of acute optic nerve compression
- Diagnosis can usually be made with close clinical observation and orbital imaging

Selected References

Jakobiec FA, Jones IS: Vascular tumors, malformations, and degenerations. In Jones IS, Jakobiec FA (eds): Diseases of the Orbit. Hagerstown, MD, Harper & Row, 1979, pp 269-308.
Iliff WJ, Green WR: Orbital lymphangiomas. Ophthalmology 86:914-929, 1979.
Jones IS: Lymphangioma of the ocular adnexa: An analysis of 62 cases. Trans Am Ophthalmol Soc 57:602-665, 1959.

Microphthalmos with Cyst

Clinical Features

- Congenital malformation resulting from incomplete closure of fetal cleft of sclera
- Usually unilateral but may be bilateral

Gross Pathology

- Thin-walled cystic structure adjacent to (and adherent to) globe
- Histologically, the eye may range from relatively normal to small and disorganized

Histopathology

- Cyst wall usually composed of fibrous tissue
- Cyst usually lined with neural elements, including gliotic retina, nonspecific glial cells, or poorly differentiated retina

Figure 20-16. Microphthalmos with cyst. A, Low-magnification view. *Black arrow* indicates orbital fat. *White arrows* show the fibrous wall of this cystic lesion. **B,** High-magnification view. *White arrow* indicates the fibrous coat of this lesion (analogous to sclera). *Black arrows* indicate neural retina.

Special Stains and Immunohistochemistry

- Primitive retinal elements within the cyst will stain with typical neural stains like synaptophysin or glial fibrillary acidic protein (glial elements)

Other Techniques for Diagnosis

- Noncontributory

Differential Diagnosis

▮ Dermoid and epidermoid cyst
- Associated with adjacent normal eye
- See "Dermoid and Epidermoid Cysts"
▮ Cephalocele
- Continuous with central nervous system
- Contains cerebrospinal fluid
- Imaging helps to differentiate
- Microphthalmos usually not present
- Neural tissue with overlying meninges present on histopathology

Pearls

- Usually a sporadic occurrence but may be associated with 13q deletion or chromosome 18 deletion

Selected References

Waring GO, Roth AM, Rodriques MM: Clinicopathologic correlation of microphthalmos with cyst. Am J Ophthalmol 82:714-721, 1976.

Mann I: Developmental Abnormalities of the Eye, 2nd ed. Philadelphia, JB Lippincott, 1957.

Solid

Orbital Rhabdomyosarcoma

Clinical Features

- Most common primary malignant orbital tumor in children

Figure 20-17. Embryonal rhabdomyosarcoma. Highly pleomorphic specimen with numerous mitotic figures.

- Found elsewhere in the body but has a predilection for the orbit (about 10% of all rhabdomyosarcomas present in the orbit)
- Average age of onset is 6 years; most occur before 10 years of age; extremely rare after age 25 years
- Usually presents as rapidly progressive proptosis or a rapidly enlarging orbital mass (progressing daily)

Gross Pathology

- Firm, rubbery, solid mass
- Arises not from extraocular muscles but from immature orbital tissue

Histopathology

- Divided into three main types
  — Embryonal
    ◆ Most common type
    ◆ Malignant rhabdomyoblasts in a loose, haphazard arrangement
    ◆ Frequent mitoses
    ◆ Round, oval, spindled, or stellate cells, some with prominent eosinophilic cytoplasm (may see cross-striations typical of striated muscle)
    ◆ Hyperchromatic, atypical nuclei with many mitotic figures
  — Alveolar
    ◆ Poorest prognosis
    ◆ Pattern resembles alveolar architecture of the lung with loosely arranged cells forming trabecular pattern
    ◆ Difficult-to-find cross-striations
  — Differentiated
    ◆ Rarest, but best prognosis
    ◆ Easily found cross-striations, fewer mitoses

Special Stains and Immunohistochemistry

- Positivity for vimentin, myosin, myoglobin, muscle-specific actin, and desmin
- Masson trichrome positive

Other Techniques for Diagnosis

- Electron microscopy may reveal typical myofibrillary differentiation; however, the classic light-microscopic appearance makes electron microscopy largely unnecessary

Differential Diagnosis

▮ Metastatic neuroblastoma
- Usually occurs late in the disease, once the primary is known
- Histopathologic findings are typical with small undifferentiated cells, Homer-Wright rosettes, pseudorosettes, and neuropil
- Can occur in up to 20% of children with adrenal neuroblastoma

▌ Leiomyoma and leiomyosarcoma
  ● Rare tumors in the orbit
  ● Electron microscopy can aid in differentiation
▌ Orbital capillary hemangioma
  ● Congenital lesion, but may become apparent later in life
▌ Orbital dermoid cyst
▌ Cephalocele
▌ Lymphangioma
▌ Orbital pseudotumor (idiopathic orbital inflammation)
  ● Uncommon in children
  ● See "Orbital Pseudotumor (Idiopathic Orbital Inflammation)"
▌ Orbital cellulitis
  ● Imaging usually reveals a periosteal abscess or adjacent sinusitis

● In most cases, does not come to biopsy, although true abscesses of the orbit are often drained

Pearls
● Survival rate of up to 90% if the tumor is confined to the orbit
● Most deaths occur within 3 years

Selected References

Jakobiec FA, Bilyk JR, Font RL: Orbit: Mesenchymal tumors—striated muscle neoplasms. In Spencer W (ed): Ophthalmic Pathology: An Atlas and Textbook, 4th ed, vol 4. Philadelphia, WB Saunders, 1996, pp 2573-2587.

Knowles DM, Jakobiec FA, Potter G, Jones IS: Ophthalmic striated muscle neoplasms: A clinico-pathologic review. Surv Ophthalmol 21:219-261, 1976.

Index

Note: Page numbers followed by f refer to figures; those followed by t refer to tables.

A

Abacterial prostatitis, chronic, 540-541
Abdomen, spindle cell tumors of, immunohistochemistry panel interpretation for, 15t
Abscess
  bone, vs. osteoid osteoma, 839
  brain, 1040-1041, 1040f
  breast
    subareolar, 701-702, 702f
    vs. diabetic mastopathy, 705
    vs. granulomatous lobar mastitis, 703
  hepatic
    bacterial, 413, 414f
    parasitic, 413
  splenic, vs. cytomegalovirus infection, 830
Acantholytic dermatosis, transient, vs. pemphigus, 75
Acanthoma, clear cell, 84, 84f
  vs. poroma, 93
Acanthosis, glycogen, of esophagus, 321-322, 322f
Acanthosis nigricans, vs. seborrheic keratosis, 83
Acid-fast bacilli, Ziehl-Neelsen staining of, 6, 7f
Acinar cell adenocarcinoma
  of prostate gland, 548-549
  vs. well-differentiated pancreatic neoplasm, 457
Acinar cell carcinoma
  of exocrine pancreas, 455, 455f
  of salivary glands, 161-162, 162f
  vs. invasive ductal adenocarcinoma, 454
  vs. pancreatoblastoma, 456
  vs. solid pseudopapillary neoplasm, 459
Acne vulgaris, 77-78, 77f
Acquired cystic kidney disease, 515-516, 515f
  vs. autosomal dominant polycystic kidney disease, 515
Acquired melanocytic nevus, 101-103, 102f
  variants of, 101-103, 102f
Acral lentiginous melanoma, 103
Actinic cheilitis, vs. leukoplakia, 193
Actinic keratosis, 85-86, 86f
Actinomycosis, vs. nocardiosis, 247
Acute bronchiolitis, 225t
Acute demyelinating encephalomyelitis, 1046
Acute hemorrhagic leukoencephalitis, 1046
Acute interstitial pneumonia, 226-227, 226f

Acute myeloid leukemia
  vs. diffuse large B-cell lymphoma, 779
  vs. Langerhans cell histiocytosis, 816-817
Acute necrotizing eosinophilic myocarditis, 955
Acute respiratory distress syndrome, 226-227, 227t
Acute thyroiditis, vs. granulomatous thyroiditis, 122-123
Adamantinoma, 871-872, 872f
  vs. osteofibrous dysplasia, 865
Addison disease, 461-462, 462f
  differential diagnosis of, 462
  primary, 461
  secondary, 461
Adenocarcinoma. *See specific type and at anatomic site.*
Adenofibroma
  endometrial, 637, 637f
  papillary, vs. endocervical polyp, 617
  vs. endometrial adenosarcoma, 638
  vs. endometrial polyp, 631
Adenohypophysis, spindle cell oncocytoma of
  vs. pituicytoma, 1030
  vs. pituitary adenoma, 1030
Adenoid cystic carcinoma
  cytoarchitectural patterns of, 160-161
  of breast, 735, 735f
  of salivary glands, 160-161, 160f
  of trachea, 214, 215f
  vs. basal cell adenoma, 158
  vs. epithelial-myoepithelial carcinoma, 166
  vs. polymorphous low-grade adenocarcinoma, 163
  vs. small cell carcinoma, 170
Adenoma. *See specific type and at anatomic site.*
Adenomatoid hamartoma, respiratory epithelial
  vs. nasal polyp, 176
  vs. sinonasal (Schneiderian) papilloma, 180
Adenomatoid nodule
  vs. Graves disease, 126
  vs. thyroglossal duct cyst, 129
Adenomatoid tumor
  fallopian tube, 691, 691f
  myometrial, 646-647, 647f
  odontogenic, 202-203, 202f
  paratesticular, 577-578, 577f
  vs. myometrial adenomyosis, 643
  vs. Sertoli cell tumor, 573

Adenomatous hyperplasia, atypical, 260-261, 260f
  prostatic, 543-544
  vs. prostatic adenocarcinoma, 550-551
  vs. prostatic basal cell carcinoma, 553
Adenomatous polyp, vs. hyperplastic gastric polyp, 339
Adenomyoma, atypical polypoid, endometrial, 636-637, 636f
Adenomyosis, myometrial, 643, 643f
Adenopathy, HIV-associated
  vs. autoimmune lymphoproliferative syndrome, 754
  vs. progressive transformation of germinal centers, 753
Adenosarcoma
  of endometrium, 637-638, 638f
  vs. endometrial adenofibroma, 637
  vs. endometrial polyp, 631
  vs. endometrial stromal sarcoma, 641-642
Adenosis
  breast, 709-710, 709f
    vs. tubular carcinoma, 730
  sclerosing. *See* Sclerosing adenosis.
  vaginal, 613, 613f
Adenosquamous carcinoma
  of pancreas, 453
  of prostate gland, 554-555
  of uterine cervix, 626-627
  poorly differentiated. *See* Glassy cell carcinoma.
  vs. metaplastic carcinoma, 732
  vs. prostatic epithelial metaplasia, 545
Adenovirus infection, in immunocompromised patients, 352-353
Adnexal carcinoma, microcystic. *See* Microcystic adnexal carcinoma.
Adrenal cortical adenoma, 466-469
  ACTH-dependent, 464
  ACTH-independent, 464
  clinical features of, 466
  Conn syndrome and, 466-467
  Cushing syndrome and, 466-467
  differential diagnosis of, 468
  histopathology of, 466-467, 467f-469f
  oncocytic, 467
  pathology of, 466, 467f-469f